OSCE IN
MEDICINE
for Postgraduates and DNB

OSCE IN
MEDICINE
for Postgraduates and DNB

Editor

Ashis Kumar Saha MD
Professor of Medicine
Academic Head of Clinical Departments
Jagannath Gupta Institute of Medical Science and Hospital
Budge Budge, Kolkata, West Bengal, India

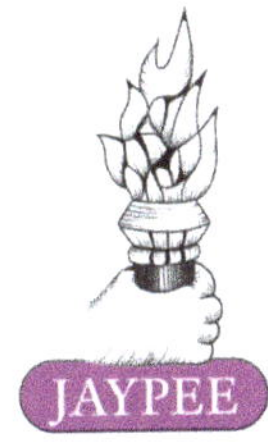

JAYPEE

JAYPEE BROTHERS MEDICAL PUBLISHERS
The Health Sciences Publisher
New Delhi | London

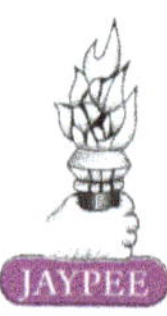

Jaypee Brothers Medical Publishers (P) Ltd

Headquarters

EMCA House
23/23-B, Ansari Road, Daryaganj
New Delhi 110 002, India
Landline: +91-11-23272143, +91-11-23272703
+91-11-23282021, +91-11-23245672
E-mail: jaypee@jaypeebrothers.com

Corporate Office

Jaypee Brothers Medical Publishers (P) Ltd.
4838/24, Ansari Road, Daryaganj
New Delhi 110 002, India
Phone: +91-11-43574357
Fax: +91-11-43574314
E-mail: jaypee@jaypeebrothers.com

Overseas Office

JP Medical Ltd.
83, Victoria Street, London
SW1H 0HW (UK)
Phone: +44-20 3170 8910
E-mail: info@jpmedpub.com

EU GPSR Authorised Representative

Logos Europe, 9 rue Nicolas Poussin
17000, La Rochelle, France
Phone: +33 (0) 6 67 93 73 78
E-mail: Contact@logoseurope.eu

Website: www.jaypeebrothers.com
Website: www.jaypeedigital.com

Inquiries for bulk sales may be solicited at: jaypee@jaypeebrothers.com

OSCE in Medicine for Postgraduates and DNB / **Ashis Kumar Saha**

First Edition: **2025**

ISBN: 978-93-5696-874-5

Preface

The Objective Structured Clinical Examination (OSCE) has become a cornerstone in the assessment of clinical skills for medical and healthcare students worldwide. This examination format, with its structured and practical approach, ensures that candidates demonstrate not only their theoretical knowledge but also their ability to apply this knowledge in real-life clinical scenarios.

The journey to mastering OSCEs can be daunting, requiring a blend of knowledge, skills, and confidence. The purpose of this book is to serve as a comprehensive guide to navigating this challenging yet rewarding path. Through carefully curated content, my aim is to demystify the OSCE process, offering students clear, practical, and effective strategies for success.

My approach in this book is threefold:

1. *Comprehensive coverage*: I have included a wide array of clinical scenarios that reflect the diverse range of cases students may encounter during their OSCEs. Each chapter is meticulously designed to cover essential clinical skills, from history-taking and physical examination and investigations in the question-answer format.
2. *Practical insights*: Recognizing that theoretical knowledge alone is insufficient, I have incorporated practical tips and real-world insights throughout the book. These are drawn from the experiences of seasoned clinicians and educators, providing readers with valuable advice on how to approach each station confidently and competently.
3. *Structured learning*: To facilitate effective learning, each section of the book follows a structured format. Clear objectives, step-by-step instructions, and detailed checklists are provided to ensure that readers can systematically develop and refine their clinical skills.

I also understand the importance of self-assessment in the learning process. Therefore, we have included numerous practice cases and mark schemes to help students gauge their progress and identify areas for improvement.

This book is the result of collaborative efforts from a team of dedicated professionals, each bringing their unique expertise and perspective to the table.

It is my hope that this book will serve as a trusted companion for all those preparing for their OSCEs. I believe that with the right preparation, determination, and support, every student can excel in their OSCEs and go on to provide exceptional care to their patients.

Wishing you success in your journey to becoming skilled, compassionate, and confident healthcare professionals.

Ashis Kumar Saha

Acknowledgments

First and foremost, I express my heartfelt gratitude to Mr Krishna Kumar Gupta, Chairman of JIMSH, whose unwavering support and vision have inspired countless endeavors in the field of medical education. His dedication to advancing medical science and education has been a guiding light for many, including myself, and I am deeply honored to have his encouragement for this book.

I extend my sincerest appreciation to Dr Balaram Gupta, Vice Chairman of JIMSH, for his insightful leadership and commitment to excellence in education. His contributions to the institution have fostered an environment of learning and innovation, and his support has been instrumental in shaping this work.

I am profoundly grateful to the students of JIMSH and various medical colleges across India, for their relentless curiosity, enthusiasm, and dedication to learning. Their thirst for knowledge and passion for the medical profession inspire educators and authors like me to contribute meaningfully to their journey. This book is a humble attempt to aid their pursuit of excellence and understanding in clinical medicine.

My heartfelt thanks go to my two sons, Subhra and Abhra, who are the very rhythm of my life. Their love, understanding, and unwavering support keep my heart beating with purpose. They have been my strength and my inspiration throughout this journey, and this work is as much theirs as mine.

I am equally grateful to my two colorful and vibrant daughters-in-law, Shilpi Saha and Tania Saha, who bring joy and warmth to our family. Their presence has enriched our lives, and their encouragement has been a beacon of positivity during the creation of this book.

I owe my thanks to my nephew, Soumya Saha, for always being there as a source of energy and optimism. His kind words and encouragement have been a silent but powerful support in my endeavors.

Finally, and most importantly, I am deeply indebted to my beloved wife, Mrs Kalyani Saha, the heartbeat of my life. Her love, patience, and unwavering belief in me have kept me going through every challenge. She is the anchor of my life, and without her presence, none of this would have been possible. She keeps my heart pumping not only with love but also with determination to achieve my dreams.

I extend my heartfelt gratitude to my one and only brother, Mr Kaushik Saha, whose constant encouragement and belief in my abilities have been a driving force behind this book. His unwavering support, wise counsel, and motivating words have always pushed me to pursue my aspirations.

I am equally thankful to wife of Kaushik Saha, Mrs Rinku Saha, for her kindness and unwavering encouragement throughout this journey. Her positivity and support have been a source of strength, and I deeply appreciate the role both of them have played in inspiring me to complete this work.

I owe a profound debt of gratitude to Mr Jitendar P Vij, who has been my philosopher and guide in the journey of writing medical books. His insightful guidance, thoughtful instructions, and visionary ideas have been the cornerstone of my work. It is under his mentorship that I have been able to explore and express my thoughts in the realm of medical literature. This book is a direct result of his brainstorming sessions and his relentless encouragement to pursue excellence. His belief in my abilities and his wisdom have been the driving force behind this endeavor, and for that, I am forever grateful.

I would like to express my sincere gratitude to Mr Sabyasachi Hazra, Associate Director—Publishing and Digital Sales, of the Kolkata branch of Jaypee Brothers Medical Publishers, for his unwavering support and invaluable contributions to this journey. His encouragement, innovative ideas, and guidance have been instrumental in shaping my endeavors to write various medical books under the esteemed banner of this publishing house. His dedication and vision have inspired me to explore new dimensions in medical writing, and I am truly thankful for your support.

Ashis Kumar Saha

Contents

Chapter 6: Geriatric Medicine   **418**

CHAPTER 1

Acid–Base Imbalance

Arterial blood gas (ABG) analysis

ABG parameters			ABG result	Calculation and interpretation		
pH	>7.45	Alkalemia		pH	pCO$_2$	Interpretation
	7.36–44	Normal				
	<7.35	Acidemia		↓	↓	Metabolic acidosis
pCO$_2$	>45	High		↑	↑	Metabolic alkalosis
	35–45	Normal		↑	↓	Respiratory alkalosis
	<35	Low		↓	↑	Respiratory acidosis
HCO$_3$	>26	High		Corrected standard anion gap (AG) for albumin		
	24 ± 2	Normal		$\dfrac{Albumin}{4} + 1.5 \times Phosphate$		
	<22	Low				
AG	>16	High		AG calculation		
	12 ± 4	Normal		$\{[Na^+] - [Cl^- + HCO_3]\} = 12 \pm 4$		
	<8	Low		Corrected Na$^+$ for AG in hyperglycemia		
Glucose	>10	High		Corrected Na$^+$ = Na + $\dfrac{Glucose - 5}{3}$		
	<2	Low				
Gap: Gap	$\dfrac{\Delta AG = AG - 12}{\Delta HCO_3\ 24 - HCO_3}$			Gap: Gap calculation for metabolic acidosis		
				<0.4	Low or normal AG metabolic acidosis	
				0.4–0.8	Normal + high AG metabolic acidosis	
Lactate	<1.9	Normal		0.8–2.0	Pure high metabolic acidosis	
	>2.0	High		>2.0	Metabolic acidosis with metabolic alkalosis/ respiratory acidosis	
pO$_2$	80–100	Normal		$PAO_2 = [713 \times FiO_2] - [pCO_2 \times 1.25]$		
	<80	Hypoxia		A-a gradient $= PAO_2 - PaO_2 = \dfrac{Age}{4} + 4$		

Compensation rules for				
Expected pCO$_2$	Metabolic acidosis		Metabolic alkalosis	
	$1.5 \times [HCO_3] + 8\ (\pm 2)$		$0.7 \times [HCO_3] + 20\ (\pm 5)$	
Expected HCO$_3$	Respiratory acidosis		Respiratory alkalosis	
	Acute	Chronic	Acute	Chronic
	$24 + \dfrac{pCO_2 - 40}{10} \times 1$	$24 + \dfrac{pCO_2 - 40}{10} \times 4$	$24 - \dfrac{40 - pCO_2}{10} \times 2$	$24 - \dfrac{40 - pCO_2}{10} \times 5$

- Respiratory acidosis: *Increased* $PaCO_2$. For every 10 mm Hg rise should have *increase* in HCO_3 by 1 (acute) or 4 (chronic) as compensation.
- Respiratory alkalosis: *Decreased* $PaCO_2$. For every 10 mm Hg rise should have *decrease* in HCO_3 by 2 (acute) or 5 (chronic) as compensation.

Every *10 mm Hg* change in $PaCO_2$ from *baseline* 40 mm Hg	HCO_3 (Baseline 24 mmol/L)	
	Acute	Chronic
↑$PaCO_2$	1	4
↓$PaCO_2$	2	5

CASE 1

An 8-year-old hypertensive man on angiotensin-converting enzyme inhibitor and normal sinus rhythm in ECG with no past history of ischemic heart disease has undergone septoplasty. During operation, there was evidence of acute depression of ST segment up to 2.5 mm and systolic blood pressure of 90 mm Hg which was revived by administration of fluid and intravenous pressor agent. Patient was transferred to intensive care unit (ICU) for monitoring. His blood pressure was 90/55 mm Hg, pulse rate of 80 beats/minute, and respiratory rate of 165 breaths/minute. Patient suddenly developed ventricular fibrillation which was reverted with single 200 Jule countershock and arterial blood gas analysis was done. His data demonstrated pH 7.26, pCO_2 56 mm Hg, pO_2 148 mm Hg, HCO_3 24.2 mmol/L, Na^+ 140 mmol/L, K^- 4.1 mmol/L, Cl^- 105 mmol/L, urea 25 mg/dL, and creatinine 0.9 mg/dL.

1. **From history what are the possibilities?**
2. **What is the interpretation of the arterial blood gas?**
3. **In spite of hypoventilation, why pO_2 is elevated?**

Answers

1. From history:
    a. Lactic acidosis, i.e., a type of metabolic acidosis resulting from the poor myocardial perfusion.
    b. Acute respiratory acidosis occurs due to:
        - Pulmonary hypoventilation
        - Respiratory depressant effect by the anesthetic agents
2. Interpretation of arterial blood gases:
    a. pH: Acidemic indicating acidosis
    b. pCO_2 is increased but HCO_3 is normal indicating respiratory acidosis.
    c. Anion gap is $138 - (103 + 24.3) = 10.7$, it is normal.
    d. Compensation: In case of acute respiratory acidosis, expected bicarbonate is $24 + 1$ mmol = 25 mmol/L. So, there is no evidence of coexistent acid–base disorder.
    e. Formulation: Acute respiratory acidosis after resuscitation from postoperative ventricular fibrillation.
3. pO_2 is elevated because patient inspired supplemented oxygen. If patient breathes room air, the alveolar pO_2 will be decreased and pCO_2 elevated.

CASE 2

A 20-year-old young insulin-dependent diabetic female with history of polyuria and polydipsia admitted into a hospital with complaint of poor compliance to medical therapy. On admission, her vitals are normal, chest is clear but there is evidence of herpes labialis as an indicator of poor nutrition. Urinalysis demonstrates 2+ ketone bodies and 4+ glucose. Her data in the blood demonstrates Na^+ 135 mmol/L, K^+ 4.9 mmol/L, Cl^- 102 mmol/L, HCO_3 10 mmol/L, urea 32 mg/dL, and creatinine 1 mg/dL. Her arterial blood gases demonstrated pH 7.25, pCO_2 15 mm Hg, pO_2 125 mm Hg, and HCO_3 7 mmol/L

1. **From which disease is the patient suffering from?**
2. **What other types of acidosis may occur in diabetic patient?**
3. **Interpret the arterial blood gas analysis and correlates with blood biochemistry.**

Answers

1. Patient has been suffering from diabetic ketoacidosis.
2. Other form of acidosis:
   a. Lactic acidosis from the poor tissue perfusion
   b. Hyperchloremic metabolic acidosis from:
      - Replacement of ketoanions which is lost in urine.
      - Resuscitation with saline administration.
   c. Respiratory acidosis from:
      - Secondary infection
      - Decreased level of consciousness
3. Arterial blood gas interpretation:
   a. pH is low indicating acidosis.
   b. Types: Bicarbonate is low indicating metabolic acidosis.
   c. Clues: Since the patient is diabetic having severe glycosuria and proteinuria, it suggests diabetic etiology.
   d. Anion gap: $135 - (102 + 10) = 135 - 112 = 23$ indicating high anion gap.
   e. Delta ratio: 0.79, since chloride level and sodium level are normal; hence, there is no evidence of anion gap concurrent metabolic acidosis. Since saline is infused during resuscitation, this may develop during treatment. Again, lactate level has not been recorded.
   f. Final diagnosis is high anion gap metabolic acidosis, most likely diabetic ketoacidosis.

CASE 3

A 21-year-old pregnant insulin-dependent female having poor compliance to antidiabetic therapy was admitted in a hospital with complaint of absent movement of the fetus and doctor diagnosed that the fetus was dead. She has a past history of recurrent admission in hospitals due to diabetic ketoacidosis. In the last admission prior to recent admission, her blood biochemical data demonstrated Na^+ 140 mmol/L, K^+ 4.3 mmol/L, Cl^- 112 mmol/L, urea 35 mg/dL, and creatinine 1.0 mg/dL. Her arterial blood gas data demonstrated pH 6.9, pCO_2 11, pO_2 135 mm Hg, and HCO_3 3 mmol/L.

1. **Interpret arterial blood gases and correlate with the serum biochemistry.**
2. **What is your final diagnosis?**

Answers

1. Arterial blood gas interpretations:
   a. pH is acidic.
   b. Type: Since bicarbonate is only 3 mmol/L and pCO_2 is low, it indicates metabolic acidosis.
   c. Since the patient suffered previously from diabetic ketoacidosis, hence this data suggests diabetic ketoacidosis.
   d. Anion gap: $140 - (112 + 3) = 140 - 115 = 25$, suggesting anion gap metabolic acidosis.
   e. Delta ratio: 0.62. Since chloride level is high, there may be concurrent anion gap metabolic acidosis.
2. Final diagnosis is high anion gap metabolic acidosis along with concurrent anion gap metabolic acidosis.

CASE 4

A 60-year-old nondiabetic, nonhypertensive woman has been admitted in a hospital with profound weakness and areflexia. Her oral intake is poor. In the hospital, sedative was given to the patient. Her serum biochemistry demonstrated Na^+ 144 mmol/L, K^+ 1.8 mmol/L, Cl^- 86 mmol/L, HCO_3 44 mmol/L, and urinary chloride 74 mmol/L. Her arterial blood gas data demonstrated pH 7.59, pCO_2 50 mm Hg, pO_2 95 mm Hg, and HCO_3 45 mmol/L.

1. **From the history what are the possibilities?**
2. **Interpret the arterial blood gases and correlate with the serum biochemistry.**
3. **What is your final diagnosis?**
4. **What are the serious complications of severe hypokalemia?**
5. **Mention few causes of metabolic alkalosis.**
6. **What caution is required during interpretation of urinary chloride in patient using diuretics?**

Answers

1. Hypokalemia is responsible for areflexia. Since there was no history of diarrhea or vomiting or polyuria, hence poor oral intake was responsible for hypokalemia. Again, poor oral intake led to dehydration resulting hypoperfusion of the blood vessels and this might produce lactic acidosis. But, here there was no increase in the respiratory effort. Hence, this history did not support the acid–base abnormality. Hypochloremia was due to increased excretion of chloride through the urine.

2. Arterial blood gases:
    a. pH: There is alkalemia.
    b. Type: There was high pCO_2 as well as high HCO_3 indicate either metabolic alkalosis or respiratory acidosis. Since there is respiratory distress, hence there is question of respiratory acidosis.
    c. Anion gap: $144 – (86 + 44) = 144 – 130 = 14$, it is normal. Increased urinary excretion of chloride suggests metabolic alkalosis.
    d. Compensation: In case of metabolic alkalosis, expected pCO_2 is $(0.7 \times 45) + 20 = 51$, it is close to actual level of pCO_2.

3. Final diagnosis is metabolic alkalosis with proper respiratory compensation with life-threatening hypokalemia.

4. Complications of severe hypokalemia:
    a. Life-threatening cardiac arrhythmias
    b. Rhabdomyolysis
    c. Renal failure

5. Causes of metabolic alkalosis:
    a. Chloride responsive metabolic alkalosis, i.e., urinary chloride is <10 mmol/L:
        - Severe vomiting in case of pyloric obstruction leading to loss of gastric juice
        - Diuretic therapy
    b. Chloride resistant metabolic alkalosis, i.e., urinary chloride is >20 mmol/L:
        - Primary aldosteronism
        - Bartter syndrome
        - Cushing syndrome
        - Other causes responsible for excess adrenocortical activity
        - Current use of diuretics

6. There is biphasic action of diuretics. Diuretics lead to increased excretion of chloride through the urine. But as the pharmacological actions of the diuretics have been passed, then chloride excretion through the urine will be diminished. So, there is constant relationship with the excretion of chloride through urine and timing of diuretic administration which will influence the data interpretation regarding urinary chloride.

CASE 5

A 62-year-old female has been admitted in a hospital with acute lobar pneumonia. Previously she was admitted for congestive cardiac failure for which she is on thiazide diuretic. On recent admission, her arterial blood gas demonstrated pH 7.64, pCO_2 30 mm Hg, pO_2 75 mm Hg, HCO_3 36 mmol/L, and K^+ 2.1 mmol/L.

1. **What is the initial assessment from clinical point of view and correlation with blood gas data?**
2. **What is your interpretation from the arterial blood gases?**
3. **What is your final diagnosis?**
4. **Why there is respiratory alkalosis?**

Answers

1. Initial assessment:
    a. Respiratory alkalosis resulting from hyper-ventilation as the patient is having breathing difficulty.
    b. Metabolic alkalosis from diuretic therapy
    c. Severe hypokalemia from diuretic therapy

2. Arterial blood gases demonstrate:
    a. pH: Alkalemia indication alkalosis.
    b. Type: pCO_2 is decreased and HCO_3 is increased suggesting both are directing in different directions from their normal ranges. As pCO_2 decreases, it suggests respiratory alkalosis and HCO_3 increases suggesting metabolic alkalosis, So, there are both respiratory as well as metabolic alkalosis.
    c. As there is severe hypokalemia and the patient is on diuretic therapy, it suggests that patient has chloride responsive alkalosis.
    d. Compensation:
        - In case of chronic respiratory acidosis, expected HCO_3 will be 22 mmol/L after

maximal compensation, but the actual value is 36 mmol/L, hence there must be metabolic alkalosis.

- Again, in case of metabolic alkalosis, the expected pCO_2 should be 46 mm Hg; but the actual value is much lower suggesting there must be respiratory alkalosis.

3. Final diagnosis: This is a case of combined respiratory alkalosis and diuretic mediated metabolic alkalosis.
4. As this patient was suffering from acute lobar pneumonia, there was decreased lung compliance; in order to get more oxygen, the patient had to hyperventilate thereby washing out the CO_2, thereby decreasing the pCO_2 resulting respiratory alkalosis.

CASE 6

An 80-year-old hypertensive old woman admitted in the intensive care unit with respiratory distress due to right anterior flail chest and fractured patella following motor vehicle accident; patient though hemodynamically stable but suffered from respiratory distress due to paradoxical movement of the flail chest and underwent intubation and mechanical ventilation with the setting of 25 mL/kg tidal volume and minute volume of 250 mL/kg. In this setting, her arterial blood gases demonstrated pH 7.57, pCO_2 26 mm Hg, pO_2 400 mm Hg, and HCO_3 20 mmol/L.

1. **What is your initial assessment?**
2. **Interpret the arterial blood gases.**
3. **What is your final diagnosis?**

Answers

1. Initial assessment: Since this is acute disorder and patient is under mechanical ventilation with above setting; so in this setting, respiratory alkalosis is obvious.
2. Arterial blood gases interpretation:
   a. pH: It is alkalemia, hence it indicates alkalosis.
   b. Type: Since pCO_2 is low and HCO_3 is low, it suggests the presence of both metabolic and respiratory alkalosis.
   c. Compensation: Since the total incidence is of sudden onset, hence it is acute disorder. In case of acute respiratory alkalosis, expected change in the HCO_3 is 21.6 mmol/L, which is very close to the actual value of 20 mmol/L.
3. The final diagnosis is acute respiratory compensation due to mechanical hyperventilation.

CASE 7

A 60-year-old woman with history of chronic obstructive lung disease has been admitted in hospital with complaint of epigastric pain in a hospital. Patient was on salbutamol and oral prednisolone 5 mg. After emergency operation for duodenal perforation, patient was transferred to intensive care unit for intubation and mechanical ventilation and in the next morning extubation was done. On the third day of operation, patient again became agitated and respiratory depressed, and on the fourth day of operation again she was ventilated and orally 1 g acetazolamide had to be started. Her serial arterial blood gas data demonstrated:

No. of analysis	First time	Second time	Third time	Fourth time	Fifth time	Sixth time	Seventh time	Eighth time
Date	Admission first day	Operation first ventilation second day	Extubation third day	Fourth day	Fourth day	Fifth day	Reintubation fifth day	Fifth day
pH	7.39	7.41	7.37	7.42	7.37	7.27	7.37	7.28
PCO_3	50	39	54.8	56	65	83	74	85
pO_2	158	132	88	62	92	80	85	100
HCO_3	30	24	30	34	37	37	41	39

1. **What is your clinical impression regarding the patient?**
2. **Interpret the blood gas data.**
3. **What is your final diagnosis?**

Answers

1. Clinical impression:
   a. As the patient has been suffering from chronic obstructive lung disease, hence blood gas analysis demonstrated evidence of chronic respiratory acidosis.
   b. As the patient had acute upper abdominal pain, there may be increase respiratory effort leading to respiratory alkalosis.
   c. Again, long-term steroid use may lead to metabolic alkalosis.
2. Interpretation of blood gases:
   a. pH: It is within the normal range as the normal range is between 7.35 and 7.45.
   b. Type:
      - On admission, pCO_2 is high because the patient is a patient of COPD.
      - On the second day, as the patient was ventilated large amount of pCO_2 was washed out leading to decrease in pCO_2.
      - On the third day as the patient was extubated, the patient again started accumulation of carbon dioxide leading gradual increase in pCO_2 up to fifth day prior to intubation when there is dipping of the level.
      - Prior to intubation and severe epigastric pain, due to hyperventilation, pO_2 was increased. But as the patient was ventilated, pO_2 was reduced to normal range.
      - Throughout the period of admission, HCO_3 was high in the range of 30–39 mmol/L as the patient is a patient of COPD.
   c. Compensation:
      - Patient has been suffering from respiratory acidosis. If this acidosis was acute the expected changes in the HCO_3 should be 25, and if it was chronic acidosis, expected value of HCO_3 was 28 mmol/L. So, the patient has been suffering from chronic respiratory acidosis.
      - Compensatory metabolic alkalosis due to retention of bicarbonate by the kidney.
3. Final diagnosis is:
   a. Chronic respiratory acidosis from chronic obstructive pulmonary disease with compensatory metabolic alkalosis.
   b. Acute abdominal pain led to increased respiratory effort resulting sudden decrease in the pCO_2.

CASE 8

A 40-year-old man has been admitted in a hospital with complaint of severe diarrhea for 3 days. On admission, the pulse was thready, blood pressure 95/60 mm Hg, and patient was severely dehydrated. His blood biochemistry demonstrated Na^+ 133 mmol/L, K^+ 2.1 mmol/L, Cl^- 111 mmol/L, HCO_3 14 mmol/L, urea 75 mg/dL, and creatinine 1.5 mg/dL. His arterial blood gases data demonstrated pH 7.30, pCO_2 32 mm Hg, pO_2 90 mm Hg, and HCO_3 15 mmol/L.

1. **What is your initial clinical assessment and correlation with blood gas data?**
2. **Interpret arterial blood gases.**
3. **What is your diagnosis?**
4. **What is the cause of severe hypokalemia?**

Answers

1. Initial clinical assessment:
   a. Patient being severely dehydrated from severe diarrhea developed prerenal failure.
   b. Patient developed acidosis with hyperchloremia.
2. Data interpretation:
   a. pH: There is acidemia, patient was suffering from acidosis.
   b. Type:
      - Bicarbonate is very low indicating metabolic acidosis.
      - pCO_2 is low indication respiratory alkalosis.

c. Anion gap: $133 - (111 + 14) = 133 - 125 = 8$, so it is normal. Though creatinine and urea in the blood was elevated but not too much extent to increase the anion gap.

d. Delta ratio: –0.4, which was slightly negative, hence combined acidosis.

e. Compensation: Respiratory compensation requires at least 12–24 hours to develop and patient already passed this time. Expected pCO_2 should be 31 mm Hg which is very close to the actual pCO_2.

3. This patient had been suffering from normal anion gap metabolic acidosis with compensatory respiratory alkalosis.

4. Severe hypokalemia occurs due to following reasons:

a. Due to severe electrolyte loss through the stool

b. Due to severe hypovolemia there is secondary hyperaldosteronism leading to increased reabsorption of sodium with increased excretion of potassium resulting severe hypokalemia.

CASE 9

A 25-year-old long-term insulin-dependent diabetic woman admitted in the intensive care unit of a hospital with severe vomiting, polyuria for 1 day as she omitted the insulin dose for last 10 days. Her blood pressure was 135/80 mm Hg, pulse rate 112 beats/min, regular, respiration rate 42 breaths/min, and temperature was normal. Patient's all the systemic examination was normal. Urine demonstrated high for ketone bodies, glucose ++++, her serum biochemistry and arterial blood gas data was supplied on admission, after 3 hours, 8 hours, and 16 hours:

Hours	On admission	3 hours	8 hours	16 hours
Sodium	133	140	135	136
Potassium	7.6	4.4	4.1	4.6
Chloride	103	120	116	111
Urea	102	70	45	28
Creatinine	2.6	2.2	1.8	1.0
Osmolarity	296	290	271	265
Glucose	540	182	148	98
Anion gap	26.8	15.5	3.5	10
pH	6.9	7.05	7.25	7.4
pCO_2	12	13.5	26	30
HCO_3	3.2	4.5	11.5	15

1. **What is your initial clinical assessment?**
2. **How can you interpret arterial blood gases?**
3. **What is your final diagnosis?**
4. **Why there was hyperchloremia during treatment?**
5. **Why there is delay in the treatment of acidosis?**
6. **What is the fallacy of treating with bicarbonate?**

Answers

1. Initial clinical assessment:

a. Patient has been suffering from the diabetic ketoacidosis.

b. There may be associated lactic acidosis which may be the consequence of poor tissue perfusion, this type of acidosis is anion gap.

c. There may be metabolic alkalosis as a result of severe vomiting but in this setting it is very difficult to differentiate it.

2. Interpretation of data:

a. pH is acidic, so the patient was suffering from acidosis.

b. Type:
   - Low pCO_2 suggesting respiratory acidosis.
   - Low HCO_3 suggesting metabolic acidosis.

c. Clues:
   - Presence of hyperglycemia, high anion gap, and high urinary ketones confirms the diagnosis of diabetic ketoacidosis.

- Creatinine may be elevated during laboratory test because ketones will interfere with this method used for measuring creatinine (Jaffe reaction), so creatinine may be falsely high.
- Level of HCO_3 was very low as compared to anion gap and expected bicarbonate level in this pH is 2.8 which nearly toward expected level suggesting absence of background metabolic alkalosis in spite of severe vomiting.

  d. Compensation:
  - Expected pCO_2 is 9.6, which is nearly similar to the actual pCO_2, so there is complete respiratory compensation.
  - Initial delta ratio was 0.71 which was changed to –0.22 which is consistent with the hyperchloremic acidosis during treatment.

3. Complete diagnosis is diabetic ketoacidosis with maximum respiratory compensation with no evidence of background metabolic alkalosis.
4. During treatment of diabetic ketoacidosis, increased anion gap metabolic acidosis was changed to anion gap metabolic acidosis because renal loss of ketoacids was replaced by chloride and this will be enhanced during treatment with normal saline.
5. During treatment, few ketoacids remained which were metabolized to generate bicarbonate, hence there is delay in the correction of acidosis.
6. If sodium bicarbonate is applied, it will produce rebound alkalosis or hyperkalemia in spite of rapid correction of blood gases.

CASE 10

A 70-year-old male developed sudden cardiac arrest in the ward following an operation. Patient was transferred to intensive coronary care unit and intubated and ventilated. Arterial blood was collected after 10 minutes for data interpretation. His data demonstrated pH 6.8, pCO_2 82 mm Hg, pO_2 200 mm Hg, and HCO_3 14 mmol/L. His blood biochemistry demonstrated sodium 138 mmol/L, potassium 4.8 mmol/L, chloride 103 mmol/L, and lactate 10 mmol/L.

1. **What is the clinical assessment?**
2. **Interpret the blood gases.**
3. **What is your final diagnosis?**
4. **Why there is high level of pO_2?**

Answers

1. Clinical assessment:
   a. As the patient suffered from hypoventilation, he developed respiratory acidosis.
   b. Due to alveolar hypoventilation, there is hypoperfusion of the tissue leading to anaerobic metabolism resulting lactic acidosis.
2. Analysis of blood gases:
   a. pH: It is acidic, so there is evidence of severe acidosis.
   b. Type:
   - pCO_2 is very high suggesting respiratory acidosis.
   - Low HCO_3 suggests metabolic acidosis.

   c. Anion gap: $138 - (103 + 14) = 138 - 117 = 21$, it suggests increased anion gap metabolic acidosis.
   d. Delta ratio: 0.9
   e. Compensation:
   - Expected pCO_2 is 31.5 mm Hg, whereas actual pCO_2 is very much high suggesting associated respiratory acidosis.
   - Since serum lactate level is high; it is lactic acidosis.
3. Final diagnosis: Patient suffered from combined lactic acidosis due to diminished tissue perfusion as a result of low cardiac output as a consequence of cardiac arrest due to high lactate level and respiratory acidosis as a result of alveolar hypoventilation.
4. High level of pO_2 occurred due to high fraction of inspired oxygen during ventilation.

CASE 11

A 57-year-old insulin-dependent diabetic woman with past history of left ventricular failure admitted in the emergency in drowsy state following several days of nonspecific illness. Patient is on digoxin and thiazide diuretic. Her arterial blood gases demonstrated pH 7.4, pCO_2 33 mm Hg, pO_2 85 mm Hg, HCO_3 18 mmol/L, and anion gap 30.

1. **What is your initial assessment?**
2. **Interpret the data?**
3. **What is your final diagnosis?**
4. **Name the situations where there are mixed metabolic acidosis and metabolic alkalosis.**

Answers

1. Initial assessment:
   a. As the diabetic patient was admitted with drowsiness, following conditions should be in the mind:
      - Diabetic ketoacidosis though drowsiness is uncommon.
      - Hyperosmolar nonketotic coma
      - Stroke
      - Subarachnoid hemorrhage
      - Head injury
      - Hyponatremia
2. Data interpretation:
   a. pH: It is normal suggesting following possibilities:
      - There is no acid–base disorder
      - There may be compensating disorders like alkalosis and acidosis together.
      - Rarely fully compensated disorder—it may occur during recovery from the primary disorder prior to the level of compensation to adjust.
   b. Type:
      - pCO_2 is lower than normal suggesting respiratory alkalosis.
      - HCO_3 is low suggesting metabolic acidosis.
   c. Clue:
      - Anion gap is very high as compared to little decease in bicarbonate suggesting background metabolic alkalosis as a result of diuretic therapy with thiazide.
      - Here delta ratio is (observed anion gap – normal anion gap)/(normal bicarbonate level – observed bicarbonate level) = (30 – 12)/(24 – 18) = 18/6 = 3, which is very high and consistent with the high anion gap metabolic acidosis in a case of preexisting metabolic alkalosis.
   d. Compensation: In this case, expected pCO_2 is (1.5 × 18 + 8) = 35 mm Hg, which is very close to actual value, so there is full compensation occurred.
3. So the diagnosis is high anion gap metabolic acidosis in case preexisting metabolic alkalosis as a consequence of diuretic therapy.
4. Following are two conditions where there are mixed metabolic acidosis and mixed metabolic alkalosis:
   a. Diabetic ketoacidosis where patients are on diuretic therapy.
   b. In patients with high anion gap metabolic acidosis having severe vomiting.

CASE 12

A 75-year-old nondiabetic male admitted with features of congestive cardiac failure in intensive care unit. There was history of repeated vomiting for >5 days but was on no medication.

Patient was hypoventilating hence given oxygen mask. His blood biochemistry demonstrated sodium 128 mmol/L, potassium 5.3 mmol/L, chloride 80 mmol/L, urea 355 mg/dL, creatinine 6.5 mg/dL, and glucose 172 mg/dL. His arterial blood gases demonstrated pH 7.6, pCO_2 20 mm Hg, pO_2 160 mm Hg, and HCO_3 18 mmol/L.

1. **What is your initial assessment?**
2. **Interpret the arterial blood gases?**
3. **What is your final diagnosis?**

Answers

1. Initial assessment:
   a. pCO_2 is 20 mm Hg suggesting respiratory alkalosis.
   b. Since the patient has been suffering from congestive cardiac failure, so there will be low cardiac output leading to diminished tissue perfusion resulting lactic acidosis.
   c. Since patient was vomiting for several days, it will lead to metabolic alkalosis.
2. Interpretation of blood gases:
   a. pH: It showed alkalemia suggesting metabolic alkalosis.
   b. Types:
      - pCO_2 is low suggesting respiratory alkalosis.
      - HCO_3 is low suggesting metabolic acidosis.
      - It is already known that if metabolic is present, primary disorder will be respiratory acidosis.
   c. Clue:
      - Anion gap is $128 - (80 + 18) = 128 - 98 = 30$ mmol/L. Since anion gap is very high, it suggests high anion gap metabolic acidosis. Since the patient is not diabetic, hence there is no question of ketoacidosis.
      - Since there is high creatinine, glomerular filtration rate is <20 mL/min resulting in hyperkalemia. As a consequence, there is decreased excretion of potassium through the kidney. Here metabolic acidosis is due to increased retention of acids.
      - There is no history of ingestion of toxins, so there is no question of toxins associated acidosis.
      - There is no result related to lactate level in the blood.
      - Delta ratio: $(30 - 12)/(24 - 18) = 18/6 = 3$, which suggests there is associated metabolic alkalosis.
   d. Compensation: In case of respiratory acidosis, expected level of HCO_3 is $(24 - 10) = 14$, but the actual HCO_3 is much higher, i.e., 18 mmol/L, which suggests there is background metabolic alkalosis.
3. Diagnosis is:
   a. High anion gap metabolic acidosis which is the consequence of prerenal failure resulting increased retention of acids as well as less tissue perfusion due to decreased cardiac output.
   b. Respiratory acidosis due to hypoventilation.
   c. Metabolic alkalosis due to severe vomiting.

CASE 13

A 65-year-old was admitted with severe dehydration due to severe loose motion for 6 days. Patient suffered from orthostatic hypotension with low blood pressure. Her circulatory blood volume electrolytes were replenished with intravenous fluid and supplementation of potassium. On admission, arterial blood and blood biochemistry demonstrated sodium 136 mmol/L, potassium 2.6 mmol/L, chloride 116 mmol/L, creatinine 4.5 mg/dL, anion gap 11 mmol/L, pH 7.1, pCO_2 18 mm Hg, pO_2 85 mm Hg, and HCO_3 5.1 mmol/L.

1. **What is your initial clinical assessment?**
2. **How can you interpret the data?**
3. **What is your diagnosis?**

Answers

1. Initial clinical assessment:
   a. Diarrhea led to hyperchloremic anion gap metabolic acidosis.
   b. There was hypokalemia due to severe diarrhea.
   c. Diarrhea led to hypovolemia which in turn reduced tissue perfusion resulting lactic acidosis.
2. Analysis of data:
   a. pH: It is acidic indicating severe acidosis.
   b. Type:
      - Since bicarbonate is very low, it suggests metabolic acidosis.
      - Since pCO_2 is very low, it suggests compensatory hyperventilation leading to respiratory alkalosis.
   c. Clues:
      - Anion gap is normal, it suggests normal anion gap metabolic acidosis.

- Delta ratio: $(11 - 12)/(24 - 5.1) = -1/18.9 = 0.05$, which is very low suggesting pure hyperchloremic acidosis.
  d. Compensation: In case metabolic acidosis, expected pCO_2 will be $(1.5 \times 5.1) + 8 = 15.7$ which is very close to actual value suggesting maximum compensation.

3. Diagnosis: This data is suggestive of hyperchloremic hypokalemic anion gap metabolic acidosis due to severe diarrhea with fully compensated respiratory alkalosis.

CASE 14

A 25-year-old was transferred to intensive care unit following a cesarean section and was on continuous intravenous infusion of morphine along with oxygen through the mask. The patient suffered from fatty liver of pregnancy. Patient was completely drowsy on the very next day. The arterial blood gases demonstrated pH 7.17, pCO_2 65 mm Hg, pO_2 120 mm Hg, and HCO_3 20 mmol/L.

1. **What is the initial assessment of the patient?**
2. **Interpret the arterial blood gases data.**
3. **What is your final diagnosis?**
4. **If there was lactic acidosis what are the causes?**

Answers

1. As the patient was on the morphine infusion, she was very drowsy indicating the opioid toxicity. So, she had respiratory depression. During pregnancy, usually a patient develops hyperventilation, so pCO_2 should be depressed and it is typical. As the patient suffered from fatty liver disease of pregnancy in the third trimester, she may develop abdominal pain, nausea, vomiting, and it may progress to fulminant liver failure along with secondary prerenal failure and disseminated intravascular coagulation leading to death unless urgent delivery is not done. But here as the cesarean section was done, hence there was no chance of hepatic failure, and pCO_2 was high, hence it was due to acute respiratory acidosis as a consequence of morphine infusion.

2. Interpretation of data:
   a. pH: There is significant acidemia indicating acidosis.
   b. Type:
      - As the pCO_2 was high, it suggests respiratory acidosis.
      - HCO_3 was decreased indicating metabolic acidosis.
      - High pO_2 was due to oxygen supplementation of oxygen through the mask.
   c. Compensation: Expected decrease of bicarbonate is $24 + (65 - 40)/10 = 24 + 2.5 = 26.5$, so it is on the high normal range. But actual HCO_3 was 22 mmol/L, lower as compared to expected level. It suggested that there was also a component of metabolic acidosis.

3. The final diagnosis is acute respiratory acidosis as a consequence of morphine-induced respiratory depression with mild metabolic acidosis that may be due to elevated lactate or prerenal failure resulting increased urea and creatinine.

4. Lactic acidosis may be due to poor perfusion due to hypovolemia.

CASE 15

A 50-year-old hypertensive man with history of indigestion came to hospital with severe upper abdominal pain and cough and received intramuscular morphine injection. But on the very next day, again pain became severe again and collapsed at midnight, ambulance was called on. Doctor of ambulance diagnosed the patient as apneic, comatose, and pulseless and started cardiopulmonary resuscitation, patient started breathing, and pulse became palpable. After admission in intensive care unit, on examination, abdomen was rigid and severely tender and systolic blood pressure of 85 mm Hg. Urgent laparotomy was done to treat perforated duodenal ulcer and peritoneal toileting.

On admission, the biochemical and arterial blood gases data are as follows: serum sodium 142 mmol/L, potassium 5.5 mmol/L, chloride 107 mmol/L, bicarbonate 6.2 mmol/L, lactate 9.3 mmol/L, creatinine 3.2 mg/dL, urea 200 mg/dL, pH 6.8, pCO_2 32 mm Hg, and pO_2 230 mm Hg.

1. **What is your initial assessment?**
2. **Analyze the arterial blood gases.**
3. **What is your final diagnosis?**

Answers

1. Initial assessment:
   a. As the patient developed cardiopulmonary arrest, there is decreased peripheral perfusion leading to anaerobic metabolism of the tissue with the generation of lactate, as a result there was metabolic acidosis.
   b. Severe abdominal pain with cardboard rigidity suggests perforated viscus.
   c. There was also prerenal failure due to cardiopulmonary arrest.
2. Interpretation of data:
   a. Types:
      - Decreased HCO_3 suggests metabolic acidosis.
      - Decreased pCO_2 suggests respiratory acidosis.
      - Increased lactate suggests lactic acidosis.
      - Anion gap: 142 – (107 + 6.2) = 142 – 113.5 = 27.5, it also suggests metabolic acidosis.
   b. Compensation: Expected pCO_2 is 1.5 × 6.2 + 8 = 17.3, but actual pCO_2 was 32 mm Hg. So, there was no time for compensation to develop and it will take at least 12–24 hours to develop.
3. So, the diagnosis is metabolic acidosis probably lactic acidosis with prerenal failure having some contribution in the metabolic acidosis without any compensation.

CASE 16

An 80-year-old hypertensive patient on metoprolol and prazosin having history of abdominal aortic aneurysm admitted in the intensive care unit with sudden severe abdominal pain with shock. On examination in intensive care unit, blood pressure was 70/50 mm Hg, respiratory rate 32 breaths/min, and abdomen was guarded and tender. Patient was taken to operation theater for urgent laparotomy with 100% moist oxygen through the mask. Prior to operation, his arterial blood gas analysis was done. The arterial blood gases pH 7.36, pCO_2 22 mm Hg, pO_2 164 mm Hg, and HCO_3 12 mmol/L.

1. **What was initial clinical assessment?**
2. **Interpret the arterial blood gases data.**
3. **What is your final diagnosis?**

Answers

1. Initial assessment of the patient:
   a. As the patient developed acute peripheral circulatory failure, there is poor tissue perfusion leading to anaerobic metabolism and development of metabolic acidosis probably due to increased lactate.
   b. As the patient developed hyperventilation, there was wash out of the carbon dioxide leading to decreased pCO_2 resulting respiratory alkalosis.
2. Arterial blood gas analysis data:
   a. pH: Here it is within the normal range, so it may be very mild acidosis or mixed acid–base disorder.
   b. Type:
      - pCO_2 is low suggesting respiratory alkalosis.
      - Bicarbonate was also low indicating metabolic acidosis.
      - So here there is mixed metabolic acidosis and respiratory alkalosis.
   c. Compensation:
      - Expected bicarbonate: 24 – [(40 – 22)/10] × 2 = 24 – 3.6 = 20.4 mmol/L. Actual bicarbonate was 12 mmol/L. This indicates that there was also a component of metabolic acidosis.
      - Again, if the metabolic acidosis is the primary disorder, then expected pCO_2: 1.5

× 12 + 8 = 26 mm Hg whereas, actual level was 22 mm Hg. So, it is slightly lower than expected value, so it may be due to near maximal compensation. But, the blood was collected within 4 hours of the incidence. During this time, it is not possible to develop maximal compensation. Hence, this actual low value indicates associated respiratory alkalosis.

3. The diagnosis is patient suffered from lactic acidosis along with respiratory alkalosis due to hyperventilation.

CASE 17

A 45-year-old normotensive, nondiabetic female was admitted in the intensive care unit with weakness, inability to elevate the lower limbs, lethargy following severe vomiting 4 days ago. Her cardiovascular and respiratory systems are normal, only power in lower limbs was 3/5, and deep tendon reflexes 1+. Her blood biochemistry demonstrated sodium 127 mmol/L, potassium 1.7 mmol/L, chloride 103 mmol/L, glucose 102 mg/dL, urea 112 mg/dL, and creatinine 2.3 mg/dL. Her arterial blood gases demonstrated pH 7.32, pCO_2 25 mm Hg, pO_2 90 mm Hg, and HCO_3 12 mmol/L

1. **What is your initial clinical assessment?**
2. **Interpret the arterial blood gases?**
3. **What is your final diagnosis?**

Answers

1. Initial clinical assessment:
   a. Severe hypokalemia leading to severe muscle weakness involving both the lower limbs which should be corrected without any delay.
   b. Severe vomiting leading to metabolic alkalosis.
   c. Severe vomiting leading to large amount of fluid loss which may be responsible for:
      • Poor tissue perfusion leading to lactic acidosis.
      • Prerenal failure
   d. There was respiratory acidosis due to weakness of the respiratory muscles.
2. Interpretation of the arterial blood gases:
   a. pH: It is acidic indicating acidosis.
   b. Type:
      • Bicarbonate was low indicating metabolic acidosis.

   • Anion gap: 127 – (103 + 12) = 127 – 115 = 12.
   • Delta ratio: (12 – 12)/(24 – 12) = 0/12 = 0.
   • So, above value indicates the normal anion gap metabolic acidosis.

   d. Compensation:
      • It is normal anion gap metabolic acidosis.
      • If hyponatremia is present, normal anion gap metabolic acidosis occurs without any elevation of chloride.
      • Expected pCO_2 in metabolic acidosis is 1.5 × 12 + 8 = 18 + 8 = 26 mm Hg, which is equal to actual value and it showed that there was full respiratory compensation as sufficient time was passed.

3. The diagnosis is normal anion gap metabolic acidosis with full respiratory compensation.

CASE 18

A 70-year-old patient with comorbidity such as chronic obstructive pulmonary disease and exercise tolerance of 100 meters and past history of restless legs syndrome was admitted with worsening of respiratory distress for 3 hours. On examination, patient was alert and orientated tachypneic, and there was bilateral wheezing. On investigation, there was leukocytosis and hyperinflated lung. Her arterial blood gases demonstrated pH 7.29, pCO_2 68 mm Hg, pO_2 53 mm Hg, and HCO_3 27 mmol/L.

1. **What is your initial assessment?**
2. **How can you interpret the arterial blood gases data?**
3. **What is your final diagnosis?**

Answers

1. Initial clinical assessment: As the respiratory distress is acute, patient was suffering from acute respiratory acidosis. Patient was also hemodynamically stable.
2. Analysis of the data:
   a. pH: It is acidemic, hence the patient was suffering from acidosis.
   b. Type:
      - HCO_3 was raised indicating metabolic alkalosis.
      - pCO_2 was raised indicating respiratory acidosis.
   c. Compensation:
      - As the history was acute, so there should be no time to compensate respiratory acidosis.
      - Expected HCO_3 level should be 24 + [(68 – 40)/10] = 24 + 2.8 = 26.8, whereas, the actual level was 27 mmol/L. Hence, it is very close to the actual vale indicating the absence of mixed acid–base disorder.
3. This patient has been suffering from respiratory acidosis with compensated metabolic acidosis in case of chronic obstructive pulmonary disease.

CASE 19

A 20-year-old boy admitted with ingestion of barium carbonate dissolved in the hydrochloric acid complained of areflexic paralysis of muscles, sialorrhea, abdominal pain, and loose motion. On examination, there was raised blood pressure. His blood biochemistry demonstrated sodium 138 mmol/L, potassium 2.2 mmol/L, chloride 95 mmol/L, and lactate 10 mmol/L. His arterial blood gases demonstrated pH 7.2, pCO_2 35 mm Hg, pO_2 70 mm Hg, and HCO_3 12 mmol/L.

1. **What is your initial assessment?**
2. **What is your interpretation regarding the blood gas data?**
3. **What is your final diagnosis?**
4. **How barium sulfate produce hypokalemia?**

Answers

1. Initial assessment:
   a. There was high lactate indicating lactic acidosis.
   b. The areflexic muscle paralysis involving respiratory muscles also leading to hypoventilation resulting respiratory acidosis.
   c. As the duration of diarrhea is of short duration, there was little time to produce hyperchloremic metabolic acidosis.
2. Interpretation of the data:
   a. pH: It is acidic indicating acidosis.
   b. Pattern:
      - Low bicarbonate indicating metabolic acidosis.
      - Low pCO_2 indicating respiratory acidosis.
      - Anion gap: 138 – (95 + 12) = 138 – 107 = 31, indicating high anion gap metabolic acidosis.
      - Delta ratio: (31 – 12)/(24 – 12) = 19/12 = 1.5.
   c. Compensation: Expected arterial pCO_2 is (1.5 × 12) + 8 = 26 mm Hg, which is very high as compared to actual bicarbonate.
3. Final diagnosis is high anion gap metabolic acidosis with minimal compensation as there is anion gap lactic acidosis.
4. Barium helps potassium from extracellular to intracellular fluid in the muscle cells due to reduced passive permeability of the muscle membrane to potassium without affecting Na^+K^+-ATPase thereby minimizing the loss of potassium from the cell. In this patient, hemodialysis rapidly falls the level of barium.

CASE 20

A 62-year-old patient with history of decompensated alcoholic cirrhosis having past history of several episodes of bleeding varices for which sclerotherapy being done admitted in intensive care unit with several bouts of hematemesis and melena for >48 hours and respiratory distress. On examination, there was evidence of peripheral circulatory failure with shock, jaundice, and signs of chronic liver disease. The serum biochemistry demonstrated sodium 132 mmol/L, potassium 4.3 mmol/L, chloride 87 mmol/L, lactate 21 mmol/L, hemoglobin 5 g/dL, urea 88 mg/dL, and creatinine 2.1 mg/dL. The arterial blood gases demonstrated pH 7.0, pCO_2 13 mm Hg, pO_2 106 mm Hg, and HCO_3 5 mmol/L.

1. **What is your initial clinical assessment?**
2. **How you interpret the data?**
3. **What is your final diagnosis?**

Answers

1. Initial clinical assessment:
   a. Peripheral circulatory failure along with continued gastrointestinal bleeding with history of decompensated cirrhosis led to lactic acidosis.
   b. As a result of severe respiratory distress, patient was hyperventilating leading to development of respiratory alkalosis.
   c. Severe vomiting may produce metabolic alkalosis if there is severe loss of gastric acid along the vomiting.
2. Interpretation of the data:
   a. pH: It is acidic suggesting acidosis.
   b. Pattern:
      - Bicarbonate is low indicating metabolic acidosis.
      - Low pCO_2 suggesting respiratory alkalosis.
      - Since pH is acidic, it suggests metabolic acidosis in this case it is compensatory response.
      - Anion gap: $132 - (87 + 5) = 132 - 92 = 40$, it indicates high anion gap metabolic acidosis.
      - As serum lactate level is high very high, there is lactic acidosis. In case of severe lactic acidosis, there may be false negative value in case urine test as acetoacetate will be converted into β-hydroxybutyrate as it cannot react with nitroprusside.
      - As the urea and creatinine were elevated, it led to renal failure resulting increased retention of anion
      - Delta ratio is $(40 - 12)/(24 - 5) = 28/19 = 1.47$, it is consistent with the diagnosis of metabolic acidosis with high anion gap.
      - Anion gap rise exceeds the bicarbonate level fall because these anion will remain extracellular. Intracellular buffering of hydrogen ion will decrease the extracellular buffering by the bicarbonate ion.
   c. Compensation:
      - Expected pCO_2 is $1.5 \times 5 + 8 = 7.5 + 8 = 15.5$ mm Hg, which is near to the actual value. It suggests nearly full compensation as sufficient time has elapsed.
3. Final diagnosis is severe lactic acidosis with full respiratory compensation in a patient suffering from decompensated alcoholic cirrhosis with peripheral circulatory failure.

CASE 21

A 35-year-old female with history of long-term laxative and diuretic abuse was admitted in a hospital with watery diarrhea, generalized weakness, and respiratory distress. Previously patient was diagnosed as a case of Sjögren's syndrome complicated by renal tubular acidosis and patient was recovered proper administration of intravenous fluid. On examination, her blood pressure was 90/60 mm Hg, pulse rate was 78 beats/min, and systemic examination was normal. Her blood biochemistry demonstrated sodium 124 mmol/L, potassium 2.7 mmol/L, chloride 100 mmol/L, glucose 102 mg/dL, urea 103 mg/dL, and creatinine 2.1 mg/dL. Her blood gas analysis demonstrated pH 7.2, pCO_2 25 mm Hg, pO_2 110 mm Hg, and HCO_3 11 mmol/L.

1. **What is your initial assessment regarding the patient?**
2. **How can you interpret the blood gases?**
3. **What your final diagnosis?**

Answers

1. Initial assessment:
   a. Chronic long-term laxative abuse leads to metabolic alkalosis.
   b. Chronic long-term diuretic abuse leads to metabolic alkalosis.
   c. Hypotension leading to decreased tissue perfusion resulting high anion gap lactic acidosis.
   d. Prerenal failure leads to high anion gap metabolic acidosis.
   e. Severe watery diarrhea leads to normal anion gap metabolic acidosis.
   f. Respiratory distress leads to hyperventilation resulting respiratory alkalosis.

2. Interpretation of arterial blood gases:
   a. pH: It is acidic indicating acidosis.
   b. Pattern:
      - Low pCO_2 indicates respiratory alkalosis.
      - Low HCO_3 indicates metabolic acidosis.
      - Anion gap: $124 - (100 + 11) = 124 - 111 = 13$ mmol/L, which is normal.
      - Serum chloride level is normal and it is associated with hyponatremia.
      - Plasma glucose is normal.
   c. Compensation: Expected pCO_2 is $1.5 \times 11 + 8 = 24.5$, which is nearly equal to the actual pCO_2 indicating nearly complete compensation. So, there is no coexistent respiratory disorder.

3. The complete diagnosis is normal anion gap metabolic acidosis with maximum respiratory compensation.

CASE 22

An 80-year-old man admitted in a hospital with persistent hiccup, drowsiness, fever, and right upper quadrant pain and subsequently diagnosed as acute calculus cholecystitis with sepsis as white blood cell count was >15,000/cc. So, patient with cholecystectomy was transferred to ICU with oxygen mask and arterial blood gas was done. But after 3 days, patient sudden became violent followed by becoming unconscious, then arterial blood gases done and the patient was ventilated. After 3 hours blood gas analysis was done again.

Item	First sample during admission	Second sample prior to intubation	Third sample postventilation
pH	7.3	6.8	7.4
pCO_2	33	103	34
pO_2	155	200	100
HCO_3	17	22	17
Sodium	128	122	130
Potassium	5.6	4.5	3.9
Urea	220	–	–
Creatinine	–	–	–

1. **What is your initial assessment from clinical pathological view?**
2. **How you interpret the arterial blood gas data?**
3. **What is your final diagnosis?**

Answers

1. Initial assessment:
   a. Patient has been suffering from acute choledo-cholithiasis with sepsis.
   b. Patient was drowsy because of hyponatremia or sepsis.
   c. Prior to intubation, patient was violent that may be due to respiratory acidosis superadded by hyponatremia.
   d. After ventilation, patient recovered from respiratory acidosis.

2. Interpretation of arterial blood gases:
   a. In the first sample:
      - Bicarbonate was low pH was acidic indicating respiratory acidosis due to prolonged hyponatremia.
      - pCO_2 was low indicating compensatory respiratory alkalosis.
   b. In the second sample:
      - pH was gradually decreased due to acidosis.
      - pCO_2 reached to very high level resulting respiratory acidosis due to severe hypo-ventilation from unconsciousness.
      - Expected bicarbonate level should be 24 + [(103 – 40)/10] = 24 + 6.3 = 30.3 mmol/L, but actual level was 22 mmol/L, so it is lower than 30.3 mmol/L. So background metabolic acidosis was present. There was also severe hyponatremia at that time which may contribute to continued unconsciousness. This continued unconsciousness may be due to difficulty in the reversal of neuromuscular blockade.
   c. In the third sample:
      - After mechanical ventilation, respiratory acidosis was corrected.
      - Bicarbonate was decreased again resulting in metabolic acidosis which may be due to renal failure of accumulation anionic acid.

3. Final diagnosis is early metabolic acidosis with compensatory respiratory alkalosis which was followed by severe respiratory acidosis with background metabolic acidosis that was corrected by mechanical ventilation with apparent metabolic acidosis.

CASE 23

A 64-year-old noninsulin-dependent diabetes mellitus (NIDDM) on metformin and glibenclamide nonalcoholic man admitted in one hospital with severe vomiting and diarrhea and severe drowsiness. On admission, the blood glucose was 25 mg/dL. His blood report demonstrated sodium 144 mmol/L, potassium 3.8 mmol/L, chloride 112 mmol/L, and lactate: 22 mmol/L. His arterial blood gases demonstrated pH 6.9, pCO_2 23 mm Hg, pO_2 90 mm Hg, and HCO_3 7 mmol/L.

1. **What is your initial assessment?**
2. **How can you interpret the blood bases?**
3. **What is your diagnosis?**
4. **What are the causes of metabolic acidosis?**

Answers

1. Initial assessment: Patient was suffering from hyperchloremic metabolic acidosis along with metabolic acidosis.

2. Interpretation of arterial blood gases:
   a. pH: There is severe acidosis.
   b. Pattern:
      - Bicarbonate level was very low indicating metabolic acidosis.
      - Low pCO_2 suggests respiratory alkalosis, i.e., respiratory compensation.
      - Anion gap: 144 – (112 + 7) = 144 – 119 = 25 mmol/L.
   c. Compensation:
      - Expected pCO_2: 1.5 × 7 + 8 = 18.5 mm Hg. But the actual level was 23 mm Hg; it indicates that there is a component of respiratory acidosis and it occurred due to central respiratory depression as a result of hypoglycemia.
      - Delta ratio: (Present anion gap – normal anion gap)/(normal bicarbonate level – present bicarbonate level) = (25 – 12)/(24 – 7) = 13/17 = 0.76, this value indicates mixed hyperchloremic and high anion gap metabolic acidosis.

3. Final diagnosis is patient suffered from hyperchloremic metabolic acidosis, phenformin-induced lactic acidosis, and mild respiratory acidosis.
4. Increased lactate level when exceeds the renal threshold of lactate, it will lead to increased loss of lactate in exchange of chloride ion leading to hyperchloremia. This will be added to the chloride present in the replaced intravenous fluid. Again diarrhea may produce hyperchloremic acidosis.

CASE 24

A 74-year-old man having past history of coronary artery bypass surgery admitted in the orthopedic department for surgery of fractured femur. During surgery, she had moderate bleeding for which he was given blood; but after giving blood, patient suddenly developed breathlessness for which he was shifted to intensive care unit.

On examination, patient was conscious, cooperative, and alert. His blood pressure was 165/105 mm Hg, moderately anemic, pulse rate 120 beats/min, regular. There was bilateral crackle in the both bases and oliguria. On laboratory investigation, his hemoglobin was 9 g/dL, leukocyte count 16,000/cc, platelet 280,000/cc, urea 120 mg/dL, and creatinine 2.5 mg/dL. His blood gas analysis demonstrated pH 7.29, pCO_2 48 mm Hg, pO_2 62 mm Hg, HCO_3^- 21 mmol/L, lactate 0.4 mmol/L, sodium 131 mmol/L, potassium 4.1 mmol/L, and chloride 102 mmol/L.

1. **How can you interpret this arterial blood gas analysis?**
2. **What are your inference and its etiology?**
3. **What is the interpretation of alveolar–arterial gradient?**
4. **Why there is anemia?**
5. **What should be the condition of the oxygen dissociation curve?**

Answers

1. Interpretation of arterial blood gas analysis:
    a. pH is suggestive of acidemia.
    b. Pattern:
    - Bicarbonate is low, it suggests primarily metabolic acidosis.
    - Secondary compensation:
        i. Expected $PaCO_2 = 1.5 \times$ bicarbonate $+ 8 = (1.5 \times 21) + 8 = 39.5$ mm Hg
        ii. Observed $PaCO_2 = 48$ mm Hg
        So, there is associated respiratory acidosis.
    - Anion gap: $Na - (Cl + HCO_3) = 131 - (102 + 21) = 131 - 123 = 8$, so it is <12.
    So it is nonanion gap metabolic acidosis.

2. So, final diagnosis is normal anion gap combined with metabolic and respiratory acidosis as a consequence of renal failure.
3. Alveolar (A)–arterial (a) gradient =
    Calculated gradient $= (150 - PaCO_2/0.8) - PaO_2 = (150 - 48/0.8) - 62 = (150 - 60) - 62 = 90 - 62 = 38$ mm Hg
    Expected A–a gradient for age $=$ (Age in years $+ 10)/4 = (74 + 10)/4 = 84/4 = 21$ mm Hg
    So, calculated A–a gradient is more than the expected A–a gradient for age, it suggests intrinsic lung disease.
4. Anemia in this case is due to the decreased oxygen carrying capacity of the blood.
5. In presence of acidic pH, the oxygen dissociation curve will be shifted to the right. It is due to:
    a. Decreased affinity for oxygen
    b. Increased delivery of the oxygen to the tissues

CASE 25

A 60-year-old type 2 diabetic, hypertensive female admitted with fever with chill and rigor for last 3 days followed by sudden onset respiratory difficulty for last few hours.

On examination, patient is fully conscious, orientated and alert, pulse rate 125 beats/min, blood pressure 150/100 mm Hg, and respiratory rate 28 breaths/min.

Laboratory examination demonstrated hemoglobin 13 g/dL, total leukocyte count 22,000/cc, platelet count 80,000/cc, glucose 398 mg/dL. Chest X-ray demonstrated:

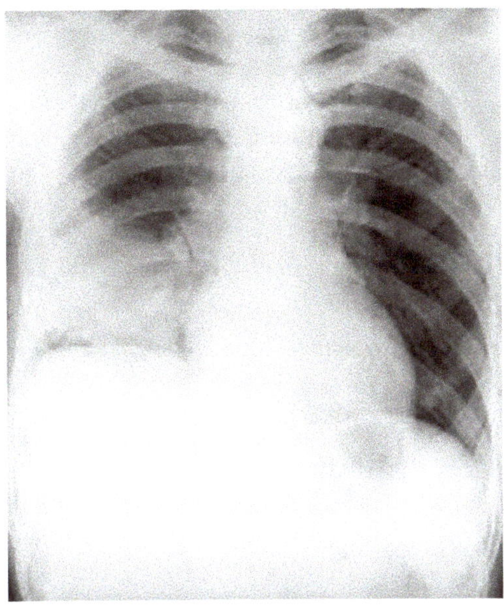

Arterial blood gas analysis demonstrated pH 7.25, $PaCO_2$ 30 mm Hg, PaO_2 55 mm Hg, HCO_3 16 mmol/L, lactate 1.1 mmol/L, sugar 330 mg/dL, sodium 128 mmol/L, potassium 3.5 mmol/L, and chloride 95 mmol/L.

1. **What is the feature in chest X-ray?**
2. **Interpret arterial blood gas analysis.**
3. **What is the etiological diagnosis?**
4. **What investigation is required to intensify the diagnosis?**

Answers

1. Chest X-ray demonstrated the evidence of homogenous shadow present in the right lower zone suggestive of right lower zone consolidation.
2. Interpretation of the blood gases:
   a. pH is 7.25 suggestive of acidemia.
   b. Pattern:
      - HCO_3 is low suggestive of metabolic acidosis.
      - Secondary compensation:
        i. Expected $PaCO_2$ = 1.5 × bicarbonate + 8 ± 2 = 1.5 × 16 + 8 ± 2 = 24 + 8 ± 2= 30–34 mm Hg.
        ii. Observed $PaCO_2$ = 30 mm Hg, which is within the range of expected value.

   So, there is adequate compensation of $PaCO_2$.
   - Anion gap: Na – (Cl + bicarbonate) = 128 – (95 + 16) = 128 – 111 = 17 mmol/L. It is higher than normal anion gap.
   - For evaluation of high anion gap delta gap has to be measured. Which is:

     (Delta anion gap – Delta bicarbonate) = (17 – 12) – (24 – 16) = 5 – 8 = –3, so it is within +6 and –6.
3. So, the diagnosis is high anion gap metabolic acidosis with fully compensatory respiratory alkalosis.
4. Proper investigation regarding the diabetic ketoacidosis should be done.

CASE 26

A 70-year-old type 2 diabetic, hypertensive on amlodipine, severely obese female having history of chronic kidney disease on maintenance hemodialysis thrice weekly has been admitted with drowsiness. She had previous history of admission with the same complaint and was diagnosed as obesity-induced obstructive sleep apnea syndrome and advised home base noninvasive ventilation strategy, but she neglected this advice.

On examination, patient was drowsy, patient responded but after small answer again became drowsy, blood pressure 130/85 mm Hg and pulse rate 90 beats/min, regular.

Laboratory investigation demonstrated hemoglobin 14 g/dL, total leukocyte count 10,000/cc, urea 100 mg/dL, and creatinine 5.2 mg/dL.

Arterial blood gas analysis demonstrated pH 7.1, $PaCO_2$ 80 mm Hg, PaO_2 48 mm Hg, HCO_3 26 mmol/L, lactate 0.8 mmol/L, sodium 136 mmol/L, potassium 3.5 mmol/L, and chloride 104 mmol/L.

1. **What are the comorbidity factors working here?**
2. **How can you interpret this arterial blood gases?**
3. **What is the etiological diagnosis?**
4. **How can you interpret alveolar–arterial gradient?**

Answers

1. This patient has following comorbidity factors:
   a. Old age
   b. Type 2 diabetes mellitus
   c. Hypertension
   d. Huge obesity
   e. Noncompliance to therapy
2. Interpretation of arterial blood gases:
   a. pH: Acidemia
   b. Since $PaCO_2$ is high, it suggests respiratory acidosis.
   c. Secondary compensation:
      - Rise in bicarbonate by 1 mmol/L for each 10 mm Hg rise in $PaCO_2$ above 40 mm Hg
      - Expected rise in bicarbonate = 24 + ($PaCO_2$ – 40)/10 = 24 + (80 – 40)/10 = 24 + 4 = 28 mmol/L
      - Observed rise in bicarbonate = 26 mmol/L
      - So, it is less than expected rise in bicarbonate, hence compensation is inadequate.
      - Anion gap = Na – (Cl + bicarbonate) = 136 – (104 + 26) = 136 – 130 = 6 mmol/L. So, this is normal anion gap.
3. The diagnosis is acute respiratory acidosis due to hypoventilation with normal anion gap mild metabolic acidosis.
4. A–a gradient:
   - Calculated gradient = (150 – $PaCO_2$/0.8) – PaO_2 = (150 – 80/0.8) – 52 = (150 – 100) – 48 = 50 – 48 = 2 mm Hg.
   - Expected gradient for this age = (Age in years + 10)/4 = (70 + 10)/4 = 20 mm Hg

      Here, calculated A–a gradient is less than the expected gradient for age, it suggests that this patient has no intrinsic lung disease. Hence, this patient has been suffering from hypoventilation syndrome.

CASE 27

A 70-year-old male has been admitted with severe respiratory distress along with productive cough for 2 days prior to admission and he was diagnosed as type 2 respiratory failure and noninvasive ventilation with FiO_2 60%. She was being treated with bronchodilators and antibiotics. Her blood report demonstrated hemoglobin 13 g/dL, total leukocyte count 11,000/cc, renal function test, and serum electrolytes were within normal. Arterial blood gas demonstrated pH 7.47, $PaCO_2$ 70 mm Hg, PaO_2 145 mm Hg, HCO_3^- 50 mmol/L, lactate 1 mmol/L, glucose 140 mg/dL, sodium 135 mmol/L, potassium 3.7 mmol/L, and chloride 100 mmol/L. Urinary creatinine is 14 mmol/L.

1. **How can you interpret this blood gases?**
2. **What is your etiological diagnosis?**
3. **How can you detect alveolar-arterial gradient?**
4. **What is our interpretation regarding A–a gradient?**
5. **What is the main mechanism of hypercapnia?**

Answers

1. Interpretation of blood gas analysis:
   a. pH: It indicates alkalemia.
   b. Bicarbonate is high; hence, it is primary metabolic alkalosis.
   c. Secondary compensation:
      - Expected rise in $PaCO_2$ = 0.7 × (bicarbonate – 24) + 40 ± 2 = 0.7 × (50 – 24) + 40 ± 2 = (0.7 × 26) + 40 = 18.2 + 40 ± 2 = 56.2–60.2 mm Hg
      - Observed rise in $PaCO_2$ = 70 mm Hg.

      So, secondary compensation by $PaCO_2$ is higher than the expected value which indicates associated respiratory acidosis.
   d. Urinary chloride is less than the normal value, i.e., <30 mmol/L.

2. The etiological diagnosis is chloride responsive metabolic alkalosis along with respiratory acidosis due to intrinsic lung disease.

3. For a given FiO_2 alveolar PaO_2 can be calculated by: $PAO_2 = (P_B – PH_2O) \times FiO_2 – PaCO_2/R$ at the sea level = (760 – 47) × 0.4 – 70/0.8 = 285.2 – 87.5 = 197.7 mm Hg

   So, alveolar – arterial gradient = 197.7 – 145 = 52.7 mm Hg

   Expected A – a gradient = (Age in years/4 + 4) + 50 (FiO_2 – 0.21) = (70/4 + 4) + 50 (0.4 – 0.21) = 21.5 + 9.5 = 31 mm Hg

4. So, respiratory acidosis is due to intrinsic lung disease as calculated gradient is higher than the expected gradient.

5. The mechanism of hypercapnia is:
   a. Haldane effect
   b. V/Q mismatch
   c. Central hypoventilation

CASE 28

A 20-year-old boy was admitted with headache, spiking fever, and vomiting along with altered conscious for 3 days. Subsequently, his cerebrospinal fluid demonstrated the feature of viral meningitis and was found as coronavirus disease 2019 (COVID-19) positive. So, treatment was initiated according to the COVID-19 protocol. But during third day of treatment, his condition deteriorated and he again developed spiking temperature. MRI brain was performed, and it showed multiple small infarcts. Chest X-ray was done, which is shown below. Laboratory investigation demonstrated hemoglobin 10 g/dL, total leukocyte count 15,000/cc with neutrophilic predominance. So, the patient was ventilated with FiO_2 60% and antibiotic was upgraded.

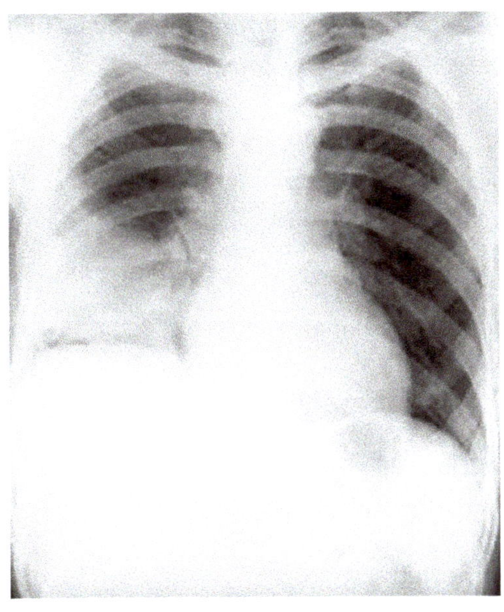

His arterial blood gas analysis was performed and it showed pH 7.40, $PaCO_2$ 33 mm Hg, PaO_2 130 mm Hg, HCO_3^- 23 mmol/L, lactate 1.4 mmol/L, glucose 110 mg/dL, sodium 135 mmol/L, potassium 3.5 mmol/L, and chloride 95 mmol/L. Urinary chloride is 14 mmol/L.

1. **Describe the above chest X-ray.**
2. **Interpret the arterial blood gases.**
3. **What is the etiological diagnosis?**

Answers

1. Chest X-ray demonstrates evidence of lower zone consolidation in the right lung.
2. Interpretation of the arterial blood gases:
   a. pH is 7.40 indicating alkalemia.
   b. $PaCO_2$ is 33 mm Hg indicating respiratory alkalosis.
   c. Secondary compensation:
      - Expected bicarbonate: $24 - [(40 - PaCO_2)/10 \times 2] = 24 - [(40 - 33)/10 \times 2] = 24 - (0.7 \times 2) = 24 - 1.4 = 22.6$ mmol/L

- Observed bicarbonate is 23 mmol/L.

So, the observed bicarbonate level is more than the expected bicarbonate level indicating additional metabolic alkalosis.

3. The diagnosis is respiratory acidosis due to pneumonia along with metabolic alkalosis, which may be due to steroid administration.

CASE 29

A 60-year-old hypertensive patient on diuretics having past history of pulmonary tuberculosis admitted in the emergency department with high fever, cough with purulent expectoration, and breathlessness. He was evaluated and diagnosed as infected bronchiectasis. So, antibiotics along with steroid were started.

His arterial blood gases demonstrated pH 7.48, $PaCO_2$ 52 mm Hg, PaO_2 60 mm Hg, HCO_3^- 40 mmol/L, Na 125 mmol/L, potassium 3.2 mmol/L, and chloride 102 mmol/L. Urinary chloride is 50 mmol/L.

1. **How can you interpret arterial blood gases?**
2. **What is your diagnosis?**
3. **From history as well as investigations what extra information can be derived?**

Answers

1. Arterial blood gas analysis:
   a. pH is 7.48 indicating alkalemia.
   b. Bicarbonate is high indicating metabolic alkalosis.
   c. Compensation:
      - Expected rise in $PaCO_2 = 0.7 \times$ (bicarbonate $- 24) + 40 \pm 2 = 0.7 \times (40 - 24) + 40 \pm 2 = (0.7 \times 16) + 40 \pm 2 = 51.2 \pm 2 = 49.1$–$53.1$ mm Hg
      - Observed rise in $PaCO_2 = 52$ mm Hg

      So, secondary compensation by $PaCO_2$ is complete.
   d. Urinary chloride is 50 mmol/L.

2. So, the etiological diagnosis is chloride resistant metabolic alkalosis due to diuretics with secondary respiratory acidosis.
3. As there is alkalemia, oxygen dissociation curve will be shifted to the right indicating the following information:
   a. Increased affinity toward oxygen
   b. Decreased delivery of oxygen to the tissues

   As a result, though the SpO_2 is normal, the patient will be hypoxemic. Hence, ABG is more reliable as compared to SpO_2.

CASE 30

A 64-year-old man with history of hypertension, diabetic, chronic obstructive pulmonary disease, and chronic kidney disease has come to emergency department with severe respiratory distress, cough, and spiking fever. He was examined and was mechanically ventilated at FiO_2 0.6. His arterial blood gases are as follows: pH 7.2, $PaCO_2$ 41 mm Hg, PaO_2 80 mm Hg, HCO_3 14 mmol/L, Na 140 mmol/L, potassium 4.5 mmol/L, chloride 100 mmol/L, lactate 4 mmol/L, and SpO_2 92%.

Laboratory investigation demonstrates hemoglobin 11 mg/dL, total leukocyte count 12,000/cc, and renal function test normal.

1. **What are the comorbidities in this case?**
2. **Interpret above blood gas analysis?**
3. **How can you interpret A–a gradient?**
4. **What is the etiological diagnosis?**

Answers

1. Following are the comorbidities:
   a. Hypertension
   b. Diabetes mellitus
   c. Chronic obstructive pulmonary disease
   d. Chronic kidney disease
2. Arterial blood gas interpretation:
   a. pH is 7.2 indicating acidemia.
   b. The bicarbonate is 14 mmol/L, indicating metabolic acidosis.
   c. Secondary compensation:
      - Calculated $PaCO_2 = 1.5 \times$ (bicarbonate) $+ 8.2 \pm 2$ mm Hg $= (1.5 \times 14) + 8 \pm 2 = 29 \pm 2 = 27–31$ mm Hg
      - Observed $PaCO_2$ is 41 mm Hg

   Observed $PaCO_2$ is more than that of calculated $PaCO_2$ indicating respiratory acidosis.

   d. Anion gap = Sodium – (chloride + bicarbonate) = 140 – (100 + 14) = 140 – 114 = 26 mmol/L.
   e. Delta ratio = (Delta anion gap) – (Delta bicarbonate) = (26 – 12) – (24 – 14) = 14 – 10 = 4, which is in between –6 and + 6.
3. Interpretation of the A–a gradient:
   For a given FiO_2, PaO_2 can be calculated as $PAO_2 = (P_B – PH_2O) \times FiO_2 – (PaCO_2/R)$ at the sea level
   $= (760 – 47)\ 0.6 – (41/0.8) = 713 \times 0.6 – 51.25 = 427.8 – 51.25 = 376.55\ mm\ Hg$
   Expected A–a gradient for FiO_2 0.6 = (age in years/4 + 4) + 50 (FiO_2 – 0.21) = (64/4 + 4) + 50 (0.6 – 0.21) = 20 + 50 × 0.39 = 20 + 19.5 = $39.5\ mm\ Hg$
   Calculated A–a gradient is more than the expected A–a gradient indicating the intrinsic lung disease along with ventilation/perfusion mismatch.
4. The etiological diagnosis is metabolic acidosis which is due to lactic acidosis with respiratory acidosis due to underlying chronic obstructive lung disease

CASE 31

A 72-year-old hypertensive male has come to emergency with severe diarrhea, cough, high fever, and respiratory distress for 3 days.

On examination, his blood pressure is 80/60 mm Hg, pulse rate 126 beats/min, respiratory rate 28 breaths/min. On laboratory investigation, his hemoglobin is 7 g/dL, total leukocyte count 12,000/cc, urea 88 mg/dL, creatinine 2.5 mg/dL. Chest X-ray is normal. Arterial blood gas analysis demonstrated pH 7.28, $PaCO_2$ 22 mm Hg, PaO_2 58 mm Hg, lactate 4.5 mmol/L, HCO_3 10 mmol/L, sodium 125 mmol/L, potassium 3.8 mmol/L, and chloride 88 mmol/L.

1. **Interpret arterial blood gases.**
2. **What is your etiological diagnosis?**

Answers

1. Interpretation of the arterial blood gases:
   a. pH indicates acidemia.
   b. HCO_3 is low indicating metabolic acidosis.
   c. Pattern of compensation:
      - Secondary compensation by $PaCO_2$ can be calculated as = 1.5 × (bicarbonate) + 8 ± 2 = 1.5 × 10 + 8 ± 2 = 15 + 8 ± 2 = 23 ± 2 = 21–23 mm Hg
      - Observed $PaCO_2$ is 22 mm Hg.

      So, observed $PaCO_2$ value is within the range of expected value indicating full respiratory compensation.

   d. Anion gap = Sodium – (chloride + bicarbonate) = 122 – (95 + 10) = 122 – 105 = 17 mmol/L.

      So, it is a case of high anion gap metabolic acidosis.

   e. Delta ratio = (Delta anion gap) – (Delta HCO_3^-) = (17 – 12) – (24 – 10) = (5 – 14) = –9. This value is suggestive of high anion gap metabolic acidosis with normal anion gap metabolic acidosis.

2. The diagnosis high anion gap metabolic acidosis due to lactic acidosis and normal anion gap metabolic acidosis as a consequence of diarrhea.

CASE 32

A 64-year-old hypertensive male admitted in the intensive care unit with fever, productive cough, sore throat for 5 days, and respiratory distress for last 1 day prior to admission. In the hospital, he was diagnosed as COVID-19 positive. On examination, his pulse rate was 124 beats/minute, blood pressure 150/100 mm Hg, and respiratory rate 28 breaths/min. Chest X-ray demonstrated pneumonic consolidation and CT severity score 16/25.

Arterial blood gas demonstrated pH 7.45, $PaCO_2$ 30 mm Hg, PaO_2 84 mm Hg, HCO_3 25 mmol/L, lactate 0.7 mmol/L, Na 136 mmol/L, K 3.8 mmol/L, Cl^- 100 mmol/L. Urine chloride is 10 mmol/L.

1. **How can you interpret this arterial blood gases?**
2. **How can you calculate A–a gradient?**
3. **What is your etiological diagnosis?**
4. **Is there any relation of urinary chloride with the acid–base imbalance?**

Answers

1. Interpretation of the blood gases:
   a. pH 7.5 indicating alkalemia.
   b. $PaCO_2$ is 30 mm Hg indicating respiratory alkalosis.
   c. Compensation:
      - Expected compensation by bicarbonate: 24 – [(40 – 30)/10/2] = 24 – (10/5) = 22 mmol/L.
      - Observed bicarbonate level is 25 mmol/L.

      So, observed bicarbonate is more than the expected value of bicarbonate indicating additional metabolic alkalosis.

   d. Anion gap = 136 – (100 + 25) = 136 – 125 = 11 mmol/L
   e. Delta ratio = (12 – 11) – (24 – 25) = 1 – 1 = 0

2. For a given FiO_2, alveolar pO_2 is calculated as:

   $PAO_2 = (P_B – PH_2O) FiO_2 – PaCO_2/R$ at the sea level = (760 – 47) × 1 – (30/0.8) = 713 – 37.5 = 675.5

   So, A–a gradient = 675.5 – 84 = 591.5 mm Hg

   Expected A–a gradient = (Age in years/4 + 4) + 50 (FiO_2 – 0.21) = (64/4 +4) + 50 (1 – 0.21)

   = 20 + 39.5 = 59.5 mm Hg

   Here, calculated A–a gradient is greater than expected or the age indicating pathological shunting.

3. The etiological diagnosis is respiratory alkalosis due to pathological shunting along with metabolic alkalosis.

4. As urinary chloride is lower than the normal range, it indicates that the metabolic alkalosis is chloride responsive.

CASE 33

A 75-year-old man has been admitted with history of progressively increasing headache, vomiting followed by deep unconsciousness and he was intubated by mechanical ventilation.

After 2 days, his arterial blood gases demonstrated pH 7.3, $PaCO_2$ 45 mm Hg, PaO_2 85 mm Hg, HCO_3^- 26 mmol/L, Na 136 mmol/L, K 3.8 mmol/L, and Cl 104 mmol/L.

1.   **What is primary disturbance in the arterial blood gas analysis?**
2.   **What is the secondary compensation?**
3.   **What is anion gap?**
4.   **What is A–a gradient?**
5.   **What is your diagnosis?**

Answers

1.   Primary acid–base disturbance is:
     a.   pH demonstrated acidemia
     b.   As $PaCO_2$ is high, hence the primary pathology is respiratory acidosis.
2.   Secondary compensation:
     a.   Expected rise in bicarbonate = $24 + [(45 – 40)/10] \times 4 = 24 + 5/10 \times 4 = 24 + 0.5 \times 4 = 26$ mmol/L
     b.   Observed rise in bicarbonate = 26 mmol/L
          So, in this chronic respiratory acidosis, the compensatory response is complete.
3.   Anion gap is $136 – (102 + 26) = 136 – 128 = 8$ mmol/L.

4.   A–a gradient:
     a.   Calculated A–a gradient = $(150 – PaCO_2/R) – PaO_2$ = $(150 – 45/0.8) – 85 = (150 – 56.25) – 85 = 93.75 – 85 = 8.75$ mm Hg
     b.   Expected A–a gradient = (Age in years + 10)/4 = $(75 + 10)/4 = 85/4 = 21.25$ mm Hg

     Here, calculated A–a gradient is less than the expected A–a gradient for age indicating absence of any intrinsic lung disease.
5.   This patient has been suffering from respiratory acidosis from alveolar hypoventilation.

CASE 34

A 68-year-old smoker opium addicted man having history of chronic obstructive lung disease has been admitted with severe respiratory distress and cough and diagnosed as acute exacerbation of the disease. On examination, the pulse rate was 120 beats/min, blood pressure 150/90 mm Hg, respiratory rate 24 breaths/min, increased jugular venous pressure, and pedal edema as he was on diuretics for few weeks.

On investigation, demonstrated total leukocyte count is 15,000/cc, hemoglobin 16 g/dL, urea 70 mg/mL, and creatinine 2 mg/mL.

His blood gases demonstrated pH 7.5, $PaCO_2$ 80 mm Hg, PaO_2 56 mm Hg, HCO_3^- 58 mmol/L, lactate 0.6 mmol/L, sodium 135 mmol/L, potassium 4.8 mmol/L, and chloride 96 mmol/L. Urinary chloride is 20 mmol/L.

1.   **What is the primary acid–base disturbance?**
2.   **What is the secondary compensation?**
3.   **What is the anion gap?**
4.   **What is A–a gradient?**
5.   **What is the etiology of primary and secondary acid–base disturbances?**

Answers

1.   Primary acid–base disturbance:
     a.   pH is 7.5, it is alkalemia.
     b.   Since bicarbonate is high, it leads to metabolic alkalosis.

2.   Secondary compensation:
     a.   Expected rise in $PaCO_2$ = $0.7 \times$ (bicarbonate) + $20 \pm 5 = 0.7 \times 58 + 20 \pm 5 = 40.6 + 20 \pm 5 = 60.6 \pm 5 = 55.6$ to 65.6 mm Hg
     b.   Observed rise in $PaCO_2$ = 80 mm Hg

So, observed rise in $PaCO_2$ is more than the expected rise suggesting associated respiratory acidosis.

3. Anion gap = $135 - (96 + 58) = 135 - 154 = -19$ mmol/L
4. A–a gradient:
   a. Calculated A–a gradient = $(150 - PaCO_2/0.8) - PaO_2 = (150 - 80/0.8) - 56 = (150 - 100) - 56 = 50 - 56 = -6$ mm Hg

   b. Expected A–a gradient for age = (Age in years + 10)/4 = $(68 + 10)/4 = 78/4 = 19.5$ mm Hg

So, here calculated A–a gradient is less than the expected A–a gradient for age suggesting absence of intrinsic pulmonary disease.

5. Respiratory acidosis is due to central hypoventilation. Metabolic alkalosis is due to use of diuretics and it is chloride responsive as urinary chloride is less normal.

CASE 35

A 74-year-old man suffering from carcinoma stomach on chemotherapy admitted in casualty department with drowsiness, spiking fever, and burning sensation in the micturition.

On examination, his pulse rate was 120 beats/min, blood pressure 90/60 mm Hg, respiratory rate 28 breaths/min. Patient is drowsy.

His arterial blood gas demonstrated pH 7.5, $PaCO_2$ 22 mm Hg, PaO_2 80 mm Hg, HCO_3^- 16 mmol/L, Na 120 mmol/L, K 3.8 mmol/L, and Cl 80 mmol/L.

1. **What is the primary acid–base disturbance?**
2. **What is the secondary compensation?**
3. **What is anion gap?**
4. **What is A–a gradient?**
5. **What is your diagnosis?**

Answers

1. Primary acid–base disorder:
   a. pH 7.5 indicating alkalemia.
   b. Since $PaCO_2$ is high indicating respiratory alkalosis.
2. Secondary compensation: Since the disease is acute
   a. Expected bicarbonate = $24 - [(40 - 22)/10] \times 2 = 24 - 1.8 \times 2 = 24 - 3.6 = 20.4$ mmol/L
   b. Observed bicarbonate = 16 mmol/L

So, observed bicarbonate level is less than the calculated bicarbonate level indicating associated metabolic acidosis.

3. Anion gap: $120 - (90 + 16) = 120 - 106 = 14$ mmol/L, so anion gap is high leading high anion gap metabolic acidosis.

4. A–a gradient:
   a. Calculated A–a gradient = $[150 - (PaCO_2/0.8)] - PaO_2 = (150 - 22/0.8) - 80 = (150 - 27.5) - 80 = 122.5 - 80 = 42.5$ mm Hg
   b. Expected A–a gradient as per age = (Age in years + 10)/4 = $(74 + 10)/4 = 84/4 = 21$ mm Hg

Here, calculated A–a gradient is more than the expected gradient for age indicating the presence of intrinsic lung disease.

5. The diagnosis is respiratory alkalosis which may be due to intrinsic lung involvement resulting from aspiration in drowsy patient along with high anion gap metabolic acidosis which may be the resultant of lactic acidosis.

CASE 36

A 78-year-old patient suffering from Parkinson's disease admitted in intensive care unit with breathlessness, productive cough for 2 days, and altered sensorium since the morning on the day of admission. Patient was ventilated in mechanical ventilation.

Laboratory examination demonstrated hemoglobin 8.5 g/dL, total leukocyte count 22,000/cc, other liver and renal parameters were normal.

Arterial blood gases demonstrated pH 7.25, $PaCO_2$ 30 mm Hg, PaO_2 82 mm Hg, bicarbonate 16 mmol/L, lactate 10 mmol/L, Na 122 mmol/L, K 4.2 mmol/L, and Cl 90 mmol/L.

1. **What is the primary acid–base disorder?**
2. **What is the secondary compensatory mechanism?**
3. **What is anion gap?**
4. **What is delta gap?**
5. **What is the etiological diagnosis?**

Answers

1. Primary acid-base disorder:
   a. pH is 7.25 indicating acidemia.
   b. Bicarbonate is 16 mmol/L indicating metabolic acidosis.
2. Secondary compensation:
   a. Calculated $PaCO_2 = 1.5 \times$ (bicarbonate) $+ 8 \pm 2 = 1.5 \times 16 + 8 \pm 2 = 24 + 8 \pm 2 = 32 \pm 2$ mm Hg.
   b. Observed $PaCO_2 = 30$ mm Hg
   So, $PaCO_2$ is in the range of compensation.
3. Anion gap $= 122 - (90 + 16) = 122 - 106 = 16$ mmol/L
   So, anion gap is high resulting high anion gap metabolic acidosis.
4. Delta gap = (Delta anion gap) – (Delta bicarbonate) $= (16 - 12) - (24 - 16) = 4 - 8 = -4$, it suggests no other associated metabolic disorder.
5. The exact diagnosis is metabolic acidosis due to lactic acidosis resulting from sepsis.

CASE 37

A 90-year-old patient with bronchial asthma and pulmonary hypertension suffering from chronic type 2 respiratory failure has been operated for fracture femur, but within 12 hours he developed altered sensorium and shifted to intensive care unit.

On examination, the pulse rate is 134 beats/min and blood pressure 90/70 mm Hg.

Laboratory examination demonstrated hemoglobin 11 g/dL, total count 12,000/cc.

Arterial blood gases demonstrated pH 7.26, $PaCO_2$ 56 mm Hg, PaO_2 58 mm Hg, bicarbonate 22 mmol/L, lactate 2.4 mmol/L, Na 142 mmol/L, K 4 mmol/L, and Cl 110 mmol/L.

1. **What is the primary acid–base disturbance?**
2. **What is the secondary compensation?**
3. **What is anion gap?**
4. **What is A–a gradient?**
5. **What is the etiological diagnosis?**

Answers

1. Primary acid-base disturbance:
   a. pH is 7.26 indicating acidemia.
   b. $PaCO_2$ is 56 mm Hg indicating respiratory acidosis.
2. Secondary compensation:
   a. Calculated bicarbonate level: $24 + (PaCO_2 - 40)/10 = 24 + (56 - 40)/10 = 24 + 1.6 = 25.6$ mmol/L
   b. Observed bicarbonate $= 22$ mmol/L
   Here, observed value of bicarbonate is less than the calculated bicarbonate level suggesting associated metabolic acidosis.
3. Anion gap $= 142 - (110 + 22) = 142 - 132 = 10$ mmol/L. So, this is a case of normal anion gap metabolic acidosis.
4. A–a gradient:
   a. Calculated A-a gradient $= (150 - PaCO_2/0.8) - PaO_2 = (150 - 56/0.8) - 58 = (150 - 70) - 58 = 80 - 58 = 22$ mm Hg
   b. Observed A–a gradient for age = (Age in years + 10)/4 $= (90 + 10)/4 = 100/4 = 25$ mm Hg
   Calculated A-a gradient is less than the observed A-a gradient indicating the presence of intrinsic lung disease.
5. Etiological diagnosis is respiratory acidosis due to hypercapnic respiratory failure normal anion gap metabolic acidosis may be due to infusion of the intravenous fluid.

CASE 38

A 30-year-old male having history of chronic kidney disease on maintenance hemodialysis came to emergency department with high fever for 2 days and progressively increasing breathlessness for 1 day. On examination, his blood pressure is 155/100 mm Hg, pulse rate 132 beats/min, respiratory rate 32 breaths/min and on auscultation there was coarse crepitation in the both lung bases. He was intubated and he was subsequently found as COVID-19 positive and CT severity score 12/25.

His arterial blood gas analysis demonstrated pH 7.36, $PaCO_2$ 30 mm Hg, PaO_2 100 mm Hg, bicarbonate 18 mmol/L, lactate 3.2 mmol/L, sodium 137 mmol/L, potassium 3.8 mmol/L, and chloride 104 mmol/L.

1. **What is the primary acid–base disturbance?**
2. **What is the secondary compensation?**
3. **What is anion gap?**
4. **What is A–a gradient?**
5. **What is the etiological diagnosis?**

Answers

1. Primary acid-base disturbance:
   a. pH indicates acidemia
   b. Bicarbonate is 18 mmol/L indicating metabolic alkalosis.
2. Following are the secondary compensation:
   a. Calculated $PaCO_2 = (1.5 \times \text{bicarbonate}) + 8 \pm 2 = 1.5 \times 18 + 8 \pm 2 = 24 + 8 \pm 2 = 32 \pm 2 = 32–34$ mm Hg
   b. Observed $PaCO_2 = 30$ mm Hg
   Here, observed $PaCO_2$ is within the range of calculated $PaCO_2$.
3. Anion gap: $137 – (104 + 18) = 137 – 122 = 15$, indicating high anion gap.
4. A–a gradient:
   a. $(150 – PaCO_2/0.8) – PaO_2 = (150 – 30/0.8) – 124 = (150 – 37.5) – 100 = 112.5 - 100 = 12.5$
   b. Observed A–a gradient for age = (Age in years +10)/4 = (30 +10)/4 = 40/4 = 10 mm Hg

So, here calculated gradient was more than the observed gradient for age indicating the hypoventilation due to intrinsic lung disease.

5. The etiological diagnosis is metabolic acidosis is due to lactic acidosis along with respiratory alkalosis in full compensation.

CASE 39

A 60-year-old male with past history of tuberculosis associated bronchiectasis came to emergency with acute worsening of shortness of breath, cough with productive sputum, and fever for last 4 days.

On examination, his pulse rate was 120 beats/min, respiratory rate 26 breaths/min, and blood pressure 120/80 mm Hg.

Laboratory investigation demonstrated hemoglobin 10.5 g/dL, total count 15,000/cc, and renal function test normal.

Arterial blood gas analysis demonstrated pH 7.54, $PaCO_2$ 68 mm Hg, PaO_2 54 mm Hg, bicarbonate 54 mmol/L, Lactate 0.6 mmol/L, sodium 140 mmol/L, potassium 2.6 mmol/L, and chloride 80 mmol/L.

1. **What is the primary acid–base disturbance?**
2. **What is the secondary compensation?**
3. **What is anion gap?**
4. **What is A–a gradient?**
5. **What is the etiological diagnosis?**

Answers

1. Primary metabolic disturbance:
   a. pH is 7.54 indicating alkalemia.
   b. Bicarbonate was 54 mmol/L indicating metabolic alkalosis.
2. Secondary compensation:
   a. Calculated $PaCO_2 = 0.7 \times$ (bicarbonate) $+ 20 \pm 5 = 0.7 \times 54 + 20 \pm 5 = 37.8 + 20 \pm 5 = 57.5 \pm 5 = 52.5$–$62.5$ mm Hg
   b. Observed $PaCO_2 = 68$ mm Hg

   Here, observed $PaCO_2$ is more than the calculated $PaCO_2$ indicating respiratory acidosis.

3. Anion gap: $140 - (80 + 54) = 140 - 134 = 6$, indicating normal anion gap.
4. A–a gradient:
   a. Calculated A–a gradient $= (150 - PaCO_2/0.8) - PaO_2 = (150 - 68/0.8) - 54 = (150 - 85) - 54 = 65 - 54 = 11$ mm Hg
   b. Observed A–a gradient for age $= (60 + 10)/4 = 70/4 = 17.5$ mm Hg

   Here, observed gradient was more than the calculated A–a gradient indicating the cause is extrinsic to lung.
5. The diagnosis is metabolic alkalosis with respiratory acidosis.

CASE 40

An 80-year-old diabetic female admitted with severe respiratory distress, productive cough, and fever for 2 days. On examination, her pulse rate was 130 beats/min and blood pressure 90/60 mm Hg. Patient was ventilated and sedated.

Laboratory investigation demonstrated hemoglobin 12 g/dL, total leukocyte count 15,000/cc, chest X-ray demonstrated:

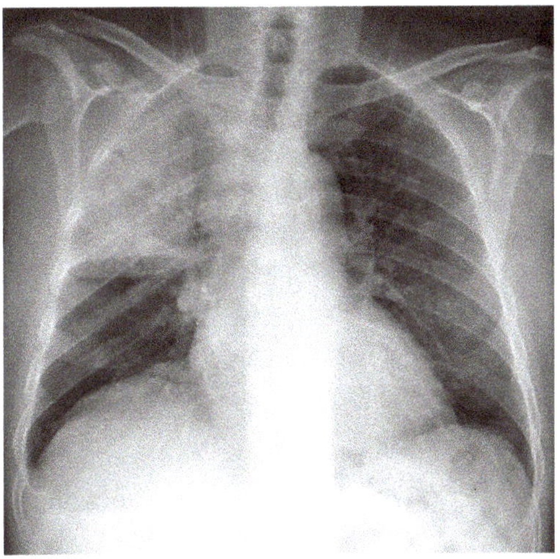

Arterial blood gases demonstrated pH 7.48, $PaCO_2$ 26 mm Hg, PaO_2 100 mm Hg, bicarbonate 19 mmol/L, lactate 6.6 mmol/L, sodium 135 mm Hg, potassium 4 mmol/L, and chloride 98 mmol/L.

1. **What is the finding in the above chest X-ray?**
2. **What is the primary acid–base disturbance?**
3. **What is the secondary compensation?**
4. **What is anion gap?**
5. **What is A–a gradient?**
6. **What is the etiological diagnosis?**

Answers

1. Above chest X-ray demonstrated consolidation involving the right upper and mid zone.
2. Primary acid–base disturbance:
   a. pH is 7.48 indicating alkalemia.
   b. $PaCO_2$ is 26 mm Hg indicating respiratory alkalosis.
3. Secondary compensation:
   a. Calculated bicarbonate = $24 - [(40 - 26)/10 \times 2] = 24 - (1.4 \times 2) = 24 - 2.8 = 21.2$ mmol/L.
   b. Observed bicarbonate = 19 mmol/L.

   Observed bicarbonate level is less than calculated bicarbonate indicating metabolic acidosis. Since serum lactate level is high, it indicates metabolic acidosis secondary to lactic acidosis.
4. Anion gap: $135 - (98 + 19) = 135 - 117 = 18$, indicating high anion gap.
5. A–a gap:
   a. Calculated A–a gradient = $(150 - 26/0.8) - 100 = (150 - 32.5) - 90 = 117.5 - 90 = 27.5$ mm Hg
   b. Observed A–a gradient = (Age in year + 10)/4 = $(80 + 10)/4 = 22.5$ mm Hg

   So, calculated A–a gradient is more than observed A–a gradient indicating the presence of intrinsic lung disease.
6. The diagnosis is respiratory alkalosis along with metabolic acidosis resulting from lactic acidosis due to hypoventilation as the patient has been suffering from intrinsic lung disease.

CASE 41

An 80-year-old patient having history of chronic obstructive lung disease admitted with progressively increasing respiratory distress, productive cough along with fever for 5 days.

On examination, the pulse rate is 120 beats/min, blood pressure 150/95 mm Hg, and respiratory rate 28 breaths/min.

Laboratory investigation demonstrated total leukocyte count 18,000/cc, hemoglobin 12 g/dL, and creatinine 1.9 mg/dL.

Arterial blood gas demonstrated pH 7.2, $PaCO_2$ 64 mm Hg, PaO_2 46 mm Hg, bicarbonate 26 mmol/L, sodium 136 mmol/L, potassium 5.2 mmol/L, and chloride 106 mmol/L.

1. **What is the primary acid–base disturbance?**
2. **What is the secondary compensation?**
3. **What is anion gap?**
4. **What is A–a gradient?**
5. **What is the etiological diagnosis?**

Answers

1. Primary acid–base imbalance:
   a. pH is 7.2 indicating acidemia.
   b. $PaCO_2$ is 64 mm Hg indicating respiratory acidosis.
2. Secondary compensation:
   a. Calculated bicarbonate = $24 + (64 - 40)/10 = 24 + 2.4 = 26.4$ mmol/L
   b. Observed bicarbonate = 26

   It indicates complete metabolic compensation.
3. Anion gap: $136 - (106 + 26) = 136 - 132 = 4$ mmol/L
4. A–a gradient:
   a. Calculated A–a gradient = $(150 - 64/0.8) - 46 = (150 - 80) - 46 = 70 - 46 = 24$ mm Hg
   b. Observed A–a gradient for age = (Age in years + 10)/4 = $(80 + 10)/4 = 22.5$ mm Hg

   Calculated A–a gradient is more than observed A–a gradient indicating intrinsic lung disease.
5. Patient has been suffering from respiratory acidosis with completely compensatory metabolic alkalosis due to hypoventilated lung resulting from intrinsic lung disease.

CHAPTER 2

Cardiology

A 41-year-old male presented with palpitation, dyspnea on exertion, and past history of rheumatic fever.

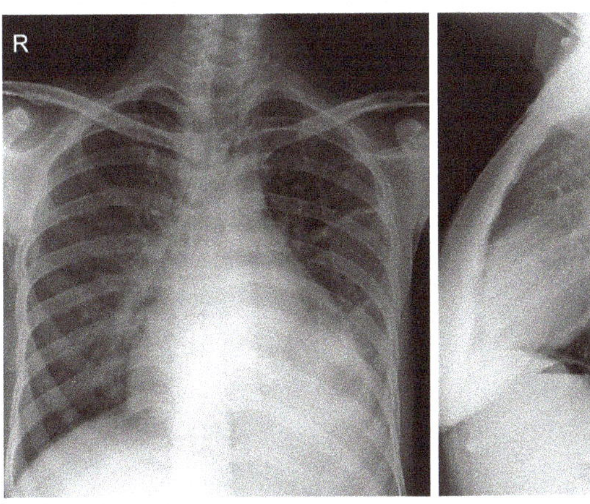

1. **Describe the picture of chest.**
2. **What are the structures that form left border of the heart?**
3. **What is your diagnosis?**
4. **How can you determine the severity of the valvular lesion?**
5. **What are the factors that determine the success of valvoplasty?**

Answers

1. Chest X-ray description:
   a. Cardiac shadow is enlarged.
   b. Straightening of the left border of the heart.
   c. Double contour right ventricle—it is formed by right border of enlarged left atrium.
   d. Splaying of carinal angle
2. Left border of the heart is formed by:
   a. Aortic knuckle
   b. Prominent pulmonary conus
   c. Concave left atrial appendages which is usually convex.
   d. Left ventricular wall

3. The diagnosis is mitral stenosis of rheumatic origin with pulmonary hypertension.
4. Following factors determine the severity of the mitral stenosis:
   a. Mild mitral stenosis:
      - Symptoms are absent.
      - Gap between the second heart sound and opening snap is >120 ms.
      - Valve area is >1.5 cm^2.
      - Pulmonary second heart sound is normal.
      - Pulmonary artery systolic pressure is <30 mm Hg.
      - Mean pressure gradient between the left atrium and left ventricle is <5 mm Hg.

b. Moderate mitral stenosis:
- Symptoms are New York Heart Association (NYHA) II to III.
- Gap between the second heart sound and opening snap is >80–100 ms.
- Valve area is 1.0–1.5 cm^2.
- Pulmonary second heart sound is loud.
- Pulmonary artery systolic pressure is 30–50 mm Hg.
- Mean pressure gradient between the left atrium and left ventricle is 5–10 mm Hg.

c. Severe stenosis:
- Symptoms are NYHA II to IV.
- Gap between the second heart sound and opening snap is <80 ms.

- Right parasternal lift
- Valve area is <1.0 cm^2.
- Pulmonary second heart sound is loud.
- Pulmonary artery systolic pressure is >50 mm Hg.
- Mean pressure gradient between the left atrium and left ventricle is <10 mm Hg.

5. Following factors determine the success of valvoplasty:
a. Good mobility of the mitral valves
b. Very little or absence of calcification
c. Minimal subvalvular disease
d. Mild mitral regurgitation

CASE 2

A 45-year-old man with past history of rheumatic fever came to outpatient department (OPD) with dyspnea of exertion, cough with expectoration, and history of paroxysmal nocturnal dyspnea demonstrated following features:

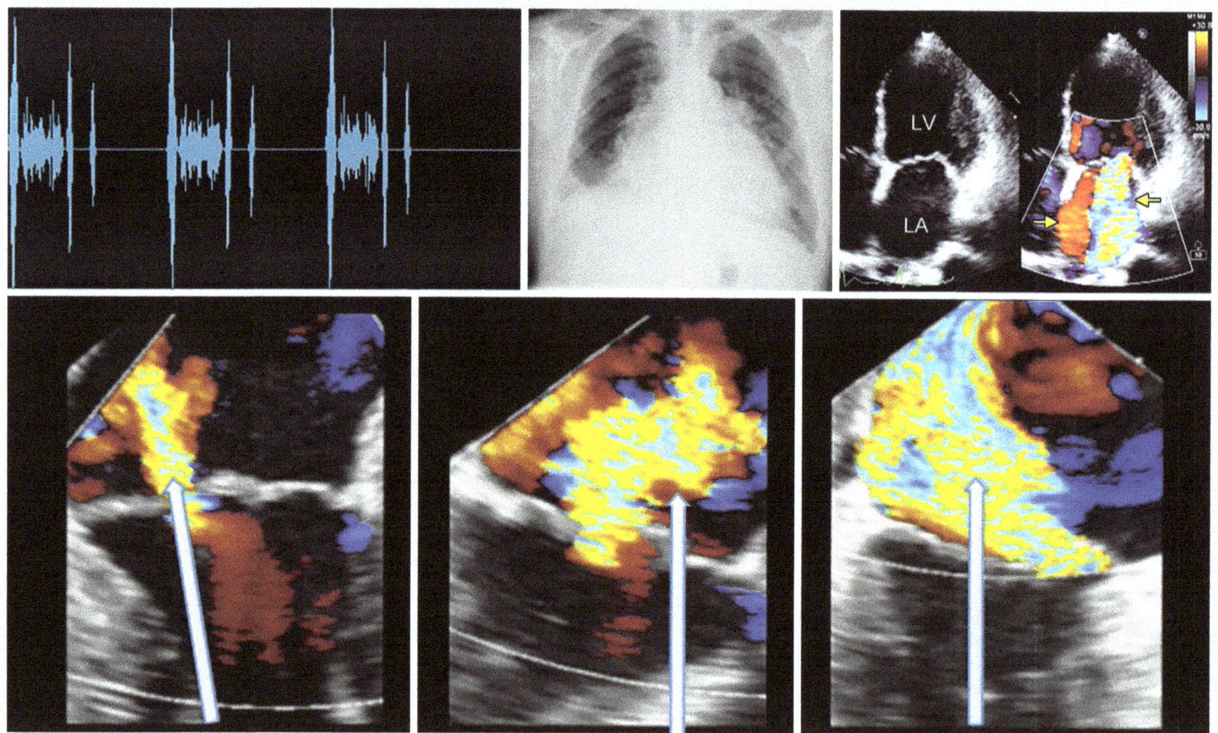

1. **What is the radiological feature?**
2. **What is the phonocardiographic feature?**
3. **What are the echocardiographic features?**
4. **What is your diagnosis?**
5. **Classify the disease?**
6. **How you can qualitatively and quantitatively estimate the severity of this disease?**

Answers

1. Description of the straight X-ray of the chest:
   a. Left atrial appendage is convex.
   b. Double contour of right ventricle or double density sign due to right side of the enlarged left atrium pushes the lung creating additional contour on the right ventricle
   c. Upper zone engorgement of vein due to pulmonary venous hypertension
   d. Bilateral hilar congestion
2. Phonocardiographic features:
   a. There is pansystolic rectangular murmur.
   b. There is presence of S3 gallop.
3. Echocardiographic features are:
   a. Enlarged left ventricle
   b. Cooptation point of the mitral leaflets point has been displaced into left ventricle.

   c. Next picture will demonstrate the severity of the regurgitation.
4. The diagnosis is mitral regurgitation.
5. This disease can be subclassified into three types based on movement of the leaflets (Carpentier's classification):
   a. Type I: Here, valve movement is normal; so, there may be perforation of leaflet or annular dilatation of the ring.
   b. Type II: Excessive movement of the leaflet such as rupture of papillary muscles.
   c. Type III: Here, the movement of the leaflet will be restricted, it will be subclassified into two types:
      i. Type IIIa: Restriction in the diastolic phase, i.e., rheumatic fever
      ii. Type IIIb: Restriction in the systolic phase, i.e., restrictive cardiomyopathy.

6. Estimation of severity:

Mild mitral regurgitation		Moderate mitral regurgitation		Severe mitral regurgitation	
Qualitative	Quantitative	Qualitative	Quantitative	Qualitative	Quantitative
Angiographic grade 1	Regurgitant volume: <30 mL/beat	Angiographic grade 2+	Regurgitant volume: <30 to 59 mL/beat	Angiographic grade 3 – 4+	Regurgitant volume: ≥ 30 mL/beat
Doppler vena contracta width 0.3 cm	Regurgitant fraction: <30%	Doppler vena contracta width 0.3–0.69 cm	Regurgitant fraction: 30–49%	Doppler vena contracta width >0.7 cm	Regurgitant fraction: ≥50%
Small central jet <4 cm^2	Regurgitant orifice area: <0.20 cm^2	Signs of mitral regurgitation are greater than mild mitral regurgitation	Regurgitant orifice area: 0.20–0.39 cm^2	• Large central jet or with wall impinging jet of any size • Swirling of left atrium	Regurgitant orifice area: ≥0.20 cm^2

CASE 3

A 65-year-old male came to OPD with exertional chest pain. His ECG was normal. His pulse demonstrated:

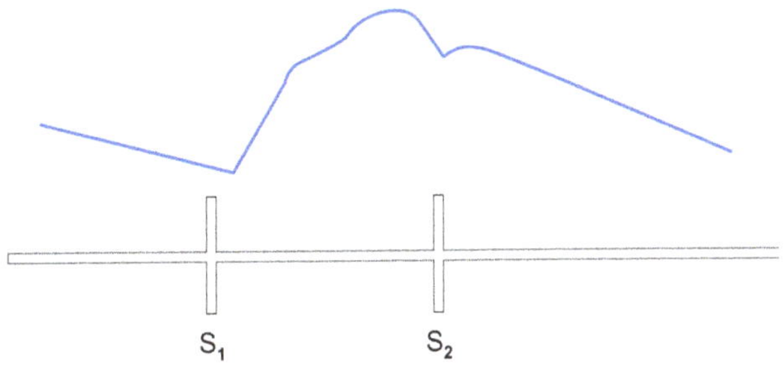

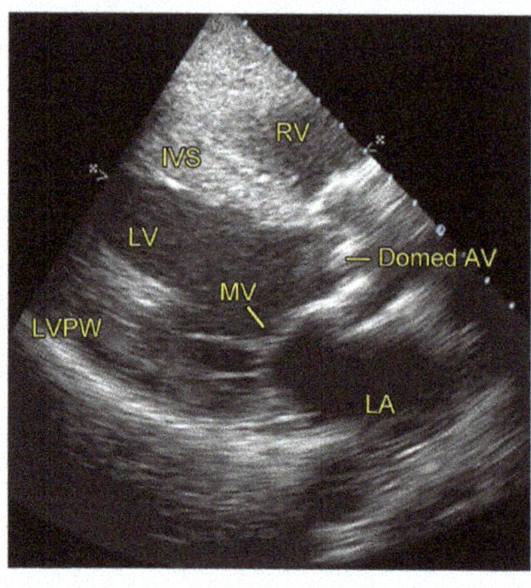

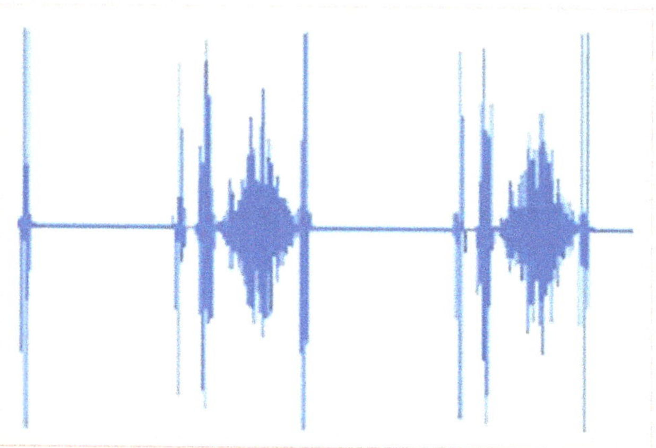

1. **Describe the pulse wave and echo picture and phonocardiography.**
2. **What is your diagnosis?**
3. **How can you determine the severity of isolated lesion of this valve?**
4. **What are the indications of echocardiography in this lesion?**
5. **What the second heart sound indicates in this lesion?**
6. **What are the relations between this lesion and bleeding into the gastrointestinal tract?**

Answers

1. Description of the above pictures:
   a. Pulse wave—anacrotic pulse—slow rise and slow decline
   b. Echocardiography picture: Paracentral long axis demonstrates calcific aortic valve doming into the aorta during systole.
   c. Phonocardiography demonstrates crescendo-decrescendo, i.e., diamond-shaped systolic murmur following ejection click immediately after first heart sound.
2. Diagnosis is aortic stenosis.
3. Severity can be diagnosed by the following measurement:
   a. Mild aortic stenosis:
      - Jet velocity: <3 m/s
      - Mean gradient: <25 mm Hg
      - Valve area: <1.5 cm^2
   b. Moderate aortic stenosis:
      - Jet velocity: 3–4 m/s
      - Mean gradient: 25–40 mm Hg
      - Valve area: 1–1.5 cm^2
   c. Severe aortic stenosis:
      - Jet velocity: >4 m/s
      - Mean gradient: >40 mm Hg
      - Valve area: <1 cm^2
      - Valve area index: 0.6 cm^2/m^2
4. Indications of echocardiography in aortic stenosis:
   a. Diagnosis and assessing the severity of the aortic stenosis
   b. It can define the level of lesion.
   c. Identification of the calcification in the aortic valve
   d. It can assess the size, function, and hemodynamics of left ventricle.
   e. In case of changing the clinical features, reevaluation of the lesion
   f. Reevaluation of the asymptomatic patients in case severe lesion
   g. It can evaluate the patient during pregnancy.
5. Second heart sound indicates:
   a. Soft second heart sound indicates the good mobility of the aortic leaflet.
   b. Single second heart sound indicates either there is fibrosis or fusion of valvular leaflets.
   c. Reverse splitting of the second heart sound indicates mechanical prolongation of the ventricular systole.
   d. Normal second heart sound indicates absence of critical aortic stenosis.
6. Abnormality of von Willebrand factor is closely associated with the severity of aortic stenosis. This factor usually circulates in the blood as large multimer which helps in coagulation of blood through the platelet aggregation. In severe aortic stenosis, this factor is subjected to sheering stress as it passes through the valve leaflet and susceptible to cleavage by metalloprotease ADAMTS13. As a result, there is chance of bleeding from gastrointestinal tract and skin.

CASE 4

A 44-year-old male came to OPD with palpitation. His pulse wave and echocardiographic feature are:

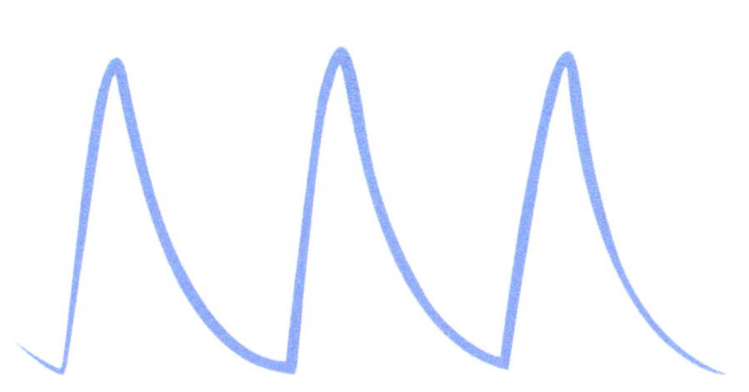 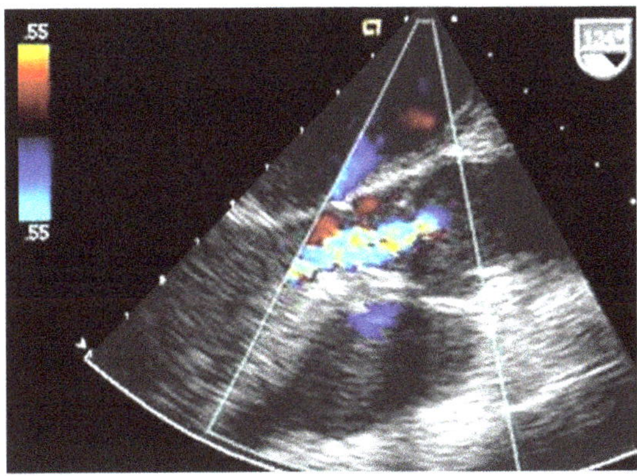

1. **Describe the pulse wave and echocardiographic picture.**
2. **What is your diagnosis?**
3. **How can you determine the severity of the lesion?**
4. **What are clinical signs of severity?**
5. **Name the indication of pupil examination in this lesion.**

Answers

1. Description of the pictures:
   a. Phonocardiographic features: Sudden rise and sudden fall of blood flow due to low diastolic pressure.
   b. Echocardiographic features: Rapid backward flow due to low diastolic pressure in the aorta.
2. The diagnosis is aortic regurgitation probably of rheumatic origin.
3. Following are the features of severity of aortic regurgitation:

Mild regurgitation		Moderate regurgitation		Severe regurgitation	
Qualitative	Quantitative	Qualitative	Quantitative	Qualitative	Quantitative
Angiographic grade 1+	Regurgitant volume: <30 mL/beat	Angiographic grade 2+	Regurgitant volume: 30–59 mL/beat	Angiographic grade 3–4+	Regurgitant volume: ≥60 mL/beat
Color Doppler jet width: Central jet is <25% of left ventricular outflow tract	Regurgitant fraction: <30%	Color Doppler jet width: Central jet is >25% but <65% of left ventricular outflow tract	Regurgitant fraction: 30–49%	Color Doppler jet width: Central jet is >65% of left ventricular outflow tract	Regurgitant fraction: ≥50%
Doppler vena contracta width: <0.3 cm	Regurgitant orifice area: 0.10 cm^2	Doppler vena contracta width: 0.3–0.6 cm	Regurgitant orifice area: 0.10–0.29 cm^2	Doppler vena contracta width: >0.6 cm	Regurgitant orifice area: ≥0.3 cm^2

4. Following are clinical signs of severity:
   a. Wide pulse pressure
   b. Soft second heart sound
   c. Austin Flint murmur
   d. Duration of the murmur
   e. Presence of left ventricular third heart sound
   f. Signs of left ventricular failure
5. Check of Argyll Robertson pupil as it may indicate the etiology as syphilitic aortic regurgitation

CASE 5

A 70-year-old man has come to your OPD with vertigo, tremor, and slow abnormal gait. His ambulatory blood pressure demonstrated the following:

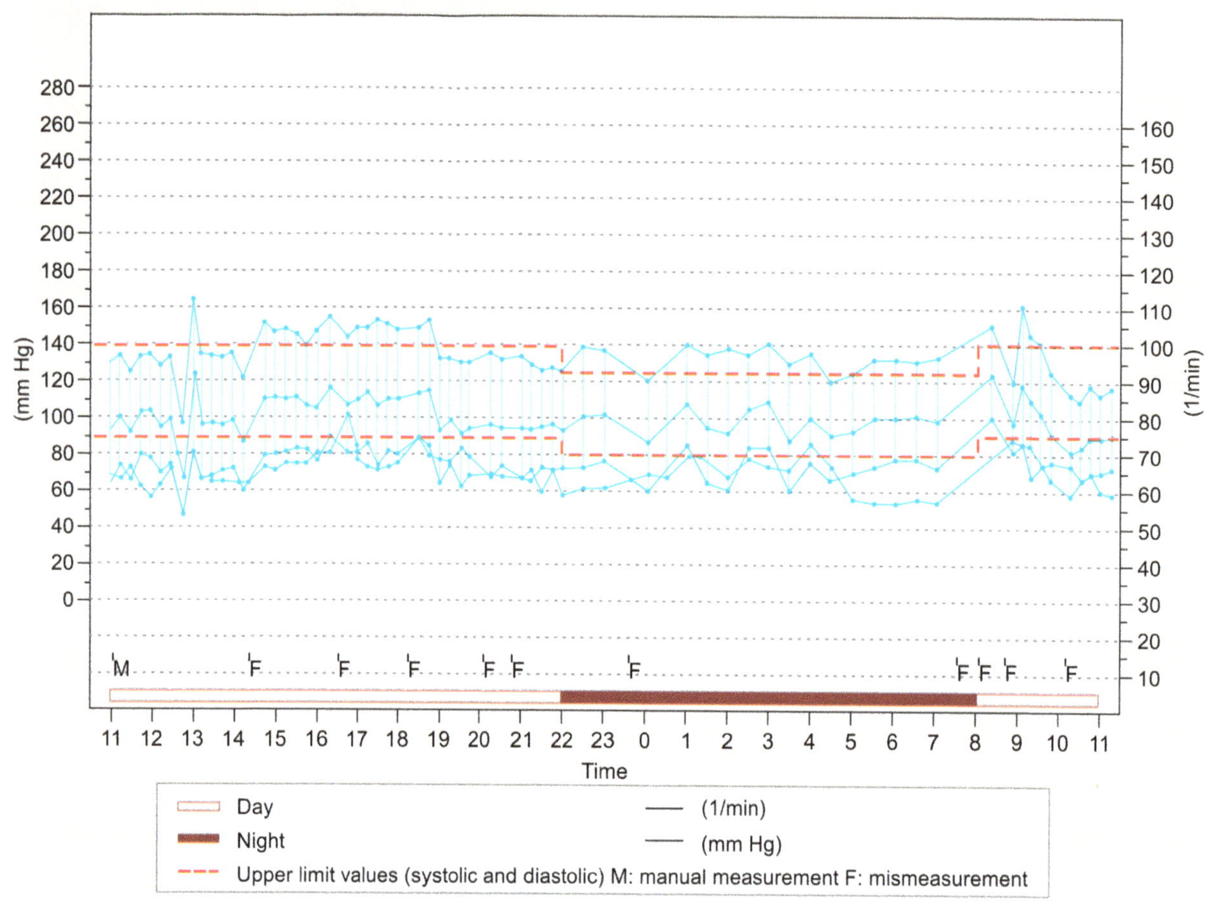

1. **Describe the report of ambulatory blood pressure recording.**
2. **What is your diagnosis?**
3. **What are the normal values of ambulatory blood pressure monitoring?**
4. **What are the indications of ambulatory blood pressure monitoring?**
5. **How can you define hypertension from ambulatory blood pressure monitoring?**
6. **Define white coat hypertension.**
7. **What may be the risk from masked hypertension?**
8. **Name five implication of masked hypertension.**
9. **Name five indications of ambulatory pressure monitoring in elderly.**

Answers

1. In this recording, there is absence of dipping of nocturnal blood pressure. This is the marker of marked orthostatic hypertension. So, it can be used to detect presence or absence of orthostatic hypotension.

2. The presence of bradykinesia, short shuffling gait, and pill-rolling tremor are suggestive of Parkinson's disease.

3. Normal value of ambulatory blood pressure:

Item	Systolic blood pressure	Diastolic blood pressure
Total average	130.7 ± 14.2 mm Hg	79 ± 10.9 mm Hg
Daytime	130 mm Hg	80 mm Hg
Night	120 mm Hg	70 mm Hg

4. Indications of ambulatory blood pressure monitoring:
   a. Exclusion of white coat hypertension
   b. Elderly patients
   c. Deciding diagnosis in case of borderline hypertension
   d. Identification of nocturnal hypertension
   e. Hypertensive patients resistant to treatment
   f. As a guide to treatment with antihypertensive drugs
   g. Hypertension in pregnancy
   h. Diagnosis of hypotension
5. Diagnosis of hypertension by ambulatory blood pressure monitoring:
   a. If the daytime blood pressure is ≥140/90 mm Hg and diastolic blood pressure is ≥125/75 mm Hg, it can be diagnosed as systemic hypertension.

6. Definition of white coat hypertension:
   a. Office blood pressure is ≥140/90 mm Hg.
   b. Daytime normal ambulatory blood pressure is <135/85 mm Hg.
7. Following are the risk from white coat hypertension:
   a. Considerably less than sustained hypertension
   b. Patient may be a state of prehypertension.
   c. It may not be an innocent condition.
8. Clinical implications of masked hypertension:
   i. It must be considered in a case of newly hypertensives.
   ii. It should be considered prior to prescription of antihypertensive drugs.
   iii. It is common in elderly and pregnancy.
   iv. It always needs follow-up and remonitoring
   v. There is presence of overall risks.
9. Following five are the indications of ambulatory pressure monitoring in elderly:
   i. White coat hypertension
   ii. Isolated systolic hypertension
   iii. Autonomic failure
   iv. Drug-induced hypotension
   v. Postural hypotension

CASE 6

A 55-year-old man attended in an OPD with occasional palpitation. His ECG demonstrated:

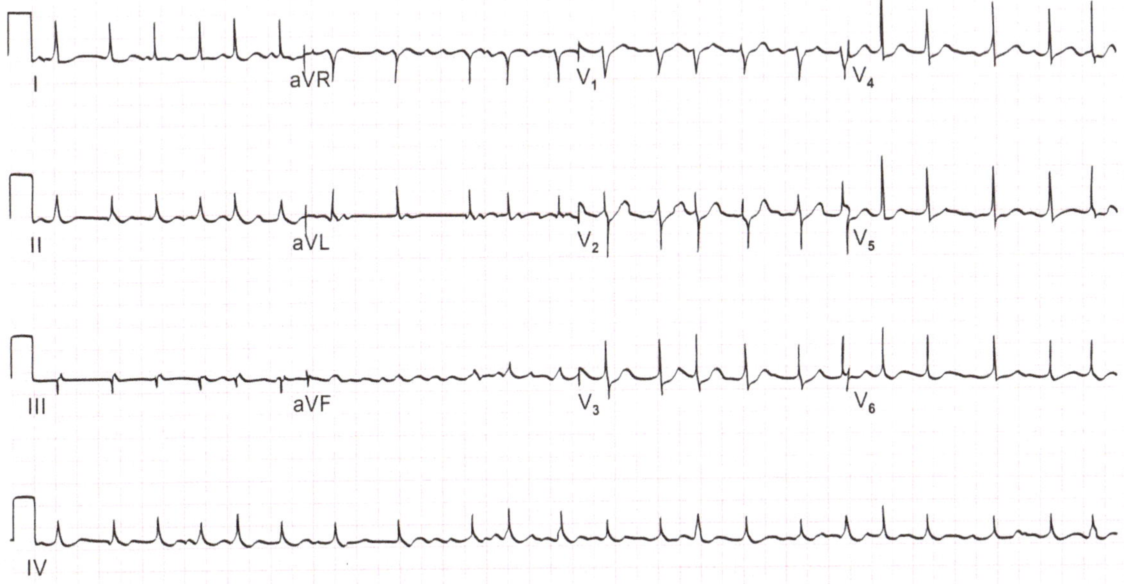

1. **Describe the ECG finding.**
2. **What are the genetic disorders associated with this disease?**
3. **What are the nonmodifiable and modifiable risk factors associated with the disease?**
4. **Classify the disease.**
5. **What are the sites of origin of ectopic foci?**
6. **What are the components of bleeding risk index?**
7. **What are the roles of surgery in the treatment of this disease?**
8. **How can you treat a case of atrial fibrillation?**

Answers

1. ECG features are:
   a. Absence of P wave.
   b. Irregular RR intervals due to irregular conduction of impulses into the ventricles.
   c. Narrow QRS complexes: It signifies normal conduction from the atria.
2. Following genetic disorders are associated with the atrial fibrillation:
   a. Familial atrial fibrillation as monogenic disease.
   b. Familial atrial fibrillation in the setting of other inherited cardiac diseases:
      - Dilated cardiomyopathy
      - Hypertrophic cardiomyopathy
      - Familial amyloidosis
   c. Inherited arrhythmic syndrome:
      - Congenital long QT syndrome
      - Brugada syndrome
      - Short QT syndrome
   d. Nonfamilial atrial fibrillation in the genetic background such as ACE gene polymorphism
3. Risk factors:
   a. Nonmodifiable risk factors:
      - Age
      - Sex
      - Ethnicity
      - Genetics
   b. Modifiable risk factors:
      - Sedentary lifestyle
      - High blood pressure
      - Tobacco
      - Obesity
      - Diabetes
      - Obstructive sleep apnea
4. Classification of atrial fibrillation:

   Based on the temporary or pattern of episodes:
   a. Paroxysmal atrial fibrillation: This is characterized by presence of atrial fibrillation persisting for <7 days and resolving spontaneously in <7 days with or without intervention. It can be subclassified into:
      - Vagotonic atrial fibrillation: This type of atrial fibrillation is induced by drugs such as digitalis or period that induces high vagal tone.
      - Adrenergic atrial fibrillation: This type of atrial fibrillation results from period of high adrenergic tone.
   b. Persistent atrial fibrillation: Here, atrial fibrillation last >7 days but <1 year.
   c. Long-lasting persistent atrial fibrillation: This type of atrial fibrillation lasts longer than a year.
   d. Permanent atrial fibrillation: Here, atrial fibrillation is present for years. This atrial fibrillation cannot be restored to sinus rhythm by cardioversion.
   e. Recent onset atrial fibrillation: This is the first diagnosed atrial fibrillation.
   f. Secondary atrial fibrillation: It occurs secondary to the following diseases:
      - Myocarditis
      - Myocardial infarction
      - Pulmonary embolism
      - Pericarditis
      - Pneumonia
      - Hyperthyroidism
      - Postcardiac surgery
      - Acute pulmonary diseases

   Based on the presence of concomitant valvular disease:
   a. Valvular atrial fibrillation: Here, atrial fibrillation occurs in mitral stenosis or other mechanical valvular disease.
   b. Nonvalvular atrial fibrillation: It includes all other forms of valvular diseases except mitral stenosis or mechanical valvular diseases.

   Based on etiology of atrial fibrillation:
   a. Atrial fibrillation secondary to structural heart diseases such as:
      - Left ventricular systolic dysfunction

- Left ventricular diastolic dysfunction
- Long-standing hypertension leading to left ventricular hypertrophy.

b. Focal atrial fibrillation: These patients have short runs, frequent, and repetitive paroxysmal atrial fibrillation.

c. Monogenic atrial fibrillation: It occurs in presence of inherited cardiomyopathies such as channelopathies.

d. Polygenic atrial fibrillation: Here, atrial fibrillation occurs in the carriers of common genetic variants in whom atrial fibrillation occurs is early in onset.

e. Postoperative atrial fibrillation: Here, atrial fibrillation occurs after major cardiac surgery that had prior sinus rhythm and no history of atrial fibrillation.

f. Valvular atrial fibrillation

g. Atrial fibrillation in athletes: Here, it occurs in athletes and it is related to duration and intensity of training.

5. Sites of origin of ectopic foci:
   a. Rapid atrial discharge from atria adjacent to pulmonary vein.
   b. Reentrant leading circle
   c. Spiral waves arising from left atrium near the pulmonary vein

6. Following are the components of bleeding risk index:
   a. Age >65 years: 1 point
   b. History of stroke: 1 point
   c. History of gastrointestinal bleeding: 1 point
   d. Any one or more can be associated (1 point):
      - Diabetes mellitus
      - Recent myocardial infarction

- Packed cell volume of <30%
- Serum creatinine of >1.5 mg/dL

Annular risk of stroke:
a. Low risk: 0 point
b. Intermediate risk: 1–2 points
c. High risk: 3–4 points

7. Role of surgery in atrial fibrillation:
   a. Maze procedure: It involves multiple incisions in the atria for preventing the reentrant loops. It is highly effective in preventing atrial fibrillation.
   b. Corridor procedure: This procedure separates left from right atrium only leaves a myocardial strip that connects sinus node to atrioventricular (AV) node. This procedure cannot prevent atrial fibrillation but can isolates fibrillating atria.

8. Treatment of atrial fibrillation: 4C approaches:
   a. Restoration of ventricular rate:
      - In case of hypertensive patient: Calcium antagonists such as verapamil and diltiazem
      - In case of hyperthyroidism: β-blocker such as propranolol
      - In case of ischemic heart disease: β-blockers such as diltiazem and verapamil
      - In case of heart failure: Digoxin and verapamil
      - In case of hypertrophic cardiomyopathy: Calcium antagonist or β-blockers
      - If the patient is intolerant or nonresponding to the drugs: Radiofrequency catheter ablation of the AV node
      - If the foci are near the pulmonary vein: Radiofrequency ablation of the pulmonary veins

CASE 7

A 56-year-old nonalcoholic and nondiabetic patient has been admitted in casualty with pedal edema, and right upper abdominal pain and orthopnea. He has neither history of liver disease nor kidney disease. His neck vein demonstrated:

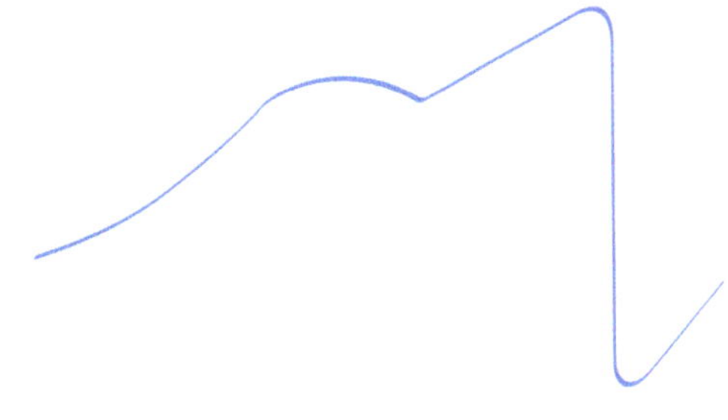

1. **Describe the wave.**
2. **What is your diagnosis?**
3. **What is hepatojugular reflux?**
4. **What are the clinical types of this disease?**
5. **What are the clinical signs of this disease?**

Answers

1. Description of the wave:
   a. Absence of x descent
   b. Increased v wave due to atrial filling during systole leading to formation of "cv" wave—it is specific but never sensitive for tricuspid regurgitation. Its amplitude increases with inspiration.
   c. "cv" is followed by deep y descent.
2. The diagnosis is tricuspid regurgitation.
3. Hepatojugular reflux:
   Physiologically:

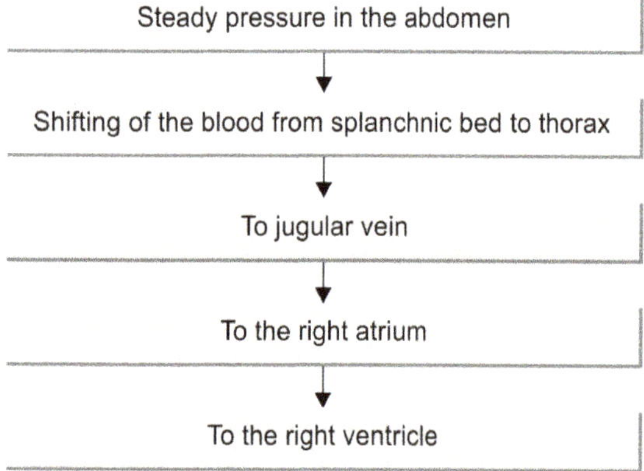

In case of slightly elevated jugular venous pressure, the raised pressure becomes overt.

Uses of hepatojugular reflux:
a. Subclinical right ventricular failure
b. Silent tricuspid regurgitation
c. Symptomatic left ventricular failure

Compression on liver during abdominojugular reflux is detrimental in patient with passive venous congestion because compression on the already stretched Glisson's capsule may elicit pain and valsalva response. Hence, compression over the periumbilical area can be done anywhere to elicit.

4. Following are the clinical types:
   a. Primary tricuspid regurgitation: It is an organic form where it may be congenital like Epstein anomaly or any infection producing damage of the valve.
   b. Secondary or functional tricuspid regurgitation: Here, valve itself may be abnormal but in any type of left-sided valvular damage, there may be malfunction of tricuspid valve.
   c. Isolated tricuspid regurgitation: Here, right atrial enlargement or may be due to prior heart surgery or prior transvenous pacemaker.
5. Following are the clinical signs:
   a. Distended jugular vein with prominent v wave
   b. Diminished volume of pulse due to decreased forward blood flow
   c. If there is left ventricular dysfunction, basal crepitation
   d. S3 gallop
   e. S4 gallop which will be increased during inspiration.
   f. Left parasternal heave due to right ventricular enlargement
   g. There may be pansystolic murmur in the tricuspid area.
   h. Ascites
   i. Enlarged tender liver
   j. Pedal edema
   k. May be jaundice
   l. There may be malabsorption leading to cachexia.

CASE 8

A 35-year-old nonhypertensive and nondiabetic man presenting with extreme fatigue, exertional dyspnea, and progressively increasing peripheral edema and abdominal swelling came to OPD. During clinical examination, neck vein and X-ray demonstrated:

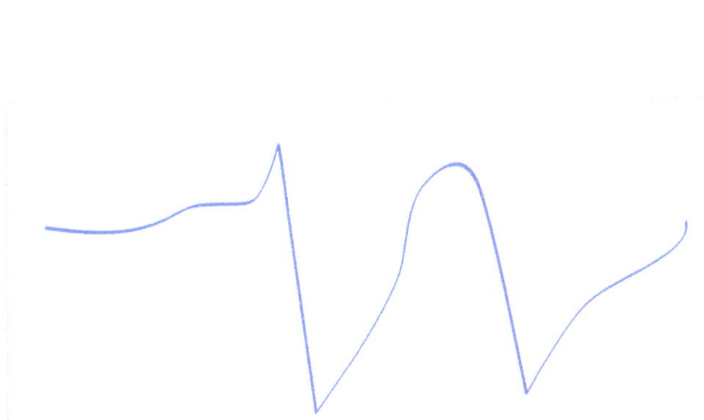

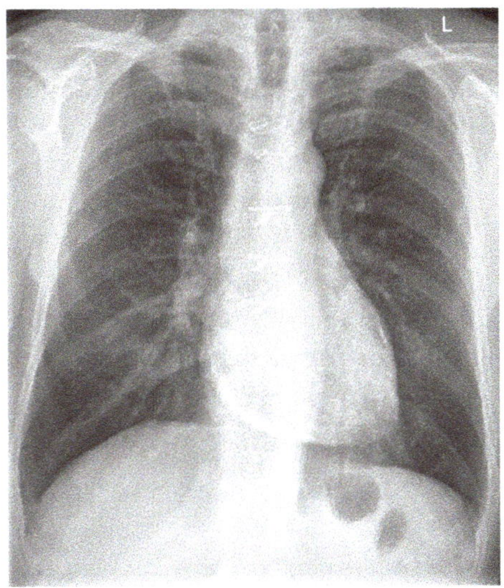

1. **What are the findings in the venous wave and chest X-ray?**
2. **What is your diagnosis?**
3. **What are the clinical signs in this disease?**
4. **What are the findings in echocardiography?**
5. **Name five important complications of this disease.**
6. **How can you differentiate it from restrictive cardiomyopathy?**
7. **How can you differentiate this disease from cardiac tamponade?**
8. **What are the similarities between this disease and cardiac tamponade?**

Answers

1. Above picture demonstrates:
   a. Venous wave demonstrates exaggerated x and y descent.
   b. X-ray picture demonstrates evidence of pericardial calcifications.
2. The diagnosis is constrictive pericarditis.
3. Clinical signs are the following:
   a. General examination reveals:
      - Increased jugular venous pressure and it is nonpulsatile. But, patient should not be examined in supine position as in this position, upper level of venous pulse will be above the angle of the jaw.
      - Decreased volume of the pulse. If pulsus paradoxus is present, it indicates systolic blood pressure drop of >10 mm Hg during inspiration and it suggests associated pericardial effusion.
      - Blood pressure will be low.
      - Tachycardia
      - Pitting pedal edema
      - Ascites
      - Hepatomegaly
   b. Cardiovascular examination reveals:
      - Heart sound may be muffled.
      - Presence of pericardial knock heard in the left sternal border high pitch—it will correspond to sudden cessation of the ventricular filling early in the diastole. It occurs earlier than third heard sound.
4. Features in echocardiography:
   a. Following features are found in M-mode echocardiography:
      - During inspiration, posterior motion of ventricular septum in early diastole
      - In inspiration, absence of increased systemic venous return.

- Due to increased right ventricular diastolic pressure as compared to pulmonary arterial pressure, premature opening of pulmonary valve.

b. Doppler echocardiography demonstrates following features:
- In early diastole, abnormal passive filling of the ventricles.
- Increased velocity of the diastolic flow across the tricuspid valve in inspiration and it will be decreased during expiration.
- Increased reduction of the velocity of the flow of blood through the pulmonary veins and mitral valve during inspiration
- Leftward shift of interventricular septum

5. Complications of constrictive pericarditis:
   a. Pulmonary hypertension
   b. Renal failure
   c. Metabolic acidosis
   d. Shock
   e. Death

6. Differences between the restrictive cardiomyopathy and constrictive pericarditis:

Item	Constrictive pericarditis	Restrictive cardiomyopathy
Respiratory variation in left-sided and right-sided pressure/flows	Exaggerated	Normal
Enhanced respiratory variation in mitral inflow velocity	>25%	≤10%
Thickness of the ventricular wall	Normal	Increased
Thickness of the pericardium	Increased	Normal
Atrial size	Left atrial enlargement	Biatrial enlargement

Continued

Continued

Item	Constrictive pericarditis	Restrictive cardiomyopathy
Doppler E' velocity	Increased	It is reduced
Speckle tracking	• Normal longitudinal restriction • Decreased circumferential restoration	• Decreased longitudinal restriction • Normal circumferential restoration
Specific area index	Greater: >1.1	Lesser: <1.1

7. The differences are the following:
   a. In case of cardiac tamponade, pericardial space is open so that it can transmit thoracic pressure in the respiratory variation to the heart; whereas, in case of constrictive pericarditis, pericardial cavity will be obliterated, as a result this cannot transmit thoracic pressure changes. This dissociation of intrathoracic and intracardiac pressure changes is responsible for hemodynamic, physical, and echocardiographic feature of constrictive pericarditis.
   b. In cardiac tamponade increased venous return during inspiration will enlarge the right side of the heart then to left heart; whereas, there is no increase in systemic venous return in constrictive pericarditis.

8. Similarities are the following:
   a. Hemodynamics of both left and right side of the heart in both the diseases are directly and highly influenced by each other, i.e., interdependence.
   b. Diastolic dysfunction
   c. Preserved ventricular ejection fraction
   d. Increased variation in respiration of ventricular inflow and outflow
   e. Equally elevated central venous pressure
   f. Equally elevated pulmonary venous pressure
   g. Ventricular diastolic pressure
   h. Mild pulmonary hypertension

CASE 9

A 42-year-old female came to OPD with fatigue, cough, and exertional dyspnea. Doctor examined her and asked to do a chest X-ray which demonstrated:

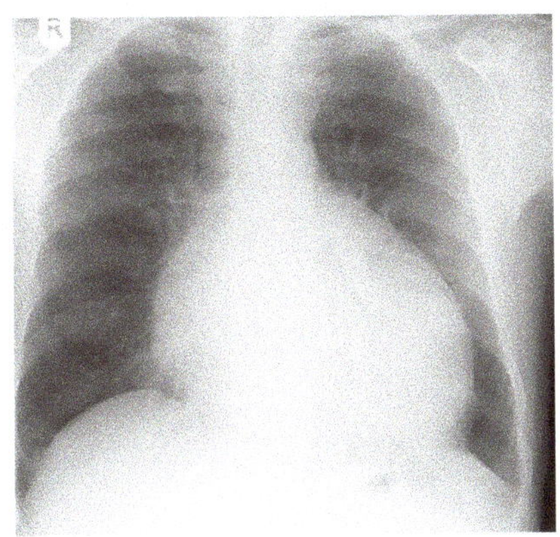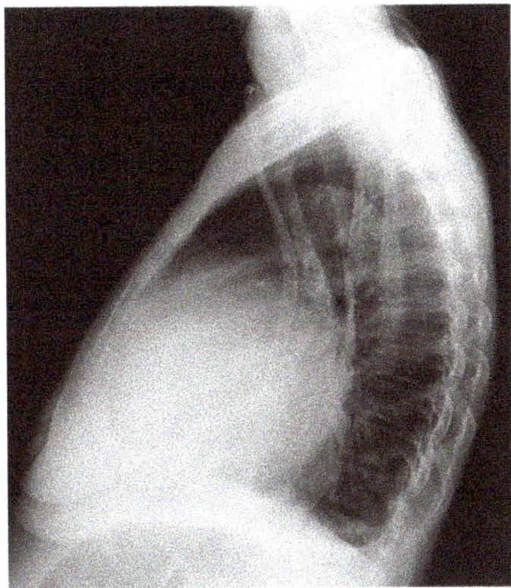

1. **What are the features present in the anteroposterior (AP) view and lateral view of X-ray chest?**
2. **What is your diagnosis?**
3. **How can you estimate the volume of the pericardial effusion?**
4. **What are the clinical signs in this case?**

Answers

1. Chest X-ray demonstrates the following:
   a. In AP view:
      - There is globular enlargement of the cardiac shadow leading to water bottle configuration.
      - There is increased cardiothoracic ratio.
      - Differential density of the cardiac border.
   b. In the lateral view:
      - There is vertical opaque line indicating pleural fluid separates vertical lucent line that is present behind the sternum which is pericardial fat anteriorly.
      - There is vertical opaque line indicating pleural fluid seperates vertical lucent line representing epicardial fat posteriorly—it is known as Oreo cookie sign.
      - There is widening of the subcarinal angle in absence of left atrial enlargement.
2. The diagnosis is pericardial effusion.
3. If the fluid is distributed throughout the pericardial cavity, depth of the effusion may be used the volume of fluid:
   a. Less than 5 mm: 50–100 of fluid
   b. 5–10 mm: 100–250 mL of fluid
   c. 10–20 mm: 250–500 mL of fluid
   d. More than 20 mm: >500 mL of fluid

But as the anatomy of the pericardium is complex, it is better to report the volume in general term:
   a. Less than 10 mm: Small pericardial effusion
   b. 10–20 mm: Moderate pericardial effusion
   c. More than 20 mm: Large pericardial effusion
4. Clinical signs in pericardial effusion:
   a. Classical Beck triad are:
      - Hypotension
      - Muffled heart sound
      - Jugular venous distention
   b. Pulsus paradoxus characterized by systolic pressure drop of >10 mm Hg during inspiration as a result of collapse of left ventricle at the expense of right ventricle with pedal edema.
   c. May be peripheral cyanosis
   d. Tachycardia
   e. Tachypnea
   f. Engorged nonpulsatile neck vein
   g. Decreased breath sound
   h. Ewart's sign:
      - Dullness on percussion beneath the angle of left scapula
      - Tubular breath sound
      - Egophony

CASE 10

A 38-year-old man has been admitted with exertional dyspnea and productive cough. He was examined thoroughly. His pulse demonstrated:

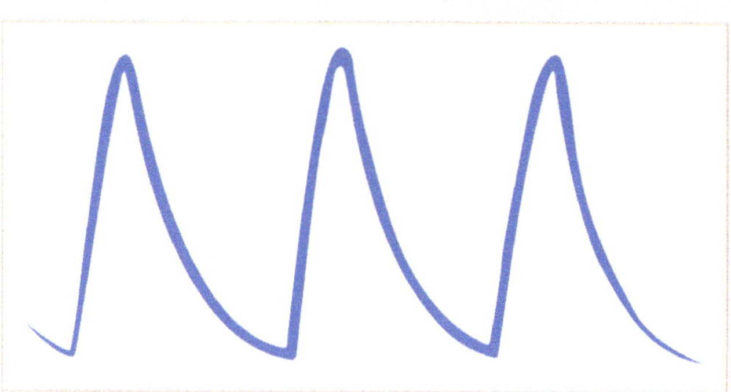

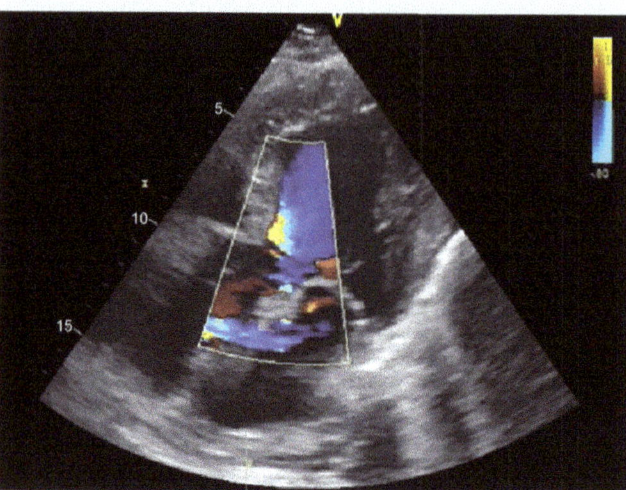

1. **Describe the picture above.**
2. **Name seven peripheral signs of aortic regurgitation.**
3. **What are the indications of echocardiography in this disease?**
4. **What are the clinical signs of severity of this disease?**
5. **What is cor bovinum?**
6. **How can you determine the severity of this disease?**

Answers

1. Descriptions of above pictures:
   a. Pulse wave demonstrates collapsing pulse, i.e., sudden rise and sudden fall of the blood column.
   b. Doppler echocardiography demonstrates:
      - Evidence of regurgitant jet extending below the left ventricular outflow tract
      - Holodiastolic reversal of flow in the descending aorta

2. Following are the seven peripheral signs of aortic regurgitation:
   i. Visible retinal arteries pulsation through the ophthalmoscope—Becker sign
   ii. Corrigan sign: Water hammer pulse with abrupt distention and quick collapse.
   iii. De Musset sign: Nodding of the head with each arterial pulsation.
   iv. Duroziez sign: Evidence of systolic murmur heard over the femoral artery when the femoral artery is compressed proximally and diastolic murmur when the femoral artery is compressed distally.
   v. Hill sign: Blood pressure is increased in the lower extremity as compared to that in the upper limb.
   vi. Mayne sign: There is 15 mm Hg of diastolic pressure drop when the arm is raised.
   vii. Quincke sign: Evidence of alternate flushing and paling at the base of the nail bed as the pressure applied at the tip of the nail.

3. Indication of echocardiography in this disease:
   a. To confirm the diagnosis of aortic regurgitation
   b. To determine the etiology of this disease
   c. To assess the morphology of the valve
   d. To estimate semiquantitatively the severity of regurgitation
   e. To assess the left ventricular dimension
   f. To assess the size of the aorta
   g. To assess the systolic function of left ventricle
   h. To estimate the degree of pulmonary hypertension
   i. To determine whether there is rapid equilibrium occurs in aortic and left ventricular pressure.

4. Following are the clinical signs of severity:
   a. Wide pulse pressure
   b. Second heart sound will be soft
   c. Presence of Austin Flint murmur
   d. Duration of the decrescendo murmur

e. Presence of left ventricular third heart sound

f. Signs of left ventricular failure

5. In case of chronic aortic regurgitation, there is evidence of progressive dilatation as well as hypertrophy of the left ventricle to attempt to normalize the stress, as a result the size of the heart becomes larger than any other form of chronic heart disease—this is known as cor bovinum or heart of ox.

6. Following can determine the severity of aortic regurgitation:

a. Mild aortic regurgitation:
   - Qualitative:
     - Grade 1+ angiographically
     - Color Doppler width of the central jet is <25% of left ventricular outflow tract obstruction.
     - Width of Doppler vena contracta is <0.3.
   - Quantitative:
     - Volume of the regurgitant is <30 mL/beat.
     - Fraction of the regurgitant is <30%.
     - Area of the regurgitant orifice is 0.10 cm^2.

b. Moderate aortic regurgitation:
   - Qualitative:
     - Grade 2+ angiographically
     - Color Doppler width of the central jet is >25% but <65% of left ventricular outflow tract obstruction.
     - Width of Doppler vena contracta is 0.3–0.6.
   - Quantitative:
     - Volume of the regurgitant is 30–59 mL/beat.
     - Fraction of the regurgitant is 30–49%.
     - Area of the regurgitant orifice is 0.10–0.29 cm^2.

c. Severe aortic regurgitation:
   - Qualitative:
     - Grade 3 to 4+ angiographically
     - Color Doppler width of the central jet is >65% of left ventricular outflow tract obstruction.
     - Width of Doppler vena contracta is >0.6.
   - Quantitative:
     - Volume of the regurgitant is ≥60 mL/beat.
     - Fraction of the regurgitant is ≥50%.
     - Area of the regurgitant orifice is ≥0.30 cm^2.

CASE 11

A 60-year-old man with history of long-standing hypertension, while attending hypertension clinic with exertional breathlessness, demonstrated dilated aortic root and severe aortic incompetence in echocardiography. Following are the pictures in this patient:

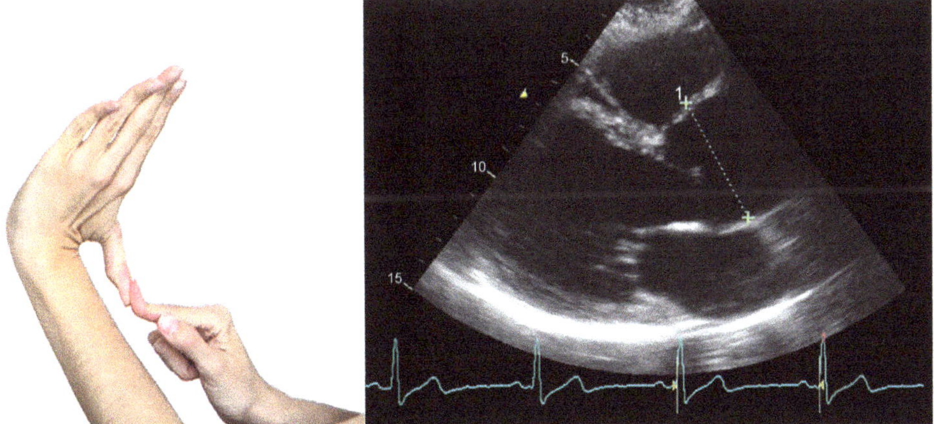

1. **Describe the pictures above.**
2. **What is your diagnosis?**
3. **What are the criteria of skeletal system involvement?**
4. **What are the criteria in ocular system involvement?**
5. **What is the indication of surgery in this patient?**

Answers

1. Description of the above pictures:
   a. Hyperextensible joint in thumb
   b. Dilated aortic root in echocardiography
2. Diagnosis is Marfan syndrome.
3. Criteria of skeletal system involvement:
   a. Major criteria:
      - Pectus excavatum
      - Reduced upper to lower segment ratio of <0.85
      - Arm span to height ratio of >1.05
      - When encircling contralateral wrist, there is overlap of thumb and index fingers—positive wrist sign.
      - Steinberg sign: When the digits held flexed in the palm, thumb will be extended beyond the ulnar border.
      - Thoracolumbar scoliosis of >20°
      - Pes planovalgus deformity due to progressive collapse of the hind foot
      - Protrusio acetabuli of any degree
   b. Minor criteria:
      - Moderately severe pectus excavatum
      - Joint hypermobility
      - High-arched palate with dental crowding
      - Facial appearance
        ○ Dolichocephaly
        ○ Malar hypoplasia
        ○ Enophthalmos
        ○ Retrognathia
        ○ Down-slanting palpebral fissure

   Two major criteria and one minor criterion or one major criterion and two minor criteria should be present to diagnose skeletal system involvement.
4. Following are the criteria of ocular system involvement:
   a. Major criterion is ectopia lentis.
   b. Minor criteria:
      - Abnormally flat cornea
      - Increased axial length of the globe in ultrasonography
      - Hypoplastic iris or hypoplastic ciliary muscle leading to myopia
5. Aortic root dilatation is indicated if the aortic root diameter is ≥45 mm.

   One major criterion and two minor criteria should be present to diagnose ocular system involvement.

CASE 12

A 60-year-old male with history of primary angioplasty in right coronary artery came to clinic with history of breathlessness without any chest pain. On examination, his blood pressure was normal and bradycardia. There was apical soft pansystolic murmur. ECG demonstrated atrial fibrillation, chest is clear. Urgent echocardiography was done:

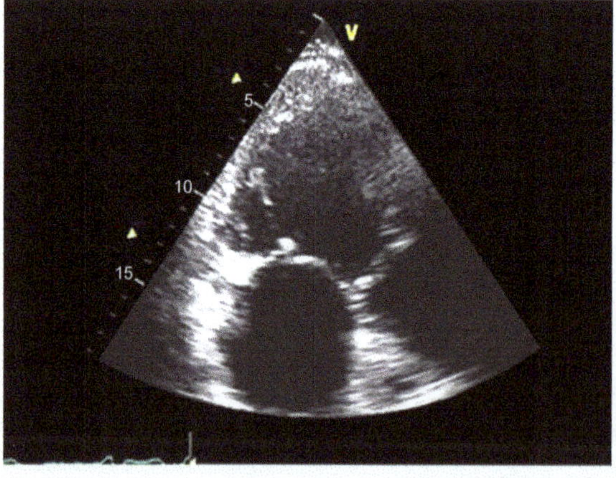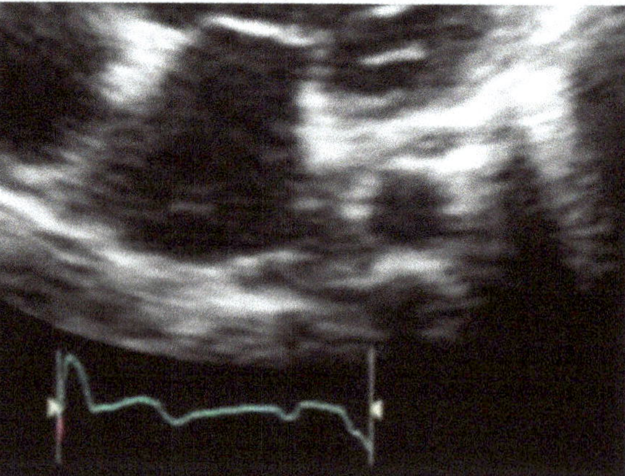

1. **What is being demonstrated in echocardiography?**
2. **What is your diagnosis?**
3. **Which is the most effective test and why?**

Answers

1. In the above echocardiography, tethering of the structural mitral valve leaflet and left ventricular hypokinesia are seen.
2. Diagnosis is acute mitral regurgitation due to tethering of posterior mitral leaflet.

3. Stress echocardiography is the most important test in this patient because ischemic mitral regurgitation is a dynamic condition and during exercise there is increase in the size of effective regurgitant orifice of ≥ 13 mm^3 which may lead to either hospitalization for cardiac decompensation or risk of sudden death.

CASE 13

An 82-year-old farmer with known history of aortic stenosis with blood pressure of 175/105 mm Hg attended in the echocardiography clinic for yearly surveillance of the condition of the heart. Echocardiography features were:

- Peak velocity has been increased from 3.7 to 4.1 m/s.
- Mean gradient across the aortic valve is 42 mm Hg.
- Aortic valve is 1 cm^2.
- Left ventricular hypertrophy
- Overall left ventricular function is good.

1. **What is the role of exercise tolerance test in this patient?**
2. **What are the complications of aortic stenosis?**
3. **What are the clinical variations may occur in the second heart sound in this case?**
4. **What are the indications of surgery in these patients?**
5. **What are the risk factors for consideration of aortic valve surgery?**

Answers

1. Exercise stress testing is not contraindicated in this patient because the patient is not symptomatic, as this test will unmask the symptoms in the physically active patient along with the fall in the blood pressure in asymptomatic patient with severe aortic stenosis. So, it should be done in this type of patients with left ventricular ejection fraction of $\geq 50\%$ and mean gradient of ≥ 40 mm Hg.
2. Complications in aortic stenosis:
   a. In patient with severe stenosis, there is risk of sudden death.
   b. Heart failure secondary to left ventricular hypertrophy and fibrosis resulting diastolic dysfunction.
   c. Chronic elevation of left ve3ntricular diastolic filling pressure leading to pulmonary hypertension.
   d. Conduction abnormalities resulting from:
      - Left ventricular hypertrophy
      - Extension of calcium from the aortic valve leaflets to interventricular septum
      - Increased risk of infective endocarditis in case of bicuspid aortic valve
      - Increased risk of gastrointestinal bleeding due to secondary von Willebrand disease
      - Calcific emboli from the aortic valve may produce cerebral emboli.

3. Variation of second heart sound in aortic stenosis:
   a. Diminished or absent aortic second heart sound
   b. In case of moderately severe aortic stenosis, second heart sound may be single due to overriding of the aortic sound to pulmonary component.
   c. Paradoxical split of the second heart sound due to delayed closure of the aortic valve in severe aortic stenosis
   d. Accentuated pulmonary component due to secondary pulmonary hypertension
4. Following are the class I recommendations of surgery in these patients:
   a. Symptomatic patients with:
      - High-grade severe aortic stenosis
      - Low-flow, low-gradient severe aortic stenosis (left ventricular ejection fraction of <50%)
      - Low-flow, low-gradient severe aortic stenosis (left ventricular ejection fraction of >50%), but aortic stenosis is the most likely cause of symptoms.
   b. Asymptomatic patients with:
      - Severe aortic stenosis with left ventricular ejection fraction of <50%
      - Severe aortic stenosis but undergoing cardiac surgery for other indications

5. Following are the risk factors for consideration of aortic valve surgery:
    a. Peak velocity is >5.5 m/s.
    b. Severe calcification of the aortic valve with progression of the velocity of ≥0.3 m/s/year.
    c. Marked elevated brain natriuretic peptide (BNP) levels
    d. Exercise induced increase in mean gradient of >20 mm Hg
    e. Excessive left ventricular hypertrophy in absence of history of hypertension

CASE 14

A 45-year-old male came to echocardiography clinic for echocardiography to assess the cardiac status as because patient has been suffering from exertional breathlessness.

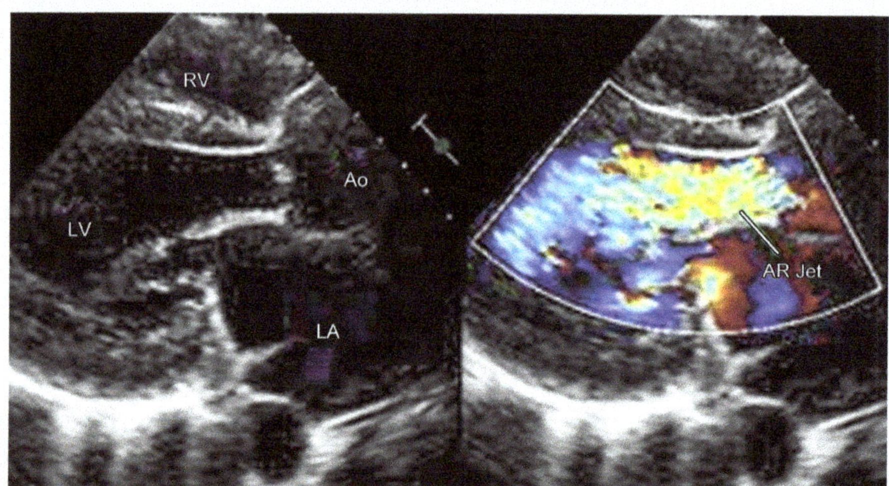

1. **What are the features in the above diagram?**
2. **What is your diagnosis?**
3. **What are the parameters that will be assessed by transthoracic echocardiography?**
4. **What are the other tests used to assess the cardiac status and why?**
5. **What are the parameters suggest severe aortic regurgitation?**

Answers

1. The following features are seen in the above echocardiography:
    a. Dilated left ventricle and left atrium, aorta
    b. Presence of opened mitral valve leaflets in-between left atrium and left ventricle
    c. Left atrium is thickened.
    d. Evidence of multicolor jet in the left ventricular outflow tract anterior to anterior mitral leaflet
    e. Presence of thickened aortic valve leaflet in-between aorta and left ventricle
2. The diagnosis is aortic regurgitation.
3. Following parameters are calculated by echocardiography:
    a. Presence of aortic regurgitation
    b. Severity of aortic regurgitation
    c. Etiology of aortic regurgitation
    d. Evaluation of the size and function of left ventricle
    e. Estimation of the pulmonary artery pressure
4. Other tests that are performed to assess the cardiac status are as follows:
    a. Cardiac magnetic resonance: It should be done because it can assess accurately:
        • Left ventricular systolic function
        • Left ventricular systolic and diastolic volumes
        • Severity of aortic regurgitation by measuring:
            ○ Left ventricular regurgitant volume
            ○ Left ventricular regurgitant fraction
    b. Left heart catheterization: It should be done in case of:
        • Any discordance of clinical findings and echocardiographic findings
        • Any contraindication of magnetic resonance

5. Following parameters suggest severe aortic regurgitation:
   a. Width of the central jet is >65% of the left ventricular outflow tract.
   b. Vena contracta is >0.6 cm.
   c. Pressure half time is <200 ms.
   d. There is reversal of holodiastolic aortic flow in the descending aorta.
   e. Moderate or greater left ventricular enlargement
   f. Amount of regurgitant volume is ≥60 mL/beat.
   g. Amount of regurgitant fraction is ≥50%.
   h. Effective regurgitant surface area is ≥0.3 cm^2.

CASE 15

A 75-year-old nondiabetic male with known case of aortic stenosis has been referred to cardiothoracic department for aortic valve replacement.

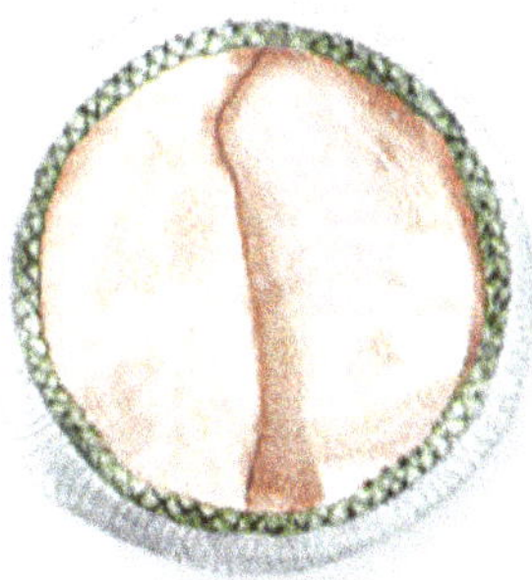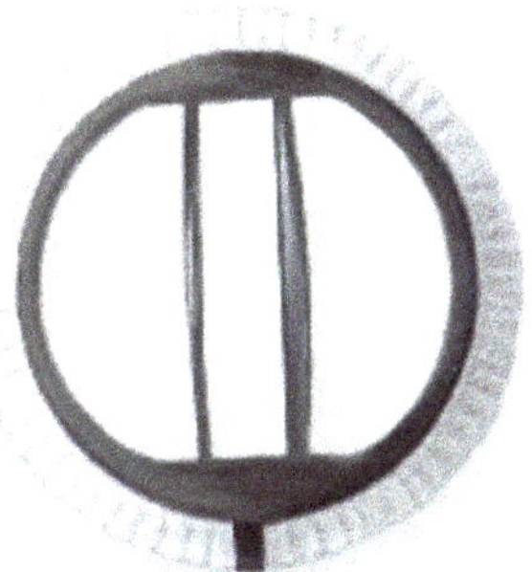

1. **Describe the above pictures.**
2. **What is the main determining factor in case of prosthesis of aortic valve?**
3. **What are the advantages of the above prosthesis?**

Answers

1. Description of the pictures:
   a. First one is the bioprosthetic valve made of human or animal tissue lasting for 12–15 years and that patient need not take the anticoagulant.
   b. Second one is the mechanical prosthetic valve made by human being, material being titanium or stainless steel. It lasts for longest time but the patient has to take blood thinning drug.
2. The determining factor being:
   a. Anticoagulant-related bleeding as well as thromboembolism in case of mechanical prosthetic valve.
   b. Risk of deterioration of the bioprosthetic valve
3. Advantages of the following valves [European Society of Cardiology (ESC) guideline 2012]:
   a. Mechanical valve:
      - Patient is already on anticoagulant because of other prosthesis.
      - Patient is on anticoagulant because of high risk of thromboembolism.
      - Desire of the informed patient and absence of contraindication for long-term anticoagulation.
      - Patients those are at high risk of accelerated structural valve deterioration including young age and hyperparathyroidism.
      - Age <60 years (aortic prosthesis) and <65 years (mitral prosthesis). In patient aged 60–65 years who receive aortic prosthesis and those between 65 and 70 years in case of mitral prosthesis, both valves are acceptable and the choices require careful analysis of factors other than age.
      - Patients with reasonable life expectancy of >10 years, for whom redo valve surgery would be high risk.
   b. Bioprosthetic valve:
      - Desire of informed consent
      - Unavailability of good quality anticoagulation (contraindication or high risk, unwillingness, compliance problem, lifestyle, and occupation)

- Reoperation of mechanical valve thrombosis despite good long-term anticoagulant control
- Patients for whom future redo valve surgery would be low risk.

- Limited life expectancy (lower than presumed durability of the bioprosthesis) or age >65 years (aortic prosthesis) or >70 years (mitral prosthesis).
- Young women contemplating pregnancy

CASE 16

A 25-year-old patient, allergic to penicillin with history of Mustard operation for transposition of the great vessels, developed baffle stenosis for which stent had been inserted. Now, he developed toothache for which he needs root canal procedure within next week by dental surgeon.

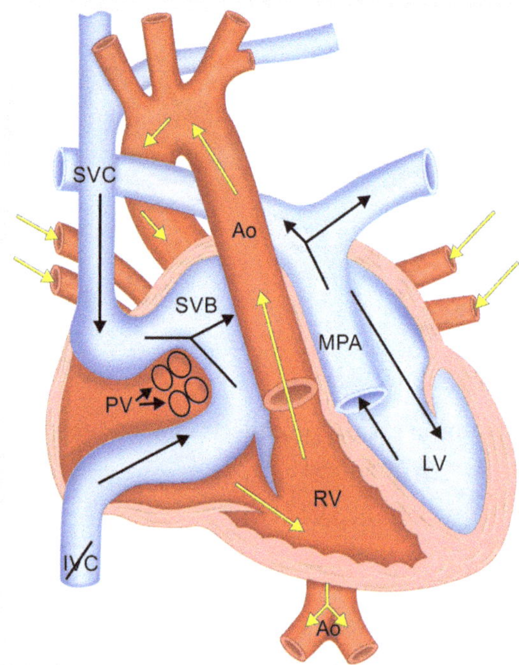

1. **What the above picture signifies?**
2. **What is the risk in this patient?**
3. **What precaution is needed for that patient?**
4. **What are the other procedures at high risk and with which organisms requiring this precaution?**
5. **Which patients are at increased risk for infective endocarditis?**

Answers

1. Above picture signifies Mustard procedure done to correct this abnormality. Here, deoxygenated blood is transported to the left ventricle through the two-way systemic venous baffles. This blood goes to the lungs. After full oxygenation, red oxygenated blood goes to the right atrium through the pulmonary venous baffle then to aorta through right ventricle.
2. There is increased risk of infective endocarditis.
3. Patient needs antibiotic prophylaxis prior to dental procedure.
4. Following are the high-risk procedures requiring antibiotic prophylaxis:
   a. Upper gastrointestinal endoscopy—infecting organisms are:
      - Coagulase-negative staphylococci
      - Streptococci
      - Diphtheroids
   b. Colonoscopy:
      - *Escherichia coli*
      - *Bacteroides*

c. Barium enema:
- Enterococci
- Aerobic and anaerobic gram-negative rods

d. Dental extraction: *Streptococcus viridans*

e. Transurethral resection of prostate:
- Coliforms
- Enterococci
- *Staphylococcus aureus*

f. Transesophageal echocardiography:
- *Streptococcus viridans*
- Streptococci
- Anaerobic organisms

5. Following patients are at high risk of infective endocarditis requiring antibiotic prophylaxis:
   a. Prosthetic valves
   b. Previous history of infective endocarditis
   c. Congenital cyanotic heart disease
   d. Congenital heart disease undergone repair with prosthetic material within 6 months
   e. Presence of residual defect after repair with prosthetic materials

CASE 17

A 40-year-old intravenous drug user was admitted with history of fever with rigor, malaise, and weakness in a hospital. On examination, there was tachycardia, tachypnea, high temperature, and pansystolic murmur at left lower sternum. Transthoracic echocardiography was performed.

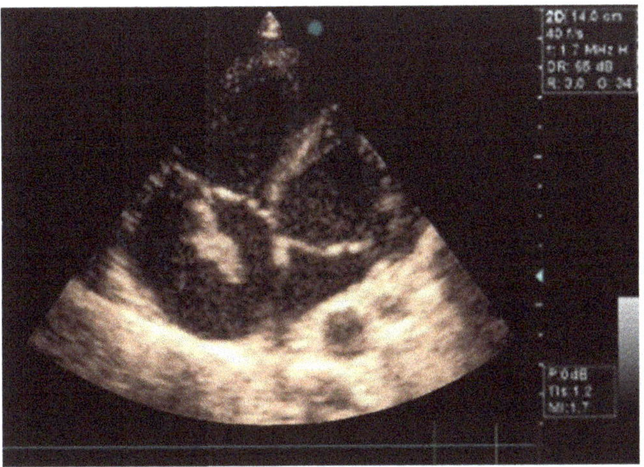 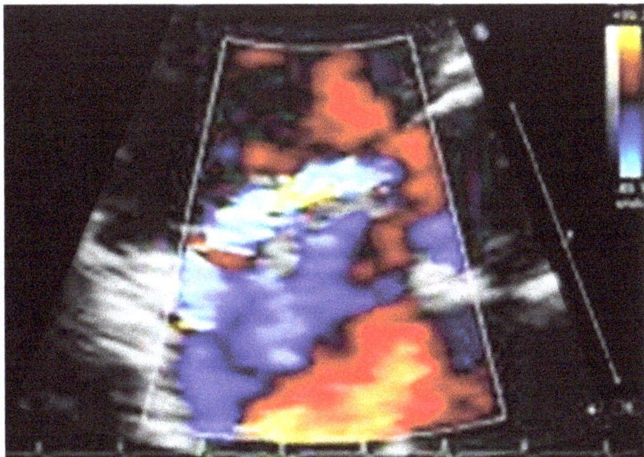

1. **Describe the above echocardiographic picture.**
2. **What is your diagnosis?**
3. **In blood culture, which organism is mostly found?**
4. **If the culture is negative, which organisms are mostly responsible?**
5. **What are the echocardiographic predictors of systemic embolization?**

Answers

1. First picture demonstrated vegetation in the tricuspid valve. Second picture demonstrated presence of severe tricuspid regurgitation from the right ventricle to right atrium.

2. The diagnosis is patient suffering from right-sided infective endocarditis as he is an intravenous drug user.

3. In blood culture, mostly *Staphylococcus aureus* is found.

4. Other group of organisms in blood culture negative patient is HACEK (*Haemophilus* species, *Aggregatibacter actinomycetemcomitans, Cardiobacterium hominis, Eikenella corrodens, Kingella kingae*). This group consists of:
   a. *Haemophilus* species
   b. *Aggregatibacter*
   c. *Cardiobacterium hominis*
   d. *Eikenella corrodens*
   e. *Kingella* species

5. Following are the predictors of systemic embolization:
   a. Large valvular vegetation of >100 in diameter
   b. Multiple vegetations
   c. Noncalcified vegetations
   d. Mobile but pedunculated vegetations
   e. Prolapsing vegetation
   f. Progressively increasing size of the vegetation

CASE 18

A 34-year-old male with history of aortic valve replacement as he suffered from aortic stenosis was admitted with fever with chill, weakness, anorexia. On examination, there was tachycardia, tachypnea, and high temperature. There are few lesions in the hand and presence of early diastolic murmur heard over the neoaortic area. Blood count is 16,000/cc with predominant neutrophils and C-reactive protein (CRP) was 100 mg/dL. His echocardiography demonstrated the following:

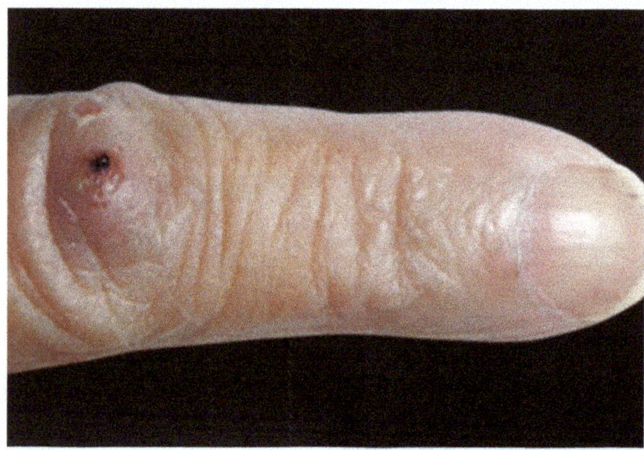
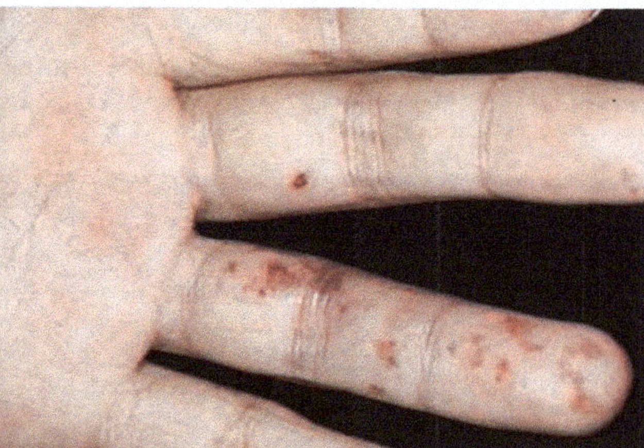

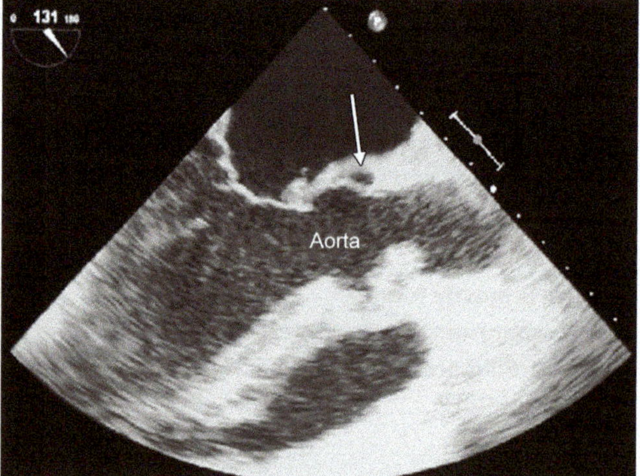

1. **Describe the pictures.**
2. **What is the pathophysiology beyond these lesions?**
3. **What is the echocardiographic feature?**
4. **What is your diagnosis?**

Answers

1. First picture is Osler nodes which is characterized by tender raised lumps with pale center found on the dorsal surface of proximal interphalangeal joints. Second picture is Janeway lesion which is characterized by nontender hemorrhagic lesions within the skin found in the plantar surface of ring finger of left hand.

2. Pathophysiology of these lesions:
   a. Skin biopsy demonstrates neutrophilic vasculitis affecting the glomus apparatus or may be the microabscesses containing bacteria in absence of vasculitis.
   b. Janeway lesion is consistent with the septic embolism containing bacteria found within the blood vessels.

3. Echocardiographic features: Aortic root abscess in patient with aortic valve raft.

4. The diagnosis is infective endocarditis involving the aortic valve leading to formation of aortic root abscess.

CASE 19

A 45-year-old man with past history of rheumatic mitral stenosis developed fever for 5 days with chill and rigor, and malaise and has been admitted in a hospital. His echocardiography demonstrated the following:

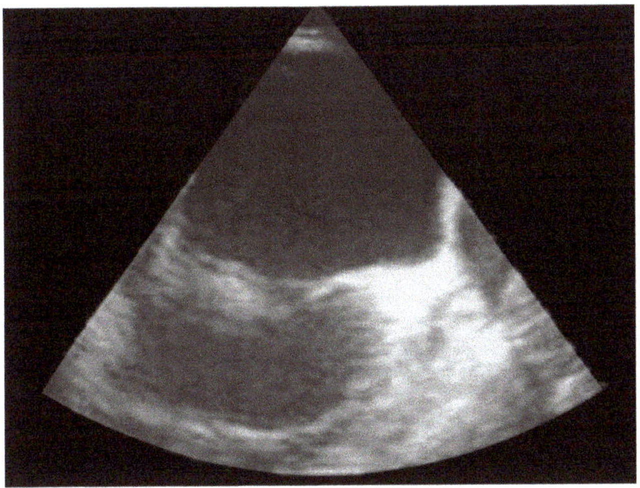 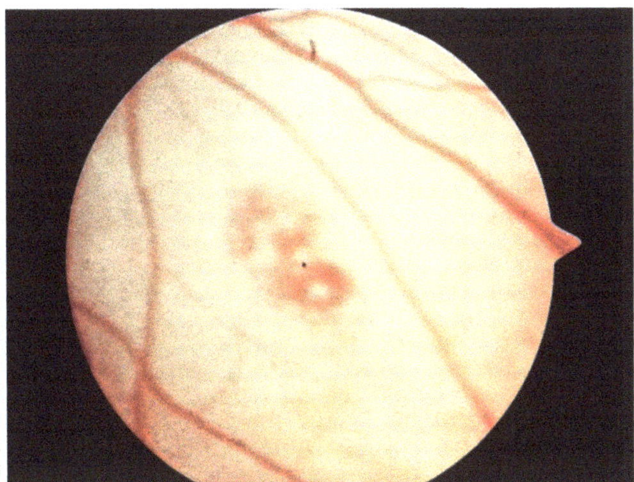

1. **What is your finding in the echocardiography?**
2. **What is the composition of this finding?**
3. **What is the spectrum of pathophysiology in the finding?**
4. **What are the predisposing cardiac lesions in this disease?**
5. **Why this disease is less likely in large ventricular septal defect (VSD)?**
6. **In case of small VSD and coarctation of aorta, in which sites this may occur?**
7. **Mention the dermatological manifestations in this disease?**
8. **What is eye finding in this disease?**
9. **What are the neurological complications?**
10. **What are the indications of surgical intervention?**

Answers

1. There is evidence of vegetation in the mitral valve.
2. Vegetation is a mass which is composed of platelet, fibrins, and infecting organisms which are held by agglutinating antibodies produced against the bacteria.
3. If the inflammation is continued, it will lead to ulceration thereby producing perforation of the cusps of the valve resulting in:
   a. Valvular incompetence
   b. Damage of the conducting pathways if the septal area is involved.

c. If aortic area is involved, there is rupture of sinus of Valsalva.

4. Following are the predisposing cardiac lesions in this disease:
   a. Rheumatic heart disease
   b. Hypertrophic cardiomyopathy
   c. Subaortic stenosis
   d. Ventricular aneurysm
   e. Congenital heart diseases:
      - Ventricular septal defect
      - Coarctation of aorta
      - Bicuspid aortic valve

5. When high pressure jets enter into the low pressure jet, the vegetation will occur, hence in case of large VSD, vegetation will not occur.

6. In case of small VSD on the right ventricular side and in case of coarctation of aorta distal to the obstruction, vegetation will occur.

7. Following are the dermatological manifestations in this disease:
   a. Osler nodes
   b. Janeway lesion
   c. Splinter hemorrhages
   d. Petechiae
   e. Clubbing

8. This is Roth spot, which is characterized by boat-shaped hemorrhages with pale center present in the retina.

9. Neurological complications:
   a. Acute confusional state
   b. Development of cerebral emboli in the middle cerebral artery leading to hemiplegia and sensory dysfunction.
   c. Mycotic aneurysm in the middle cerebral artery leading to subarachnoid hemorrhage if ruptures.

10. Following are the indications of surgical intervention:
    a. Valve obstruction
    b. Paravalvular abscess
    c. Prosthetic valve endocarditis due to *S. aureus* or other resistant organisms
    d. Aortic regurgitation not responding to medical therapy
    e. Mitral regurgitation not responding to medical therapy
    f. Fungal endocarditis
    g. Development of sinus of Valsalva aneurysm
    h. Multiple embolic episodes
    i. Progressive heart failure due to destruction of valve
    j. Oscillating vegetation of >1 cm in diameter

CASE 20

A 50-year-old man has been admitted with low-grade fever and weight loss. His transthoracic echocardiography demonstrated 0.6 × 0.4 cm echogenic mass attached with the aortic cusp, CRP was 56 mg/mL, but multiple blood culture was negative.

1. **What are the causes of constantly negative blood culture?**
2. **In case of culture negative cases, what are the investigations should be done?**
3. **What are the criteria that determine suitability of outpatient parenteral antibiotic therapy for infective endocarditis?**

Answers

1. Following are the causes of culture negative cases:
   a. *Coxiella burnetii*
   b. *Bartonella*
   c. *Chlamydia*
   d. *Tropheryma whipplei*
   e. HACEK group of organism
   f. Brucella
   g. Fungi
   h. Nutritionally variant streptococci

2. In these cases, following investigations should be started:
   a. Serologic testing
   b. Cell culture
   c. Gene amplification

3. Following are the criteria determining the suitability of outpatient parenteral antibiotic therapy for infective endocarditis:
   a. Critical phase (0–2 weeks): As complications will occur in this phase, inpatient is preferred in this phase. This therapy is preferred if the patient is stable having no complication.
   b. Continuation phase (beyond 2 weeks): This therapy is done if the patient is stable and the patient has no feature of heart failure, no neurological sign of impairment of renal function.

CASE 21

A 50-year-old patient with no evidence of comorbidity and known case of heart failure with preserved ejection fraction (>65%) was admitted in the cardiac unit with breathlessness of NYHA class III. He had bradycardia, blood pressure of 120/70 mm Hg, and no pedal edema. He was on bisoprolol and ramipril daily. His electrolytes and urea/creatinine levels are normal, but his BNP level is 3,000 pg/dL.

1. **What is the goal of blood pressure in this patient?**
2. **What should be the drug of choice in this patient?**
3. **What should be the precaution in starting the above drug?**
4. **What is the use of implantable hemodynamic monitoring?**
5. **Is there any specific advantage of using interarterial device therapy?**

Answers

1. Blood pressure goal in this patient is similar to blood pressure goal in normal population. If this patient has uncontrolled symptoms of heart failure despite of control of blood pressure, goal of the blood pressure should be reduced by monitoring the dose of antihypertensive.

2. In patient with preserved ejection fraction, sodium-glucose cotransporter-2 (SGLT-2) inhibitor should be started first followed by administration of mineralocorticoid 2 weeks later if the patient can tolerate the therapy.

3. SGLT-2 inhibitor should be avoided in following cases:
   a. All the patients with type 2 diabetes mellitus
   b. Prior history of diabetic ketoacidosis or conditions predisposing to diabetic ketoacidosis in diabetic patients like prolonged fasting and addiction to alcohol.
   c. Symptomatic hypotension
   d. Estimated glomerular filtration rate (GFR) is <20 mL/min/m^2. There is a history of complicated genitourinary tract infection.
   e. Risk factors for foot amputation:
      - Neuropathy
      - Nephropathy
      - Vascular disease
      - Deformity of foot
      - Previous history of foot ulcer

   In case of mineralocorticoid antagonist if the serum potassium level is >4.5 mEq/L, this drug should be avoided.

4. In case of highly selected patient with heart failure and preserved ejection fraction with NYHA III and repeated hospitalization, pulmonary artery pressure can be monitored by remote wireless pulmonary artery pressure monitoring device.

5. Interarterial shunt device in this patient will reduce the pressure in the left atrium at rest or during exercise.

CASE 22

A 75-year-old man with exertional chest pain and shortness of breath has been admitted with features of pulmonary edema and renal impairment with effective GFR of <40 mL/min. His echocardiography demonstrated:

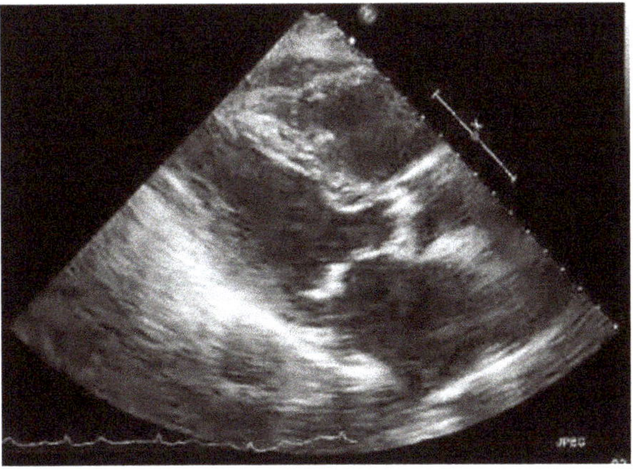

1. **What is the feature in echocardiography?**
2. **Which drug is contraindicated in this disease with heart failure?**
3. **Which drug is used in chest pain?**
4. **What are the grades of aortic stenosis?**

Answers

1. Echocardiography demonstrated severe aortic stenosis.
2. Angiotensin-converting enzyme inhibitor is contra-indicated in this disease.
3. β-blocker is used to relieve chest pain.
4. Grades of aortic stenosis:
   a. Mild aortic stenosis:
      - Jet velocity: <3 m/s
      - Mean gradient: <25 mm Hg.
      - Valve area: <1.5 cm^2
   b. Moderate aortic stenosis:
      - Jet velocity: 3–4 m/s
      - Mean gradient: 25–40 mm Hg
      - Valve area: 1–1.5 cm^2
   c. Severe aortic stenosis:
      - Jet velocity: >4 m/s
      - Mean gradient: >40 mm Hg
      - Valve area: <1 cm^2
      - Valve area index: 0.6 cm^2/m^2

CASE 23

A 36-year-old type 2 diabetic admitted with history of progressively increasing breathlessness in cardiac emergency department and was diagnosed as acute heart failure. On next day, echocardiography demonstrates global hypokinesia with ejection fraction of 22%, medication with diuretics, ramipril, and bisoprolol made him stabilize.

1. **What are the biochemical investigations should be done urgently?**
2. **What invasive investigation is of choice if the hematological and biochemical investigations are normal except NT-proBNP which was high?**
3. **What is the next choice of investigation?**

Answers

1. Following are the hematological investigations should be of choice:
   a. Hematological investigations are:
      - Total count to detect any precipitating infections
      - Erythrocyte sedimentation rate (ESR) for any infections or any autoimmune infection
      - Hemoglobin for detecting any chronic infections or any background kidney disease
      - Platelet counts to detect background liver disease
   b. Biochemical tests are:
      - Pro-BNP and NT-proBNP
      - Renal function test
      - Liver function test
      - Lipid profile to detect metabolic syndrome
      - Troponin T and troponin I to detect background heart failure
      - Creatine phosphokinase (CPK) and CPK-MB to detect any evidence of background myocardial infarction.
2. The probable diagnosis is dilated cardiomyopathy in a case of diabetes-related ischemic heart disease leading to heart failure.
3. Next investigation of choice is coronary angiography.

CASE 24

A 56-year-old type 2 diabetic man has been admitted with progressive breathlessness. Urgently the patient has been resuscitated and echocardiography done which demonstrated type 2 diastolic dysfunction.

1. **What is diastolic dysfunction?**
2. **What are the pathophysiological factors that may be related to heart failure in this case?**

3. **In contrast to heart failure with reduced ejection fraction, which factors are not related here?**
4. **Who are at highest risk of heart failure with preserved ejection fraction?**
5. **What are the risk factors in case of heart failure with preserved ejection fraction?**
6. **What are the morbidity as well as mortality in this case?**

Answers

1. Diastolic dysfunction is either due to increased viscoelastic stiffness of the cardiac chambers or impaired relaxation of the ventricles or combination of both.
2. Following pathophysiological factors may be related in this case:
    a. Systemic inflammation
    b. Disruption of cardiometabolic metabolism
    c. Microvascular dysfunction
    d. Reduced compliance of left ventricle
3. Following factors are not related in this case of heart failure with preserved ejection fraction:
    a. Pathological left ventricular remodeling
    b. Neurohormonal activation
    c. Impairment of systolic function
4. Elderly person as already reduced left ventricular compliance will contribute to excess risk of heart failure with preserved ejection fraction.

5. Risks factors associated with heart failure with preserved ejection fraction:
    a. Hypertension
    b. Metabolic syndrome
    c. Physical inactivity
    d. Coronary artery disease
    e. Atrial fibrillation
    f. Stenosis or incompetence of mitral or aortic valve
    g. Chronic kidney disease
    h. Excess central obesity
    i. Type 2 diabetes mellitus
    j. Sarcopenia
    k. Skeletal myopathy
    l. Frailty
6. In hospital mortality in this case is 2.4–4.9%. After admission, the 5 years mortality will be 40%. Following factors are associated with increased in-hospital mortality:
    a. Renal insufficiency
    b. Elevated BNP
    c. Reduced right ventricular function

CASE 25

A 45-year-old type 2 diabetic hypertensive patient recently discharged from the hospital diagnosed as a case of heart failure with preserved ejection fraction. The patient has come to OPD with breathlessness and irregular heart rate.

1. **What are the precipitating causes of recurrence?**
2. **How the heart failure with preserved ejection fraction can be diagnosed?**
3. **How can you workup this case after the diagnosis?**
4. **Describe the algorithm for the diagnosis of left ventricular diastolic function in the patient with normal ejection fraction.**

Answers

1. Following are precipitating factors for recurrences:
    a. Appearance of atrial fibrillation leading to loss of atrial contraction which is responsible for major contribution during diastolic filling.
    b. Rapid ventricular rate
    c. Acceleration of his preexisting hypertension
    d. Whether the patient is adhered to diuretics.
    e. Further ischemia to the heart that can be diagnosed by echocardiography
    f. Infection
    g. Renal dysfunction that can be diagnosed by renal function test.
2. Following are the approaches of diagnosis:
    a. Assessment of volume status, signs, and symptoms such as exertional dyspnea, orthopnea or history of paroxysmal nocturnal dyspnea, raised jugular vein, bilateral pedal edema, and basal crepitations suggests the diagnosis of heart failure.

b. Noninvasive testing and stress testing should be done, if the ejection fraction is ≥50%. Then secondary causes of heart failure to detect heart failure with preserved ejection fraction should be excluded like:
   - Uncorrected valvular disease
   - Pericardial disease
   - Isolated right-sided heart failure
   - Primary cardiomyopathy
   - High output states

c. When the secondary causes are ruled out, then assessment of risk should be done based on:
   - Comorbid conditions
   - Abnormal transthoracic echocardiography
     - Left ventricular hypertrophy
     - Left ventricular volumes
     - Left atrial volumes
   - Functional testing:
     - 6-minute walk test
     - Cardiopulmonary exercise test
   - Brain natriuretic peptide

d. Further assessment should be done by using diagnostic scores for heart failure with preserved ejection fraction of "Heart failure Association" or European Society of Cardiology"
   - In case of low probability, other etiology can be considered.
   - In case of intermediate probability, further workup testing is considered:
     - Right heart catheterization at rest and with exercise to assess increased left ventricular filling pressure at rest as well as during exercise.
     - Echocardiography tissue Doppler study with exertion to assess the increased left ventricular filling pressure.

3. Following should be done as workup:
   a. Sophisticated workup such as MRI should be done for detection of:
      - Myocardial scar
      - Myocardial edema
      - Microvascular dysfunction
      - Myocardial fibrosis
   b. Technetium pyrophosphate scintigraphy
   c. Endomyocardial fibrosis to detect amyloidosis
   d. Genetic testing

4. In case of patient with normal left ventricular ejection fraction:
   a. Average E/e' <14
   b. Septal e' velocity <7 cm/s or lateral e' velocity <10 cm/s
   c. Tricuspid regurgitation (TR) velocity is <2.8 m/s
   d. Left atrial volume index is >34 mL/m^2.
      - >50% positive: Indicates normal diastolic function
      - 50% positive: Indeterminate
      - >50% positive: Diastolic dysfunction

CASE 26

A 56-year-old type 2 diabetic man has been admitted with progressive breathlessness. Urgently the patient has been resuscitated and echocardiography done which demonstrated type 2 diastolic dysfunction.

1. **What is your diagnosis?**
2. **How can you treat this patient?**

Answers

1. Acute decompensated heart failure with preserved ejection fraction.
2. Following are the line of treatment of this patient with heart failure with preserved ejection function:
   a. Volume management:
      - Loop diuretics
      - Thiazide diuretics should be added to enhance diuresis.

      Caution:
      - There should not be overdiuresis because it may result in hypotension or acute kidney injury especially who has small volume of the left ventricle.
      - During diuretic use, renal function and electrolytes and clinical parameter of volumes loss should be tested.
   b. Control blood pressure to maintain the level at 130/80 mm Hg because high afterload will lead to:
      - Elevated left atrial pressure
      - Elevated left ventricular diastolic pressure
      - Pulmonary capillary wedge pressure

c. Reversal of precipitating factor:
- In case of cardiac ischemia, cardiac catheterization followed by revascularization.
- As atrial fibrillation with rapid ventricular rate will lead to impairment of diastolic filling through reduction of diastolic filling time as well as reduction of atrial kick, so following drugs can be given to reduce the ventricular rate:
  - β-blockers
  - Digoxin
  - Nondihydropyridine calcium-channel blockers.
- Rhythm control by antiarrhythmic drugs or by DC cardioversion.
- Amyloid or sarcoid cardiomyopathies can be treated by specific drugs.

CASE 27

A 49-year-old patient has been admitted with increasing breathlessness and he was properly resuscitated. He has history of reduction of exercise tolerance which has been limited to 120 yards in spite of being on bisoprolol. On examination, his pulse is double peak, apex is forceful, and murmur is midsystolic, no edema and basal fine crepitation. His echocardiography demonstrated following features:

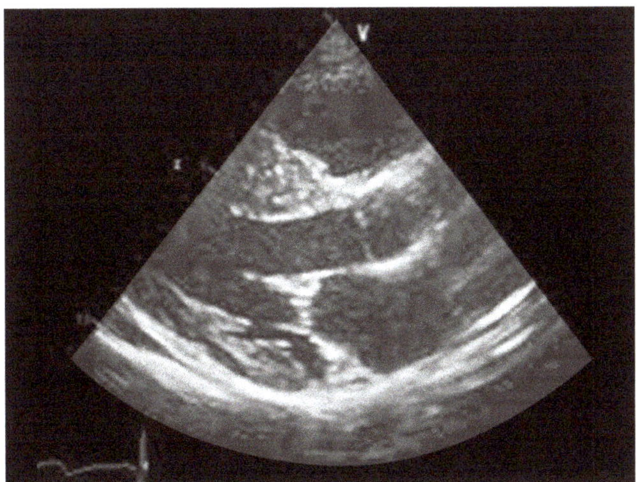

1. **What is the echocardiographic feature above?**
2. **What is your diagnosis?**
3. **What type of disease it is?**
4. **Is there any genetic mutation linked with this disease?**
5. **What should be screened in this disease?**
6. **At which age screening should be started in this?**

Answers

1. Echocardiography demonstrated:
    a. Asymmetric septal hypertrophy affecting anteroseptal wall extending toward apex
    b. At midseptal area, the thickness of left ventricular wall is 18 mm.
2. The diagnosis is hypertrophic cardiomyopathy.
3. This disease is known as "sarcomeric disease"—autosomal dominant disease.
4. Following genetic mutations occurring in the cardiac protein in this disease:
    a. Cardiac troponin T
    b. Cardiac troponin I
    c. Myosin regulatory light chain
    d. Myosin essential light chain
    e. Cardiac myosin-binding protein C
    f. α-cardiac myosin heavy chain
    g. β-cardiac myosin heavy chain

h. Cardiac α-actin
i. α-tropomyosin
j. Titin
k. Muscle LIM protein

5. First-degree relative should be screened by doing following:
   a. History
   b. Physical examination
   c. 12-lead echocardiography
   d. Two-dimensional (2D) echocardiography
6. At following ages screening should be done:
   a. In <12 years of old patient:

- It is optional unless:
  o Malignant family history of premature death in case of hypertrophic cardiomyopathy or other adverse complications
  o Onset of symptoms
  o In case of athlete in an intensive program
- 12–21 years old: Every 12–18 months
- More than 21 years:
  o Approximately every 5 years
  o Less than 5 years in case of positive family history of late onset of this disease with or without malignant clinical course.

CASE 28

A 49-year-old patient has been admitted with increasing breathlessness and he was properly resuscitated. He has history of reduction of exercise tolerance which has been limited to 120 yards in spite of being on bisoprolol. On examination, his pulse has been demonstrated below, apex is forceful, and murmur is midsystolic, no edema and basal fine crepitation. His echocardiography demonstrated following features:

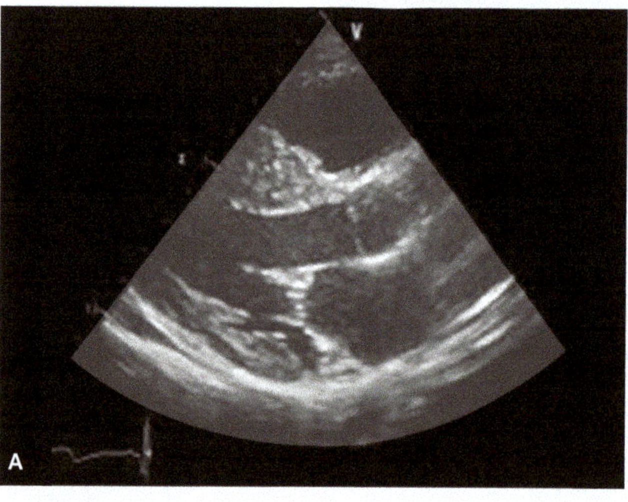
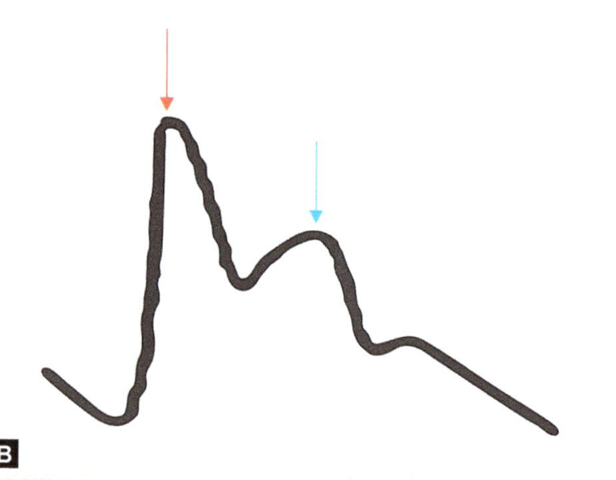

1. Describe the above pictures A and B.
2. What is your diagnosis?
3. How the pulse in this disease differs from the pulse in aortic stenosis?
4. What are the common phenotypes in this disease?
5. What are the common symptoms in this patient?
6. How can you differentiate this disease from this disease?
7. What are the causes of angina pectoris in this disease?

Answers

1. Following are the features:
   a. Echocardiography demonstrated:
      - Asymmetric septal hypertrophy affecting anteroseptal wall extending toward apex
      - At midseptal area, the thickness of left ventricular wall is 18 mm.
   b. Carotid pulse demonstrated spike and dome pattern
2. The diagnosis is hypertrophic cardiomyopathy.
3. In case of hypertrophic cardiomyopathy, there is initial brisk rise in the carotid pulse followed by midsystolic decline due to left ventricular outflow tract obstruction and this is followed by second rise. In contrast in case of aortic stenosis due to fixed obstruction, amplitude of carotid upstroke will be delayed
4. Following are the two types of hypertrophic cardiomyopathy:
   a. Two-thirds of patients demonstrate mechanical impedance of left ventricular outflow as a result of subaortic septal thickening interacting with mitral valve or muscle thickening itself.
   b. In one-third of patients, there is unobstructed outflow all the times which is known as nonobstructive hypertrophic cardiomyopathy.
5. Most common symptoms:
   a. Respiratory distress due to diastolic dysfunction of the left ventricle along with impaired filling as a result of:
      - Increased stiffness of the cardiac chambers
      - Abnormal relaxation of cardiac muscles
   b. Angina pectoris occurring in both obstructive as well as nonobstructive cardiomyopathy due to mismatch in the demand and supply of myocardial perfusion
   c. Syncope or presyncope due to decreased cardiac output as a result of:
      - Left ventricular outflow tract obstruction
      - Small size of the left ventricular cavity during diastole
      - Cardiac arrhythmias

6. Following are the point of differentiation between hypertrophic cardiomyopathy and athlete heart:

Parameters	Hypertrophic cardiomyopathy	Athlete heart
Left ventricular wall thickness	>16 mm	<16 mm
Hypertrophic pattern	<ul><li>Irregular</li><li>Asymmetric</li><li>Apical</li></ul>	Symmetric
Left ventricular end-diastolic dimension	<45 mm	>55 mm
Size of the left atrium	Enlarged	Normal
Filling pattern of left ventricle	Impaired relaxation	Normal filling
On cardiac MRI, areas of fibrosis	Present	Absent
Family history of hypertrophic cardiomyopathy	Present	Absent
Mutation of sarcomeric protein	Present	Absent
Response to deconditioning	None	Decrease in left ventricular wall thickness
ECG features	<ul><li>QRS voltage is high</li><li>Presence of Q waves</li><li>Deep negative Q waves</li></ul>	Criteria of left ventricular hypertrophy

7. Following are the causes of angina pectoris:
   a. Increased muscle mass
   b. Increased wall stress
   c. Decreased perfusion of the coronary arteries secondary to obstruction of left ventricle
   d. Elevated diastolic filling pressure
   e. Systolic compression of the intramural coronary arteries
   f. Inadequate capillary density
   g. Impaired vasodilatory reserve
   h. Abnormally narrowed small intramural coronary arteries

CASE 29

A 49-year-old patient has been admitted with increasing breathlessness and he was properly resuscitated. He has history of reduction of exercise tolerance which has been limited to 120 yards in spite of being on bisoprolol. On examination, his pulse has been demonstrated below, apex is forceful, and murmur is midsystolic, no edema and basal fine crepitation. His echocardiography demonstrated following features:

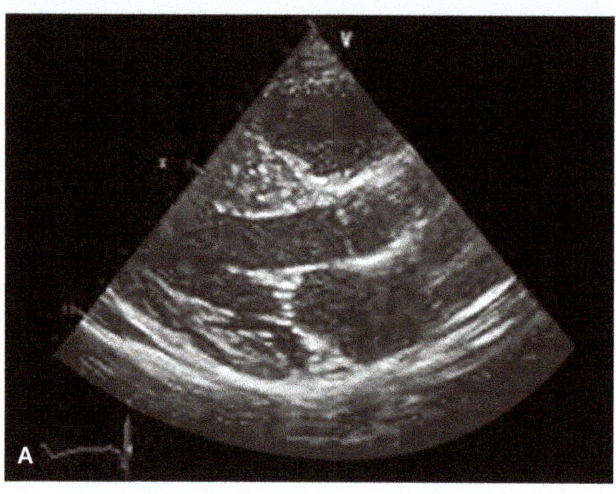
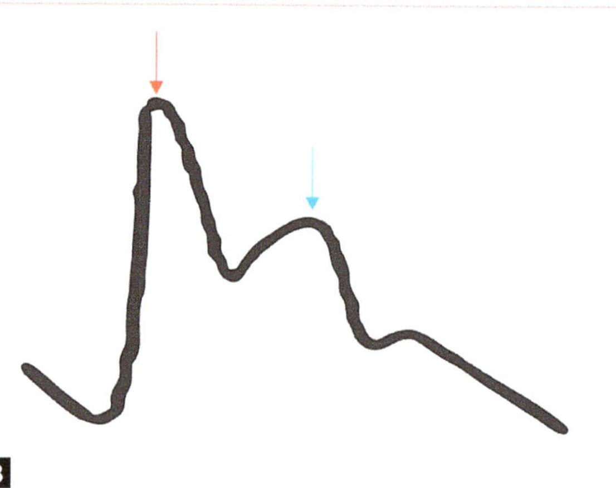

1. **Describe the above pictures a and b.**
2. **What is your diagnosis?**
3. **Describe the murmur in this case.**
4. **What are the bedside provocative maneuvers should be performed to differentiate this disease from other diseases?**
5. **What are the ECG changes in this disease?**
6. **What are the typical echocardiographic findings in this disease?**
7. **What are the causes of systolic anterior motion of anterior mitral leaflet?**
8. **What are the mechanisms of left ventricular outflow tract obstruction?**
9. **What are the indications of implantable cardioverter defibrillator in this disease?**

Answers

1. Following pictures demonstrated:
   a. Echocardiography demonstrated:
      - Asymmetric septal hypertrophy affecting anteroseptal wall extending toward apex.
      - At midseptal area the thickness of left ventricular wall is 18 mm.
   b. Carotid pulse demonstrated spike and dome pattern

2. It is a case of hypertrophic cardiomyopathy.
3. It is crescendo-decrescendo midsystolic murmur heard in the apex and the left sternal border radiating to axilla but not toward great vessels. As it is a case of dynamic obstruction, different provocative maneuvers should be done to differentiate from other diseases.

4. Following provocative maneuvers should be performed to differentiate this from other diseases by examining the augmentation or suppression of murmur:

Maneuvers	Hypertrophic cardiomyopathy	Aortic stenosis	Mitral regurgitation	Ventricular septal defect
Valsalva maneuver	Augmented	Decreased	Decreased	Decreased
Handgrip method	Decreased	Decreased	Augmented	Augmented
Squatting	Decreased	Augmented	Augmented	Augmented
Amyl nitrate	Augmented	Augmented	Decreased	Decreased
Leg rise	Decreased	Augmented	Augmented	Augmented

5. Following are the ECG changes in this disease:
   a. ST-segment and T-wave changes
   b. Voltage criteria for left ventricular hypertrophy
   c. Presence of Q wave in LII, LIII, aVF, and V_2 to V_6
   d. Left axis deviation
   e. Enlargement of left atrium
   f. In case of apical hypertrophic cardiomyopathy, giant negative T-wave in precordial leads.
6. Following are the typical echocardiographic features in this disease:
   a. Diastolic thickness of left ventricular wall is 15 mm or more with left ventricular hypertrophy.
   b. Septal to posterior wall ratio is ≥1:3 in case of asymmetric septal wall hypertrophy
   c. Small left ventricular cavity
   d. Reduced septal wall motion and thickening
   e. Normal or increased motion of the posterior wall
   f. Systolic anterior motion of mitral leaflets
   g. Midsystolic and late systolic mitral regurgitation
   h. Partial midsystolic closure of the aortic valve with coarse fluttering of the leaflets in the phase of left systole
   i. Reduction of left ventricular longitudinal systolic shortening
7. Following are the causes of systolic anterior motion of anterior mitral leaflet:
   a. Anterior mitral leaflet will be drawn toward the septum due to venture effect produced by lower pressure in the left ventricular outflow tract. It occurs due to flow of blood through the narrowed outflow tract.
   b. Anterior mitral leaflet is pushed against the ventricular septum due to abnormal attacking by the flow of blood from behind.
8. Following are the mechanisms of left ventricular outflow tract obstruction:
   a. Systolic anterior motion of anterior mitral leaflet
   b. Midsystolic contract with hypertrophic ventricular septum
      Magnitude of subaortic gradient is directly related to duration of contact in-between the mitral leaflet and interventricular septum.
9. Following are the indications of implantable cardioverter defibrillator in this disease:
   a. Secondary prevention in survivors of cardiac arrest in case of sustained ventricular tachycardia.
   b. In patients with one risk factor for sudden cardiac death according to American guidelines.
   c. In case of no risk factor, decision should be individualized. Here age of the patient, strength of the risk factors, and acceptability to the patient as well as patient's party.
   d. In case of end stage of hypertrophic cardiomyopathy, which are characterized by:
      - Systolic dysfunction of left ventricle
      - Thinning of the left ventricular wall
      - Dilatation of the left ventricular chamber
   e. Risk calculation algorithm proposed by European Society of Cardiology

CASE 30

A 25-year-old woman without any symptom accidentally detected in the clinic. The presence of midsystolic murmur in echocardiography demonstrated septal wall thickness of 18 mm and small left ventricular outflow gradient.

1. **What should be the next approach to this patient?**
2. **Is pregnancy is safe in this patient?**
3. **In this patient, how atrial fibrillation can be managed?**

Answers

1. As the patient is symptom free, she should not require any therapy. But following mechanisms are taken for risk stratification:
   a. Annual exercise test to detect presence of any exercise-induced arrhythmia such as ventricular tachycardia or atrial fibrillation
   b. Rise in blood pressure of <20 mm Hg
   c. 24 hours Holter monitoring to detect ventricular tachycardia at a rate of 3 beats at a rate of 120 beats/min.
   d. Presence of atrial fibrillation
2. Pregnancy is safe in this patient leading to normal vaginal delivery under guidance of both cardiologist as well as gynecologist.
3. Atrial fibrillation should be managed by:
   a. Verapamil
   b. β-blockers
   c. Amiodarone
   d. Anticoagulant

CASE 31

A 50-year-old male presented with lethargy as well as tiredness. On examination, his blood pressure is 100/70 mm Hg, raised jugular venous pressure, and pedal edema. Echocardiography demonstrated thickened left ventricle and thickness of the septal wall was 16 mm. E/A ratio was 1.4 and in the tissue Doppler E/E' ratio was 12. His ECG demonstrated duration of PR interval is 200 ms and duration of QRS was 147 ms with poor progression of R wave.

1. **What is your diagnosis?**
2. **What are the points in favor of your diagnosis?**
3. **Why the etiology is amyloidosis?**
4. **How cardiac amyloidosis can be diagnosed?**
5. **What are the differences in the cardiac catheterization between constrictive pericarditis and this disease?**
6. **What are the similarities during cardiac catheterization in constrictive pericarditis and the disease?**
7. **What are drugs responsible for this disease?**
8. **If the etiology is idiopathic, what are the factors governing the disease?**
9. **How can you treat this case?**
10. **What are the drugs contraindicated in this disease?**

Answers

1. The diagnosis is restrictive cardiomyopathy secondary to amyloidosis.
2. Following points are in the favor of this diagnosis:
   a. Clinical features of right-sided heart failure
   b. Thickened left ventricle
   c. Evidence of restrictive filling:
      - Reversed E/A ratio
      - Increased E/E' ratio
3. Following features are in favor of amyloid deposition:
   a. Conduction abnormalities
   b. Amplitude of QRS is small in presence of echocardiographic evidence of left ventricular hypertrophy.
4. Following are the clues to the diagnosis of cardiac amyloidosis:
   a. Red flag signs for cardiac amyloidosis:
      - Left ventricular thickening along with low voltage ECG
      - Thickening of right ventricle, valves, and atria
      - Intolerance of angiotensin-converting enzyme inhibitor/angiotensin receptor blockers (ACEI/ARBs), β-blockers, sacubitril, or valsartan
      - Evidence of low blood pressure in patient with past history of hypertension
      - History of:
        - Bilateral carpal tunnel syndrome
        - Lumbar tunnel stenosis
        - Rupture of biceps tendon
   b. Clues to the diagnosis of transthyretin cardiac amyloid:
      - Heart failure with preserved ejection fraction with carpal tunnel syndrome or spinal stenosis
      - Heart failure with preserved ejection without history of hypertension
      - Recent diagnosis of hypertrophic cardiomyopathy in older patient
      - Recent diagnosis of low-flow, low-gradient aortic stenosis in elderly
      - Presence of family history of transthyretin cardiac amyloidosis
   c. Clues to the presence of primary cardiac amyloidosis:
      - Heart failure with preserved ejection fraction with nephrotic syndrome
      - Macroglossia
      - Periorbital purpura
      - Peripheral neuropathy
      - Orthostatic hypotension
5. Points in favor of restrictive cardiomyopathy in the cardiac catheterization laboratory are:
   a. Difference of diastolic pressure between right and left ventricle is >5 mm Hg.
   b. Pulmonary artery systolic pressure is >50 mm Hg.
   c. Ratio of right ventricular diastolic to systolic pressure is <1.3.
   d. Absence of ventricular interdependence during inspiration

6. What are the similarities in the findings during the cardiac catheterization between this disease and constrictive pericarditis:
   a. Diastolic "dip and plateau" sign
   b. "Square root" sign
7. Following drugs are responsible for restrictive cardiomyopathy:
   a. Methysergide
   b. Serotonin
   c. Ergotamine
   d. Busulfan
   e. Mercurial agent
   f. Chloroquine
   g. Hydroxychloroquine
8. Following factors govern this disease if the disease is idiopathic:
   a. Age >70 years
   b. Advanced NYHA class
   c. Left atrial diameter is >6 cm.

9. Treatment options in this cardiac amyloidosis:
   a. Specific treatment options:
      - Stem cell transplantation
      - Tafamidis—transthyretin stabilizer
      - *Transthyretin* gene stabilizer
   b. Symptomatic treatment: Diuretics
10. Following drugs should be avoided in this disease:
    a. Heart rate lowering drugs because increased heart rate is responsible for maintaining cardiac output because in this disease cardiac output is fixed.
       - Nondihydropyridine group of drugs like calcium-channel blockers
       - β-blockers
    b. ACEI and ARBs because these drugs produce hypotension.
    c. Digoxin by increasing the intracellular calcium worsens the cardiac function.

CASE 32

A 65-year-old chronic alcoholic for >12 years presented with severe breathlessness. On examination, there was tachycardia and basal crepitations. His ECG demonstrated wide QRS complexes, broad left bundle branch block, and sinus rhythm. Echocardiography subsequently demonstrated ejection fraction of <30%.

1. **What is your diagnosis?**
2. **Is there any cutoff value of alcohol in this patient?**
3. **What is the risk factor in this disease?**
4. **What are the postulated mechanisms for this disease?**
5. **What are the different types of mitochondrial damage seen in alcoholic cardiomyopathy?**
6. **Mention the criteria for diagnosing alcoholic cardiomyopathy.**
7. **Mention five complications in this disease.**
8. **Which diuretic is used in this case?**
9. **When cardiac resynchronization therapy (CRT) is indicated?**

Answers

1. Diagnosis is alcoholic cardiomyopathy.
2. There is no cutoff value of alcohol consumption and alcoholic cardiomyopathy.
3. Daily intake of 80 g of alcohol for >5 years may lead to development of alcoholic cardiomyopathy. But, all chronic alcoholic develops this disease.
4. Following are the postulated mechanisms for alcoholic cardiomyopathy:
   a. Increased fragmentation of mitochondria leading to its damage.
   b. Increased concentration of reactive oxygen species in the myocytes leading to oxidation of lipids, protein, and DNA resulting cardiac dysfunction.
   c. Apoptosis of cardiac myocytes resulting from:
      - Direct toxicity of alcohol
      - Indirectly from damage by the metabolites of alcohol and acetaldehyde.
   d. Thiamine deficiency
5. Following types of mitochondrial damage seen in alcoholic cardiomyopathy:
   a. Changes in the mitochondrial reticulum
   b. Cluster formation of mitochondria
   c. Disappearance of intermitochondrial junction
   d. Appearance of minor mitochondria
   e. Appearance of septate mitochondria

6. Criteria for diagnosis of alcoholic cardiomyopathy:
   a. Dilated cardiomyopathy seen in 2D echocardiography.
   b. End-diastolic dimension of left ventricle >2 SD above the normal left ventricular ejection fraction <50%.
   c. Exclusion of hypertensive, valvular, and ischemic heart disease
7. Following are the five complications in this disease:
   i. Heart failure
   ii. Cachexia
   iii. Cardioembolism
   iv. Arrhythmias
   v. Death
8. In this case, the following diuretic is used: Spironolactone is used in patient with <35% ejection fraction and NYHA class III symptoms.
9. CRT is indicated in symptomatic patient with QRS duration of >150 ms and dyssynchrony in echocardiography.

CASE 33

A 45-year-old man was treated for stage II lymphoma by radiotherapy in the mediastinal region. On examination, there was pedal edema, tachycardia, and pulsus paradoxus. After 10 years, patient developed breathlessness and admitted in the emergency department.

1. **What are the risk factors responsible for postradiotherapy cardiac involvement?**
2. **What are the effects of radiotherapy in cardiovascular system?**
3. **What is your diagnosis?**
4. **What is the dose of radiation in case of lymphoma?**
5. **What is treatment in this case?**

Answers

1. Following are the risk factors responsible for postradiotherapy cardiac involvement:
   a. Higher doses of radiation
   b. Young age at radiation
   c. During radiation in the mediastinum, no cardiac protection
   d. Cardiac volume exposed to irradiation
   e. Increasing interval from the time of radiation
   f. Preexisting cardiovascular risk factors
2. Following are the effects of cardiac involvement postradiotherapy:
   a. Acute cardiac injury:
      - Acute myocarditis
      - Acute pericarditis
   b. Late cardiac injury:
      - Constrictive pericarditis
      - Restrictive cardiomyopathy
      - Coronary artery disease
      - Valvular disease: Left-sided valves are mostly involved for some unknown reason.
      - Conduction disturbances mainly sick sinus syndrome
   c. Medium or late vessel vasculopathy:
      - Thoracic aortic calcification (porcelain aorta)
      - Stenosis of carotid or axillary or subclavian artery
3. The diagnosis is constrictive pericarditis.
4. The radiation dose in case of lymphoma is involved field radiotherapy 35 Gy.
5. The treatment in this case is pericardiectomy.

CASE 34

A 25-year-old man came to an echocardiography clinic for routine preanesthetic checkup for hydrocele operation. The Doppler echocardiography demonstrated:

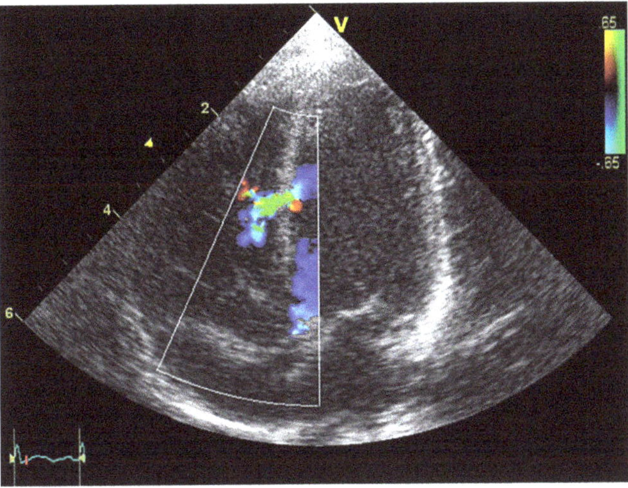

1. **What is shown in above Doppler echocardiography?**
2. **What may be the associated features in this case?**
3. **What are the risk factors associated with this disease?**
4. **What are the subtypes in this disease?**
5. **How it can be classified according to size?**
6. **How can describe the murmur in this disease?**

Answers

1. Doppler echocardiography demonstrated small VSD.
2. Following abnormalities are associated with VSD:
    a. Atrial septal defect
    b. Patent ductus arteriosus
    c. Right aortic arch
    d. Pulmonary stenosis
    e. Coarctation of aorta
    f. Subaortic stenosis
3. Following risk factors are associated with this disease:
    a. Congenital factors:
        - *TBX* genetic mutation
        - Polygenic inheritance
    b. Acquired risk factors:
        - Maternal infection: Rubella and influenza
        - Maternal diabetes mellitus
        - Phenylketonuria
        - Exposure to different toxins:
            o Alcohol
            o Cocaine
            o Marijuana
        - Certain medications:
            o Metronidazole
            o Ibuprofen
4. Following are the subtypes in this disease:
    a. Type 1 or infundibular defect: This defect is present below the aortic or pulmonary valves but above the crista supraventricularis in the outlet system.
    b. Type 2 or membranous defect: This defect is present in the membranous part of the septum below crista supraventricularis.
    c. Type 3 or AV canal: This defect is present just inferior to mitral or tricuspid valve in the inlet part of right ventricular septum.
    d. Type 4 or muscular defect: This defect is present in the muscular part of septum located in the apical, central, or outlet parts of the septum.
5. This defect can be classified according to the size of aortic annulus:
    a. Small defect: The size is ≤25% of aortic annulus.
    b. Moderate defect: The size is ≥25% but <75%.
    c. Large defect: The size is ≥75%.

6. The description of spectrum of murmur in this disease:
   a. Pansystolic murmur best heard in the lower left sternal border, it is harsh in small defect but as the size of the defect is gradually increasing murmur becomes soft.
   b. Hand grip increases the strength of this murmur
   c. In case of infundibular type, the murmur can be heard in the pulmonary area.
   d. In case of aortic regurgitation, there will decrescendo diastolic murmur.

CASE 35

A 35-year-old man presented with syncope and diagnosed as AV block. Subsequently, echocardiography demonstrated A-V and V-A discordance.

1. **What is A-V discordance?**
2. **What is V-A discordance?**
3. **In which condition there is presence of this type of discordance?**
4. **In which condition there is A-V concordance but V-A discordance?**

Answers

1. A-V discordance means connection between atria and ventricle where right atrium connects with left ventricle through the mitral valve and left atrium connects with right ventricle through the tricuspid valve.

2. V-A discordance means connection between ventricle and atria where left ventricle connects with pulmonary artery and right ventricle connects with aorta.

3. In congenitally corrected transposition of the great vessels, this type of discordance will be found.

4. In transposition of the great vessels, there is A-V concordance but V-A discordance.

CASE 36

A 56-year-old diabetic male having past history of joint pain in childhood has come to emergency department with respiratory distress. On examination, the pulse rate was 112 beats/min, low volume, irregularly irregular, and blood pressure 100/60 mm Hg. On auscultation, there was presence of murmur that has been depicted in the phonocardiography. ECG was done immediately. After 1 day, echocardiography was performed. Patient is already on anticoagulant.

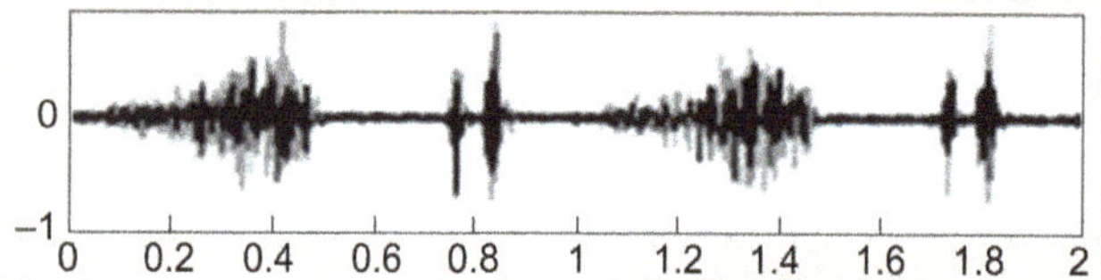
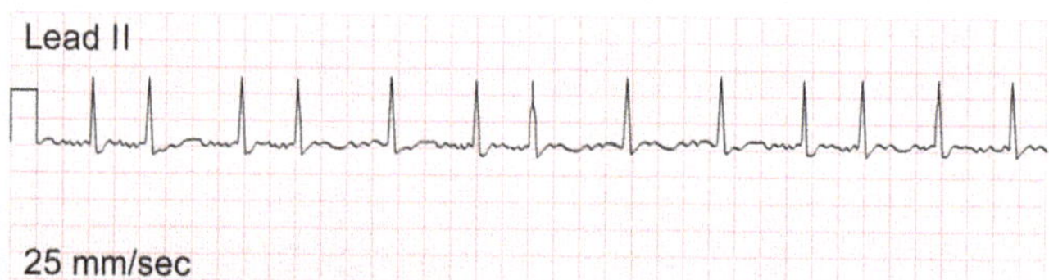

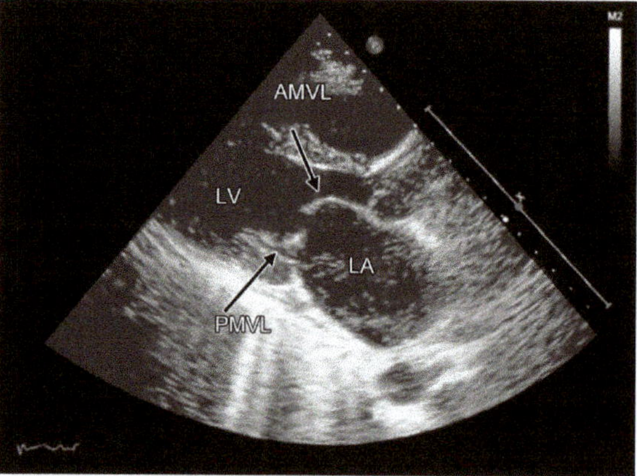

(AMVL: anterior mitral leaflet; LA: left atrium; LV: left ventricle; PMVL: posterior mitral leaflet)

1. **What are the findings in the above pictures?**
2. **What is your diagnosis?**
3. **Classify the types of this cardiac irregularity?**
4. **What are the modifiable risk factors in this type of cardiac irregularity?**
5. **What is CHA_2DS_2-VASc score and why it is used?**
6. **Patient is on anticoagulant. How can you assess the bleeding risk?**
7. **What are the alternative treatments in place of anticoagulation to prevent stroke as well as systemic embolism in atrial fibrillation?**
8. **Following are the options present for the rate control in case of atrial fibrillation:**
9. **If the patient requires cardioverter, is anticoagulation needed?**
10. **In case of failure of cardioversion, what can be done?**
11. **What do you know about "pulmonary vein isolation"?**
12. **What are the complications of catheter ablation?**

Answers

1. Above picture demonstrates:
    a. Phonocardiography demonstrated presence of an opening snap followed by mid-diastolic murmur. As the pulse is irregular, there is absence of presystolic accentuation.
    b. ECG demonstrated:
        - Absence of P wave
        - R-R interval is irregular.
    c. Parasternal long-axis view in echocardiography demonstrated presence of:
        - Diastolic doming of the anterior mitral valve leaflet
        - Thickened and restricted posterior valve leaflet
2. The most likely diagnosis is mitral stenosis probably of rheumatic origin complicated by atrial fibrillation.
3. According to current classification of atrial fibrillation:
    a. Paroxysmal atrial fibrillation: This type terminates spontaneously or by any intervention within 7 days of onset.
    b. Persistent atrial fibrillation: This type will persist or sustained for >7 days.
    c. Long-standing persistent atrial fibrillation: Continuous atrial fibrillation persisting for >12 months.
    d. Permanent atrial fibrillation: In this type, patient and clinicians will jointly decide to stop further attempt to restore the sinus rhythm.
4. Following are the modifiable risk factors in the atrial fibrillation:
    a. Assessment as well as treatment of sleep apnea
    b. Hypertension
    c. Hyperlipidemia
    d. Alcohol abuse
    e. Tobacco use
    f. Glucose intolerance
5. CHA_2DS_2-VASc score:

CHA_2DS_2-VASc risk	Score
Left ventricular ejection fraction ≤40%	1
Hypertension	1
Age ≥ 75 years	2
Diabetes	1
Stroke/transient ischemic attack (TIA)/thrombo-embolism	2
Vascular disease	1
Age 65–74 years	1
Female	1
Maximum score	9

This score is required for:
    a. Stratification of stroke risk in case of atrial fibrillation
    b. Who will be benefited from anticoagulation?
6. Patient is on anticoagulant. So, HAS-BLED score uses following risk factors to assess the bleeding risk (1 point each):
    a. Hypertension having systolic blood pressure of >160 mm Hg (H)
    b. Abnormal liver function (A)
    c. Abnormal renal function (A)
    d. History of stroke (S)
    e. History of bleeding or anemia (B)
    f. Labile international normalized ratio (INR) [>60% time therapeutic (L)]

g. Elderly: >65 years of age (E)
h. Drugs such as nonsteroidal anti-inflammatory drugs (NSAIDs) or antiplatelet agents (D)
i. Alcohol (D)

Following are the percentage of risk of bleeding:

Score	Percentage of bleeding risk
0	1
1	2
2	3
3	4
4	9
≥5	13

7. Following are the alternative treatments to oral anticoagulation:
    a. WATCHMAN device, a self-expanding metal frame which covered with a membrane, is placed in the left atrial appendages subcutaneously.
    b. Surgical occlusion of the left atrial appendages at the time of mitral valve surgery
8. Following are the options present for the rate control in case of atrial fibrillation:
    a. β-blockers
    b. Dihydropyridine group of calcium-channel blockers such as verapamil and diltiazem
    c. Digoxin in case of sedentary patients and in case of reduced left ventricular function
    d. Amiodarone in patients refractory to other therapy
    e. Pacemaker with AV ablation in patient refractory to medical therapy.
9. At the time of cardioversion:
    a. If atrial fibrillation is of <48 hours duration, cardioversion can be done without any prior anticoagulation.
    b. If atrial fibrillation is of >48 hours duration:
        - The patient should be treated with oral anti-coagulation for 3 weeks prior to cardioversion and should be continued for another 4 weeks after cardioversion.
        - Transesophageal echocardiography should be done to detect any thrombus in the atrium and the patient is on oral anticoagulant therapy. If the thrombus is present, then oral anticoagulant should be continued for 4 weeks.
10. In case of failure of cardioversion, energy delivery should be improved by following methods:
    a. Increasing the strength of the shock
    b. Use of biphasic waveform rather than monophasic waveform
    c. Altering the electrode pad leading to change in the shock vector
    d. Pressing the anterior electrode pad during delivery of shock
    e. Use of ibutilide prior to delivery of energy
11. As electrical triggers originate from pulmonary vein where it joins with left atrium, radiofrequency ablation or cryoablation in this area isolates the electrically active sleeves in the myocardium present at the pulmonary vein leading to "pulmonary vein isolation".
12. Following are the complications of catheter ablation:
    a. Access site complication
    b. Cardiac tamponade
    c. Pericarditis
    d. Stroke
    e. Paralysis of phrenic nerve
    f. Pulmonary vein stenosis
    g. Esophageal fistula
    h. Reentrant and focal left atrial tachycardia

CASE 37

A 67-year-old man having history of known ischemic heart disease came to emergency department with palpitation, diaphoresis, anginal pain, and chest discomfort. Urgently ECG was done and demonstrated below:

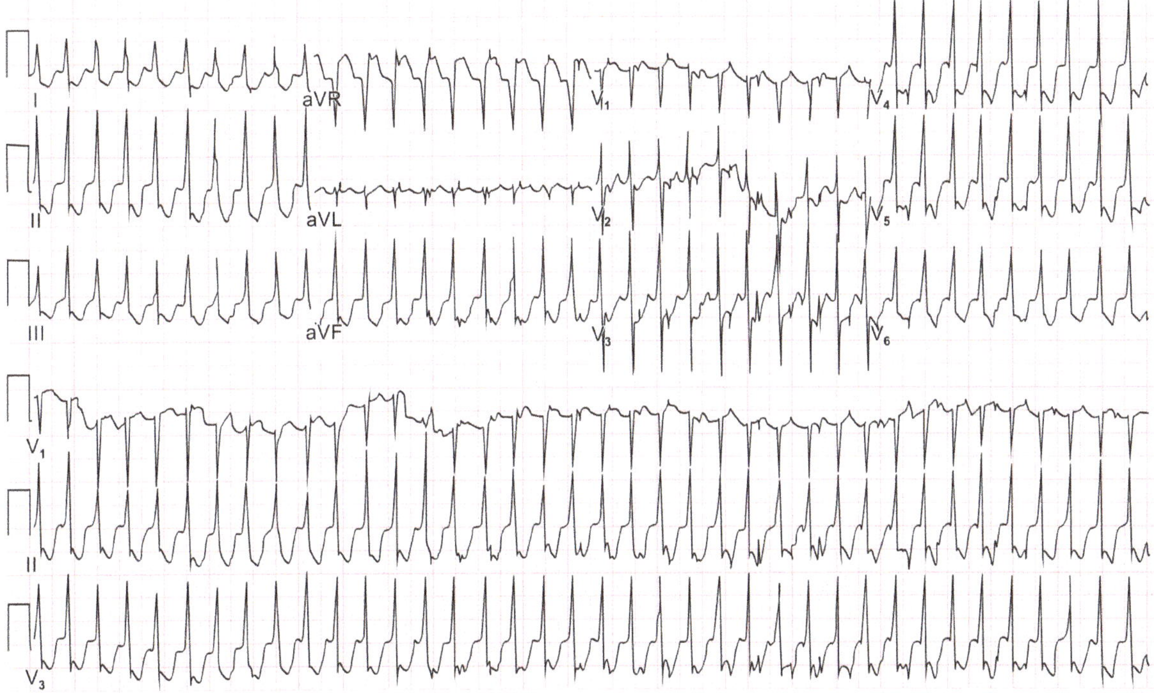

Within 15 minutes the patient's ECG was reverted to sinus rhythm, but the chest pain was continued.

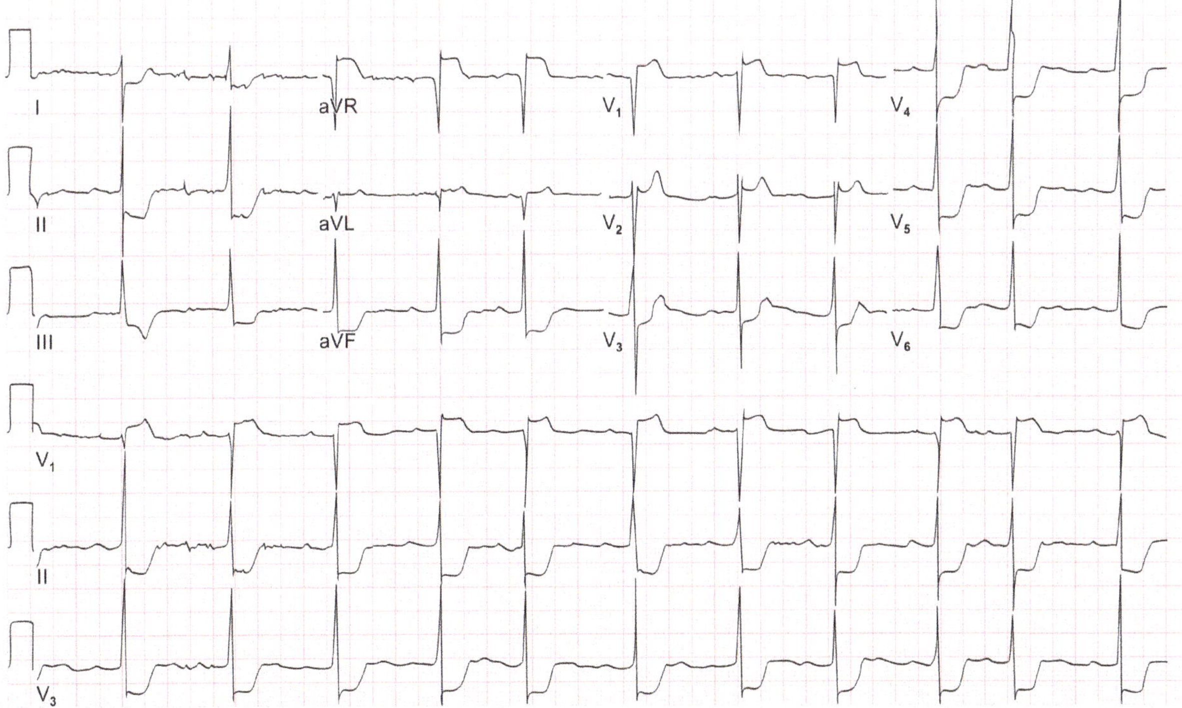

1. **What is your interpretation?**
2. **What does it indicate?**
3. **What will be the next immediate step?**
4. **If this step is normal but troponin is elevated, what will be the conclusion?**
5. **What should be the clinical presentation in this case?**
6. **What are the causes of narrow complex tachycardia?**
7. **If the patient is hemodynamically unstable and the ECG will not turn into sinus rhythm, in that case what should be the treatment of choice?**

Answers

1. Above first ECG demonstrated:
   a. Heart rate 220 beats/min
   b. ST-segment elevated in aVR
   c. Diffuse ST-segment depression in other leads
   Second ECG demonstrated:
   a. ST segment was elevated in aVR, V1, and V2.
1. It may indicate lesion in the left anterior descending artery.
2. Next step is obviously coronary artery angiography and serum troponin estimation.
3. If the coronary angiography is normal but troponin is elevated, in that case it may be due to leak of troponin in case of supraventricular tachycardia.
4. Patient with supraventricular tachycardia presents with:
   a. Palpitation
   b. Lightheadedness
   c. Diaphoresis
   d. Dyspnea
   e. Chest pain

   It will be more pronounced in case of structural heart disease and in case of elderly.

   In case of AV nodal reentrant tachycardia simultaneous contraction of atria and ventricle leading to contraction of atria against closed AV valve resulting canon waves in the jugular venous pulse. It is also known as "frog sign". During this time patient complains of "neck pounding".
5. Causes of narrow complex tachycardia with fixed R-R interval:
   a. Sinus tachycardia
   b. Atrial tachycardia
   c. Atrial flutter with fixed AV conduction
   d. AV nodal reentrant tachycardia
   e. AV reentrant tachycardia
   f. Sinoatrial (SA) nodal reentrant tachycardia
   Causes of narrow complex tachycardia with irregular R-R interval:
   a. Multifocal atrial tachycardia
   b. Atrial flutter with "variable conduction"
   c. Atrial flutter
   d. Junctional tachycardia
6. The algorithm to diagnose narrow complex tachycardia is:
   a. Regular QRS complexes:
      - Normal P waves: Normal sinus rhythm
      - Abnormal P waves prior to QRS complexes: Atrial tachycardia
      - Flutter waves: Atrial flutter
      - No P waves or evidence of atrial activity after QRS complexes:
        - AV nodal reentrant tachycardia
        - Atrioventricular reentrant tachycardia
   b. Irregular QRS complexes:
      - Evidence of multiple P wave morphologies prior to QRS complexes
      - Evidence of atrial flutter with variable conduction: Atrial flutter with variable block
      - Absence of P wave or no atrial activity: Atrial fibrillation
7. If the ECG will not turn into sinus rhythm and the patient demonstrates the following feature of hemodynamic instability, synchronized cardioversion:
   a. Hypotension
   b. Acutely altered mental status
   c. Signs of shock
   d. Chest pain

CASE 38

A 35-year-old normotensive nonsmoker male has been admitted with transient weakness of right upper limb. He has neither any similar past history nor any similar family history. His ECG and MRI brain were normal, but echocardiogram demonstrated following features:

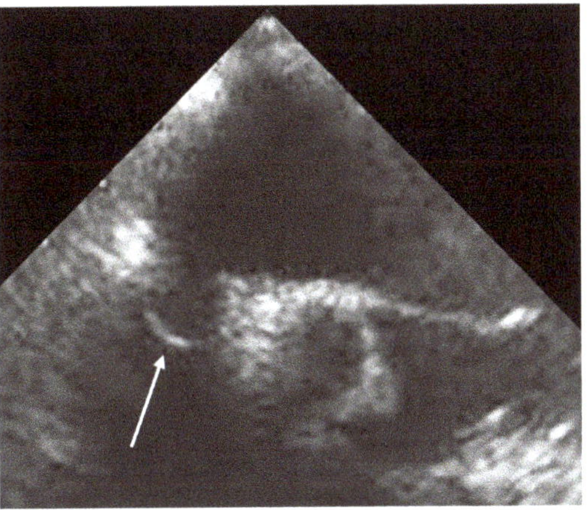

1. **What has been demonstrated in the above picture and how can you describe it?**
2. **What is your diagnosis?**
3. **What is the investigation of choice?**
4. **What is the suspected pathophysiology in this case?**

Answers

1. Echocardiography demonstrated the evidence of aneurysmal dilatation of the intra-atrial septum.
2. The most likely diagnosis is transient ischemic attack due to lodgment of the paradoxical embolus from right atrium to left atrium through the fenestration present in the intra-atrial septum.
3. The investigation of choice is well-formed bubble contrast echocardiogram with both sniff as well as valsalva as it can detect the right-to-left atrial shunt.
4. As there is common association of multiple fenestrations in the aneurysmal intra-atrial septum which will lead to high incidence of stroke.

CASE 39

A 60-year-old type 2 diabetic male has been admitted with ST-elevated myocardial infarction and was thrombolyzed. Echocardiography demonstrated global hypokinesia with ejection fraction of 40%. Within 4 hours coronary angiography demonstrated 70% block in left anterior descending artery. Optical coherence tomography (OCT) demonstrated the following feature. He was started parenteral anticoagulant and after 5 days repeat OCT was performed and it showed the resolution of the lesion.

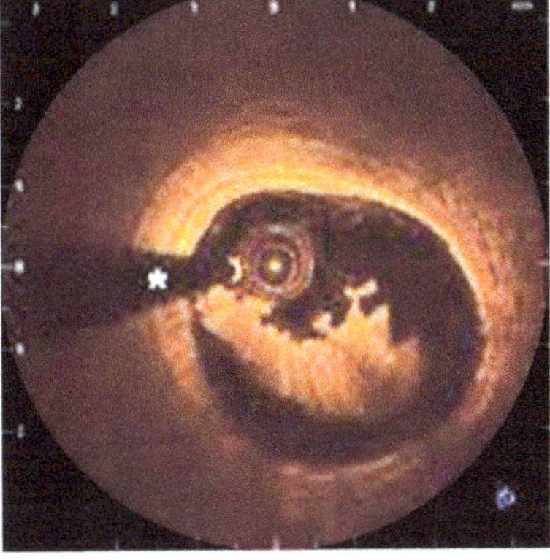
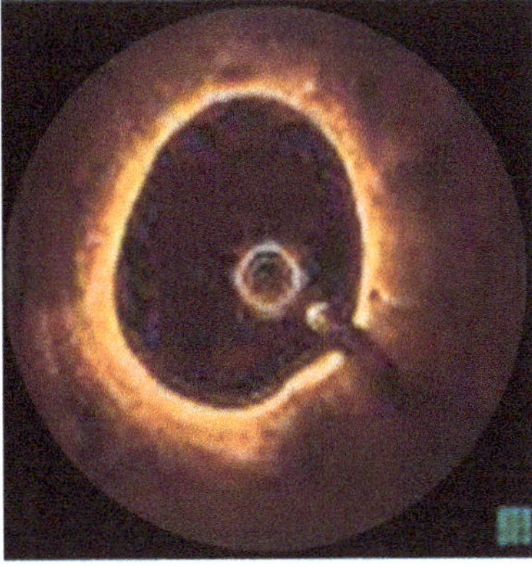

1. **What do the above pictures demonstrate?**
2. **How can it demonstrate plaque within the coronary artery?**
3. **What are the limitations of coronary angiography as compared to OCT?**
4. **What is vulnerable plaque?**
5. **How can you classify plaques of acute coronary syndrome by OCT?**

Answers

1. Above pictures demonstrate:
   a. First picture demonstrates the presence of thrombus within the coronary artery.
   b. Second picture demonstrates the resolution of the thrombus from within the coronary artery.
2. In the OCT:
   a. Fibrous plaque is demonstrated as homogeneous high signal region having low attenuation.
   b. Lipid-rich plaque is demonstrated as region of low signal having diffuse border.
   c. Calcified plaque is demonstrated as region of low signal having sharp border.
3. Coronary artery:
   a. Is two-dimensional silhouette of three-dimensional coronary artery.
   b. Has limited ability to assess the composition as well as dimension of the plaque.
   c. It has low sensitivity in detecting the calcium.
   d. Can underestimate the severity of the coronary artery lesion in presence of uniform narrowed lumen resulting from diffuse atherosclerosis.
   e. Can miss the atherosclerotic lesion growing outward with preservation of the lumen size—known as Glasgow effect.
   f. Cannot determine the morphology of the lesion as well as status of fibrous cap.
4. Vulnerable plaques are found in those:
   a. Who are prone to rupture
   b. Have thinned-out fibrous cap which is rich in macrophages overlying the lipid pool.
5. Classification of plaques by OCT:
   a. Disrupted fibrous cap:
      - Underlying lipid laden plaque—leading to rupture of the cap.
      - Underlying calcium laden plaque—it is OCT-calcified cap. It may be in the following forms:
        ○ Protruding nodular calcium
        ○ Calcium attached to thrombus
        ○ Having presence of calcium superficially
        ○ Presence of calcium proximal and distal to the lesion
   b. Intact fibrous cap:
      - Definite: Thrombus + intact underlying plaque is visualized.
      - Probable:
        ○ Thrombus (–) having irregular surface.
        ○ Thrombus (+)—underlying plaque neither visualized nor superficial lipid and presence of calcium proximal and distal to the lesion.

      It is OCT—visualized lesion.
   c. Others—it may be:
      - Tight stenosis
      - Dissection
      - Hematoma
      - Fissure
      - Coronary spasm

CASE 40

A 45-year-old woman having recurrent history of anginal pain along with hypotension in spite of oral antiplatelet drugs has been admitted with acute inferior wall myocardial infarction. Rescue percutaneous transluminal coronary angioplasty (PTCA) done within 2 hours which demonstrated the evidence of anomalous origin of the right coronary artery from left coronary sinus and there is evidence of near-total occlusion of this artery. All the catheters failed to be introduced into this anomalous artery, only Tiger guide catheter done this job successfully.

1. **What are the factors responsible for diagnosis of this type of anomaly?**
2. **What do you mean by the potentially benign and malignant course of this anomaly?**
3. **What is the importance of malignant course?**
4. **What are the mechanisms by which it may lead to severe termination in young?**
5. **What are the different sites of origin of the anomalous coronary artery?**

Answers

1. Following factors are responsible for the diagnosis of anomalous aortic origin of coronary arteries:
   a. Types of diagnostic modalities used
   b. What are the criteria used to define the anomalies
   c. Study population characteristics
2. Benign course can be defined as the anomaly which is not responsible for any hemodynamic impairment or abnormalities in the myocardial perfusion in the absence of atherosclerosis.

   Malignant course can be defined when the course of the anomalous artery is in-between the aorta and right ventricular outflow tract or pulmonary artery.
3. Importance of the malignant course of this anomalous origin of right coronary artery because it may lead to development of:
   a. Anginal syndrome
   b. Arrhythmias
   c. Myocardial infarction
   d. Sudden death in young
4. Following mechanisms are responsible for ischemia-induced sudden cardiac death in young:
   a. Acute angulation as well as kinking at the ostium of the coronary artery
   b. Abnormal slit-like opening
   c. Vasospasm of the anomalous artery
   d. As the artery passes in-between the aorta and pulmonary artery, it may lead to mechanical compression during exertion.
   e. Intramural course of the anomalous artery may lead to sudden cardiac death.
5. Following are the different sites of the origin of the anomalous coronary artery:
   a. Origin of the artery from the aorta above the sinotubular plane
   b. Origin of the artery from below the ostium of the left coronary artery
   c. Origin of the artery along the midline
   d. Origin of the artery between the midline and the origin of the left coronary artery below the sinotubular plane

---

CASE 41

A 70-year-old poorly controlled type 2 diabetic having glycated hemoglobin (HbA1c) of 8.5%, hypertensive, and smoker man was admitted with chest pain and hypotension. Urgent ECG was performed and it demonstrated recent acute anterior wall myocardial infarction. On examination, his systolic blood pressure was <80 mm Hg and fine crepitations in the both basal areas of the lungs.

1. **What is the definition of cardiogenic shock both clinically and hemodynamically?**
2. **What are the clinical features in favor of cardiogenic shock?**
3. **If the patient admitted in the non-PCI center, what are the points to be remembered prior to thrombolysis?**
4. **What are the points to be remembered prior to administration of vasopressors?**
5. **What are the critical points to be remembered prior to management of this patient?**
6. **What is the classification of the Society of Cardiovascular Angiography and Interventions for shock pyramid?**

Answers

1. Clinically, cardiogenic shock can be defined as presence of critical tissue hypoperfusion as well as hypoxia resulting from cardiac cause and absence of adequate response to volume replacement.

   Hemodynamically cardiogenic shock can be defined as sustained decrease in systolic blood pressure of <90 mm Hg, cardiac index of <2.2, and pulmonary capillary wedge pressure lower than 15 mm Hg.
2. Following are the features of the cardiogenic shock:
   a. Systolic blood pressure is lower than 80 mm Hg.
   b. Presence of persistent hypotension for >30 minutes
   c. Reduced systolic cardiac function due to old inferior as well as recent acute anterior wall myocardial infarction
   d. Evidence of hypoperfusion such as:
      - Oliguria
      - Cold extremities
      - Confusion
   e. Increased left ventricular filling pressure in the form of high pulmonary capillary wedge pressure as evidenced by basal crepitation in the both bases of the lungs.

3. Following points should be remembered during thrombolysis in non-PCI center:
   a. Bolus thrombolysis should be required.
   b. Thrombolytic reperfusion rate is time dependent. It means time from the symptom onset to presentation as it is very critical.
   c. In patient with cardiogenic shock, reperfusion rate is lower and rate of reocclusion is higher.
4. Following points have to be remembered prior to administration of vasopressin:
   a. Drug of choice is norepinephrine. But if the blood pressure is still low, then vasopressin or epinephrine should be added.
   b. If the mean arterial pressure is >65 mm Hg, then dobutamine should be added as ionotropes.
   c. If the patient is on β-blocker, then phospho-diesterase inhibitor III can be used.
   d. In case of catecholamine resistant shock, levosi-mendan should be administered.
5. Following critical points should be remembered during management of this patient:
   a. Correction of acidosis
   b. Diabetes mellitus should be treated with infusion of insulin.
   c. Sepsis if present should be treated.
   d. Renal function should be monitored.
   e. Arrhythmia should be treated.
6. The uniform classification of Society of Cardiovascular Angiography and Intervention for shock pyramid:
   a. Stage A: Patient is at development of shock, currently there is symptoms of shock.
   b. Stage B: There is presence of hypotension and tachycardia but no feature of tissue hypo-perfusion.
   c. Stage C: It is the stage of classical shock along with decreased tissue perfusion and it requires management beyond resuscitation of fluid.
   d. Stage D: In this stage, there is clinical deterioration and nonresponse to initial intervention.
   e. Stage E: In this stage, patient may experience cardiac arrest requiring extracorporeal membrane oxygenation (ECMO) or cardiopulmonary resuscitation (CPR).

CASE 42

A 65-year-old diabetic nonhypertensive woman has been admitted with acute onset chest pain and subsequently diagnosed as inferior wall myocardial infarction for which PTCA was performed, but after 2 days patient developed sudden respiratory distress of NYHA class IV.

On examination, patient is diaphoretic, pulse rate 120 beats/min, blood pressure 70/50 mm Hg, and respiratory rate 26 breaths/min. On cardiovascular examination, grade 2 systolic murmur of late onset heard at the apex and basal crepitations at the both lung bases.

On laboratory examination, cardiac biomarkers were near normal, but BNP level 1,024, serum electrolytes were within normal limit.

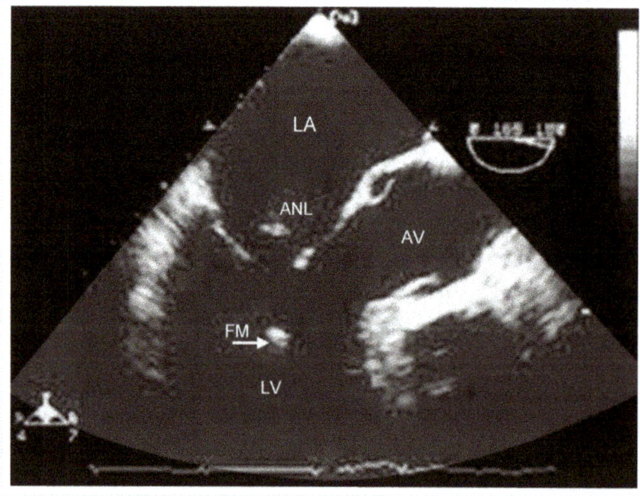

1. **What has been described in the above picture?**
2. **What is the most likely diagnosis?**
3. **What are the causes of acute mitral regurgitation?**
4. **What are the structures of the mitral valve?**
5. **Which valve leaflet is more vulnerable to rupture and why?**
6. **After how many days this type of injury occurs and why?**
7. **What are the features found in chest X-Ray?**

Answers

1. The above picture demonstrates the presence of undulating mass moving with anterior mitral leaflet during systole.
2. The most likely diagnosis is acute mitral regurgitation due to ischemic injury of the papillary muscles leading to rupture of the papillary muscles.
3. Following are the causes of acute mitral regurgitation:
   a. Papillary muscle rupture—it may be partial or complete.
   b. Rupture of chordae
   c. Acute change in the left ventricular geometry
4. Following are the structures of the mitral valve:
   a. Mitral leaflets
   b. Mitral annulus
   c. Chordae tendineae
   d. Papillary muscles
   e. Ventricular wall
   f. Atrial wall
5. Posteromedial wall is more vulnerable to rupture because it is supplied by the single coronary artery but anterolateral leaflet has dual blood supply.
6. After 2–7 days, this complication may occur and it is due to:
   a. Postinfarct ischemic injury
   b. Infarct-related extension injury
   c. Reperfusion injury
7. Following are the features in the chest X-ray:
   a. Bilateral alveolar or interstitial edema
   b. If the flow of blood is eccentric, i.e., direction of flow toward pulmonary veins leading to pulmonary edema.
   c. In absence of severe left ventricular dysfunction, there is no cardiomegaly.

CASE 43

A 50-year-old diabetic and hypertensive patient with history of allograft renal transplantation 4 months back from living donor with end-to-side anastomoses between right external iliac artery of the recipient and renal artery of the donor and was on mycophenolate mofetil, tacrolimus, and prednisolone came to transplantation clinic with headache. He was examined and revealed that his blood pressure was 200/105 mm Hg not controlled by three antihypertensive medications.

Doppler ultrasonography revealed peak systolic velocity of 300 cm/s at the anastomotic site with delayed deceleration time.

1. **What is your diagnosis?**
2. **When this complication can occur?**
3. **What are the features of this transplant-related complication?**
4. **What is the main pathophysiology in this case?**
5. **What are the common sites of stenosis of renal artery of the graft?**
6. **What is the initial diagnostic tool in this case and why?**
7. **What is the gold standard method of diagnosis in this case?**
8. **What are the lines of treatment in this case?**

Answers

1. The most likely diagnosis is transplant-related renal artery stenosis.

2. This complication occurs between 3 months to 2 years, frequently within 6 months.

3. Following are the features of transplant-related complication:
   a. Worsening of hypertension
   b. Treatment of refractory hypertension
   c. Evidence of fluid retention
   d. Dysfunction of the graft without rejection of the graft

4. The main pathophysiology in this case is activation of renin-angiotensin-aldosterone system leading to:
   a. Sodium and fluid retention
   b. Pedal edema
   c. Congestive cardiac failure
   d. Recurrent episodes of pulmonary edema

5. Following are the sites of anastomoses:
   a. End-to-side right external iliac artery of the recipient to allograft renal artery of the donor.
   b. End-to-end right internal iliac artery of the recipient to allograft renal artery of the donor

6. The initial diagnostic tool Doppler is ultrasonography because:
   a. Acceleration time in the renal and intrarenal arteries of the transplanted kidney is ≥0.1 second.
   b. In the transplanted renal artery, peak systolic velocity is >200 ms.
   c. Resistive index in the post-stenotic intrarenal arteries is >1.8.
   d. Ratio of peak systolic velocity between transplant renal and iliac arteries is >1.8.

7. The gold standard method of diagnosing this case is either conventional angiography or digital subtraction angiography. But, it should be done when the noninvasive procedure can suspect this diagnosis.

8. The treatment modalities in this case are:
   a. Medical therapy with ACEIs or ARBs with continuous monitoring of serum creatinine and potassium
   b. Percutaneous transluminal renal angioplasty with stenting
   c. Surgical revascularization:
      - Resection and reversion of the anastomoses
      - Saphenous venous bypass graft of the stenotic segment
      - Patch graft
      - Localized endarterectomy

CASE 44

A 56-year-old hypertensive patient with history of PTCA of left anterior descending artery and left circumflex artery 3 months ago has come to cardiology OPD with fever with chill, anorexia, and weight loss of >10 kg in last 2 months.

Laboratory investigation demonstrated white blood cell count of 16,000/cc, highly raised ESR, and blood culture demonstrated evidence of *Pseudomonas aeruginosa*.

Transthoracic echocardiography demonstrated:

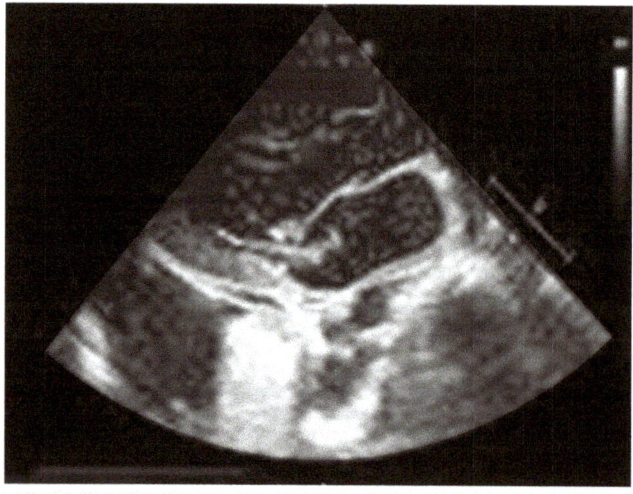

1.   **What is your finding in the above echocardiographic feature?**
2.   **What is your diagnosis?**
3.   **What are the criteria for this diagnosis?**
4.   **What are the possible mechanisms of this diagnosis?**
5.   **What are the risk factors for stent infection?**

Answers

1.   The above echocardiography demonstrated presence of vegetation on the anterior mitral leaflet.
2.   The most likely diagnosis is post-percutaneous coronary intervention-related infective endocarditis.
3.   Three of the following criteria should be fulfilled for this diagnosis:
     a.   Coronary stent placement within previous 4 weeks of intervention
     b.   Performing multiple procedures through the same arterial sheath
     c.   Evidence of significant fever
     d.   Presence of bacteremia
     e.   Leukocytosis having no other cause
     f.   Acute coronary syndrome
     g.   Positive cardiac imaging
4.   Following are the possible mechanisms of this infection:
     a.   Infection within 2 weeks of placement of stent
     b.   Hematogenous spread from another source of infection
     c.   In case of drug-eluting stent, absence of neointimal growth that leads to uncovering of the uncovering of the stent intraluminally.
5.   Following are the risk factors for infection of the stent:
     a.   Imperfect sterility during the procedure
     b.   Prolonged use of indwelling catheter
     c.   Extensive changing of wires

CASE 45

A 30-year-old nonhypertensive patient having past history of pulmonary tuberculosis and completed course of antitubercular drugs of 6 months has attended the OPD with history of progressively increasing abdominal swelling without any abdominal pain, nausea and vomiting or fever for 1 year, dry cough for 1 year, and swelling of legs for 5 months. He had no history of chest pain, orthopnea, palpitation or syncope or paroxysmal nocturnal dyspnea, no history of radiation therapy, or cardiac therapy.

On examination, the blood pressure was 105/80 mm Hg, jugular venous wave demonstrated prominent X and Y descent, and Kussmaul sign is positive.

1.   **What is your most probable diagnosis?**
2.   **What should be expected in the cardiological examination?**
3.   **What should be the feature in abdominal examination?**
4.   **What are the findings in the ECG?**
5.   **What should be the features in the chest X-ray?**
6.   **What are the features in the M-mode echocardiography?**
7.   **What are the features in the cardiac catheterization?**

Answers

1.   The most probable diagnosis is constrictive pericarditis.
2.   Following features should present in the cardiological examination:
     a.   Apical impulse is present in the left fifth intercostal space of 2.5 cm inside the midclavicular line.
     b.   First heart sound is normal.
     c.   Second heart sound intensity is normal, but there may be widening of the second heart sound because of aortic component of second heart sound may occur early due to shortening of the left ventricular systole starting at the onset of inspiration and lasting for 1 or 2 beats only.
     d.   Skoda's sign: It is characterized by systolic retraction of fifth intercostal space in the midclavicular line.

e. Broadbent's sign: It is characterized by retraction of the 10th and 11th intercostal space in the posterior axillary line.

f. Pericardial knock: It is a diastolic sound which is best heard on the left sternal border or at the cardiac apex.

3. Abdominal examination demonstrated:
   a. Hepatomegaly
   b. Horseshoe-shaped ascites

4. ECG features demonstrated:
   a. Low-voltage QRS complexes
   b. Nonspecific T-wave abnormalities
   c. P mitrale due to enlargement of left atrium
   d. In one-third of patients presence of atrial fibrillation

5. Following are the features in the chest X-ray:
   a. Evidence of pleural effusion
   b. Pericardial calcification may be present
   c. Pencilling of the heart borders
   d. Pulmonary vascular congestion in case of markedly elevated left-sided filling pressures.

6. Following are the features in the M-mode echocardiography:
   a. Thickening of the pericardium
   b. In early diastole, abrupt posterior motion of the interventricular septum—it is known as echo pericardial knock.
   c. In the atrial systole, abrupt posterior motion of interventricular septum
   d. Reduced amplitude of the left ventricular posterior wall motion as a result of reduced left ventricular filling during diastole
   e. Premature opening of the pulmonary valve due to high left ventricular end-diastolic pressure.

7. Following are the features in cardiac catheterization:
   a. Right mean arterial pressure of >10 mm Hg
   b. Pressure in the all cardiac chambers will be elevated to 20 mm Hg with equalization of end-diastolic pressure in all the chambers within 5 mm Hg.
   c. In the right and left ventricular pressure trace, demonstrate dip and plateau or square root sign. It can also be seen in the restrictive cardiomyopathy.
   d. Increased variation of left and right ventricular pressure trace during respiration.
   e. Ratio of right and left ventricular pressure times area during inspiration versus expiration is >1.1—suggests constrictive pericarditis.
   f. Systolic pressure in the right ventricle and pulmonary artery pressure are mildly elevated or normal.

CASE 46

A 30-year-old woman came to OPD with exertional breathlessness for 5 years along with exertional fatigue and weakness of left upper and both lower limbs for last 3 years. Patient had past history of low-grade fever, weight loos, and hemoptysis for which she was treated antibiotics and symptomatic drugs. She had no significant family history. Her menstruation is irregular.

On examination, pulse volume in the left upper and both lower limbs were very low except right upper limb where it is high volume. Blood pressure in the right upper limb is 150/95 mm Hg where in the left upper limb it was 110/70 mm Hg and in both lower limbs it was nonrecordable.

On inspection of the chest, there was suprasternal pulsation, and apical impulse was visible in the left sixth intercostal space outside the midclavicular line.

On palpation, there was suprasternal pulsation and left carotid thrill.

On auscultation, loud second heart sound with narrow split, presence of third heart sound, and grade 2 pansystolic murmur in the left sixth intercostal space with the diaphragm with radiation toward axilla. There is also carotid bruit.

1. **What is the most likely diagnosis?**
2. **What are the features in the chest X-ray?**
3. **What are the features in the ultrasonography?**
4. **What are the features in the angiography?**
5. **What are the features in the photoplethysmography?**
6. **What are the features of pulmonary involvement?**

7. **What are the eye changes in this disease?**
8. **What are the indications of endovascular intervention?**
9. **What are the surgical procedures in this disease?**
10. **What are the complications in the surgery of aortoarteritis?**
11. **Discuss two criteria in this disease?**
12. **Classify this disease according to involved vessels.**

Answers

1. The most likely diagnosis is inflammatory arteritis involving left carotid, left subclavian, aortic arch, thoracic and abdominal aorta with moderate mitral regurgitation, and pulmonary hypertension. Patient is in chronic phase.
2. Following are the features in the chest X-ray:
   a. Sharp definition of descending aorta is lost.
   b. Scalloped or wavy appearance of descending aorta
   c. Enlargement of the hilar region
3. Following features are present in the ultrasonography:
   a. Thickening of the circumferential thickening of the vessel is identified and measured.
   b. In the early stage, carotid and subclavian artery can be detected.
   c. Macaroni sign: It is characterized by involvement of long segment with midechoic circumferential thickening of the arterial wall.
4. Following are the features to be measured in the angiography:
   a. Thickness of the wall of the descending thoracic aorta
   b. Thickness of the two pleural layers
   c. Thickness of the periaortic inflammation
5. Following parameters are measured in the photo-plethysmography:
   a. Peak-to-peak time
   b. Crest time
   c. Reflection index to assess the vascular age and arterial compliance.
   d. Maximum systolic and diastolic slope
   e. Height of the pulse
   f. Pulse transit time
   g. Area under the pulse
6. Following are the features of pulmonary involvement:
   a. Chest pain
   b. Pleural effusion
   c. Hemoptysis
   d. Pulmonary hypertension
   e. Midsystolic murmur in the pulmonary area
   f. Involvement of right upper lobe of the lung is more than that in the left.
   g. Rarely dilatation of the pulmonary artery
7. Following are the eye changes in this disease:
   a. Hypertensive retinopathy:
      - Arteriosclerotic retinopathy:
         o Arteriolar narrowing
         o Arteriovenous nipping
         o Silver wiring
      - Neuroretinopathy:
         o Arteriolar narrowing
         o Papilledema
         o Exudates
   b. Mixed retinopathy
   c. Ischemic retinopathy:
      - Stage I: Dilatation of small vessels
      - Stage II: Microaneurysm
      - Stage III: AV anastomoses
      - Stage IV: Ocular complications
8. Following are the indications of endovascular interventions:
   a. Uncontrolled hypertension as a result of renal artery stenosis
   b. Severe symptomatic coronary artery disease
   c. Severe symptomatic cerebrovascular disease
   d. Severe aortic regurgitation
   e. Severe coarctation of the aorta
   f. Stenotic or occlusive arterial lesions leading to ischemia in the limbs
   g. Aneurysm
   h. Rupture of the aorta
9. Following are the different surgical procedures:
   a. Thoracothoracic bypass
   b. Supradiaphragmatic disease
   c. Anterior thoracoabdominal bypass
   d. Thromboendarterectomy
   e. Posterior thoracoabdominal bypass
   f. Aorta-renal anastomoses
10. Complications of surgery in this disease are:
    a. Pseudoaneurysm
    b. Anastomotic restenosis

    c. Thrombotic blockage of the graft

    d. Gastric fistula

    e. Intestinal fistula

    f. Peritonitis

11. Following are the diagnostic criteria in this disease:

    a. Ishikawa criteria:
- Obligatory: Age < 40 years
- Major criteria:
  - Left midsubclavian lesion
  - Right midsubclavian lesion
- Minor criteria:
  - Unexplained high ESR
  - Hypertension
  - Tender common carotid artery
  - Aortic regurgitation/annuloaortic ectasia
  - Lesions in the pulmonary artery
  - Left mid-common carotid lesion
  - Lesions in the distal brachiocephalic trunk
  - Lesions in the descending thoracic aorta
  - Lesions in the abdominal aorta

Diagnostic points: Obligatory + two major or one minor + two minor or more than four minor criteria.

    b. American College of Rheumatology criteria: Here, three out of six criteria must be present.
- Age < 40 years
- Claudication of the extremities
- Decreased pulse in the brachial artery
- Difference in the blood pressure is >10 mm Hg.
- Presence of bruit over the subclavian artery or aorta
- Abnormality in the arteriogram

12. Following are the types of this disease according to the vessels involved:

    a. Type I: Branches of the aortic arch only

    b. Type IIa: Ascending aorta, arch of aorta and its branches

    c. Type IIb: Type IIa + descending thoracic aorta

    d. Type III: Distal thoracic aorta, abdominal aorta, and renal artery

    e. Type IV: Abdominal aorta and/or renal arteries

    f. Type V: Type IIb + type IV

CASE 47

A 48-year-old nonhypertensive, nondiabetic, hypothyroid male on eltroxin came to emergency department with exertional respiratory distress.

On physical examination, patient is acyanotic, having no clubbing, and vitals were normal. Cardiovascular system examination demonstrated normal first heart sound, wide and fixed split of the second heart sound, presence of grade 3 or 6 systolic localized murmur in the pulmonary area, grade 3 or 6 flow murmur in the tricuspid area. SPO_2 after 6-minute walk test was reduced to 6%.

Abdominal examination revealed nonpalpable liver and spleen.

1. **What is your clinical diagnosis?**
2. **What will be shown in ECG?**
3. **What will be demonstrated in the chest X-ray?**
4. **What will be revealed in the echocardiography?**
5. **What are the types of this disease?**
6. **What is patent foramen ovale?**
7. **What is Holt–Oram syndrome?**
8. **What is the mechanism of wide and fixed split?**
9. **What are the complications of atrial septal defect?**
10. **What is the relation of atrial septal defect with pregnancy?**

Answers

1. The most likely clinical diagnosis is atrial septal defect progressing toward right ventricular overload leading to right-sided heat failure.
2. ECG demonstrated the following:
   a. Right axis deviation
   b. Right ventricular hypertrophy
   c. Right bundle branch block
3. X-ray chest demonstrated the following:
   a. Enlarged cardiac shadow
   b. Increased cardiothoracic ratio of 0.6
   c. Prominent main pulmonary artery conus
   d. Increased lung vascularity progressing toward periphery
4. Following are the features in the echocardiography:
   a. Presence of ostium secundum
   b. Dilated right atrium
   c. Dilated right ventricle
   d. Evidence of moderate tricuspid regurgitation
   e. Estimated pressure in the pulmonary artery is 80 mm Hg by jet of tricuspid regurgitation
   f. Paradoxical motion of the interventricular septum
5. Following are the types of atrial septal defect:
   a. Ostium secundum defect occurring in the middle portion of the interatrial septum having 2–4 mm in diameter.
   b. Sinus venosus type defect present just below the entrance of superior vena cava into right atrium.
   c. Ostium primum defect occurring in the lower part of septum occurring in the cleft in-between the mitral and tricuspid valves.
6. Foramen ovale is oblique valvular opening through which right and left atria communicate with each other; it will persist in the fetus till birth. After birth, as the left atrium starts receiving the blood from the lung, the pressure within the left atrium will increase as compared to right atrium leading closure of the foramen.
7. Holt–Oram syndrome is an autosomal dominant defect consisting of:
   a. Ostium type atrial septal defect
   b. Hypoplastic thumb
   c. Accessory phalanx
8. In normal person during inspiration, there is widening of the components of second heart sound due to delayed closure of the pulmonary valve. In atrial septal defect, effect of the respiration will be eliminated because of communication between the left and right atria.
9. Following are the complications of atrial septal defect:
   a. Atrial arrhythmias
   b. Pulmonary hypertension
   c. Eisenmenger syndrome
   d. Paradoxical embolus
   e. Infective endocarditis
   f. Recurrent pulmonary infection
10. In case of uncomplicated atrial septal defect, pregnancy is well tolerated. But in case of associated pulmonary hypertension, there is increased chance of morbidity and mortality; hence in case of Eisenmenger syndrome pregnancy should be avoided. Hence in uncomplicated case, closure of the defect should be done prior to pregnancy.

CASE 48

A 20-year-old hypertensive, nondiabetic male came to OPD with history of repeated respiratory infection and exercise intolerance.

On examination, pulse rate was 90 beats/min, apical impulse was laterally displaced, and there was evidence of palpable systolic thrill, which was accompanied by pansystolic murmur on the left lower sternal border. 2D echocardiography and Doppler echocardiography demonstrated:

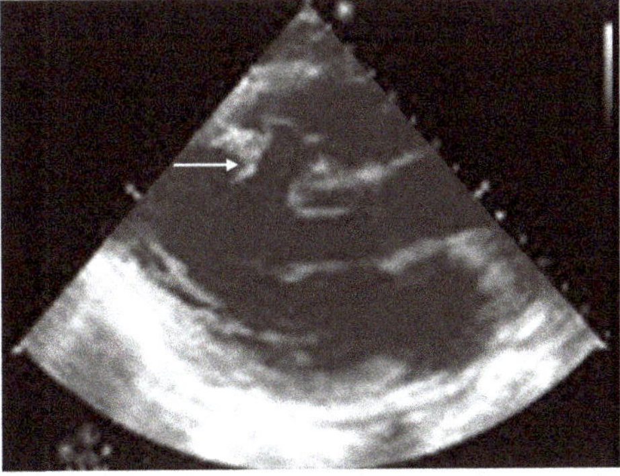 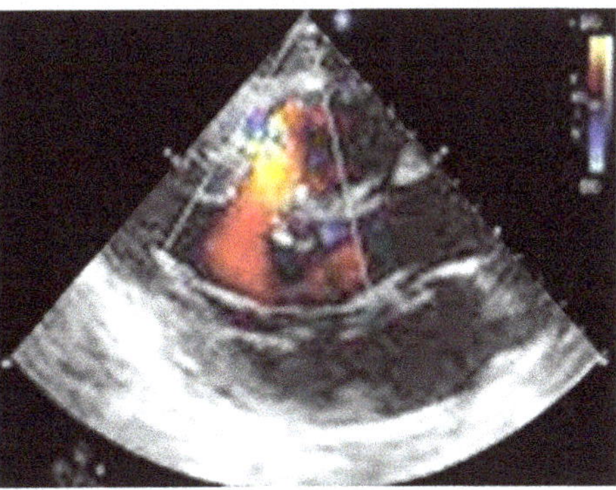

1. **What is the finding of echocardiography in the above?**
2. **What is your diagnosis?**
3. **Classify this disease.**
4. **What are the features that may be developed in late?**
5. **What are the conditions that may be associated with this disease?**
6. **Is there any effect of this disease on pregnancy?**
7. **What are the conditions from which the patient may get benefit from surgery?**
8. **How can you manage this disease?**

Answers

1. Following are the features:
   a. 2D echocardiography demonstrated the evidence of VSD
   b. Doppler echocardiography demonstrated evidence of arterial blood entering from the left ventricle to right ventricle through the defect in the interventricular septum.
2. The diagnosis is patient has been suffering from defect in the interventricular septum.
3. Classification of the VSD:
   a. Supracristal type: It is defect below the pulmonary valve and right coronary cusp of aortic valve.
   b. Infracristal defect: This defect occurs either in the upper membranous part or lower muscular part. It is of following types:
      - Maladie de Roger defect or small defect
      - Multiple small defect or Swiss cheese appearance
      - Large defect
      - Gerbode defect, i.e., defect opening into right atrium
4. The late features of VSD:
   a. On inspection: Bounding apical impulse in the apical area
   b. On palpation:
      - Apical impulse is laterally displaced and is hyperdynamic.
      - Palpable thrill in the left lower sternal border, but it may be abolished in case of right ventricular hypertrophy with pulmonary hypertension.
      - Left parasternal heave
      - Pulmonary second sound is palpable.
   c. On auscultation:
      - Loud first heart sound
      - Pansystolic high-frequency murmur presents in the left lower sternal border.
      - In the pulmonary area, there may be loud pulmonary component of second heart sound. In that case, systolic murmur may be absent in the lower left sternal border.
      - In severe case, the patient may be cyanosed due to reversal of shunt.
5. Following conditions are associated with VSD:
   a. In the following conditions, VSD is the essential feature:
      - Fallot's tetralogy
      - Double-outlet right ventricle
      - Truncus arteriosus
      - Atrioventricular canal defect
   b. In the following conditions, VSD is not the essential feature:
      - Pulmonary stenosis
      - Patent ductus arteriosus
      - Secundum type arterial septal defect
      - Tricuspid atresia
      - Coarctation of aorta
      - Pulmonary atresia
      - Transposition of the great vessels
6. Effect on pregnancy:
   a. In case of small defect, there should be no problem.
   b. In case of moderate size defect along with pulmonary hypertension, the patient may develop right ventricular failure along with rapidly developing pulmonary hypertension. In that case pregnancy should be avoided.
7. Following are the conditions from which patient may get benefit from surgery:
   a. Recurrent infective endocarditis
   b. Development of aortic regurgitation as a result of the prolapse of right coronary cusp

c. Left ventricular overload leading to progressive dilatation of left ventricle

d. Acute rupture of the ventricular septum

8. Management varies according to the size of the defect as well as development of pulmonary hypertension.

This patient having a small defect may not require surgical closure, but there may be recurrence of infective endocarditis; hence this patient will require antibiotics for prophylaxis against infection. But large defect requires surgical closure.

CASE 49

A 30-year-old male came to cardiology OPD with recurrent chest pain and occasional syncope and palpitation. He has family history of sudden death. On examination, the carotid pulse demonstrated following type of pulse. On palpation, there is double apical impulse. M-mode, two-dimensional echocardiography, and after Valsalva maneuver M-mode echocardiography demonstrated the following:

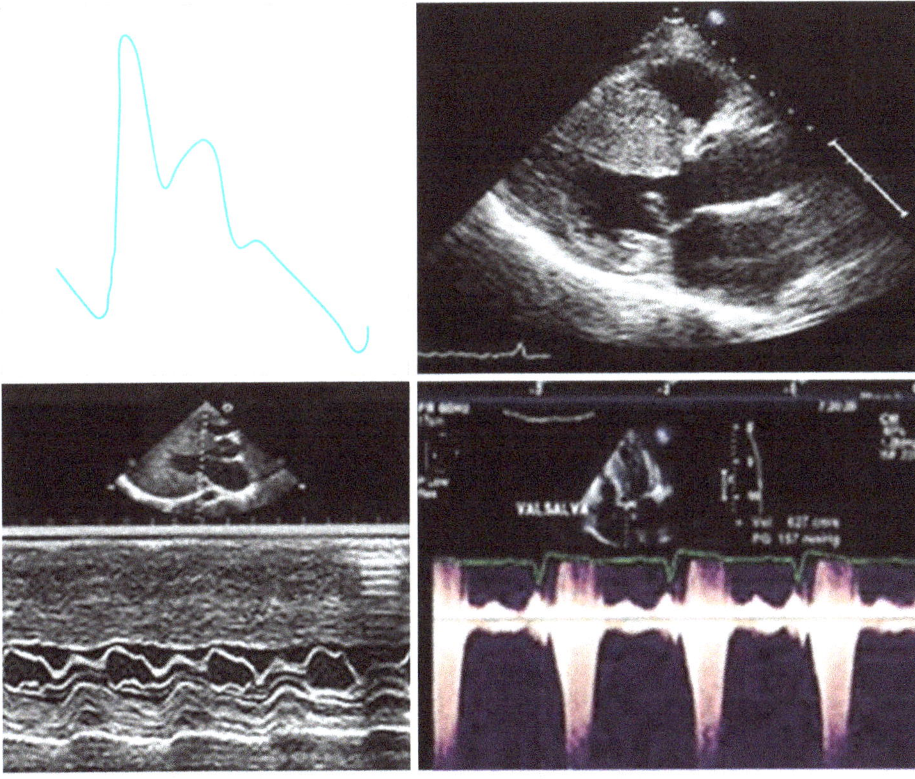

1. **What do the above pictures demonstrate?**
2. **What is your diagnosis?**
3. **What are the complications of this disease?**
4. **Which neurological condition is associated with this disease?**
5. **Mention the most important pathophysiological abnormality in this disease?**
6. **What are the relations of genetic mutation with this disease?**
7. **What are the predictors of risk of sudden death in this disease?**

Answers

1. Demonstration of the following pictures:

   a. Pulse wave demonstrated spike and dome pattern

   b. First echocardiographic picture in parasternal view demonstrates asymmetrical septal hypertrophy.

   c. Second M-mode echocardiographic picture demonstrates systolic anterior motion of the anterior mitral leaflet.

   d. Third echocardiographic picture demonstrates after the Valsalva maneuver there is late-peaking dynamic left ventricular tract obstruction.

2. Patient has been suffering from hypertrophic cardio-myopathy.
3. Following are the complications of the disease:
   a. Atrial fibrillation
   b. Sudden death
   c. Infective endocarditis
   d. Systemic embolization
4. Friedreich's ataxia is associated with hypertrophic cardiomyopathy.
5. Most important pathophysiological abnormality in this disease is diastolic dysfunction.
6. At least nine genes have been identified in this disease.
   a. Mutation of gene for β-heavy chain myosin is associated with obstruction of the left ventricular outflow.
   b. Mutation of gene for troponin T is associated with thickening of the left ventricular wall.
   c. Mutation of gene for myosin-binding protein C is associated with onset in late adult life.
   d. Mutation of arginine amino acid is associated with worse prognosis.
7. Following are the predictors of sudden death in this disease:
   a. History:
      • Exertional syncope or recurrent syncope or presyncope
      • Family history of sudden death
      • Known malignant genotype
   b. Diagnostic evaluation:
      • Severe left ventricular hypertrophy
      • Nonsustained ventricular tachycardia
      • Abnormal hemodynamic response to exercise—failure to augment systolic blood pressure by at least 20 mm Hg.

CASE 50

A 30-year-old female having past history of rubella in the first trimester of pregnancy gave birth a neonate of low birth weight. This male neonate at the age of 20 years developed dyspnea during exertion and recurrent chest infection.

On examination, pulse is collapsing, presence of both systolic and diastolic thrill, and on auscultation, there was presence of machinery murmur in the upper sternal border. His chest X-ray demonstrated:

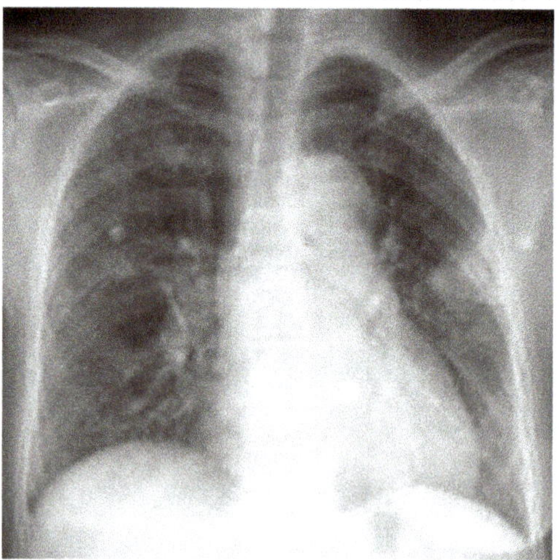

1. **What are the findings in the chest X-ray?**
2. **What is your diagnosis?**
3. **What are causes of collapsing pulse?**
4. **What are the causes of continuous murmur?**
5. **What are the associated lesions with this disease?**
6. **What are the complications?**
7. **Upon which the disease progression will depend?**
8. **What are the congenital cardiac lesions dependent on this disease?**
9. **How can you manage it percutaneously?**

Answers

1. Chest X-ray demonstrates:
   a. Pulmonary plethora
   b. Dilatation of the proximal pulmonary artery
   c. Prominent ascending aorta
2. The diagnosis is patent ductus arteriosus probably of congenital origin.
3. Causes of collapsing pulse:
   a. Systemic causes:
      - Anemia
      - Beriberi
      - Paget's disease
      - Thyrotoxicosis
      - Fever
   b. Cardiogenic causes:
      - Patent ductus arteriosus
      - Complete heart block
      - Aortic regurgitation
4. Following are the causes of continuous murmur:
   a. Mitral regurgitation with aortic regurgitation
   b. Pulmonary arteriovenous fistula
   c. Rupture of sinus of Valsalva
   d. Ventricular septal defect with aortic regurgitation
   e. Venous hum
5. Following are the associated lesions:
   a. Ventricular septal defect
   b. Pulmonary stenosis
   c. Coarctation of aorta
6. Following are the complications:
   a. Congestive cardiac failure
   b. Infective endocarditis
   c. Infective endarteritis
   d. Pulmonary hypertension with reversal of shunt
   e. Substantial right-to-left heart shunt
   f. Ductus may be aneurysmal and may be calcified leading to its rupture.
7. Disease progression depends upon volume-pressure relationship which is as follows:

   $$\text{Volume} = \text{pressure/resistance}$$

   Increased volume of blood in the pulmonary blood vessels leads to increased pressure in the pulmonary artery resulting the changes in the endothelium and the muscles in the vessel wall. These changes ultimately will culminate pulmonary vascular obstructive disease that may be irreversible.
8. Following are the congenital cardiac lesions depend upon patent ductus arteriosus:
   a. Complex coarctation of aorta
   b. Hypoplastic left heart syndrome
   c. Critical congenital aortic stenosis
9. Patent ductus arteriosus can be closed by two means:
   a. Administration of coils:
      - Gianturco-Grifka vascular occlusion device
      - Nit-occlud PDA occluder
   b. Occluders: Amplatzer PDA occluder

CASE 51

A 21-year-old male came to medical OPD with exertional fatigue and fainting attack. On examination, pulse rate was 88 beats/min, raised jugular venous pressure. On auscultation, pulmonary component is soft, there is ejection click followed by ejection systolic murmur heard in the pulmonary area increased during inspiration radiating toward left shoulder.

1. **What is the diagnosis?**
2. **What are the points in favor of this diagnosis?**
3. **What are the main causes of this disease?**
4. **How can you determine the severity of the stenosis?**
5. **What are the complications in this condition?**
6. **Classify the disease.**
7. **What are the syndromes associated with this disease?**
8. **What is the cause of cyanosis in this case?**
9. **How can you manage this case?**

Answers

1. It is a case of pulmonary stenosis.
2. Points in favor of this diagnosis are:
   a. Raised jugular venous pressure
   b. Presence of ejection click
   c. Presence of ejection systolic murmur
3. The causes are:
   a. Congenital
   b. Carcinoid tumor of the small bowel
4. Severity of the lesion:
   a. In mild case:
      - Valvular area larger than 1 cm^2/m^2
      - Transvalvular gradient < 50 mm Hg
      - Peak right ventricular systolic pressure < 75 mm Hg
   b. Moderate case:
      - Valvular area 0.5–1.0 cm^2/m^2
      - Transvalvular gradient is 50–80 mm Hg
      - Right ventricular systolic pressure 75–100 mm Hg
   c. Severe case:
      - Valvular area < 0.5 cm^2/m^2
      - Transvalvular gradient > 80 mm Hg
      - Peak right ventricular systolic pressure > 100 mm Hg
5. Following are the complications of pulmonary stenosis:
   a. Right-sided heart failure
   b. Infective endocarditis
6. Following are the classification of this disease:
   a. Valvular
   b. Supravalvular
   c. Subvalvular
7. Following syndromes are associated with this disease:
   a. Noonan syndrome characterized by:
      - Short stature
      - Webbed neck
      - Downward slanting eyes
      - Hypertelorism
      - Low-set ears
      - Low hairline
      - Mental retardation
      - Pulmonary stenosis
   b. Wilson syndrome—it is characterized by:
   c. Café au lait spot:
      - Mental retardation
      - Pulmonary stenosis
   d. Williams syndrome—it is characterized by:
      - Pulmonary stenosis
      - Supravalvular aortic stenosis
8. Due to pulmonary stenosis, right atrial pressure will be increased leading to patent foramen ovale which is usually closed during infancy; as a result deoxygenated blood will be shifted from right to left atrium resulting central cyanosis.
9. Management of this case:
   a. Mild case usually does not require treatment.
   b. Moderate case should be managed medically followed by pulmonary balloon valvoplasty.
   c. Severe case should be managed surgically.

CASE 52

A 40-year-old man came to OPD with fatigue and pain in the left hand during heavy work loading. On examination, there was low volume pulse in the radial pulse of left hand and femoral arteries of lower limb. Left hand was also cold as compared to right hand. There was also radioradial and radiofemoral delay. Blood pressure of the left arm and both lower limb was also decreased.

1. **What is your diagnosis?**
2. **What are the common causes of this disease?**
3. **If the left sided radial pulse will be absent, what are the causes?**
4. **What are the causes of differential pulse and blood pressure in both upper and lower limb?**
5. **What are the causes of radiofemoral delay?**
6. **What is Adson's test? How can you test it?**
7. **What is reverse Adson's test?**
8. **What is Allen test and how can you demonstrate it?**

Answers

1. It is case of coarctation of aorta, site of coarctation being preductal area.

2. Common causes are:
   a. Preductal coarctation of aorta
   b. Aortoarteritis

3. If the pulse of left radial artery will be absent, the causes are:
   a. Aberrant radial artery
   b. Surgical cut down of the left radial artery
   c. Stenosis of left subclavian artery
   d. Catheterization of left brachial artery
   e. Cervical rib
   f. Takayasu arteritis
   g. Blalock–Taussig shunt surgery
   h. Embolization of left radial artery

4. Causes of differential pulses between both radial and femoral pulses:
   a. Aortic stenosis leading to low volume pulses in all the four limbs
   b. Preductal coarctation leading differential pulses in-between the upper limbs and between upper and lower limbs
   c. Postductal coarctation of aorta between the upper and lower limbs
   d. Dissecting aneurysm of aorta
   e. Thoracic outlet syndrome
   f. Cervical rib
   g. Occlusion of artery supplying the lower limbs

5. Causes of radiofemoral delay:
   a. Postductal coarctation of aorta
   b. Aortoarteritis

6. Adson's test is characterized by absent of radial pulse due to compression of the axillary artery by scalene anterior muscle.
   a. Radial artery should be palpated.
   b. Arm has to be abducted slightly.
   c. The patient is asked to hyperextend the neck followed by turning the face to the affected side and inhaling slowly.
   d. Effect:
      • Paresthesia of the affected hand
      • Absent or weak pulse on the affected side

7. Reverse Adson's test: It is just opposite to the Adson's test and it can be done by turning the patient's head to the affected side.

8. Allen's test is used to determine the patency of ulnar and radial artery and it should be done prior to cannulation of radial artery. The procedures are the following:
   a. While the patient raising the hand and making fist, radial and ulnar will be occluded.
   b. Effect: There is blanching of the finger when the patient is asked to extend the finger.
   c. But after release of the compression on the radial artery, color of the fingers will return to normal. If the pulse will not return to normal even after 10 seconds, then it may be suspected as a case of thrombotic occlusion of the artery.

CASE 53

A 35-year-old diabetic male occasional drinker has been admitted with history progressively increasing respiratory distress, orthopnea, and productive cough following fever for 3 days. On examination, patient is cyanotic, features of congestive cardiac failure such as raised jugular venous pressure, tender hepatomegaly, and pedal edema. Cardiological examination demonstrated displacement of apex beat downward and outward, presence of parasternal heave, pulsation in the epigastrium indicating the right ventricular hypertrophy, pansystolic murmur in the lower right parasternal area as well as apical area, and end-expiratory basal crepitation in the both lung bases. Chest X-ray demonstrated:

1. **What the chest X-ray has been demonstrated?**
2. **What is the most likely diagnosis?**
3. **What are the points in favor this diagnosis?**
4. **Is it a case of mitral regurgitation of rheumatic etiology?**
5. **What are the causes of this disease?**
6. **Why it is not due to alcohol intake?**
7. **What are the cardiac biomarkers testing in this case?**
8. **What are the factors determining the prognosis in this disease?**

Answers

1. Chest X-ray demonstrated enlarged cardiothoracic ratio indication dilated cardiomyopathy.
2. The most likely diagnosis is dilated cardiomyopathy leading to congestive cardiac failure.
3. Following are the points in favor of the diagnosis:
   a. Patient is middle aged.
   b. Features of congestive cardiac failure
   c. Displacement of apex downward and outward.
   d. Features of mitral and tricuspid regurgitation which usually occur in dilated cardiomyopathy.
4. This is not a case of rheumatic mitral regurgitation because, there is absence of features of pulmonary hypertension like loud pulmonary second sound, and ejection systolic murmur or Graham Steell murmur.
5. The causes of this disease are:
   a. Idiopathic
   b. Alcohol
   c. Ischemic cardiomyopathy
   d. Peripartum cardiomyopathy
   e. Viral myocarditis
   f. Diabetic cardiomyopathy
   g. Drug induced:
      - Doxorubicin
      - Cyclophosphamide
      - Cocaine
   h. Friedrich's ataxia

6. It is not alcoholic cardiomyopathy because:
   a. There is no feature of alcoholic stigmata.
   b. There is absence of arrhythmia.
   c. Patient is not heavy drinker.
   d. There are all the features of congestive cardiac failure.
7. Following are the cardiac biomarkers used in this case:
   a. BNP
   b. NT-proBNP
   c. Troponin I
   d. Troponin I
   e. Cystatin C
   f. Galectin-3
   g. Soluble ST2
8. Following factors determine the prognosis of this disease:
   a. Ejection fraction
   b. Dimension of left ventricle
   c. Left ventricular mass: Eccentric hypertrophy can be defined as mass of left ventricle of >95 g/m^2 in case of female and >115 g/m^2 in case of male along with regional wall thickness of ≤0.42.
   d. Myocardial performance index of >0.77 indicates high morbidity and mortality.
   e. Diastolic dysfunction measurement

CASE 54

A 60-year-old patient having history of chronic kidney disease on maintenance hemodialysis has come to emergency department with history of central chest pain increased on lying down position and relieved on sitting position and stopping forward, no history of trauma, no joint pain, or skin rash. On examination, pulse rate was 112 beats/min and blood pressure 160/95 mm Hg. On auscultation, there is presence of grating sound which was increased after giving pressure with diaphragm of stethoscope and having no relation with respiration or coughing suggestive of pericardial rub.

ECG demonstrated:

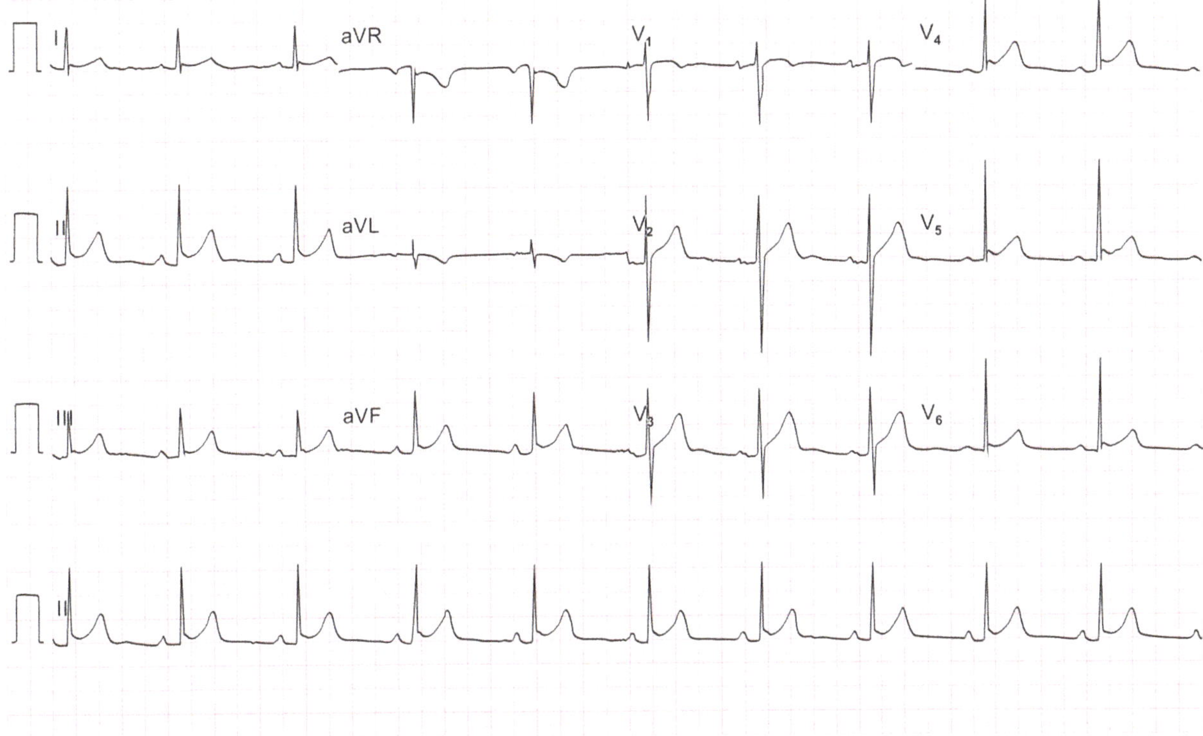

1. **What has been demonstrated in ECG?**
2. **How can you differentiate this ECG from ECG of myocardial infarction?**
3. **What is the most likely diagnosis?**
4. **What are the points in favor of this diagnosis?**
5. **How can you differentiate this pericardial rub from pleuropericardial rub?**
6. **How can you differentiate this pericardial rub from continuous murmur?**
7. **What are the factors for disappearance of this pericardial rub?**
8. **What are the causes of painless pericarditis?**
9. **Mention the causes of recurrent pericarditis.**
10. **What is postpericardiotomy syndrome?**
11. **What is myopericarditis?**

Answers

1. ECG demonstrated elevation of ST segment with concavity upward and depression of the PR segments in lead II, III, and aVF.
2. In ST elevated acute inferior myocardial infarction, ST segments are elevated with convexity upward, but in acute pericarditis elevated ST segments have concavity upward.
3. The most likely diagnosis is acute pericarditis in a case of chronic kidney disease on maintenance hemodialysis.
4. Points in favor of this diagnosis are:
   a. History of central pain aggravated in lying down position and relieved in sitting and stooping forward.
   b. On auscultation, there is evidence of grating sound aggravated on pressure of the diaphragm of stethoscope.
   c. In ECG, ST segment is elevated with concavity upward.
5. In case of pericardial rub, the sound is rubbing or grating in quality, having three components like

presystolic, systolic, and early diastolic components and this sound has no relation with respiration or coughing.

6. Difference between the pericardial rub and continuous murmur:

Pericardial rub	Continuous murmur
Scratching in quality	Machinery in quality
It may be heard in systole or diastole	It is heard in both phase of systole as well as diastole
It is best heard in sitting position with stooping forward	It can be heard in any position
It may disappear for the time being	It should not disappear

7. Following are the causes of disappearance of pericardial rub:
   a. During appearance of massive pericardial effusion
   b. With the development of chronic calcific pericarditis

8. Following are the causes of painless pericarditis:
   a. Drug-induced pericarditis
   b. Diabetes mellitus
   c. Uremia
   d. Amyloidosis

9. Following are the causes of recurrent pericarditis:
   a. Uremia
   b. Tuberculosis
   c. Radiation
   d. Neoplasia
   e. Collagen vascular disorders
   f. Autoimmune disease

10. Postpericardiotomy syndrome is an autoimmune syndrome characterized by symptoms of pericarditis 1–6 months after surgery due to development of autoimmune antibodies against pericardial tissues resulting from surgery, trauma, or irritation by the blood products.

11. Myopericarditis is characterized by features of acute pericarditis along with secondary increase in the myocardial biomarkers in absence of any impairment of left ventricular function.

CASE 55

A 40-year-old man with past history of pulmonary tuberculosis was admitted in emergency department with palpitation for last 2 days, progressive distention of the abdomen, and swelling of feet and right upper abdominal pain for 2 months. On examination, there was tachycardia and bipedal pitting edema; neck vein is demonstrated in the picture below picture. Cardiological examination demonstrated nonpalpable apical impulse. There is presence of a sound along the left sternal border which increased during inspiration. Cardiac sounds are distant and Kussmaul sign is present.

Chest X-ray demonstrated:

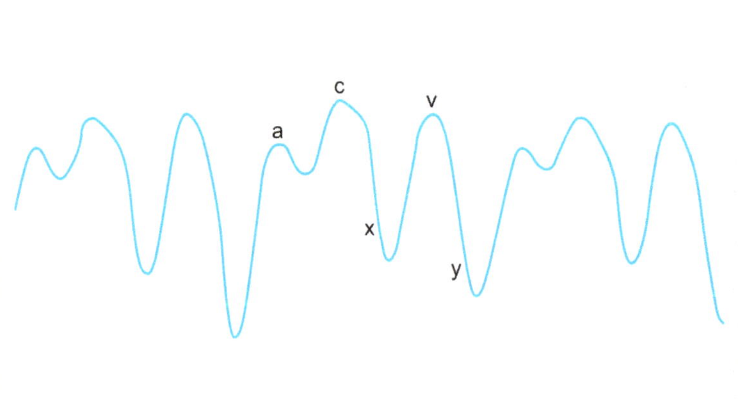

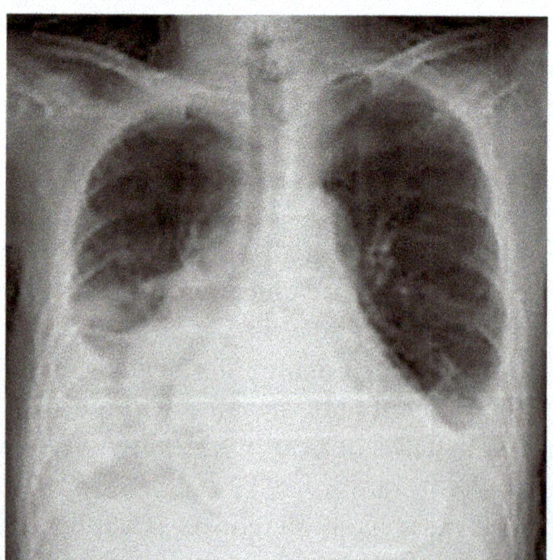

1.   **What do the above pictures demonstrate?**
2.   **What is your diagnosis?**
3.   **Why it is called chronic constrictive pericarditis?**
4.   **How can you differentiate this disease from restrictive cardiomyopathy?**
5.   **What is the sound that is heard at the left sternal border which is increased during inspiration?**
6.   **What is pulsus paradoxus?**
7.   **What are the other early diastolic sounds that are heard during cardiological examination?**
8.   **What are the similarities between the cardiac tamponade and this disease?**
9.   **What are the differences between this disease and cardiac tamponade?**
10. **What are the findings that can be demonstrated in 2D echocardiography?**
11. **What are the findings that can be demonstrated by Doppler echocardiography?**

Answers

1.   Above pictures demonstrate:
     a.   Deep X and Y descent in the right internal jugular vein.
     b.   Chest X-ray demonstrates calcification along the border of pericardium.
2.   The most likely diagnosis is chronic constrictive pericarditis.
3.   This disorder results from obliteration of the pericardial cavity by formation of granulation tissue leading to scar formation encasing heart resulting from healing of:
     a.   Acute fibrinous pericarditis
     b.   Acute serofibrinous pericarditis
     c.   Chronic pericardial effusion
4.   Differentiation between chronic constrictive pericarditis and restrictive cardiomyopathy:

Features	Constrictive pericarditis	Restrictive cardiomyopathy
Pulsus paradoxus	Absent	Present
Deep Y descent	Present	Absent
Kussmaul sign	Present	Absent
Third heart sound	Absent	Rare
Pericardial knock	Present	Absent

5.   The sound that is heard in the left sternal border is pericardial knock.
6.   Pulsus is characterized by the inspiratory decline in the systolic arterial pressure > 10 mm Hg and this can be measured by subtracting the systolic pressure heard during expiration only from the sound of systolic pressure heard during throughout the respiratory cycle provided either tachypnea or tachycardia should be absent.

7.   Differential diagnosis of early diastolic sound:
     a.   Pericardial knock
     b.   Early diastolic murmur
     c.   Opening snap
     d.   Tumor plop
     e.   S3 gallop
8.   Following are the similarities between the constrictive pericarditis and cardiac tamponade:
     a.   Greatly enhanced ventricular interdependence where hemodynamics of right and left heart chambers are influenced by each other
     b.   Diastolic dysfunction
     c.   Preserved ventricular ejection fraction
     d.   Respiratory variation of ventricular inflow as well as outflow is increased.
     e.   Equal elevation of:
          •   Central venous pressure
          •   Pulmonary venous pressure
          •   Ventricular diastolic pressure
     f.   Mild pulmonary hypertension
9.   Following are the dissimilarities between the constrictive pericarditis and cardiac tamponade:
     a.   In case tamponade pericardial cavity is open, so it can transmit the respiratory variation in the thoracic pressure to the heart. But in case of constrictive pericarditis, the pericardial cavity is obliterated, so it cannot transmit the respiratory variation in the thoracic pressure to the heart.
     b.   In cardiac tamponade, inspiratory increase in systemic venous return enlarges the right side of the heart and encroaches to the left side of the heart. In case of chronic constrictive pericarditis, there is no inspiratory increase in the venous return, so right side of the heart will not increase.
     c.   In cardiac tamponade, there is impairment of early ventricular filling but in constrictive pericarditis early ventricular filling will be enhanced.

10. Following features are demonstrated in 2D echocardiography:
    a. Increased thickness of the pericardium
    b. Abrupt posterior motion of the ventricular septum in early diastole during inspiration
    c. Plethora of the inferior vena cava and hepatic veins
    d. Enlarged atria
    e. Abnormal contour between posterior left ventricular walls and left atrial posterior wall

11. Following features are demonstrated in Doppler echocardiography:
    a. High E velocity of left and right ventricular inflow and rapid deceleration
    b. Normal or increased tissue Doppler E'
    c. 25–40% fall in the transmitral flow
    d. Highly increased blood through the tricuspid valve in first beat after inspiration

CASE 56

A 45-year-old man was admitted with fever, respiratory distress, dry cough, and hoarseness of voice. On examination, pulse rate was 100 beats/min, pulsus paradoxus, blood pressure 100/70 mm Hg, jugular venous pressure as demonstrated below, pedal edema, and tender hepatomegaly. Cardiovascular examination demonstrated nonpalpable apical impulse, increased area of cardiac dullness in percussion, and there was bronchial breathing in the interscapular area and heart sounds were muffled. Chest X-ray demonstrated the following:

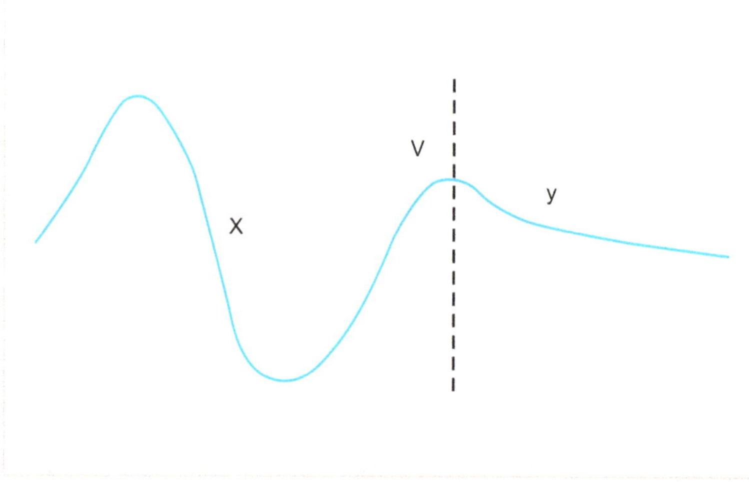

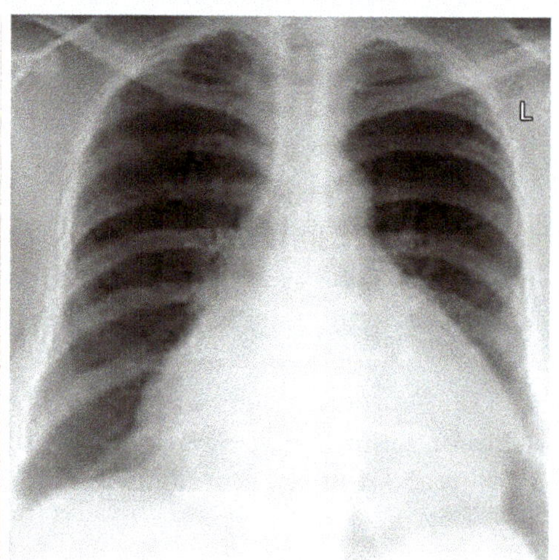

1. What are demonstrated in the above pictures?
2. What is the most likely diagnosis?
3. What are the points in favor of this diagnosis?
4. What are the two specific signs found in this case?
5. How can you differentiate this disease from dilated cardiomyopathy?
6. What are the features in ECG in this case?
7. How can you classify pericardial effusion?
8. What feature can be seen in the transthoracic echocardiography?
9. How features of effusion can be characterized by cardiac CT?
10. When pericardial effusion will turn into pericardial tamponade?
11. Is there any role of echocardiography in case of pericardial tamponade?

Answers

1. The above picture demonstrates:
   a. Deep X descent and loss of Y descent because decrease in intrapericardial pressure during ventricular ejection but systolic atrial filling is maintained
   b. Chest X-ray demonstrated the water bottle configuration of the heart
2. The most likely diagnosis is pericardial effusion.
3. Following points are in favor of this diagnosis in this case:
   a. Presence of fever
   b. Evidences of congestive cardiac failure
   c. Low volume pulse
   d. Pulsus paradoxus
   e. Absence of pericardial rub
   f. Nonpalpable apical impulse
   g. Distant or muffled heart sound
   h. Presence of bronchial breath sound in the interscapular region
4. Following are the two signs:
   a. Rotch's sign: It is characterized by presence of dullness on the right side of the sternum in the fifth intercostal space.
   b. Edward's sign: It is characterized by dullness in the interscapular region and presence of bronchial breath sound. It is due to compression of the base of the lung.
5. Differences between the dilated cardiomyopathy and pericardial effusion:

Features	Pericardial effusion	Dilated cardio-myopathy
Pulse	• Pulsus paradoxus • Narrow pulse pressure	• Absent pulsus paradoxus • Low volume pulse
Jugular venous pressure	Raised with deep X descent	• Raised • Y collapse
Early diastolic sound	Pericardial knock	Third heart sound
Heart sounds	Absent or muffled	Feeble
Apical impulse	Not palpable	Palpable and heaving in character
Murmur	Absent	May be present
Lung on auscultation	Normal	Basal crepitations present

6. ECG demonstrated the following features:
   a. In case of small effusion, nonspecific ST changes
   b. In case of large effusion, presence of electrical alternans which is characterized by QRS of varying heights which corresponds to back-and-forth motions of the heart in the pericardial cavity.
   c. If the pericardial effusion is due to acute pericarditis—depressions of PR segments or diffuse elevation of ST segments.
7. Classifications of pericardial effusion:
   a. According to onset:
      • Acute onset: <3 months
      • Chronic onset: >3 months
   b. Size of effusion:
      • Mild: 50–100 mL having echofree space of <10 mm
      • Moderate: 100–500 mL having echofree space of 10–20 mm
      • Large: >500 mL having echofree space of >20 mm
   c. Location of effusion:
      • Loculated effusion
      • Circumferential effusion
   d. Composition of effusion:
      • Transudate
      • Exudate
      • Hemopericardium
      • Pyopericardium
   e. According to hemodynamic impact:
      • None
      • Effusive-constrictive
      • Tamponade
8. Following features can be evidenced by transthoracic echocardiography:
   a. Persistence of echofree space in the intra-pericardial area throughout the cardiac cycle—it is associated with effusion of >50 mL of fluid.
   b. Presence of small fluid posteriorly distal to AV ring having echofree space of <10 mm
   c. Moderate effusion associated with echofree space of 10–20 mm
   d. Large effusion having echofree space of >20 mm.
   e. To differentiate anterior epicardial fat from anterior small effusion based on:
      • Higher echo density as compared to myocardium
      • Movement in synchrony with the heart
9. Cardiac CT can characterize the pericardial fluid based on the attenuation:
   a. Simple transudative effusion: <10 HU
   b. Purulent, malignant, or myxedematous effusion: 20–60 HU
   c. Hemopericardium or chylopericardium: 60 HU

10. Cardiac tamponade is characterized by equal elevation of both atrial and the pericardial pressure and this can be diagnosed during:
    a. Severity of the pericardial effusion
    b. Time course of the development of the pericardial effusion
11. Echocardiographic features in case of cardiac tamponade are the following:
    a. Hemodynamic compromise resulting from reversal of right atrial as well as right ventricular diastolic transmural pressure
    b. Respiratory variation in the tricuspid and mitral flow velocities will be greatly increased and will be out of phase.
    c. Reduction of the diameter of the already dilated inferior vena cava during inspiration indicating markedly elevated central venous pressure
    d. Abnormal right-sided flow of venous blood, i.e., systolic predominance and expiratory diastolic reversal.

CASE 57

A 45-year-old man presented in the emergency department with fever, arthralgia, dry cough, backache and palpitation for 3 days, and respiratory distress for 1 day. On examination, patient had raised temperature, raised pulsatile jugular venous pressure, tachycardia, and tender hepatomegaly. On cardiological examination, apical impulse was feeble; On auscultation, there was feeble heart sound and presence of pansystolic murmur in the apical area. On auscultation of chest, there was basal crepitation on both sides.

1. **What is your diagnosis?**
2. **What are the points in favor of your diagnosis?**
3. **What are the causes of this disease?**
4. **What are the effects of demography on myocarditis?**
5. **What are the clinical spectrums of pathophysiology in this disease?**
6. **What are the blood tests for detecting this diagnosis specifically?**
7. **Is there any role of endomyocardial biopsy in this disease?**
8. **What are the limitations of endomyocardial biopsy?**
9. **What are the procedures increase the sensitivity of biopsy?**

Answers

1. The most probable diagnosis is myocarditis probably of viral etiology.
2. Points in favor of this diagnosis are:
    a. Fever
    b. Constitutional symptoms such as backache and arthralgia
    c. Sore throat
    d. Features of congestive cardiac failure
    e. Feeble cardiac sounds
    f. Pansystolic murmur may be of papillary muscle dysfunction.
    g. Bilateral basal crepitations
3. Causes of myocarditis are:
    a. Viral:
        - Coxsackie B
        - Cytomegalovirus
        - Epstein–Barr virus
        - Hepatitis virus
        - Influenza virus
        - Human immunodeficiency virus (HIV)
    b. Rickettsial causes:
        - Q fever
        - Spotted fever
        - Typhus fever
    c. Bacterial myocarditis:
        - Diphtheria
        - Meningococci
        - *Salmonella*
        - *Mycoplasma*
    d. Protozoal causes:
        - Trypanosomiasis
        - Malaria
        - *Toxoplasma*
    e. Fungal causes:
        - *Aspergillus*
        - *Candida*
        - *Histoplasma*

  f. Hypersensitivity:
- Antibiotics—penicillin, chloramphenicol, and tetracycline
- Antiepileptic
- Sulphonylurea
- Amphotericin

  g. Toxic:
- Cocaine
- Catecholamine

  h. Irradiation

  i. Poison: Snake bites

4. Effects of demography on myocarditis are:
  a. Incidence and the severity of myocarditis are higher in males.
  b. Testosterone exacerbates myocarditis
  c. There are two peaks of myocarditis:
- One in the first year of life
- Second one between the age of puberty and at the age of 40 years

  d. Death rate is higher in the first year of life.
  e. After the age of 15 years, the number due to death is higher in males as compared to females.

5. Acute viral myocarditis progresses to the stage of chronic dilated cardiomyopathy through the three phases:
  a. Phase 1 or acute viral injury: Following viral infection, there is proliferation of the myocardium leading direct injury of cardiac tissue signaling innate immunity system.
  b. Phase 2 or activation of innate immunity leading to formation of adaptive immune response which is characterized by:
- Upregulation of inflammatory mediators
- Antigen specific T and B cell responses

  c. Phase 3 or remodeling to dilated cardiomyopathy:
- Initial injury leading to fibrosis with or without chronic inflammation

- Persisting viral antigen triggers the remodeling of the ventricular wall in the susceptible individuals.

6. Following blood tests should be done to detect the etiology:
  a. Inflammatory markers which are elevated in this disease:
- CRP
- ESR

  b. Cardiac biomarkers which are elevated in this disease:
- CPK-MB—if it is >29.5 ng/mL, indicates higher mortality.
- Troponin I

7. Endomyocardial biopsy is highly specific but less sensitive.
  a. Focal involvement indicates:
- Lymphocytic myocarditis
- Sarcoidosis

  b. Immunostatins for detecting specific cell types increase the incidence of positivity.
  c. Electrocardiography may act as guide in case of suspected:
- Arrhythmogenic right ventricular cardio-myopathy
- Sarcoidosis

8. Two main limitations of endomyocardial biopsy are:
  a. Limited availability of this procedure
  b. Low sensitivity

9. Following procedures increase the sensitivity of the endomyocardial biopsy:
  a. Prior cardiac imaging to localize the site of abnormality
  b. Intracardiac electrogram can identify the site of inflammation or fibrosis.

CASE 58

A 46-year-old diabetic male has been admitted with fever, productive cough for 5 days, respiratory distress, and pain in the right upper abdomen for 2 days. On examination, patient is orthopneic, engorged pulsatile neck vein, tachycardia, central cyanosis, pedal edema, and tender hepatomegaly. Cardiovascular system demonstrated apical impulse was down and out, presence of left parasternal heave, low pitch heart sound and low-pitched systolic murmur the mitral area, and bilateral basal crepitations.

Chest X-ray demonstrated:

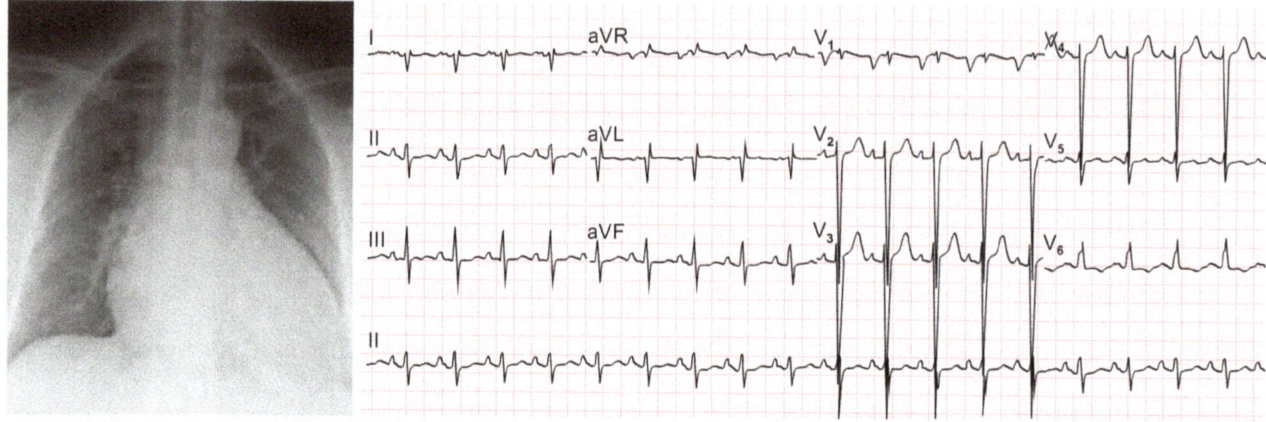

1. **What do the above pictures demonstrate?**
2. **What is the most likely diagnosis?**
3. **What are the points in favor of your diagnosis?**
4. **Mention the pathophysiology of this disease.**
5. **What are the advantages and disadvantages of cardiac MRI in diagnosing this disease?**
6. **What are the indications of endomyocardial biopsy in this case?**
7. **What is prognostic significance of cardiac biomarkers in dilated cardiomyopathy with left ventricular dysfunction?**

Answers

1. Chest X-ray demonstrates:
    a. Cardiomegaly
    b. Pulmonary venous congestion
    c. Interstitial edema
2. Most likely diagnosis is dilated cardiomyopathy following viral infection associated congestive cardiac failure.
3. Following are the points in favor of this diagnosis:
    a. Middle-aged male
    b. Progressively increasing dyspnea
    c. Features of congestive cardiac failure
    d. Shifting of apical impulse down and out
    e. Presence of parasternal heave
    f. Absence of pulmonary hypertension
    g. Low-pitched pansystolic murmur indicative of mitral regurgitation
    h. Cardiomegaly and pulmonary congestion
    i. Bilateral crepitations
4. Pathophysiology of disease is dilated cardiomyopathy: Initial neurohumoral response will activate the sympathetic nervous system and renin–angiotensin–aldosterone system for maintaining the systemic perfusion through renal vasoconstriction and sodium and water conservation respectively. But prolonged activation of the system leads to:
    a. Adverse cardiac remodeling
    b. Increased cardiac fibrosis
    c. Inexorable progression of the disease
5. Advantages of cardiac MRI in diagnosis of dilated cardiomyopathy are:
    a. It will assess the left ventricular ejection fraction and left ventricular volume.
    b. It will avoid foreshortening of the images.
    c. It is responsible for superior assessment of the right ventricular function.
    d. It can detect:
        • Cardiac fibrosis
        • Cardiac scars
        • Cardiac infiltration
    e. It can assess the myocardial viability in ischemic cardiomyopathy.
    f. There is no radiation.
    g. Its diagnostic value is superior to endomyocardial biopsy for infiltrative diseases.

Disadvantages of cardiac MRI in the diagnosis of dilated cardiomyopathy are:
    a. It is not widely available.
    b. It is expensive.

c. It is time consuming.

d. In case of pacemaker, special precaution should be taken.

e. In case of effective GFR of <30 mL, there is chance of fibrosis of kidney tissue if gadolinium is used.

6. There are two indications of endomyocardial biopsy in this case:

a. If patients present with acute heart failure of <2 weeks with evidence of hemodynamic compromise.

b. In case of new heart failure between 2 weeks and 3 months duration with evidence of dilated cardiomyopathy who have:
   - New ventricular arrhythmias or
   - High-degree AV block and/or
   - Failure to respond to specific medical care

7. Prognostic significance of cardiac biomarkers in dilated cardiomyopathy: The cardiac biomarkers are BNP and proBNP generated and secreted by the cardiac myocytes during excessive stretching of the myocardium.

a. These will diagnose as well as guide the prognosis of this disease.

b. In case of heart failure, its elevated level is associated with worse prognosis and decreased level is associated with improved outcome.

c. Increased level of BNP is found in:
   - Renal failure
   - Age
   - Sepsis
   - Atrial fibrillation

d. Decreased level of BNP is associated with obesity.

CASE 59

A 36-year-old diabetic female in the 32 weeks of gestation has been admitted with productive cough for 5 days, respiratory distress, and pain in the right upper abdomen for 2 days. On examination, patient is orthopneic, engorged pulsatile neck vein, tachycardia, pedal edema, and tender hepatomegaly. Cardiovascular system demonstrated apical impulse was down and out, presence of parasternal heave, low pitch heart sound and low-pitched systolic murmur in mitral area, and bilateral basal crepitations. She has 32 weeks gravid uterus.

Chest X-ray demonstrated:

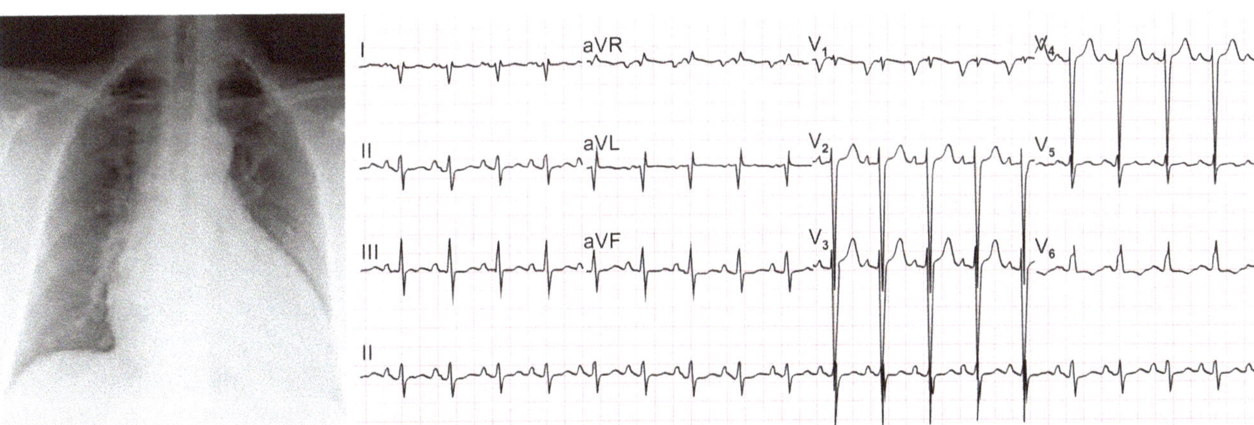

1. **What do the above pictures demonstrate?**
2. **What is the most likely diagnosis?**
3. **What are the points in favor of your diagnosis?**
4. **Mention the pathophysiology of this disease.**
5. **What are the characteristics of this disease?**
6. **What are the risk factors for this disease?**
7. **What are the drugs contraindicated in this disease prior to delivery and in postpartum period what is contraindicated?**
8. **What is the chance of occurrence during next pregnancy?**
9. **What is the rate of recovery in this case?**

10. **What are the drugs contraindicated during lactation period?**
11. **What are the drugs safe to be administered during pregnancy?**
12. **What are the good prognostic factors in this disease?**
13. **What are the bad prognostic factors in this disease?**
14. **What are the possible complications in this disease?**

Answers

1. Chest X-ray demonstrated:
   a. Cardiomegaly
   b. Pulmonary venous congestion
   c. Interstitial edema
2. Most likely diagnosis is dilated cardiomyopathy during third trimester of pregnancy leading to congestive cardiac failure.
3. Following are the points in favor of this diagnosis:
   a. Middle-aged male
   b. Progressively increasing dyspnea
   c. Features of congestive cardiac failure
   d. Shifting of apical impulse down and out
   e. Presence of parasternal heave
   f. Absence of pulmonary hypertension
   g. Low-pitched pansystolic murmur indicative of mitral regurgitation
   h. Cardiomegaly and pulmonary congestion
   i. Bilateral crepitations
4. Pathophysiology of this disease is peripartum cardiomyopathy:
   a. During pregnancy, there is increase in the red blood cells as well as blood volume leading to increase in the cardiac output by 20–30% and stroke volume by 15–25% in the first and second trimester but patient will not be symptomatic in absence of heart disease. But if these symptoms occur during peripartum, it will lead to great hemodynamic stress.
   b. It may be due to viral myocarditis as there may be viral genome in the biopsy of the patients in case of peripartum cardiomyopathy.
   c. It may occur due to hormonal changes:
      • Toxic hormonal environment that will be generated during pregnancy.
      • Genetic factor associated with the hormonal changes leads to development of peripartum cardiomyopathy.
      • Prolactin will be increased in the late pregnancy and puerperium stage. An enzyme in the myocardium protects the heart from the reactive oxygen species which if increased secretes peptidase, cathepsin D, and it will cleave the prolactin into N-terminal prolactin fragment leading to promotion of apoptosis of endothelial cells and cardiomyocyte.
      • Proinflammatory state may be responsible for cardiomyopathy due to increased level of cytokines such as tumor necrosis factor-α (TNF-α) and interleukin-6.
      • Autoimmunity may be a cause of this disease.
5. Following are the characteristics of peripartum cardiomyopathy:
   a. Development of congestive cardiac failure during third trimester of pregnancy or 6 months after delivery.
   b. Other causes of the heart failure will be absent.
   c. Systolic dysfunction of the left ventricle leading to left ventricular ejection fraction of <45%.
   d. Left ventricle may or may not be dilated.
6. Following are the risk factors of peripartum cardiomyopathy:
   a. African American race
   b. Pregnancy-related hypertension
   c. Preeclampsia
   d. Multigestational pregnancy
   e. Older maternal age
   f. Multiparity
   g. Obesity
   h. Chronic hypertension
   i. Prolonged use of tocolytics
7. Following two drugs are contraindicated during pregnancy because of their well-known teratogenic effect:
   a. Angiotensin-converting enzyme inhibitor
   b. Angiotensin receptor blockers
   c. β-blockers
   d. Nitroprusside
8. Patients with peripartum cardiomyopathy will recover from this disease and improve the left ventricular ejection fraction, in the subsequent pregnancy patient may again develop this disease; hence the patient should be counseled accordingly. But if the left ventricular ejection fraction cannot improve, in that case subsequent pregnancy should be discouraged.

9. This disease can recover within 3–6 months as compared to other forms of heart failure but in case of African American patients rate of recovery will be slower.
10. Following drugs are contraindicated during pregnancy:
    a. Angiotensin-converting enzyme inhibitor
    b. Angiotensin receptor blockers
    c. β-blockers
11. Following drugs are safe during pregnancy:
    a. Carvedilol
    b. Digoxin
    c. Hydralazine
    d. Minoxidil
    e. Hydrochlorothiazide
    f. Thiazides
12. Following are the good prognostic factors in the peripartum cardiomyopathy:
    a. Diastolic dimension of the left ventricle is <5.5 cm.
    b. At the time of diagnosis, left ventricular ejection fraction is 30–35%.
    c. At the time of diagnosis, fractioning of shortening is >20%.
    d. Absence of elevation of troponin
    e. Absence of thrombus in the left ventricle
    f. Ethnicity is non-African American.
13. Following are the poor prognostic factors in this disease:
    a. Duration of QRS is >120 ms.
    b. Delayed diagnosis
    c. High NYHA class
    d. African descent
    e. Multiparity
14. Following are the complications in this disease:
    a. Maternal complications:
       • Arrhythmias
       • Thromboembolism
       • Progressive heart failure
       • Misdiagnosed as preeclampsia
    b. Fetal complications: Hypoxia resulting from fetal distress

CASE 60

A 47-year-old nondiabetic, normotensive nonsmoker male was admitted with sudden respiratory difficulty and chest pain. Patient had past history of open cholecystectomy. On examination, there was tachycardia, tachypnea, and chest examination was normal. ECG demonstrated elevated ST segment in the anterior wall and cardiac enzymes were elevated. Urgent coronary angiography was normal. Echocardiography demonstrated basal hyperkinesias of the left ventricular mid-segments. But after 3 days, patient was completely normal, ECG demonstrated no abnormal wave, and echocardiograph became normal.

1. **What is your diagnosis?**
2. **What are the criteria for this diagnosis?**
3. **What is the pathophysiology behind this disease?**
4. **What are the theories regarding this disease?**
5. **What are the risk factors for this disease?**
6. **What are the complications in this disease?**
7. **What is the prognosis in this disease?**

Answers

1. The diagnosis is Takotsubo's cardiomyopathy.
2. The criteria for this diagnosis are:
   a. Transient dyskinesia, akinesia, or hyperkinesias of the left ventricular mid-segments with or without apical involvement. Abnormalities of regional wall-motion extend beyond the single epicardial vascular distribution; stressful trigger may or may not be present.
   b. Absence of obstructive coronary artery disease or angiographic evidence of acute rupture of plaque.
   c. New abnormalities in ECG (either elevation of ST segment and/or inversion of T wave) or modest rise in cardiac troponin level.
   d. Absence of pheochromocytoma or myocarditis
3. Pathophysiology in this disease: Normal myocardium utilizes the 90% of its energy from aerobic oxidation of fatty acids. But in case of ischemia, there is suppression of this pathway with shifting toward glucose pathway leading impaired cardiac function. Most important factor is stress-related release of catecholamine with toxicity followed by subsequent myocardial stunning.

4. There are many theories have been proposed against this disease:
    a. Multivessel coronary artery spasm
    b. Impaired metabolism of myocardial fatty acids
    c. Impaired cardiac microvascular function
    d. Underlying dysfunction of coronary endothelium
    e. Acute coronary syndrome with reperfusion injury
    f. Endogenous catecholamine-induced stunning of myocardium as well as microinfarction.
5. Risk factors for this disease:
    a. Bad financial news
    b. Legal problems
    c. Surgery
    d. Stay in the intensive care unit
    e. Collision with motor vehicles
    f. Natural disasters
    g. Newly diagnosed significant medical problems
    h. Learning of a death of a loved one
    i. Seizures
6. Following are the complications developed in 20% patients with this disease:
    a. Cardiogenic shock
    b. Mitral regurgitation
    c. Left ventricular outflow tract obstruction
    d. Failure of the left side of the heart with or without pulmonary edema
    e. Rupture of the left ventricular free wall
    f. Ventricular arrhythmias
    g. Mural thrombus formation within the left ventricle
    h. Death
7. Prognosis in this disease:
    a. Left ventricular ejection fraction will be recovered within 1–2 weeks, maximum within 6 weeks.
    b. 20% patient recurs within 10 years.

CASE 61

A 60-year-old diabetic hypertensive woman attended the cardiology clinic with chest pain and respiratory distress. Patient had history of breast cancer for which she was irradiated and is now under daunorubicin. ECG demonstrated low voltage complexes.

1. **What is the most likely diagnosis?**
2. **What are the risk factors for this disease?**
3. **What are the mechanisms involved in this case?**
4. **What are the relations of this disease with anthracycline?**

Answers

1. The most likely diagnosis is anthracycline-induced cardiomyopathy.
2. Following are the risk factors in this disease:
    a. Genetic predisposition
    b. Female sex
    c. Black ethnicity
    d. Below the age of 4 years or at old age
    e. Preexisting cardiac disease
    f. Nutritional deficiencies
    g. Total cumulative dose
    h. Diabetes
    i. Dyslipidemia
    j. Physical inactivity
    k. Smoking
    l. Hypertension
    m. Concomitant radiotherapy
    n. Abnormal cardiac imaging or abnormal cardiac biomarkers
3. Following are the mechanisms of anthracycline-induced cardiac disease:
    a. Iron complexes formation followed by reaction with O_2 to form O_2^- which in turn dismutates to hydrogen peroxide.
    b. Increased production of reactive oxygen species or reactive nitrogen species
    c. Lipid peroxidation
    d. Induced apoptosis of cardiomyocyte
    e. Inflammation
    f. Interstitial fibrosis
    g. Abnormal signaling of the epidermal growth factor and β-arrestin
    h. Inhibition of nuclear topoisomerase IIβ
4. Relation of cardiomyopathy with anthracycline:
    a. Early during the commencement of the therapy
    b. 10–20 years after commencement of therapy
    c. This disease is partly dose-dependent.

CASE 62

A 34-year-old male came with recurrent syncope, palpitation, and exertional respiratory distress for 2 months. There was family history of sudden death of his brother 10 years ago.

On examination, there was bifid pulse, neck vein demonstrated prominent "a" wave, and blood pressure 150/60 mm Hg.

Cardiovascular examination demonstrated double apical impulse, and left parasternal heave. On auscultation, presence of pansystolic murmur in the mitral area, presence of fourth heart sound, and presence of ejection systolic murmur along the left sternal border accentuated by standing and Valsalva maneuver.

1. **What is your diagnosis?**
2. **What are the histological characteristics in this disease?**
3. **What are the clinical strategies in the detection of this disease?**
4. **What are the common types of this disease?**
5. **What are the characteristics in the pulse in this disease?**
6. **What is the mechanism of systolic anterior motion of the mitral leaflet?**
7. **What is the mechanism of left ventricular outflow tract obstruction in this disease?**
8. **What are the factors for the sudden death in this disease?**
9. **Which medications are contraindicated in this disease?**
10. **What is Brockenbrough–Braunwald sign?**
11. **Mention the nonpharmacological treatment in this case.**

Answers

1. This patient has been suffering from hypertrophic obstructive cardiomyopathy.
2. Histological characteristics in this disease are:
   a. Hypertrophy of cardiac myocytes
   b. Disarray of the myocardial fibers located in the middle layers of myocardium
   c. Increase in the amount of collagen fibers in the interstitial area
   d. Disorganized arrangement of the components of matrix
3. Clinical screening strategies in the diagnosis of this disease are:
   a. Less than 12 years old: Optional unless—
      • Family history of sudden death due to this disease
      • Competitive athlete in the intense training program
      • Clinical suspicion in case of early left ventricular hypertrophy
   b. 12–18 years old: Every 1 year to 1.5 years
   c. More than 18 years old: Every 5 years or more frequently in case of late onset of hypertrophic cardiomyopathy or malignant clinical course.
4. There are two phenotypes of hypertrophic cardiomyopathy:
   a. It occurs in two-thirds of cases during any provocation like exercise. Outflow of the left ventricle is impeded mechanically as a result of thickening of the subaortic septum interacting with the mitral valve. It is obstructive cardiomyopathy.
   b. It occurs in one-third of cases and the outflow is unobstructed completely. It is known as unobstructive cardiomyopathy.
5. Characteristics of the pulse in this disease are:
   a. There is initial brisk rise
   b. Midsystolic decline due to left ventricular outflow tract obstruction
   c. Second rise
   But in case of fixed obstruction as in case of aortic stenosis, the rise is slow and amplitude will be diminished.
6. Abnormal anterior displacement of the anterior mitral leaflet toward the interventricular septum in the midsystole due to the following mechanism:
   a. Anterior leaflet of the mitral valve is drawn toward the interventricular septum as a result of Venturi effect produced as a result of lower pressure in the left ventricular outflow tract. It results from the accelerated flow of blood in the narrow outflow tract.
   b. As the flow of blood attacks the mitral valve from behind, anterior mitral valve leaflet will be pushed against the hypertrophied interventricular septum or due to maloriented papillary muscles.

7. Mechanism of left ventricular outflow tract obstruction:
   a. Systolic anterior motion of the anterior mitral leaflet
   b. Midsystolic contact with the hypertrophied ventricular septum:
      Magnitude of the subaortic gradient depends upon the provocative maneuvers as this gradient is dynamic.
   c. Obstruction is also present at the midcavity level between the interventricular septum and thickened papillary muscles.
8. Following are the factors of sudden death:
   a. Ventricular arrhythmia
   b. Prior cardiac arrest or sustained ventricular tachycardia
   c. Family history of sudden cardiac death
   d. Unexplained syncope
   e. Massive thickness of the left ventricular wall of >30 mm
   f. Left ventricular aneurysm
   g. Impaired left ventricular ejection fraction
   h. Hypotensive blood pressure response to exercise
   i. On ambulatory monitoring presence of sustained ventricular tachycardia
   j. High-risk mutant genes
   k. Magnitude of the left ventricular outflow gradient
   l. Diameter of left atrium
9. Following medications are contraindicated in this disease:
   a. Preload reducing agents like diuretics should be used cautiously in case of persistent heart failure or volume overload.
   b. Afterload reducing agent, like:
      • Dihydropyridine calcium-channel blockers
      • Nitroglycerin
      • Angiotensin-converting enzyme inhibitor
      • Angiotensin receptor II blockers
   c. Increased contractility producing medications, like:
      • Digoxin
      • Dobutamine
      • Phosphodiesterase inhibitors, i.e., milrinone
10. Following premature ventricular contraction, in case of subsequent sinus beat ventricular contractility as well as stroke volume will be increased leading to increase in the systolic blood pressure and thus increase in the pulse pressure. But in case of hypertrophic cardiomyopathy after premature ventricular contraction, increased left ventricular contractility will lead to increased left ventricular outflow tract obstruction resulting decreased in the stroke volume leading to decrease in the systolic blood pressure as well as pulse pressure. This paradoxically reduces the stroke volume and aortic pulse pressure despite the increased LV systolic pressure. This is known as Brockenbrough–Braunwald sign.
11. Following nonpharmacological treatments are available in this case:
   a. Septal myectomy or Morrow procedure where small amount of muscles from the septum will be resected through the transaortic approach.
   b. Alcohol septal ablation where 3 mL of alcohol is injected into the perforator branch of the left anterior descending coronary artery to produce a small area of septal infarction.
   c. Dual-chamber pacing for improving the symptoms

CASE 63

A 56-year-old woman having neither any history of uneventful pregnancy nor family history of hypertension came to cardiology OPD with history of headache, exertional respiratory distress, and palpitation for nearly 5 years. On examination, her face was normal, no finger staining, no thyromegaly, pulse rate 112 beats/min, and blood pressure 170/120 mm Hg in sitting position having no gross variation in the lower limbs.

Laboratory investigation demonstrated that renal and liver function tests were normal and hematological tests were also normal.

1. **What is the most probable diagnosis?**
2. **Classify this disease?**
3. **What are the conditions responsible for discrepancy in the blood pressure in upper and lower abdomen?**
4. **What are the indications of ambulatory blood pressure monitoring?**
5. **What is white coat hypertension?**
6. **What is masked hypertension?**

7. **What is hypertensive emergency?**
8. **What is hypertensive urgency?**
9. **What are the investigations to be performed to detect secondary causes?**
10. **What antihypertensive drugs should be prescribed in case hypertension in African American people?**
11. **Which part of blood pressure is powerful predictor of cardiovascular complication?**
12. **What is resistant hypertension?**
13. **What are the risk factors for resistant hypertension?**

Answers

1. Most probable diagnosis is idiopathic systemic hypertension.
2. According to Eighth Joint National Committee (JNC-8) guideline:

Stages	Systolic blood pressure (mm Hg)	Diastolic blood pressure (mm Hg)
Normal	<120	<80
Stage I or pre-hypertension	120–139	80–89
Stage II	140–159	90–99
Stage III	>160	≥100

3. Conditions responsible for discrepancy in the blood pressure in upper and lower abdomen:
   a. Coarctation of aorta
   b. Thoracic inlet syndrome
   c. Patent ductus arteriosus
   d. Dissection aneurysm of aorta
   e. Supravalvular aortic stenosis
   f. Aortoarteritis
   g. Stenosis of the subclavian artery
   h. Thrombotic occlusion of bifurcation of aorta
4. Following are the indications of ambulatory blood pressure monitoring:
   a. Hypertension resistant to three or more drugs
   b. To exclude white coat hypertension
   c. If the blood pressure is unusually variable
   d. If the symptoms of the patient suggestive of hypertension
5. If a normotensive patient develops high blood pressure in the Doctor's clinic but otherwise normal, it is known as white coat hypertension and the patient may require ambulatory blood pressure monitoring.
6. Masked hypertension can be defined as such type of hypertension where office blood pressure is <140/90 mm Hg but the ambulatory or home blood pressure is within the normal range.

7. Hypertension emergency is characterized by a state where severely elevated blood pressure of >200/130 mm Hg is associated with features of different organ dysfunctions like nephropathy, retinopathy, or encephalopathy requiring intravenous therapy under close supervision in the intensive care unit.
8. Hypertension urgency is characterized by a state where severely elevated blood pressure of >200/120 mm Hg is not associated with any organ dysfunction and which blood pressure can be controlled by oral antihypertensive therapies.
9. Following investigations should be done to detect secondary causes of hypertension:
   a. To exclude kidney disease:
      • Blood urea and creatinine
      • Intravenous pyelography and ultrasonography to detect adult polycystic kidney diseases
      • Digital subtraction angiography to detect renal artery stenosis
   b. 24 hours urine catecholamine or vanillylmandelic acid for detecting pheochromocytoma
   c. To detect Cushing's syndrome, urinary cortisol and dexamethasone suppression test
   d. To detect Conn's syndrome, plasma aldosterone level and plasma renin activity
   e. To detect coarctation of aorta, MR angiography or plain angiography
10. In African and American people with hypertension, the drug of choice is thiazides or calcium-channel blockers.
11. Systolic and diastolic blood pressure is independent predictor of cardiovascular complication, but isolated systolic blood hypertension is the more powerful predictor of cardiovascular complication.
12. Resistant hypertension is a state when the blood pressure cannot be controlled despite of taking three different classes of antihypertensive drugs.

13. Following are the risk factors associated with resistant hypertension:
    a. Older age
    b. Obesity
    c. Diabetes mellitus
    d. Excessive ingestion of salts
    e. High baseline blood pressure
    f. Chronic kidney disease
    g. Female
    h. African American ethnicity
    i. Left ventricular hypertrophy
    j. Residents of Southeastern United States

CASE 64

A 36-year-old man came to cardiac clinic with history of recurrent episodes of headache, severe sweating, and palpitations. He had past history of admission four times in the hospital and diagnosed as hypertensive crisis. In the office, his blood pressure was always in the range of 130/70 mm Hg.

Laboratory investigation demonstrated blood sugar 231 mg/dL.

1. **What is the most likely diagnosis?**
2. **Why there is palpitation?**
3. **Which process may trigger the hypertension?**
4. **What do you mean by rule of 10 in this disease?**
5. **How can you diagnose this case?**

Answers

1. The most likely diagnosis is pheochromocytoma.
2. High level of catecholamine in the serum will lead to paroxysms.
3. Gentle palpation of the abdomen may lead to trigger the hypertensive crisis.
4. The rule of 10 in this disease:
    a. 10% of all the cases are familial.
    b. 10% cases are bilateral.
    c. 10% cases are due to malignant adrenal tumor.
    d. 10% cases may recur.
    e. 10% cases are extra-adrenal cases.
    f. 10% cases occur in children.
    g. 10% cases are associated with multiple endocrine neoplasia.
    h. 10% cases present with stroke as initial presentation.
5. By following processes, this case can be diagnosed:
    a. Urine testing for:
       - Metanephrine
       - Fractionated catecholamine

       It can diagnose the presence of catecholamine-secreting tumor.
    b. Next step is the localization of the tumor. In 90% cases, it is found in the adrenal medulla and in 10% cases it is found in the enterochromaffin tissues found throughout the body.

CASE 65

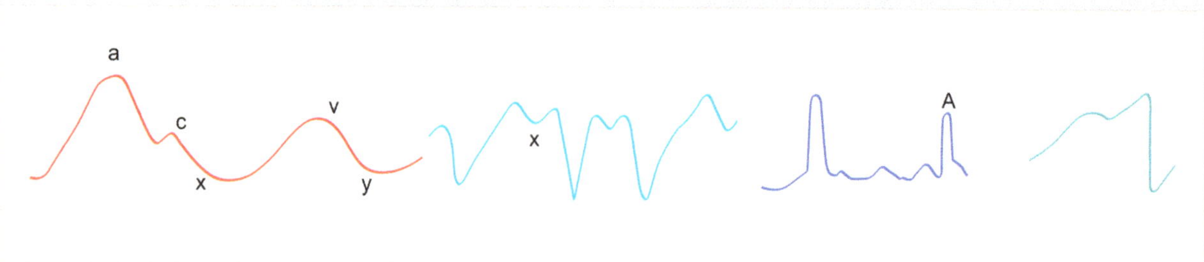

1. **Describe the above pictures. What is the importance of different positive and negative waves in different pictures described above?**
2. **What are the other causes of the third picture described above?**
3. **What are the causes of increased "y" descent?**

Answers

1. Description of the above pictures:
   a. First picture is normal jugular venous waves:
      - "*a*"-positive wave: Forceful right atrial contraction prior to first heart sound.
      - "*c*"-positive wave: It occurs due to bulging of the tricuspid valve into the right atrium due to increased pressure in the right ventricle.
      - "*v*"-positive wave: It increased volume of blood into the right atrium during the phase of ventricular systole when the tricuspid valve is closed.
      - "*x*"-negative wave: It occurs due to relaxation of the atrium.
      - "*y*"-negative: It occurs due to opening of the tricuspid valve leading to rapid inflow of the blood into right ventricle.
   b. Second picture demonstrates absence of "*a*" wave indicating presence of atrial fibrillation.
   c. Third picture demonstrates giant "*a*" wave indicating presence of AV block.
   d. Fourth picture demonstrates "*cv*" wave indicating severe tricuspid regurgitation.
2. Causes of third picture described above:
   a. Causes of prominent "*a*" wave:
      - Pulmonary hypertension
      - Pulmonary stenosis
      - Tricuspid stenosis
   b. Giant "*a*" wave:
      - Complete heart block
      - Junctional tachycardia
      - Ventricular tachycardia
3. Following are the causes of increased "*y*" descent:
   a. Sharp "*y*" descent:
      - Constrictive pericarditis
      - Right-sided heart failure
   b. Slow "*y*" descent:
      - Tricuspid stenosis
      - Right atrial myxoma

CASE 66

A 63-year-old man presented with fatigue, occasional syncope, and exercise intolerance in the OPD.

ECG demonstrated:

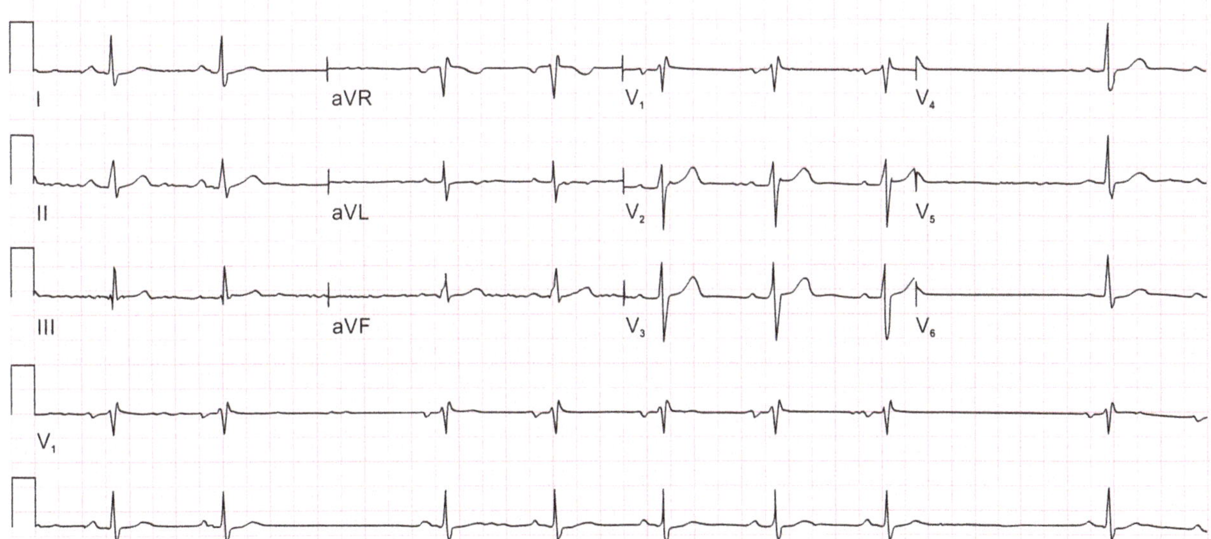

The patient was admitted for management. The ECG showed the following after management:

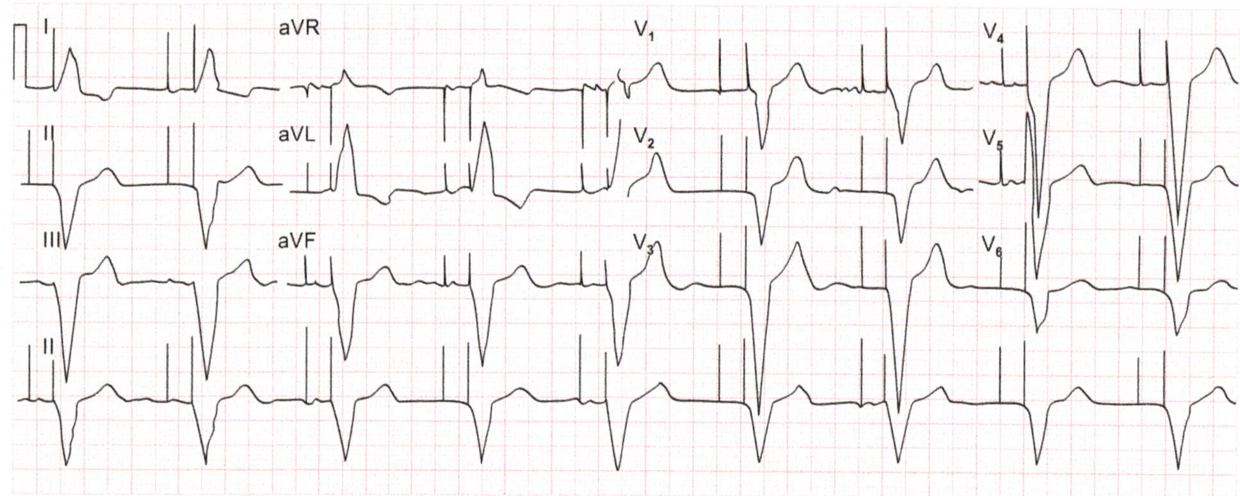

1. **What is the correlation in the above two ECGs?**
2. **Define this disease?**
3. **What are the causes of the disease?**
4. **What are the cells responsible for the function of the sinus node?**
5. **What are the types of blocks in the sinus node?**
6. **What is Tachy-brady syndrome?**
7. **What is chronotropic incompetence?**
8. **What is the treatment in this disease?**

Answers

1. The first picture demonstrated the feature of sick sinus syndrome as evidence of recurrent sinus pause.
2. Sick sinus syndrome is characterized by a spectrum of sinus node abnormalities ranging from the generation of impulse to propagation of impulse as evidenced by sinus pause, sinus bradycardia, paroxysmal sinus arrest, and sinus node exit block of insufficient chronotropic effect.
3. Causes of the disease:
   a. Intrinsic pathology of the sinus node resulting from the nodal tissue fibrosis:
      - Congenital disorders from mutation of ion channels leading to familial or congenital form block.
      - Infiltrative diseases:
        - Sarcoidosis
        - Amyloidosis
        - Hemochromatosis
        - Collagen vascular disease
        - Metastatic cancer
      - Surgery:
        - During correction of congenital heart disease
        - Correction of the valvular disease
   b. Extrinsic causes affecting pacing function of the SA node:
      - Increased vagal tone:
        - Carotid sinus hypersensitivity
        - Vasovagal syncope
        - Autonomic dysfunction
      - Metabolic derangements:
        - Hypothyroidism
        - Hyperkalemia
        - Hypokalemia
        - Hypoxia
        - Hypothermia
        - Hypocalcemia
      - Obstructive sleep apnea leading to profound hypoxia resulting depression of the nodal function.
      - Increased intracranial pressure (Cushing reflex)

- Drugs:
  - Antiarrhythmic drugs
  - Digoxin
  - Lithium
  - Sympatholytic medications
4. There are two types of cells in the sinus node:
   a. Pacemaker "P" cells: These cells are responsible for generation of the impulses in the sinus node.
   b. Transitional "T" cells: These cells are responsible for propagation of the impulse into the right atrium.
5. There are three types of block in the sinus node:
   a. First-degree SA block: It is subclinical and can be detected by only ECG.
   b. Second-degree SA block: It is of two types:
      - Type I block: It is characterized by progressive shortening of PP interval followed by drop of P wave.
      - Type II block: It is characterized by drop of P wave without any preceding changes PP interval.
   c. Third-degree SA block: It is characterized by complete failure of SA node in transmitting the impulses to the right atrium as evidenced by absence of P wave in the ECG.
6. Tachy-brady syndrome is characterized by bradycardia which is alternating with supraventricular tachyarrhythmias mostly atrial fibrillation resulting from abnormal automaticity and abnormal conduction within the atrial tissue.
7. Chronotropic incompetence is characterized by inappropriate bradycardia resulting from inability to meet metabolic demand.
8. The treatment in this case are:
   a. Correction of the reversal factors
   b. Placement of permanent pacemaker.

CASE 67

A 65-year-old man came to cardiology clinic with history of recurrent blackout, the last episode being on the last day, and chest pain for last 2 months following an event of acute inferior wall myocardial infarction. He was urgently advised ECG which demonstrated:

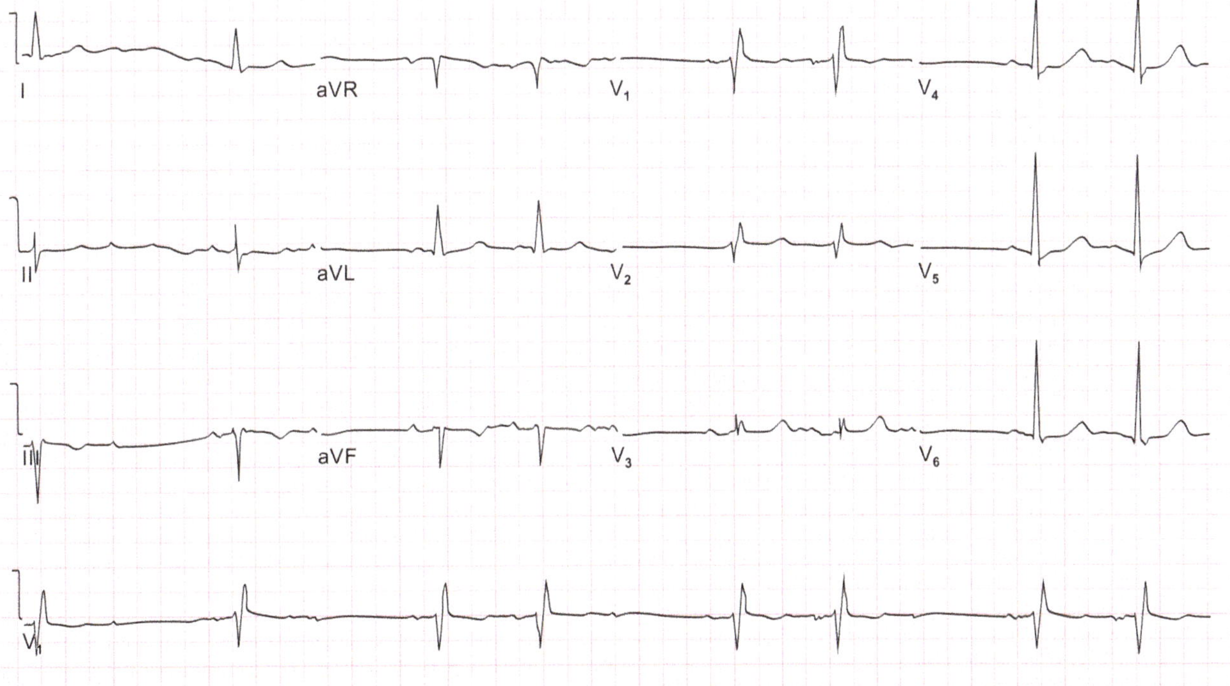

1. **What is the feature described here?**
2. **What is the most probable diagnosis?**
3. **Classify this disease.**
4. **What are the sites of involvement in each type?**
5. **What is the clinical significance in each type of disease?**
6. **What is prognosis in this disease?**

Answers

1. The ECG demonstrated:
   a. Constant PP intervals
   b. Constant RR intervals
   c. Constant PR interval
   d. One atrial impulse fails to conduct to ventricle after two subsequent conducted beats.
2. The most likely diagnosis is Mobitz type II secondary heart block.
3. This disease can be classified into following types:
   a. First-degree heart block:
      - PR interval is prolonged—more than 0.2 second without any dropped beat.
      - 1:1 AV conduction
   b. Second-degree heart block: It is of two types:
      - Mobitz type I block: It is characterized by progressively increasing PR interval culminating eventually nonconducted P wave, but PP interval will not change.
      - Mobitz type II block: It is characterized by:
         - No progressively increasing PR interval
         - PR interval remain constant
         - P wave occurs at constant rate
         - PP interval will be constant.
         - RR interval surrounding the dropped beat is the multiple of the preceding RR interval and it will remain unchanged.
   c. Second-degree high-grade AV block: It looks like second-degree incomplete block, but here two or more P wave will be blocked, so it looks like third-degree heart block.
   d. Third-degree or complete heart block: Here, as there is no conduction from AV node, hence P wave never correlates with QRS wave leading to complete dissociation between atria and ventricles.
4. Following are the sites of involvement:
   a. In case of first-degree AV block: Here, the defect is the delay in conduction of the entire P wave, so PR interval will be prolonged but all the impulses will conduct to AV node.
   b. In case of Mobitz type I second-degree heart block: Here, AV nodal cells will be fatigued, so that they fail to conduct the impulse to AV node leading to generation of dropped beat.
   c. In case of Mobitz type II second-degree heart block: Here, the defect occurs below the AV node along the entire fascicles of His bundle, both bundle branches, and three fascicles.
   d. In case third-degree heart block: It can occur in any site of the conduction tissue.
5. Clinical significance:
   a. First-degree heart block is clinically not significant as it will never produce hemodynamic instability and pacemaker will never be required.
   b. Second-degree Mobitz type I heart block:
      - It is benign.
      - It will not produce hemodynamic instability.
      - Patient will be asymptomatic.
      - Progression to third-degree heart block is rare.
      - Patient will respond to atropine.
      - Permanent pacemaker will not be required.
   c. Second-degree Mobitz type II block:
      - It is associated with severe bradycardia.
      - It will produce hemodynamic instability.
      - It will either progress to third-degree heart block or complete asystole.
      - It can lead to syncope or sudden cardiac death.
      - Patient must require permanent pacemaker.
   d. High-grade second-degree heart block:
      - It will produce hemodynamic instability.
      - It will either progress to third-degree heart block or complete asystole.
      - It can lead to ventricular tachycardia or sudden cardiac death.
      - Patient must require permanent pacemaker.
   e. Third-degree heart block:
      - It will produce hemodynamic instability.
      - It will progress to complete asystole.

- It can lead to syncope or sudden cardiac death.
- Patient must require permanent pacemaker.

6. Prognosis in this disease:
   a. Older age

b. Diabetes mellitus
c. Chronic kidney disease
d. Underlying heart disease
e. Type of AV block

CASE 68

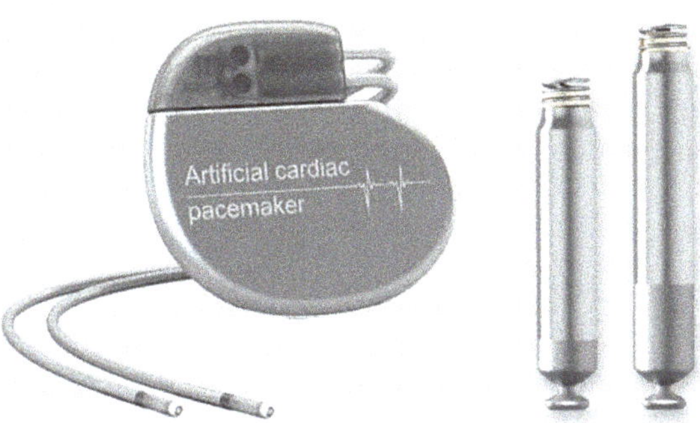

1. **What are the pictures described above?**
2. **What are the components in the first picture?**
3. **What are the indications of using these?**
4. **What are the accepted nomenclatures for the different modalities of these devices?**
5. **What are the characteristics of the second picture?**
6. **What are the complications of using this instrument?**
7. **What are syndromes related to this device?**
8. **Is right ventricular pacing is deleterious?**

Answers

1. The two pictures are:
   a. Artificial cardiac pacemaker
   b. Leadless pacemaker
2. Components of artificial pacemaker:
   a. Pulse generator: It is implanted in the upper left chest area.
   b. Pacing leads: These are implanted either atria or ventricle or both based on the indication for implantation.
3. Following are the indications of implantation of pacemaker:
   a. Class I indications:
      - Sinus node disease like sinus block, sinus pause, and SA block.
      - Mobitz type II, second-degree heart block
      - High-grade second-degree heart block
      - Third-degree heart block
      - Persistent atrial fibrillation with asymptomatic pauses of ≥5 seconds
      - Ventricular tachycardia with long QT syndrome
      - Recurrent syncope as a result of carotid sinus hypersensitivity
   b. Class II indications:
      - Symptomatic disease of sinus node
      - Unexplained syncope
      - Chronic bifascicular block
      - Pacemaker syndrome
      - High-risk patient having long QT syndrome
      - Hypertrophic cardiomyopathy
4. Following are the accepted nomenclatures of these devices:
   a. Letter 1: Chamber to be paced:
      - A: Atria
      - V: Ventricle
      - D: Dual chamber

b. Letter 2: Chamber to be sensed:
- A: Atria
- V: Ventricle
- D: Dual chamber
- 0: None

c. Letter 3: Response to the sensed event:
- I: Inhibited pacing
- T: Triggered pacing
- D: Dual response
- 0: None

d. Letter 4: Rate response feature which is characterized by response to body movement and increases the rate of pacing according to programmable algorithm.
- R: Rate response pacemaker
- 0: None

e. Letter 5: Chamber that is paced in multisite pacing:
- A: Atria
- V: Ventricle
- D: Dual chamber.

5. Characteristics of the leadless pacemaker:
a. It is placed into the heart directly without the help of pacing leads.
b. It is much smaller as compared to conventional pacemaker.
c. It comprises pulse generator that includes:
- Battery: Placed intracardiac
- Leads: Placed intracardiac
d. It will remove the subcutaneous pocket-related complications of standard pacemaker.
e. It will achieve high degree of AV synchrony pacing.

6. Complications of pacemaker implantation:
a. Complications at the time of implantation:
- Bleeding
- Infection
- Hemothorax
- Pneumothorax
- Cardiac perforation
- Arrhythmias
- Diaphragmatic pacing
- Phrenic nerve pacing
- Pocket hematoma
- Trauma to coronary sinus
- Prolonged exposure to radiation

b. Late complications:
- Erosion of the pacer through the skin
- Lead malfunction:
  - Lead fracture
  - Break in the insulation
  - Dislodgment of the leads
- Electromagnetic interference
- Device failure
- Infection
- Endless-loop tachycardia

7. Following are the pacemaker-related syndromes:
a. Pacemaker syndrome: This syndrome is characterized by worsening of the congestive cardiac failure due to single-chamber ventricular pacing resulting asynchronicity in the ventricular pacing and inappropriately timed contraction of the atrium and this can be corrected by both dual-chamber pacing as well as proper selection of pacing mode.
b. Twiddler's syndrome: This rare complication of implantation of pacemaker is caused by unintentional and repetitive twisting of the generator leading to either lead fracture or lead dislodgment resulting pacemaker failure observed mostly in patients with behavioral disorders.

8. If the patient has left ventricular dysfunction with heart failure and right ventricular pacing may lead to intraventricular dyssynchrony leading to worsening of ventricular function and overall worse outcome.

CASE 69

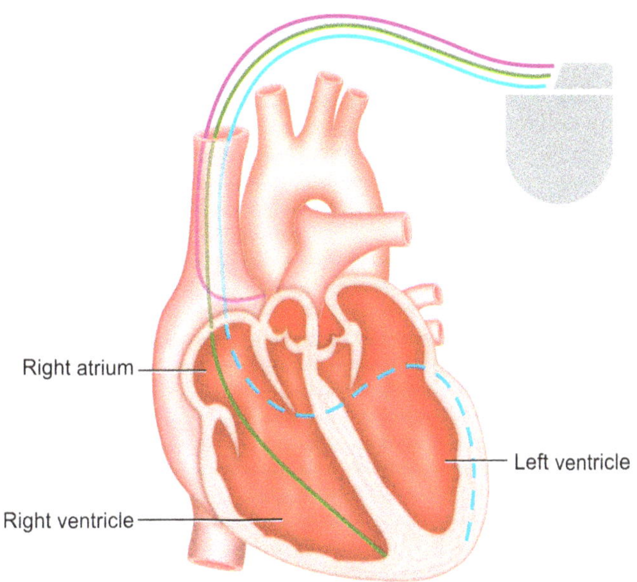

1. **What do you mean in the above picture?**
2. **What do you mean by this?**
3. **What are the potential benefits in this therapy?**
4. **What are the indications of this pacing?**
5. **Who will respond to this therapy?**
6. **What do you mean by multipoint pacing in this therapy?**
7. **What do you mean by para-Hisian pacing?**

Answers

1. Above picture demonstrates the biventricular pacing. It is method of CRT.
2. Rationale of CRT is that any intraventricular delay in conduction or presence of bundle branch block may worsen the systolic heart failure by dyssynchronization of the both ventricles thereby decrease in the efficiency of the ventricular contraction. Pacing of the left ventricle can be achieved by:
   a. Placement of the lead in the lateral venous system through the coronary sinus
   b. Placement of the epicardial left ventricular lead
   c. Permanent pacing of the His bundle with recruitment of left bundle branch
   d. Direct left bundle pacing
3. Potential benefits in CRT are as follows:
   a. Improved contractile function of the heart:
      - Increase in the ejection fraction
      - Increase in the cardiac index
      - Decrease in the pulmonary capillary wedge pressure
   b. Reverse ventricular remodeling:
      - Reduction in the left ventricular end-systolic dimension
      - Reduction in the end-diastolic dimension
      - Severity of mitral regurgitation
      - Reduction of left ventricular mass
4. Indications of CRT are as follows:
   a. Severe left ventricular systolic dysfunction having:
      - Ejection fraction of <35%
      - Intraventricular conduction delay of QRS of >120 ms in case of left bundle branch block
      - Intraventricular conduction delay of QRS of >150 ms in case of non-left bundle branch block.
      - High percentage of ventricular pacing is >40%.
   b. Wide QRS complex with NYHA class I or with atrial fibrillation
   c. Patient with sinus rhythm treated by goal-directed medical therapy presenting with heart failure.

5. Factors for responding to CRT are:
   a. Female gender
   b. Nonischemic cardiomyopathy
   c. Wide QRS complex
   d. Left bundle branch block
6. Multipoint pacing allows capture of more left ventricular tissue through the delivery of two pacing pulses thereby:
   a. Improving CRT response
   b. Improving left ventricular electrical activation
   c. Reducing the left ventricular dyssynchrony
   d. Decreasing the end-systolic volume
   e. Improving function of left ventricular function
7. Permanent para-Hisian pacing is characterized by activation of His bundle by pacemaker leading to ventricular activation to prevent dyssynchrony and negative inotropic effect that can be seen in case of right ventricular apical pacing.

CASE 70

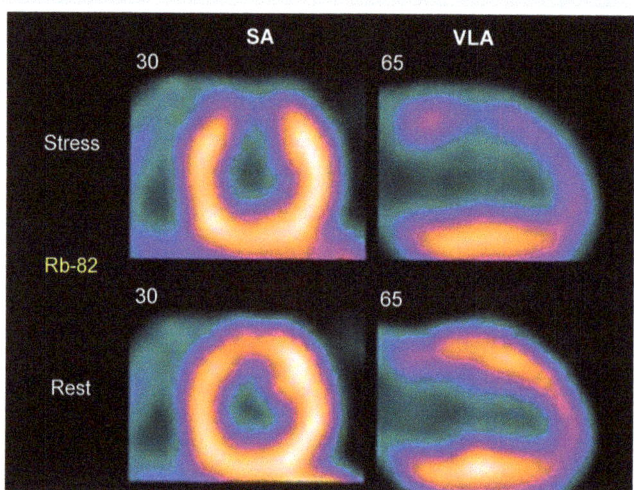

1. **What is the above picture?**
2. **What are the other tracers used in this positron emission tomography (PET)?**
3. **What are advantages of it over single photon emission computed tomography?**
4. **How can you estimate the coronary flow reserve by this scan?**
5. **What is the radiopharmaceutical used in case of cardiac PET?**
6. **What other cardiac infectious diseases can be diagnosed by this method?**
7. **What do you mean by perfusion and metabolism mismatch?**

Answers

1. Above picture demonstrates the use of rubidium-82 to detect the myocardial perfusion at rest as well as in stress.
2. Other tracers used in this case are as follows:
   a. Nitrogen-13
   b. C-11 acetate (Krebs cycle)
   c. C-11 palmitate (fatty acid metabolism)
   d. C-11 lactate (utilization of lactate)
   e. C-11 phenylephrine (presynaptic catecholamine uptake and metabolism)
   f. F-18 fluorodeoxyglucose
   g. F-18 florbetaben
   h. F-18 florbetapir
3. Advantages of PET myocardial perfusion over single photon emission computed tomography are:
   a. It is more sensitive and specific.
   b. It is cost-effective.
   c. It results in the lower dose of radiation.
   d. It can quantify the myocardial blood flow absolutely in mL/min/g of tissue.
4. Estimation of coronary blood flow reserve: It can be calculated by maximum blood flow to the myocardium by baseline myocardial blood flow at rest in a given coronary artery.

Maximum as well as resting myocardial blood flow can be derived by processing radionuclide activity-based data that is collected under vasodilator stress and resting PET scan respectively.

5. Radiopharmaceutical F-18 fluorodeoxyglucose is used as radiotracer.

6. Other cardiac infectious diseases can be diagnosed by this method:
   a. Myocarditis
   b. Endocarditis with large vegetations of >6 mm
   c. Cardiac and paracardiac masses
   d. Perivalvular abscesses
   e. Cardiac device pocket infection

7. Perfusion and metabolism mismatch can be diagnosed if the area of decreased perfusion shows normal or increased uptake of the tracer like FDG-18 which is consistent with the area of hibernating viable myocardial tissue.

CASE 71

A 54-year-old type 2 diabetic male patient came to emergency department with orthopnea, having history of paroxysmal nocturnal dyspnea, swelling of legs, and palpitation.

On examination, pulse rate 112 beats/min, pedal edema, and auscultation demonstrated presence of third and fourth heart sound heard with the bell of the stethoscope.

Pulse demonstrated:

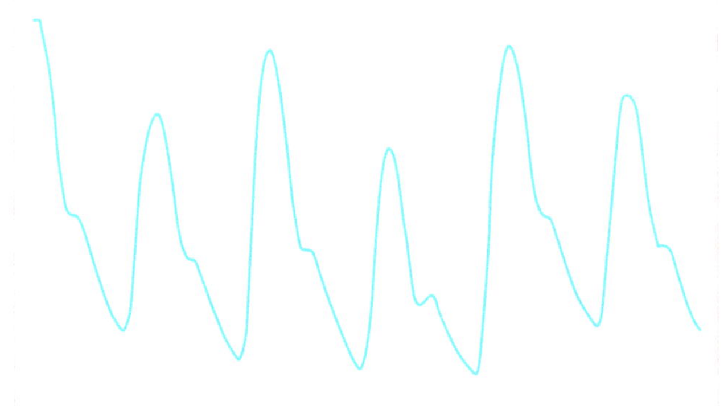

1. **Describe the pulse and the cause of this pulse.**
2. **What is your diagnosis?**
3. **What are the causes of third and fourth heart sound?**
4. **Name the causes of third heart sound.**
5. **Name the causes of fourth heart sound.**
6. **How can you differentiate between fourth heart sound and first heart sound or ejection click?**

Answers

1. This pulse is characterized by high volume and low volume. It is known as pulsus alternans.

2. Patient has been suffering from incipient heart failure having gallop rhythm and tachycardia.

3. Third heart sound is caused by rapid ventricular filling during the diastolic phase. Fourth heart sound is produced by forceful contraction of atria during the last phase of diastole.

4. Causes of left ventricular third heart sound:
   a. Physiologically in children
   b. Pathologically:
      - Left heart failure
      - Left ventricular dysfunction
      - Left-to-right heart shunt with rapid inflow in the left ventricle

   Causes of right ventricular third heart sound:
      - Right ventricular failure
      - Right ventricular dysfunction

5. Causes of fourth heart sound:
   a. Physiologically in elderly patient
   b. Pathologically:
      - Hypertension
      - Aortic stenosis
      - Pulmonary stenosis
      - Acute myocardial infarction
      - Hypertrophic cardiomyopathy

6. Differences between the fourth heart sound and first heart sound are:
   a. Fourth heart sound is heard by the bell of stethoscope but first heart sound or ejection click is heard by the diaphragm of the stethoscope.
   b. Fourth heart sound is low pitched but first heart sound and ejection click are high-pitched sound.
   c. Fourth heart sound can be obliterated pressure over the chest wall with the stethoscope but first heart sound and ejection click cannot be heard.

CASE 72

A 34-year-old male patient came to OPD with recurrent nasal discharge and productive cough. He has past history of recurrent sneezing, cough with purulent expectoration, and fever for last 6 years. He had no issue as his sperm was demonstrated as dysmotile due to ciliary dysfunction.

On examination, tender maxillary sinus, third-degree clubbing, cardiovascular system demonstrated absent apical impulse on the left fifth intercostal space, but it was present on the right fifth intercostal space and heart sound was prominent on the right side. Gastrointestinal examination demonstrated upper border of liver dullness on the fifth right intercostal space.

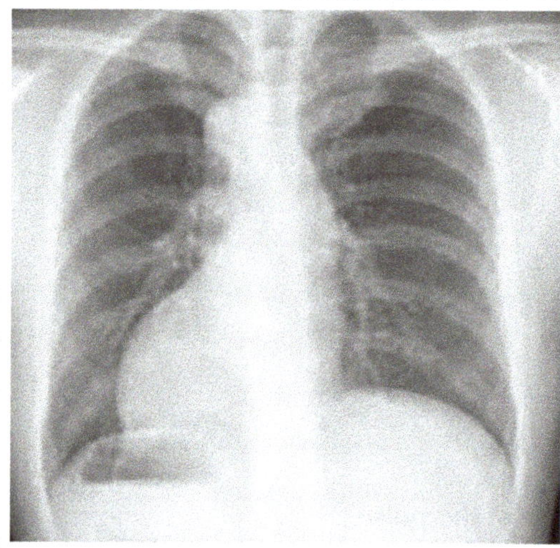

1. **What are the findings present in the chest X-ray?**
2. **What is your diagnosis?**
3. **What are the points in favor of your diagnosis?**
4. **What will be the early manifestation in this case?**
5. **What are the other manifestations in the high-resolution computed tomography (HRCT) in this case?**
6. **What should be the findings in the ECG?**
7. **What do you mean by pseudodextrocardia?**
8. **What do you mean by dextroversion and what are its causes?**
9. **What are the extracardiac abnormalities associated with dextrocardia only?**
10. **What are other abnormalities associated with dextrocardia?**
11. **What is levoversion?**

Answers

1. Chest X-ray demonstrated the following suggestive of dextrocardia:
   a. Cardiac apex is on the right side.
   b. Gas bubbles suggestive of stomach are on the right side of the chest.
   c. Aortic knuckle and thoracic aorta are in the right side of the chest.
   d. Left dome of the diaphragm is more elevated as compared to the right dome.
2. The patient has been suffering from Kartagener's syndrome.

3. Following are the points in favor of this diagnosis:
   a. Clinical and radiological features in the chest suggestive of dextrocardia
   b. Tender maxillary sinus suggestive of maxillary sinusitis
   c. Recurrent cough with purulent sputum
   d. Infertility as indicated by dysmotile cilia
4. The early manifestation in the chest X-ray is thickening of the bronchial wall.
5. Other manifestations in the HRCT are as follows:
   a. Focal air trapping
   b. Atelectasis
   c. Extent of bronchiectasis
6. Following findings are observed in the ECG:
   a. Negative P and QRS in L1 and aVL
   b. Positive P and QRS in aVR
   c. Negative QRS and T waves in all the precordial leads
7. In case of technical dextrocardia or pseudo-dextrocardia:
   a. Inadvertent interchange of the right arm and left arm electrodes leading to production of technical dextrocardia only in the limb leads
   b. Inversion of P, QRS-T complexes in L1, and aVL where positive deflection in the aVR

8. Dextroversion means shifting of the mediastinum to the right side without any change of position of chambers of the heart like left-sided aorta and left-sided stomach cavity due to:
   a. Removal of left lung
   b. Removal of the part of the lung
   c. Collapse or atelectasis of the right lung
9. Following are the extracardiac abnormalities associated with dextrocardia:
   a. Abnormal bilobed lungs
   b. Abnormal gallbladder
   c. Bilateral symmetrical liver
10. Following are the other abnormalities associated with dextrocardia:
    a. Ventricular septal defect
    b. Corrected transposition of the great vessels
    c. Single ventricle
    d. Single atrium
    e. Endocardial cushion defect
    f. Pulmonary hypoplasia
    g. Right aortic arch
    h. Aortic atresia
11. Levoversion is characterized by the following features:
    a. Left-sided apex
    b. Right-sided descending aorta
    c. Right-sided stomach

CASE 73

A 20-year-old male having history of congenital cardiac disease came to emergency department with complaints of effort intolerance, respiratory distress, palpitation, and pedal swelling.

On examination, there was tachycardia, central cyanosis, raised pulsatile neck vein with prominent "*a*" wave, enlarged tender liver, and pedal edema.

Cardiovascular examination demonstrated left parasternal heave and epigastric pulsation indicating right ventricular hypertrophy, and palpable pulmonary component. On auscultation, there was loud pulmonary second sound, single second heart sound, and presence of early diastolic murmur suggestive of pulmonary regurgitation, and pansystolic murmur in the tricuspid area.

1. **What is your provisional diagnosis?**
2. **What are the features in favor of this diagnosis?**
3. **How can you define this disease?**
4. **What are the other causes of congenital heart disease?**
5. **What are the possible complications in this disease?**
6. **What are the factors responsible for deleterious to pulmonary hypertension?**
7. **What are the bad prognostic factors in this patient?**
8. **Why phlebotomy has been restricted in this patient as a method of treatment?**

Answers

1. The provisional diagnosis is Eisenmenger's syndrome in a case of patent ductus arteriosus with pulmonary hypertension.
2. Following are the points in favor of this diagnosis:
   a. Past history of congenital heart disease
   b. Presence of clubbing and central cyanosis
   c. Pedal edema
   d. Loud pulmonary component
   e. Murmur of pulmonary regurgitation
   f. Single second heart sound
   g. Pansystolic murmur in the tricuspid area
3. Eisenmenger's disease is characterized by pulmonary hypertension with reversal of shunt in case of congenital heart diseases such as atrial septal defect, VSD, and patent ductus arteriosus.
4. The name of the congenital heart diseases other than Eisenmenger's syndrome:
   a. Fallot's tetralogy
   b. Transposition of the great vessels
   c. Common atrium
   d. Persistent truncus arteriosus
   e. Total anomalous pulmonary venous connections
5. Following are the possible complications in this disease:
   a. Polycythemia due to central cyanosis
   b. Hemoptysis due to pulmonary infarction resulting from paradoxical embolism
   c. Right ventricular failure
   d. Tricuspid regurgitation
   e. Hyperuricemia
   f. Infective endocarditis
   g. Abnormal hemostasis resulting bleeding
   h. Paradoxical embolism
   i. Cerebrovascular thrombosis due to increased viscosity
6. Following are the factors responsible for deleterious to pulmonary hypertension:
   a. Dehydration
   b. Fluid overload
   c. Pregnancy
   d. Hepatic dysfunction
   e. Renal dysfunction
   f. Arrhythmias
   g. Systemic hypertension
   h. Acute infection
   i. Increased viscosity due to hypercoagulable state
   j. Hypoxia resulting from smoking
7. Following are the bad prognostic factors:
   a. Right ventricular systolic dysfunction
   b. Recurrent syncopal attack
   c. Low cardiac output
   d. Polycythemia
   e. Hypoxemia
8. In this patient, phlebotomy can be done to decrease the symptoms of hyperviscosity such as headache, dizziness, or fatigue because in this disease hypoxia stimulates bone marrow to stimulate production of red blood cells and thereby increases blood viscosity. On the other hand, phlebotomy leads to iron deficiency and decreases exercise tolerance. Hence, phlebotomy should be restricted only to those patients who are suffering from features of hyperviscosity syndrome.

CASE 74

A 20-year-old male came with following features and exertional dyspnea which was relieved after squatting and syncopal attack. On auscultation, second heart sound is single and ejection systolic murmur in the pulmonary area.

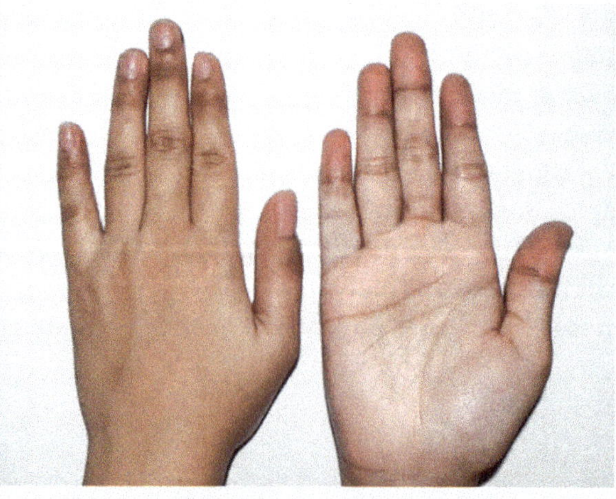

1. **What is the most probable diagnosis?**
2. **What are the components of this disease?**
3. **What are the features of Fallot's pentalogy and Fallot's trilogy?**
4. **Why squatting relieves respiratory distress?**
5. **What are the associated anomalies in this disease?**
6. **Why the murmur will not be present in the tricuspid area?**
7. **What is the most important complication in this disease?**

Answers

1. The most probable diagnosis is Fallot's tetralogy.
2. The components of the Fallot's tetralogy are:
   a. Right ventricular hypertrophy
   b. Infundibular pulmonary stenosis
   c. Ventricular septal defect
   d. Overriding of the aorta
3. Fallot's pentalogy includes:
   a. Right ventricular hypertrophy
   b. Infundibular pulmonary stenosis
   c. Ventricular septal defect
   d. Overriding of the aorta
   e. Atrial septal defect
   Fallot's trilogy includes:
   a. Ventricular septal defect
   b. Atrial septal defect
   c. Pulmonary stenosis
4. Squatting:
   a. Increases the peripheral vascular resistance
   b. Reduce the venous return of the unsaturated blood to the right side of the heart.

All the factors the above factors:
   a. Reduce the right-to-left heart shunting of the desaturated blood
   b. Improve cerebral oxygenation
   c. Reduce the cyanotic spells
5. Following may be the associated anomalies in this case:
   a. Anomalies of coronary artery
   b. Atrial septal defect
   c. Double aortic arch
   d. Right-sided aortic arch and left-sided superior vena cava
   e. Hypoplasia of the pulmonary arteries
6. In this disease, shunt at the level of VSD is more or less balanced without much blood flow across the defect. Hence, the pansystolic murmur will not be present in the tricuspid area.
7. The most important complication in this disease is right ventricular dysfunction and exercise tolerance resulting from pulmonary insufficiency.

CASE 75

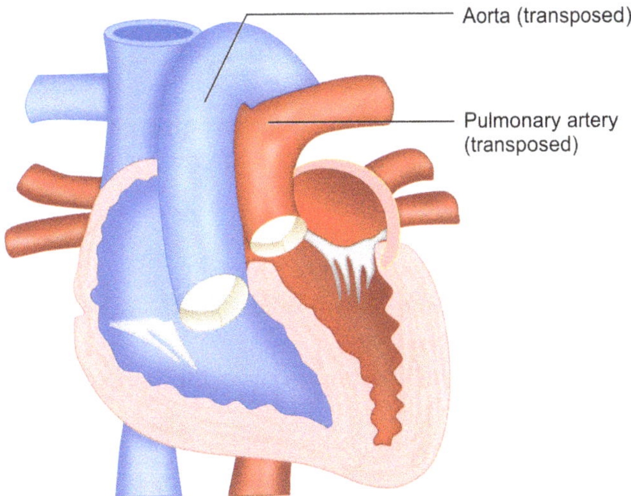

1. **Describe the picture.**
2. **What is your diagnosis?**
3. **What are the predisposing factors for this disease?**
4. **What are the symptoms in this baby?**
5. **What are the auscultatory findings in this disease?**
6. **What is the operation of choice in this disease?**
7. **What are the late potential complications in this operation?**

Answers

1. This is the flow pattern:
   a. Deoxygenated blood flows from the right atrium to right ventricle then to aorta.
   b. Oxygenated blood flows from the left atrium to left ventricle then to lung bed.

   This is incompatible with life unless there are bidirectional shunts at the following levels:
   a. At the atrial level, atrial septal defect
   b. At the ventricular level, ventricular septal defect
   c. At the level of great vessels, patent ductus arteriosus
2. The diagnosis is complete transposition of the great vessels.
3. Following are the predisposing factors in this disease:
   a. Maternal age is >40 years
   b. Insulin-dependent type 1 pregnancy during pregnancy
   c. Poor nutrition during pregnancy
   d. Ingestion of the drugs like benzodiazepines during pregnancy
   e. Infection of varicella or other virus during pregnancy

4. Following features are:
   a. In absence of VSD, the baby will be blue after birth.
   b. In presence of VSD, the baby will be blue few weeks after birth.
   c. Breathing will be rapid.
   d. Anorexia
   e. Poor gain in weight
   f. In first few weeks after birth, the heart size is normal but it will be gradually increased.
5. The auscultation in the heart demonstrated:
   a. First heart sound is normal.
   b. Second heart sound is single.
   c. In absence of VSD—grade I/II systolic murmur
   d. In presence of VSD—grade III/IV systolic murmur
6. The operation of choice is arterial switch.
7. Potential late complication after this operation:
   a. Arrhythmias
   b. Sudden cardiac death
   c. Endocarditis
   d. Tricuspid regurgitation
   e. Pulmonary hypertension
   f. Right ventricular dysfunction
   g. Baffle obstruction or leak

CASE 76

A known patient with history of AV septal defect with Eisenmenger complex, trisomy 21 was advised complete blood count as he had past history of venesection for hemoglobin of 25 g/cc with history of headache. Recent hemoglobin was also 26 g/dL but no history of headache or dizziness.

1. **What is the cause of previous headache in this patient?**
2. **What will be the advice to be given to the patient now?**
3. **What is the cause of persistent rise in hemoglobin in this patient?**
4. **What are the features of hyperviscosity syndrome?**
5. **Why headache or other neurological manifestations occur in this patient?**
6. **What are the ocular features occur in this patient?**

Answers

1. The cause of the headache is very high hemoglobin which led to hyperviscosity of the blood resulting this feature.
2. As this patient has no feature suggestive of hyperviscosity syndrome, he will not be advised to do repeat phlebotomy.
3. Chronic cyanosis leads to stimulation of bone marrow to increase red blood cell production, so that proper amount of oxygen can be supplied to the patient. This increased amount of red blood cells leads to hyperviscosity syndrome. The fluid within the vessel is thicker and travels very slowly. On the other hand, hyperviscosity will change the shape of the red blood cells leading to red blood cells aggregation.
4. Features of hyperviscosity syndrome are as follows:
   a. Bleeding manifestations
   b. Neurological manifestation
   c. Ocular manifestations
   d. Cardiopulmonary manifestations
5. Neurological manifestations occur due to:
   a. Decreased blood flow to the central nervous system
   b. Deposition of the paraproteins within the myelin sheath of the peripheral nerves
6. Ocular manifestations in this disease:
   a. Sausage link or boxcar engorgement of the retinal veins
   b. Papilledema
   c. Flame-shaped hemorrhage
   d. Exudates

CASE 77

A 25-year-old man with previous history of surgical repair for Fallot's tetralogy has recently developed features of transient presyncope. Echocardiography demonstrated severe pulmonary regurgitation with right ventricular outflow tract obstruction. ECG demonstrated first-degree AV block with right bundle branch block with QRS interval of 190 ms.

1. **What is the risk in this patient?**
2. **What should be the treatment of choice in this patient?**
3. **What types of ventricular tachycardia may occur in this patient?**

Answers

1. In patient with previous history of repair for Fallot's tetralogy, QRS duration of >180 ms is risky to develop ventricular tachycardia, and sudden cardiac death.
2. The treatment of choice is administration of intracardiac device along with pulmonary valve intervention as there is severe pulmonary regurgitation along with right ventricular outflow tract obstruction.
3. Ventricular tachycardia is of right ventricular origin. Nonsustained ventricular tachycardia will not lead to sudden cardiac death. So, antiarrhythmic drugs are not prescribed in asymptomatic patient. Only sustained ventricular tachycardia requires treatment.

CASE 78

A 46-year-old hypertensive man having history of stroke had no carotid atheroma in Doppler study, but Holter monitoring demonstrated asymptomatic atrial fibrillation. He was advised bubble contrast echocardiography which demonstrated complete left heart opacification with Valsalva release. Size of left atria was 31 cm^2. Patient was on antiplatelet therapy.

1. **What are the possible causes of stroke in this case?**
2. **What should be the immediate strategy in this case from cardiac point of view?**
3. **What may be the cause of atrial fibrillation in this case and how it can be eliminated?**
4. **If the bubble echo suggests the possibility of patent foramen ovale, what is the modality of choice to confirm this foramen?**

Answers

1. The possible causes of stroke here are:
   a. Left atrial thrombus as a result atrial fibrillation
   b. Paradoxical embolus from right atrium through the patent foramen ovale
2. The immediate strategy is administration of anticoagulant to protect embolus originating from both the sources.
3. Atrial fibrillation may be due to uncontrolled hypertension which can be treated by the use of ACE inhibitors.
4. Transesophageal echocardiography is the modality of choice to confirm the presence of patent foramen ovale.

CASE 79

A 35-year-old nonsmoker, nondiabetic slim male came with progressively increasing breathlessness as well as intermittent palpitations. Transthoracic echocardiogram demonstrated dilated right heart with normal valves but systolic pressure in the right ventricle was 32 mm Hg. There was no abnormality in the Doppler study.

1. **Which side is involved in this patient?**
2. **What are the defects can be detected in this patient by echocardiography?**
3. **What are the cardiac defects cannot be detected by echocardiography?**
4. **What is the most common abnormality suspected in this case and why?**
5. **Where is that defect?**
6. **The defect that cannot be detected by transthoracic echocardiography can be detected by which methods?**
7. **If this defect is not corrected, what may be the remote complications?**

Answers

1. Right side of the heart is involved in this case.
2. Following defects can be detected by echocardiography:
   a. Atrial septal defect
   b. Ventricular septal defect
   c. Patent ductus arteriosus
3. Anomalous pulmonary venous drainage and sinus venosus type atrial septal defect cannot be detected by echocardiography.
4. As the right side of the heart is involved and right ventricular systolic pressure is high, hence this patient has anomalous pulmonary venous drainage along with sinus venosus defect.
5. This defect is present at the entrance of superior vena cava into the right atrium.
6. This anomalous venous drainage and sinus venosus defect can be detected by:
   a. Transesophageal echocardiography
   b. CT scan
   c. MRI
7. If the defect is uncorrected, there will be the following remote complications:
   a. Irreversible right heart dysfunction
   b. Pulmonary hypertension
   c. Development of the atrial arrhythmias

CASE 80

A 38-year-old female with history of mechanical mitral valve replacement having one child after several miscarriages has come to take a doctor for taking information regarding contraception.

1. **Which is the most effective contraception?**
2. **What is the opinion regarding the use of condom in this patient?**
3. **What is the opinion regarding the combined pill in this patient?**
4. **Whether warfarin can be used in this patient while using contraception?**

Answers

1. The most effective contraception in this patient is progesterone pill including morning-after pill as it is safe for all the cardiac conditions.
2. As there is high incidence of failure rate in condom use, it should not be used in this case.
3. Combined pills should not be used in this patient as the clotting is hazardous in the following conditions:
   a. Dilated cardiomyopathy
   b. Fontan operation
   c. Mustard operation
   d. Senning operation
   e. Atrial flutter
   f. Atrial fibrillation
   g. Previous clot
   h. Cyanosis
   i. Presence of shunt
   j. Pulmonary hypertension
   k. Mechanical valves
4. Regarding use of warfarin:
   a. If the patient is using mini pill or depot pill, there is chance of excessive bleeding or irregular bleeding.
   b. If the patient is using mini pill or depot pill, there is chance of heavy painful bruising at the injection sites.
   c. Warfarin should be used if the patient will use Mirena coil.

CASE 81

A 35-year-old pregnant female having no family history of hypertension developed headache and was referred to medicine department for checkup and there she was diagnosed as pregnancy-induced hypertension.

1. **What are the categories of hypertensive medicines to be used in case of pregnant mother and fetus?**
2. **Which drug is mostly effective in pregnancy?**
3. **What is your opinion regarding β-blockers in pregnant woman?**
4. **What is your opinion regarding ACE inhibitors?**
5. **What is your opinion regarding thiazide diuretics?**

Answers

1. Categories of hypertensive medicines are as follows:
   a. Category A drug is safe in pregnancy but no drug is in this category.
   b. Category B drug is in the experimental stage but there is no evidence of harmful effect in animal and human being.
   c. Category C drugs: These groups of drugs have been shown as harmful in case of animal but not in case of human being.
   d. Category D drugs: These groups of drugs have harmful effect on the fetus but effective to the mother which outweighs the risk to fetus.
   e. Category X drugs: These groups of drugs have harmful effect on the fetus but effective to the mother which does not outweigh the risk to fetus.
2. Methyldopa is the most effective first-line drug used in pregnancy. It is a category B drug.
3. β-blockers are category B and C drugs which affect fetus and neonates in the following manner:
   a. Intrauterine growth retardation
   b. Neonatal hypoglycemia
   So, these groups of drugs are used with growth scan four weekly.
4. ACE inhibitors are the category D drugs, these drugs may cause following abnormalities in fetus:
   a. Oligohydramnios
   b. Limb contractures
   c. Renal abnormalities
5. Thiazide diuretics are teratogenic and responsible for the following abnormalities:
   a. Neonatal thrombocytopenia
   b. Hyponatremia
   c. Jaundice
   d. Bradycardia

CASE 82

A 26-year-old female with history of mechanical mitral valve replacement and on warfarin has come to medical doctor to take his opinion regarding using warfarin during pregnancy because she wants to take pregnancy.

1. **What is the opinion regarding the use of warfarin in pregnancy?**
2. **What is your opinion regarding the use of heparin?**
3. **Why pregnancy is a hypercoagulable state?**
4. **Which drug can be safely used in this case?**

Answers

1. Warfarin has the following effects during pregnancy:
   a. Warfarin crosses placenta to produce:
      - Spontaneous abortion
      - Stillbirth
      - Prematurity
      - Neonatal death
   b. Following teratogenic effects like warfarin embryopathy in 6–9 weeks of pregnancy:
      - Nasal hypoplasia
      - Saddle-shaped nasal bridge
      - Skeletal defects
      - Short fingers and toes
      - Low birth weight
      - Delay in development

   But, if the dose of warfarin is <5 mg/day, incidence of embryopathy is nearly zero.
2. Heparin though cannot cross the placenta, but it can produce valve thrombosis leading to maternal death.
3. Pregnancy is a hypercoagulable state leading to production of mitral valve thrombosis due to activation of:
   a. Prothrombin 1 and 2
   b. Thrombin–thrombin complex
   c. D-dimer
4. Warfarin should be continued throughout the pregnancy at a low dose but should be stopped several weeks prior to delivery to avoid the risk of neonatal intracranial hemorrhage.

CASE 83

A 31-year-old female with 18 weeks of pregnancy came to emergency department with progressively increasing breathlessness and cough. Transthoracic echocardiography demonstrated ejection fraction of 24% and left ventricular end-diastolic diameter 6 cm.

1. **What is the most important nonpharmacological treatment in this case and why?**
2. **What are the causes of early termination in this case?**
3. **What are the hemodynamic changes in pregnancy in the second trimester?**

Answers

1. The most important nonpharmacological treatment is complete bed rest, the aim being to reach the fetus as much viable as possible without compromising the mother.
2. The causes of termination of pregnancy in this case are:
   a. Pulmonary edema
   b. Intractable heart failure
   c. Stroke
   d. Fetal loss
3. Following are the hemodynamic changes in pregnancy in the second trimester:
   a. Blood volume: Increase in the red blood cell mass leading to increased cardiac output
   b. There is peak in the cardiac output in this trimester.
   c. There is decrease in the peripheral vascular resistance due to:
      - Circulating prostaglandin
      - Circulating other gestational hormones
      - Low resistance vascular bed in the placenta

   Hence, the blood pressure will come to normal in the second trimester.

CASE 84

A 35-year-old female developed sudden respiratory distress and orthopnea 3 hours after delivery. On examination, there was tachycardia, tachypnea, blood pressure 140/90 mm Hg, and on auscultation of the chest there was crepitations.

1. **What is the most possible diagnosis?**
2. **What are the hemodynamic changes after delivery?**
3. **When the hemodynamic change will be recovered?**
4. **What effect of amniotic fluid during delivery may occur?**

Answers

1. The patient has been suffering from peripartum cardiomyopathy which is characterized by cardiac dysfunction at the time of extreme increased in the workload.
2. Following are the hemodynamic changes in the peripartum period:
   a. At the time of labor and during delivery, cardiac output and blood pressure are increased:
      - Due to pain during labor
      - Due to uterine contraction
   b. Just after labor, cardiac output will be increased due to:
      - Relief from compression of the inferior vena cava
      - Autotransfusion from the contracted and emptied uterus
3. All the hemodynamic changes will be resolved within 2 weeks of postpartum period.
4. During delivery, amniotic fluid embolism leads to:
   a. Shortness of breath
   b. Hypotension
   c. Central cyanosis
   d. Cardiac arrest

CASE 85

A 35-year-old female containing 38 weeks of pregnancy has come with palpitation. Her ECG demonstrated:

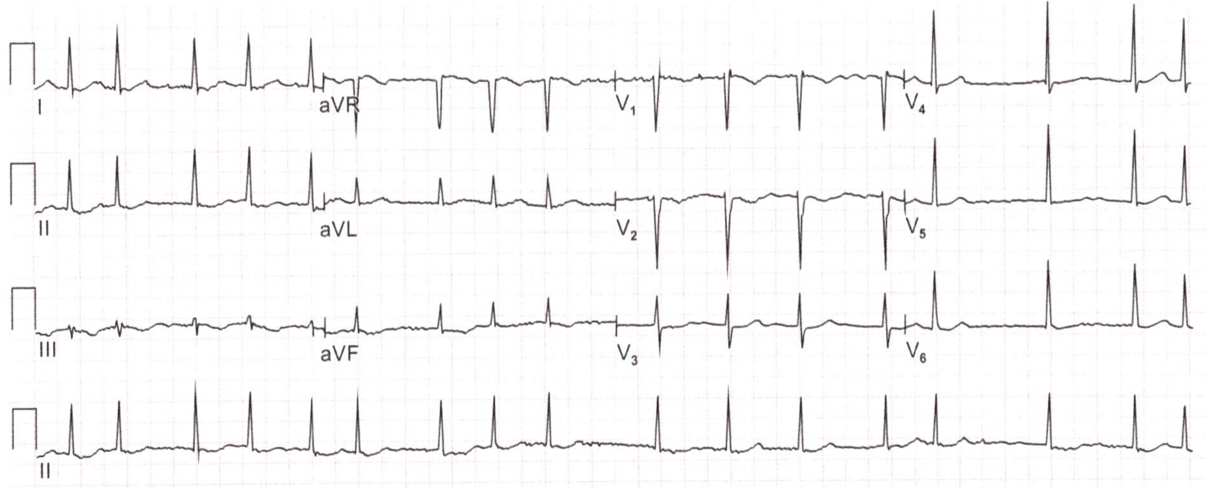

1. **What is the ECG feature in this patient?**
2. **What is the medication required in this case and why?**
3. **What are the drugs can be given in this context to the pregnant patient?**
4. **What are the precautions should be taken in the above drugs?**
5. **Why amiodarone is not safe in this case?**

Answers

1. The patient has been suffering from atrial fibrillation which is consistent with the palpitation.
2. As the pregnancy is a hypercoagulable state, hence low molecular weight heparin should be administered until 4 weeks after restoration of sinus rhythm.
3. Following drugs can be given in this patient:
   a. Flecainide
   b. Digoxin
   c. β-blockers
4. Following precautions should be taken in this patient:
   a. Dose should be increased as the glomerular filtration will be increased.
   b. In case of any suspected toxicity to the fetus, the drug level in the blood should be checked.
5. Amiodarone is not safe because:
   a. It causes problem with thyroid in fetus
   b. It is responsible for intrauterine growth retardation.

CASE 86

A 42-year-old female came to medicine OPD with brassy cough and there is swelling in the left infraclavicular region. She was recommended chest X-ray which demonstrated the following. Then CT thorax was done which demonstrated the following:

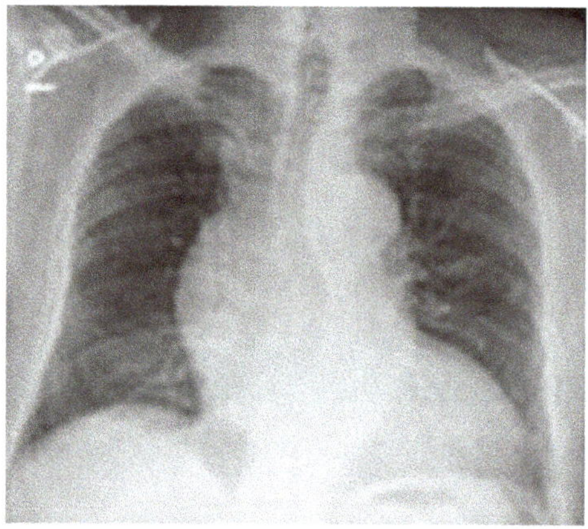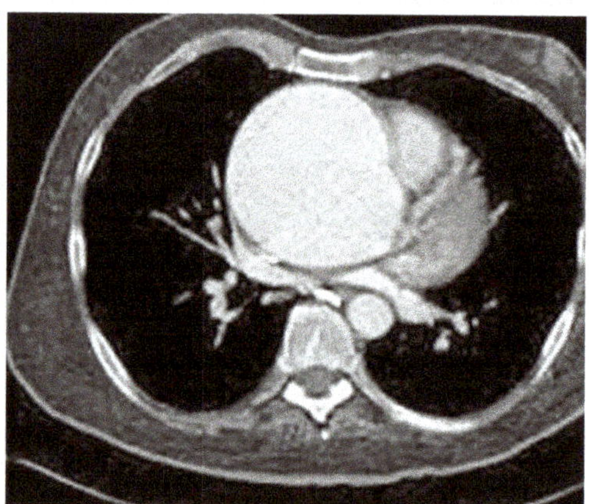

1. **Describe the above pictures.**
2. **What is your diagnosis?**
3. **What is the genetic predisposition in this disease?**
4. **Defined the disease.**
5. **What are the compression features can be seen?**
6. **If this involves thoracic part, what findings are clue to the diagnosis?**
7. **What are the causes of aneurysm of the ascending aorta?**
8. **Classify this disease.**
9. **Which factor is important pathophysiologically in this case and why?**
10. **What is the annual risk complication of aortic aneurysm?**
11. **What is cystic medial necrosis?**
12. **Which type of Ehlers–Danlos syndrome is associated with this disease?**

Answers

1. Straight X-ray demonstrated:
   a. Widening of the mediastinum
   b. Enlargement of the aortic knob
   c. Displacement of the aorta from the midline

   CT scan of chest demonstrated:
   a. Huge dilatation of the ascending aorta
2. The most likely diagnosis is aneurysm of the ascending aorta.

3. Following genetic abnormalities are associated with this disease:
   a. Marfan syndrome
   b. Loeys–Dietz syndrome
   c. Ehlers–Danlos syndrome
4. Definition: This disease can be defined as ≥50% or increase in diameter as compared to normal containing all the three layers of arteries. False aneurysm can be defined as disrupted aortic wall and all the three layers are not present.
5. Following structures are compressed:
   a. Compression of trachea—stridor
   b. Brassy cough—compression over the bronchus
   c. Facial puffiness along with edema of the neck and arms—superior vena caval obstruction.
   d. Hoarseness of voice—pressure on the recurrent laryngeal nerve
6. If this disease will involve, following clinical features are clue to the diagnosis:
   a. Edematous and plethoric face—compression of superior vena cava
   b. Height and weight proportions—clue to Marfan syndrome
   c. Hyperextensibility of the joints and increased elasticity of the skin—Ehlers–Danlos syndrome
   d. High volume pulse along with wide pulse pressure, water hammer pulse, and dancing carotid—suggest aortic regurgitation
   e. Expansible pulsation in the suprasternal notch
7. Causes of aneurysm of ascending aorta aneurysm are:
   a. Atherosclerosis
   b. Connective tissue disorders:
      • Marfan syndrome
      • Ehlers–Danlos syndrome
      • Cystic medial necrosis
   c. Trauma
   d. Syphilitic aneurysm
   e. Mycotic infections

8. Classification of the disease:
   a. Stanford classification:
      • Any dissection involving the ascending aorta
      • Any dissection not involving the ascending aorta
   b. DeBakey classification:
      • Entry point in the ascending aorta extends to the aortic arch and beyond
      • Confined entirely to the ascending aorta
      • Entry into the descending aorta distal to subclavian artery and extends distally or proximally
9. Bicuspid aortic valve has ninefold higher risk of aortic dissection in the ascending aorta because of the following reasons:
   a. Cystic medial degeneration
   b. Impaired fibrillin-1
   c. Infiltration of lymphocytes in the aortic wall
10. Annual risk complication of aortic aneurysm depends upon the size of the aneurysm.

Size of aneurysm	Risk of rupture annually (%)	Annual risk of death (%)
>4 cm	0.3	4.6
>5 cm	1.7	4.8
>6 cm	3.6	10.8

11. Aorta wall is composed of three layers: (1) adventitia, (2) media, and (3) intima. In case of aortic dissection, all the layers will be interrupted leading to flow of blood in-between the adventitia and media. Since the media is responsible for the strength of the aortic wall, so weakening of this wall will lead to formation of aneurysm.
12. Ehlers–Danlos syndrome type IV is associated with this disease because the associated gene encoding the synthesis of collagen type III (*COL3A1*) gene will be defective. This disease is dominant.

CASE 87

A 60-year-old smoker hypertensive man came to emergency department with severe and sudden tearing pain with radiation in-between the shoulder blades in the central part of the chest in the anterior part.

On examination, patient was very restless, blood pressure difference was 25 mm Hg in the both arms, wide pulse pressure, and pulses in the lower limbs were feeble. On auscultation, there was presence of early diastolic murmur in the neoaortic area.

Urgent chest X-ray demonstrated:

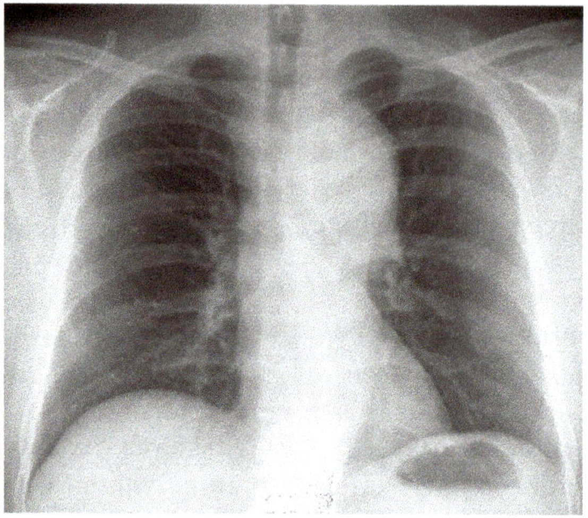

1. **What does the above picture demonstrate?**
2. **What is your diagnosis?**
3. **What are the features in the chest X-ray demonstrate in this disease?**
4. **What should be the CT scan in the chest finding in this disease?**
5. **What should be the transthoracic echocardiography in this disease?**
6. **What should be the medical treatment in this disease?**

Answers

1. The above chest X-ray demonstrates:
   a. Presence of left apical pleural cap
   b. Widening of the upper mediastinum
   c. Enlarged aortic knob
   d. Displacement of the trachea to the left
   e. Clear lungs
   f. Cardiac shadow is not enlarged.
2. The patient has been suffering from acute aortic dissection.
3. Following are the classical features in the chest X-ray:
   a. Left apical flap
   b. Pleural effusion
   c. Deviation of the esophagus
   d. Deviation of the trachea to the right
   e. Depression of the left main stem bronchus
   f. Loss of paratracheal stripe
4. Following are the CT scan of chest findings:
   a. Intimal dissection flap
   b. Double lumen
   c. Aortic dilatation and hematoma
   d. Regions of malperfusion
   e. Leak of contrast leading to rupture of aorta
5. Findings in the transthoracic echocardiography are:
   a. Dissection flap and differential Doppler flow
   b. Thrombosis in the false lumen
   c. In the ascending aorta, presence of true as well as false lumen
   d. Pericardial effusion
   e. Central displacement of intimal calcification
6. Medical treatment of the disease:
   a. Adequate analgesia
   b. Administration of short-acting intravenous β-blockers to maintain the heart rate at 60 beats/min.
   c. In case of contraindication to β-blockers, nondihydropyridine calcium-channel blockers can control the heart rate.
   d. In case of sustained rise in blood pressure, intravenous nitroprusside should be given to maintain the systolic blood pressure of 100–120 mm Hg.
   e. In case of hypotension, intravenous fluid should be given.
   f. Vasopressin can be added.
   g. Surgical therapy:
      • Excision of intimal tear
      • Obliteration of the entry of blood into the false lumen proximally
      • Reconstitution of aorta with interposition of synthetic vascular graft

CASE 88

A 40-year-old patient has been admitted with acute sharp right paravertebral pain. ECG demonstrated features of left ventricular hypertrophy according to voltage criteria in presence of sinus rhythm. CT scan demonstrated no feature of dissection but only the presence of thrombus in the left subclavian artery.

1. **What is the cause of the intravascular hematoma in this patient?**
2. **What is the progression of this hematoma?**
3. **What should be the process of treatment?**

Answers

1. This hematoma is the precursor of dissection as it occurs due to rupture of vasa vasorum within the media along with communication with the lumen due to infarction of the aortic wall.
2. In nearly 47% of cases, it will progress to dissection of the aorta.
3. Methods of treatment:
   a. If it involves ascending aorta, it should be treated surgically because medical management may lead to worse outcome.
   b. If it involves descending thoracic aorta, wait and watch should be the policy.

CASE 89

A 34-year-old woman having known history of Marfan syndrome in childhood but untreated during teenager time, now wants to take child. Her blood pressure is 140/80 mm Hg. Her CT scan of chest demonstrated 44 mm.

1. **What are the risks in this patient when the CT scan diameter of aneurysm is 44 mm?**
2. **What is your advice to the patient?**
3. **What is the risk in this patient based on the diameter of the aneurysm?**
4. **When cesarean section is recommended?**

Answers

1. Following are the risks in this patient:
   a. Patient has increased risk of aortic dissection and aortic aneurysm.
   b. If the diameter is >45 mm, it is a threshold of aortic root replacement.
   c. If annulus and valves are affected, in that case total aortic valve has to be replaced otherwise this valve should be preserved to prevent long-term oral anticoagulation.
2. In case of pregnancy, there is increase in the stroke volume as well as plasma volume. Again, hormonal change will lead to physiological changes in the wall of vessels. These physiological changes make the patient at high risk as aortic root will already been dilated in the last trimester of pregnancy and early postnatal period. Hence, the aortic valve has to be replaced.
3. If the diameter is <40 mm, the risk is 1% and if the diameter is >40 mm, the risk is 10%.
4. Cesarean section is recommended if the diameter is >45 mm.

CASE 90

A 70-year-old man was admitted with sudden onset acute severe back pain for 8 hours followed by sudden weakness. On examination, pulse was 120 beats/min, regular, blood pressure 90/50 mm Hg, and jugular venous pressure elevated. Immediate CT scan done and it demonstrated dissection in aortic arch extending from sinus of Valsalva along with moderate pericardial effusion.

1. **Do you want to drain pericardial effusion immediately?**
2. **Why there is hypotension in this case?**
3. **What is the incidence of mortality after surgical repair?**
4. **What is the incidence of mortality without surgical repair?**

Answers

1. As patient requires urgent surgery, so pericardial effusion drainage will delay to operate which will lead to death of the patient.
2. Hypotension in this is due to the following:
   a. Hemopericardium
   b. Pericardial tamponade
   c. Bleeding into the mediastinum diameter of aneurysm
   d. Acute aortic insufficiency as a result of aortic arch dilatation
   e. Lactic acidosis
   f. Spinal shock
   g. Rupture of aorta
3. Mortality after surgical repair:
   a. 10% on first day
   b. 12% on second day
   c. 20% after 2 weeks
4. Mortality without surgical repair:
   a. 24% on first day
   b. 29% on second day
   c. 20% at 20 weeks

CASE 91

A 66-year-old smoker came to clinic repeated times and blood pressure was 160/95 mm Hg, but home blood pressure monitoring demonstrated 130/80 mm Hg always.

1. **What is the cause of increased clinic blood pressure?**
2. **What is masked hypertension?**
3. **How this type of blood pressure variation can be resolved?**
4. **How can you define hypertension?**
5. **What are the major medications according to JNC-8 guideline?**
6. **What are the lifestyle modifications to be done in this patient?**

Answers

1. White coat hypertension can be defined as the presence of high blood pressure in the clinic but the home blood pressure is normal.
2. Masked hypertension can be defined as occurrence of hypertension in the home or any other setting but increased blood pressure at doctor's clinic.
3. This type of blood pressure variation can be resolved by ambulatory blood pressure monitoring because it can assess the variation in blood pressure over the extended period of time.
4. Definition of hypertension:
   According to JNC-7 guideline:
   a. Normal: <120/80 mm Hg
   b. Prehypertension: 120–139/80–89 mm Hg
   c. Stage 1 hypertension: 140–159/90–99 mm Hg
   d. Stage 2 hypertension: ≥160/100 mm Hg
   Changes in the JNC-8 guideline:
   a. In a patient of ≥80 years old who is nondiabetic and non-CKD, the blood pressure is <150/90 mm Hg.
   b. Patient with ≥18–59 years having no major comorbidities and in patients of >60 years old diabetic or chronic kidney disease, patients blood pressure <140/90 mm Hg.
5. Treatment schedule according to JNC-8 guideline:
   a. First line and later line of treatment:
      - Thiazides
      - Calcium-channel blockers
      - ACEI
      - ARBs
   b. Second and third line of treatment: High dose or combination of ACEI, ARBs, thiazides and calcium-channel blockers.
   c. Alternative drugs in the later line:
      - β-blockers
      - α-blockers
      - α1/β-blockers
      - Vasodilators
      - Central α2-adrenergic agonists
      - Direct vasodilators
      - Loop diuretics
      - Aldosterone antagonists
      - Peripherally acting adrenergic antagonists
6. Following are the lifestyle modifications:
   a. Weight loss—per 10 kg weight loss systolic blood pressure will decrease by 5–20 mm Hg.
   b. Alcohol intake should be limited—less than 30 mL/day in case of male and <15 mL of alcohol daily in case of woman. It will decrease the systolic blood pressure by 2–4 mm Hg.

c. Reduction of daily sodium intake by 6 g decreases of the systolic blood pressure by 2–8 mm Hg.

d. Dietary potassium intake should be 90 mmol/day.

e. Adequate amount of calcium and magnesium should be taken.

f. Smoking should be stopped.

g. Saturated fat and cholesterol should be reduced to improve cardiovascular health.

h. Aerobic exercise 30 minutes daily for most of the days reduces the systolic blood pressure by 4–9 mm Hg.

CASE 92

A 60-year-old diabetic hypertensive man came to hypertensive clinic with headache and vision disturbance. On examination, the blood pressure was 180/105 mm Hg.

1. **What are the characteristics of patients associated with resistant hypertension?**
2. **What are the medications that interfere with decrease in blood pressure?**
3. **What are the features associated with secondary causes of hypertension?**

Answers

1. Following are the characteristics of the patients associated with resistant hypertension:
   a. African American race
   b. Southeastern United States
   c. Older age
   d. Female
   e. Diabetes mellitus
   f. Left ventricular hypertrophy
   g. Female gender
   h. High blood pressure
   i. Excessive ingestion of dietary salt
   j. Chronic kidney disease
   k. Left ventricular hypertrophy

2. Following are the medications interfere with decrease in blood pressure:
   a. Oral contraceptives
   b. Erythropoietin
   c. Nonnarcotic analgesic
   d. NSAIDs
   e. Alcohol
   f. Natural licorice
   g. Sympathomimetic drugs
   h. Cyclosporine
   i. Selective cyclooxygenase-2 (COX-2) inhibitors

3. Following are the features associated with secondary hypertension:

Clinical symptoms and signs	Secondary cause
Female of <35 years of age	Renal artery stenosis due to fibromuscular dysplasia

Continued

Continued

Clinical symptoms and signs	Secondary cause
• Age >55 years • Atherosclerotic patient • Exaggerated drop in blood pressure after starting the ACEI • Abdominal bruit	Renal artery stenosis
Hypokalemia, generalized weakness, high dose of diuretics	Primary hyperaldosteronism

• Use of:
  ○ Birth control pills in younger woman
  ○ Licorice by adult
  ○ Laxatives by older adults
	Mineralocorticoid effect

• Headache • Paroxysm of palpitation • Sweating	Pheochromocytoma
• Raised calcium • Presence of renal calculi	Hyperparathyroidism leading to obstructive uropathy
• Abdominal striae • Truncal obesity	Cushing's syndrome
High blood pressure in the arms and diminished blood pressure in lower limb	Coarctation of aorta
• Polycystic kidney disease • Worsening of kidney function • Small kidney in ultrasound	Chronic kidney disease
• Facial puffiness • Periorbital swelling	Acute glomerulonephritis
• Recurrent urinary tract infection • Inadequately treated urinary tract infection	Chronic pyelonephritis

CASE 93

A 45-year-old smoker and chronic alcoholic male having no past significant history has come to clinic with headache and blood pressure measured was 180/100 mm Hg and body mass index 36. To exclude secondary cause, urinary cortisol was measured and was found increased. At once low-dose dexamethasone test was performed, but it was found to be normal.

1. **Why low-dose dexamethasone suppression test is done?**
2. **In case of positive low-dose dexamethasone suppression test, what test has to be done to confirm this etiology?**
3. **What are the causes of raised level of cortisol?**
4. **In this patient, if low-dose suppression test is normal, what it suggests?**

Answers

1. Low-dose dexamethasone suppression test is done to detect whether the high cortisol level is endogenous.
2. High-dose dexamethasone suppression test should be done to detect whether the source of cortisol is from adrenal gland or pituitary gland.
3. Raised level of cortisol is found in:
   a. Pseudo-Cushing syndrome
   b. Obesity
   c. Depression
4. Normal value of low level dexamethasone suppression test is suggestive of pseudo-Cushing's disease.

CASE 94

A 75-year-old women having history of recurrent pulmonary emboli but no comorbidity has come to emergency department with recurrent respiratory distress for 3 months, she cannot climb more than one stair now along with fluctuation swelling of lower limbs in last 1 month. Her liver function and INR were normal. Echocardiography demonstrated:

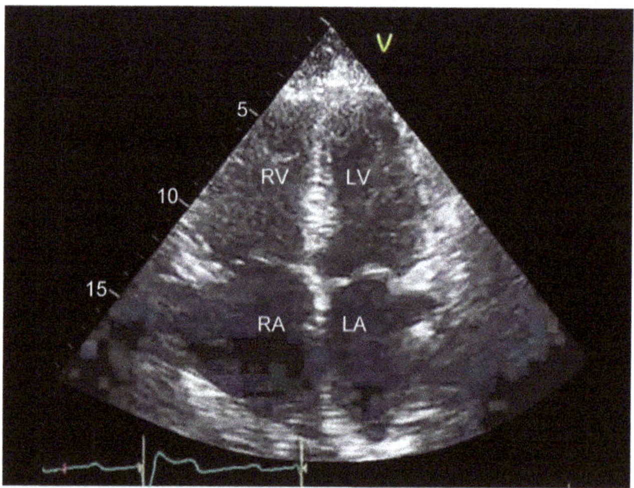

1. **What are the features demonstrated in the echocardiographic picture?**
2. **What is your most likely diagnosis?**
3. **Define this disease.**
4. **Classify pulmonary hypertension.**
5. **How WHO classify the functional status of the patient with this disease?**
6. **What is the hemodynamic definition of this disease?**
7. **What are the factors responsible for survival of pulmonary hypertension?**
8. **How can you treat this patient?**

Answers

1. The above echocardiographic picture demonstrated the following features:
   a. Increased right ventricular to left ventricular ratio
   b. Enlarged right atrium
2. The most likely diagnosis is patient has been suffering from primary pulmonary hypertension.
3. Pulmonary hypertension can be defined as the increase in the mean arterial pressure of ≥25 mm Hg due to cellular proliferation along with luminal narrowing of the small- and medium-sized vessels resulting in increased the vascular resistance thus causing reduced blood flow through the arteries.
4. According to WHO, pulmonary hypertension can be classified into five broad groups:
   a. Group 1: Pulmonary arterial hypertension:
      - Idiopathic variety
      - Inherited causes due to genetic mutation:
         - *BMPR2*
         - *Alk1*
         - *ENG*
         - *SMAD9*
         - *CAV1*
         - *KCNK3*
      - Drugs and toxins
      - Congenital heart disease
      - Collagen vascular disease
      - HIV
      - Portal hypertension
      - Schistosomiasis
      - Persistent pulmonary hypertension
      - Veno-occlusive diseases
   b. Group 2: Pulmonary hypertension as a consequence of left heart diseases
      - Systolic dysfunction
      - Diastolic dysfunction
      - Valvular heart diseases
      - Congenital cardiomyopathy
   c. Group 3: Pulmonary hypertension as a consequence of lung diseases
      - Chronic obstructive lung disease
      - OSA
      - Chronic exposure to high altitude
      - Interstitial lung disease (ILD)
      - Alveolar hypoventilation
      - Developmental anomalies
   d. Group 4: Chronic thromboembolic pulmonary hypertension
   e. Group 5: Pulmonary hypertension with unclear multifactorial mechanisms
      - Hematologic disorders:
         - Chronic hemolytic anemia
         - Myeloproliferative disorders
         - Splenectomy
      - Metabolic disorders:
         - Gaucher disease
         - Glycogen storage disease
         - Thyroid disorders
      - Systemic disorders:
         - Sarcoidosis
         - Lymphangioleiomyomatosis
         - Neurofibromatosis
5. Classification of the functional status in patient with pulmonary hypertension:
   a. Class I: Patient with pulmonary hypertension but without resulting limitation in the physical activity. Ordinary physical activity does not cause undue dyspnea or fatigue, chest pain, or near syncope.
   b. Class II: Patient with pulmonary hypertension resulting in slight limitation of physical activity. They are comfortable at rest. Ordinary physical activity causes undue dyspnea or fatigue, chest pain, or near syncope.
   c. Class III: Patient with pulmonary hypertension resulting marked limitation in the physical activity. They are comfortable at rest. Less than ordinary activity causes undue dyspnea or fatigue, chest pain, or near syncope.
   d. Class IV: Patient with pulmonary hypertension with inability to carry out any physical activity without symptoms. These patients manifest signs of right-sided heart failure. Dyspnea or fatigue may be present even at rest. Discomfort increases by any physical activity.
6. Hemodynamic definition of pulmonary hypertension:

Type of PH	Hemodynamics	Groups of PH
Pulmonary hypertension	Mean pulmonary arterial pressure >25 mm Hg.	Group 1–4
Precapillary pulmonary hypertension	- Mean pulmonary arterial pressure >25 mm Hg - Pulmonary capillary wedge pressure <15 mm Hg - Normal or reduced cardiac output	Group 1, 3, and 4

Continued

Continued

Type of PH	Hemodynamics	Groups of PH
Postcapillary pulmonary hypertension	• Mean pulmonary arterial pressure >25 mm Hg • Pulmonary capillary wedge pressure >15 mm Hg • Normal reduced or increased cardiac output	Group 2

7. Following factors are responsible for survival of pulmonary hypertension:
   a. Increased risk:
      • Demography:
         ○ Male
         ○ Age > 65 years
      • Functional capacity:
         ○ Higher WHO or NYHA class
         ○ Lower 6-minute walk distance
      • Laboratory biomarkers:
         ○ Higher BNP
         ○ Increased creatinine level
      • Echocardiography: Pericardial effusion
      • Lung function test: Lower than predicted diffusion capacity of lung for carbon monoxide.
      • Hemodynamic:
         ○ Higher mean arterial pressure
         ○ Lower cardiac output or cardiac index
         ○ Higher pulmonary vascular resistance or pulmonary vascular resistance index
   b. Decreased risk:
      • Functional capacity:
         ○ Lower WHO/NYHA class
         ○ Higher 6-minute walk test
      • Laboratory data: Lower BNP
      • Lung function test: Higher than predicted diffusion capacity of lung for carbon monoxide.
      • Hemodynamics: Higher cardiac output and cardiac index

8. Following are the approved therapies in this disease:
   a. Endothelin receptor antagonist: Endothelin 1 acts through the differential activation of ETA and ETB receptors leading to pulmonary vasoconstriction and endothelial cell proliferation. Drugs used are:
      • Bosentan and macitentan are the antagonists of both the above receptors.
      • Ambrisentan is the antagonist of ETA receptor.
   b. Prostacyclin agonist: Prostacyclin is the product of arachidonic acid pathway in the vascular endothelium will lead to:
      • Inhibit the proliferation of the smooth muscle cells
      • Promote pulmonary vascular relaxation
   Drugs that are the prostacyclin agonist:
      • Epoprostenol
      • Treprostinil
      • Iloprost
      • Selexipag
   c. Phosphodiesterase-5 inhibitor pathway: Phosphodiesterase-5 inhibitor increases the activity of endogenous nitric oxide resulting from the breakdown of cyclic guanosine monophosphate in the vascular endothelium leading to pulmonary vasodilatation. The phosphodiesterase inhibitors are:
      • Sildenafil
      • Tadalafil
   d. Guanylate cyclase stimulant pathway: These stimulators stimulate nitric oxide receptor and soluble guanylate synthetase thereby performing dual actions:
      • It will increase the sensitivity of soluble guanylate synthetase to endogenous nitric oxide leading to pulmonary vasodilatation.
      • It will also stimulate the receptor thereby mimicking the action of nitric oxide.

CASE 95

A 45-year-old smoker diabetic male having history of amputation of the right leg came to medicine OPD with complaint of intermittent pain during walking for 6 months which progressed to pain in the lower legs when at rest for the last 2 weeks along with presence of ulcer at the left great toe.

On examination, the skin is cold and calm, hair loss on the left leg, painful ulcer along with gangrene of the left great toe, and peripheral pulses are all feeble.

1. **What is the provisional diagnosis?**
2. **What are the points in favour of your diagnosis?**
3. **Define this disease.**
4. **What is the possible pathophysiology of this disease?**
5. **What is the classical radiographic sign found in this disease?**
6. **What are the other causes of gangrene of left great toe?**
7. **What are the diagnostic triad in this disease?**

Answers

1. This patient has been suffering from Buerger's disease.
2. Points in favor of this diagnosis are:
   a. Male sex
   b. Smoker
   c. History of amputation of his right leg
   d. Feeble peripheral pulses
   e. Presence of gangrene along with ulcers on left great toe.
3. Buerger's disease or thromboangiitis obliterans can be defined as progressive, inflammatory segmental vascular disease affecting upper as well as lower limbs.
4. This disease is the result of immunological dysfunction and hypersensitivity to tobacco intake leading to:
   a. Increased cellular sensitivity to two types of collagen—type 1 and type 3.
   b. Impaired endothelium-dependent relaxation of vascular endothelium
   c. Increased titers of antiendothelial antibody
   There may be genetic association in this disease as there is increased prevalence of HLA-A9 and HLA-B5.

As a result:
   a. There is thrombosis in the small as well as medium size arteries and veins.
   b. Aggregation of polymorphonuclear leukocytes
   c. Microabscesses
   d. Presence of multinucleated giant cells
5. The characteristic arteriographic signs in this disease are:
   a. Nonatherosclerotic segmental vascular occlusion involving small and medium size arteries such as tibioperoneal, radioulnar, and digital arteries.
   b. Characteristic "corkscrewing" or "pigtailing" sign: It is characterized by presence of small collateral arteries around the occluded arteries.
6. Other causes of gangrene in this disease are as follows:
   a. Peripheral vascular disease
   b. Bacterial endocarditis
   c. Repeated atheroembolism
   d. Sickle cell anemia
   e. Small vessel vasculitis
7. Classical triad in this disease:
   a. Intermittent classification involving extremities
   b. Raynaud's phenomenon
   c. Migratory superficial vein thrombophlebitis

CASE 96

A 34-year-old male was admitted with severe retrosternal pain radiating to left hand and subsequently diagnosed as acute myocardial infarction and treated with percutaneous coronary intervention. There was family history of premature cardiovascular disease in his father. His lipid profile demonstrated cholesterol level 455 m/dL and low-density lipoprotein (LDL) 282 mg/dL.

On general survey, there was tendon xanthoma.

1. **What is the most likely diagnosis?**
2. **Which genetic mutations responsible for this disease?**
3. **What are genetic types of this disease?**
4. **What are the types of genetic defect in the LDL receptor?**
5. **What is the spectrum of presentations suspicious of this?**

Answers

1. The most likely diagnosis is familial hypercholesterolemia.
2. Following genetic mutations are responsible for this disease:
   a. Defect in the LDL receptor
   b. Defect in the apolipoprotein B
   c. Proprotein convertase subtilisin/kexin type 9

   Each mutation will lead to LDL receptor impairment resulting reduced uptake of LDL cholesterol thereby increasing the concentration of LDL cholesterol.
3. There are two subgroups of this genetic disease:
   a. Autosomal dominant
   b. Codominant transmission with 90% or more penetrance
4. Following are the types of genetic defect in the LDL receptors:
   a. Class 1: Null, this defect is due to defect in the synthesis of LDL receptor.
   b. Class 2: Defective transport where impairment of transport of LDL receptor from the endoplasmic reticulum to Golgi in the cells.
   c. Class 3: There is defect in binding where there is dysfunction of LDL receptor to bind LDL.
   d. Class 4: Defect in the internalization where LDL receptor does not cluster in the clathrin-coated pits thereby minimizing the internalization of LDL by the hepatocytes.
   e. Class 5: Defect in the recycling where LDL receptor is no recycling to cell membrane.
5. Following is the spectrum of presentation in this disease:
   a. In patient of ≤20 years old, fasting serum LDL level ≥ 160 mg/dL or non-HDL cholesterol ≥ 190 mg/dL.
   b. In patient of >20 years old, fasting serum LDL cholesterol ≥ 190 mg/dL or serum non-HDL level ≥ 220 mg/dL.
   c. Presence of familial hypercholesterolemia in the family member or total cholesterol level >240 mg in either parent.
   d. Presence of tendon xanthoma at any age, presence of arcus senilis in patient <45 years of age and yellow orange xanthelasma or tuberous xanthoma in patient having age in-between 20 and 25 years.

CASE 97

A 60-year-old man presented in the medical clinic with chronic nonproductive nonprogressive cough and chest pain for 2 years. His vitals are normal. Cardiovascular and respiratory system examinations were normal. CT scan demonstrated:

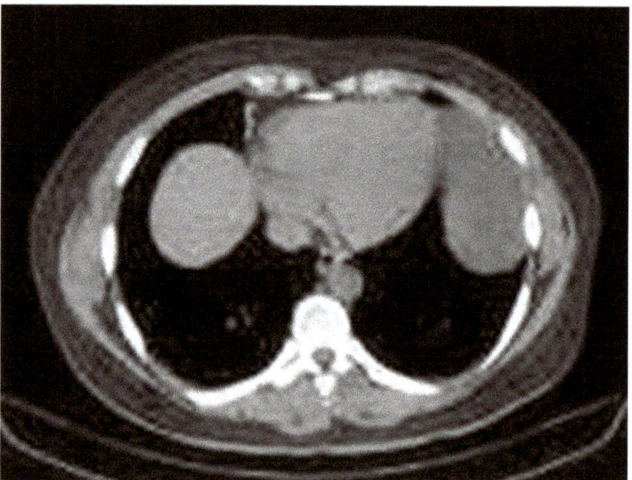

1. **What is the finding in the CT scan of chest?**
2. **What is your diagnosis?**
3. **How this disease is produced?**
4. **What are the complications in this disease?**

Answers

1. This CT scan of chest demonstrated a large well-defined nonenhancing fluid attenuated rounded mass next to pericardium.
2. The most probable diagnosis is pericardial cyst.
3. It is a congenital abnormality where incomplete fusion of pericardial folds in embryogenic development leading to herniation of the pericardial sac looking like diverticulum. But, if the communication with the pericardial cavity will be obliterated, it will form pericardial cyst.
4. Following are the complications in this disease:
   a. Asymptomatic presentation
   b. Compression of the lung due to obstruction of the right main stem bronchus
   c. Compression of the adjacent lobe of the lung
   d. Pericarditis due to infection of the cyst
   e. Rupture of the pericardial cyst leading to:
      - Pneumonitis
      - Pleuropericarditis
   f. Erosion of the cyst into:
      - Superior vena cava
      - Wall of the right ventricle leading to recurrent syncope
   g. Torsion of pericardial cyst leading to chest pain

CASE 98

A 45-year-old man presented in the cardiology OPD with syncope and respiratory distress following several episodes of presyncope for 5 months. Holter monitoring demonstrated the correlation of the syncopal attack with the complete AV dissociation. Then transthoracic echocardiography demonstrated a mass of nearly 20 mm present at the inferior aspect of right atrium.

1. **What is your diagnosis?**
2. **Where it is usually located?**
3. **How it can be demonstrated better?**
4. **What are the complications of this mass?**

Answers

1. The most likely diagnosis is cystic tumor of the AV node known as tawarioma.
2. This rare tumor is multicentric nodule located in the:
   a. Atrioventricular region
   b. Triangle of Koch
   c. Right side of the intra-atrial septum in front of the coronary sinus
3. It can be better demonstrated by angiogram which may demonstrate "tumor flush" or abnormality in the course of AV nodal artery.
4. Following are the complications of this mass:
   a. Sudden death in 10% patients
   b. Complete block in 75% patients
   c. Incomplete heart block in 15% patients

CASE 99

A 60-year-old man came to emergency department with progressively increasing shortness of breath and low-grade fever for 2 months. Urgent chest X-ray was done which demonstrated massive pericardial effusion along with multiple nodular lesions in both the lungs.

Effusion was drained and fluid was yellow colored showing poorly differentiated cells. Urgent CT scan of chest was performed and it again demonstrated a lobulated immobile nonpedunculated mass projecting into right atrium compressing inferior vena cava. At once CT-guided biopsy was performed from that tissue which demonstrated:

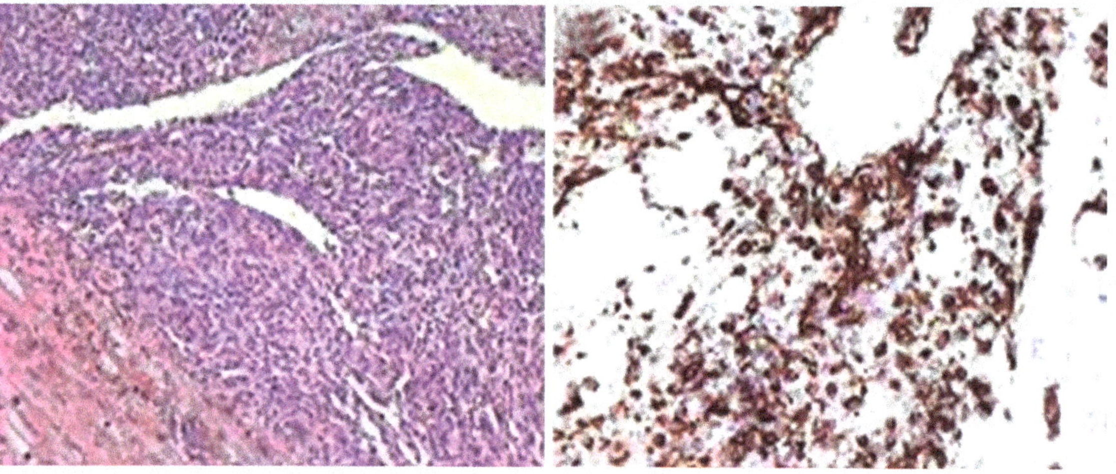

1. **What are the features demonstrated in the biopsy?**
2. **What is your diagnosis?**
3. **What are the symptoms may be presented in this patient?**
4. **What is the most common site of this mass?**
5. **Which is the definite mode of diagnosis?**
6. **What is the mode of differentiation of this mass?**
7. **Is there is any relation of mutation with this disease?**
8. **What are endothelial cell antigens expressed on the tumor?**

Answers

1. Biopsy demonstrated:
   a. Cells are atypical with hyperchromatic nuclei.
   b. These cells are present along the poorly formed immature vessels.
   c. Immunochemical stain CD31 demonstrated endothelial nature of the above tumor cells
2. Patient has been suffering from primary cranial tumor angiosarcoma.
3. Following symptoms may be present in this patient:
   a. Swelling of the lower limbs and congested neck veins with or without abdominal distention.
   b. Features of accumulation of the pericardial fluid such as chest pain, breathing difficulty, and palpitations
   c. Blocking of the distant blood vessels in the different distant organs by the tiny pieces of cardiac tumors depending upon sides of originating tumors.
   d. Arrhythmias
   e. Congestion of faces
   f. Fever
   g. Weight loss
   h. Night sweat
   i. Malaise
   j. Raynaud's phenomenon
4. The most common site of tumor is right atrium.
5. Endomyocardial biopsy is the definite method of diagnosis.
6. Nature of the differentiation is either poorly differentiated or moderately differentiated tumor.
7. Mutations of *TP53* and *KRAS* gene are associated with this disease.
8. Following expression of endothelial cell antigen are present in this tumor:
   a. Factor VIII
   b. Von Willebrand factor
   c. CD31
   d. CD34

CHAPTER 3

Electrocardiogram Cases

A 45-year-old man has been admitted with severe retrosternal pain. Immediately, his electrocardiogram (ECG) was done which demonstrated:

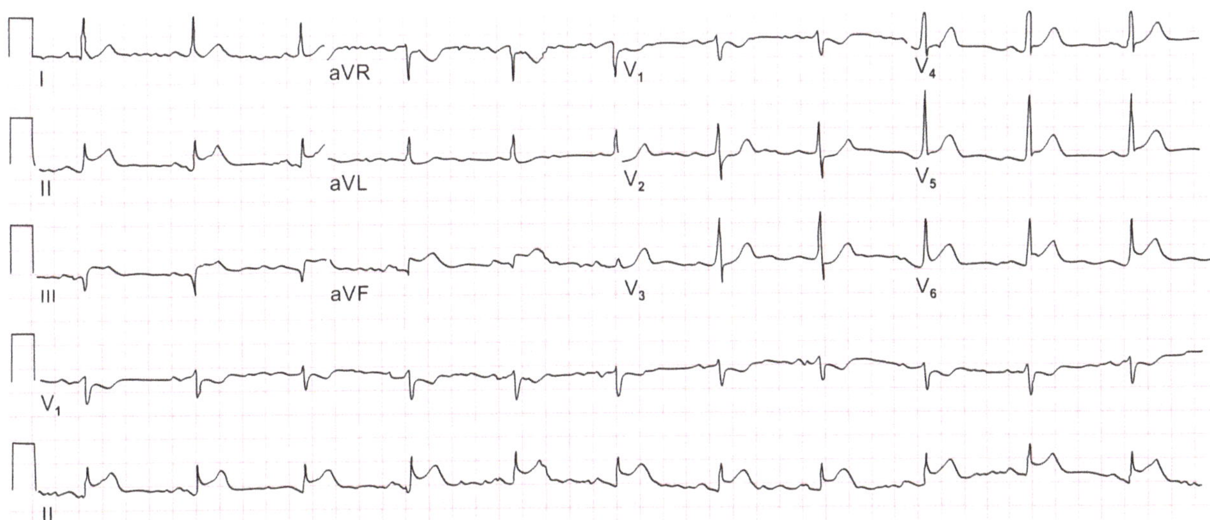

1. **Describe the ECG.**
2. **What is your conclusion?**
3. **Which vessel is the culprit for producing this lesion?**

Answers

1. Description of the ECG:
   a. Rate: 62 beats/min
   b. Rhythm: Regular
   c. Axis: Normal
   d. PR interval: 0.1 second
   e. P wave morphology: Normal
   f. QRS morphology:
      - Q wave is present in LII and aVF.
      - Tall R wave in VII to VIII
   g. ST segment is elevated in LII, LIII, aVF, V_5, and V_6 and depression in V_2 to V_3.
2. Conclusion: Inferolateral infarction
3. Culprit vessel is right circumflex artery.

CASE 2

A 50-year-old woman has been admitted with left-sided chest pain with vomiting. Immediately, her ECG was done which demonstrated:

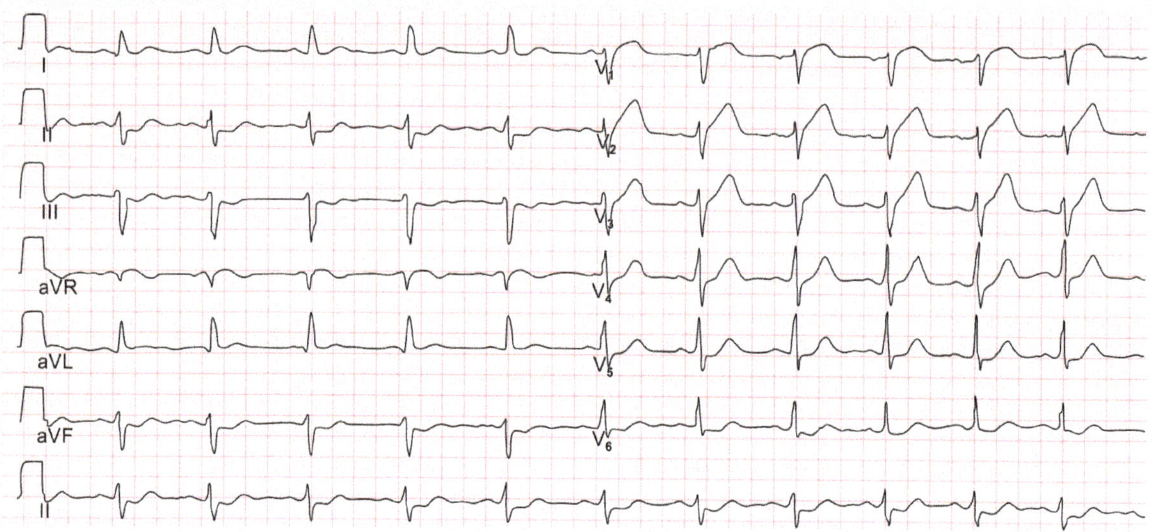

1.   **Describe the ECG.**
2.   **What is your conclusion?**
3.   **Which vessel has been involved?**

Answers

1.   Description of ECG:
    a.   Rate: 75 beats/min
    b.   Rhythm: Regular rhythm
    c.   Axis: Left axis deviation
    d.   P wave: Normal
    e.   PR interval: Normal
    f.   QRS interval: 0.12 second
    g.   QT interval: Normal
    h.   ST segment is elevated in V_1, V_2, V_3, and aVR and reciprocal depression in LII, LIII, and aVF.
2.   Conclusion: Acute anterior wall ischemia with reciprocal changes in inferior wall.
3.   Culprit artery is left main coronary artery.

CASE 3

A 50-year-old man has been admitted with retrosternal pain in intensive coronary care unit. His ECG was done which demonstrated:

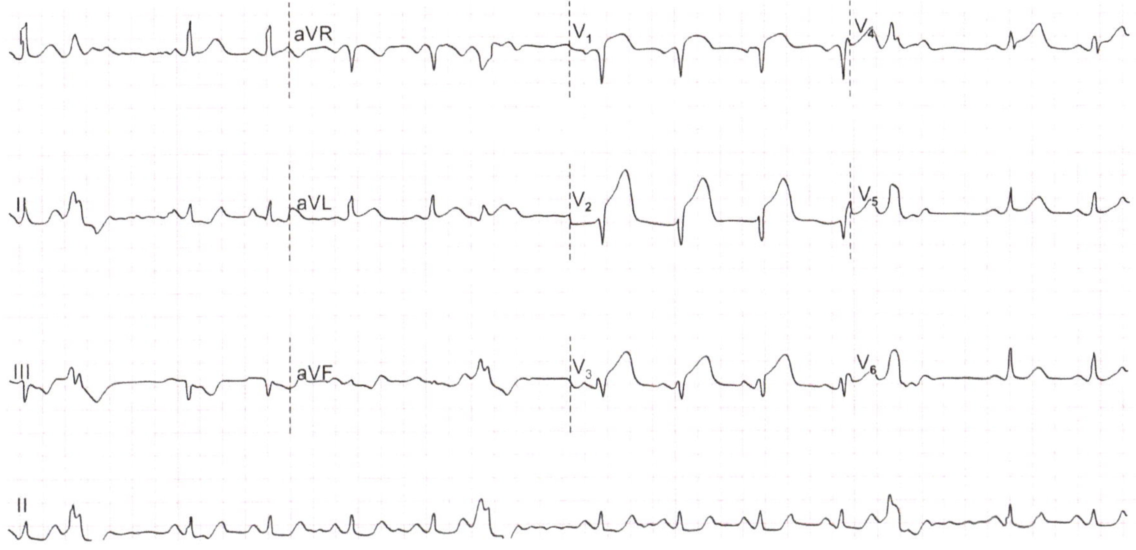

1. **Describe the ECG.**
2. **What is your conclusion?**
3. **Which is the culprit vessel?**

Answers

1. Description of ECG:
   a. Rate: 82 beats/min
   b. Rhythm: Regular with three ventricular ectopic beats
   c. P wave morphology: Normal
   d. PR interval: Normal
   e. QRS morphology:
      - Presence of Q in V_1
      - Poor progression of the R wave
   f. ST segment:
      - Elevation in V_1, V_2, V_3, and V_4
      - Reciprocal depression in LII, LIII, and aVF
2. Conclusion: Acute anterior wall myocardial infarction with reciprocal changes in inferior wall.
3. Culprit vessel is proximal part of left anterior descending artery.

CASE 4

A 57-year-old woman was admitted in intensive coronary care unit with severe chest pain. Her ECG demonstrated:

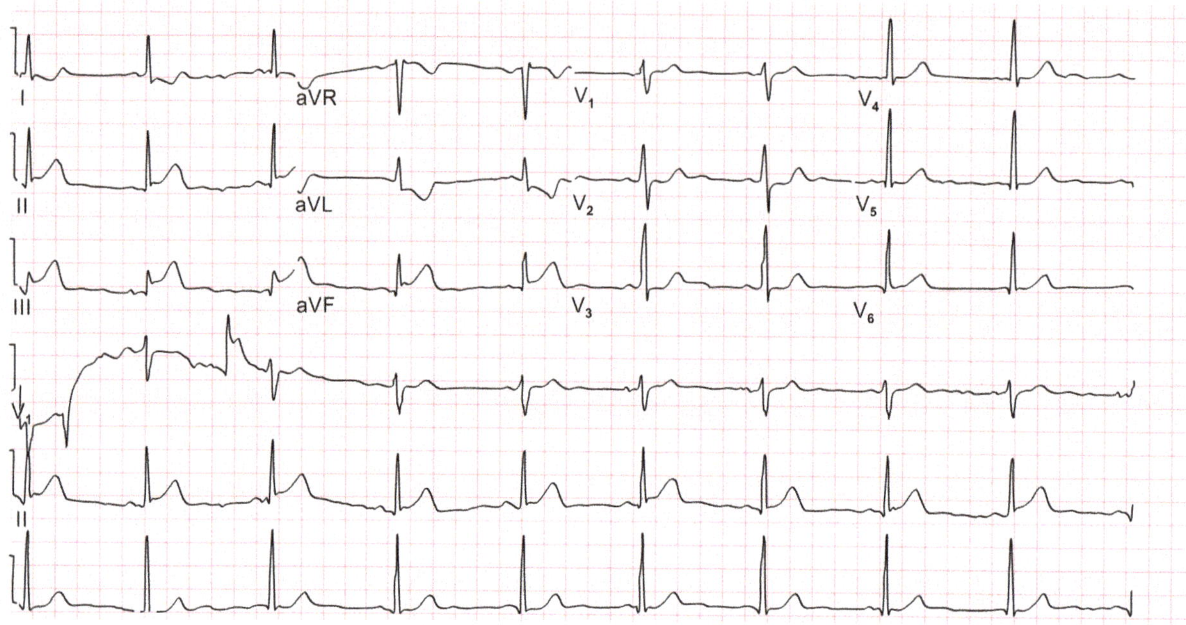

1. **Describe the ECG.**
2. **What is your conclusion?**
3. **Which coronary vessel is involved?**

Answers

1. Description of ECG:
   a. Rate: 56 beats/min
   b. Rhythm: Regular
   c. PR interval: Normal
   d. P wave morphology: Normal
   e. Axis: Normal axis
   f. QRS morphology: Normal
   g. ST segment:
      - Elevated in LII and LIII with more elevation in LIII
      - ST-segment depression in LI, aVL, and V_2
2. Conclusion: Posteroinferior myocardial infarction
3. Culprit vessel is right coronary artery.

CASE 5

A 62-year-old woman has been admitted with severe chest pain with severe headache. Her ECG was done and it was demonstrated:

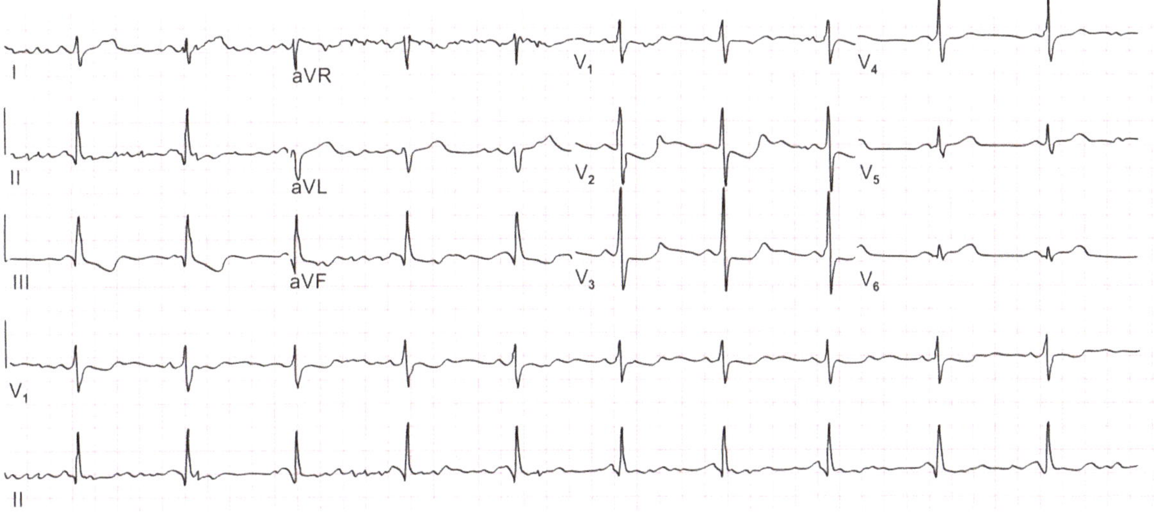

1. **Describe the ECG.**
2. **Derive your conclusion.**
3. **Which vessel is the culprit?**

Answers

1. Description of ECG:
   a. Rate: 62 beats/min
   b. Rhythm: Regular
   c. Axis: Normal
   d. P wave morphology: Normal
   e. PR interval: Normal
   f. QRS morphology: Tall R wave is seen in V_1 and V_2
   g. ST segment:
      - It is elevated in LI and aVL.
      - It is depressed in LII and aVF and V_2 and V_3.
2. Conclusion: Posterolateral myocardial infarction.
3. The culprit vessel is right coronary artery.

CASE 6

A 56-year-old lady has been admitted with severe retrosternal pain in intensive coronary care unit. Her ECG demonstrated:

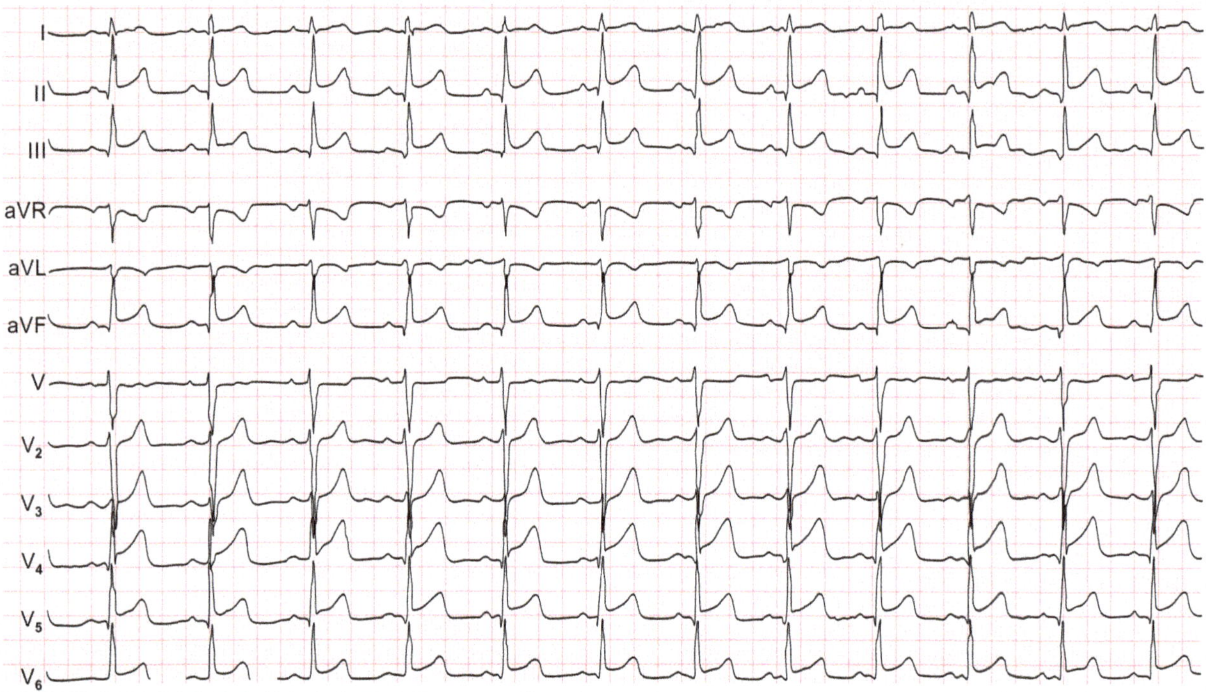

1. **Describe the ECG.**
2. **What is your conclusion?**
3. **Which artery is the culprit artery?**

Answers

1. Description of the artery:
   a. Rate: 74 beats/min
   b. Rhythm: Regular
   c. Axis: Normal
   d. P wave morphology: Normal
   e. PR interval: Normal
   f. QRS morphology: Normal
   g. ST segment:
      - Elevated in LII, LIII, aVF, V_4, V_5, and V_6.
      - Depressed in aVR
2. Conclusion: Inferolateral myocardial infarction.
3. Culprit vessel is distal part of left anterior descending artery.

CASE 7

A 51-year-old smoker has been admitted in intensive care unit (ICU) with postprandial retrosternal pain in ICU. His ECG demonstrated the following:

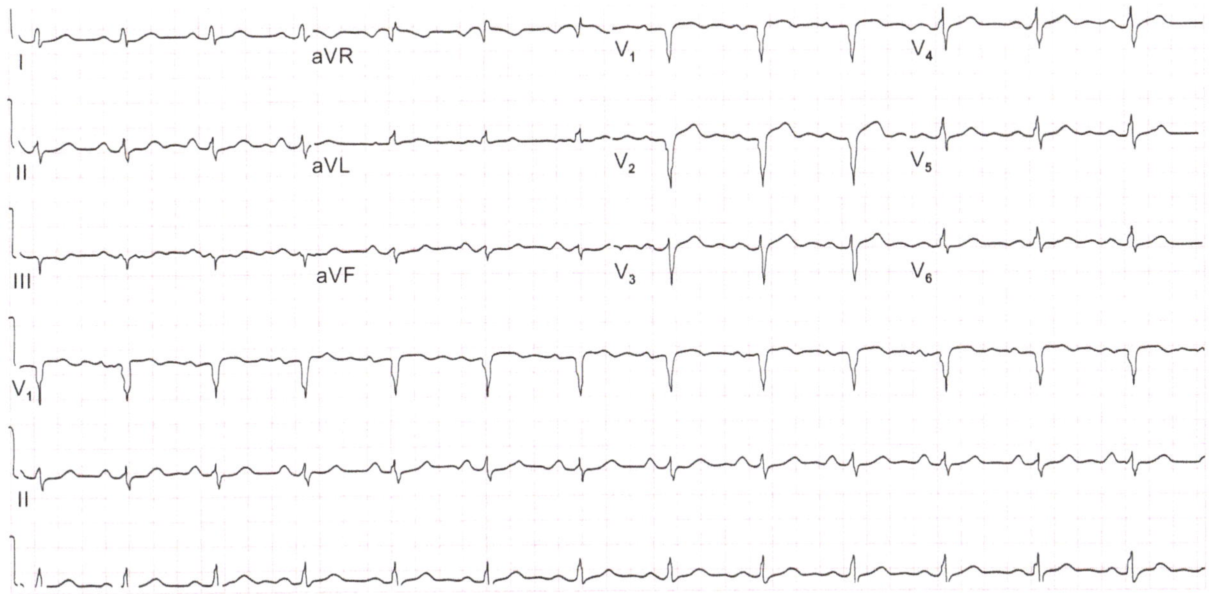

1. **Describe the ECG.**
2. **What is your conclusion?**
3. **Which vessel is the culprit?**

Answers

1. Description of the ECG:
   a. Rate: 75 beats/min
   b. Rhythm: Regular
   c. Axis: Normal
   d. PR interval: Normal
   e. P wave morphology: Normal
   f. QRS morphology: QS pattern in V_1 and V_2.
   g. ST segment: It is elevated in V_1 to V_4.
2. Conclusion: Anteroseptal myocardial infarction.
3. Culprit vessel is left anterior descending artery.

CASE 8

A 65-year-old man was admitted with pain in the retrosternal region. His ECG demonstrated the following:

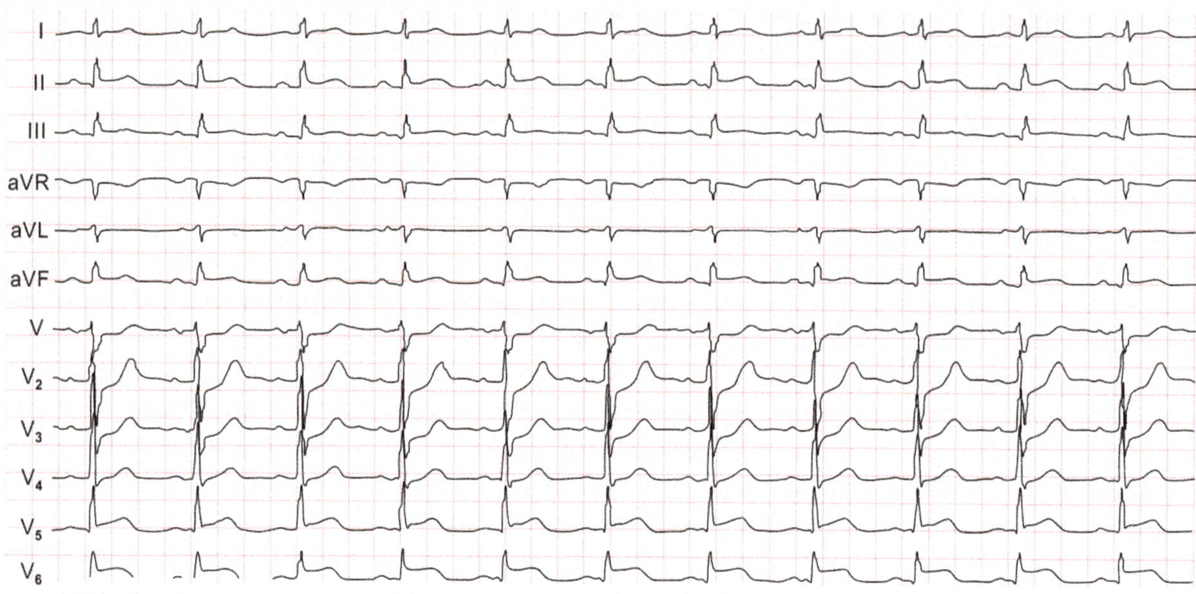

1. **Describe the ECG.**
2. **What is your conclusion?**
3. **Which vessel is the culprit?**

Answers

1. Description of ECG:
   a. Rate: 76 beats/min
   b. Rhythm: Regular
   c. Axis: Normal
   d. P wave morphology: Normal
   e. PR interval: Normal
   f. QRS morphology: Tall R in V_2 and V_3
   g. ST segment:
      - Elevated in LII, LIII, aVF, V_5, and V_6
      - Depressed in V_1, V_2, V_3, and V_4
2. Conclusion: Inferolateral myocardial infarction.
3. Culprit artery is right circumflex artery.

CASE 9

A 78-year-old woman was admitted in the hospital with severe chest pain. Her ECG demonstrated:

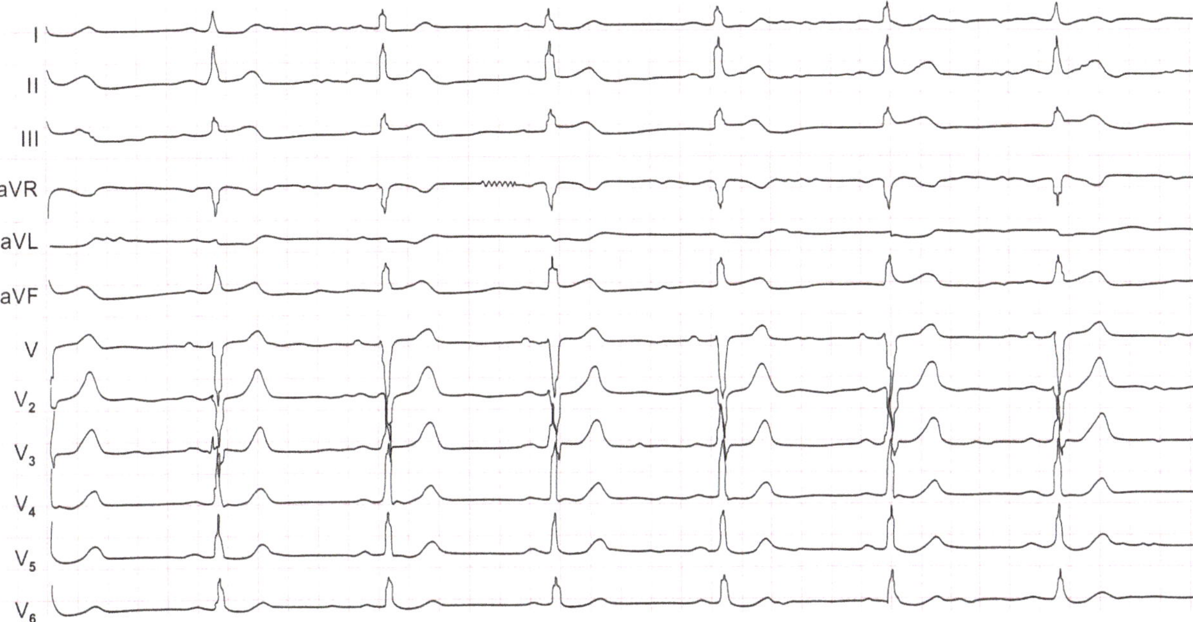

1. **Describe the ECG.**
2. **What is your diagnosis?**
3. **Which vessel is the culprit?**

Answers

1. Description of ECG:
   a. Rate: 55 beats/min indicating sinus bradycardia
   b. Rhythm: Regular
   c. Axis: Normal
   d. P wave morphology: Normal
   e. PE interval: Normal
   f. QRS morphology: Normal
   g. ST segment:
      - Elevated in LII, LIII, and aVF
      - Depressed in LI, aVL, V_4, V_5, and V_6
2. Inferior wall myocardial infarction with reciprocal changes in the anterior wall.
3. Culprit vessel is right coronary artery.

CASE 10

A 59-year-old man has been admitted in the intensive coronary care unit with following ECG:

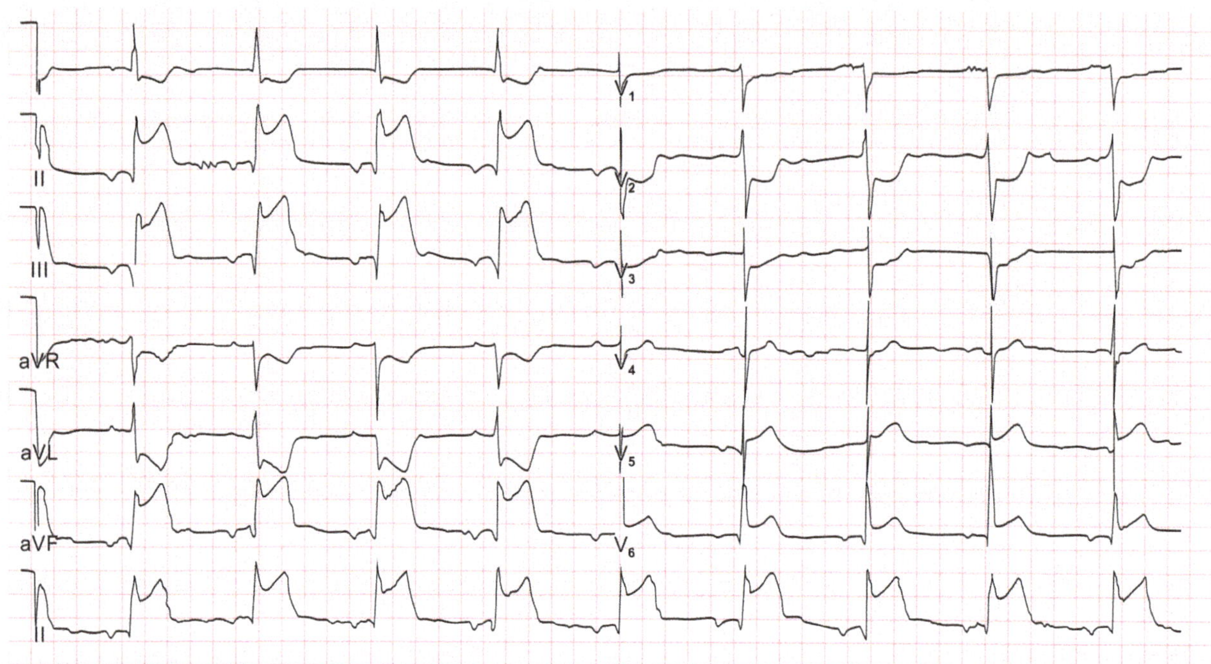

1. **Analyze the ECG.**
2. **What is your diagnosis?**
3. **Which coronary artery has been involved?**

Answers

1. Description of the ECG:
   a. Rate: 58 beats/min indicating sinus bradycardia
   b. Rhythm: Regular
   c. Axis: Normal
   d. P wave morphology: Normal
   e. PR interval: Normal
   f. QRS morphology: Normal
   g. ST segment:
      - Elevated in LII, LIII, aVF, V_5, and V_6
      - Depressed in LI and aVL
2. Diagnosis is inferior wall myocardial infarction with reciprocal changes in the anterior wall.
3. Artery involved is right coronary artery.

CASE 11

A 45-year-old smoker male was admitted with severe left-sided chest pain radiating to the left arm. His ECG demonstrated:

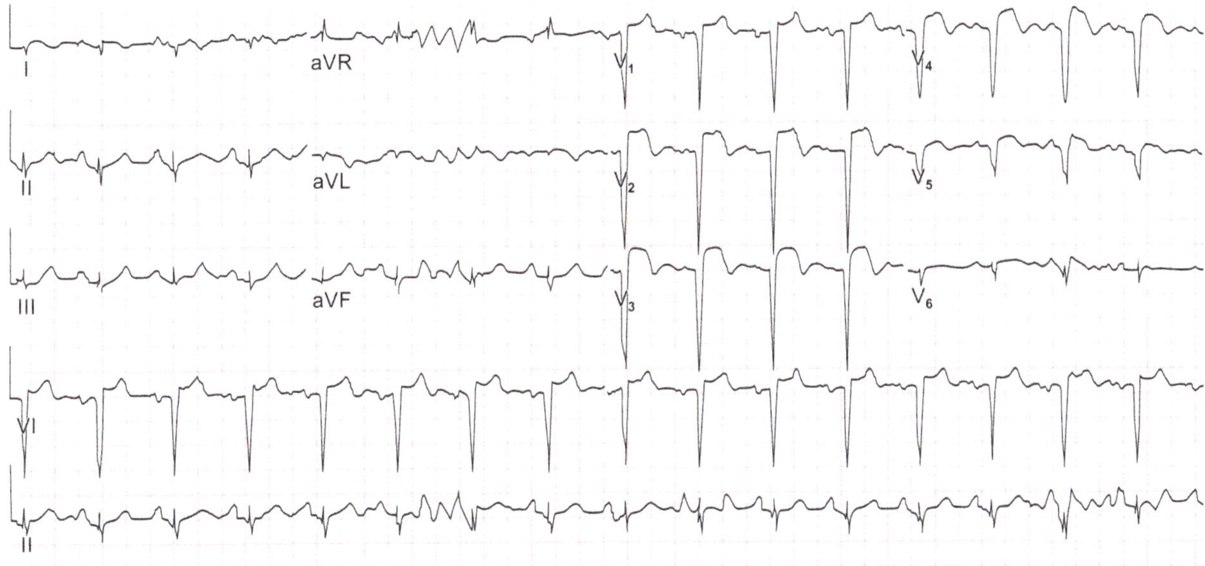

1. **Interpret the ECG.**
2. **What is your conclusion?**
3. **Which artery has been involved?**

Answers

1. Interpretation of ECG:
    a. Rate: 102 beats/min indicating sinus tachycardia
    b. Rhythm: Regular
    c. Axis: Normal
    d. P wave morphology: Tall in lead II indicating right atrial dilatation
    e. PR interval: Normal
    f. QRS morphology:
        - Loss of R wave in V_1 to V_6
        - QS wave in V_5 and V_6
    g. ST segment: Elevated in V_1 to V_5

2. Conclusion: Extensive anterior wall myocardial infarction.

3. Culprit coronary artery is left anterior descending artery.

CASE 12

A 65-year-old male has been admitted in the hospital with left-sided chest pain. His ECG demonstrated:

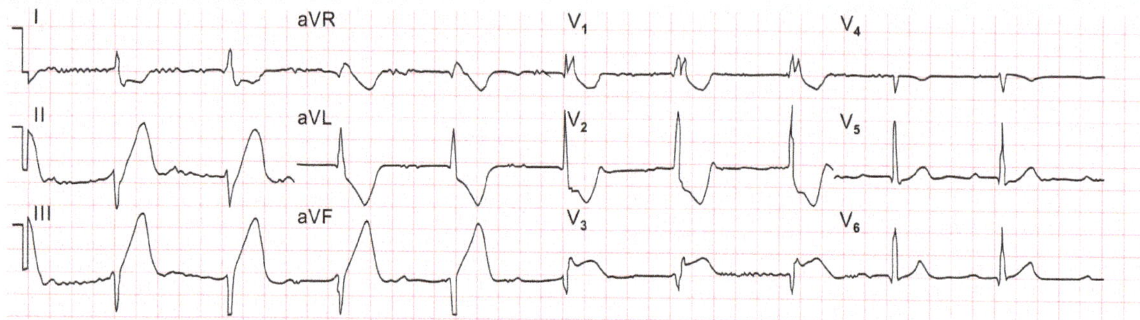

1. **Interpret the ECG?**
2. **What is your diagnosis?**
3. **Which artery is involved?**

Answers

1. Interpretation of ECG:
   a. Rate: 58 beats/min
   b. Rhythm:
      - In V_1 to V_3, there is no relation between P and QRS waves indicating ventricular escape rhythm
      - There is RsR' pattern in V_1.
      - In V_4 to V_6, the QRS waves are preceded by P waves indicating normalization to sinus rhythm.
   c. P wave morphology:
      - In V_4 to V_6: Normal
      - In aVF: It is positive.
      - In aVR: It is negative.
   d. QRS morphology:
      - Right bundle branch block pattern in V_1
   e. QRS duration: 0.11 seconds but in case of wide complexes it is 0.16 seconds.
   f. Axis: There is left axis deviation.
   g. QT interval: 400 ms
   h. ST segment:
      - Elevated in LII, LIII, and aVF
      - Depressed in LI, aVL, V_1, and V_2
   i. T wave: It is hyperacute in LI, aVL, V_1, and V_2.
2. Diagnosis:
   a. Inferior wall myocardial infarction with reciprocal changes in anterior wall
   b. Transient atrioventricular (AV) block with ventricular escape rhythm followed by sinus rhythm.
   c. Right bundle branch block pattern
   d. Left axis deviation
3. Coronary artery involved is right coronary artery.

CASE 13

A 60-year-old man was admitted with right-sided chest pain with severe sweating. His ECG was given as below:

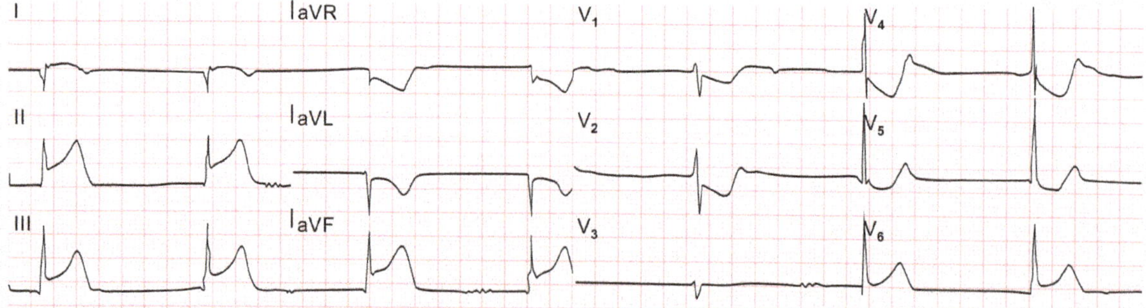

1. **Interpret the above ECG.**
2. **What is your diagnosis?**
3. **Which artery has been involved?**

Answers

1. Interpretation of ECG:
   a. Rate: 40 beats/min
   b. Rhythm:
      - Regular
      - Absence of P wave
      - Narrow QRS complexes indicating nodal escape rhythm
   c. Axis: Right axis deviation
   d. P wave: It is completely absent
   e. QRS morphology:
      - Absence of pathological Q wave
      - Normal progression of R wave in the precordial leads
      - Presence of a notch at the terminal part of QRS complexes in V_5 and V_6
   f. ST segment:
      - Elevated in LI, LII, LIII, and aVF
      - Depression in aVL and V_1 to V_5
2. Diagnosis:
   a. Inferolateral myocardial infarction with reciprocal changes in the anterior wall
   b. Escape nodal rhythm at regular rhythm
3. Artery involved: Right circumflex artery.

CASE 14

A 45-year-old male has come to emergency department with palpitation and syncope. His ECG demonstrated:

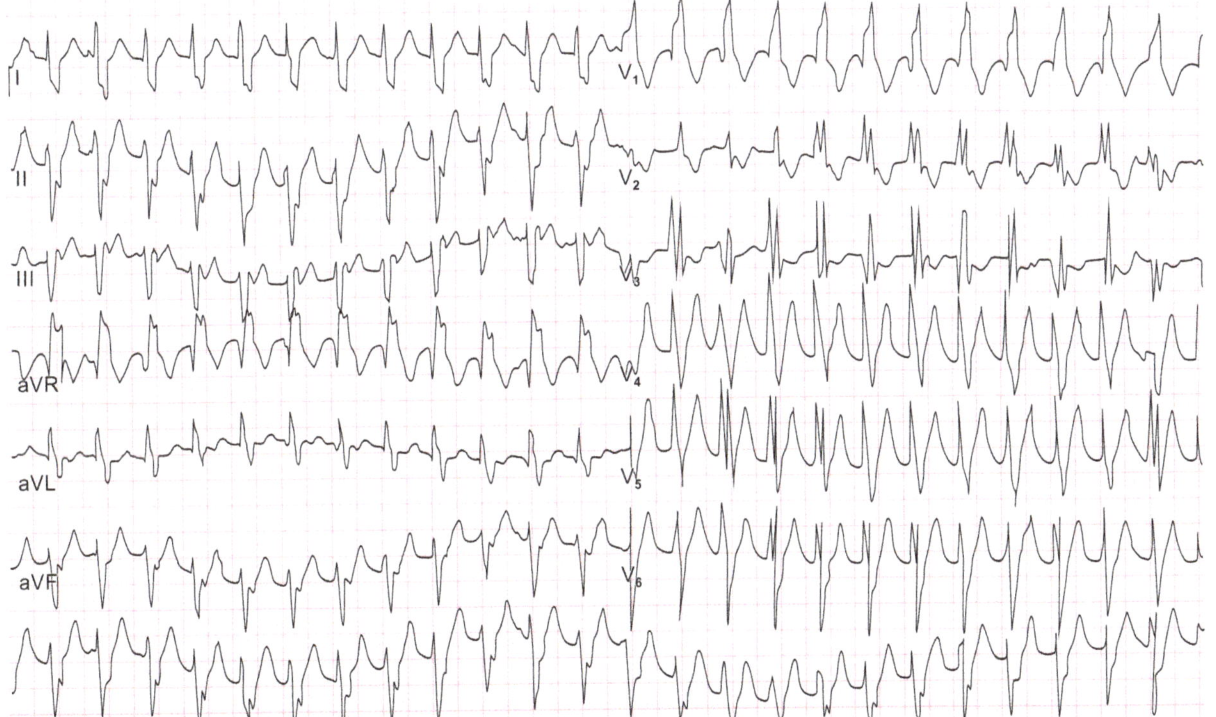

After administration of calcium channel blocker:

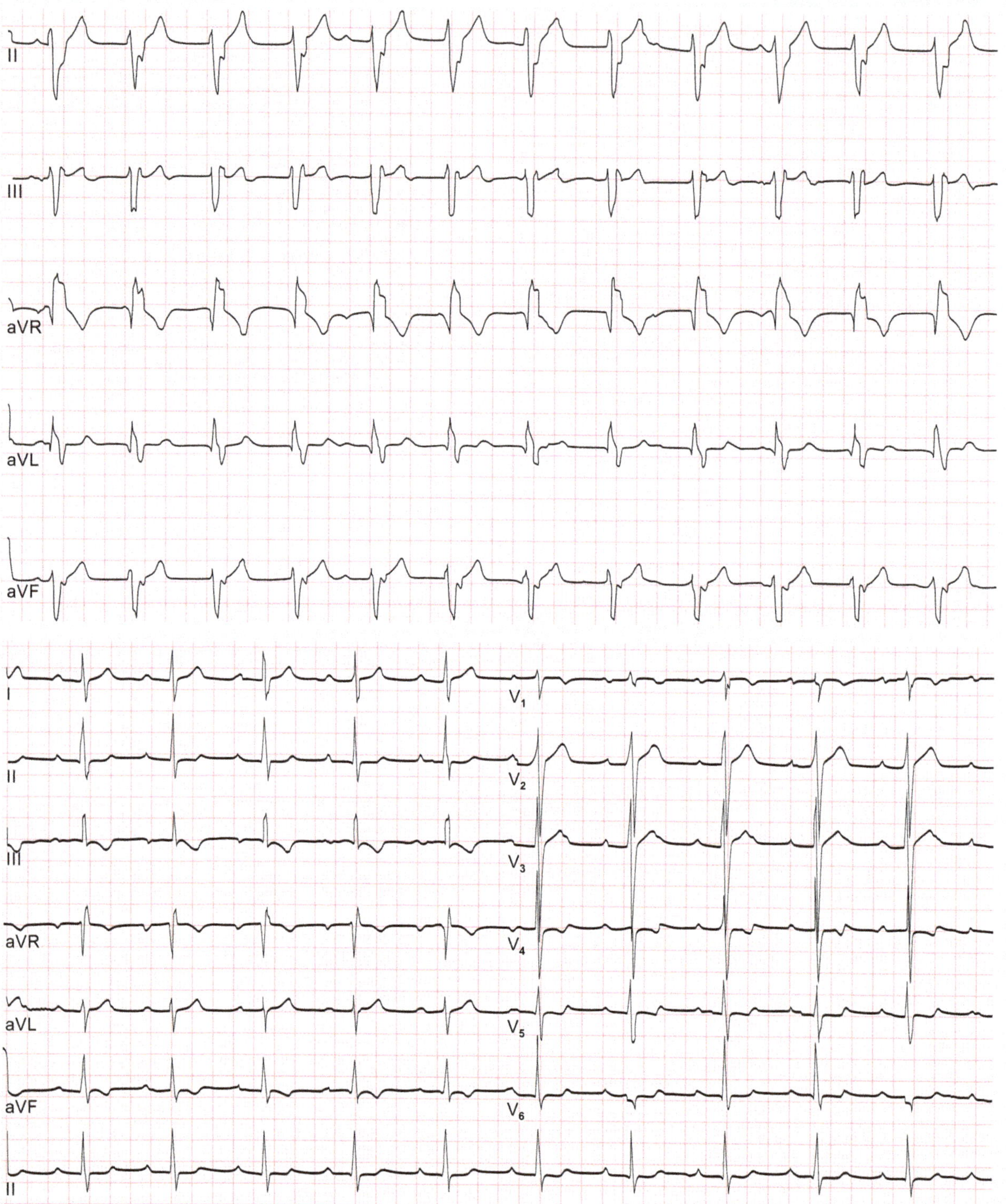

1.   **Interpret the above serial ECGs.**
2.   **What is your interpretation?**

Answers

1.   *Above first picture demonstrates*:
     a.   Rate: 160 beats/min
     b.   Rhythm: Regular
     c.   Axis: Extreme axis
     d.   In V_1, right bundle branch block pattern
     e.   R to S ratio is not >100 ms.
     f.   Absence of fusion beats
     g.   There is complete dissociation.
2.   Conclusion: Ventricular tachycardia.

In the second picture after administration of vera-pamil:
a.   There is slowing of ventricular tachycardia.
b.   Atrioventricular dissociation is more evident.

In the third picture:
a.   There is sinus rhythm.
b.   All Ps are evident.
c.   Each P is followed by QRS wave.
d.   PR interval is normal.
e.   Duration of QRS is normal.

CASE 15

An 80-year-old patient has been admitted with palpitation having not under medication and no significant past history. On examination, pulse is irregularly irregular with pulse deficit of 20 beats/min.

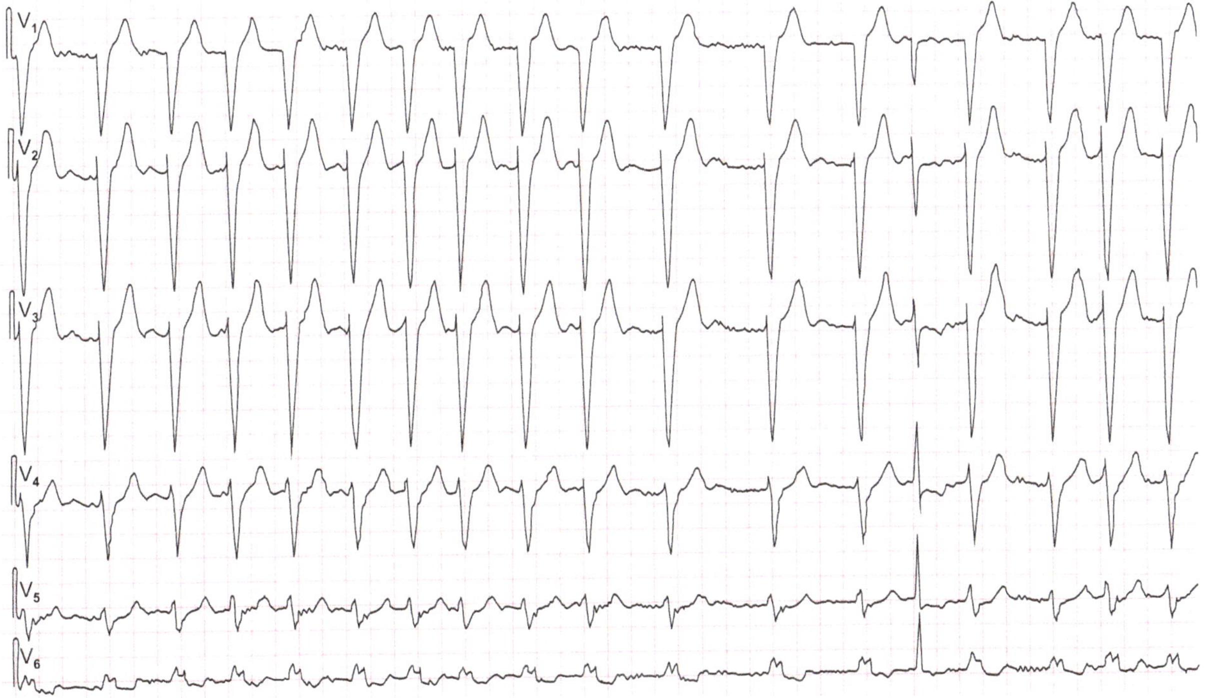

1.   **Interpret the ECG.**
2.   **What are the explanations of this QRS complexes?**

Answers

1.   Interpretation:
     a.   P wave is absent.
     b.   QRS demonstrates left bundle branch block pattern. But, the morphology of QRS complexes is narrow.
2.   Following are the two explanations of this type of QRS complexes:
     a.   It may be due to aberrant conduction through the right bundle branch with slowing of conduction through the left bundle which occurs during longest RR interval in case of atrial fibrillation.
     b.   Appearance of ventricular ectopy in the left bundle during that time when impulse already passes through the right bundle.

Hence in both cases, QRS morphology looks like normal.

CASE 16

A 5-year-old male has come to emergency department with palpitation. Two years ago, the patient developed irregular pulses with tachycardia for which he was prescribed digoxin for controlling the faster heart rate. Physical examination revealed only irregular pulses. Chest X-ray and echocardiography were normal. His ECG demonstrated:

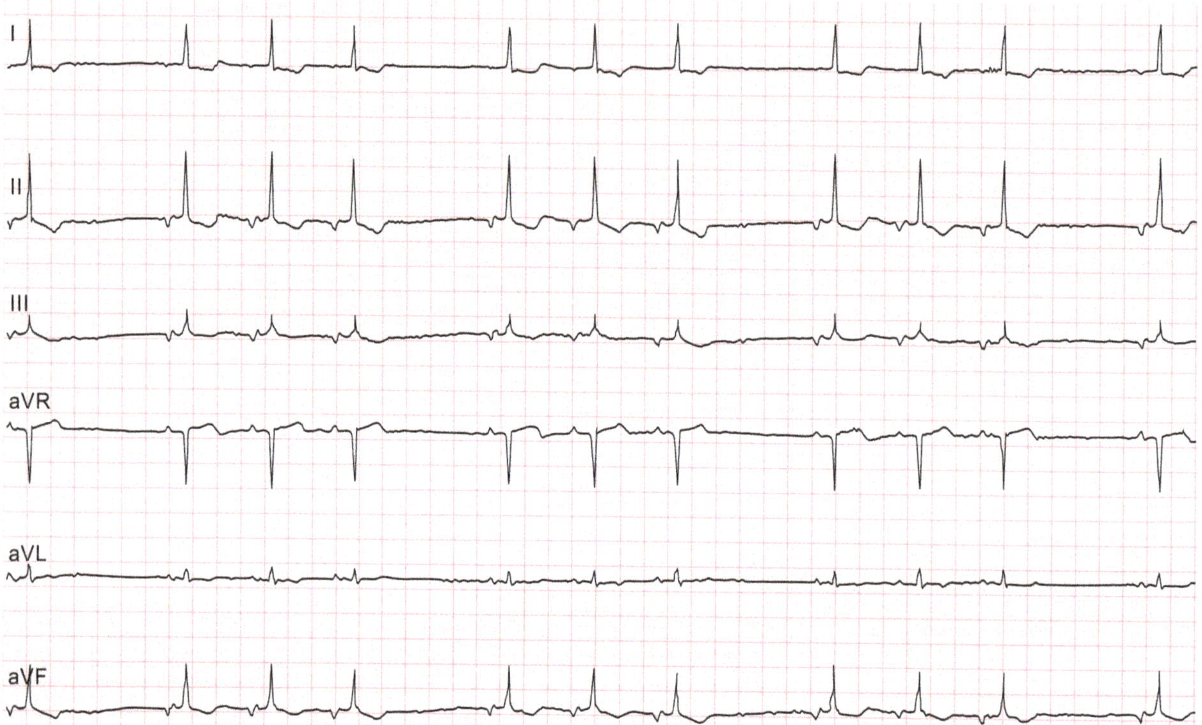

1. **Interpret the ECG findings.**
2. **What is your diagnosis?**
3. **What is the effect of digoxin here?**
4. **How this feature can be reverted?**

Answers

1. Interpretation of ECG:
   a. Rate: 42–96 beats/min
   b. Rhythm: Irregular
   c. Morphology of P wave: Negative deflection in the LI, LI, LIII, aVF leads and positive in aVR—it indicates that P wave originates from left atrium.
   d. After every fourth beat, atrial impulse fails to originate as there is no P wave.
   e. Conduction and the AV and ventricular level are normal.
2. Diagnosis is ectopic focus from left atrium with pause after every third ventricular complexes.
3. There is no evidence of AV block, hence effect of digoxin cannot be considered as the cause of this ECG feature.
4. This can be reverted by cardioversion.

CASE 17

A 60-year-old male came to outdoor with complaint of recurrent syncope having no triggering factor. He had no other medical history. On physical examination, only pulse rate was 42 beats/min, no other abnormal systemic findings were noted. His ECG finding was:

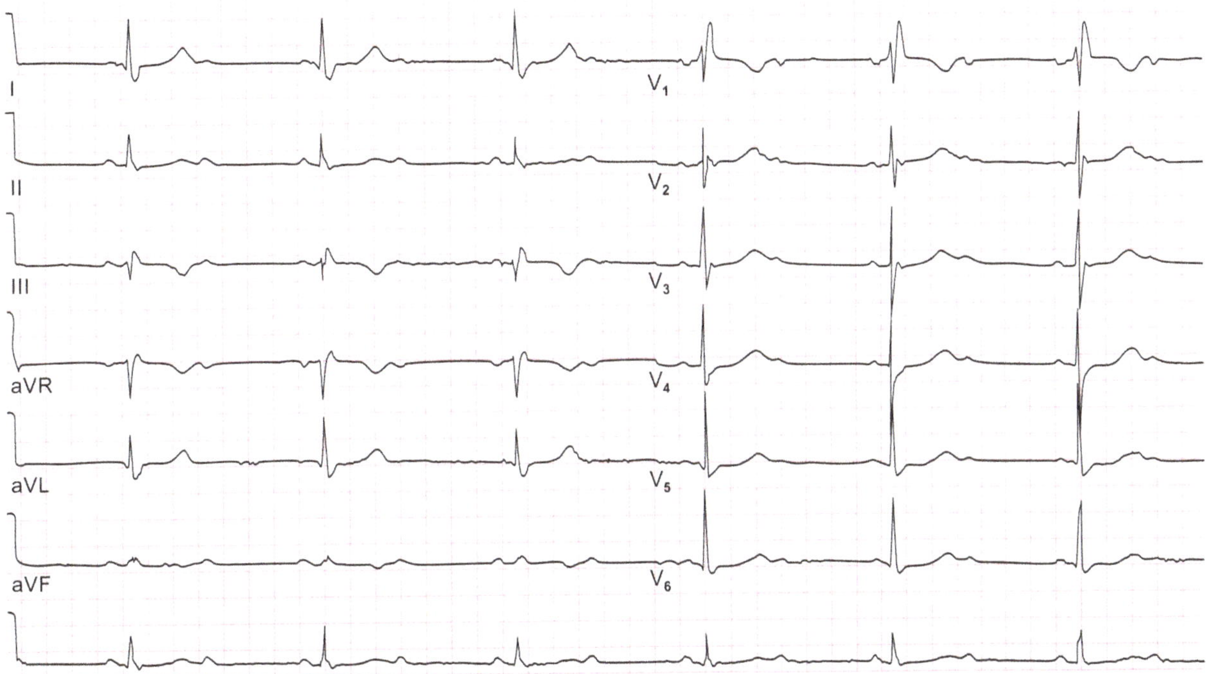

1. **How can you interpret this ECG?**
2. **What is your diagnosis?**
3. **What should be definite therapy?**

Answers

1. Interpretation of ECG:
   a. Rate:
      - Ventricular rate: 38 beats/min
      - Atrial rate: 75 beats/min
   b. Rhythm: There is 2:1 block; hence the rhythm is regularly irregular.
   c. In all the leads except V_1, the P wave following QRS wave can be accepted as U wave, but in the V_1, P wave is clearly visible.
   d. There is RSR' pattern seen in V_1.
2. Diagnosis is fixed second-degree heart block with right bundle branch block.
3. As the patient developed symptomatic bradycardia in the form of syncope, permanent pacemaker should be done in this patient.

CASE 18

A 56-year-old man with history of smoking and family history of ischemic heart disease was suddenly collapsed after 2 hours of anginal pain in the hospital. Instant ECG demonstrated ventricular fibrillation which was reverted by defibrillator. Just after reversion ECG was taken:

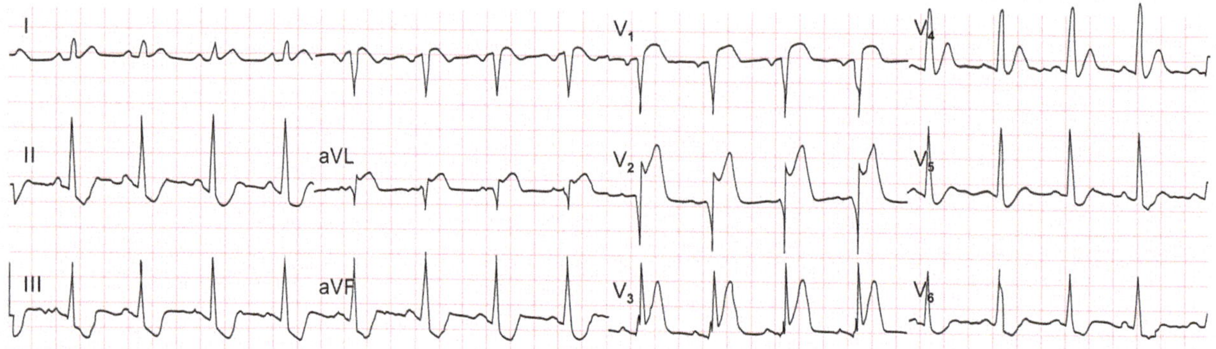

1. **Interpret this ECG.**
2. **Which artery is the culprit?**

Answers

1. Interpretation of ECG:
   a. Rate: 135 beats/min
   b. Rhythm: Regular
   c. Axis: Normal
   d. P wave morphology: Normal
   e. PR interval: Normal
   f. QRS morphology: Normal
   g. ST segment:
      - Elevated with pathological Q waves in the right precordial leads
      - Elevated in LI and aVL.
      - Reciprocal depression in LII, LIII, and aVF
2. All the features are suggestive of occlusion of left anterior descending artery.

Second ECG demonstrates:

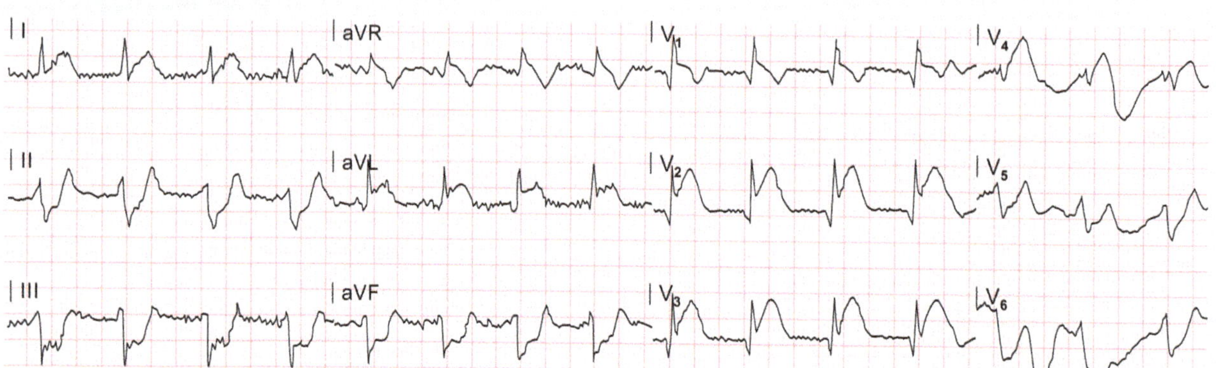

1. **Interpret the second ECG.**
2. **Which artery is involved?**

Answers

1. Interpretation:
   a. Rate: 100 beats/min
   b. Rhythm: Regular
   c. Axis: Left axis deviation
   d. P wave is absent.
   e. QRS complexes:
      - Widened
      - In V_1, there is RSR' pattern.
      So there is bifascicular block.
2. Right bundle branch block along with involvement of left anterior fascicle suggests septal branch of proximal left anterior descending artery.

CASE 19

A 30-year-old corporate worker after a bout of heavy drinking at weekend has come to emergency room with sudden palpitation.

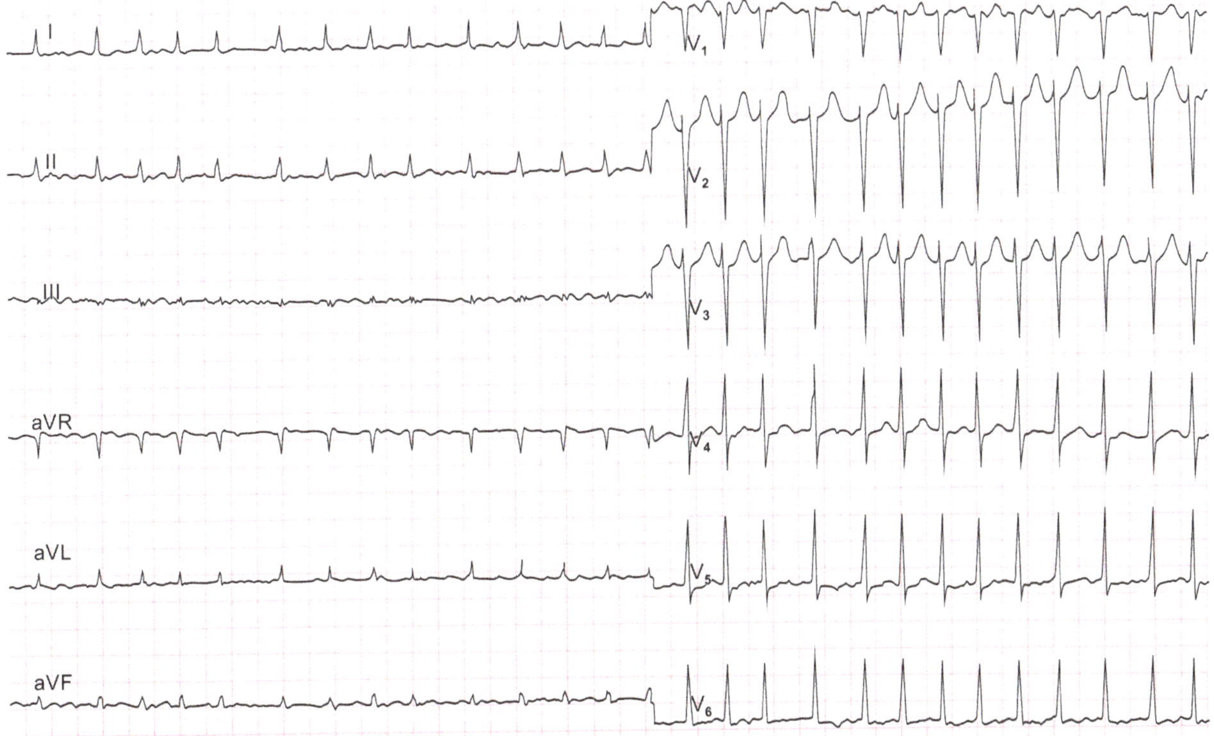

1. **Interpret ECG.**
2. **What is your diagnosis?**

Answers

1. Interpretation:
   a. Rate: 100–152 beats/min
   b. Rhythm: It is highly irregular.
   c. Axis: Normal axis
   d. P wave: It is not present.
   e. PR interval: As there is P wave, there is no question of PR interval.
   f. QRS complex: Normal
   g. T wave: Normal
   h. ST segment: Normal
   i. QTc: Normal
2. Diagnosis: Atrial fibrillation with rapid ventricular rate—indicative of "holiday heart syndrome".

CASE 20

A 60-year-old male was admitted in intensive care unit with palpitation and dizziness with Glasgow Coma Scale of 14, blood pressure of 90/50 mm Hg, and heart rate of 180 beats/min. His ECG demonstrated:

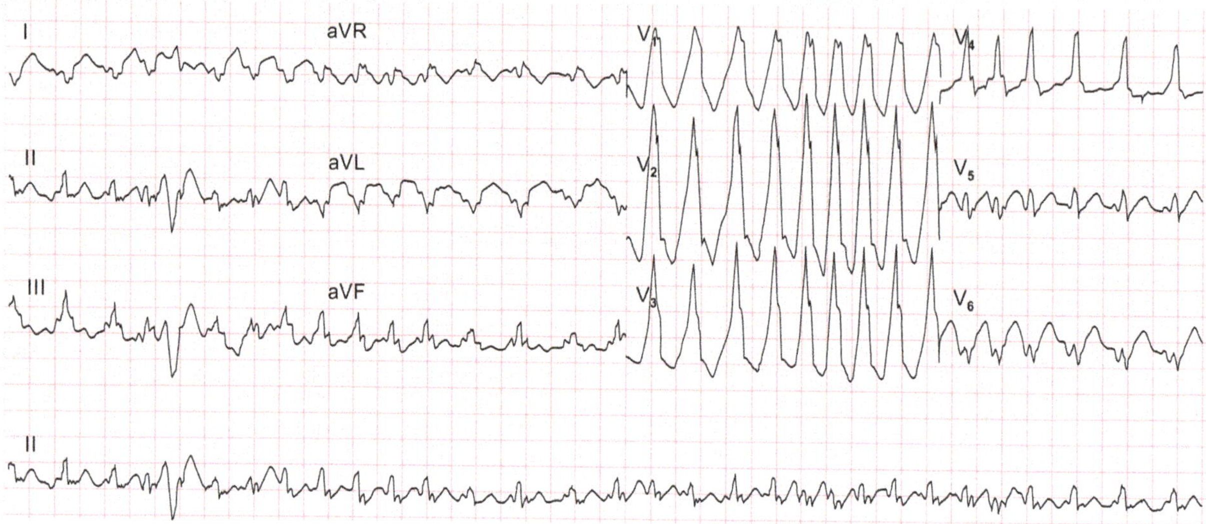

1. **Interpret the ECG.**
2. **What is your diagnosis?**
3. **Is there are any point in favor of preexcitation?**
4. **After what treatment, ECG has been changed to following?**

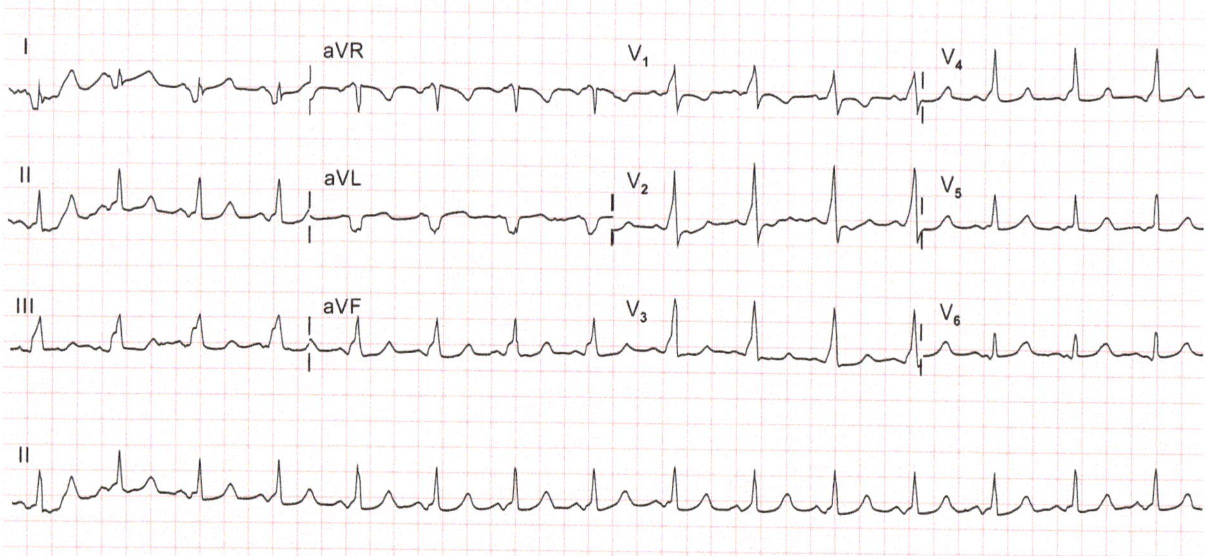

5. **What is the interpretation in ECG?**
6. **Why AV nodal blocking is contraindicated in this patient?**

Answers

1. Interpretation of ECG:
   a. Rate: 185 beats/min
   b. Rhythm: Irregularly irregular complexes
   c. Complexes are broad.
   d. P wave: Not clearly visible
   e. QRS morphology demonstrates right bundle branch block pattern
   f. There is ST-T wave changes.
2. Diagnosis: Atrial fibrillation with delayed conduction due to right bundle branch block or preexcitation.

3. Yes:
   a. Ventricular rate is 300 beats/min, which is not conducted through the AV node.
   b. There are variations in the QRS complex morphology.
4. DC cardioversion can reverse this to sinus rhythm making the hemodynamics stable.
5. Second ECG demonstrates the following features:
   a. Rate: 90 beats/min
   b. Rhythm: Regular
   c. P wave morphology: Normal
   d. Axis: Right axis deviation
   e. PR interval: <0.12 seconds
   f. QRS morphology:
      - Wide with slurred upstrokes indicating the appearance of delta wave
      - Tall R wave in V_1 indicates left-sided accessory pathway—suggests type A Wolff–Parkinson–White (WPW) syndrome.

- Delta wave is negative in aVL—it mimics Q wave in lateral infarction—it is known as pseudoinfarction.
- In right precordial leads, R wave is tall mimicking right ventricular hypertrophy.

6. Adenosine, β-blocking agents, and calcium channel blocker are contraindicated because:
   a. As the refractory period in the accessory pathway is shorter as compared to AV nodal pathway, there is chance of very rapid ventricular rate.
   b. Antegrade conduction passes through the both accessory pathway and AV nodal pathway to fuse in the ventricles. Conduction through the AV node is a brake on the conduction through the accessory pathway thereby propagation path in the ventricle will be blocked.

CASE 21

A 45-year-old female has been admitted with right-sided chest pain radiating to shoulder and diaphoresis for 3 hours. On examination, heart rate is 72 beats/min and blood pressure is 170/80 mm Hg. Her ECG demonstrated:

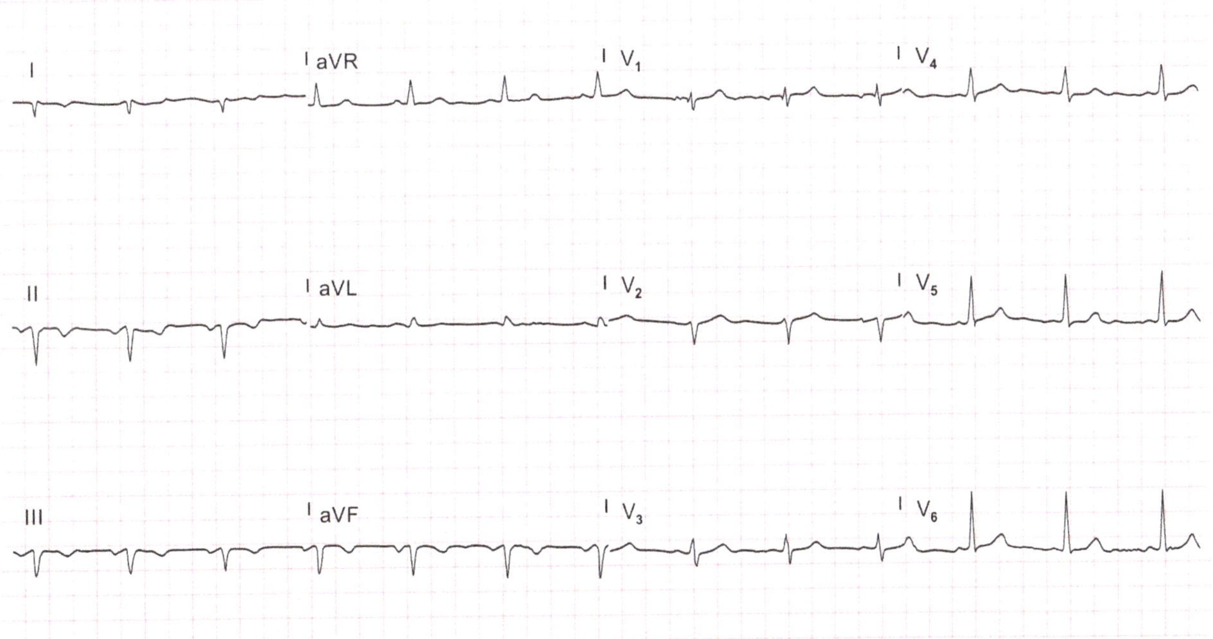

1. **What is your interpretation in ECG?**
2. **What is your inference?**
3. **What are the causes of this axis?**

Answers

1. Interpretation of ECG:
   a. Rate: 75 beats/min
   b. Rhythm: Regular
   c. Axis: Northwest axis
   d. Axis of P wave:
      - Upright in aVR
      - Negative in LII
   e. QRS wave: Q wave is present in LI, LII, LIII, and aVF.
   f. T wave: It is inverted in LI, LII, LIII, and aVF.

2. The inference is reversal of leads in right and left hands. Because, axis is northwest but precordial leads are normal—it is of no sense.

3. Causes of northwest axis:
   a. Dextrocardia
   b. Hyperkalemia
   c. Extreme right axis deviation
   d. Ventricular rhythm

CASE 22

A 60-year-old man has been admitted with chest pain following melena for 2 days. On examination, heart rate is 102 beats/min, blood pressure of 80/60 mm Hg, SpO_2 of 90 mm Hg, and hemoglobin was 5 g/dL. His ECG showed:

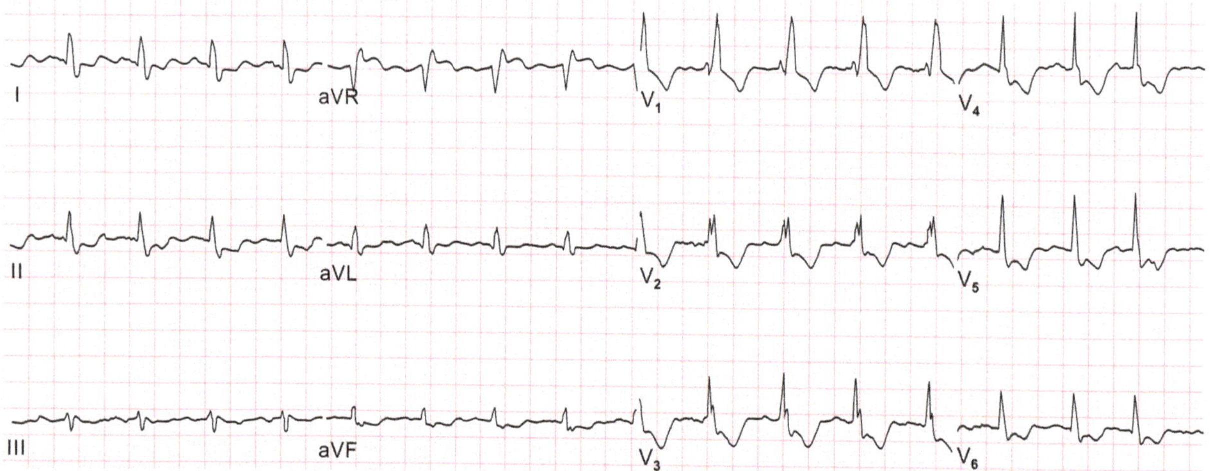

After resuscitation and two units of blood transfusion, the ECG was done again:

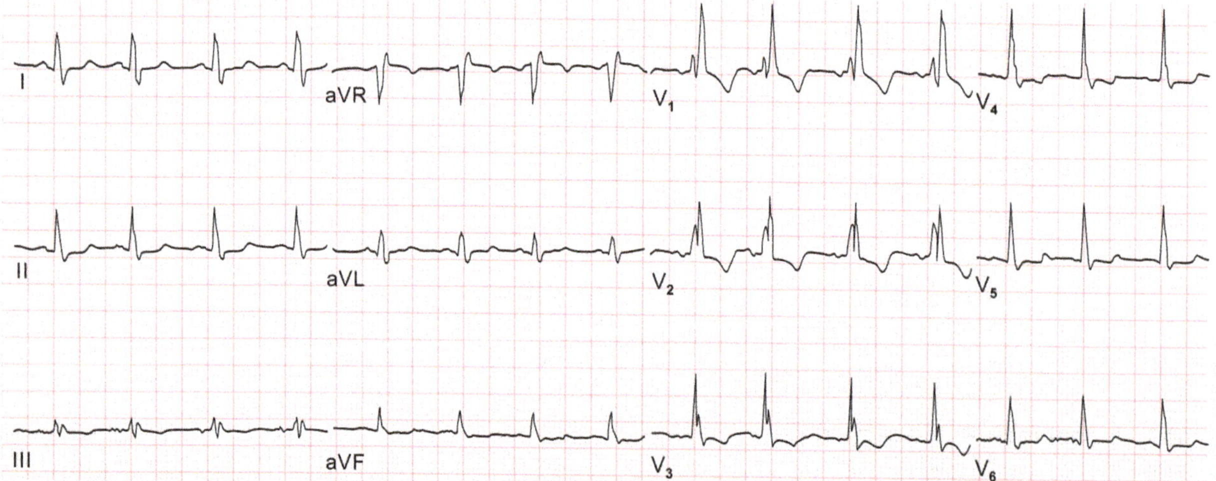

1. **Interpret the first and second ECG.**
2. **What is your inference?**

Answers

1. Interpretation ECG:
    In the first ECG
    a. Rate: 100 beats/min
    b. Rhythm: Regular
    c. Depression of ST segment in LII and V_4 to V_6
    d. RSR' pattern in V_1 and V_2
    e. ST-segment depression in V_2 and V_3
    f. ST segment is elevated in aVR.
    In the second ECG:
    a. Rate: 100 beats/min
    b. Rhythm: Regular
    c. Axis: Normal
    d. QRS morphology:
        - RSR' pattern in V_1 and V_2—right bundle branch block
    e. ST segment become isoelectric.
2. Inference: This widespread depression of ST segment is due to mismatch between oxygen demand and oxygen supply and it is due to decrease in the hemoglobin content in the blood and it is due to melena for 2 days. This ST depression has been reverted after transfusion of two units of blood, hence the ECG becomes normal.

CASE 23

An 80-year-old man complained for palpitation with blood pressure of 130/70 mm Hg and SpO_2 of 99%. His ECG demonstrated:

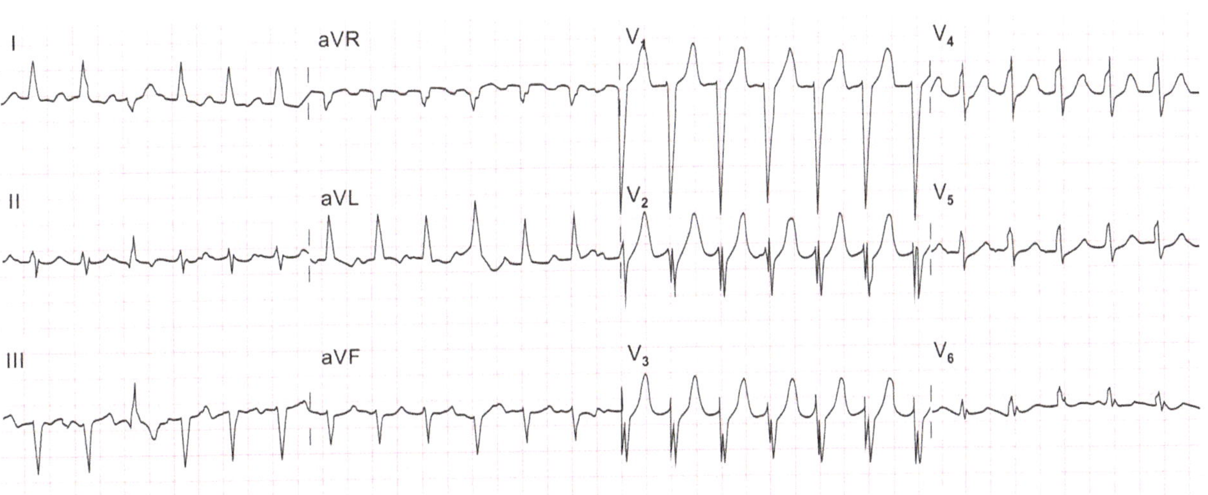

After administration of a drug the ECG was transformed into sinus rhythm.

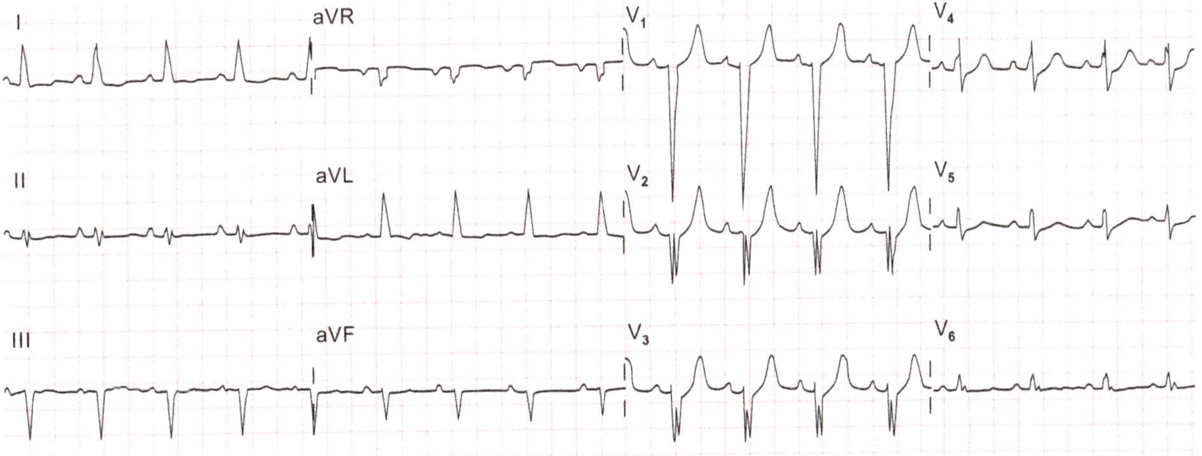

1. **Describe the first ECG.**
2. **What are the differential diagnoses?**
3. **How can you confirm it?**
4. **Which drug is responsible for transforming this rhythm to sinus rhythm?**
5. **What is your final diagnosis?**

Answers

1. Interpretation of ECG:

   First ECG:
   a. Rate: 150 beats/min
   b. Rhythm: Regular
   c. Axis: Left axis
   d. RS pattern in LII, LIII, and aVF
   e. ST depression in V_2 to V_5
   f. P wave is buried in T wave of LII and aVL. In LII and aVL, P wave is upright.
   g. P wave axis moves toward left.
   h. There is single ventricular ectopic in the third beat.

   Second ECG:
   a. Rate: 100 beats/min
   b. Rhythm: Regular
   c. P wave morphology: Normal
   d. Left anterior fascicular block
   e. P wave axis is normal.

2. Differential diagnoses:
   a. Atypical AV nodal reentrant tachycardia
   b. Focal atrial tachycardia (FAT)
   c. Permanent junctional reciprocal tachycardia

3. In atypical AV nodal reentrant tachycardia and permanent junctional reciprocal tachycardia, P wave is retrograde from a focus near AV node. So, P wave is negative in the LII, LIII, and aVF. But, here P wave is upright in lead LII. So, it is diagnosed as FAT.

4. Adenosine 12 mg was given intravenously to convert it to sinus rhythm.

5. Adenosine reverts the rhythm in some cases of FAT, but vagal maneuver should be the first option in the management of FAT.

CASE 24

A 70-year-old hypertensive, diabetic male having history of chronic kidney disease has been admitted with history of acute gastroenteritis for 12 hours. His ECG showed:

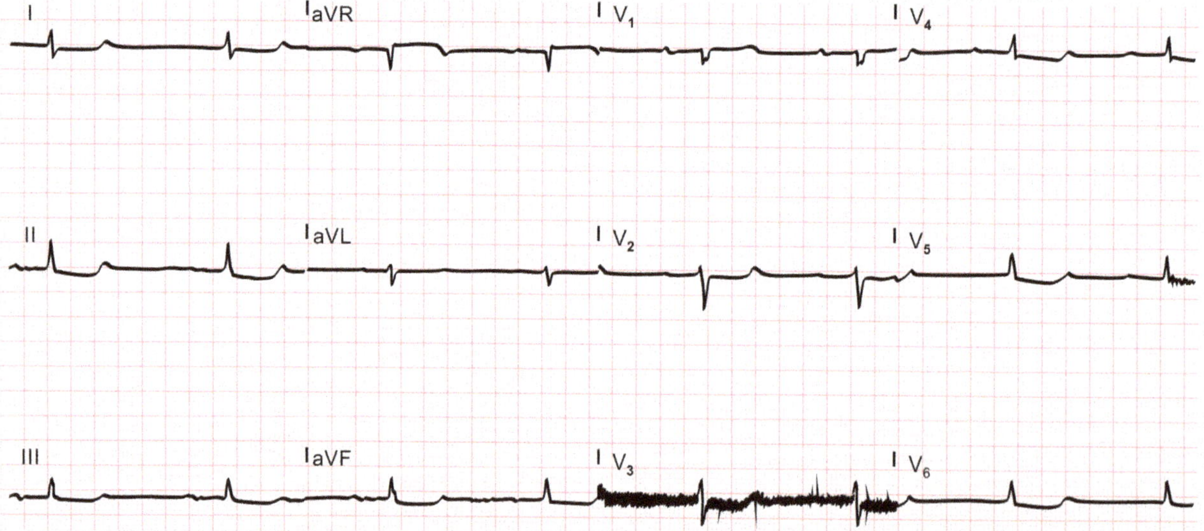

1. **Interpret the ECG.**
2. **What are the causes of this type of rhythm?**
3. **What is your diagnosis and why?**

Answers

1. Interpretation:
   a. Rate: 45 beats/min
   b. Rhythm: Sinus rhythm
   c. Axis: Normal
   d. PR interval: Prolonged
   e. Nonspecific changes in ST segment like depression in the inferior leads
2. The possible diagnoses:
   a. Inferior wall myocardial infarction
   b. Hyperkalemia

   c. AV nodal blocking drugs
   d. Increased intracranial pressure
3. Since the patient has history of chronic kidney disease and hypertension. The patient has been suffering from severe diarrhea. Patient may develop hypotension leading to renal hypoperfusion thereby further aggravating the kidney damage. In that case patient may develop hyperkalemia which is responsible for this ECG changes. Again patient may be under AV nodal blocking drugs. So, in this case, the probable diagnosis may be either hyperkalemia or AV nodal blocking drugs such as β-blocker and calcium channel blockers.

CASE 25

A 36-year-old diabetic male presented with respiratory distress and abdominal pain in the emergency department. His arterial blood gases demonstrated diabetic ketoacidosis and his ECG demonstrated:

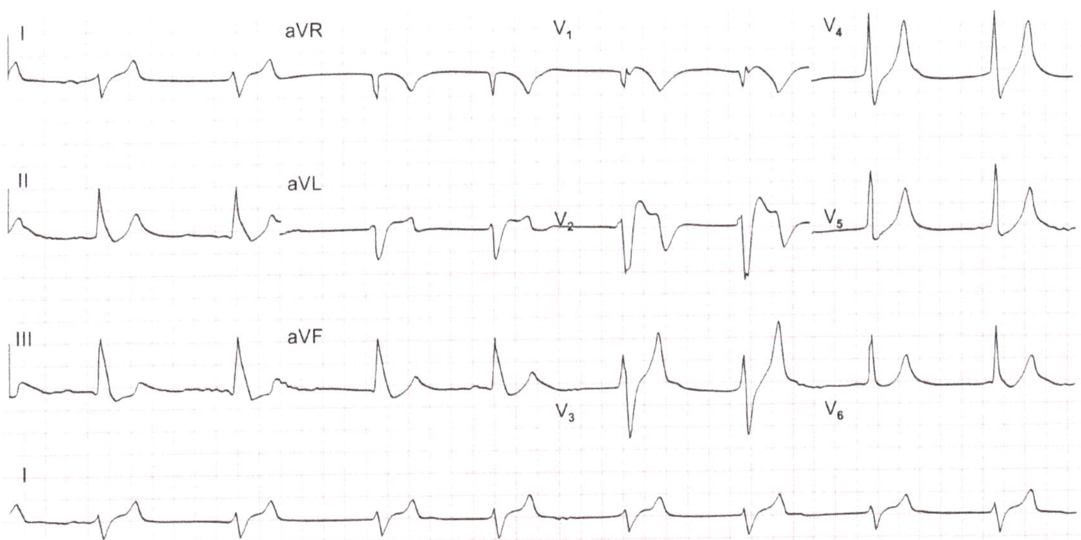

After treatment of ketoacidosis, following ECG was taken and it demonstrated:

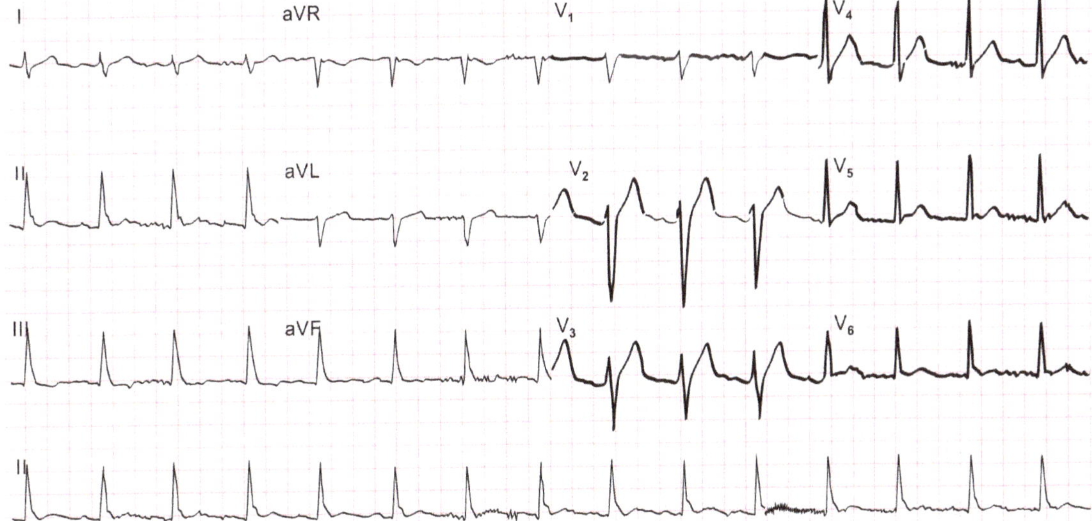

1. **Interpret the ECG.**
2. **What are the differential diagnoses?**
3. **What is the clinical outcome?**

Answers

1. Interpretation:
   a. Rate: 50 beats/min
   b. Rhythm: Regular
   c. Axis: Right axis deviation
   d. P wave: Absent
   e. QRS duration: Prolonged and bizarre-shaped
   f. ST segment:
      - Elevated in LI, aVL, V_1, V_2, V_3, and V_4
      - Depressed in LIII and aVF
      - Prominent T in V_3 to V_6

2. Differential diagnoses are as follows:
   a. Acute myocardial infarction
   b. Hyperkalemia
   c. Drug toxicity
3. Any abnormality in ECG in a diabetic patient with abdominal pain suggests the possibility of hyperkalemia. Again in case of diabetes, there may be precipitation of cardiac ischemia leading to development of hypercoagulable state.

CASE 26

A 65-year-old man presented in the emergency department with history of 1 hour exertional central chest pain. His ECG demonstrated:

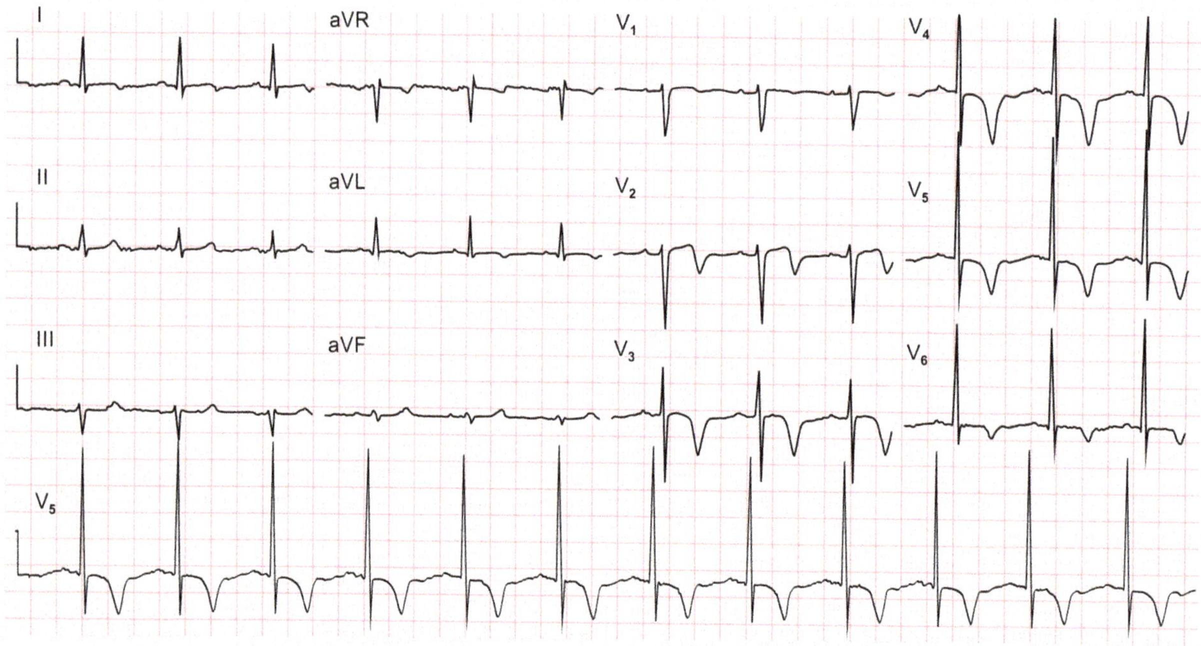

Now suddenly patient developed chest pain and during that time ECG was taken and it showed:

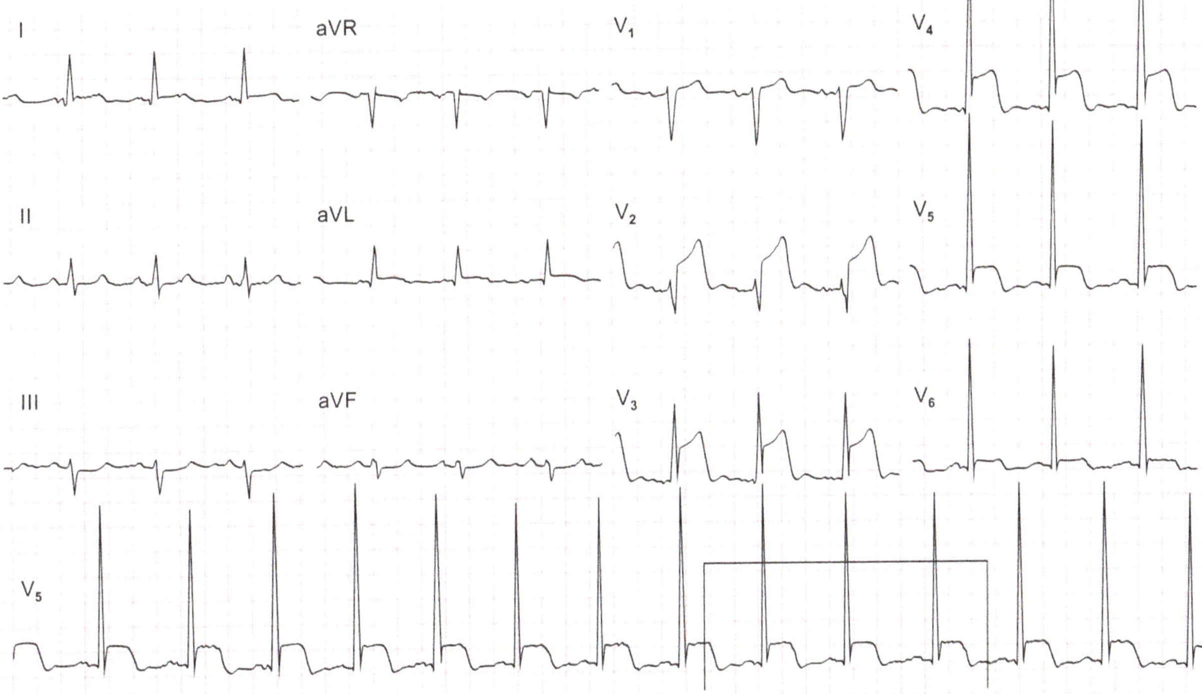

1. **Describe the first ECG.**
2. **What is your interpretation?**
3. **What it suggests?**
4. **Now describe the second ECG.**
5. **Now what is your interpretation?**

Answers

1. Description of first ECG:
   a. Rate: 73 beats/min
   b. Rhythm: Regular
   c. Axis: Normal
   d. PR interval: Normal
   e. P wave: Normal
   f. QRS morphology: Normal
   g. QT interval: Normal
   h. ST segment: Elevated in V_1
   i. T wave:
      - Biphasic in V_2
      - Inversion in LI, aVL, and V_3 to V_6
      - According voltage criteria, there is feature of left ventricular hypertrophy.
2. Interpretation: Differential deep inversion with broad shape of T wave in absence of pain suggests Wellens syndrome.
3. It suggests lesion in the left anterior descending artery.
4. Description of second ECG:
   a. Rate: 85 beats/min
   b. Rhythm: Regular
   c. Axis: Normal
   d. P wave: Normal
   e. PR: Normal
   f. QRS morphology: Normal
   g. ST segment: Elevated in following forms:
      - <1 mm in LI
      - 1 mm in aVL and V_2
      - 6 mm in V_2
      - 7 mm in V_3 and V_4
      - 4 mm in V_5
      - 1 mm in V_6

      Depressed in LII and aVF
   h. T wave:
      - No resolution of T wave inversion
      - Hyperacute T wave in V_2 and V_3
   i. According to voltage criteria, there is presence of left ventricular hypertrophy.
5. Interpretation is anterolateral ST segment elevated myocardial infarction.

CASE 27

A 29-year-old woman presented in emergency department with acute onset severe respiratory distress, cyanosis, and shock. Her ECG was like below:

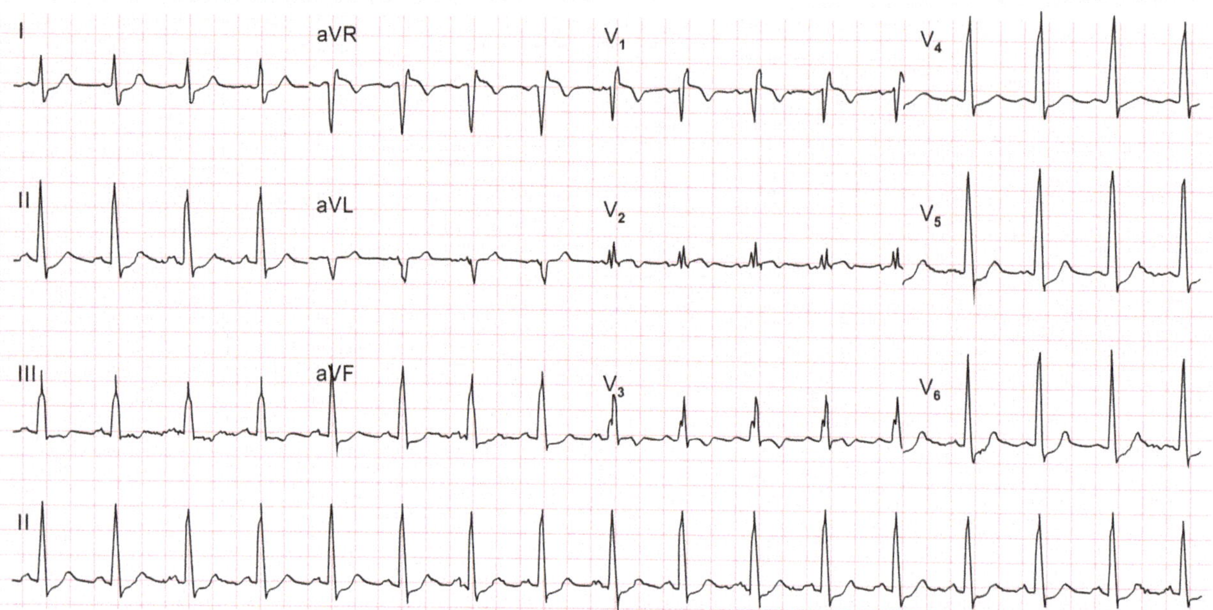

1. **Describe the ECG.**
2. **What is your impression?**

Answers

1. Description of ECG:
   a. Rate: 100 beats/min
   b. Rhythm: Regular
   c. Axis: Normal
   d. P wave: Normal
   e. PR interval: Normal
   f. QRS duration:
      - Prolonged
      - Small Q wave in LII, LIII, and aVF
      - RSR' pattern in V_1 and V_2
   g. QT interval: Normal
   h. ST segment:
      - Elevated in aVR, V_1, and V_2
      - Depressed in LI, LII, LIII, and V_4 to V_6
   i. T wave inverted in: LIII, aVR, and V_1 to V_3
2. The differential diagnoses are:
   a. Pulmonary embolism
   b. Acute coronary syndrome

But correlated with the history; this ECG was suggestive of pulmonary embolism.

CASE 28

A 30-year-old female was admitted in the emergency department with severe occipital headache. Her ECG demonstrated the following:

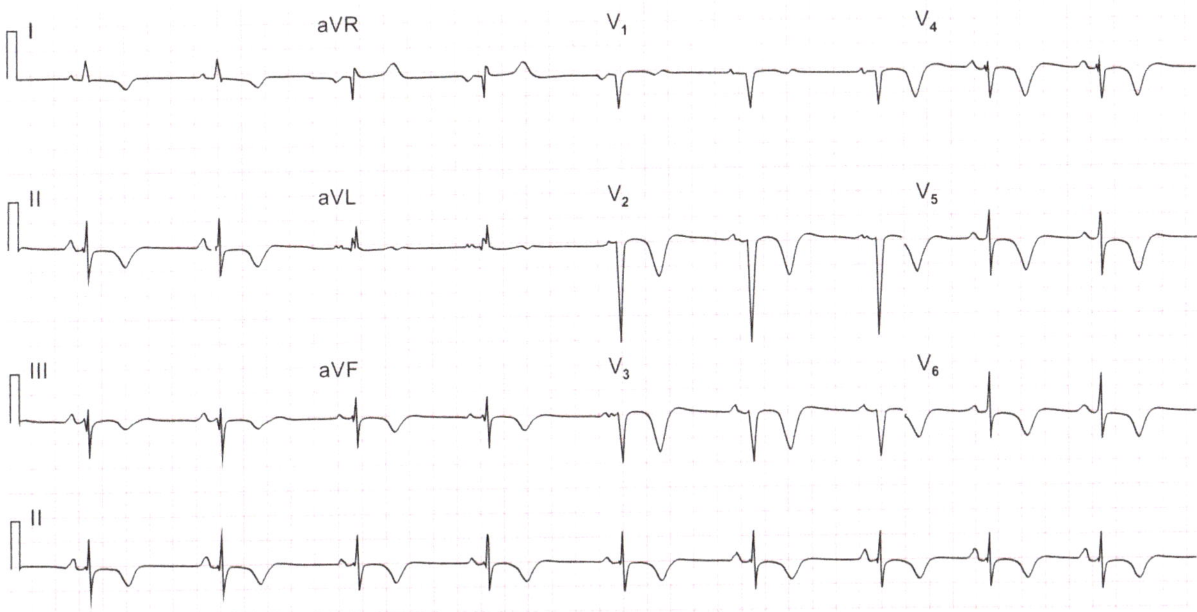

1. **Describe the ECG.**
2. **What is the correlation of history with ECG pattern?**

Answers

1. Description of ECG:
   a. Rate: 55 beats/min
   b. Rhythm: Regular
   c. Axis: normal
   d. P wave: Normal
   e. PR interval: Normal
   f. QRS morphology: Normal
   g. QT interval: Normal
   h. T wave: Inversion in LI, LII, LIII, aVF, and V_2 to V_6
2. There is sinus bradycardia. Since the patient presented with severe occipital headache and CT scan demonstrates subarachnoid hemorrhage. This ECG is suggestive of increased intracranial tension.

CASE 29

A 40-year-old man presented with pain in right shoulder with severe diaphoresis. His blood pressure is 170/80 mm Hg.

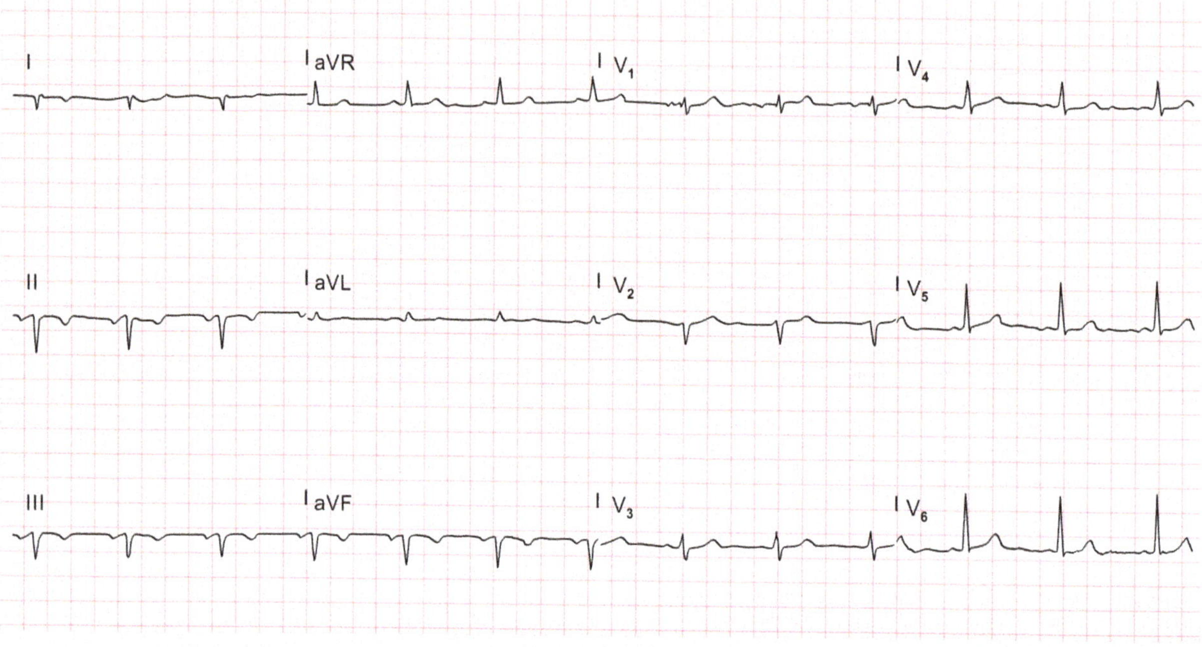

1. **Describe the ECG.**
2. **What is your inference?**
3. **What are the differential diagnoses?**
4. **Why it is not hyperkalemia?**
5. **Why it is not a case of extreme right axis deviation?**
6. **Why it is not a case of dextrocardia?**

Answers

1. Description of ECG:
   a. Rate: 80 beats/min
   b. Rhythm: Regular
   c. Axis: Northwest axis
   d. P wave:
      - Upright in aVR
      - Negative in LII
   e. Q waves: Present in LII, LIII, and aVF.
   f. T wave inversion in LII, LIII, and aVF
   g. R wave is progressed normally in precordial leads.

2. This is the result of limb lead reversal. Northwest axis in presence of normal precordial leads os of no sense.

3. The differential diagnoses are:
   a. Hyperkalemia
   b. Dextrocardia
   c. Ventricular rhythm
   d. Extreme right axis deviation

4. This ECG is not suggestive of hyperkalemia because:
   a. Northwest axis is very late sign.
   b. Presence of "sine wave" configuration suggestive of ventricular conduction delay with abnormal QRS complex.

5. It is not a case of extreme right axis deviation because it is associated with chronic obstructive pulmonary disease having following features:
   a. Right ventricular strain
   b. P pulmonale
   c. Dominant R wave in V_1 suggestive of right ventricular hypertrophy

6. It is not a case of dextrocardia because:
   a. Absence of R wave progression in precordial leads
   b. Sometimes R wave reversal because lateral precordial leads will proceed further away from the right side of heart.

CASE 30

A 45-year-old male was presented to the emergency ward with vomiting for >2 weeks. He is under sotalol and rivaroxaban for treatment of paroxysmal atrial fibrillation.

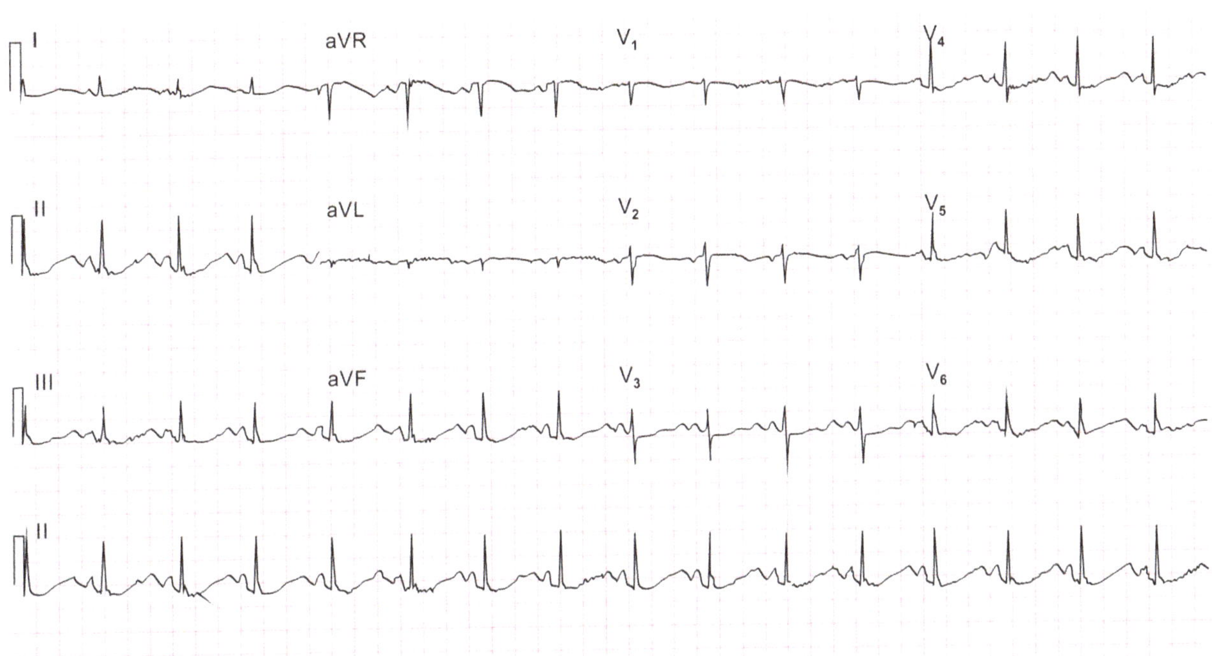

Suddenly patient became completely unconscious. ECG was taken and it demonstrated:

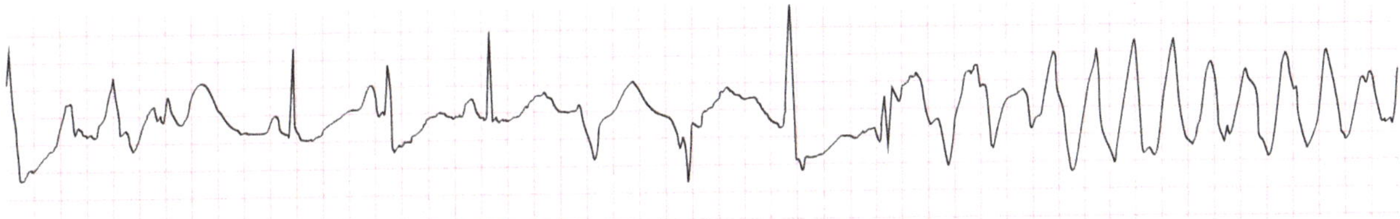

1. **Describe the first ECG.**
2. **What is your interpretation?**
3. **Describe the second ECG.**
4. **What should be the acid–base interpretation?**

Answers

1. Description of ECG:
   a. Rate: 98 beats/min
   b. Rhythm: Regular
   c. Axis: Normal
   d. P wave: Normal
   e. PR segment: Normal
   f. QRS: Normal
   g. QT duration: Prolonged
   h. ST segment: Depressed in LII, LIII, aVF, and V_4 to V_6
   i. Prominent U wave in V_3 to V_5

2. Marked QT prolongation and U wave suggestive of:
   a. Hypokalemia
   b. Hypomagnesemia
   c. Sotalol administration

3. Description of second ECG: Presence of paroxysmal ventricular tachycardia with R on T phenomenon which ultimately transformed into polymorphic ventricular tachycardia.

4. Acid–base interpretation should demonstrate metabolic alkalosis with hypokalemia.

CASE 31

A 35-year-old man was admitted with severe vomiting with vertigo. His ECG was done:

His venous blood gas analysis demonstrates: pH 7.5, pCO_2 55 mm Hg, PO_2 30 mm Hg, HCO_3 65 mmol/L, Na 136 mmol/L, K 4.4 mmol/L, chloride 80 mmol/L, and glucose 105 mg/dL.

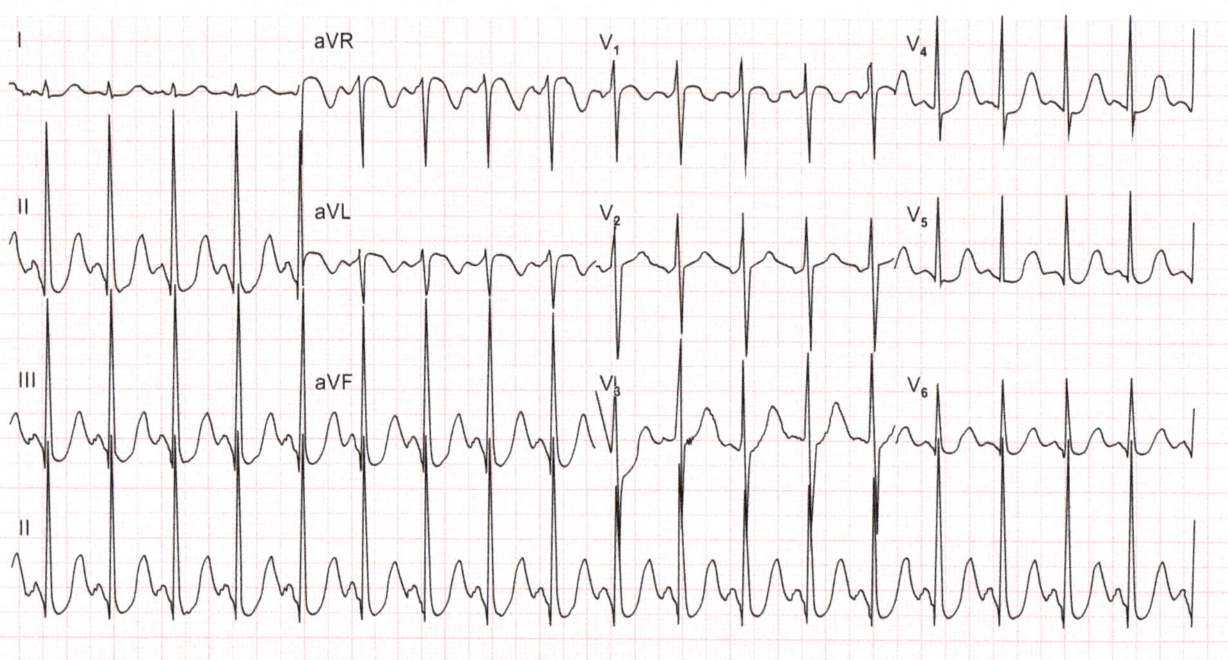

1. **Describe the ECG.**
2. **What is the inference regarding venous blood gases?**
3. **What is your inference?**

Answers

1. Description of ECG:
    a. Rate: 108 beats/min
    b. Rhythm: Regular
    c. Axis: Normal
    d. P wave morphology: Normal
    e. PR interval: Normal
    f. QRS morphology: Normal
    g. QT interval: Prolonged
    h. ST segment:
        - Elevated in V_1, aVL, and aVR
        - Depressed in LII, LIII, and aVF
2. Venous blood gases demonstrate evidence of metabolic alkalosis
3. Inference: QT prolongation along with ST changes in the background of metabolic alkalosis is suggestive severe metabolic alkalosis.

CASE 32

A 28-year-old male came to outpatient department with palpitation. His blood pressure was 120/75 mm Hg. His ECG demonstrated following:

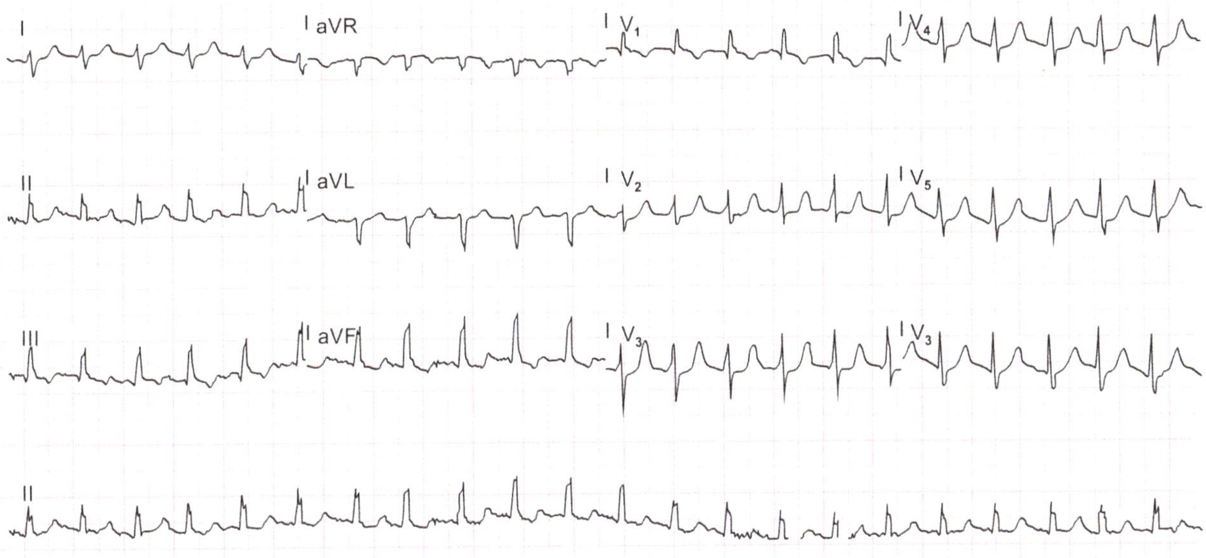

1. **Describe the ECG.**
2. **What is your impression?**
3. **What is your diagnosis?**

Answers

1. Description of ECG:
   a. Rate: 130 beats/min
   b. Rhythm: Regular
   c. Axis: Right axis
   d. P wave morphology: Normal, absence of flutter wave.
   e. PR interval: Normal
   f. QRS morphology:
      - Dominant R wave in V_1
      - Presence of pseudo R' wave at the terminal portion of QRS complex in V_1
   g. ST segment: In the isoelectric line in V_1. Absence of rate-related ischemia.
   h. There is presence of notch at the apex of QRS complexes in LII, LIII, and aVF—Crochetage sign.
2. Following are the important points:
   a. Dominant R wave suggests right ventricular hypertrophy.
   b. Pseudo R' wave at the terminal portion of QRS complex in V_1, isoelectric baseline and absence of atrial flutter waves indicate AV nodal reentrant tachycardia.
3. Presence of Crochetage sign is suggestive of atrial septal defect with 92% specificity.

CHAPTER 4

Endocrinology

A 60-year-old type 2 diabetic man on oral hypoglycemic drugs came to diabetic clinic with anorexia, vomiting, gross weight loss, and postural dizziness for 4 months.

On examination, his blood pressure was 135/85 mm Hg on lying down and 110 mm Hg on standing, pulse rate 88 beats/min, and body mass index (BMI) 20 kg/m². Buccal mucosa demonstrated as below:

Chest X-ray was normal, CT scan of abdomen demonstrated as below.

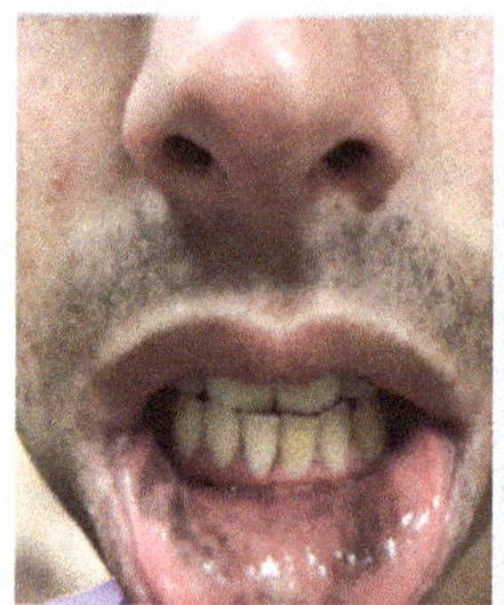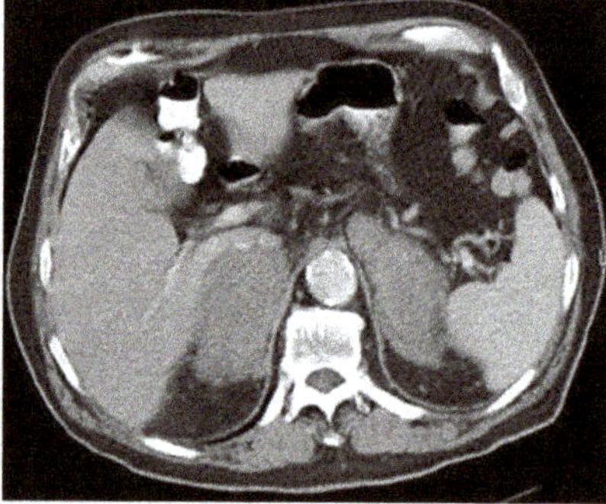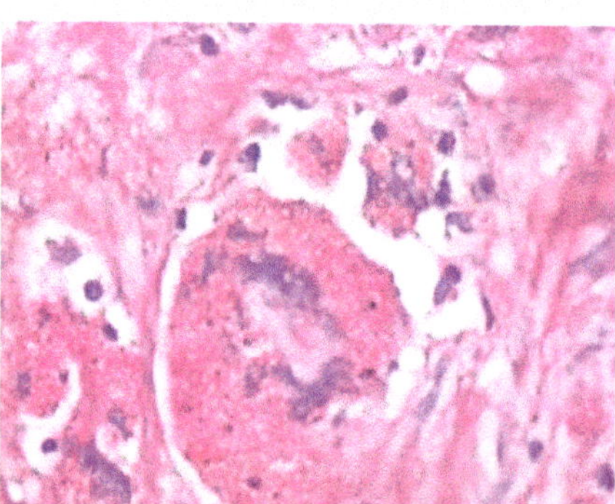

Laboratory investigation demonstrated serum sodium 128 mEq/L, potassium 2.8 mEq/L, fasting blood sugar 180 mg/dL, serum cortisol 4.8 μg/dL, adrenocorticotropic hormone (ACTH) 200 pg/mL, and dehydroepiandrosterone (DHEA) sulfate 11 μg/dL.

1. **What do the above pictures demonstrate?**
2. **What is your diagnosis?**
3. **What are the points in favor of your diagnosis?**
4. **What are the types of this disease?**
5. **Why sodium level is low in this case?**
6. **Why there is hypotension?**
7. **Why there is hyperpigmentation in the buccal mucosa?**
8. **What are the autoimmune causes of this disease?**
9. **What are the investigations to be done here?**
10. **What is the modality of treatment?**

Answers

1. The above pictures demonstrate:
   a. First picture: Pigmentation in the inner side of buccal mucosa.
   b. Second picture: CT scan of abdomen demonstrated bilateral enlargement of the adrenal glands.
   c. Third picture of fine needle aspiration cytology demonstrated:
      - Presence of inflammatory cells
      - Small yeast cells extracellularly and intracellularly showing the morphology of *Histoplasma*.
      - Presence of necrosis
2. Diagnosis is Addison's disease due to bilateral adrenal histoplasmosis.
3. Following are the points in favor of this diagnosis:
   a. History suggestive of weight loss, nausea, vomiting, and postural dizziness
   b. Wide gap between the blood pressure during lying down and standing position
   c. Low BMI
   d. Pigmentation in the buccal mucosa
   e. CT scan demonstrating bilateral adrenal gland involvement
   f. Fine needle aspiration cytology demonstrating the features suggestive of histoplasmosis
4. Three types adrenal insufficiency are as follows:
   a. Primary causes:
      - Infective:
         ○ Tuberculosis
         ○ Histoplasmosis
         ○ Cryptococcosis
         ○ *Cytomegalovirus*
      - Autoimmune
      - Bilateral adrenal hemorrhage
      - Genetic:
         ○ Congenital adrenal hyperplasia
         ○ Adrenal hypoplasia
         ○ Adrenoleukodystrophy
   b. Secondary causes: Defect at the level of pituitary
   c. Tertiary causes: Defect at the hypothalamic level
5. Serum sodium level is low due to:
   a. Aldosterone deficiency leading to loss of sodium
   b. Increased release of antidiuretic hormone due to absence of cortisol negative feedback at the level of hypothalamus.
6. Hypotension is due to:
   a. Deficiency of mineralocorticoid leading to extracellular volume contraction
   b. Loss of vascular tone due to impaired ability of catecholamine to exert
7. In case of primary adrenal insufficiency, there is increased level of ACTH. There is presence of melanocyte-stimulating hormone (MSH) in the ACTH molecule, so high level of ACTH will bind to MSH receptor leading increased production of melanin production resulting increased pigmentation in the buccal mucosa, friction areas, and in the skin creases.
8. Autoimmune causes of Addison's disease are as follows:
   a. Type I autoimmune polyglandular syndrome: It is characterized by—
      - Hypoparathyroidism
      - Addison's disease
      - Mucocutaneous candidiasis
   b. Type II polyglandular syndrome: It is characterized by—
      - Autoimmune thyroiditis (Schmidt syndrome)
      - Type 1 diabetes (Carpenter syndrome)
      - Autoimmune conditions such as pernicious anemia and vitiligo
      - Addison's disease
9. Following investigations should be done:
   a. Serum cortisol level: <3 µg/dL (normal level is ≥ 19 µg/dL)
   b. Serum ACTH level:
      - Increased level: Primary adrenal insufficiency
      - Low level: Secondary adrenal insufficiency
   c. Corticotropin stimulation test:
      - In primary cause: No increase in the serum level of cortisol
      - In secondary cause: Increased response of serum cortisol level
   d. Serum aldosterone level: Decreased in primary cause
   e. Plasma renin activity: Decreased in primary cause
   f. Serum thyroid-stimulating hormone (TSH) level is low because:
      - Decreased level of cortisol
      - Abnormal TSH circadian rhythm
   g. Anti-21-hydroxylase antibodies: Anti-21-hydroxylase is required for the synthesis of cortisol in adrenal cortex.
10. Treatment of histoplasmosis:
    a. Administration of itraconazole and amphotericin B
    b. Replacement of glucocorticoids and mineralocorticoids

CASE 2

A 60-year-old man came to medical emergency department with history of right upper abdominal pain for 6 months, but no other history such as anorexia, nausea, vomiting, fever, yellow discoloration in the eye, palpitation, and any abnormal pigmentation or abdominal striae are found.

On examination, his pulse rate was 80 beats/min, blood pressure 125/80 mm Hg without any postural drop, no jaundice, and no clubbing.

Laboratory investigation demonstrated that all the hematological, biochemical like testosterone, DHEA, and 24 hours urinary metepinephrine are within normal limit but urinary normetepinephrine was 4,035 µg/24 hour.

CT scan demonstrated the following:

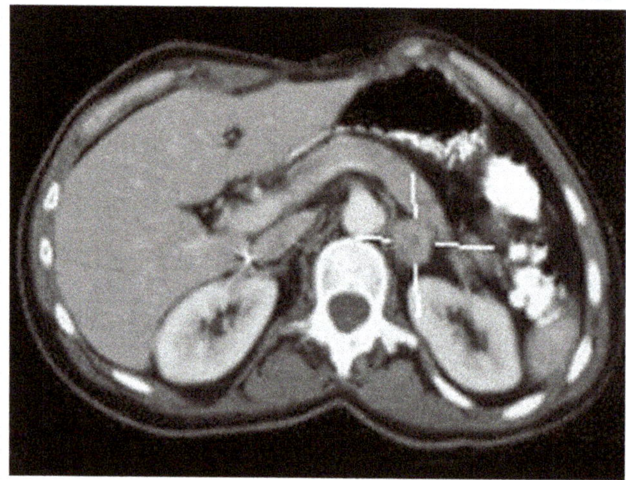

1. **What is the finding of the above CT scan of abdomen?**
2. **What is your diagnosis?**
3. **How can you evaluate this diagnosis?**
4. **What are the CT scan criteria for this diagnosis?**
5. **What are the indications of surgery in this case?**

Answers

1. CT scan feature of the abdomen demonstrated low attenuated noncontrast, i.e., <10 HU mass and size is <4 cm.
2. The diagnosis is adrenal incidentaloma.
3. Following are the process of evaluation:
   a. Primary hyperaldosteronism:
      - Clinical features:
        - High blood pressure
        - Low potassium
        - High plasma renin activity
      - Biochemical test: Plasma aldosterone to renin ratio
   b. Pheochromocytoma:
      - Clinical features:
        - High blood pressure with postural drop
        - Headache
      - Biochemical abnormality:
        - Plasma free metanephrines
        - Urinary free metanephrines
   c. Cushing syndrome or silent Cushing syndrome:
      - Clinical features: Features of Cushing syndrome
      - Biochemical features: Overnight 1 mg dexamethasone test
   d. Adrenocortical carcinoma:
      - Clinical features:
        - Features of virilization
        - Features of feminization
      - Biochemical feature:
        - Urinary 17-ketosteroids
        - 17α-estradiol in male
        - Serum level of testosterone and androstenedione
        - 17α-hydroxyprogesterone or progesterone

4. CT scan criteria for the diagnosis of this case are:
   a. Homogeneous mass along with low attenuation before the administration of the contrast of <10 HU suggests benign adenoma.
   b. If the tumor size is <4 cm.
5. Following are the indications of surgery in adrenal incidentaloma:
   a. 20% cases may develop the features of hormonal excess, the excess hormone is cortisol.
   b. Features of biochemical evidence of pheochromocytoma
   c. If the diameter of the mass is >4 cm
   d. If there is associated high level of corticosteroids
   e. If the diameter of the mass is >6 cm.
   f. If there are features of malignancy in imaging like:
      - Lack of clear circumscribed margin
      - Vascular invasion

CASE 3

A 30-year-old male was attended the medicine outpatient department with severe recurrent headache, tiredness for last 2 months. On enquiry, there was no evidence of snoring, no feature of urinary complaint, nonsmoker, nondiabetic, and lean.

On examination, there was no jaundice or clubbing, blood pressure in sitting position 170/110 mm Hg, BMI 20 kg/m^2, pulse rate 80 beats/min, regular, no radio-radial or radio-femoral inequalities of pulses, volume are normal in all the arteries, and no tremor.

Laboratory investigation demonstrated that electrolytes were normal, renal and liver function test were normal, and chest X-ray and echocardiography and polysomnography were normal.

1. **What is your diagnosis?**
2. **What are the possibilities?**
3. **What should be the precaution taken as the patient is on antihypertensive drug?**
   If plasma aldosterone was 13.6 ng/dL and plasma renin activity was 0.3 ng/mL/hour.
4. **What is the plasma aldosterone/renin ratio? What is the value and what is the interpretation?**
5. **What are the confirmatory tests for this diagnosis?**

Answers

1. The diagnosis is renin activity—secondary hypertension.
2. The possibilities of secondary hypertension are:
   a. Renal parenchymal disease—but it has been excluded as there was no history of abnormalities and inequality of pulse, and renal function test was normal.
   b. Obstructive sleep apnea—but this has been excluded because of no suggestive history.
   c. Renal artery stenosis—but all the peripheral pulses were normal and there was no inequality of pulses.
   d. Endocrine causes:
      - Primary hyperaldosteronism
      - Paraganglioma
      - Pheochromocytoma
3. As the patient was on antihypertensive drugs, these drugs have to be stopped for at least 4–6 weeks before taking samples from the blood for plasma aldosterone and plasma renin activity.
4. Plasma aldosterone was 13.6 ng/dL and plasma renin activity 0.3 ng/mL/hour. So, the plasma aldosterone to plasma renin activity ratio is 45.33 ng/dL per ng/mL/hour. So, the ratio is very high. So, the diagnosis is primary hyperaldosteronism.
5. The confirmatory tests are as follows:
   a. Intravenous saline loading test
   b. Oral salt loading test
   c. Captopril challenge test
   d. Fludrocortisone suppression test

CASE 4

A 60-year-old new-onset hypertensive woman on hydrochlorothiazide came to medicine outpatient department with chronic nonproductive cough and multiple ecchymosis on the body.

On examination, patient was overweighed, centripetal obesity, and striae on the central and lower part of abdomen.

Laboratory examination demonstrated serum potassium was 2 mEq/L, serum cortisol 88 µg/dL, and ACTH 245 pg/dL; after 8 mg overnight; dexamethasone suppression test demonstrated serum cortisol was 76 µg/dL and ACTH 200 pg/dL. Her straight X-ray demonstrated the following picture. Her bronchoscopy demonstrated:

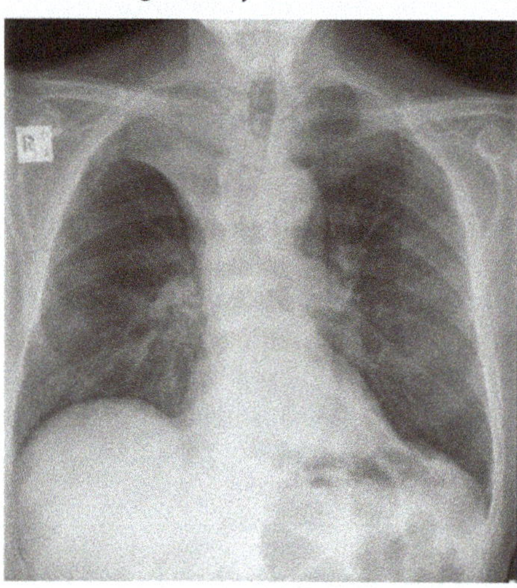
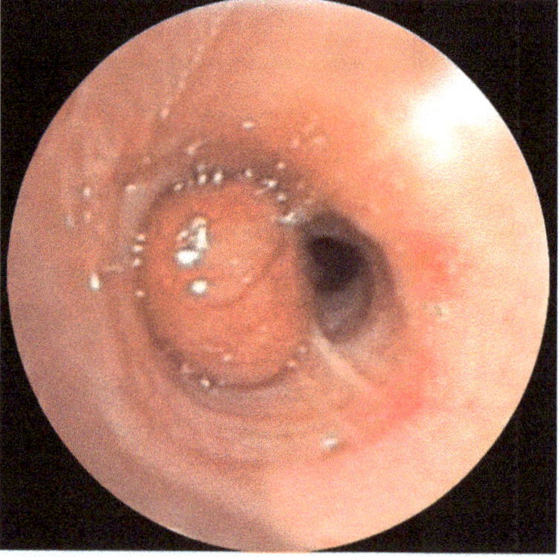

1. **What do the above pictures demonstrate?**
2. **What is your diagnosis?**
3. **What are the points in favor of your diagnosis?**
4. **What are the drugs producing the false-negative results of 1 mg overnight dexamethasone suppression test?**
5. **What is the normal response to 1 mg overnight dexamethasone suppression test?**
6. **What are the conditions responsible for incomplete suppression of cortisol in the dexamethasone suppression test?**
7. **What is the importance of salivary cortisol?**
8. **What are the causes responsible for falsely positive salivary cortisol?**

Answers

1. The above pictures demonstrate:
   a. Chest X-ray demonstrated radiopaque shadow having definite lower border concavity downward seen in the right apical region indicating collapse of right upper lobe.
   b. Bronchoscopy demonstrated a round well-circumscribed tumor seen in the right main bronchus.
2. The patient has been suffering from Cushing syndrome due to ectopic secretion of ACTH from the carcinoid tumor in the right bronchus.

3. Following are the points in favor of this diagnosis:
   a. Presence of centripetal obesity
   b. Presence of abdominal striae
   c. Presence of ecchymosis
   d. High serum cortisol and ACTH
   e. Failure of suppression with 1 mg overnight dexamethasone suppression test.
   f. Presence of bronchial carcinoid
4. Following are the drugs producing the false-negative results of 1 mg overnight dexamethasone suppression test:
   a. Nifedipine
   b. Rifampin

c. Hydantoin
d. Carbamazepine
e. Phenobarbital
f. Tamoxifen
g. Topiramate

5. Normal response to 1 mg overnight dexamethasone suppression test is <1.8 µg/dL.

6. Following are the conditions responsible for incomplete suppression of cortisol in the dexamethasone suppression test:
    a. In chronic renal failure due to decreased clearance of cortisol

b. High estrogen states:
    • Pregnancy
    • Consumption of estrogen containing drugs

7. Salivary cortisol level of >4.3 nmol/L suggests hypercortisolism.

8. Following are the causes responsible for falsely positive salivary cortisol elevation:
    a. Men >60 years of age
    b. Obese
    c. Hypertension
    d. Diabetes mellitus
    e. Critically ill patients

CASE 5

A 42-day-old exclusively breastfed female presented with vomiting and anorectic. On examination, patient was malnourished, dehydrated, and blood pressure of 70/50 mm Hg. Her genitalia demonstrated ambiguous, hyperpigmented, and partially fused labia majora with rugosity. Her elder brother was healthy.

Laboratory investigation demonstrated that serum sodium was 120 mEq/L, potassium 2 mEq/L, and chloride 84 mEq/L. Serum hydroxyprogesterone was 65,000 ng/dL. She is karyotypically XX.

1. **Do you know the phenotypic sex in this female patient?**
2. **What is the most likely diagnosis?**
3. **What is the pathophysiology in this disease?**
4. **How can you diagnose this case?**
5. **What will be the level of the 17-hydroxyprogesterone at baseline and after stimulation?**
6. **What is the molecular genetics in this disease?**
7. **How can you treat this patient?**

Answers

1. It is very difficult to know the sex of this patient phenotypically.

2. The most likely diagnosis is salt-losing variety of 21-hydroxylase deficiency caused by autosomal recessive disorder due to defective 21-hydroxylase allele inheritance.

3. Pathophysiology in this disease: Failure of conversion of progesterone and 17-hydroxyprogesterone to 11-deoxycorticosterone and 11-deoxycortisol respectively by 21-hydroxylase leading to increased formation of androstenedione, testosterone, dihydro-testosterone, and estradiol resulting increased ACTH and adrenal hyperplasia and development of ambiguous genitalia and salt wasting.

4. Diagnosis is based on the following:
    a. Elevated baseline of ACTH
    b. ACTH-stimulated serum level of 17-hydroxypro-gesterone and androstenedione
    c. Urinary metabolites of pregnanetriol and 17-ketosteroids to confirm the diagnosis
    d. Decreased ratio of aldosterone to plasma renin activity ratio
    e. In case of nonclassic form of this disease, baseline level of 17-hydroxyprogesterone is not so high or may be normal, but after stimulation with ACTH, the level will be 2,000–10,000 ng/dL.

5. Level of 17-hydroxyprogesterone:
    a. At baseline, 10,000–100,000 ng/dL
    b. After ACTH stimulation, 25,000 to >100,000 ng/dL

6. Most of the mutations are the combinations between active *CYP21A2* and inactive *CYP21A1P* genes leading to deficiency of 21-hydroxylase resulting less mineraloconversion.

7. Management/treatment of this disease is as follows:
    a. Glucocorticoids: In case of adult, 0.25 mg of dexamethasone should be administered during hour of sleep. In case of children, 8–12 mg/m^2 has to be started.
    b. Mineralocorticoids in the form of 9-fludro-cortisone should be administered at a dose of

    0.1–0.3 mg daily in patient with overt or subtle salt wasting.

c. 1–3 mg sodium chloride should be administered in infants with salt-wasting syndrome to adequately replace the salt.

d. Replacement of sex hormones at puberty in patients with gonadal steroid deficiency to develop secondary sexual characteristics.

e. Surgical correction of the ambiguous genitalia should be performed in the first year of life in clinically stable patients.

CASE 6

A 40-year-old man came to medical outpatient department with progressively increasing gain in weight, easy fatigability, and difficulty in raising up from sitting position in the chair and headache.

On examination, the face was round and chubby and plethoric, pulse rate 80 beats/min, regular, respiration rate 18 breaths/min, and blood pressure 155/90 mm Hg. Abdominal skin demonstrated:

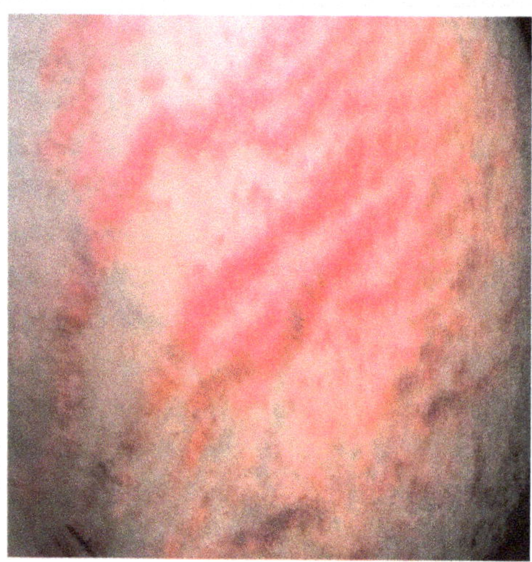

Laboratory investigation demonstrated that fasting plasma glucose was 202 mg/dL, serum cortisol at 8 AM 700 nmol/L, 1 mg overnight dexamethasone suppression test 452 nmol/L and 8 mg dexamethasone suppression test demonstrated 120 nmol/L, TSH 2.1 nmol/L, and follicle-stimulating hormone (FSH) and luteinizing hormone (LH) 2 and 1.2 nmol/L, respectively.

Contrast-enhanced computed tomography (CECT) scan abdomen demonstrated presence of a mass in the left adrenal gland. Inferior petrosal sinus sampling demonstrated increased secretion of ACTH from the right petrosal sinus.

1. **What is your diagnosis?**
2. **What is the cause of this feature?**
3. **What are the causes in this hypercortisolemia where the striae will be absent?**
4. **What are the causes of abdominal striae in absence of this disease?**
5. **What are the causes of weight loss in this disease?**
6. **What are the other causes of hypercortisolemia?**
7. **What is pseudovariation of this disease and what is the pathophysiology?**
8. **In case of obesity, what is the alteration of the cortisol dynamics?**
9. **What is cyclical Cushing's syndrome?**
10. **What do you mean by subclinical variety of this disease?**
11. **What are the causes of headache in this disease?**
12. **What are the dermatological manifestations in this disease?**
13. **What are the causes of proximal muscle weakness in this patient?**
14. **What are the causes of hypertension in this disease?**

Answers

1. The above picture demonstrates the abdominal striae along with centripetal obesity.
2. In the Cushing syndrome:
   a. Striae in the abdomen occurs due to:
      - Dilatation of the venules due to loss of support of perivenular collagen
      - Thinning of the dermis due to breakdown of dermal collagen
   b. Central distribution of fat is due to:
      - Increased expression of the glucocorticoid receptors
      - Elevated activity of 11β-hydroxylase activity in the omental fat
3. Following are the causes in this hypercortisolemia where the striae will be absent:
   a. Childhood Cushing's syndrome
   b. Adrenocortical carcinoma
   c. Ectopic Cushing's syndrome
   d. Hypercortisolemia associated with excess androgen
4. Following are the causes of abdominal striae in absence of hypercortisolemia:
   a. Rapid gain in weight during puberty
   b. Pregnancy
   c. Pseudo-Cushing's states
5. Following are the causes of weight loss in this disease:
   a. Adrenocortical carcinoma
   b. Ectopic Cushing's syndrome
   c. Uncontrolled diabetes mellitus
   d. Concurrent infections like tuberculosis
   e. Endogenous depression
   f. Concurrent ACTH- or TSH-secreting adenoma
   g. McCune–Albright syndrome
6. Following are the causes of hypercortisolemia:
   a. Stress is due to:
      - Hospitalization
      - Surgery
      - Pain
   b. Intense chronic exercise
   c. Anorexia nervosa
   d. Malnutrition
   e. Excess cortisol-binding globulin
7. Pseudovariation of this disease is characterized by signs of Cushing's syndrome and hypercortisolism but anomalous response to dexamethasone suppression test. The causes are:
   a. Morbid obesity
   b. Depression
   c. Alcoholism
   d. Metabolic syndrome
   e. Poorly controlled diabetes mellitus
   f. Polycystic ovarian disease (PCOD)

   Chronic stress will lead to cytokine release as well as overactivity of the neurotransmitter leading to activation of hypothalamic-pituitary-adrenal axis resulting hypercortisolemia.
8. In case of obesity:
   a. Loss of circadian rhythm of cortisol
   b. Normal serum cortisol
   c. Mildly increased serum cortisol
   d. Variable response to overnight dexamethasone suppression test
   e. Increased turnover of serum cortisol
   f. Increased clearance of cortisol
   g. Increased synthesis of cortisol due to inhibition of insulin growth factor-1 mediated inhibition of hepatic 11β-hydroxysteroid dehydrogenase type 1 leading to decreased peripheral conversion of cortisol from cortisone.
9. Cyclical Cushing's syndrome can be defined biochemically as the presence of three peaks and two troughs over a period of weeks to months resulting from periodic genesis requiring frequent monitoring of urinary free cortisol or late night salivary cortisol but not the dexamethasone suppression test for establishing the diagnosis.
10. Subclinical Cushing's syndrome can be defined as absence of clinical features of this disease in presence of autonomous secretion of glucocorticoids, suppressed DHEA sulfate, and ACTH in patients with obesity, hypertension, or type 2 diabetes mellitus. Diagnostic cutoff in this disease following 1 mg overnight dexamethasone suppression test is >5 μg/dL as compared to >1.8 μg/dL in case of Cushing's syndrome.
11. Causes of headache in this disease:
    a. Adrenal adenoma
    b. Sinusitis
    c. Thrombosis of the cortical veins
    d. Benign intracranial hypertension
    e. Glaucoma
12. Following are the dermatological manifestations in this disease:
    a. Bruise, striae, and plethora due to loss of dermal collage, and plethora due to increased erythropoiesis.
    b. Cuticular atrophy due to atrophy of the stratum corneum

c. Purpura due to qualitative abnormalities of the platelets function

d. Hyperpigmentation due to excess of ACTH

e. Acne or hirsutism due to excess secretion of androgen.

13. Causes of proximal muscle weakness in this patient are:

a. Decreased synthesis of the muscle proteins due to suppression of synthesis of muscle proteins by inhibiting insulin-like growth factor-1 (IGF-1) and Akt1 signaling in the myocytes

b. Increased catabolism of the muscle protein

c. Apoptosis of the myocytes

d. Hypokalemia

e. Hypophosphatemia

f. Hypomagnesemia

g. Deficiency of vitamin D

h. Hypogonadism

14. *Causes of hypertension in this syndrome are*:

a. Increased vasoreactivity to circulating vasoconstrictors like endothelin 1, catecholamine, and angiotensin II

b. Decreased activity of endothelial nitric oxide synthase

c. Augmented production of renin in the liver

d. Action of excess cortisol and mineralocorticoid receptors

e. Retention of sodium and water due to hyperinsulinemia or insulin resistance

f. Increased intravascular fluid volume

g. Accelerated catabolism of renal vasodilatory prostaglandin

h. ACTH-mediated increased secretion of deoxycorticosterone acetate

CASE 7

A 35-year-old man came to emergency department with complaints of palpitation, epistaxis, severe headache, and diaphoresis. On examination, his blood pressure was 185/110 mm Hg, pulse rate 100 beats/min, and respiratory rate 28 breaths/min. Laboratory investigation demonstrated that fasting serum glucose was 256 mg/dL. His blood pressure could not be controlled despite of giving calcium channel blocker, diuretics, and angiotensin receptor blockers (ARBs).

1. **What is the provisional diagnosis and why?**
2. **How can you confirm the diagnosis?**
3. **Which serum level is better?**
4. **What should be the level in this case?**
5. **What are the differential diagnoses in this case?**
6. **What are the clinical clues to the diagnosis in this case?**
7. **How can you differentiate this disease from paraganglioma?**
8. **What do you mean by "rule of 10" in this disease?**
9. **Is there any interaction between the adrenal medulla and cortex?**

Answers

1. The provisional diagnosis is pheochromocytoma which is based on the following features:

a. Diaphoresis

b. Severe headache

c. Palpitation

d. Hypertension

2. Following tests should be done to confirm the diagnosis:

a. 24 hours urine for:
   - Catecholamines
   - Vanillylmandelic acid (VMA)
   - Metanephrines
   - Normetanephrines

b. Plasma for:
   - Free metanephrines
   - Free normetanephrines

3. Metanephrines and normetanephrines measurement are better than the catecholamine measurement because these can differentiate anxiousness from the pheochromocytoma where:

a. Low metanephrines high catecholamine in case of anxious patient

b. High metanephrines and high catecholamine in true pheochromocytoma

4. In pheochromocytoma:
   a. Plasma free metanephrines >0.5 mmol/L
   b. Plasma free normetanephrine >09 mmol/L
   c. Urinary VMA is >9 mg/dL in 24 hours.
5. Following are the differential diagnoses:
   a. Renal artery stenosis
   b. Pheochromocytoma
   c. Paraganglioma
   d. Primary aldosteronism
   e. Cushing's syndrome
   f. Glucocorticoid resistance syndrome
6. Following are the processes of evaluation in this case:
   a. Renovascular hypertension:
      - Recurrent flush pulmonary edema
      - Renal bruit
      - Abnormal urine analysis
      - After administration of angiotensin-converting enzyme inhibitor (ACEI) or ARBs, there is rise in creatinine of ≥30% from the baseline level.
   b. Pheochromocytoma:
      - History suggestive of palpitation, diaphoresis, and headache
      - Presence of postural drop of blood pressure
      - Marfanoid features
      - Evidence of mucosal neuroma
      - Neurofibroma
      - Café-au-lait spots
   c. Primary aldosteronism:
      - Evidence of hypokalemia
      - Diastolic hypertension
      - Metabolic alkalosis
   d. Cushing's syndrome:
      - Features of Cushing's syndrome
      - Hypokalemia

   e. Glucocorticoid resistance syndrome:
      - Clinical features of androgen excess
      - Hypokalemia
      - Hypertension
7. Differences between pheochromocytoma and sympathetic and parasympathetic paraganglioma:

Features	Pheochromocytoma	Sympathetic paraganglioma	Parasympathetic paraganglioma
Functionality	Functional	Functional	Rarely functional
Location of the tumor	Adrenal medulla	• Abdomen • Pelvis • Mediastinum	• Head • Neck
Inheritance	Sporadic	Commonly familial	Familial
Chance of malignancy	Low	High	High

Rule of 10 in this disease are:
   a. 10% are extra-adrenal.
   b. 10% in children
   c. 10% are familial
   d. 10% multiple or bilateral
   e. 10% recurs after surgical removal
   f. 10% are malignant
   g. 10% are detected in the incidentaloma.
9. Norepinephrine is converted to epinephrine in the adrenal medulla by the enzyme phenylethanolamine N-methyltransferase induced by cortisol which is secreted from the adrenal cortex. So, all the tumor responsible for secretion of epinephrine will arise from adrenal medulla whereas paraganglioma only secrete norepinephrine as there is lack of that enzyme or lack of induction of this enzyme by cortisol.

CASE 8

A 26-year-old female after her onset of menarche at 13 years developed menorrhagia for which she was started with oral contraceptive pills for about 1 year after which she developed oligomenorrhea. So, she continued the pill intermittently. For the recent 8 months, she had secondary amenorrhea with progressive growth of hair throughout the body along with increasing weight gain. So, she was started with laser treatment but without much effect. She had no history of easy bruisability, proximal muscle weakness or galactorrhea, nonhypertensive and nondiabetic, and no significant family history.

On examination, her vitals were normal, no acne and temporal recession of hair, and no abdominal striae. She had clitoromegaly, male torso, and absence of features of defeminization.

Laboratory investigations demonstrated renal and liver function tests and electrolytes were normal, thyroid function tests, cortisol levels, overnight dexamethasone suppression tests, FSH and LH were 15 mIU/ML (3.5–12.5) and 10 mIU/L (1.7–8.6), testosterone was 11 nmol/L (0.2–2.9 nmol/L), DHEAS 965 µg/dL (144–407 µg/dL), and

17-hydroxyprogesterone 2.4 ng/dL (<2 ng/dL). 24 hours metepinephrine and normetanephrine were normal. CECT abdomen demonstrated:

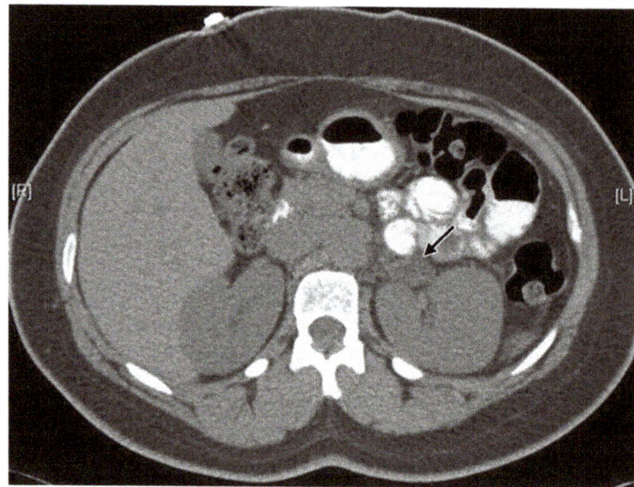

1. **What does the above picture demonstrate?**
2. **Why menorrhagia is followed by oligomenorrhea?**
3. **What are the possibilities in this case?**
4. **How can you exclude the differential diagnoses?**
5. **High level of testosterone and DHEA suggests what diagnosis?**
6. **Why FSH and LH are high in this case?**
7. **What is the source of androgen in female?**
8. **What are the disorders of androgen excess?**
9. **What is hirsutism?**
10. **What are the features of defeminization?**
11. **What are the types of hair in human being?**
12. **What are the nonandrogen-dependent hair?**
13. **What are the areas where androgen excess produces excess hair and what is the area where androgen excess reduces the hair?**

Answers

1. The above picture demonstrates an evidence of a well-defined mass in the left adrenal gland, nearly 70% washout within 10 minutes, absence of necrosis, calcification or hemorrhage suggest—adrenal adenoma.

2. History of menorrhagia followed by oligomenorrhea is suggestive of:
   a. Polycystic ovarian syndrome which is most common in adolescent girl.
   b. Late onset congenital adrenal hyperplasia due to 21-hydroxylase deficiency with features of hirsutism, acne as well as virilization.

3. Following features are the process of exclusion:
   a. Androgen-secreting ovarian or adrenal malignant tumor can be excluded by slow and progressive development of evidences of virilization in absence of defeminization as well as palpable pelvic or abdominal mass.
   b. Ovarian hyperthecosis can be excluded as the patient is in postmenopausal period and severe features of hyperandrogenism.
   c. Cushing's syndrome can be excluded by absence of:
      • Features of protein catabolism
      • Acne
      • Bruise
      • Proximal muscle weakness

4. The differential diagnoses are:
   a. Androgen-secreting adrenal tumor
   b. Ovarian tumor
   c. Ovarian hyperthecosis
   d. Cushing's syndrome
   e. Use of androgen or androgenic progestins

5. High level of testosterone suggests:
   a. Adrenal or ovarian neoplasia
   b. Peripheral conversion of DHEA to testosterone
   High level of DHEA suggests and confirms the diagnosis of adrenal neoplasia.
6. High serum levels of FSH and LH are due to inhibition of estrogen-mediated negative feedback by high testosterone in the serum interfering with the binding of estrogen to the receptor in the hypothalamic-pituitary axis.
7. High levels of androgen are secreted from adrenal gland and the ovary. 50% of testosterone is secreted from the adrenal gland and the ovary directly. Rest 50% is produced from the peripheral conversion of weaker androgens secreted by ovary and adrenal gland like DHEA, androstenedione, and DHEA sulfate.
8. Following are the causes of androgen excess:
   a. Polycystic ovarian disease
   b. Late onset congenital adrenal hyperplasia
   c. Idiopathic hirsutism
   d. ACTH-dependent Cushing's syndrome
   e. Glucocorticoid resistance syndrome
   f. Hyperprolactinemia
   g. Virilizing ovarian tumor
   h. Virilizing adrenal tumor
9. Hirsutism can be defined as growth of excessive hair in male pattern in the androgen-dependent area in female.
10. Features of defeminization include:
    a. Breast atrophy
    b. Oligomenorrhea
    c. Amenorrhea
    d. Loss of gluteofemoral obesity
11. There are two types of hair in the human being:
    a. Terminal hair which is thick, course as well as pigmented and it is present in the androgen-dependent areas.
    b. Vellus hair which is thin, nonpigmented, and fine and present all over the body.
12. Following hairs are nonandrogen dependent:
    a. Eyebrows
    b. Eyelashes
    c. Nostrils
    d. Lateral scalp hair
    e. Occipital scalp hair
13. In the following areas, growth of hair requires androgen excess:
    a. Hair in the upper lip
    b. Chin
    c. Chest
    d. Upper arms
    e. Abdomen
    f. Back
    g. Thigh
    Scalp hairs require regression in case of androgen excess.

CASE 9

An 18-year-old normotensive well-nourished male came to medicine department with short stature but no dysmorphic feature. He had neither past history of chronic illness nor chronic medications. He was full-term delivered vaginally. He was up-to-date in his study.

On examination, his weight was 41 kg, height 150 cm, no thyromegaly, noted to be tanner 1 for prepubertal testicle as well as pubic hair.

Laboratory investigation demonstrated FSH 0.50 mIU/mL, LH 0.09 mIU/mL, testosterone <2.4 ng/dL, serum cortisol 4.5 μg/dL, upon stimulation cortisol 15 μg/dL, and TSH level 0.2 mIU/L, fT4 0.5 ng/dL, and growth hormone 4 ng/dL.

1. **What should be the expected changes in this patient during puberty?**
2. **What do you mean by delayed puberty?**
3. **What are the causes of delayed puberty?**
4. **What is your diagnosis in this case?**
5. **What are the causes of short stature?**
6. **How can you differentiate constitutional delay of growth and puberty (CDGP) from this disease?**
7. **How can you treat constitutional delayed puberty?**
8. **If the patient is female, in that case what is the suggested hormone replacement?**
9. **What are the forms in which the testosterone can be administered?**

Answers

1. Expected changes in this patient during puberty:
   a. Secondary sexual characteristics:
      - Testes: More than 4.4 mL, normal in volume and length >2.5 cm longitudinally
      - Thinning of the scrotum
      - Pigmentation of the scrotum
      - Growth of the penis will be increased
      - Breaking of the voice
      - Axillary hair and facial hair growth
      - Acne
   b. Prepubertal spurt of growth: Maximum growth occurs at the genital stage of IV and V.
   c. Spermaturia

2. Delayed puberty can be defined as failure in the manifestation of the initial signs of the sexual maturation by the age of >2–2.5 standard deviation scores above the mean in case of boys of >14 years which is characterized by testicular enlargement.

3. Causes of delayed puberty:
   a. Central causes that lead to secondary or tertiary hypogonadotropic hypogonadism
   b. Peripheral or gonadal or primary hypogonadotropic hypogonadism
   c. Constitutional delay in the growth as well as puberty

4. The diagnosis is hypogonadotropic hypogonadism.

5. Causes of pathologic short stature:
   a. Disproportionate short stature:
      - Osteochondrodysplasia
      - Achondroplasia
      - Hypochondroplasia
      - Other osteochondrodysplasia:
        - Epiphyseal dysplasia
        - Metaphyseal dysplasia
        - Dysplasia with defective bone mineralization
        - Spondylometaphyseal dysplasia
        - Acromelic or acromesomelic dysplasia
      - Disproportionate short stature with rickets:
        - Vitamin D deficiency rickets
        - Hypophosphatemic rickets
   b. Proportionate short stature:
      - Intrauterine growth retardation
      - Russell–Silver syndrome
      - Beckwith–Wiedemann syndrome
   c. Proportionate short stature with postnatal onset:
      - Nutritional causes of growth failure

- Chronic organ system disease:
  - Gastrointestinal disease and malabsorption
  - Cardiovascular causes
  - Hematological disorders
  - Pulmonary disorders
  - Infections
- Voluntary restriction of nutrition
- Involuntary restriction of calorie
- Genetic causes:
  - Turner syndrome
  - Noonan syndrome
  - SHOX deficiency
  - Prader–Willi syndrome
  - Down syndrome
  - 18q deletion syndrome

6. Constitutional delay of growth and puberty can be differentiated from hypogonadotropic hypogonadism by:
   a. Serum level of inhibin B is >35 pg/mL—suggests CDGP
   b. Anti-Müllerian hormone is >110 pmol/L—suggests CDGP
   c. Response of gonadotropin to gonadotropin-releasing hormone—absent in hypogonadotropic hypogonadism
   d. Response of testosterone to human chorionic gonadotropin—absent in hypogonadotropic hypogonadism

7. Constitutional delayed puberty can be treated by 50–100 mg of testosterone enanthate or cypionate or propionate should be administered every 4 weeks for 3–6 months, and same dose can be repeated if required.

8. If the patient is girl:
   a. Hormonal replacement should be started at 11–12 years of age.
   b. 5 µg ethinyl estradiol orally or 0.3 mg conjugated estrogen should be administered orally daily for 4–6 months, or, 0.1 µg/kg/day estradiol should be given transdermally with gradual increase in the dose over next 2 years to adult dose of 20 µg estradiol daily or 1.25 mg conjugated estrogen or 100 µg estradiol transdermally.
   c. After 2 years or when breakthrough bleeding will start, progestin should be added. Then estrogen should be given cyclically for 21 days followed by 200–300 mg micronized progesterone should be given orally for next 12 days of that month from day 10–21. So, next 7-day pill free period will lead to the breakthrough bleeding.

9. Following forms of testosterone can be found:
    a. Testosterone enanthate or cypionate should be administered intramuscularly every 2–4 weeks.
    b. Testosterone undecanoate: A long-acting intramuscular injection should be given at every 3 months.
    c. Testosterone gel
    d. Transdermal testosterone patches
    e. Testosterone pellet—subcutaneously placed

CASE 10

A 31-year-old female was admitted with history of menorrhagia, abdominal pain, progressively increasing weight, and secondary growth of hair in the face and acne.

Laboratory investigation demonstrated that LH became high. Ultrasound of the abdomen demonstrated:

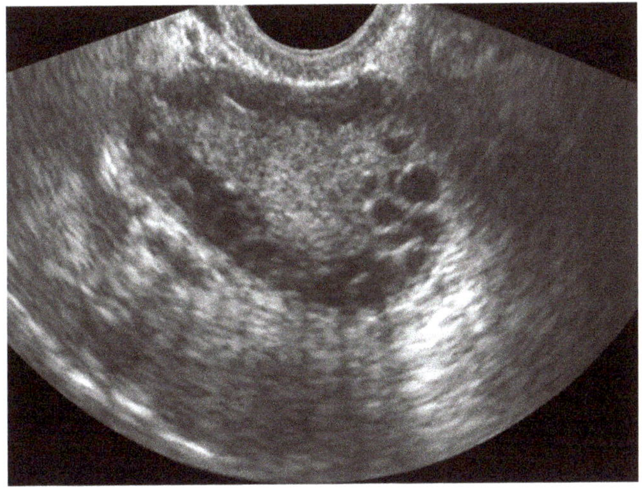

1. **What does the above picture demonstrate?**
2. **What is the definition of this disease?**
3. **What are the clinical manifestations in this disease?**
4. **In which age this disease will present?**
5. **What are the unusual presentations in this disease?**
6. **Why this disease will produce the female infertile?**
7. **How can you differentiate this disease from ovarian hyperthecosis?**
8. **What are the causes of secondary cause of this disease?**

Answers

1. The above picture demonstrates multiple cysts in the ovary.
2. This disease is characterized by clinical and/or biochemical features of hyperandrogenism, menstrual abnormalities, and polycystic ovaries along with insulin resistance.
3. Clinical manifestations in this disease:
    a. Menstrual irregularities:
        -   Oligomenorrhea
        -   Secondary amenorrhea
        -   Primary amenorrhea
        -   Menorrhagia
    b. Normal anovulatory cycles
    c. Hirsutism in 60% patients
    d. Acne in 20% patients
    e. Obesity
    f. Android distribution of fat
    g. Features of insulin resistance:
        -   Acanthosis nigricans
        -   Skin tags
4. This disease is common in the three phases of life:
    a. Peripubertal phase—most common in this phase
    b. Peripartum phase
    c. Perimenopausal phase

During these phases:
a. There is maximum perturbation of gonadotropin-releasing hormone pulse activity.
b. Increase in the adipose tissue mass
c. Psychological disturbances

Slow pulse of this hormone is related to stimulation of FSH whereas fast pulse is related to stimulation of LH hormone. During these phases, there is fast pulsatility of gonadotropin-releasing hormone and there is increased secretion of LH as compared to FSH secretion leading to hyperplasia of theca and anovulation.

5. Following are the unusual presentations in this disease:
a. Primary amenorrhea with normal development of secondary sexual characteristics. These patients have high androgen level, increased incidence of metabolic syndrome, delayed pubarche, and lack of withdrawal bleeding due to estrogenized endometrium and lack of secretion of progesterone.
b. Menorrhagia occurs due to endometrial hyperplasia
c. Galactorrhea due to hyperprolactinemia
d. Virilization

6. Following are the causes of infertility in this disease:
a. Chronic anovulation
b. Presence of senescent ova
c. Hostile cervical mucus
d. Unfavorable endometrial environment

7. Ovarian hyperthecosis is characterized by:
a. Severe hyperandrogenism
b. Insulin resistance
c. Postmenopausal woman
d. Presentation should be:
   - Acne
   - Hirsutism
   - Features of virilization

This disease is characterized by
a. Younger woman
b. Mild hirsutism
c. Menstrual abnormalities
d. Lack of features of virilization

8. Secondary causes of this disease:
a. Hypothyroidism
b. Acromegaly
c. Cushing's syndrome
d. Hyperprolactinemia
e. Thyrotoxicosis
f. Congenital adrenal hyperplasia

CASE 11

A 24-year-old man came with difficulty in deglutition in the ENT department. ENT specialist demonstrated:

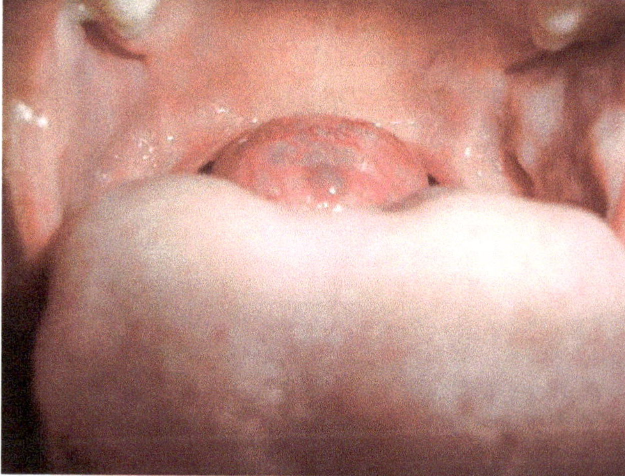

1. **What does the above picture demonstrate?**
2. **How the thyroid gland is developed?**
3. **What are the developmental abnormalities in the thyroid gland?**
4. **What are the muscles surround the thyroid gland?**
5. **Describe the arterial supply of this gland.**

Answers

1. The above picture demonstrates the presence of lingual thyroid.
2. Thyroid gland has been developed in-between first and second pharyngeal pouches at the root of the tongue as an analage. During the development, thyroid is connected with foramen cecum via thyroglossal duct in the mouth. With the development, the gland descends inferiorly to its normal position in front of the thyroid cartilage along with the obliteration of the thyroglossal duct.
3. The developmental abnormalities are:
   a. Thyroglossal cyst due to failure of obliteration of the thyroglossal duct
   b. If the thyroid gland not at all descends, it will produce lingual thyroid.
   c. If the thyroid gland moves more inferiorly to the retrosternal position, it will produce retrosternal thyroid.
4. The muscles surround the thyroid gland are:
   a. Omohyoid muscle
   b. Sternohyoid muscle
   c. Sternothyroid muscle
   d. Thyrohyoid muscle
5. Following are the arterial supply of the thyroid gland:
   a. Superior thyroid artery from the external carotid artery
   b. Inferior thyroid artery from the thyrocervical trunk arising from the first part of subclavian artery.

CASE 12

A 28-year-old strictly vegetarian female, mother of one child came to medicine outpatient department with progressively increasing weight, lethargy, and joint pain. She used sunscreen with sun protecting factor of 50. On examination, thyroid examination demonstrated as below. Her TSH level was 8.5 mIU/L and T4 6 µg/dL. Her thyroid peroxidase (TPO) antibody was above 1,300 U/L.

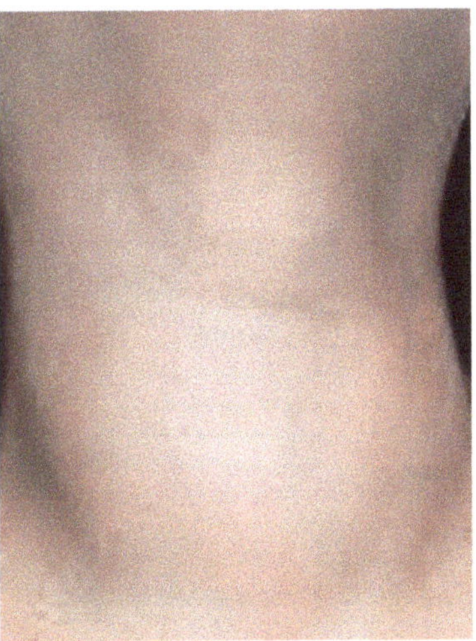

1. **Describe the above picture.**
2. **What is the diagnosis and why?**
3. **What are the normal ranges of TSH level?**
4. **What are the autoimmune diseases associated with this disease?**
5. **What should be the normal level of TSH if the patient becomes pregnant?**
6. **When anti-TPO antibody should be measured?**
7. **What are the indications of treatment in this disease?**
8. **What is the proper gap between the drug ingestion and the diet?**
9. **If the patient becomes pregnant, which is the best monitoring tool in this days?**

Answers

1. The above picture demonstrates generalized enlargement of thyroid gland which is smooth and rubbery in consistency.
2. The diagnosis is Hashimoto thyroiditis because:
   a. Serum TSH is high.
   b. Serum T4 is low or low normal.
   c. Serum antithyroid peroxidase antibody is high.
   d. Thyroid gland is enlarged.
3. Normal range of TSH level in the serum: Normal range will change with age of the patient.
   a. TSH level will be lowest in the late afternoon and highest around the hour of sleep.
   b. In elderly, the mildest elevation of TSH suggests subclinical hypothyroidism or it may be a part of the normal aging.
4. Following are the autoimmune diseases associated with this disease:
   a. Pernicious anemia
   b. Type 1 diabetes mellitus
   c. Myasthenia gravis
   d. Celiac disease
   e. Rheumatoid arthritis
   f. Addison's disease
   g. Systemic lupus erythematosus (SLE)
5. If this patient is pregnant, the levels of TSH are the following:

Trimesters	Levels of TSH in mIU/L
First trimester	• If TPO is negative—up to 4 • If TPO is positive, level is 2.5 • High-risk pregnancy

Continued

Continued

Trimesters	Levels of TSH in mIU/L
Second trimester	• If TPO is negative—up to 4 • If TPO is positive, level is 3 • High-risk pregnancy
Third trimester	• If TPO is negative—up to 4 • If TPO is positive, level is 3 • High-risk pregnancy

In following cases anti-TPO antibodies should be measured:
   a. If the patient will suffer from subclinical hypothyroidism, anti-TPO antibodies should be measured for diagnosing Hashimoto thyroiditis.
   b. If the patient has history of recurrent abortions.
   c. If there is history of infertility.
7. Following are the indications of treatment in this disease:
   a. Hypothyroidism with positive anti-TPO antibody
   b. Atherosclerotic cardiovascular disease
   c. Heart failure
   d. If the patient is pregnant.
   e. If there is planning for conception.
8. The drug should be taken 1 hour prior to breakfast or 4 hours after the last meal, and this tablet should be taken with water.
9. If the patient is pregnant, serum T4 should be measured as compared to FT4, because there is alteration serum proteins during pregnancy leading to low value of FT4.

CASE 13

A 34-year-old female came to medicine outpatient with progressive weight loss, menorrhagia, and palpitation. On examination, there was tachycardia, tremor on the outstretched hand, and hand was warm and moist. Eye demonstrated grittiness with following features:

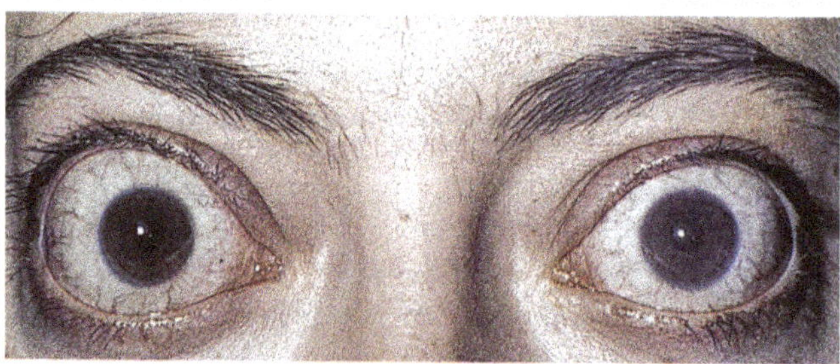

1. **What does the above picture demonstrate?**
2. **What is your diagnosis?**
3. **How can you differentiate this disease clinically from subacute thyroiditis and toxic multinodular goiter?**
4. **What is the principle of radioiodine uptake study in this disease?**
5. **What is the absolute contraindication of radioiodine uptake in this case?**
6. **Thyrotoxicosis is either due to thyroiditis or other causes—explain.**
7. **Is technetium-99 scanning is same as that of radioiodine?**
8. **How do you monitor the patient who is on antithyroid drug?**
9. **What is Jod-Basedow phenomenon?**
10. **What is Wolff–Chaikoff effect?**
11. **Mention the cause of Wolff–Chaikoff effect.**

Answers

1. The above picture demonstrates proptosis. Eyes are red. There is retraction of the both eyelids leading to exposure of the conjunctiva above the pupil.
2. The working diagnosis is primary hyperthyroidism.
3. Following features will give clue to the diagnosis:
   a. Duration of the symptoms
   b. Thyroid gland—its size and shape
   c. Tenderness over the thyroid gland
   d. Extrathyroidal features of Graves' disease.

   Graves' disease:
   a. Presence of family history
   b. Patient becomes symptomatic for several weeks to months.
   c. Presence of diffuse goiter
   d. Presence of extrathyroidal manifestation like ophthalmopathy, increased grittiness in the eyes.

   Toxic multinodular goiter:
   a. Patient is generally older.
   b. Presence of multiple nodules in the thyroid gland
   c. Patient will be symptomatic for months.
   d. Absence of extrathyroidal manifestation.

   Subacute thyroiditis:
   a. Any age
   b. Symptoms for days to weeks
   c. Gland is firm but tender.
   d. Erythrocyte sedimentation rate (ESR) is >50 mm in 1st hour.
4. To detect the cause of hyperactivity of the thyroid gland, radioactive iodine uptake should be done:
   a. If the uptake is high, it is either Graves' disease or toxic multinodular goiter.
   b. If the uptake is close to zero, it is thyroiditis.

   The pattern of uptake:
   a. If the uptake is generalized, it is Graves' disease.
   b. If the uptake is localized, it is either nodular goiter or there is presence of fibrosis.
   c. If the uptake is focal with suppressed uptake in the surrounding tissue or contralateral tissue, it is thyroid adenoma.
5. Absolute contraindication to radioiodine uptake is pregnancy.
6. In case of thyroiditis, it is due to release of thyroid hormone secondary to destruction of the glandular tissue for 1–3 months which can be managed by β-blockers but antithyroid drugs are not required in thyroiditis. So, diagnosis is required as it will affect the treatment.
7. Iodine and technetium are taken up by the thyroid gland by sodium-iodide symporter present in the glandular tissue. The advantages of technetium over the radioiodine are:
   a. Imaging within 20 minutes
   b. Lesser exposure to iodine
   c. Easy accessibility as compared to radioiodine
8. After administration of the antithyroid drugs, serum T3 and T4 are to be obtained 2–4 weeks after initiation of the therapy and dose of the drug should be adjusted. When the patient becomes euthyroid, dose of the drug should be decreased by 30–40% and repeated serum testing should be done in 4–6 weeks.
9. In the iodine deficient area, supplementation of iodine leads to development of hyperthyroidism—this is known as Jod-Basedow phenomenon. This phenomenon may be due to:
   a. Autonomous nodule which is usually seen in elderly individual
      or,
   b. Presence of TSH receptor stimulating antibodies present in case of diffuse goiter in younger patient—it is also known as "latent Graves".

So in these cases, supplementation with iodine may lead to development of thyrotoxicosis. So, administration of radioiodinated contrast or amiodarone can lead to development of this phenomenon.

10. Exposure to excess iodine inhibits oxidation and organification in the synthesis of thyroid hormone will lead to formation of organic iodocompound along with suppression of TPO activity—this is known as Wolf–Chaikoff effect. Minimum dose of organic iodide compound to produce this effect is 2,000 µg.

11. Causes of the persistent Wolf–Chaikoff effect: Persistent effect results in permanent hypothyroidism and it can occur in patients with underlying thyroid disease like:
    a. Autoimmune thyroiditis
    b. Past history of postpartum or subacute thyroiditis
    c. Previous therapy with radioiodinated iodine in case of Graves' disease
    d. In case neonate due to failure of downregulation of sodium-iodine symporter.

CASE 14

A 45-year-old female having family history of thyroid disease came to endocrinology clinic with palpitation and amenorrhea and anorexia. On examination, there was tachycardia, bilateral conjunctival congestion and tearing, and weakness on the lateral gaze bilaterally. On neck examination, the thyroid gland was enlarged diffusely. In the lower extremity, the skin lesion demonstrated as below:

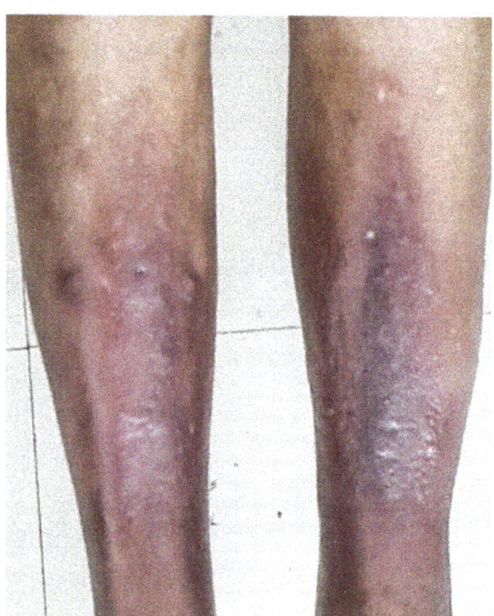

1. **Describe the above picture.**
2. **What is the working diagnosis?**
3. **What is the classical triad in this disease?**
4. **What are the three common causes of this disease?**
5. **What are the differentiating features in the different causes of thyrotoxicosis?**
6. **Mention the unusual manifestations in this disease?**
7. **Mention the monosymptomatic presentation in this disease?**
8. **What are the causes of anorexia?**
9. **What are the manifestations in the hand in this disease?**
10. **What are the menstrual abnormalities in this disease?**
11. **What are the mechanisms responsible for these types of menstrual abnormalities?**
12. **How can you treat this disease?**
13. **What are the types of liver dysfunction developed with above drugs?**
14. **What types of glucose-insulin abnormalities in this disease?**
15. **In which conditions propylthiouracil can be given?**
16. **Which is the preferred drug in this disease?**
17. **Mention the autoimmune disorders associated with this disease.**

Answers

1. The above picture demonstrates brownish red discoloration in the pretibial area along with darkening around the hair follicles.
2. The working diagnosis is Graves' disease.
3. The classical triad in this disease is:
   a. Diffuse toxic goiter
   b. Infiltrative ophthalmopathy
   c. Infiltrative dermopathy
4. Following are the three common causes of this disease:
   a. Subacute thyroiditis
   b. Graves' disease
   c. Toxic micronodular goiter

5. The above causes can be differentiated by following methods:

Features	Subacute thyroiditis	Graves' disease	Toxic multinodular goiter
Age	Any age	20–40 years	>40 years age
Sex	Any gender	Female: Male ratio 10:1	Female: Male ratio 4–10:1
Duration	Days to weeks	Weeks to months	Months to years
Neck pain	Present	Absent	Absent
Symptoms	Very severe	Severe	Mild to moderately severe
Thyroid enlargement	Asymmetrically enlarged	Diffusely enlarged	Firm nodule
Thyroid function tests	• TSH is very low • T4 very high • T3 normal/high	• TSH low • T4 high • T3 very high	• TSH low • T4 high • T3 very high
TSH receptor stimulating antibodies	Absent	Present	Absent
Radio uptake/technetium scan	Uptake is low	Diffusely high uptake	Scattered uptake
Ultrasonography	Enlarged mildly with very low echogenicity	Enlarged diffusely with mildly reduced echogenicity	Multiple nodule with scattered variable echogenicity
Color Doppler study	Vascularity is decreased, but during recovery phase increased vascularity	Increased vascularity	Variable vascularity

Following are the unusual manifestations in this disease:

Unusual features	Causes of the manifestations
Apathetic hyperthyroidism	• Elderly in age-related neuropathy • Relative resistance of the tissue to thyroid hormone
Sinus bradycardia	• Sick sinus syndrome • Patient is on β-blocker
Weight gain	• Young patient • Patients is on glucocorticoids in patients with thyroid-associated neuropathy • Congestive cardiac failure
Pyrexia of unknown origin	• Graves' disease • Subacute thyroiditis
Isolated thyroid-associated orbitopathy	It may precede Graves' disease
Isolated thyroid-associated dermopathy	It may precede orbitopathy or Graves' disease
Periodic paralysis	• Hyperkalemia • Hypokalemia
Rhabdomyolysis	Severe thyrotoxicosis
Hypercalcemia	Severe resorption of bone
Hypoglycemia	• Autoimmune disease • Methimazole administration
Gynecomastia	Altered T/E2 ratio

Monosymptomatic presentation in this disease:
- a. Lone atrial fibrillation
- b. Pyrexia of unknown origin
- c. Malabsorption syndrome
- d. Hypokalemic periodic paralysis
- e. Hyperkalemic periodic paralysis
- f. Apathetic hyperparathyroidism
- g. Hyperpigmentation
- h. Gynecomastia
- i. Pruritus

In case of children:
- a. Attention-deficit/hyperactivity disorders
- b. Tall stature

8. Causes of anorexia are:
   - a. Thyrotoxic cardiomyopathy
   - b. Apathetic hyperthyroidism
   - c. Thyrotoxicosis-induced hypercalcemia
9. Features in the hand in case of thyrotoxicosis:
   - a. Tachycardia
   - b. Fine tremor
   - c. Palmar erythema
   - d. Warm and moist hand
   - e. Onycholysis
   - f. Thyroid acropathy
   - g. Knuckle hyperpigmentation
   - h. Vitiligo
   - i. Thyroid-associated dermopathy
10. Following are the types of menstrual abnormalities in this disease:
    - a. Oligomenorrhea
    - b. Hypomenorrhea
    - c. Polymenorrhea
    - d. Rarely amenorrhea
11. The mechanisms responsible for the above menstrual abnormalities are:
    - a. Increased serum sex hormone-binding globulin
    - b. Decreased free estradiol
    - c. Impaired surge of LH
    - d. Secondary polycystic ovarian disease
    - e. Increased catabolic state in this disease
12. Patient has to be treated with methimazole or propylthiouracil. The later drug blocks the T4 to T3 conversion by the enzyme type 1 deiodinase.

Methimazole is given once a day and propylthiouracil can be given twice a day.

Radioiodine can be given in this disease but it may make the eye disease worse.

13. Carbimazole and methimazole are responsible for cholestatic jaundice.

    Propylthiouracil and methylprednisolone are responsible for hepatocellular disease.
14. Patient may develop glucose intolerance due to following mechanisms:
    - a. Increased absorption of glucose from the intestine
    - b. Enhanced hepatic neoglucogenesis
    - c. Rapid clearance of insulin from the blood
    - d. Resistance of insulin at the receptor level
    - e. Elevated levels of counterregulatory hormones like catecholamine and glucagon
    - f. High level of lactate due to enhanced anaerobic glycolysis
15. In following conditions, propylthiouracil can be administered in this disease:
    - a. First trimester of pregnancy, it can be administered because of its increased binding with the albumin it cannot cross the placental barrier.
    - b. It should be given in thyroid storm because it will prevent peripheral conversion of T4 to T3.
16. Carbimazole is the preferred drug in this disease and should be given as once daily dose. This prodrug that will be converted into methimazole in the liver. Though its serum half-life is 6–8 hours, but it will be concentrated in the thyroid gland 16 times more than that in the plasma, hence it is given as once daily dose and makes the patient euthyroid early as compared to propylthiouracil.
17. Following autoimmune disorders are associated with pregnancy:
    - a. Myasthenia gravis
    - b. Type 1 diabetes mellitus
    - c. Pernicious anemia
    - d. Celiac disease
    - e. Vitiligo
    - f. Autoimmune thrombocytopenia
    - g. Autoimmune hepatitis
    - h. SLE
    - i. Autoimmune hypoglycemia

CASE 15

A 35-year-old female having history of thyroid disease came to surgical department with large swelling in front of neck but without any symptom. On examination, her vitals were normal, thyroid was diffusely enlarged, nontender, and rubbery in consistence. Her ankle jerk relaxation time was delayed.

Laboratory investigation demonstrated that serum T4 was 0.4 ng/dL and TSH 35 mIU/L.

1. **What is the working diagnosis?**
2. **What are the other investigations should be done to confirm the diagnosis?**
3. **What type spectrum of clinical features is seen in this disease?**
4. **How can you treat this case?**
5. **What are the common drugs that interfere with thyroxine absorption?**

Answers

1. The working diagnosis is subclinical hypothyroidism.
2. The following investigations should be done in this case:
   a. Antithyroid peroxidase antibody
   b. Antithyroglobulin antibody
   As these antibodies combine with the complement to produce complement-dependent antibody mediated cytotoxicity.
3. In case of early inflammation, there is transient thyrotoxicosis which is also known as hashitoxicosis. This is followed by development of permanent hypothyroidism.
4. Average replacement dose is oral thyroxine 112 µg daily, but it should be adjusted with the level of TSH. The aim is to maintain the TSH level to normal.
5. Following drugs interfere with the absorption of thyroid drugs:
   a. Bile acid resin
   b. Proton pump inhibitors
   c. Iron sulfate
   d. Calcium carbonate

CASE 16

A 68-year-old male came to emergency department with high fever, sore throat, and chest pain for which angiography was done which was found as insignificant. So, he was started nitroglycerin along with metoprolol. His blood pressure was 135/60 mm Hg, pulse rate 92 beats/min, respiratory rate 20 breaths/min, and temperature 101°F. There was tenderness in front of the neck, mild tremor but no eye involvement was noted. Blood examination demonstrated raised ESR and leukocytosis, chest X-ray demonstrated no infiltrate.

1. **What is the most probable diagnosis?**
2. **What are the cardiac manifestations in Graves' disease that are reversible with treatment?**
3. **What are the characteristics of hypertension in this disease?**
4. **What are blood tests should be done in this patient?**
5. **What are the additional investigations should be done to come to a diagnosis?**
6. **How can you treat this patient?**

Answers

1. The most likely diagnosis is painful thyroiditis.
2. The cardiac manifestations in Graves' disease which are reversible with treatment:
   a. Mitral valve prolapse
   b. Sick sinus syndrome
   c. Pulmonary hypertension
   d. Rate-related cardiomyopathy
   e. Pleuropericardial friction rub
3. Following are the characteristics of hypertension in this disease:
   a. Systolic hypertension due to:
      • Increased cardiac output
      • Increased contractility of myocardium

b. Decreased diastolic blood pressure due to:
  - Peripheral vasodilatation due to:
    o Direct effect of thyroid hormone on the vessels
    o Increased production of nitric acid
c. Wide pulse pressure

4. Following blood tests are done:
   a. T4—increased
   b. FT4—mildly increased
   c. TSH—not detectable
   d. Serum thyroglobulin—increased
   e. Radioiodine uptake—absent
   f. Urinary iodine level should be done to exclude high level of iodine in the body where there is decreased radioiodine uptake.

5. This patient has been suffering from early phase or destructive phase of thyroiditis. There are three phases:
   a. First phase or destructive or hyperthyroid phase
   b. Euthyroid phase
   c. Hypothyroid phase

6. The patient can be treated by:
   a. Anti-inflammatory drugs to get relief from pain and fever.
   b. Glucocorticoid should be given to decrease the inflammation of the thyroid gland.
   c. Parenteral antibiotics should be given urgently to prevent abscess formation

CASE 17

A 45-year-old female having family history of thyroid disease came to endocrinology clinic with palpitation and amenorrhea and anorexia. On examination, there was tachycardia, bilateral conjunctival congestion and tearing, weakness on the lateral gaze bilaterally, and proptosis. On neck examination, the thyroid gland was enlarged diffusely.

1. **What is your diagnosis?**
2. **Grade the goiter.**
3. **What is the cause of nodular goiter?**
4. **Why in some cases there is increased level of T3 as compared to T4 in the blood?**
5. **Why thyroid profile should be done in thyrotoxicosis at the time of diagnosis?**
6. **Why recovery of the serum TSH level is delayed during the treatment of Graves' disease?**
7. **What are the predictors of remission in case of Graves' disease?**
8. **Which patients with Graves' disease fail to get remission with antithyroid treatment?**
9. **Mention the indications of beta-blockers in thyrotoxicosis?**

Answers

1. The diagnosis is Graves' disease.
2. Grading of goiter:
   a. Grade 0: No palpable thyroid gland
   b. Grade 1: In the extended neck, thyroid gland is palpable and/or visible.
   c. Grade 2: In the neutral position of the neck, the thyroid gland is palpable and/or visible.
   d. Grade 3: Thyroid gland is visible from distance.
   e. Grade 4: Monstrous goiter
3. The intermittent therapy in case of Graves' disease leads to fluctuation in the level of serum TSH resulting in the development of the nodule in the thyroid gland.
4. Graves' disease, toxic adenoma, or toxic multinodular goiter may be associated T3-toxicosis as there is increase in the serum level of T3 due to increased extrathyroidal as well as intrathyroidal conversion of T4 to T3 as a result of activation of the enzyme type 1 deiodinase. Again, during treatment of hyperthyroidism, the methimazole inhibits the oxidation of iodine peroxidase and organification in the thyroid gland, the gland is unable to utilize the intrathyroidal iodine leading to relative higher secretion of T3.
5. In thyrotoxicosis, there is increased level of free T3, free T4, and TSH. Subclinical hyperthyroidism, thyrotropinoma, and resistance to thyroid hormone may be missed if free T4 and free T3 are measured. So, all cases of hyperthyroidism total thyroid profile should be measured.
6. Recovery of TSH level in the blood during the treatment of Graves' disease will be delayed due to:
   a. Prolonged inhibitory effect of plasma T3 and T4 on the thyrotropes

b. Suppressive effect of intrapituitary cytokines on the thyrotropes leads to increased conversion of T4 to T3

7. Following are the predictors of remission in Graves' disease on treatment:
   a. Young age
   b. Female sex
   c. Small goiter
   d. T3-toxicosis
   e. Decrease in the size of goiter during treatment
   f. Normalization of TSH
   g. Declined level of thyroid receptor antibodies in the blood

8. Following patients with Graves' disease fail to get remission with treatment:
   a. Older age
   b. Male sex
   c. Chronic smoker
   d. Grade III or more the size of the goiter
   e. If thyrotoxicosis associated with the level of T3 >9 ng/dL
   f. If the treatment duration is <18 months
   g. Inability to taper the dose of the antithyroid drugs to 5–10 mg of carbimazole in 18–24 months
   h. Lack of normalization of TSH
   i. Development of nodularity in the thyroid gland
   j. Persistence of thyroid receptor antibodies in the blood

9. Indications of β-blockers in thyrotoxicosis:
   a. Atrial fibrillation with rapid ventricular rate
   b. Rate-related heart failure
   c. Thyrotoxic periodic paralysis
   d. Thyroid storm

CASE 18

A 45-year-old female having two sons came to medical outpatient department with two small nodules on both sides in front of the neck and thyroid cartilage which moved up and down with deglutition.

Laboratory examination demonstrated T4 1.5 ng/dL and TSH 1 mU/L

1. **What is the working diagnosis?**
2. **What initial imaging should be done in this case?**
3. **Mention the characteristics of suspicious malignancy in the nodule in ultrasound.**
4. **What is the role of radioiodine uptake in this case?**
5. **What is the next step of investigation in this case?**
6. **Mention the clinical pointers toward malignancy in this nodule.**

Answers

1. Thyroid nodule
2. Initial imaging in this case should be thyroid ultrasound which will detect hypoechoic solid nodules on both sides of the neck. ^{18}F-FDG-PET detected thyroid nodule is likely to be malignant.
3. Following characteristics of suspicious malignant nodule can be seen in the thyroid ultrasound:
   a. Hypoechogenicity
   b. Solid nodule
   c. Increased intranodular vascularity
   d. Irregular infiltrative margins
   e. Microcalcifications
   f. Absent halo
   g. Shape of the thyroid is taller than width.
4. As the thyroid function test is normal, radioiodine uptake is not required in this case. If the serum level of TSH is low, in that case this test is required to differentiate thyroiditis from thyrotoxicosis.
5. Next step of investigation will be fine needle aspiration cytology to detect the presence of malignancy.
6. Following are the clinical pointers toward malignancy in the thyroid nodule:
   a. Extremes of ages
      - <20 years of age
      - >65 years of age
   b. Male sex
   c. Family history of thyroid carcinoma
   d. History of exposure to radiation in the childhood
   e. Sudden increase in the size of the nodule
   f. If the nodule is fixed to the deeper structure.
   g. Paralysis of the recurrent laryngeal nerve
   h. Cervical lymph node enlargement

CASE 19

A 45-year-old female having family history of hypothyroidism came to outpatient department with history of only swelling in front of the neck but no other manifestation. On examination, her vitals are normal, in the neck there were two nodules present on the left side of the neck and left-sided enlarged cervical lymph node.

Thyroid function test was normal. Ultrasonography of the neck demonstrated hypoechoic rounded nodule with foci of calcification.

Fine needle aspiration cytology from the thyroid nodule was performed which demonstrated:

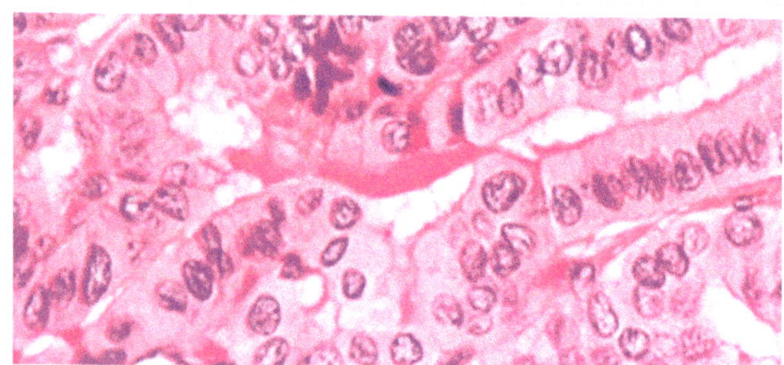

1. **What was demonstrated in the histological picture?**
2. **What is your diagnosis?**
3. **Is radioiodine uptake is helpful in this case?**
4. **What should be the treatment in this case?**
5. **What should be the recommended target of TSH in different risk groups?**

Answers

1. Histological picture demonstrated elongated follicles of columnar cells along with palisading oval nuclei containing eosinophilic cytoplasm as well as papillary nuclear features and psammoma bodies.
2. The patient has been suffering from papillary carcinoma of thyroid.
3. As the thyroid nodule is cold, radioiodine uptake is not at all helpful. But if the nodule is hyperfunctioning, TSH is depressed and T4 is high, in that case radioiodine is indicated and hot nodule never be malignant.
4. Definite treatment is total thyroidectomy along with central block dissection of cervical lymph node because of the potential of the metastasis. Levothyroxine should be started to suppress the TSH secretion to maintain below the normal range. But, if the tumor size is <1 cm having no extrathyroidal extension.
5. Recommended target of TSH in different risk groups:
   a. High-risk patients: <0.1 mU/L
   b. Intermediate-risk patient: <0.1–0.5 mU/L
   c. Low-risk patient: 0.5–2.0 mU/L

CASE 20

A 26-year-old female having history of grade III diffuse goiter and thyrotoxicosis now euthyroid on carbimazole 15 mg daily became pregnant. During first-trimester, due to worsening of symptoms, her vitals were T3 2.9 ng/mL, T4 19 µg/dL, and TSH 0.001 µIU/mL. The dose of the carbimazole was increased to 30 mg daily, but in the second-trimester she became euthyroid and dose was reduced to again 15 mg daily. She delivered a full-term baby having birth weight of 2.4 kg with normal thyroid function test and discharged.

But at third week, following lower respiratory tract infection, there was weight loss of 500 mg in spite of normal feeding and pulse rate of 165 beats/min. Thyroid function test revealed 3.6 ng/mL, T4 24 µg/mL, and TSH 0.005 µIU/mL. Methimazole was started along with propranolol. After 6 weeks, thyroid functions returned to normal thereby dose of the methimazole was reduced.

Two months after postpartum, she again became thyrotoxic and grade III diffuse goiter. Thyroid function test revealed T4 18 µg/dL, T3 1.9 ng/dL, and TSH 0.04 µIU/mL. So, dose of the carbimazole was increased to 30 mg/day.

1. **In the first trimester, why the dose of the drug was increased?**
2. **Why the reference level of thyroid hormone is high during pregnancy?**
3. **Why in the mid trimester, the serum level of thyroid receptor antibody level is tested?**
4. **In spite of transplacental passage of thyroid receptor antibody, why fetal thyrotoxicosis will not develop?**
5. **Is the neonatal thyrotoxicosis is permanent or transient?**
6. **Why there is exacerbation of symptom in postpartum period?**
7. **Which hormone can cross the placenta and why?**
8. **What are the important molecules in thyroid that can cross the placenta?**
9. **Why the requirement of iodine is increased during pregnancy?**
10. **Who are at risk of developing thyroid dysfunction during pregnancy?**
11. **What are the features which can help to suspect fetal thyrotoxicosis?**
12. **What are the causes of goiter in fetus?**
13. **What are the conditions when estimation of thyroid receptor antibodies is essential?**
14. **What are the bad effects of administration of β-blockers in pregnancy?**
15. **What is thionamide embryopathy?**
16. **What are the indications of surgery in Graves' disease during pregnancy?**

Answers

1. In the first trimester, the dose of the drug was increased due to:
   a. Raised level of human chorionic gonadotropin that stimulates the thyroid gland to secrete thyroid hormone
   b. Quiescence Graves' disease as a result of suppression of autoimmunity due to increased level of progesterone and estradiol
2. During pregnancy, the reference level of the hormone is increased because of estrogen-mediated rise in the thyroid-binding globulin in the blood.
3. In the mid trimester, serum level of thyroid receptor antibody has to be tested because there is risk of developing thyrotoxicosis in fetus. There is close fetal monitoring which is required if this antibody is positive.
4. In spite of transplacental passage of thyroid receptor antibody, why fetal thyrotoxicosis will not develop because of:
   a. Transplacental passage of antithyroid drug into the fetus and thereby preventing development of neonatal hyperthyroidism.
   b. Increased concentration of TSH-blocking antibodies as compared to TSH-stimulating antibodies.
5. Neonatal thyrotoxicosis is transient because within 3–12 weeks thyroid receptor antibodies will disappear. But if it is persistent, the alternate diagnoses are:
   a. McCune–Albright syndrome
   b. Mutation of TSH receptor activator

6. In the postpartum period, there is exacerbation of symptoms because:
   a. Withdrawal of estrogen and progesterone after 6 weeks of postpartum
   b. It may develop postpartum thyroiditis between 8 and 24 weeks of postpartum.
7. Two hormones can cross the placenta:
   a. Thyrotropin-releasing hormone (TRH)
   b. T4
   Maternal TRH will responsible for development of fetal hypothalamic-pituitary-thyroid axis.
   T4 is helpful for fetal neural growth and development.
8. Following molecules can cross the placenta:
   a. Iodine can cross the placenta because syncytiotrophoblast will express sodium iodide symporter. Iodine will help:
      - Fetal thyroid growth as well as development
      - The biosynthesis of thyroid hormone
      - Fetal neural growth and development
   b. TSH receptor antibodies:
      - Thyroid-stimulating immunoglobulin
      - TSH-binding inhibitory immunoglobulin
   c. Antithyroid drugs leading to development of hypothyroidism and goiter:
      - Carbimazole
      - Methimazole
      - Propylthiouracil
9. Following are the causes of increased requirement of thyroid hormone during pregnancy:
   a. During pregnancy:

- Increased synthesis of thyroid hormone:
    - Rising level of human chorionic gonadotropin (hCG)
    - Increased level of thyroid-binding globulin
- Increased secretion of iodine through urine due to increased glomerular filtration rate (GFR) during pregnancy
- Increased utilization of iodine by the fetus due to:
    - Thyroid hormone synthesis
    - Neurocognitive development

10. Following patients are at risk of developing thyroid dysfunction during pregnancy:
    a. Age >30 years
    b. Presence of goiter
    c. Patient is positive for TPO.
    d. Bad obstetric history
    e. BMI is >40 kg/m^2
    f. Personal history of autoimmune disease
    g. Family history of autoimmune disease
    h. Presence of iodine deficiency
    i. Prior thyroid surgery
    j. Amiodarone or lithium use

11. Following features can help to suspect fetal thyrotoxicosis:
    a. Persistent tachycardia or pulse rate >170 beats/min
    b. Intrauterine growth retardation
    c. Congestive cardiac failure
    d. Hydrops fetalis
    e. Accelerated maturation of bone

12. Following are the causes of goiter in fetus:
    a. Use of antithyroid drugs during pregnancy
    b. Use of iodine containing preparations during pregnancy
    c. Maternal Graves' disease along with trans-placental passage of thyroid receptor antibodies

    d. Fetal thyroid dyshormonogenesis
    e. TSH receptor activating mutations

13. Following are the conditions when estimation of thyroid receptor antibodies is essential:
    a. Active Graves' disease
    b. History of radioablative therapy for Graves' disease prior to pregnancy
    c. History of surgery for Graves' disease prior to pregnancy
    d. History of previous neonate with Graves' disease
    e. Elevation of thyroid receptors prior to pregnancy

Hence, thyroid receptor antibodies should be measured between 22 and 26 weeks as this is the time when fetal TSH receptors are very much responsive to these antibodies.

14. β-blockers are bad during pregnancy because it produces:
    a. Fetal bradycardia
    b. Intrauterine growth retardation
    c. Poor lung maturation
    d. Neonatal hypoglycemia

15. Thionamide embryopathy is characterized by the following:
    a. Choanal atresia
    b. Esophageal atresia
    c. Omphalocele
    d. Abnormalities in omphalomesenteric duct
    e. Aplasia cutis

16. Following are the indications of surgery during pregnancy:
    a. Intolerant to antithyroid drugs
    b. Serious drug-related adverse effects
    c. Requirement of high dose of antithyroid drugs
    d. Noncompliant to therapy

Surgery should be done in the second trimester.

CASE 21

A 26-year-old female having history of grade III diffuse goiter and thyrotoxicosis now euthyroid on carbimazole 15 mg daily became pregnant. During first trimester, due to worsening of symptoms, her vital were T3 2.9 ng/mL, T4 19 µg/dL, and TSH 0.001 µIU/mL. The dose of the carbimazole was increased to 30 mg daily, but in the second trimester she became euthyroid and dose was reduced to again 15 mg daily. She delivered a full-term baby having birth weight of 2.4 kg with normal thyroid function test and discharged.

But at third week, following lower respiratory tract infection, there was weight loss of 500 mg in spite of normal feeding and pulse rate of 165 beats/min. Thyroid function test revealed 3.6 ng/mL, T4 24 µg/mL, and TSH 0.005 µIU/mL. Methimazole was started along with propranolol. After 6 weeks, thyroid functions returned to normal thereby dose of the methimazole was reduced.

Two months after postpartum, she again became thyrotoxic and grade III diffuse goiter. Thyroid function test revealed T4 18 µg/dL, T3 1.9 ng/dL, and TSH 0.04 µIU/mL, So, dose of the carbimazole was increased to 30 mg/day.

1. **What is subclinical and overt hypothyroidism during pregnancy?**
2. **Why free T4 is estimated during pregnancy?**
3. **What are the risk of abnormalities in mother and fetus in case of subclinical hypothyroidism?**
4. **Mention the causes of bad obstetric history in hypothyroidism?**

Answers

1. If the TSH level is above the trimester-specific range with normal free T4, it is diagnosed as subclinical hypothyroidism during pregnancy.

   If the TSH level is above the reference level but below 10 µIU/mL along with low T4 or TSH level of >10 µIU/mL irrespective of any level of T4, it indicates overt hypothyroidism during pregnancy.

2. Total T4 level is increased because:
   a. Thyroid-binding globulin will be increased and remain increased throughout the pregnancy.
   b. Estrogen-mediated increased production of thyroid hormone
   c. Decreased clearance of thyroid hormone due to sialylation.

   Hence, free T4 has to estimate during pregnancy.

   Alternative method is to multiply normal reference range of total T4 of nonpregnant mother by 1 and half time.

3. Following are the risks during pregnancy in case of subclinical hypothyroidism:
   a. Maternal risk factors:
      - Miscarriage
      - Preterm delivery
      - Stillbirths
   b. Fetal risks:
      - Low birth weight
      - Impaired neurocognitive development

4. Causes of bad obstetric history in hypothyroidism:
   a. Recurrent miscarriage due to:
      - Impaired folliculogenesis
      - Defect in the luteal phase
      - Fertilization of senescent ova
   b. Presence of secondary ovarian disease
   c. Hyperprolactinemia
   d. Impaired surge of LH
   e. Altered metabolism of estrogen
   f. Gestational hypertension
   g. Placental abruption

CASE 22

A 30-year-old female came to medicine outdoor with the following:
Thyroid function test was done which demonstrated raised T4, FT3, and very low TSH.

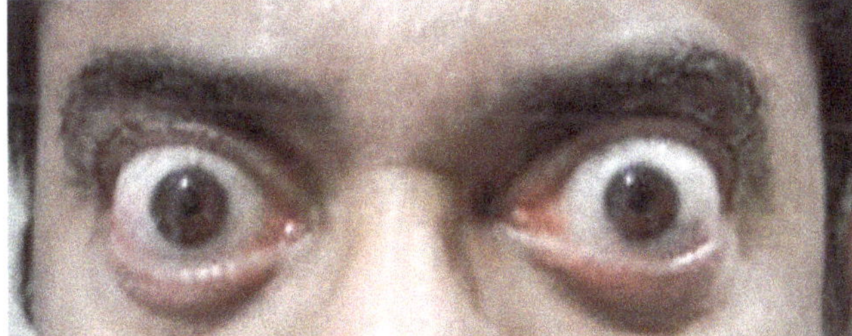

1. **What is your diagnosis?**
2. **What are the five important signs in this disease?**
3. **Mention the classifications of the eye signs in the thyroid disease.**
4. **How can you calculate the clinical activity score in this disease?**
5. **What are the eye signs in this disease?**
6. **Describe the pathogenesis in the lid lag.**

7. **How can you treat this disease?**
8. **Is there any difference between the thyroid-associated ophthalmopathy and Graves' orbitopathy?**
9. **What are the endocrine causes of proptosis?**
10. **Why there is proptosis in case of Graves' disease?**
11. **What is frozen globe?**
12. **What are the causes of ptosis in Graves' disease?**
13. **What are the indications of orbital decompression?**

Answers

1. The patient has been suffering from Graves' ophthalmopathy.
2. Five important signs in ophthalmopathy are:
   a. Swelling of the eyelids
   b. Chemosis
   c. Redness of the eyelid
   d. Redness of the conjunctiva
   e. Inflammation of the caruncle
3. Classifications of the eye signs in this disease:
   a. 0: No sign or symptom
   b. 1: Only sign, i.e., lid lag or lid retraction, but no symptom
   c. 2: Involvement of the soft tissue, i.e., pretibial myxedema
   d. 3: Presence of proptosis
   e. 4: Involvement of the extraocular muscles, i.e., diplopia
   f. 5: Corneal involvement
   g. 6: Loss of sight
4. Clinical activity score depending upon the presence or absence of seven characteristics:
   a. Presence of spontaneous retrobulbar pain
   b. Pain on eye movements
   c. Redness of the eyelids
   d. Redness of the conjunctiva
   e. Chemosis of the conjunctiva
   f. Swelling of the eyelids
   g. Swelling of the plica or caruncle
5. Following are the eye signs in this disease:
   a. Von Graefe's sign: If the patient is asked to look upward while the patient's face is inclined downward, there is absence of wrinkling.
   b. Gifford's sign: Absence of manual retraction of upper eyelids
   c. Kocher's sign: Stare looking
   d. Naffziger's sign: There is evidence of protrusion from the supraciliary ridge.
   e. Dalrymple's sign: There is visibility of the upper sclera.
   f. Moebius sign: Failure to converge the eyeballs
   g. Ballet's sign: Evidence of weakness of one extraocular muscle
   h. Rosenbach's sign: There is evidence of tremor while closing the eyelids.
   i. Jendrassik's sign: There is evidence of paralysis of extraocular muscles.
   j. Stellwag's sign: There are evidences of:
      • Stare looking
      • Infrequent blinking
      • Widening of the palpebral fissure
6. Pathogenesis of lid lag:
   a. Overactivity of the Müller's muscle due to sympathetic stimulation.
   b. Overactivity of the superior rectus and levator muscles due to myopathy of the inferior rectus muscle
   c. Restrictive myopathy of the levator palpebrae superioris
7. Treatment of the Graves' ophthalmopathy:
   a. In severe disease:
      • Corticosteroids
      • Orbital irradiation
      • Plasma exchange
      • If no improvement with above treatment, surgical decompression of the orbit
      • Use of rituximab
   b. Moderate disease: Symptomatic treatment by:
      • Elevation of the head at night
      • To reduce retrobulbar edema diuretics
      • To protect from the sun, wind tinted glasses can be used.
      • Administration of methylcellulose in the eye to treat corneal grittiness and dryness
      • To treat exposure keratitis, lateral tarsorrhaphy should be done.
      • Smoking should be stopped.
      • If the ophthalmopathy becomes worsen, steroids, orbital irradiation as well as orbital decompression should be done.

8. Thyroid associated with ophthalmopathy is an autoimmune thyroid disease like Graves's disease or Hashimoto thyroiditis. Graves' ophthalmopathy means orbitopathy associated with Graves' disease.

9. Following are the endocrinal causes of proptosis:
    a. Cushing's syndrome
    b. Acromegaly
    c. Morbid obesity
    d. Primary hyperthyroidism

10. Proptosis denotes the protrusion of the eyeball that measures the corneal position in relation to the lateral margin of the orbit. Normal value is <17 mm in case of Asian adult. If it is >20 mm, it can be described as moderate-to-severe proptosis. The causes of proptosis are:
    a. Proliferation of the retro-orbital fibroblast and adipocytes
    b. Deposition of glycosaminoglycans in the retro-bulbar spaces as well as extraocular muscles

11. Frozen globe can be described as restriction of eyeball movement in all the quadrants due to involvement of ocular nerve, but can occur due to involvement of extraocular muscles without involvement of the cranial nerve.

12. Following are the causes of proptosis in Graves' disease:
    a. Myasthenia gravis
    b. Superior orbital fissure syndrome
    c. Orbital apex syndrome
    d. Mechanical failure of levator palpebrae superioris as a result of long-standing proptosis

13. Following are the indications of orbital decompression:
    a. Dysthyroid optic neuropathy
    b. Breakdown of the cornea not responding to methylprednisolone
    c. Globe subluxation not responding to methylprednisolone
    d. Active disease intolerant to glucocorticoids

CASE 23

A 30-year-old female came to outpatient department with holocranial mild headache without vomiting or seizures or any focal neurological feature for last 1 and half years. Neuroimaging demonstrated sellar mass with suprasellar extension. She had no visual abnormality. Laboratory investigation demonstrated low T4, T3, but very high TSH and prolactin and cortisol. She developed amenorrhea.

On examination, her hair was dry, coarse skin, hoarse voice, delayed relaxation time of ankle jerk, and galactorrhea. Ultrasound demonstrated polycystic ovarian disease.

1. **What is the working diagnosis?**
2. **What are the features in favor of your diagnosis?**
3. **What is the effect of levothyroxine in this case?**
4. **What are the monosymptomatic presentations in this case?**
5. **What are the causes of weight loss in this disease?**
6. **What are the causes of tachycardia in this disease?**
7. **What are the causes of anemia in this disease?**
8. **Mention the causes of anemia without pallor in this disease.**
9. **What are the causes of delayed relaxation of deep tendon reflexes in this disease?**

Answers

1. The diagnosis is primary hypothyroidism, thyrolactotrope hyperplasia, and nonfunctioning pituitary tumor.

2. Following are the points in favor of your diagnosis:
    a. In spite of low T3 and T4, there is high level of TSH indicating thyrotropic hyperplasia
    b. Hyperprolactinemia indicating lactotrope hyperplasia
    c. Presence of amenorrhea which may be due to:
        - Concurrent hyperprolactinemia
        - Central hypogonadism due to mass effect
        - PCOD

3. Levothyroxine can be administered to reduce the thyrotropic hyperplasia either in step up or step down manner. Step up means the drug has to be started in low dose and gradually increased, whereas step down approach means the drug has to be started in high dose then gradually decreased to low dose.

4. Following are the monosymptomatic presentations in this case:
    a. Weight gain
    b. Menorrhagia

  c. Infertility
  d. Galactorrhea
  e. Recurrent miscarriage
  f. Pericardial effusion
  g. Multicystic ovaries
  h. Sinus bradycardia
  i. Refractory anemia
  j. Dyslipidemia
  k. Dementia
  l. Carpal tunnel syndrome
  m. Ataxia

5. Following are the causes of weight loss in this disease:
   a. Recovery phase of subacute thyroiditis
   b. Secondary hypothyroidism with multiple pituitary hormone deficiency
   c. Hypothyroidism associated with polyglandular endocrine failure
   d. Overtreatment with levothyroxine

6. Common causes of tachycardia in this disease:
   a. Overtreatment with levothyroxine
   b. Cardiac tamponade
   c. Congestive cardiac failure
   d. Concurrent presence of anemia

7. Following are the causes of anemia in this disease:
   a. Menorrhagia:
      • Coagulation abnormalities
      • Dysfunction of platelet
      • Increased capillary fragility
      • Deficient secretion of progesterone
   b. Impaired absorption of the nutrients such as folic acid, vitamin B12, and iron due to:
      • Reduced output of gastric acid
      • Decreased motility of the gut
   c. Poor intake
   d. Erythropoietin deficiency
   e. Concurrent celiac disease
   f. Pernicious anemia
   g. Blind loop syndrome

8. Following are the endocrine causes of pallor without anemia:
   a. Hypogonadism resulting decreased cutaneous vascularity as a result of deficiency of testosterone
   b. Cutaneous vasoconstriction in hypothyroidism in hypometabolic state
   c. Reduced production of melanin from the melanocytes in deficiency of ACTH in secondary hypoadrenalism

9. Following are the causes of delayed relaxation of deep tendon reflexes in this disease:
   a. Selective atrophy of type 2 along with compensatory hypertrophy of type 1 muscle fibers
   b. Decreased activity of Na^+/K^+-ATPase
   c. Reduced expression of myosin ATPase
   d. Impaired contractility of actin-myosin complex
   e. Defective sarcolemmal depolarization

CASE 24

A 39-year-old male came to medical outpatient department with history of progressively increasing headache, tonic-clonic seizures, and diabetes having poor control.

On examination, following facies was found along with diffuse hyperpigmentation, hyperhidrosis, and seborrhea, but dehydrated with HbA1c 16% and fasting blood sugar 488 mg/dL. Arterial blood gases demonstrated anion gap metabolic acidosis. There was serum T4 3.2 µg/dL, TSH 1.3 µIU/mL, morning cortisol 604 nmol/L, ACTH 35 pg/mL, prolactin 19 ng/mL, testosterone 1.1 nmol/L, growth hormone 118 ng/mL, and IGF-1 776 ng/mL.

Eye examination demonstrated bitemporal hemianopia.

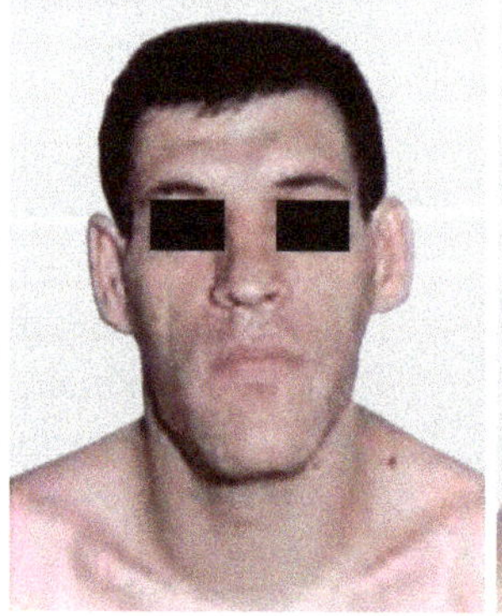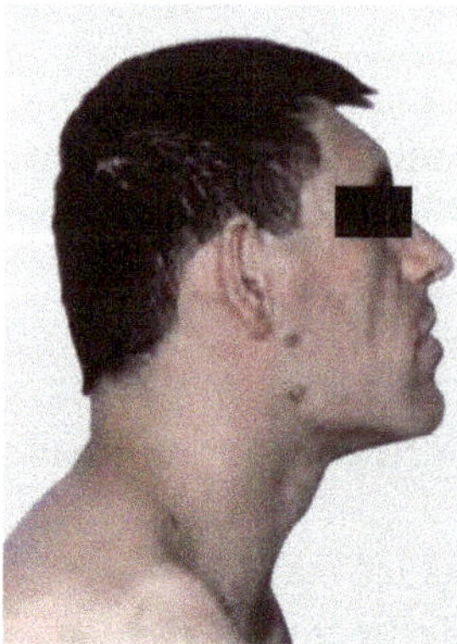

1. **What is your diagnosis?**
2. **What are the features of active acromegaly present here?**
3. **What type of diabetes is present here and why?**
4. **In this patient, why there was incidence of seizures?**
5. **Why there was hyperpigmentation in this patient?**
6. **Mention the causes of this disease with subtle facial features.**
7. **What do you mean by fugitive acromegaly?**
8. **What is pseudovariety of this disease?**
9. **Why ectopic growth hormone-releasing tumor is more common as compared to ectopic growth hormone-secreting tumor?**
10. **What are the familial types of this disease?**
11. **What are the causes of autosomal dominant form of familial disease?**
12. **Describe the correlation between histological phenotype and clinical features.**
13. **What are the unusual presentations in case of acromegaly?**
14. **What are the emergency conditions in this disease?**
15. **What are the causes of headache in this disease?**

Answers

1. The diagnosis is acromegaly.
2. Following features of acromegaly present here are:
    a. Progressing worsening of the headache
    b. Hyperhidrosis
    c. Seborrhea
    d. Uncontrolled blood glucose control
    e. New-onset visual abnormality
3. This patient has been suffering from secondary diabetes because:
    a. Young age of onset
    b. Lack of family history of diabetes
    c. Severe and resistant hyperglycemia
4. This patient suffered from tonic-clonic seizures due to cerebral dehydration because of diabetic ketoacidosis.
5. Diffuse hyperpigmentation in this patent is due to:
    a. Direct effect of growth hormone on melanocytes
    b. Growth hormone
    c. ACTH co-secreting tumor
    d. Diffuse acanthosis nigricans
6. Following are the causes of acromegaly with subtle facial features:
    a. McCune–Albright syndrome
    b. Adolescent acromegaly
    c. Mild acromegaly
    d. Concurrent thyrotoxicosis
    e. Fugitive acromegaly
    f. Sarcopenia associated with poorly controlled diabetes mellitus

7. Fugitive acromegaly is characterized by:
    a. Subtle features of acromegaly
    b. Normal or mildly raised growth hormone
    c. Suppressible growth hormone after glucose load
    d. Marginally elevated IGF-1.
8. Pseudoacromegaly is characterized by features of acromegaly in absence of excess growth hormone. The causes are the following:
    a. Severe diabetes resistant to insulin
    b. Pachydermoperiostitis
    c. Hypothyroidism
    d. Insulin-like growth factor-2-secreting tumor
    e. Insulinoma
    f. Drugs—minoxidil and phenytoin
9. Growth hormone-releasing hormone (GHRH) is smaller peptide containing 44 amino acid residues as compared to growth hormone having 191 amino acids. So, it will be easier to dedifferentiated cells in the tumor to such peptide containing smaller number of amino acids, hence GHRH-secreting tumor is more common as compared to growth hormone-secreting tumor.
10. What are the features suggestive of familial acromegaly:
    a. Age of onset is <30 years
    b. Tumor is aggressive.
    c. Presence or development of multiple endocrine neoplasia
    d. Family history of pituitary tumor

11. Causes of autosomal dominant familial acromegaly are:
    a. Carney's complex
    b. Familial isolated pituitary adenoma
    c. Multiple endocrine neoplasia like MEN1 and MEN4
    d. Paraganglioma associated with SDH mutation
12. Following are the correlations between the clinical phenotype and the histological features in the somatotropinoma:

Histological subtypes	Hormone secreted	Clinical presentations
Densely granulated	Growth hormone	It is mild disease responding to treatment
Granulated sparsely	Growth hormone	Rapidly progressive responding poorly to treatment
Mammosom-atotropinoma	Growth hormone Prolactin hormone	It occurs in children Features of gigantism
Acidophil stem cell adenoma	Growth hormone Prolactin hormone	Fugitive acromegaly Hyperprolactinemia is predominant

13. Following are the unusual presentations in acromegaly:
    a. Malocclusion of jaw
    b. Diabetic ketoacidosis
    c. Pituitary apoplexy
    d. Cerebrospinal fluid (CSF) rhinorrhea
    e. Facial asymmetry like facial dysplasia in McCune–Albright syndrome
    f. Tonsillomegaly
    g. Recurrent nasal obstruction
    h. Severe hirsutism
    i. Entrapment neuropathy
    j. Dilated cardiomyopathy
    k. Cutis verticis gyrata
    l. Frontal lobe syndrome
14. Emergencies in this patient are:
    a. Pituitary apoplexy
    b. Subarachnoid hemorrhage
    c. Status epilepticus from:
       • Hyponatremia
       • Raised intracranial hypertension
       • Cerebral invasion
    d. Paraplegia resulting from prolapse of intervertebral disk
    e. Accelerated hypertension
    f. Diabetic ketoacidosis
    g. Gastrointestinal bleeding from colonic polyposis or carcinoma
    h. Cardiac arrhythmias
    i. Acromegalic cardiomyopathy
15. Following are the causes of headache in this disease:
    a. In case of microadenoma due to raised intrasellar pressure as the tumor grows in closed space
    b. In case of macroadenoma due to stretching of the dura which is supplied by ophthalmic division of the trigeminal nerve.
    c. Suprasellar extension of the tumor
    d. Cavernous sinus invasion leading to involvement of trigeminal nerve
    e. Periosteal stretch due to calvarial thickness
    f. Osteoma
    g. Recurrent sinusitis
    h. Secretion of analgesic peptides by the tumor tissue

Causes of acute onset headache:
    a. Pituitary apoplexy
    b. Aneurysmal rupture
    c. Raised intracranial tension

CASE 25

The pictures of a 35-year-old hypertensive woman having blood pressure of 160/90 mm Hg on antihypertensive medication:

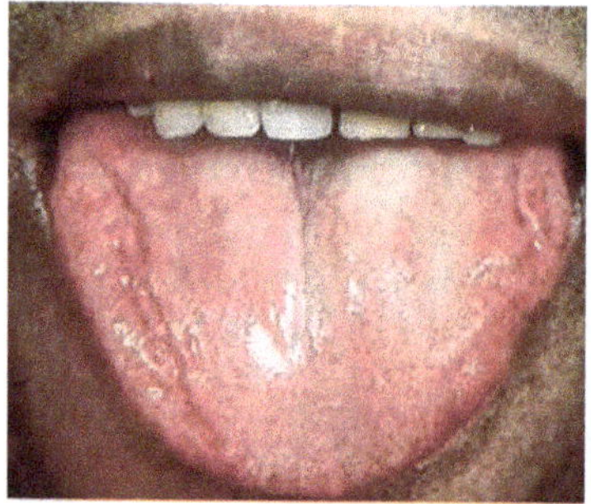
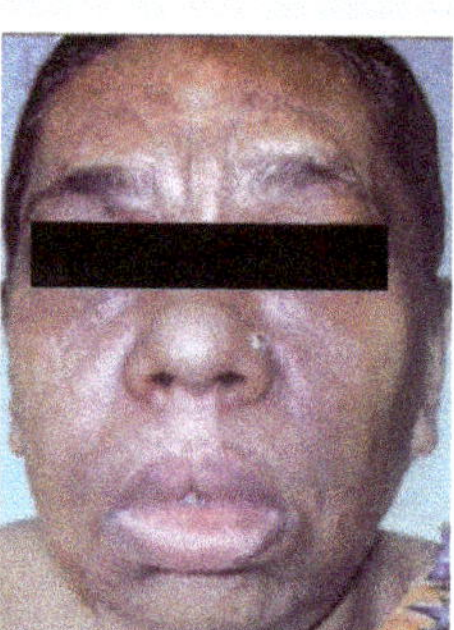

1. **What is your diagnosis?**
2. **What are the causes of this conditions of the tongue?**
3. **What are the dermatological manifestations in this disease?**
4. **How growth hormone affects the thyroid function?**
5. **Mention the cardiovascular features of this disease.**
6. **What are the reasons for increased cardiovascular risk in this disease?**

Answers

1. The patient has been suffering from acromegaly.
2. The causes of macroglossia are:
   a. Acromegaly
   b. Primary hypothyroidism
   c. Down syndrome
   d. Amyloidosis
   e. Hemangioma
   f. Lymphangioma
   g. Cancer of tongue
3. Following are the dermatological manifestations in this disease:
   a. Hyperhidrosis
   b. Seborrhea
   c. Hirsutism
   d. Acanthosis nigricans
   e. Skin tag of >3—indicates associated colonic polyp
   f. Hyperpigmentation
   g. Cutis verticis gyrata
   h. In case of McCune–Albright syndrome, café-au-lait macules
   i. In case of MEN1 syndrome, lipoma and angiofibroma
4. Growth hormone can potentiate T3 and T4 neogenesis by:
   a. Activation of 5′-monodeiodinase
   b. Decreased thyroxine-binding globulin
   c. Inhibition of TSH through increased tone of somatostatin
5. Following are the cardiovascular manifestations in this disease:
   a. Cardiomyopathy
   b. Heart failure
   c. Asymmetric septal hypertrophy
   d. Arrhythmias
   e. Coronary artery disease
6. Following are the reasons for increased cardiovascular risk in this disease:
   a. Hypertension
   b. Obstructive sleep apnea
   c. Increased left ventricular mass
   d. Atherogenic lipid profile
   e. Hyperfibrinogenemia
   f. Increased concentration of plasminogen activator inhibitor-1
   g. Insulin resistance
   h. Hyperinsulinemia

CASE 26

A 40-year-old female having features of acromegaly and MRI features of macroadenoma, IGF-1, and growth hormone post-glucose load was performed.

1. **Why these tests were done?**
2. **What are the causes of discordant growth hormone and IGF-1 values?**
3. **When IGF-1 will be more reliable as compared to growth hormone?**
4. **After confirmation of the diagnosis, what are the investigations should be done?**
5. **What is the primary modality of therapy in this patient?**
6. **What are the factors associated with poor response to therapy?**

Answers

1. Both the investigations are required for:
   a. Confirmation of the diagnosis
   b. It can differentiate active versus inactive disease.
2. The causes of discordant growth hormone and IGF-1 values are:
   a. Nonsuppressed growth hormone and low or normal IGF-1 values:
      - Hepatic failure
      - Renal failure
      - Hyperthyroidism
      - Use of oral contraceptive pill (OCP)
      - Poorly controlled diabetes mellitus
      - Therapy with dopamine agonists
      - Therapy with somatostatin analog
   b. Suppressed growth hormone and high IGF-1 values:
      - Hyperthyroidism
      - Postradiotherapy
      - Mild acromegaly
      - Immediate postoperative period
3. IGF-1 is more reliable as compared to growth hormone level in following cases:
   a. Patient with poorly controlled diabetes mellitus
   b. Those patients received previous radiotherapy
   c. Monitoring the response to therapy normalization of IGF-1 values as compared to growth hormone level after glucose load
   d. It is better predictor of active disease.
   e. Treatment with pegvisomant should be monitored only by this IGF-1 value.
4. Following investigations are required after confirmation of the diagnosis of acromegaly:
   a. Serum calcium
   b. Serum phosphorus
   c. Lipid profile
   d. Blood glucose
   e. Hormone profile includes:
      - Serum T3
      - Serum T4
      - Serum TSH
      - 8 AM serum cortisol
      - Serum testosterone
      - Serum estradiol
      - Prolactin
   f. MRI of the sella should be done for localizing the source of the growth hormone.
   g. CT scan of the sella in case of children for demonstrating the pneumatization of the sella as well as fibrous dysplasia.
   h. Visual acuity and visual field have to be detected.
   i. X-ray of the spine should be done to detect kyphoscoliosis.
   j. DEXA is required to evaluate osteoporosis.
   k. ECG should be done in all the patients.
5. Transsphenoidal surgery is the primary modality of therapy in this patient.
6. Risk factors associated with the poor response to therapy are:
   a. Younger age of onset
   b. Large and invasive tumor—cavernous sinus invasion
   c. Serum growth hormone is >40 ng/mL
   d. Mutation of *AIP* gene
   e. On histology, sparsely granulated tumor
   f. Oversuppression of tumor indices like p53 and Ki67
   g. Pituitary tumor transforming gene
   h. Reduced expression of somatostatin receptor subtype 2 and 5 by the tumor

CASE 27

A 30-year-old nonhypertensive man having no history of vertigo, fever, seizures, headache or visual deficit or no head injury, decreased libido, and cranial nerve palsy came to emergency department with sudden history of severe headache, projectile vomiting, and dizziness.

On examination, his blood pressure was 110/70 mm Hg, pulse rate 80 beats/min, regular, no features of acromegaly, Cushing's syndrome, but sparse beard. Ophthalmic examination demonstrated bitemporal hemianopia.

Laboratory examination demonstrated serum T3, T4, and TSH were within normal limit. LH and FSH were in lower level of normal and testosterone was 6 nmol/L. Prolactin level was 22,345 ng/mL and 8 AM serum cortisol level was 240 nmol/L.

CT scan demonstrated:

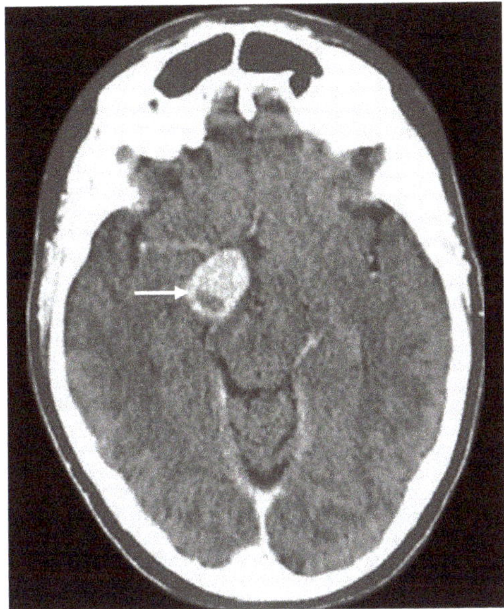

1. **What does the above picture demonstrate?**
2. **What is your diagnosis?**
3. **What are the points in favor of your diagnosis?**
4. **Patient is in hypocortisolic state. Give reasons.**
5. **What are the differential diagnoses in this case?**
6. **What is the definite point against the nonfunctioning pituitary adenoma?**
7. **What is the important role of prolactin?**
8. **Mention the causes of nontumor high prolactin level.**
9. **Mention the causes of this disease in hypothyroidism.**
10. **What are the clinical features of hyperprolactinemia?**
11. **How hyperprolactinemia leads to gonadal dysfunction in women?**
12. **How hyperprolacteinemia produces hypogonadism in men?**

Answers

1. CT scan demonstrates hemorrhage within macro-prolactinoma.
2. Diagnosis is macroprolactinoma with pituitary apoplexy.
3. Points in favor of the diagnosis are:
    a. Sudden severe headache
    b. Projectile vomiting
    c. Ophthalmic examination demonstrated bitemporal hemianopia
    d. Serum prolactin level is very high.
4. Patient is in hypocortisolic state because:
    a. Serum cortisol is low, i.e., <900 nmol/L.
    b. Blood pressure was low.
    c. History of dizziness

5. The differential diagnoses in this case are:
    a. Hemorrhage
    b. Meningioma
    c. Lymphoma
    d. Granuloma
    e. Craniopharyngioma
6. Very high prolactin level is the main differentiating point against nonfunctioning pituitary adenoma.
7. Prolactin has important role in:
    a. Galactopoiesis
    b. Mammogenesis
    c. The immune system
    d. Gonadal dysfunction
8. Nontumor causes of hyperprolactinemia:
    a. Antidopaminergic drugs like:
        • Haloperidol

- Chlorpromazine
- Domperidone
- Sulpiride
    b. Cimetidine
    c. Antidepressants:
    - Imipramine
    - Amitriptyline
    d. Antihistaminic—α-methyldopa
    e. Estrogen
    f. Phenytoin
    g. Calcium channel blockers
    h. Primary hyperthyroidism
    i. Hepatic dysfunction
    j. Renal dysfunction
    k. PCOD
    l. Chest lesion
9. Causes of hyperprolactinemia in case of hypo-thyroidism:
    a. Lactotroph hyperplasia due to increased drive of TSH
    b. Decreased clearance of prolactin
    c. Suppressed dopaminergic tone
    But the level of prolactin is never >100 ng/dL.
10. Clinical features in hyperprolactinemia:
    a. In women:
    - Menstrual irregularities
    - Galactorrhea
    - Infertility
    b. In men:
    - Decreased frequency of shaving
    - Reduced libido
    - Erectile dysfunction
    - Infertility
    - But absence of galactorrhea due to absence of breast tissue
11. Prolactin produces gonadal dysfunction in women by the following processes:
    a. Inhibition of kisspeptin neuron which is present in hypothalamus.
    b. Direct suppression of gonadotropin secretion from the pituitary
    c. Impairment of folliculogenesis
    d. Exertion of inhibitory effects on the granulosa cells leading to decreased production of estradiol.
    e. Interference with ovulation
12. Hyperprolactinemia produces hypogonadism in men by the following mechanisms:
    a. Inhibition of gonadotropin-releasing hormone pulse generator activity
    b. Inhibition of gonadotropin secretion
    c. Dysfunction of the Leydig cells leading to decreased secretion of testosterone
    d. Direct inhibitory effect on developing spermatogonia leading to Inhibition of spermatogenesis

CASE 28

A 30-year-old female presented with secondary amenorrhea, acromegalic features, and galactorrhea. Her IGF was normal and post-glucose load growth hormone has been suppressed.

1. **What is your working diagnosis and how can you exclude it?**
2. **Now the serum prolactin level was 465 ng/mL, but serum cortisol and T4 were within normal limit and CT scan of brain revealed microadenoma. What is your diagnosis now?**
3. **Why the patient developed acromegalic feature?**
4. **How the acromegalic feature can be regressed?**

Answers

1. The working diagnosis is somatostatinoma because of secondary amenorrhea, galactorrhea, and acromegalic features. But as the serum IGF level was normal and post-glucose load growth hormone has been suppressed, the diagnosis of somatostatinoma will be excluded.
2. The diagnosis is macroprolactinoma.
3. As there is intrinsic growth hormone like activity of the prolactin in case macroprolactinoma because of homology between the growth hormone and prolactin.
4. Administration of cabergoline leads to decreased level of prolactin level resulting regression of the acromegalic features.

CASE 29

A 32-year-old woman came to medicine outpatient department with history of oligomenorrhea, galactorrhea, and infertility. Repeated estimation of serum prolactin demonstrated 8–10 ng/mL. MRI of brain demonstrated 5 mm hypotense lesion seen on the right pituitary.

1. **What is your working diagnosis?**
2. **Why serum prolactin level is normal?**
3. **How can you get the original serum level of prolactin?**

Answers

1. The working diagnosis is hyperprolactinemia.
2. Serum prolactin level was normal because of the hook effect—it means low estimation serum prolactin in spite of its high level in the serum, which is due to saturation of antibodies used in immunoradiometric assay.
3. For rectification of this hook effect, serum prolactin should be measured in dilution method (1:100). If the test demonstrates high level in the serum, the diagnosis is confirmed.

CASE 30

A 28-year-old female presented with serum prolactin level of 110 ng/mL, but no galactorrhea and menstrual cycles were normal.

1. **What is your instant diagnosis?**
2. **How this can be diagnosed?**
3. **What may be the other possibility?**

Answers

1. The instant diagnosis or suspicion is macro-prolactinemia.
2. Macroprolactin can be diagnosed polyethylene glycol precipitation method.
3. Macroprolactinemia are developed as a result of:
   a. Binding of prolactin with IgG antibody
   b. Prolactin binds with antiprolactin antibodies

   As a result the molecular weight of this macroprolactin will be >150 kD. This macroprolactin will interfere with prolactin assay resulting high value of this.

CASE 31

A 65-year-old nonhypertensive nonsmoker male having past history of extraction of renal stone came to outpatient department with intermittent moderately severe epigastric pain, anorexia, and constipation associated with nausea and vomiting and weight loss for 8 months. He had no history of bone pain or fracture.

On examination, his blood pressure was 95/65 mm Hg, pulse rate 120 beats/min, regular, and dehydrated. Abdominal examination revealed epigastric mass. Ultrasonography demonstrated pancreatic mass with peripancreatic collections. CT scan chest demonstrated bilateral hilar adenopathy.

Laboratory examination demonstrated serum corrected calcium 14.5 g/mL, phosphate 3.1 mg/dL, iPTH 8.2 pg/mL, and $1,25(OH)_2$ 65 pg/mL. Chest X-ray revealed hilar bilateral lymphadenopathy.

1. **What is your diagnosis?**
2. **What are the points in favor of hyperthyroidism?**
3. **What are the points suggestive of parathyroid-independent hypercalcemia?**
4. **What are the differential diagnoses of parathormone-dependent hypercalcemia?**
5. **What are the investigations to be done to detect the etiology?**
6. **What is the suspected etiology in this case?**

7. **What is the weight loss in this case?**
8. **What is the cause of pancreatitis in this case?**
9. **What are the causes of hypercalcemia in this case?**
10. **How can you administer zoledronic acid?**
11. **Why glucocorticoid should be given in this case?**
12. **Why vitamin D should not be given in this case?**
13. **What are the precautions to be taken during estimating serum calcium?**
14. **How can you estimate corrected serum calcium?**
15. **What are the causes of pseudohypercalcemia?**
16. **What are the correlations between the serum calcium and parathormone?**
17. **What are the causes of parathormone-dependent hypercalcemia?**

Answers

1. The diagnosis is parathyroid hormone-independent hypercalcemia along with pancreatitis.
2. Following points are in favor of hyperparathyroidism:
   a. History of extraction of renal stones
   b. Pancreatitis with peripancreatic collection
3. Presence of hypercalcemia in presence of iPTH suggestive of parathyroid-independent hypercalcemia
4. Following are the differential diagnoses of parathormone-dependent hypercalcemia:
   a. Malignancy:
      - Lung
      - Breast
      - Kidney
      - Lymphoma
      - Multiple myeloma
   b. Drugs:
      - Lithium
      - Thiazide
      - Vitamin D
      - Calcium-containing antacids
5. Following investigations should be done to detect the etiology:
   a. Chest X-ray
   b. CT scan of chest and abdomen
   c. Serum protein electrophoresis
   d. Urine protein electrophoresis
   e. ACE levels
   f. $1,25(OH)_2$ vitamin D3
   g. 25 vitamin D3
6. The suspected etiology in this case is sarcoidosis.
7. Cause of weight loss and nausea in this case is due to secretion of interleukin-6 and interferon-γ.

8. Pancreatitis in this case is due to:
   a. Severe hypercalcemia
   b. Possible involvement of the pancreas by sarcoid granuloma
9. Hypercalcemia in this case is due to marked intravascular volume depletion as a result of:
   - Vomiting
   - Pancreatitis
   - Nephrogenic diabetes insipidus
10. Zoledronic acid can be administered in this patient with following GFR:
    a. If effective GFR is >60 mL/min, this drug should be safely administered.
    b. If effective GFR is between 30 and 60 mL/min, this drug can be given in full dose but at reduced rate.
    c. If the effective GFR is <30 mL/min, this drug should be avoided.
11. Glucocorticoid should be given in this case because:
    a. They inhibit the macrophage-1α hydroxylase.
    b. Decrease the production of parathyroid hormone-related protein (PTHrP) and interferon-γ
    c. Decrease the production of bone resorbing cytokines
12. Vitamin D should not be given in this chronic granulomatous disorder because:
    a. Increased risk of developing hypercalcemia as a result of upregulation of the activity of 1α-hydroxylase in the macrophages
13. Following precautions should be taken during estimation of serum calcium:
    a. Hydration status
    b. Application of tourniquet
    c. Serum albumin
    d. Analytic method

14. Corrected serum calcium (mg/dL):
    a. $0.8 \times [0.4 - \text{serum albumin (g/dL)}]$ + measured total calcium (mg/dL)
15. Causes of pseudohypercalcemia:
    a. Severe dehydration
    b. Paraproteinemia
16. Following are the correlations between serum calcium and parathormone:
    a. Raised parathormone along with hypercalcemia suggests PTH-dependent hypercalcemia
    b. In 10% to 20% cases, serum parathormone level is within the reference range in presence of hypercalcemia.
    c. If the parathormone level is <20 pg/mL, it suggests parathormone-independent hypercalcemia.
17. Following are the causes of parathormone-dependent hypercalcemia:
    a. Primary hyperthyroidism
    b. Tertiary hyperparathyroidism
    c. Familial hypocalciuric hypercalcemia
    d. Lithium therapy
    e. Anti-CaSR antibody-mediated hyperparathyroidism

CASE 32

A 40-year-old female having no family history of endocrine disease came to orthopedic department with swelling of the upper part of right tibia for last 1 year, which was found to be lytic lesion and treated bony curettage along with fibular graft implantation and histopathologically it showed a giant cell tumor. Whole body scan demonstrated multiple similar lytic bony lesions.

On laboratory investigation, her serum calcium was 15.8 mg/dL, phosphate 2.3 mg/dL, iPTH 1,565 pg/mL, alkaline phosphatase 869 IU/mL, creatinine 1.2 mg/dL, urinary creatinine 654 mg, and prolactin 16 ng/mL.

Ultrasonography of abdomen and neck demonstrated bilateral nephrolithiasis left inferior parathyroid adenoma. This patient has been treated with intravenous zoledronic acid prior to parathyroidectomy.

1. **What are the differential diagnoses in this case?**
2. **What are close differential diagnoses and which estimation can clench the diagnosis?**
3. **What are the features in favor of the diagnosis of hyperparathyroidism and osteitis fibrosa cystica in this case?**
4. **How can you know that the patient's disease is sporadic?**
5. **Why this patient should be treated with intravenous zoledronic acid preoperatively?**
6. **What are the classical pentad of this disease?**
7. **Mention the unusual presentation in this disease.**
8. **How this disease can produce rickets in child?**
9. **Why hyperparathyroidism occurs in postmenopausal woman?**
10. **What are the radiological manifestations of osteitis fibrosa cystica?**

Answers

1. The differential diagnoses are:
    a. Osteoclastoma
    b. Osteitis fibrosa cystica
    c. Fibrous dysplasia
    d. Simple bone cyst
    e. Aneurysmal bone cyst
    f. Osteosarcoma
2. The close differential diagnoses are:
    a. Osteoclastoma
    b. Osteitis fibrosa cystica

    These two can be differentiated by estimation of corrected serum calcium as it favors the diagnosis of primary hyperparathyroidism leading to formation of osteitis fibrosa cystica, whereas eucalcemia favors the diagnosis of osteoclastoma.
3. Following are the features in favor of the diagnosis of osteitis fibrosa cystica:
    a. Hypercalcemia
    b. Raised alkaline phosphatase
    c. Bilateral nephrolithiasis
    d. Normal effective glomerular filtration rate
    e. High iPTH

f. Hypophosphatemia

g. Osteoporosis

h. Multiple cystic lesion in the bone

4. The disease is sporadic as:
   a. She has no family history of primary hyperparathyroidism
   b. Serum prolactin level is normal.

5. This patient should be treated with intravenous zoledronic acid preoperatively because:
   a. It will reduce the serum calcium effectively.
   b. It will reduce the postoperative risk of hungry bone syndrome.

6. The classical pentad in this disease are:
   a. Stones—renal stones
   b. Bones—fracture and osteitis fibrosa cystica
   c. Groans—pancreatitis, gall stones, and acid peptic disease
   d. Moans—disorder of mood
   e. Overtones—myalgia and myopathy

7. Following are the unusual presentations in this disease:
   a. Rickets
   b. Distal tubular acidosis
   c. Facial asymmetry
   d. Proptosis
   e. Anemia
   f. Recurrent pancreatitis

8. By following mechanisms, this disease produces rickets:
   a. High serum level of phosphate leading to:
      • Increased wasting of phosphate through the kidney
      • Increased turnover of the bone

All these factors result as decrease the effective mineralization of the matrix.
   b. Poor oral intake due to:
      • Hypercalcemia-induced anorexia
      • Increased demand of calcium during puberty

9. In postmenopausal woman, there is estrogen deficiency. As estrogen inhibits the action of parathyroid by:
   a. Interfering with the postreceptor signaling
   b. Antagonizing the cytokine-mediated resorption of bone

So in postmenopausal woman, action of parathormone will be unopposed leading to development of hyperparathyroidism.

Lack of estrogen leads to tumorigenesis.

Estrogen deficiency leads to lack of 1α-hydroxylase activity resulting increase in the proliferation of parathyroid cells.

There is upregulation of the estrogen receptors in the parathyroid cells leading to potentiation of the generation of IGF-1 resulting proliferation of parathyroid cells.

10. Following are the radiological manifestations of osteitis fibrosa cystica:
    a. Resorption of the subperiosteal phalangeal bone
    b. Acrosteal resorption of the terminal phalanx
    c. Brown tumor seen in the:
       • Ribs
       • Jaw
       • Pelvis
       • Trabecular portion of the long bones
       • Vertebrae rarely
    d. Salt and paper appearance in the skull bones
    e. Bone cysts
    f. Fracture

CASE 33

A 54-year-old female having family history of hypercalcemia in her brother came for checkup after she found her serum calcium level 12 mg/dL. She was physically unremarkable. But, her intact parathormone level was 130 pg/mL and 24 hours urinary excretion of calcium was 42 mg.

1. **What is your diagnosis?**
2. **What are the points in favor of your diagnosis?**
3. **Mention the pathophysiology of this disease.**
4. **What should be the level of calcitriol and why?**

Answers

1. The most likely diagnosis is familial hypocalciuric hypocalcemia.
2. Following are the points in favor of this diagnosis:
   a. Family history of elevated serum calcium
   b. Mildly elevated serum calcium
   c. Low 24 hours urinary calcium
3. This disease occurs from CaSR defect which is present in the kidney and parathyroid glands. As a result of mutation of the receptors that lead to the defect in the receptors which misread the calcium. So, there is increased secretion of parathormone from the parathyroid gland leading to inappropriate absorption of calcium in the kidney resulting decreased secretion of the calcium in the urine.
4. Vitamin calcitriol is high or high normal in case of primary hyperparathyroidism. But in this disease, parathormone level is much lower and so the calcitriol level.

CASE 34

An 88-year-old poor edentulous female living in closed poorly ventilated room came to outpatient department with history of taking only soup only because of difficulty in chewing. She was no medication.

On examination, there was wasting in the temporal region, dry mucous membrane, and left-sided facial droop. Patient expressed pain during movement of extremities.

Laboratory examination demonstrated serum calcium level of 8 mg/dL, raised alkaline phosphatase, and phosphorus 1.9 mg/dL. X-ray of pelvis demonstrated appearance of pseudofracture in the pelvic rami.

1. **What is the most likely diagnosis?**
2. **Why serum calcium and phosphorus both were low and alkaline phosphatase is high?**
3. **Which is single diagnostic test that can confirm the diagnosis?**

Answers

1. The most likely diagnosis is osteomalacia due to lack of:
   a. Sunlight as she was staying in the closed poorly ventilated room
   b. Poor diet
2. Serum calcium and phosphorus levels are low due to reduced production of $1,25(OH)_2D$. Serum alkaline phosphatase is high indicating increased bone turnover.
3. Estimation of calcidiol or $25(OH)D$.

CASE 35

A 75-year-old hypertensive male having history of smoking of >60 packs/day and chronic obstructive lung disease came to chest outdoor with history of chronic cough and recurrent hemoptysis.

On examination, there was clubbing, pulse rate 110 beats/min, blood pressure 110/75 mm Hg, and respiratory rate 28 breaths/min. On auscultation, the breath sound was diminished in the left base and coarse crepitation.

Laboratory investigation demonstrated that serum calcium was 12 mg/mL and phosphorus 1.9 mg/dL.

1. **What is the most likely diagnosis?**
2. **What is the most likely mediator of this hypercalcemia?**
3. **The parathormone level will be low in this patient. Why?**

Answers

1. The most likely diagnosis is squamous cell carcinoma of lung leading to development of paraneoplastic syndrome.
2. In squamous cell carcinoma of lung hypersecretion of PTHrP leads to development of hypercalcemia.
3. High serum calcium will suppress the production of endogenous parathormone from the chief cells of the parathyroid gland.

CASE 36

A 30-year-old pregnant woman having past history of operation for follicular thyroid adenoma and taking thyroid hormone postoperatively came to outpatient department with new-onset of spasm of the hand and positive Chvostek and Trousseau signs. Laboratory examination demonstrated serum calcium of 8 mg/dL.

1. **During estimation of serum calcium, what other measures you will take?**
2. **In presence of hypocalcemia, how the pregnant patient will present?**
3. **What is the relation of serum calcium, phosphate, and parathormone?**

Answers

1. In case of estimation of total serum calcium, serum albumin level will have to be measured. Because in case of pregnant woman, serum albumin level should be measured to make correction of serum calcium.
2. Parathyroid glands are present within the thyroid gland. So, these are very vulnerable to be traumatized during surgery. So during operation, complete damage to the parathyroid gland will lead to decreased release of parathormone. But if the gland is damaged incompletely, the parathormone level will be low normal and the patient may not develop the hypocalcemic symptoms. But in pregnant woman due to stress and also for the maturation of the fetal skeleton, the calcium requirement will be increased. So during this time, the hypocalcemia will be obvious and the patient will develop the symptoms of hypocalcemia.
3. After surgery, serum parathormone, calcium will be low and serum phosphate level will be high.

CASE 37

A 55-year-old hypertensive man having past history of renal stones came to medical outdoor with history of progressively worsening of fatigue, bone pain, and weakness for last 5 months. Laboratory investigations demonstrated that all the metabolic panels were normal except serum calcium 12 mg/dL.

1. **What is the most likely diagnosis and how can you confirm it?**
2. **^{99m}Tc-sestamibi scan demonstrated the uptake by the single parathyroid gland. What is your diagnosis?**
3. **What is the treatment in this patient?**

Answers

1. The most likely diagnosis is hyperparathyroidism. This diagnosis is confirmed by the simultaneous measurement of serum calcium and parathormone level. At the same time family history of familial hypocalciuric hypercalcemia should be excluded by estimating 24 hours urinary calcium.
2. The diagnosis is parathyroid adenoma.
3. The definite treatment is excision of parathyroid adenoma, but other parathyroid glands should also to be inspected.

CASE 38

The mother of 2-year-old infant came to pediatric outpatient department with complaint of inability to grow properly. Patient was exclusively breastfed for 1 year twice daily, but rarely took other dairy products. On examination, patient's weight was <5% of his age and height <5% of his age. There was frontal bossing, anterior fontanel was open, and bowlegged. Radiologically, there was cupping of the distal end of the both radius and ulna.

1. **What is your diagnosis?**
2. **What should be the level of 25(OH)D and 1,25(OH)$_2$D in the nutritional and vitamin D-dependent rickets?**
3. **How can you treat it?**
4. **What are the tests to performed to rule out the chronic disease?**

Answers

1. The most likely diagnosis is nutritional rickets.
2. In vitamin D-deficient rickets type 1, there is absent or reduced 1α-hydroxylase. In this case, the level of 25(OH)D is high but level of 1,25(OH)$_2$ is low. Whereas, in vitamin D-deficient rickets type 2, the defect is the mutation of the vitamin D receptor. So, in this case, the level of 25(OH)D may be normal, high, or low depending upon the dietary intake of vitamin D or synthesis of vitamin D in the skin, but 1,25(OH)$_2$ level will be high and this can differentiate the nutritional rickets from vitamin D-deficient rickets type 1.
3. This patient should be treated with vitamin 60,000 IU weekly or daily dose of 4,000 IU in case of nutritional rickets. Type 1 vitamin D deficiency rickets should be treated by 1,25(OH)$_2$D, whereas type 2 vitamin D deficiency rickets can be treated with high dose of 1,25(OH)$_2$D or may be resistant to vitamin D.
4. a. Blood test:
     - Serum calcium to rule out hypocalcemia in this disease.
     - Serum phosphorus to rule out hypophosphatemia present in the defective mineralization of bone.
     - Alkaline phosphatase which is elevated due to increased activity of osteoblast.
     - Serum parathyroid hormone which is found due to secondary hyperparathyroidism.
     - Serum vitamin D3: Decreased in case of to less than 20 ng/mL.
   b. Urine test:
     - Calcium excretion—decreased in this disease.
     - Phosphorus—increased in case of renal tubular disorder.
     - Urine pH to assess the renal tubular acidosis.
   c. Radiological test:
     - X-ray of long bones widened, cupped and frayed metaphyses.
     - Thinning of the cortical bones. Thinning of the cortical bones.
     - Bone mineral density.
   d. Following tests to rule out the chronic disease:
     - Renal function test to rule out secondary hyperparathyroidism.
     - Liver function test to rule out liver disease as liver is involved in the conversion of vitamin D.
     - Celiac serology as this disease is involved in case calcium and phosphorus absorption.
     - Thyroid function test as hyperparathyroidism is responsible for bone demineralization.
     - Inflammatory markers as these are the sign of chronic inflammatory disease.

CASE 39

A mother came to pediatric outdoor for evaluation of her 8 years baby girl for poor growth in spite of good health, good appetite, and on healthy food. Karyotyping from amniocentesis was normal. Height of father and mother were 5 ft 8 inch and 5 ft 4 inch tall respectively and health was good. Other two brothers are of good health and their height were average.

On examination, patient's height was below third percentile and weight 23 kg. Sexual development was prepubertal.

Serum IGF-1 was 150 ng/mL (normal 45–358 ng/mL) and bone age.

1. **What is the most likely diagnosis?**
2. **What are the causes of delayed bone age?**
3. **Is there any importance of bone age?**
4. **What are the tests to be performed to rule out chronic disease?**

Answers

1. The most likely diagnosis is:
   - Familial short stature
   - Deficiency of growth hormone
2. Following are the important causes of delayed bone age:
   a. Chronic disease
   b. Constitutional delay
   c. Hypothyroidism
   d. Deficiency of growth hormone
3. Bone age can be delayed in the different diseases. Familial short stature is unlikely because this patient was near 50% at 3.5 years of age. She already crossed several percentiles prior to coming to the attention of parents. So, bone age will help in the diagnosis.

4. Following tests are performed to rule out the chronic disease:
   a. Complete blood count
   b. ESR
   c. Liver and renal function tests
   d. Thyroid profile
   e. To exclude celiac disease, antiendomysial antibodies
   f. For Cushing's syndrome, urinary cortisol level
   g. Provocative test for growth hormone—after arginine/L-dopa stimulation, maximum release of growth hormone is 5.1 ng/mL.
   h. MRI brain is required to detect growth hormone deficiency.

CASE 40

A 42-year-old male came to medical outdoor with chief complaints of erectile dysfunction and decreased libido having no gynecomastia or fatigue. He had no change in the size of finger not under medication. Patient also complained of bitemporal hemianopia. Laboratory investigation demonstrated serum prolactin level 608 µg/mL (value <15 µg/mL).

1. **What is your working diagnosis?**
2. **What should be the next radiological examination of choice?**
3. **Is there any importance if estimating thyroid hormone as well as IGF-1 in the blood?**

Answers

1. The most likely diagnosis is macroprolactinoma as the serum prolactin level is very high and there is evidence of visual field defect.
2. MRI of the brain is required to detect the size of the mass and the monitoring of the treatment.
3. Thyroid hormone should be checked because in hypothyroidism hypothalamic, TRH promotes secretion of the prolactin hormone. But, here the level of prolactin is >200 µg/mL which is not only due to thyroid hormone alone. It may be due to conjoint effect of both thyroid hormone and growth hormone. The excess growth hormone can be diagnosed by suppressing test of growth hormone by oral glucose tolerance test.

CASE 41

A 29-year-old female came to medicine outdoor with complaints of hyperhidrosis, paresthesia, fatigue, and enlargement of the acral parts of the body for last 7 months along with chronic cough. She also had history of persistent galactorrhea and amenorrhea after the delivery of the healthy child.

Laboratory investigation demonstrated that serum IGF-1 was 500 ng/mL and prolactin 41 µg/mL. Chest X-ray showed a small opacity in the left lung. Bronchoscopy demonstrated an endobronchial tumor which was biopsied: CT scan demonstrated symmetric enlargement of the pituitary gland.

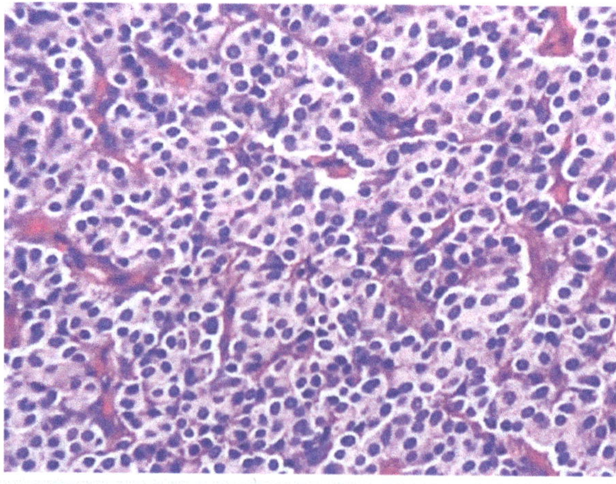

1. **What is the histopathological diagnosis?**
2. **From which disease the patient has been suffering from?**
3. **What is the reason for increased level of prolactin?**
4. **What is the cause of increased level of growth hormone?**
5. **What is the final etiology in this case?**

Answers

1. Histopathology demonstrated nest and cords of small round and uniform cells suggestive of bronchial carcinoid tumor.
2. The patient has been suffering from acromegaly.
3. As a result of stretching of the stalk or compression of the stalk from enlargement of the pituitary gland, prolactin level will be increased.
4. As the CT scan demonstrated the pituitary hyperplasia, hence the cause of increased level of growth hormone due to either centrally from pituitary hyperplasia or peripherally from tumor of lung or pancreas.
5. The final etiology is bronchial carcinoid which is responsible for secretion of GHRH which is easily measured in the blood. After resection of the tumor, this hormone will be undetectable.

CASE 42

A 9-year-old female child, product of consanguineous marriage, came with mother with chief complaints of recurrent hypoglycemia and extreme short stature. Her parents were at 37% and 25% for adult height. Her facies demonstrated depressed nose and small chin.

Laboratory investigation demonstrated that IGF-1 level was 4 ng/mL, serum growth hormone 30 ng/mL which was increased to 45 ng/mL after administration of provocative stimuli.

1. **Why the level of growth hormone was increased before provocative stimuli?**
2. **What is the most likely diagnosis?**
3. **Why there is several incidence of hypoglycemia?**
4. **How can you treat this patient?**

Answers

1. Due to deficiency of IGF-1 level, there is lack of negative feedback on the growth hormone leading to high level of the growth hormone in the blood.
2. The most likely diagnosis is insensitivity of growth hormone due to growth hormone receptor mutation or Laron dwarfism.
3. Mutation or absence of the growth hormone receptor leading to absent action of growth hormone resulting in recurrent hypoglycemia in this patient.
4. This patient can be treated by recombinant IGF-1. If the treatment is started early with the patient, she will achieve the height early. This recombinant IGF-1 can also improve the insulin resistance.

CASE 43

A 32-year-old man having karyotyping of 46XY came to outpatient department with tall stature, early growth of the pubic hair at 11 years and starting shaving at 15 years. On enquiry, his father was 71 inches and mother was 65 inches.

On examination, his height is 81 inches, fully bearded, gross pubic hair, normally descended testes, and normal genitalia.

Laboratory investigation demonstrated that serum testosterone was normal, but FSH and LH were 35 IU/L (normal 2–15 IU/L) and 38 IU/U (normal 2–20 IU/L), respectively. His bone age is 15 and bone density is >2 SD.

X-ray knee demonstrates nonfusion of the epiphyses.

1.   **Is the timing of the puberty of the patient is correct?**
2.   **What is Tanner staging?**
3.   **How can you calculate the stature of the patient?**
4.   **Patient's upper segment is 96 cm and lower segment is 108 cm. What is your interpretation?**
5.   **What is the most likely diagnosis based on the hormone measurement and delayed bone age?**
6.   **Is there any normal feedback by testosterone in this patient?**

Answers

1.   Normal starting age in male is 12 years. His Tanner staging is 5 for testes and pubic hair.
2.   Tanner staging:

Tanner Stage	Breasts	Pubic hair	Growth	Other
1	Elevation of papilla only	Vellus hair only	2–2.4 Inches per year	Adrenarche and ovarian growth
2	Breast bud under the areola, areola enlargement	Sparse hair along the labia	2.8–3.2 inches per year	Clitoral enlargement, labia pigmentation, growth of uterus
3	Breast tissue grows but has no contour or separation	Coarse hair curled pigmented covers the pubes	3.2 inches per year	Axillary hair, acne
4	Projection of areola and papilla, secondary mound formation	Adult hair, does not spread to the thigh	2.8 inches per year	Menarche and development of menses
5	Adult-type contour, projection of papilla only	Adult hair, spreads to the medial thigh	Cessation of linear growth	Adult genitalia

Tanner stage	Genitalia	Pubic hair	Growth	Other
1	Testes <2.5 cm	Vellus hair only	2.0–2.4 inches per year	Adrenarche
2	Testes 2.5–3.2 cm thinning and reddening of the scrotum	Sparse hair at penis base	2.0–2.4 inches per year	Decreases in body fat
3	Testes 3.3–4.0 cm Increase of penis length	Thicker curly hair spreads to the pubis	2.8–3.2 inches per year	Gynecomastia, voice break, increased muscle mass
4	Testes 4.1–4.5 cm, penis growth darkening of scrotum	Adult hair does not spread to thighs	4.0 inches per year	Axillary hair, voice change, acne
5	Testes >4.5cm, adult genitalia	Adult hair spreads to medial thigh	Deceleration, cessation	Facial hair, muscle mass increases

3.   Calculation of the height of a person: Midparental height, a good predictor of adult height can be calculated from the adult height:
     a.   Midparental height for girls: [(Father's height – 5 inches) + Mother's height]/2
     b.   Midparental height for boy: [(Mother's height + 5) + Father's height]/2.
4.   Upper segment to lower segment ratio helps to evaluate the stature of a patient whether the patient is tall or short. This ratio is decreases from 1.7 to 0.9 before puberty because lower limb will grow more as compared to spine of the child. As the patient reaches puberty, growth of the spine increases more due to effect of the steroids. So, normal ratio in adult is 1. In this patient, the ratio is 96/107 or 0.9. So, the patient is tall. Most important cause of tall stature is Klinefelter syndrome, women, and African-American people. This patient has been suffering from estrogen resistance or mutation of the estrogen receptor.
5.   Due to mutation of the estrogen receptor, there is resistance to estrogen. As a result though the level of estradiol level is high, but due to estrogen receptor resistance on the bone, there is nonfusion of the bony epiphysis leading to decreased density of the bone.
6.   Central feedback of testosterone is mediated through estrogen. In this patient, level of testosterone is normal, but FSH and LH levels are high indicating absence of negative feedback.

CASE 44

A 6-year-old female came to outpatient department with development of breast. Her mother started menstruation at the age of 10 years. On examination, she is 122 cm in height, her development of the pubic hair and breast were Tanner stage 2 and 3, respectively. Growth graph demonstrated 8 cm increase in the last year. Her bone age was approximately 8 years.

Laboratory investigation demonstrated that serum estradiol level was 42 pg/mL and LH and FSH level were 7 and 2 IU/L even after gonadotropin-releasing hormone stimulation test.

1. **What do you mean by bone age mentioned here?**
2. **What is the most likely diagnosis?**
3. **Is there any requirement of MRI in this patient?**
4. **What is the treatment in this patient?**
5. **If the patient is not treated, what will be the fate in this patient?**

Answers

1. Bone age and velocity of growth are closely related to precocious puberty as compared to chronological age. Here, the patient's bone age, pubertal growth, and advanced pubertal signs are the signs of precocious puberty.
2. The most likely diagnosis is central precocious puberty.
3. The cause of central precocious puberty depends upon the gender. In case of female, the cause is rarely central rather than the common cause is idiopathic. On the other hand, the cause in case of boys is due to structural cause in the brain. Since this patient is female, so there is usually no need of doing the MRI of the brain.
4. Gonadotropin-releasing hormone agonist should be administered continuously to suppress the axis. So that pubertal growth can be stopped and normal growth will start.
5. If this patient should not be treated, the high estradiol level will fuse the epiphysis early and the patient will be short stature.

CASE 45

A 4-year-old boy came to pediatrician with large phallus. On enquiry, the height of father and mother was 63 cm and 68 cm, respectively. No history of intake of steroid for the cosmetic reason.

On examination, his height as well as weight were >95% for the age. On examination, his phallus and pubic hair were Tanner 4.

Laboratory investigations demonstrated that serum testosterone was 610 ng/mL and undetectable LH and FSH level and the bone age was 6 years.

1. **In which category this patient will fall?**
2. **What is your diagnosis?**
3. **Why females are not affected in this disorder?**
4. **How can you treat this patient?**

Answers

1. This patient will fall in the region where there is precocious puberty but gonadotropin level is undetectable.
2. The most likely diagnosis is familial male-related precocious puberty or familial testotoxicosis due to autosomal dominant mutation of the LH receptor.
3. A precocious pubertal girl requires estrogen. In this disorder, estrogen is not elevated. But androstenedione liberated from the theca cells will be increased. Combined action of gonadotropin is required to synthesize estradiol. Hence, females are not affected in this disorder.
4. Combinations of ARBs along with aromatase inhibitor like testolactone, letrozole, or anastrozole are given. For bone maturation, aromatization from testosterone to estradiol is required, this reaction is irreversible. Along with the above drugs, ketoconazole is required which can be the synthesis of testosterone in the testes. But as this drug also blocks, the adrenal gland leading to many side effects.

CASE 46

A 14-year-old boy came to medical clinic with complaints of enlarged and tender breast and impulsive behavior in the school, but IQ level was normal, height as well as weight within the 98% of reference. Physical examination demonstrated gynecomastia, Tanner stage 2 for pubic hair and Tanner 3 for testes, and upper-to-lower segment ratio was 0.79.

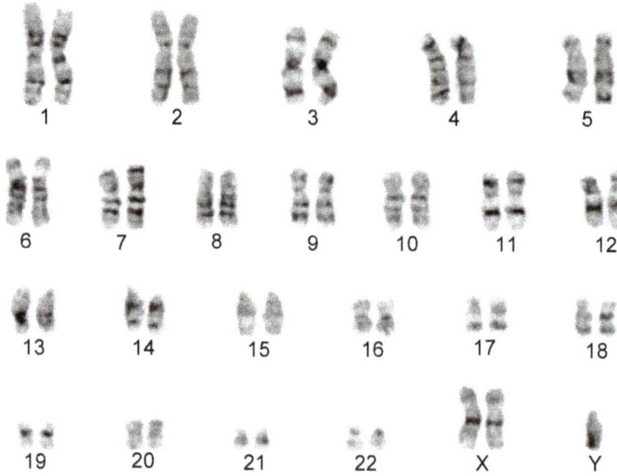

1. What the chromosome study demonstrated?
2. Why there is gynecomastia in this patient?
3. What should be the diagnosis from the hormone point of view?
4. What should be treatment in this patient?

Answers

1. The chromosome study demonstrated the XX and Y. So, the diagnosis is Klinefelter syndrome.
2. Sertoli cells have aromatase, whereas Leydig cells suppress the expression of aromatase in the Sertoli cells. Since the production of testosterone will be reduced in this patient, more estradiol hormone is produced leading to development of gynecomastia in males and enlargement of breast in the females.
3. In this patient, testosterone level is low but gonadotropin level is high. So, testosterone level in this patient is <200 ng/mL or total level is higher but free testosterone will be low. So, this is a case of hypergonadotropic hypogonadism.
4. In this patient, testosterone in the form of intramuscular injection or transdermal patch. Counseling is also needed to correct the impulsive and irritated behavior.

CASE 47

A 20-year-old female having short stature came to emergency department with recurrent seizures and was since then she was on antiepileptic for last 8 months. In spite of that again seizures developed.

On examination, her blood pressure was 90/50 mm Hg, pulse rate 112 beats/min, regular, and respiratory rate 22 breaths/min. During blood pressure measurement, the following features were seen.

Laboratory investigation demonstrated serum calcium 5.5 mg/dL, phosphorus 1.4 mg/dL, and parathormone 522 pg/mL.

Noncontrast CT scan demonstrated calcification in the basal ganglia and pineal gland.

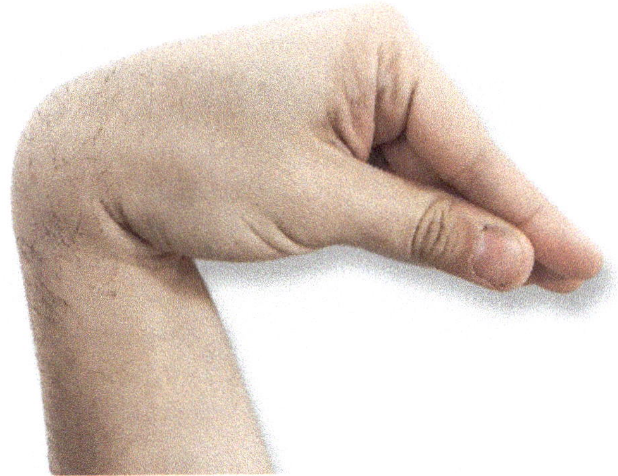

1. **What is the provisional diagnosis?**
2. **What are the causes of hypocalcemia in patient with high blood level of parathyroid hormone?**
3. **How can you classify the pseudohypoparathyroidism?**
4. **What is the function of ionized calcium in the body?**
5. **Is magnesium measurement is necessary in this case?**
6. **What are the causes of hypocalcemia in alkalosis?**
7. **What are the cardiovascular manifestations of hypocalcemia?**
8. **How can you measure serum corrected calcium?**

Answers

1. The provisional diagnosis: Patient has been suffering from hypocalcemic seizures in the background of hyperparathyroidism, but seizures may be due to vitamin D loss as a result of anticonvulsant therapy.
2. The causes of hypocalcemia in the face of high parathormone are:
   a. Vitamin D deficiency:
      - Inadequate intake:
        - Inadequate exposure to sunlight
        - Malabsorption
      - Accelerated loss:
        - Increased enterohepatic circulation
        - Anticonvulsant therapy
        - Impaired hydroxylation due to liver disease
        - Impaired 1α-hydroxylation due to kidney disease
      - Vitamin D-resistant rickets type 1
      - Oncogenic osteomalacia
      - Vitamin D-resistant rickets type 2
      - Phenytoin administration
   b. Parathormone resistance:
      - Hypomagnesemia
      - Renal failure
      - Pseudohypoparathyroidism
   c. Loss of calcium from the circulation:
      - Acute pancreatitis
      - Sepsis
      - Hyperphosphatemia
      - Tumor lysis syndrome
      - Osteoblastic metastasis
      - Acute respiratory alkalosis
3. Pseudohypoparathyroidism can be defined as end organ resistance to parathormone. It is classified into two types:
   a. Type I: Pseudohypoparathyroidism has been subdivided into three types:
      - Type Ia: It occurs due to reduced Gsα-protein characterized by:
        - Hypocalcemia
        - Features of Albright's hereditary osteo-dystrophy:
          - Short stature
          - Mental retardation

- – Obesity
- – Brachymetacarpia
- – Brachymetatarsia
- – Subcutaneous formation of bones
- – Round facies
  - Type Ib: Autosomal mode of inheritance
  - Type Ic: Autosomal mode of inheritance having features of Albright syndrome but short stature
  b. Type II: Here, the defect lies in the failing to rise the serum calcium or urinary secretion of phosphate, features suggestive of vitamin D deficiency but this feature cannot be corrected by administration of vitamin D.
4. Ionized calcium in the neuromuscular system:
   a. Facilitates nerve conduction
   b. Contraction of the muscles
   c. Relaxation of the muscles
5. Magnesium measurement is essential in case of hypocalcemia because if the serum magnesium is low, serum level of calcium cannot be corrected without correction of serum magnesium level.
6. Following are the causes of hypocalcemia in patient with acid–base imbalance:
   a. Hyperventilation-induced alkalosis
   b. Hypokalemia
   c. Emotional stress-induced epinephrine
7. Following are the cardiovascular manifestations in hypocalcemia:
   a. Prolongation of QT interval
   b. Hypotension
   c. Arrhythmias
8. Calculation of corrected calcium in the serum:

$$[0.8 \times (\text{Normal albumin} - \text{Pt's Albumin})] + \text{Serum Ca in mg}$$

CHAPTER 5

Gastroenterology

A 40-year-old female after taking a heavy fried chicken suddenly developed right upper abdominal pain associated with nausea and vomiting.

1. **What are the differential diagnoses?**
2. **How can you conclude your diagnosis?**

Answers

1. Differential diagnoses are the following:
   a. Gastric ulcer
   b. Duodenal ulcer
   c. Cholelithiasis
   d. Acute hepatitis
2. The diagnosis is acute cholecystitis because:
   a. Pain of duodenal ulcer will be diminished after taking food and the pain is not acute.
   b. Pain of gastric ulcer is not acute in onset and the pain may radiate toward back.
   c. Pain of acute hepatitis is dull aching and not acute. There may be associated jaundice.
   d. Pain of acute cholecystitis is of acute onset after ingestion of spicy fatty food; hence, the diagnosis is acute cholecystitis.

A 30-year-old male presented with chronic burning abdominal pain mainly in empty stomach which is relieved by taking food or antacids but without any previous history of gastrointestinal bleeding or anemia or intake of nonsteroidal anti-inflammatory drugs (NSAIDs).

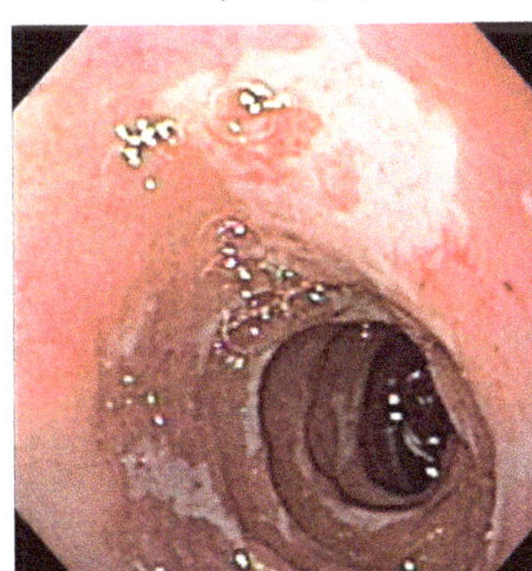 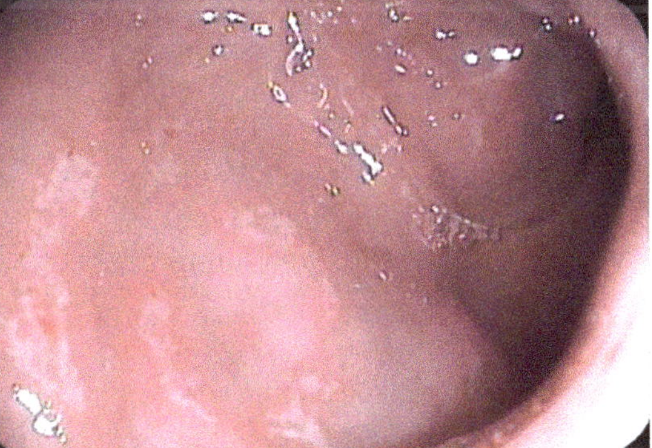

1. **What is your diagnosis?**
2. **Describe the endoscopic pictures.**
3. **What are the red flag symptoms that are not present in this disease?**

Answers

1. The diagnosis is active duodenal ulcer.
2. Endoscopic finding of the first picture: Multiple superficial ulcers with white, sloughed bases without any bleeding points seen on the anterior and posteromedial wall of the duodenal bulb.

   Second picture demonstrates multiple tiny superficial aphthous ulcers seen involving all the walls of the duodenum.

3. Red flag symptoms in this case are:
   a. Young age
   b. Weight loss
   c. Bleeding
   d. Anemia
   e. Chronicity of the symptoms

CASE 3

A 34-year-old man came to the outpatient department with dysphagia to liquid and solid. He was advised upper gastrointestinal endoscopy which demonstrated:

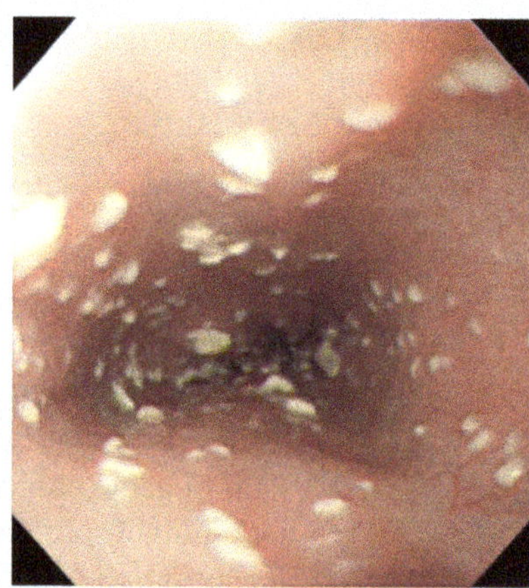 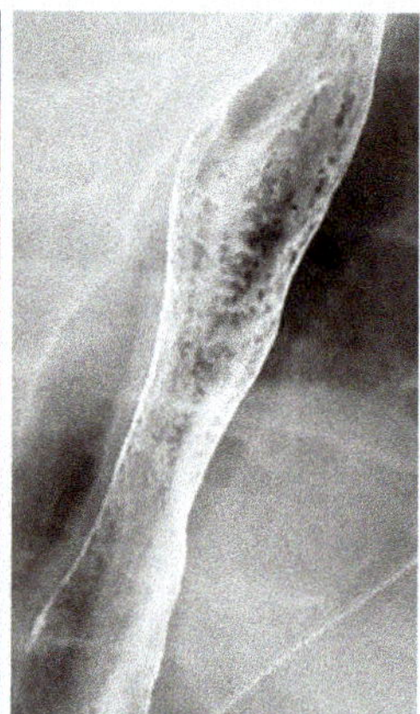

1. **Describe the endoscopic picture and air esophagogram.**
2. **What is your diagnosis?**
3. **Name five common causes of this disease.**
4. **Which is the hallmark of this disease?**
5. **What should be the CD4$^+$ count in case of HIV infection?**
6. **Mention the grading of this disease.**
7. **Name five complications of this disease.**

Answers

1. Description of the endoscopic picture: It demonstrates multiple whitish plaques scattered all over the mucosa of the esophagus.

   Description of the esophagogram: Double-contrast esophagogram in upright position demonstrates multiple filling defects present in the upper thoracic esophagus.

2. The diagnosis is esophageal candidiasis.
3. Five important causes of esophageal candidiasis:
   a. Impaired cell-mediated immunity:
      • HIV infection
      • Patients on radiation to neck region
      • Patients on chemotherapy
   b. Chronic systemic or local corticosteroid therapy
   c. Advanced age
   d. Diabetes mellitus
   e. Adrenal insufficiency
4. The hallmark of esophageal candidiasis is odynophagia.
5. CD4$^+$ count is <200/cc.
6. Grading of candida esophagitis:
   a. Grade 1: Few raised whitish plaques of nearly 2 mm in size but no ulceration.
   b. Grade 2: Multiple raised white plaques of >2 mm in diameter but no ulceration.

c.   Grade 3: Confluent linear, nodular, and elevated plaques with ulcers.

d.   Grade 4: Grade 3 plus narrowing of the lumen.

7.   Complications are:

a.   Esophageal bleeding

b.   Weight loss

c.   Esophageal perforation

d.   Candidemia

e.   Esophageal stricture

CASE 4

A 42-year-old man presented with dysphagia, upper abdominal pain, and diarrhea.

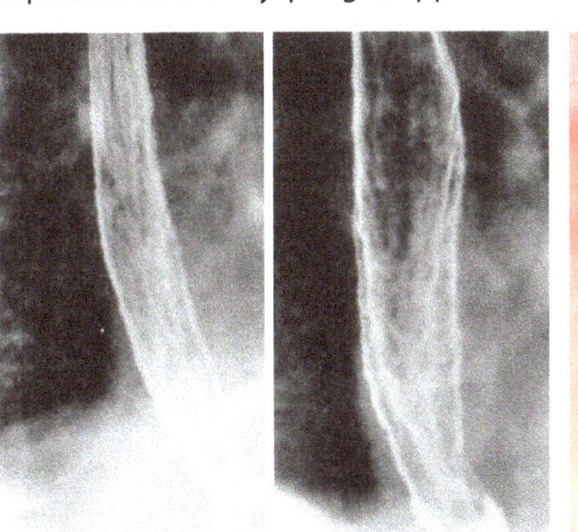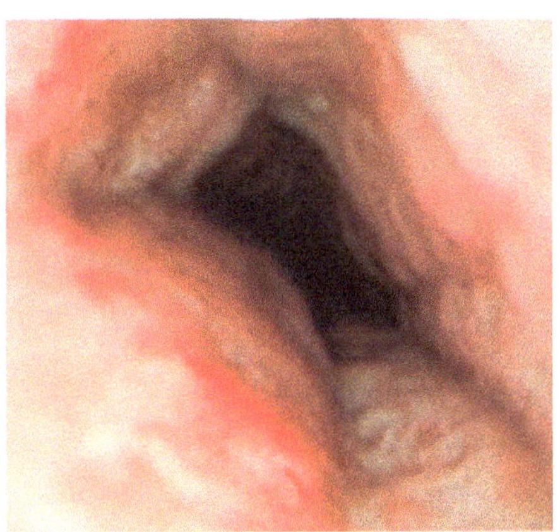

1.   **Describe the lesion in the above pictures.**
2.   **What is your diagnosis?**
3.   **What are the histopathologic features of the biopsy from that lesion?**
4.   **What are the patterns of this infection?**
5.   **What are other four organs involved by this infection?**
6.   **Name three complications in this disease.**

Answers

1.   Endoscopic picture demonstrated evidence of vertical and horizontal shallow and few deep ulcers with surrounding edema and nodularity with intervening normal mucosa seen in the mid and lower esophagus.

Double-contrast esophagogram demonstrated multiple giant-shaped flat and some deep mucosal filling defect suggestive of ulcers with some satellite filling defect suggestive of ulcer seen in the mid and lower esophagus.

2.   The diagnosis is cytomegalovirus esophagitis.

3.   Classical histopathologic features are:

a.   25–35 µm giant cells with *Cytomegalovirus*

b.   Large, ovoid, or pleomorphic nuclei containing basophilic inclusions which are known as owl's eye as they are separated from the nuclear membrane by cytoplasmic halo.

4.   There are three patterns of this disease:

a.   First pattern, where the patient has not been exposed to this organism before, but will be infected by a seropositive patient.

b.   Second pattern, where the patient is seropositive but the infection is latent, but will be activated when the patient is immunocompromised.

c.   Third pattern, where the patient is already seropositive for *Cytomegalovirus*, but again receives latently infected cells from another already infected patient. So, it is a type of superinfection.

5.   Following diseases may occur:

a.   Cytomegalovirus retinitis

b.   Cytomegalovirus adrenalitis

c.   Cytomegalovirus pneumonia

d.   Cytomegalovirus colitis

6.   Potential complications are the following:

a.   Stricture formation

b.   Periesophageal pseudoaneurysm

c.   Rarely perforation

CASE 5

A 35-year-old male suffering from acute myeloid leukemia receiving chemotherapy presented with dysphagia and nausea and vomiting. Endoscopy of upper gastrointestinal tract and double-contrast esophagogram was performed.

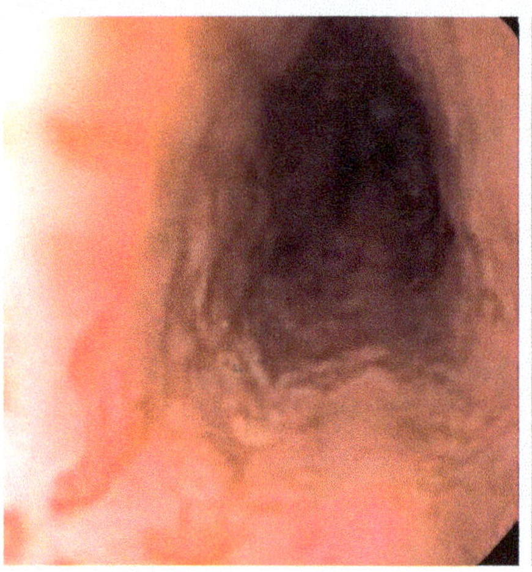
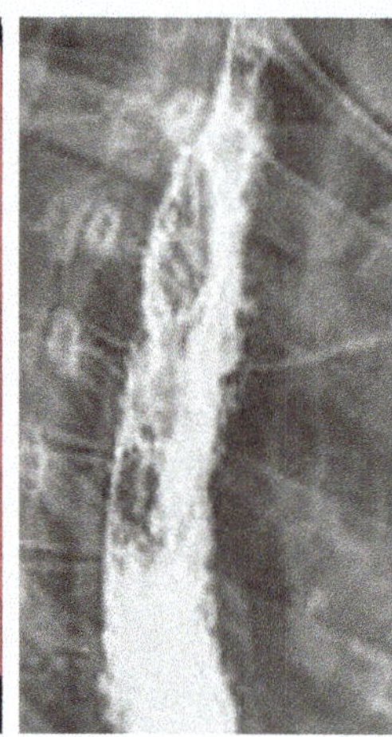
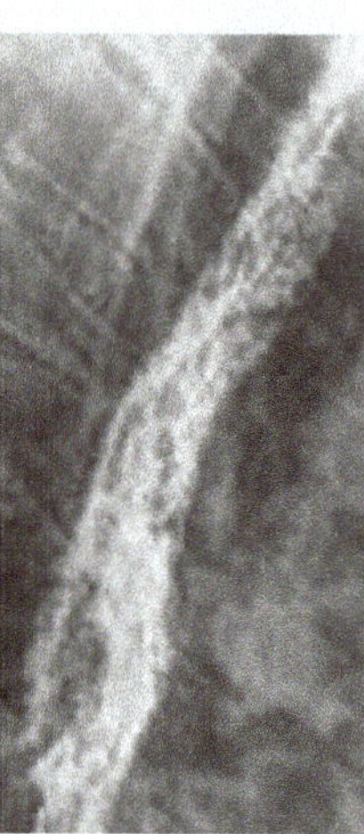

1. **Describe the above pictures.**
2. **What is your diagnosis?**
3. **Classify this disease.**

Answers

1. Upper gastrointestinal endoscopy demonstrated multiple punched-out longitudinal or transverse ulcers with intervening normal mucosa seen in the mid and lower esophagus. In some areas, there is presence of 1–3 mm round vesicles in the mid esophagus.

   Double-contrast esophagogram demonstrated multiple punctate, linear, or satellite filling defects with intervening radiolucent mounds of edema seen in the mid and distal esophagus.

2. The diagnosis is Herpes simplex esophagitis.

3. Classification of this disease:
   a. Type I lesion: Presence of small punched-out lesion having slightly yellow-colored fibrin exudates present in the mid and lower esophagus.
   b. Type II lesion: Presence of small punched-out lesion, no color, and absence of exudation. These are present in the mid and lower third of esophagus.
   c. Type III lesion: Presence of multiple confluent ulcers like map present throughout the esophagus.

CASE 6

A 35-year-old man presented with retrosternal pain, chronic cough which was aggravated during sleep, and hoarseness of voice. His endoscopy was done. Later on upper gastrointestinal endoscopy was done which demonstrated:

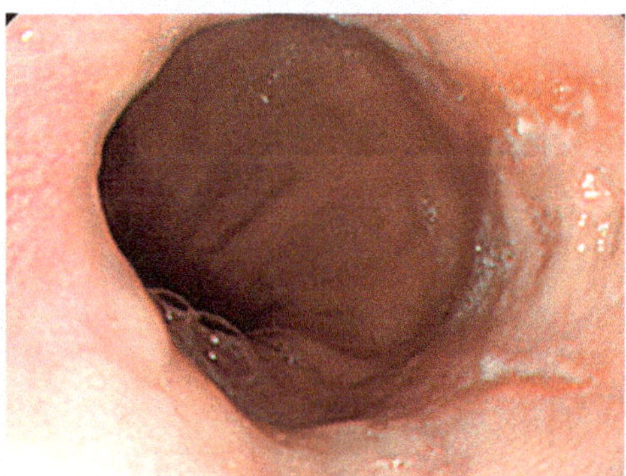
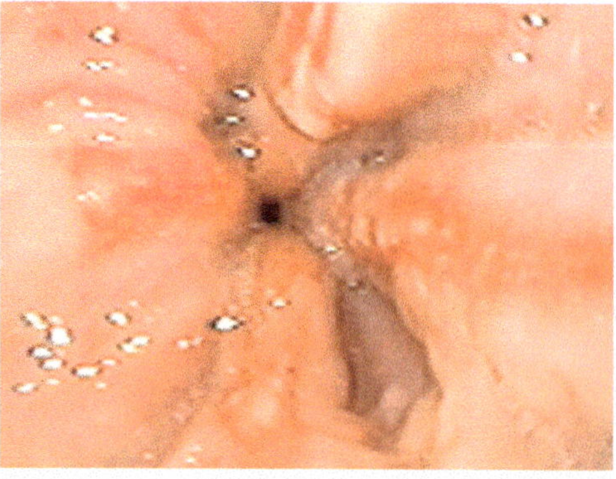

1. **Describe the endoscopic findings.**
2. **What is your diagnosis?**
3. **Mention current endoscopic staging of this disease.**
4. **What is the major pathophysiological factor in this disease?**
5. **Name five dietary factors which are responsible for this disease.**
6. **Name five medications which are responsible for gastroesophageal reflux disease (GERD).**
7. **Name five important complications of this disease.**
8. **What is rumination syndrome?**

Answers

1. Description of the endoscopic findings:
   a. Two linear erosions seen at the lower end of esophagus extending upward in first endoscopic picture and length of erosion is <5 mm in length—stage I esophagitis.
   b. Four linear erosions of >5 mm in length are present at the lower end of esophagus with cicatricial changes in the mucosa—stage II of reflux esophagitis.
2. The diagnosis is reflux esophagitis.
3. Los Angeles staging of esophagitis:
   a. Grade A: 5 mm mucosal damage in the mucosal fold.
   b. Grade B: Damage is >5 mm in the mucosal folds but no continuity between the folds.
   c. Grade 3: Mucosal damage is continuous between two or more mucosal folds but not all around.
   d. Grade 4: All-around mucosal damage involving >75% of the esophageal lumen.
4. The most important pathophysiological factor is transient lower esophageal sphincter relaxations (TLESRs) which can be defined as transient lower esophageal sphincter relaxation in response of gastric distention lasting for 10–30 seconds leading to physiologic gastroesophageal reflux. But in patients with GERG, this TLESR is increased in number as well as duration is also increased.

5. Following five dietary factors are responsible for lowering of lower gastroesophageal sphincter:
   a. Acidic foods
   b. Caffeine
   c. Alcohol
   d. Chocolate
   e. Peppermint
6. Following five medications are responsible for lowering of lower gastroesophageal sphincter:
   a. Calcium channel blockers
   b. Progesterone
   c. β-adrenergic drugs
   d. Nitrates
   e. Barbiturates
7. Following are the five complications of GERD:
   a. Esophageal stricture
   b. Barrett esophagus
   c. Esophageal ulcers with or without bleeding
   d. Adenocarcinoma
   e. Pulmonary manifestation
8. Rumination syndrome is characterized by the following:
   a. Regurgitation of the undigested food following consumption
   b. There is absence of nausea, abdominal pain, and heart pain.
   c. Diagnosis is based on history and clinical diagnosis.

CASE 7

A 45-year-old man came to the outpatient department with postprandial heartburn for years and aggravated at night during sleep for which he has to get up from the bed. He was advised to perform pH monitoring in the esophagus which is described below:

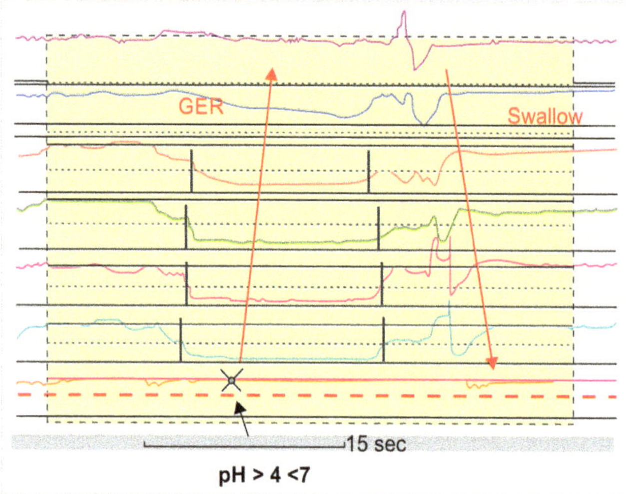

1. **What is this method and for which it is usually done?**
2. **Is the proton pump inhibitor (PPI) therapy continued during the procedure?**
3. **What are the indications of this method?**
4. **What are the types of reflux?**
5. **What is reflux hypersensitivity?**
6. **What is functional heartburn?**
7. **What are the two indices which are required to assess the association of the patient's symptoms with gastroesophageal reflux episodes?**

Answers

1. This is a method for assessing the correlation between patient's symptoms with the gastroesophageal reflux episodes. The name of the method is multichannel intraluminal impedance–pH monitoring.

2. Whether to continue the PPI therapy or not depends upon the indications. In case of patient's symptoms refractory to treatment who has history of GERD, the drug can be continued. In this case, it is done to detect the weak acid or nonacid reflux. Patient should be on PPI for at least 1 week prior to this procedure. But if it is not clear that the symptoms are due to GERD, in that case PPI therapy should be discontinued 1 week prior to this procedure to diagnose GERD.

3. Indications for this procedure are:
   a. For quantifying and characterizing the gastro-esophageal reflux who are refractory or nearly refractory to PPI therapy.
   b. For evaluation of patients with atypical symptoms of gastroesophageal reflux

   c. For evaluation of reflux symptoms and achlorhydria
   d. For evaluation of reflux symptoms postgastrectomy
   e. For evaluation of postprandial symptoms in patients
   f. For evaluation of reflux symptoms and ingestion of meals frequently

4. There are three types of acid reflux:
   a. Acidic: <4
   b. Weakly acidic: pH is 4–7.
   c. Weakly alkaline: pH is >7.

5. Reflux hypersensitivity:
   a. This can be diagnosed when all Rome IV criteria are met for the last 3 months with symptomatic onset for at least 6 months prior to diagnosis:
      - Retrosternal symptoms such as heartburn and chest pain
      - Eosinophilic esophagitis or normal endoscopy is ruled out.

- Absence of any major esophageal motor disorder
- In spite of normal exposure to acid on pH monitoring or normal pH–impedance monitoring

6. Functional heartburn: This can be diagnosed when all Rome IV criteria are met for the last 3 months with symptomatic onset for at least 6 months prior to diagnosis with frequency of twice per week:
   a. Retrosternal burning or pain
   b. In spite of adequate antireflux therapy, no relief of symptom
   c. Absence of major esophageal motor disorders

7. Two indices are required to assess the association of the patient's symptoms with gastroesophageal reflux episodes:
   a. Symptoms index: It can be defined as number of symptoms associated with reflux episodes occurring in the preceding 5 minutes interval which is divided by total number of symptoms recorded by the patient during the period of monitoring.

- If it is >50%, it is considered as positive and the patient is considered to have symptomatic reflux episodes in spite of PPI therapy.
- If the index is <50%, it is considered as negative and the patient if presents with persistent symptoms in spite of PPI therapy, in that case it is due to causes other than gastroesophageal reflux.

   b. Symptom-association probability: Total measuring time divides into 2 minutes interval. Contingency table having four fields will assess the correlation with the Fisher exact test:
   - Number of intervals with gastroesophageal reflux and symptoms
   - Number of intervals with gastroesophageal reflux without symptoms
   - Number of intervals without gastroesophageal reflux with symptoms
   - Number of intervals without gastroesophageal reflux without symptoms

Positive symptom-association probability of >95% has been considered as statistically significant.

CASE 8

A 40-year-old man resident of Brazil came to the outpatient department with history of dysphagia to liquid but later on also to solid, along with postprandial vomiting. He was advised upper gastrointestinal endoscopy followed by barium swallow of esophagus.

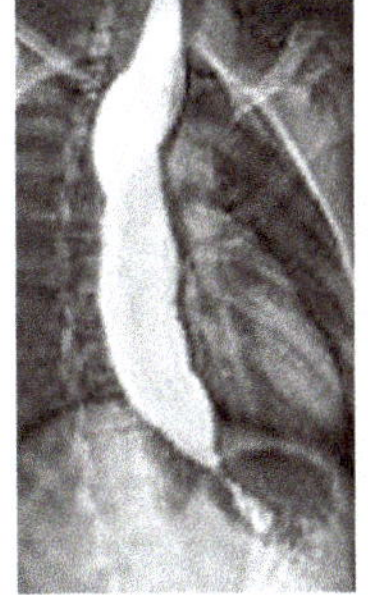 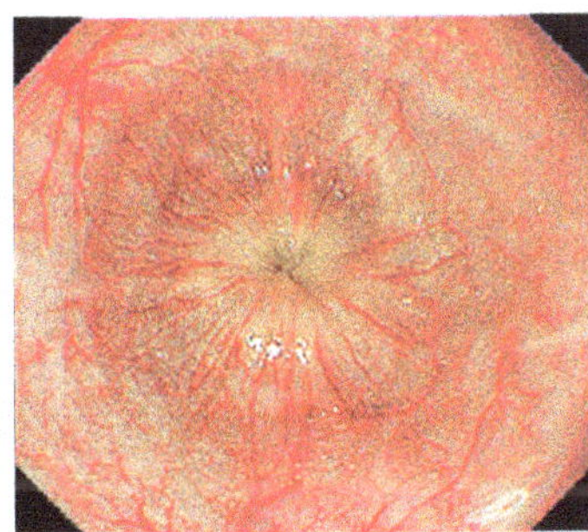 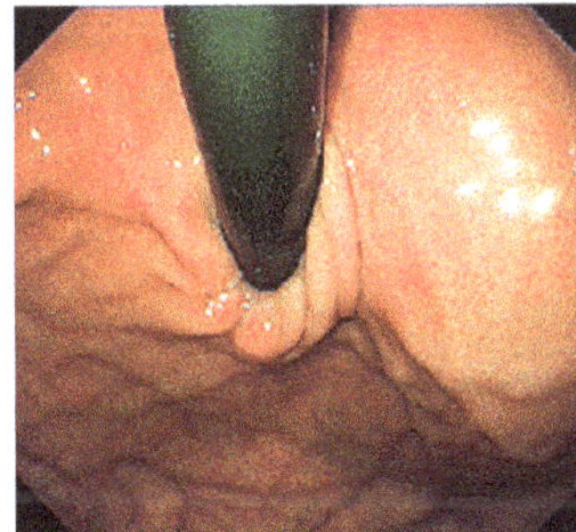 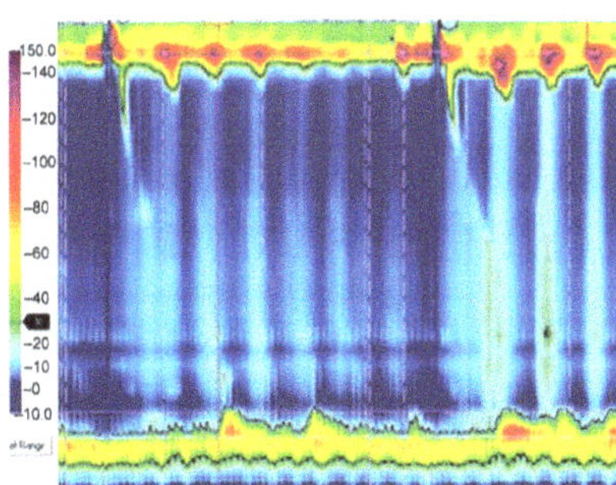

1. **Describe the above pictures.**
2. **What is your diagnosis?**
3. **What is the pathophysiology behind this disease?**
4. **What are the types of the disease?**
5. **How can you quantify the types? What is its importance?**
6. **How can you differentiate this disease from dysphagia due to scleroderma?**
7. **How can you treat the disease?**
8. **What is the importance of ethnicity here?**

Answers

1. Description of the above pictures:
   a. Barium swallow of the esophagus demonstrated:
      - Esophagus appeared dilated
      - Absence of esophageal peristalsis
      - Failure of the relaxation of lower esophageal sphincter
      - Distal esophagus is narrowed resembling the bird's beak appearances.
   b. Upper gastrointestinal endoscopy demonstrated:
      - Functional stenosis at the lower gastro-esophageal junction
      - Wrapping around the esophagogastric junction
   c. Esophageal manometry demonstrated:
      - Absence of distal pressurization of >30 mm Hg
      - No evidence of contraction of the esophageal cavity
2. The diagnosis is classical achalasia cardia.
3. Pathophysiology of achalasia cardia:
   a. Immune-mediated ganglionitis due to viral infection or toxins resulting in decrease in number or absence of myenteric neurons leading to aperistalsis or impaired relaxation of the lower esophageal sphincter. Antibodies against myenteric neurons may be demonstrated in the serum.
   b. There is association between the genetic polymorphism in HLA class II molecules and achalasia cardia. These HLAs are HLA-DQA1*0103 and DQB1*0603 allels.
4. There are three types of achalasia:
   a. Type I: Classical achalasia, there is no evidence of pressurization.
   b. Type II: Achalasia with compression or compartmentalization in distal esophagus of >30 mm Hg.
   c. Type III: Achalasia with two or more contractions.
5. Quantification of lower esophageal sphincter relaxation is "integrated relaxation pressure".
   a. Type I achalasia: Upper limit of normal is 10 mm Hg.
   b. Type II achalasia: Upper limit of normal is 15 mm Hg.
   c. Type III achalasia: Upper limit of normal is 17 mm Hg.
   It can differentiate achalasia from nonachalasic subject and diffuse esophageal spasm.
6. In scleroderma:
   a. There is hypoperistalsis or aperistalsis of the esophagus.
   b. Hypotensive of lower esophageal sphincter
7. Treatment:
   a. Pharmacologic treatment:
      - Nitrates: It will inhibit the normal contraction of the lower esophageal sphincter by dephosphorylation of the light chain of myosin.
      - Nifedipine: It will inhibit the contraction of the lower esophageal sphincter muscles by inhibiting cellular uptake of calcium.
      - Botulinum toxin A: It inhibits the release of acetylcholine from the nerve terminal.
   b. Pneumatic dilatation of the lower esophageal sphincter muscle by Rigiflex balloon dilator—it is available in three diameters: 30, 35, and 40 mm.
   c. Surgical approach: Nowadays, Heller myotomy should be done. Advantages of this method are:
      - Shorter duration of stay
      - Postoperative complications should be minimal.
      - Response rate is >90%.
   But during this procedure, intraoperative endoscopy should be done for confirming the position of the anatomical position of the myotomy.
   The only complication of this procedure is gastroesophageal reflux which can be covered by fundoplication, but it should not be too tight to produce dysphagia again.
8. As the patient came from Brazil, he probably suffered from Chagas disease. In this case, antibodies to this organism should be performed.

CASE 9

A 47-year-old chronic alcoholic male came to the emergency department with a history of esophageal reflux and occasionally dysphagia. He had undergone upper gastrointestinal endoscopy and biopsy was taken from the reddened area in the esophagus.

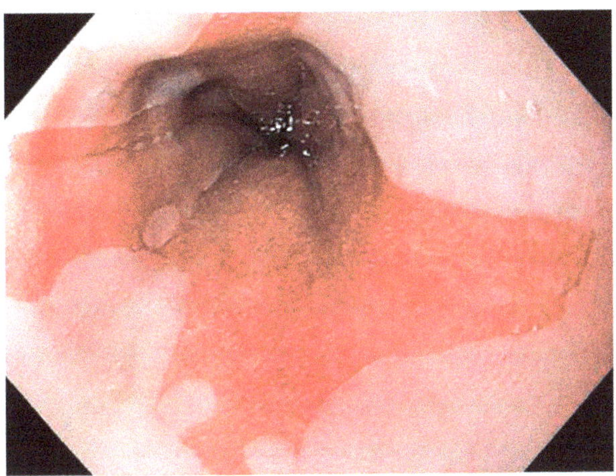
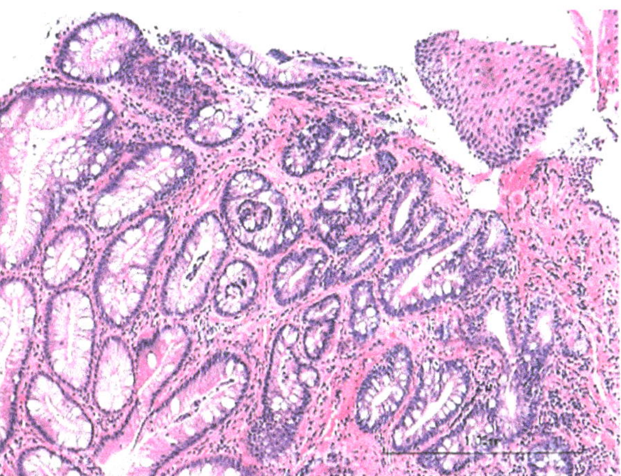

1. **What is the finding in the upper gastrointestinal endoscopy?**
2. **What is the feature in the biopsy?**
3. **What is your diagnosis?**
4. **What is the diagnostic algorithm in Barrett's esophagus?**
5. **What are the types of Barrett's esophagus and how can they be differentiated?**
6. **What are the complications that may occur in this case?**
7. **What is the management in this patient?**
8. **What should be the surveillance interval in case of Barrett's esophagus?**

Answers

1. Endoscopic feature is salmon-colored patch extending above the gastroesophageal junction, i.e., Z line, above which there is white-colored mucosa indicating squamous epithelium.

2. Histology demonstrates: Evidence of intestinal metaplasia in the lower end of esophagus in patient with reflux esophagitis.

3. The diagnosis is Barrett esophagus.

4. Diagnosis of Barrett's esophagus depends upon the both endoscopic and histological findings:
   a. First step: Clear identification of gastroesophageal junction, i.e., visualization of the proximal margin of the gastric folds in a minimally distended esophagus.
   b. Second step: Identification of the salmon-colored mucosa, i.e., columnar-lined esophagus along with identification of the length as well as circumference of this area.
   c. Third and final step: Presence of specialized intestinal metaplasia seen in the area of the columnar-lined mucosa. In this case, biopsy should be taken from the all four quadrants of the Barrett's segment to exclude the presence of dysplasia or cancer.

5. There are two types of Barrett esophagus:
   a. Long-segment Barrett esophagus of >3 cm in diameter.
   b. Short-segment Barrett esophagus of <3 cm in diameter.

   Special features in two types of Barrett esophagus:
   a. In long-segment Barrett esophagus:
      - Longer duration of symptoms of reflux
      - During 24 hours esophageal pH monitoring, there are evidence of severe pattern of reflux in both erect and supine position.
      - Reduced lower esophageal sphincter pressure
      - Patient is less sensitive to direct acid exposure.
   b. In case of short-segment Barrett esophagus:
      - Shorter duration of reflux

- During 24 hours esophageal pH monitoring, there are evidence of severe pattern of reflux in both erect positions.
  - Normal lower esophageal sphincter pressure
  - Patient is more sensitive to direct acid exposure.
6. Complications of Barrett esophagus:
   a. Adenocarcinoma of esophagus—it occurs in patients with GERD.
   b. Squamous cell carcinoma of esophagus: It occurs in patient on alcohol, cigarette, and tobacco product.
7. Treatment of Barrett esophagus:
   a. In case of high-grade dysplasia, surveillance endoscopy with intensive biopsy at every 3 months interval till the appearance of malignancy.
   b. Endoscopic ablation—goal is to remove all neoplasia as well as Barrett mucosa.
   c. Radiofrequency ablation: It is done to perform circumferential followed by focal ablation of dysplasia.

   d. Surgical resection: It can be done but it cannot regress the Barrett esophagus.
8. Surveillance interval of the Barrett's esophagus:
   a. Intestinal metaplasia without any evidence of dysplasia:
      - Endoscopy as well as biopsy should be repeated in 1 year.
      - If there is no dysplasia, in that case endoscopy with biopsy should be repeated every 3 years.
   b. Low-grade dysplasia:
      - Upper gastroesophageal endoscopy should be done within 6 months.
      - It should be repeated at 1 year interval until the absence of any dysplasia.
   c. High-grade dysplasia:
      - Upper gastrointestinal endoscopy should be performed within 3 months.
      - In case of high-grade dysplasia, endoscopic resection of any irregular mucosa
      - Ablation of any flat mucosa

CASE 10

A 32-year-male came to the outpatient department with dysphagia to bolus liquid and solid and retrosternal pain radiating to back. Barium swallow of esophagus and manometry have been advised.

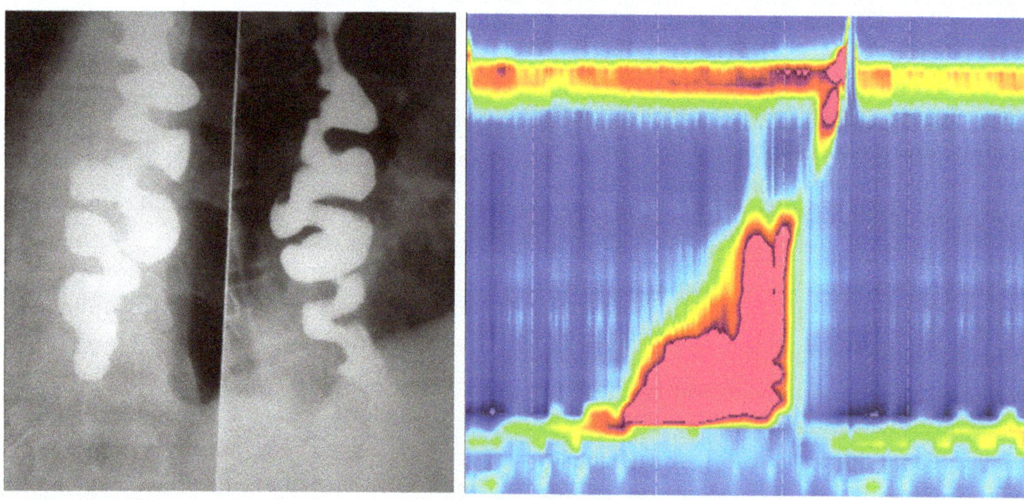

1. **What is the finding in the barium swallow esophagus?**
2. **What is the finding in manometry?**
3. **What is your diagnosis?**
4. **What are the possible pathophysiological factors in this disease?**
5. **How can you treat the disease?**

Answers

1. Barium swallow demonstrates:
   a. Poor progression of the bolus
   b. Evidence of disordered simultaneous contraction in the esophagus and tertiary contraction mimicking the appearance of diverticula.
2. Esophageal manometry demonstrates:
   a. Evidence of aperistalsis in >30% of wet swallows
   b. 20% simultaneous contraction
   c. Amplitude of contractions in the distal three-fifths of esophagus is >30%.
3. The diagnosis is diffuse esophageal spasm.
4. Possible pathophysiology in diffuse esophageal spasm is:
   a. Increased release of acetylcholine in the myoneural junction
   b. Elevated basal metabolic rate
   c. Hyperglycemia
   d. Hyperlipidemia
5. Treatment:
   a. First line of treatment:
      - Calcium channel blocker
      - Nitrates
   b. Second line of therapies:
      - Endoscopic injection of botulinum toxin
      - Pneumatic dilatation
   c. Surgical therapy:
      - Myotomy involving the whole length of involved segment that can be found by esophageal manometry. It involves several centimeter above the proximal border of the spastic region for preventing remnants of the spasticity.
      - In case of refractory patient, Heller myotomy can be done.

CASE 11

A 60-year-old man presented with intermittent dysphagia to both solid and liquid and history of choking during swallowing without any weight loss. He has also evidence of mild left-sided weakness but does not take any medication.

1. **What are the differential diagnoses?**
2. **What is the definite diagnosis and why?**
3. **The diagnosis can be established by which investigation?**

Answers

1. Differential diagnoses are:
   a. Reflux esophagitis
   b. Squamous cell carcinoma of esophagus
   c. Esophageal adenocarcinoma
   d. Neurologic dysfunction
2. Diagnosis is neurologic dysfunction because this patient has a history of oropharyngeal dysphagia which may be secondary to stroke because he has also evidence of mild left-sided weakness. Any type of esophageal cancer is associated with weight loss and progressively increasing dysphagia. In case of reflux esophagitis, there should be history of heartburn, painful deglutition, acid regurgitation, and dysphagia to solid and liquid will not be present.
3. This type of dysphagia can be detected by videoradiographic study to observe the process of deglutition. Whereas esophageal dysphagia can be detected by either upper gastrointestinal endoscopy or barium esophagogram. Reflux esophagitis can be detected by pH testing.

CASE 12

A 20-year-old man came to an emergency department with painful swallowing on solid food and odynophagia and intermittent retrosternal chest pain. Patient was on steroid inhaler to treat asthma and oral doxycycline for treating acne. He has no history of weight loss. He has a family history of gastric cancer. His physical examination is within normal limit.

1. **What are the five common differential diagnoses?**
2. **What is the definite diagnosis and why?**
3. **Any other medications are responsible for this disease?**
4. **What are the risk factors of pill-induced esophagitis?**

Answers

1. Differential diagnoses are:
   a. Esophageal cancer
   b. Erosive gastritis
   c. Pill-induced esophagitis
   d. Candida esophagitis
   e. Achalasia cardia
2. Definite diagnosis is "doxycycline" pill-induced esophagitis.
   a. Achalasia is not the diagnosis because achalasia does not produce symptom acutely.
   b. As the patient's age is only 20 years, hence esophageal cancer is very unlikely at this age.
   c. As there is no preceding history of reflux symptom, hence this is not a case of reflux esophagitis.
   d. Candida infection is unlikely as this patient is immunocompetent.
3. The medications responsible for pill-induced esophagitis:
   a. Direct toxicity which is drug induced—tetracycline
   b. Through the production of caustic acid:
      • Ascorbic acid
      • Ferrous sulfate
   c. Through the production of caustic alkali: Bisphosphonate
   d. Through the production of hyperosmolar solution: Potassium chloride
   e. Indirect injury mediated by the effects on the esophageal motility like stasis or through facilitating reflux: Calcium channel blockers
4. Following are the risk factors that predispose to medication-induced esophagitis:
   a. Decreased production of saliva:
      • Sicca syndrome
      • Anticholinergic medication
   b. Disorders of esophageal motility:
      • Achalasia
      • Stricture
      • Ineffective motility
      • Aging
   c. Disorder of the local anatomy:
      • Aortic aneurysm
      • Enlarged left atrium
   d. Medication formulation:
      • Capsule
      • Large tablets
      • Sustained-release formulation
   e. Drugs affecting the lower esophageal sphincter:
      • Benzodiazepines
      • Calcium channel blockers
      • Opioid antagonists
      • Theophylline
      • α-adrenergic agonists
   f. Intake of medicines in supine position

CASE 13

A 40-year-old man on NSAID for treatment of osteoarthritis developed upper abdominal pain. He used to take 15 cigarettes per day. His endoscopic picture and biopsy from the antrum demonstrated:

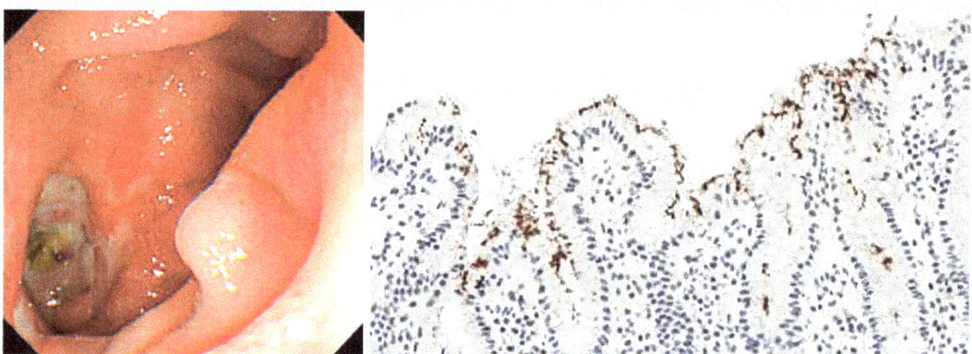

1. **Describe both the pictures.**
2. **What is your diagnosis?**
3. **Name five risk factors for developing this ulcer.**
4. **Here according to you, which factor in this patient is responsible for decreasing the incidence of NSAIDs-induced peptic ulcer disease?**

Answers

1. Endoscopic picture demonstrated a deep punched-out ulcer having white, sloughed base and surrounding the erythematous mucosa seen on the medial wall of the bulb.

   Biopsy from the antral mucosa demonstrated brown-shaped elongated bodies seen on the inner surface of the mucosal lining in the antrum.

2. The diagnosis is chronic active duodenal ulcer due to *Helicobacter pylori* infection.

3. Five risk factors for duodenal ulcer are:

   a. Age > 60 years

   b. Concomitant use of glucocorticoids

   c. Use of multiple doses or high doses of NSAIDs

   d. Prior history of peptic ulcer disease

   e. Oral anticoagulant use

4. In any patient with *H. pylori*-induced duodenal ulcer, eradication of *H. pylori* cannot decrease the incidence of NSAIDs-induced duodenal ulcer; but, cessation of smoking will decrease the incidence of NSAIDs-induced peptic ulcer disease. Hence, cessation of smoking may reduce the incidence of NSAID-induced peptic ulcer disease.

CASE 14

A 6-year-old child with a history of allergy to prawn and family history of asthma came to the outpatient department with retrosternal burning and rashes. His upper gastrointestinal endoscopy and biopsy done which demonstrated:

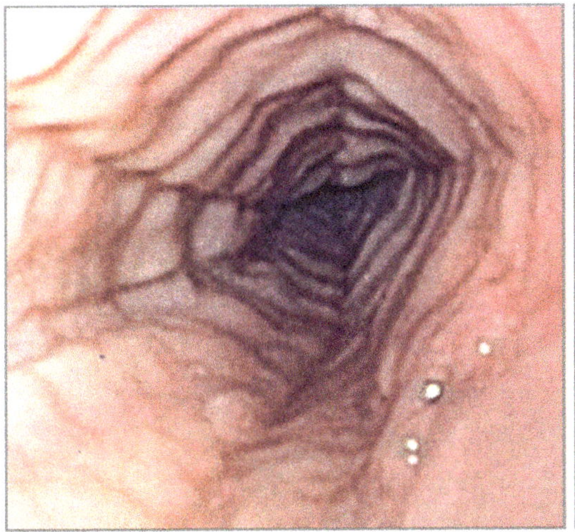
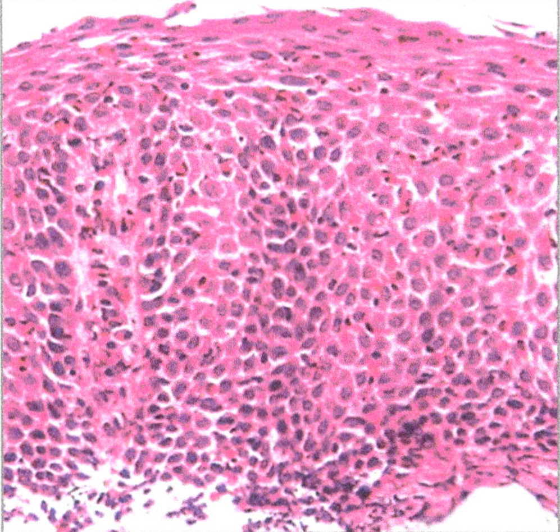

1. **Describe the above pictures.**
2. **What is your diagnosis?**
3. **What is the pathophysiology behind this disease?**
4. **How can you grade the endoscopic grade of this disease?**
5. **What is the treatment rationale in this disease?**

Answers

1. Endoscopic picture of esophagus showed:
   a. Edema of the esophageal mucosa
   b. Corrugated esophageal mucosa
   c. Concentric fixed ring and furrows in the esophageal mucosa leading to trachealization
   d. Whitish mucosal exudates

   Histological section demonstrated:
   a. Infiltration of the mucosa with abundant number of eosinophils
   b. Basal cell hyperplasia
   c. Superficial layering with eosinophils
   d. Elongated papillae reaching into top one-third of the epithelial layer
   e. Extracellular eosinophilic granules

2. History, endoscopic picture, and biopsy findings are suggestive of eosinophilic esophagitis.

3. Pathophysiology behind the eosinophilic esophagitis:
   a. No single agent is responsible for this disease. There is an inverse relation between *H. pylori*

infection and eosinophilic esophagitis. There is an association of celiac disease with eosinophilic esophagitis.

b. Environmental aeroallergen and pollen have a role in this disease.

c. Loss of function of a skin structural barrier protein filaggrin is associated with the incidence of atopic dermatitis and eosinophilic esophagitis. Expression of filaggrin is downregulated by interleukin-13 in the esophagus, as a result the barrier function of the epithelium in the esophagus will be lost. So, antigen will be taken up by esophagus leading to further inflammation.

d. Vigorous T helper 2 cells immune response along with the activated eosinophils leads to increased tissue damage.

e. As a result of increased concentration of the activated eosinophils in the epithelial cells and increased concentration of interleukin-13 which leads to increase in eotaxin-3.

f. Upregulation of interleukin-5 occurs as a result of increased response of T helper 2 cells to antigen which leads to increased response of eosinophils to eotaxin-3.

g. Desmoglein 1, an intracellular adhesion molecule, is downregulated in this disease.

h. Local inflammation leads to:
   - Increased immunoglobulin E (IgE) production
   - Migration of mast cells
   - Fibrosis

i. In high concentration eosinophil:
   - Secretes chemokine and cytokines
   - Release cytotoxic granules
   - Creates mitochondrial DNA trap upon their death resulting trapping of bacteria in the extracellular matrix

4. Endoscopic grade of eosinophilic esophagitis:
   a. Grade 1: Mucosal edema, mucosal ring, and furrow
   b. Grade 2: Presence of exudate
   c. Grade 3: Stricture

5. Treatment in eosinophilic esophagitis is based on the symptomatology as well as findings in the upper gastrointestinal endoscopy:
   a. In case of patient with symptoms related to GERD, PPIs may be given.
   b. In case of findings like furrow, plaques, and exudates, administration of local and systemic steroids based on the severity of the symptoms.
   c. If the patient has a strong history of atopy, asthma or food allergies, patch testing, or skin prick test should be done.

CASE 15

A 70-year-old male with severe dysphagia both to solid and liquid underwent endoscopy which showed 4 cm ulcerated polypoidal lesion in the distal third of esophagus and diagnosed as esophageal cancer. Endoultrasonography and computerized tomography demonstrated no regional lymphadenopathy and distant metastasis respectively. Following operation was done which demonstrated:

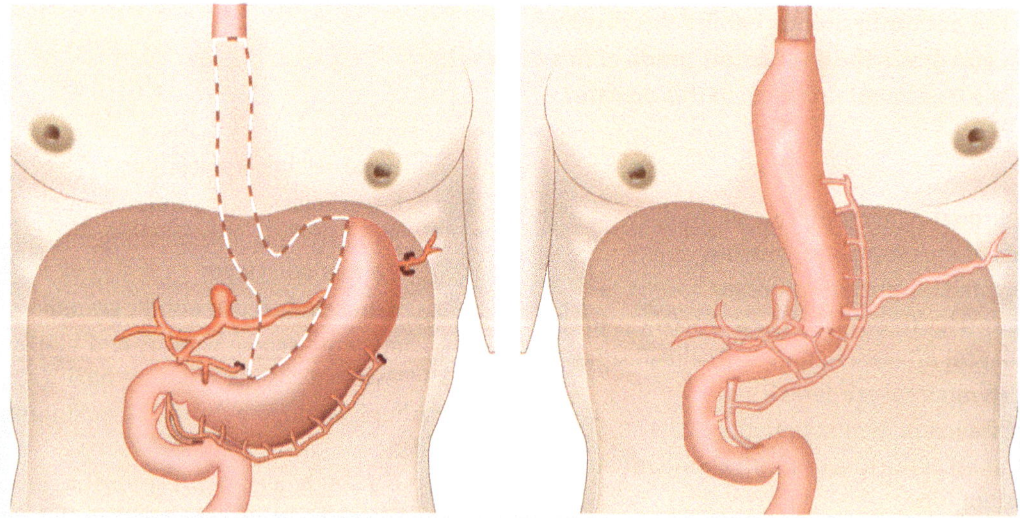

1. **What operation was done in this patient?**
2. **What are the approaches that can be done?**
3. **What extra operation should be done during esophageal resection?**
4. **Name five indications of this procedure.**
5. **Name three complications of this operation.**

Answers

1. Esophagectomy followed by gastric tube reconstruction surgery.
2. There are four approaches of operation:
    a. Transhiatal approach
    b. Ivor Lewis approach
    c. Three-hole or McKeown approach
    d. Laparoscopic approach
3. As the vagus nerve was damaged during the resection of the esophagus, to improve the gastric emptying, pyloroplasty should also be done. Feeding jejunostomy should also be required to improve nutrition during the period of recovery.
4. Following are the indications of this operation:
    a. Malignant neoplasm in the esophagus
    b. High-grade dysplasia in the Barrett's esophagus
    c. Perforation of the esophagus
    d. Severe caustic damage of the esophagus
    e. Rarely in case of achalasia cardia, scleroderma, and diffuse esophageal spasm
5. Three complications of this operation are:
    a. Early postoperative complications:
        - Bleeding due to inadequate hemostasis
        - Arrhythmias
        - Atelectasis
        - Pneumonia
    b. Within 2–3 days of operation, ischemia of the conduit as manifested by tachycardia due to poor oxygenation.
    c. Leak in the site of anastomosis:
        - Thoracic anastomosis presenting with sepsis
        - Cervical anastomosis leading to drainage of the turbid fluid from the wound in the neck

CASE 16

A 40-year-old patient presented with recurrent retrosternal burning and diagnosed as reflux esophagitis and was on daily PPI, but the symptom recurred in spite of maximum dose of antisecretory medication. Repeat endoscopy demonstrated Los Angeles class B esophagitis along with presence of small hiatal hernia. Manometry also demonstrated decreased pressure in the lower esophageal sphincter. So, patient was undergone the following operation:

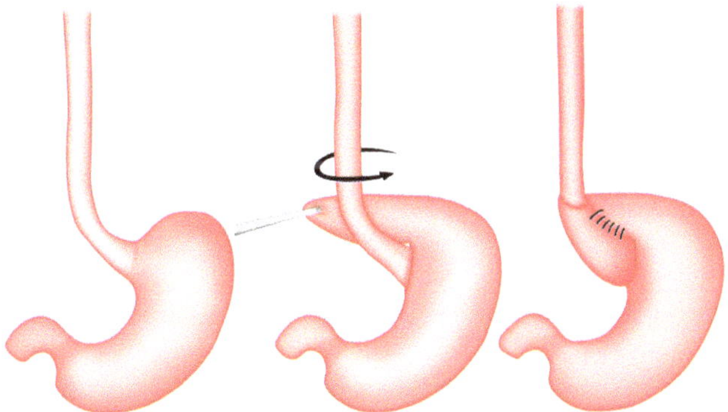

1. **What is this operation?**
2. **Describe the procedure.**
3. **What are the other types of operation in reflux esophagitis with hiatal hernia?**
4. **What are the indications of this operation?**
5. **What are the complications in this procedure?**

Answers

1. This operation is Nissen fundoplication.
2. Nissen fundoplication procedure involves:
   a. Division of short gastric vessels attached with the spleen
   b. Entire gastric fundus should be mobilized to deliver it behind the gastroesophageal junction creating 360° wrap around the distal 3–4 cm of the esophagus thereby increasing the pressure in the lower esophageal sphincter.
3. Other types of operation in reflux esophagitis:
   a. Dor partial fundoplication involving 180° anterior fundal wrap
   b. Toupet partial fundoplication involving 270° posterior fundal wrap
   c. Belsey Mark IV fundoplication involving 240° anterior partial fundoplication along with plication of the crura to narrow esophageal hiatus
4. Following are the indications of the fundoplication:
   a. Refractory gastroesophageal reflux in spite of maximum dose of medical therapy
   b. Large hiatal or paraesophageal hernia to reposition the stomach back into the abdominal cavity
   c. In nongastrointestinal features of GERD
   d. Morbid obese patient is suffering from the GERD.
5. Complications of this operation are:
   a. Gas-bloat syndrome
   b. In 20% patients, dysphagia in early postoperative period can be managed by dietary modification.
   c. Persistent dysphagia can occur in 15% patients that should be managed by:
      - Frequent dilatation
      - Converting the 360° wrap to 270° wrap or 180° wrap

CASE 17

A 25-year-old female came to the outpatient department with history of progressive weight loss of more than 4 kg. Endoscopy demonstrated dilated esophageal cavity along with retained food in the esophageal cavity. Barium swallow also demonstrated hugely dilated esophagus with bird beak of lower esophageal sphincter. Esophageal manometry demonstrated aperistalsis of the esophagus along with highly elevated lower esophageal sphincter. So, patient underwent the following operation:

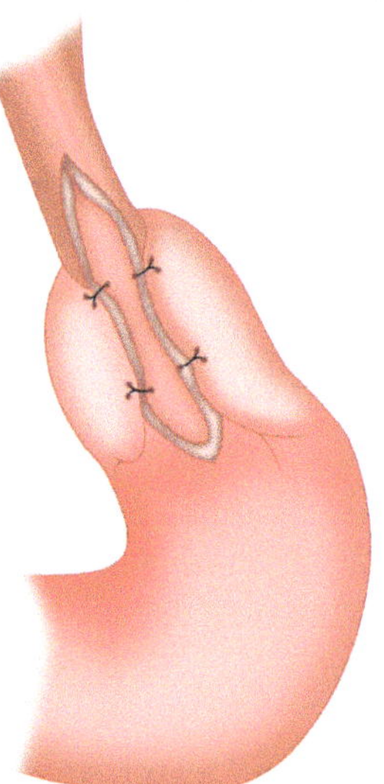

1. **Name the operation done here.**
2. **Describe in short the operative procedure.**
3. **Mention few complications of this procedure.**

Answers

1. Heller cardiomyotomy
2. Procedure:
   a. Mobilization of the lower esophagus and entire gastric fundus
   b. Before closing the diaphragmatic crura both muscular layer of the lower esophagus and seromuscular layer of gastric cardia should be closed but keeping the muscular layer intact.
   c. To prevent incomplete myotomy, myotomy should be extended. It should be extended 6 cm above and 2 cm below the squamocolumnar junction.
   d. After that crura should be closed.
   e. In some cases, partial fundoplication should be done to prevent the gastroesophageal reflux.
3. Complications:
   a. Immediate postmyotomy complication:
      - Gastric perforation
      - Esophageal perforation
   b. Persistent dysphagia resulting from incomplete myotomy or postoperative adhesion
   c. In 40% cases of GERD
   d. In case of long-lasting reflux, Barrett's esophagus may develop.

CASE 18

A 58-year-old man with history of upper abdominal discomfort and progressive weight loss of more than 5 kg in 1 month came for upper gastrointestinal endoscopy which demonstrated adenocarcinoma in the stomach. Endoscopic ultrasonography revealed neither lymphadenopathy nor submucosal invasion of the tumor. Computerized scan demonstrated thickening of the antrum. Patient was operated.

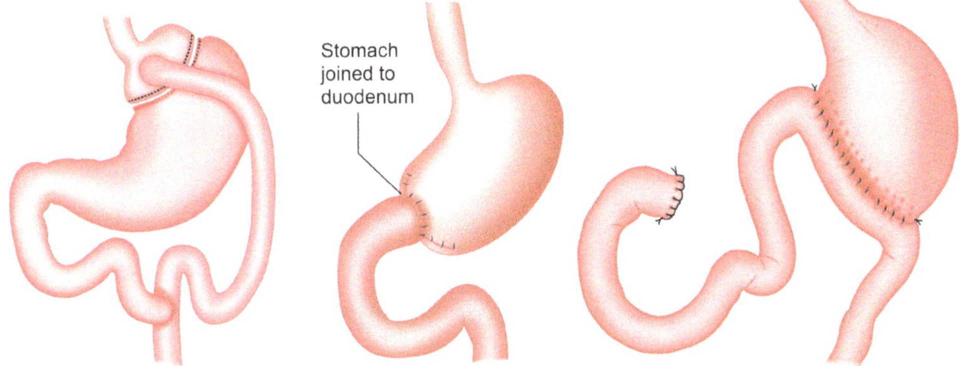

1. **What are the operations shown here?**
2. **What are the procedures involved here?**
3. **In case of malignancy, is there any requirement of excision of other organ?**
4. **In case of gastric adenocarcinoma, why is vagotomy not required?**
5. **What are the complications of this operation?**

Answers

1. Following are the operations shown here:
   a. Roux-en-Y procedure
   b. Billroth I gastroduodenostomy
   c. Billroth II gastroduodenostomy
2. The procedures involved here are:
   a. Roux-en-Y gastrojejunostomy:
      - Gastrojejunal or Roux limb of the jejunum has to be anastomosed with the biliopancreatic limb of the jejunum.
      - Subtotal or partial gastrectomy followed by end-to-end gastrojejunal anastomosis
   b. Billroth I procedure or end-to-end gastroduodenostomy:
      - Small portion of the gastric body, pylorus and antrum, and duodenal bulb are resected.
      - Anastomosis should be done inbetween the gastric remnant and the remaining part of duodenum.
   c. Billroth II procedure or end-to-side gastrojejunostomy:
      - Partial gastrectomy is done.
      - Proximal portion of the duodenum is resected.

- Anastomosis should be done inbetween the remaining portion of the stomach and remaining portion of the duodenum containing ampulla of Vater as afferent limb and loop of the jejunum with the stomach as efferent loop in the form of end-to-side.

3. Yes, in case of gastric malignancy, total lymph node resection should be done from pyloric, portal, celiac, splenic, and cardiac region.

4. In case of gastric adenocarcinoma, vagotomy is not required because patient is achlorhydric.

5. Complications:

   a. Anastomotic leak: It is a dreaded complication because it may lead to:
      - Peritonitis
      - Septic shock

      If above complications occurs in Billroth I procedure, one should shift to Billroth II procedure

   b. Postgastrectomy syndrome:
      - Postvagotomy diarrhea due to excess bile acids as well as bile salts which are not absorbed in the small intestine.
      - Alkaline reflux gastritis resulting from the reflux of bile acids into the gastric remnant and this can be treated by sucralfate, cholestyramine, and PPI. If it is refractory to medical therapy, gastrojejunostomy should be converted into Roux-en-Y anastomosis.

- Dumping syndrome characterized by post-prandial lightheadedness, hypoglycemia, palpitation, and diarrhea. It can be of two types:

   1. In early dumping syndrome: It occurs 15–30 minutes after taking the meals resulting from the rapid shift of intravascular fluid into the small intestine as hyperosmolar chyme enters into the small intestine.

   2. Late dumping syndrome: It occurs 2–3 hours after taking food resulting from the hyperinsulinemia from high carbohydrate diet.

- Afferent loop syndrome: It results from preventing of the biliary and pancreatic secretion into the stomach resulting from afferent limb obstruction by kinking, stricture, adhesion, or narrowing of the anastomotic area.

- Roux stasis syndrome: It is characterized by abdominal pain, nausea, vomiting, and early satiety resulting from Roux stasis, delayed gastric emptying, or both.

CASE 19

A 50-year-old type 2 diabetic and hypertensive obese woman with history of hyperlipidemia came to the outpatient department with joint pain that restricted her physical activities. She was asked by a dietitian to lose weight but without any effect. Hence, she came here for reduction of body weight by operative procedure.

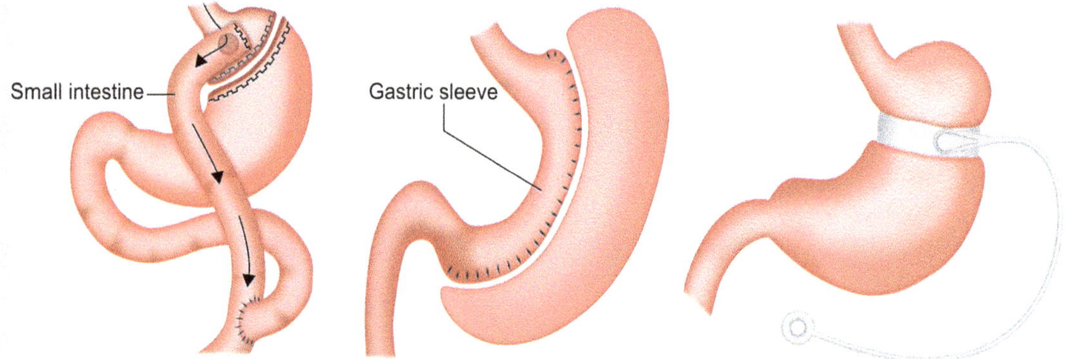

1. **What are the operations usually done as depicted in above pictures?**
2. **Describe the procedure in short.**
3. **What are the complications of these operations?**

Answers

1. The operations are the following:
   a. Roux-en-Y gastric bypass procedure
   b. Laparoscopic adjustable gastric banding procedure
   c. Sleeve gastrectomy
2. Procedures involved here:
   a. Roux-en-Y gastric bypass procedure:
      - A small pouch of stomach has to be separated from the rest of the stomach remnants.
      - Then small pouch has to anastomose with the jejunum to produce gastrojejunal anastomosis.
      - The Roux limb of this gastrojejunostomy has to connect with the biliopancreatic limb to produce Roux-en-Y configuration.
   b. Sleeve gastrectomy: This is a restrictive procedure where greater portion of the stomach cavity is removed, as a result the stomach cavity becomes tubular.
   c. Laparoscopic adjustable gastric banding:
      - On the cardia of the stomach band has to be placed around the cardia of the stomach circumferentially creating a small reservoir.
      - This band now is connected with a reservoir port and this has to be placed under the abdominal skin pad.
      - Now this port can be accessed by a saline containing needle.
      - The band can be loosened or tightened to enlarge or constrict the stomal size respectively.
3. Complications of these procedures are:
   a. Vitamin and mineral deficiencies:
      - As the fundus of the stomach is removed in Roux-en-Y gastric bypass procedure, intrinsic factor which is responsible for absorption of vitamin B_{12} from the small intestine will not be present.
      - Iron is absorbed from the proximal duodenum and acid is required for its absorption. Hence, Roux and sleeve procedure will lead to loss of proximal duodenum and loss of parietal cells respectively leading to iron malabsorption.
      - Calcium is also absorbed from the proximal duodenum. Operation that bypass the proximal duodenum will lead to malabsorption of the calcium.
      - Disruption of the enterohepatic circulation will lead to malabsorption of vitamin A and D.
   b. Roux procedure will lead to:
      - Anastomotic leak
      - Internal hernias
      - Ulceration
      - Stomal stenosis
   c. Laparoscopic adjustable gastric banding lead to slipping of the band leading to either GERD or dysphagia.

CASE 20

A 31-year-old man came with history of retrosternal pain to liquid along with postprandial vomiting and dysphagia. Barium swallow of esophagus was performed which demonstrated the following features:

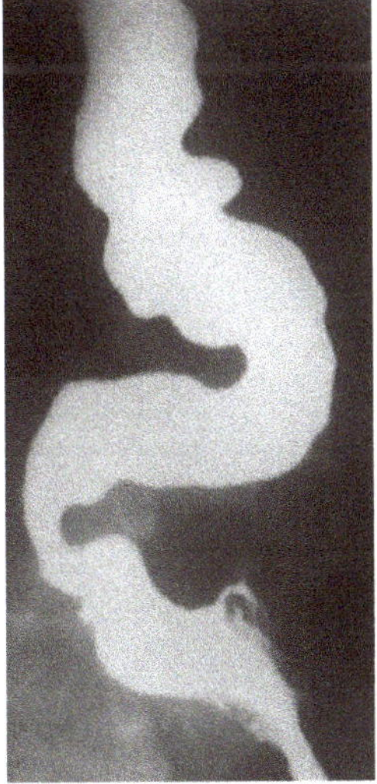

1. **Describe the barium swallow of esophagus.**
2. **What is the diagnosis?**
3. **Describe the disease.**
4. **What are the muscles of esophagus involved to produce what specific symptoms?**
5. **What is the specific treatment of this disease?**

Answers

1. Barium swallow of esophagus demonstrates uncoordinated contraction of the esophageal muscles.
2. The diagnosis is nutcracker esophagus or jackhammer esophagus.
3. Description of nutcracker esophagus: It can be defined as having mean amplitude of the contraction of the esophagus of 180 mm Hg, i.e., >2 standard deviations over the 10 consecutive wave of contractions. It is a type of hypertensive peristalsis as here, the contraction will proceed in coordinated manner but the amplitude of contraction is excessive.
4. Muscles of esophagus:
   a. Muscles of the upper esophageal sphincter involve striated muscles involving cricopharyngeus muscles including upper esophageal zone. Disorder of this muscle is responsible for aspiration pneumonia.
   b. Middle zone includes both striated and smooth muscles. Both outer longitudinal and inner circular muscle layers work conjointly to produce coordinated contraction of the esophagus downward.
   c. Lower zone involves lower esophageal sphincter produced by the smooth muscles that contract to prevent the reflux of gastric content. Disorder of this muscle is responsible for gastroesophageal reflux or thoracic dysphagia.
5. Specific treatment is:
   a. Calcium channel blocker
   b. Botulinum toxin: It will bind to the acetylcholine receptor in the nerve endings leading to less release of acetylcholine.
   c. Proton pump inhibitor is used to decrease the symptoms of reflux.
   d. Tricyclic depressant to decrease the stress

CASE 21

A 36-year-old corporate worker after a birthday party complained of severe retching or "dry heaving" followed by severe and several bouts of hematemesis. Immediately that patient was admitted and upper gastrointestinal endoscopy was performed which demonstrated the following:

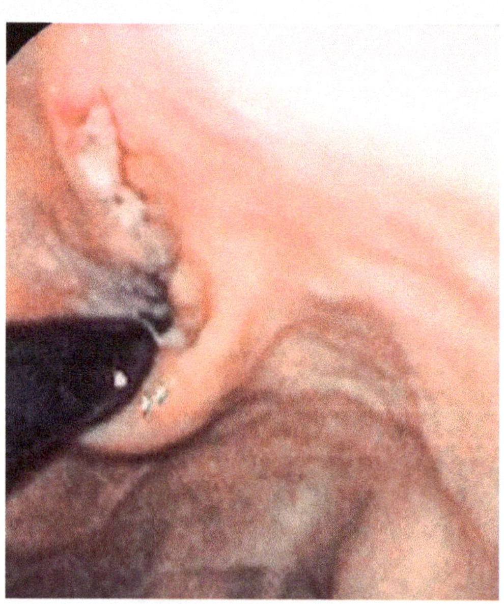

1. **Describe the picture.**
2. **What is your diagnosis?**
3. **What is the pathophysiology behind this disease?**
4. **What are the other causes of this disease?**
5. **What are the differential diagnoses?**
6. **What is the treatment?**
7. **What are the complications of this disease?**

Answers

1. Upper gastrointestinal endoscopy demonstrated a linear erosion at the lower end of esophagus in the retroflexed view of esophagus.
2. Diagnosis is Mallory–Weiss tear of esophagus.
3. As a result of increased gradient between intra-abdominal and intrathoracic pressure forceful vomiting causes shearing forces in direct proportion to luminal diameter at the gastroesophageal junction as well as proximal stomach at the point of diaphragmatic hiatus leading to esophageal tear.
4. Other causes of esophageal tear:
   a. Valsalva maneuver
   b. Forceful coughing
   c. Forceful retrograde passage of air during upper gastrointestinal endoscopy
   d. Transesophageal echocardiography
   e. Cardiopulmonary resuscitation
5. Differential diagnoses are:
   a. Boerhaave syndrome
   b. Peptic ulcer
   c. Esophageal cancer
   d. Esophageal varices
   e. Arteriovenous malformation
6. Specific treatment:
   a. Proton pump inhibitor to decrease the gastric acidity as the acid hinders the healing of ulcer
   b. If there is no bleeding as evidenced during the endoscopy, no further intervention is needed.
   c. 1:10,000 diluted epinephrine can be injected to induce vasoconstriction.
   d. Multipolar electrocoagulation
   e. Injection of sclerosing agent
   f. Argon plasma coagulation
   g. Through the angiography transcatheter gel embolization to obliterate left gastric artery or superior mesenteric artery
   h. Rarely endoscopic oversewing of the esophageal tear
7. Complications of this disease are:
   a. Hypovolemic or hemorrhagic shock
   b. Metabolic disturbances
   c. Myocardial infarction
   d. Rarely esophageal perforation

CASE 22

A 60-year-old woman came to outpatient department with severe epigastric pain.

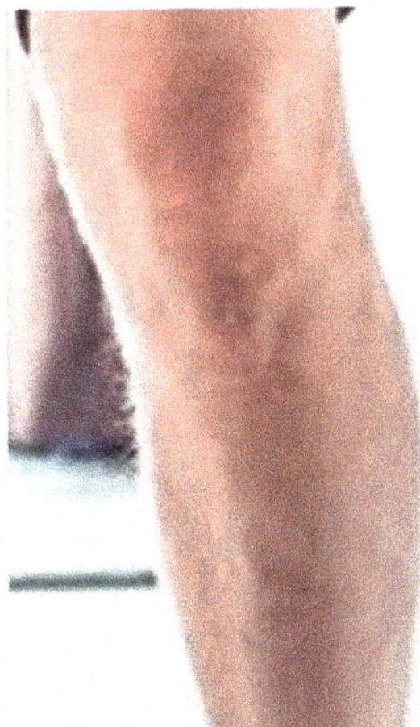
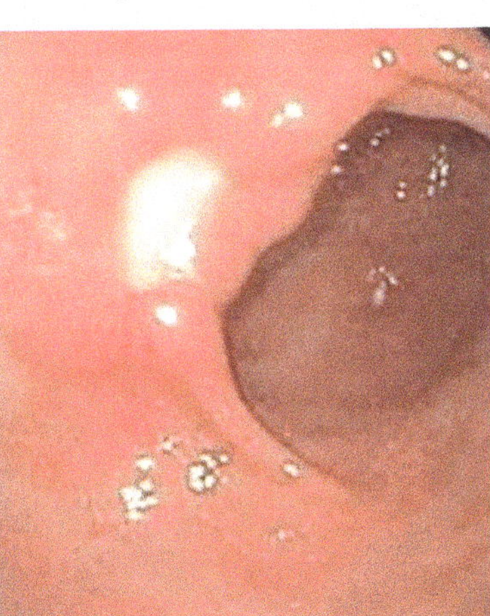
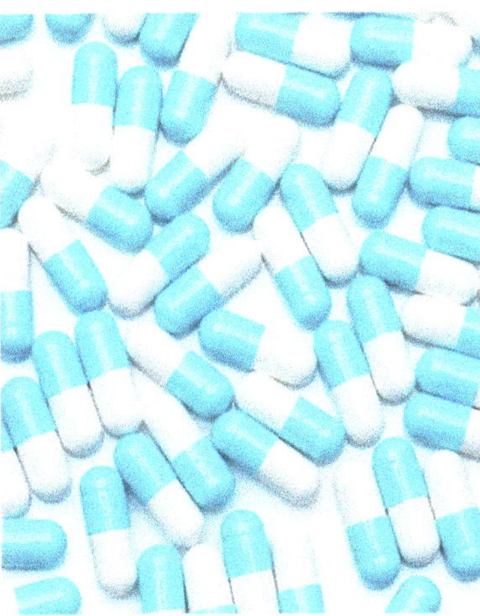

1.   **Mention the correlation between the above three pictures.**
2.   **What is your diagnosis?**
3.   **Mention the pathophysiology behind this endoscopic abnormality.**

Answers

1.   Patient has been suffering from osteoarthritis of the left knee for which she used to take NSAIDs. Due to the long-term use of this drug, the patient developed abdominal pain and through upper gastrointestinal endoscopy gastric ulcer has been demonstrated. The ulcer is deep seated having white sloughed base and surrounding edematous mucosa.

2.   The diagnosis is chronic gastric ulcer which is NSAIDs induced.

3.   There are two isoforms of this enzyme. COX-1 isoform is distributed throughout the gastric body but COX-2 isoform is expressed in response to proinflammatory cytokines. NSAID blocks both the isoenzymes. COX-1 isoform inhibits the formation of prostaglandin from the arachidonic acid which is highly protective to the gastroduodenal mucosa, whereas COX-2 isoenzyme has little role in the synthesis of prostaglandin and hence little role in the damage of the gastroduodenal mucosa.

CASE 23

A 24-year-old male presented in the outpatient department with upper abdominal pain and occasional vomiting. Following tests were done in this patient.

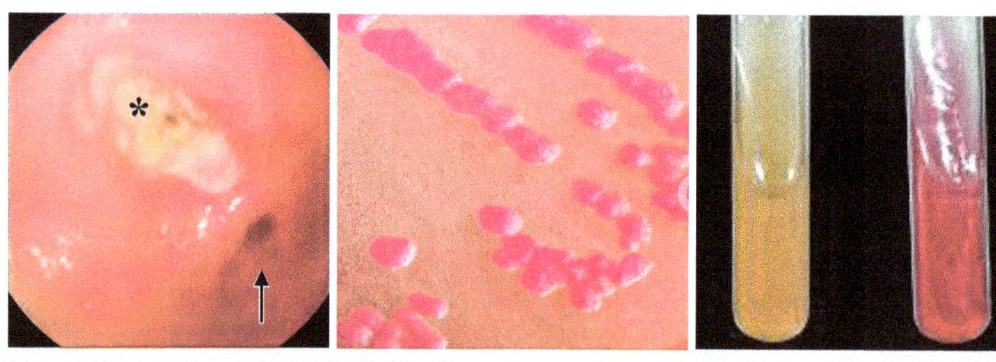

1.   **Describe the correlation between the above three pictures with the history.**
2.   **What is your diagnosis?**
3.   **What is the pathophysiology behind this disease?**
4.   **What is the treatment schedule for this disease?**

Answers

1.   The correlations are the following:
     a.   Endoscopic picture demonstrated a deep-seated punched-out ulcer having white sloughed base and surrounding edematous mucosa present in the antral mucosa near the pyloric orifice.
     b.   Mucosa taken from the antrum was sent for culture and culture demonstrated gram-negative elongated bacteria suggestive of *H. pylori*.
     c.   Urease test done here: Here, these bacteria liberate urease enzyme that breaks the urea in the solution to release ammonium ions thereby activating the pH indicator to change the color of the medium from yellow to red looking like onion peel. It usually occurs within 2 hours.

2.   The patient has been suffering from *H. pylori*-induced antral ulcer.

3.   Pathophysiology of this ulcer:
     a.   These bacteria produce urease creating an alkaline environment. It will burrow into the protective mucus gel to adhere to the gastric epithelial surface glycoprotein through varieties of adhesives present in the outer membrane protein like SabA and BabA and colonize.

b. As a result of adhesion, *H. pylori* secretes toxins, among which two toxins are mostly pathogenic:
- CagA toxin is the 60–70% toxins which translocate into the epithelial cells and lymphocytes leading to:
  - Cytokine production
  - Inhibition of apoptosis
  - Promotion of carcinogenesis
- VacA toxin inserts into the:
  - Endosomal membrane resulting in osmotic swelling
  - Apoptosis affecting the mitochondrial membrane

4. Treatment of *H. pylori*-induced peptic ulcer:
a. Current recommended regimen:
- Standard triple therapy:
  - Proton pump inhibitor twice daily
  - Amoxicillin 1 g twice daily, in case of allergy to penicillin, metronidazole
  - Clarithromycin 500 mg twice daily
  Total duration of therapy is 10–14 days.
- Levofloxacin-based therapy:
  - Proton pump inhibitor twice daily
  - Levofloxacin 500 mg daily
  - Amoxicillin 1 g twice daily
  Total duration of therapy is 14 days.
- Bismuth-based therapy:
  - Bismuth subsalicylate 2 tablets four times daily
  - Metronidazole 250 mg thrice daily
  - Tetracycline 500 mg four times daily
  - Proton pump inhibitor twice daily
b. Newer proposed therapy:
- First quadruple therapy:
  - Proton pump inhibitor twice daily and amoxicillin 1 g twice daily from day 1 to 5th day followed by PPI twice daily, clarithromycin 500 mg twice daily, and metronidazole 500 mg twice daily for 6th to 10th day.
  - Proton pump inhibitor twice daily and amoxicillin 1 g twice daily from 1st to 5th day followed by PPI twice daily, amoxicillin 1 g twice daily, clarithromycin 500 mg and metronidazole 500 mg thrice daily from 6th to 10th day.
  - Concomitant therapy of all the above drugs (metronidazole twice daily) for 14 days.
- Optimized bismuth therapy:
  - Bismuth 2 tablets four times daily
  - Tetracycline 500 mg four times daily
  - Metronidazole 500 mg thrice daily
  - Proton pump inhibitor twice daily
  Total duration of therapy is 14 days.
- Optimized levofloxacin-based therapy:
  - Proton pump inhibitor twice daily and amoxicillin 1 g twice daily from 1st to 5th day.
  - Proton pump inhibitor twice daily, levofloxacin 500 mg daily, and metronidazole 500 mg twice daily from 6th to 10th day.
c. Salvage therapy:
- First time failure: If the above regimen fails, the new regimen should have at least 1 new drug.
- Second time failure: If all the above regimen fails, antibiotic sensitivity should be obtained.
  - Experimental therapy:
    - Rifabutin 150 mg twice daily, amoxicillin 1 g twice daily and PPI twice daily for 10 days.
    - Nitazoxanide 500 mg, levofloxacin 250 mg, and omeprazole 40 mg every morning and nitazoxanide 500 mg, doxycycline 100 mg everyday in afternoon for 10 days.
    - Furazolidone 200 mg twice daily, levofloxacin 250 mg twice daily, and lansoprazole 30 mg twice daily for 7 days.

CASE 24

A 50-year-old man came to the outpatient department with vague upper abdominal pain and advised upper gastro-intestinal endoscopy. Following are the pictures:

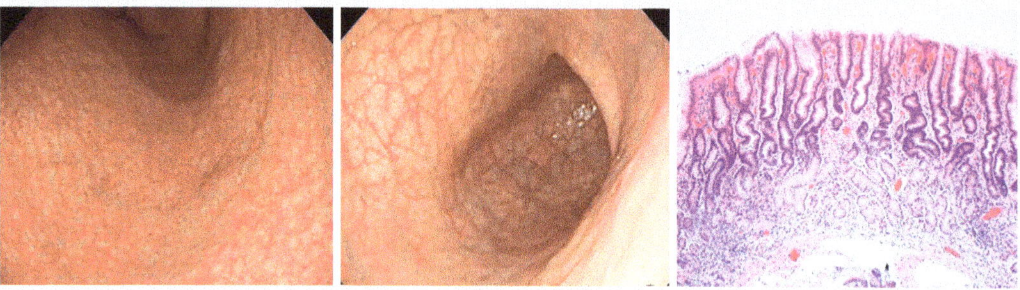

1. **Describe the above pictures.**
2. **What is your diagnosis?**
3. **How can you differentiate this disease from environmental metaplastic gastritis?**
4. **What is the spectrum of *H. pylori* involvement in the stomach mucosa?**

Answers

1. Description of the above pictures:
   a. Endoscopic picture demonstrates patchy smooth mucosa involving the gastric body with few prominent vascularity in the first endoscopic picture and in the second picture there is smooth pale mucosa with more prominent vascularity.
   b. Histological features are:
      - Patchy lymphocytic infiltrate in the lamina propria
      - Destruction of the oxyntic glands along with pseudopyloric metaplasia and replaced by intestinal metaplasia.
2. The diagnosis is chronic atrophic gastritis with metaplasia probably of autoimmune etiology.
3. Autoimmune metaplastic gastritis is autosomal dominant, female-to-male ratio of 3:1 having immune response against oxyntic mucosa leading to atrophy followed by intestinal metaplasia in the gastric body and fundus. This disease is associated with type 1 diabetes mellitus, thyroid disease, and polyglandular endocrine syndrome. This is associated with pernicious anemia and iron-deficiency anemia. Serum demonstrates:
   a. Increased gastrin
   b. Decreased ratio of pepsinogen I/pepsinogen II
   c. Vitamin B_{12} deficiency
   d. Antiparietal cell antibodies
   e. Anti-intrinsic factor antibodies

   Environmental metaplastic atrophic gastritis is caused by external factors like *H. pylori* or diet. This is patchy in distribution. Here, serum gastrin level will be normal, absence of antiparietal cell, and anti-intrinsic factor antibodies.
4. As *H. pylori* is a antrum predominant infection, so in this early phase gastrin secretion will be increased leading to development of duodenal ulcer. But, as the infection progresses, there will be cessation of function of gastrin-producing cells leading to gastric atrophy followed by intestinal metaplasia.

   In the next phase, bacteria migrate to gastric body and fundus leading to development of corpus gastritis followed by gastric ulcer and gastric cancer.

CASE 25

A 68-year-old hypertensive, diabetic, and dyslipidemic patient came to the outpatient department with 6–8 watery, floating, and malodorous bowel movements associated with cramping abdominal pain and bloating for 7 days after returning from a trip in Germany with his friends. His vitals are normal, distended, and tympanic but nontender abdomen and hyperactive bowel sounds. Complete blood count and metabolic profile are normal. Stool culture and ova and parasite count in the stool are pending.

1. **What is your diagnosis?**
2. **What antibiotic should be prescribed?**
3. **What are the causes of this type of diarrhea?**
4. **After 4 weeks, patient again came with similar type of presentation with rectal tenesmus and rectal urgency but no blood. Stool culture for enteric pathogens, ELISA test for** *Clostridium difficile* **is negative but ELISA test for trophozoites are positive. In that case, what investigation you will suggest and why?**

Answers

1. Since the patient was on a trip to Germany for several days and stool is floating and malodorous, the patient has been suffering from *Giardia lamblia*-infected acute diarrhea.
2. The antibiotic prescribed is metronidazole.
3. Other causes of watery but not floating diarrhea are:
   a. *Escherichia coli*
   b. *Vibrio cholerae*
   c. *Staphylococcus aureus*
   d. *Clostridium perfringens*
   e. *Giardia lamblia*
   f. *Cryptosporidium* species

4. I have to perform serum immunoglobulins. Due to infection with *G. lamblia*, immunoglobulin G (IgG) and secretary IgA are produced against the parasite in the body of the host, the latter one prevents the organism from adhering with the epithelial cells in the wall of the intestine. But, if the patient has selective deficiency of IgA, the patient fails to develop IgA-mediated immune response leading to persistence of infection of *Giardia* trophozoites and at the same time it is very difficult to clear with the antibiotics. Hence, in this case since there is relapse of giardia infection, the immunoglobulin level should be assessed.

CASE 26

A 60-year-old nonhypertensive, nondiabetic male was brought to emergency room with progressively increasing difficulty in walking and standing, oropharyngeal dysphagia, retrothoracic burning, and double vision following an episode of loose motion and fever 7 weeks ago lasting for 7 days after taking raw milk and poultry foods. On examination, there is tachypnea, tachycardia, and oxygen saturation at room air of 88%.

1. **What is your diagnosis and why?**
2. **What is the pathogenesis in this disease?**
3. **What is the specific treatment of this disease?**
4. **What are the complications in this disease?**

Answers

1. Past history of fever and diarrhea 7 weeks prior to this present episode indicates that the pathogen is invasive and it leads to development of ascending paralysis and weakness of the eye muscles progressing to respiratory failure which is consistent with Guillain–Barré syndrome. So, the diagnosis is *Campylobacter jejuni*-induced diarrhea leading to this neurological abnormality.
2. The pathogenesis is the molecular mimicry producing autoantibodies against peripheral nerve gangliosides GM1 and GM1a that react also with bacterial polysaccharides.
3. Specific treatment is macrolide antibiotics due to development of progressive resistance of this bacteria against many antibiotics as a result of injudicious and irrelevant use of antibiotics in the firm animals.
4. Following are the complications in this diarrhea:
   a. Guillain–Barré syndrome
   b. Cardiac complications:
      - Myocarditis
      - Pericarditis
   c. Acute oligoarthritis to disabling polyarthritis involving knee, ankles, and small joints
   d. Gastrointestinal manifestations:
      - Gastroesophageal reflux disease
      - Barrett's disease
      - Esophageal adenocarcinoma
      - Immunoproliferative small intestinal disease

CASE 27

A 60-year-old man came to the outpatient department with fever with chills and bloody diarrhea for 2 days following a course of ampicillin for treating chronic otitis media. His white blood cell count is 20,000/cc. Following are the pictures of long colonoscopy and barium enema in this case:

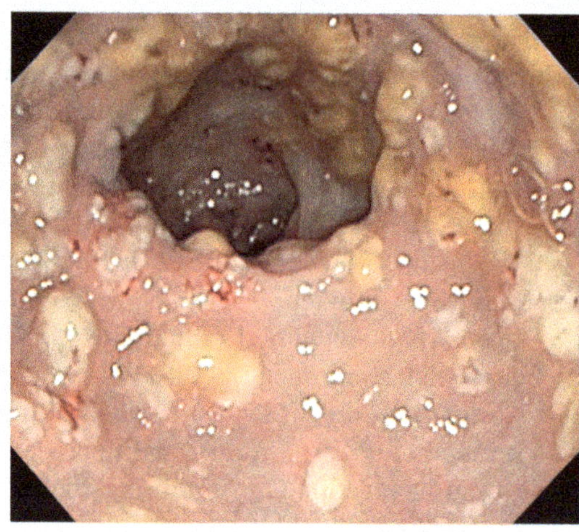 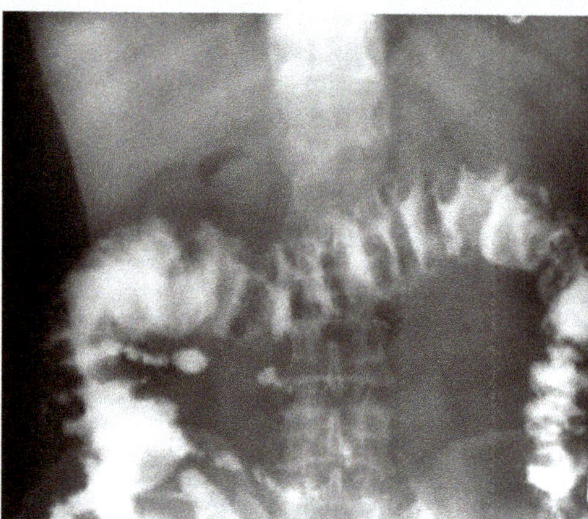

1. **Describe the above pictures.**
2. **What is your diagnosis?**
3. **What is the pathogenesis behind the disease?**
4. **Why the mortality from the disease has been increased recently?**
5. **What are the risk factors for this disease?**
6. **What is volcano lesion?**
7. **How can you treat the disease?**

Answers

1. Description of the above pictures:
   a. Colonoscopy demonstrates raised yellowish plaques having diameter of 2–10 mm distributed over the colonic mucosa in scattered manner.
   b. Barium enema demonstrates serrated appearance of the barium column as a result of trapped barium in-between the edematous mucosal folds and plaques like membrane of pseudomembranous colitis.
2. The diagnosis is pseudomembranous colitis.
3. *Clostridium difficile* bacteria liberate two types of toxins:
   a. Toxin A or enterotoxin
   b. Toxin B or cytotoxin

Both the toxins bind to the specific receptors on the intestinal wall epithelial cells. These receptor-bound toxins catalyze the specific alteration in the Rho protein namely glutamyl transpeptidase-binding protein that assists polymerization of actin and cell movement to enter the cells.

Toxin B induces senescence in the enteric glial cells which help in future development of irritable bowel syndrome (IBS) via persistent inflammation inflammatory bowel disease.

NAP1 hypervirulent strains of *C. difficile* may produce fulminant colitis.

4. Prevalence and the mortality of *C. difficile*-induced diarrhea have increased due to emergence of virulent strain NAP1/027 of this organism as it harbors mutations conferring resistance to the quinolone

antibiotics resulting increased production of both the toxins as well as facilitation of the sporulation of the bacterium.

5. Following are the risk factors in this disease:
   a. Antimicrobial therapy
   b. Increasing age
   c. Hospitalization
   d. Chemotherapy
   e. HIV infection
   f. Inflammatory bowel disease
6. Constellation of the following histological findings in this disease covering the area of ulceration is known as "volcano lesion":
   a. Eruption of inflammatory cells
   b. Necrotic debris
7. Treatment:
   a. Metronidazole 400 mg orally 3–4 times daily for 10–14 days in case of mild-to-moderate colitis.
   b. Vancomycin 125–500 mg orally four times daily for 10–14 days in case of severe colitis or in the following patients:
      - Unable to tolerate metronidazole
      - Pregnant women
      - Children of <10 years of age
      - If the diarrhea cannot be improved by metronidazole.
   c. In case of relapse of this disease:
      - Metronidazole or vancomycin in tapering schedule
      - Probiotics containing *Saccharomyces boulardii* or *Lactobacillus* species with metronidazole or vancomycin
      - Intravenous immunoglobulin
      - Rifampin
      - Cholestyramine with vancomycin and fidaxomicin

CASE 28

A 30-year-old nondiabetic male has been admitted with high fever with chill and drowsiness. On examination, temperature is 102°F, tachycardia, tachypnea, neck rigidity, and positive Kernig sign following history of abdominal pain, fever with chills, and bloody diarrhea 3 weeks back after intake of poultry food and ground beef.

1. **What is your diagnosis and why?**
2. **What is the type of diarrhea in typhoid?**
3. **How can you treat typhoid diarrhea?**
4. **Diarrhea lasts for how long?**

Answers

1. History of bloody diarrhea with fever and chill and rigor suggests invasive nature of the organism. Patients develop evidence of meningitis. The organism which is invasive and at the same time involves nervous system indicates *Salmonella* species. So, the diagnosis in this spectrum of infection is due to *Salmonella* infection.
2. In this diarrhea, stool is green liquid containing polymorphonuclear leukocytes and protein.
3. Typhoid diarrhea can be treated by fluoroquinolone in male and nonpregnant female. Second drug of choice is chloramphenicol.
4. With treatment, diarrhea will be relieved within 3–5 days. Without treatment, the disease will get worse within few weeks leading to development of different types of complications.

CASE 29

A 20-year-old male has been admitted with loose stool 6–8 times per day along with fever, vomiting, and abdominal pain within 10 hours of intake of tropical fish from a hotel. On examination, there is bradycardia, raised temperature, myalgia, arthralgia, perioral paresthesia, pruritus, and hypotension.

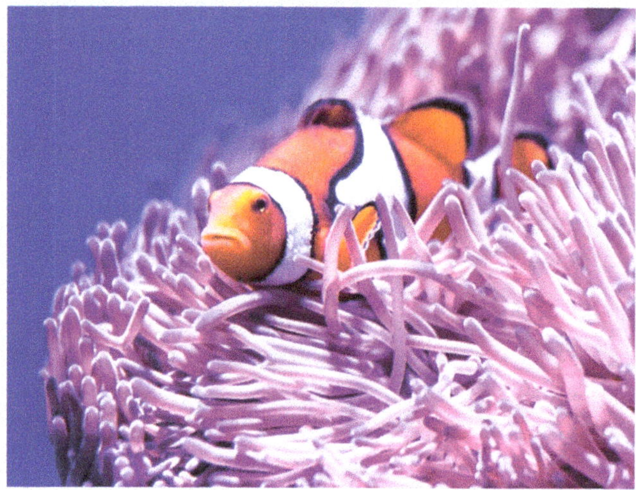

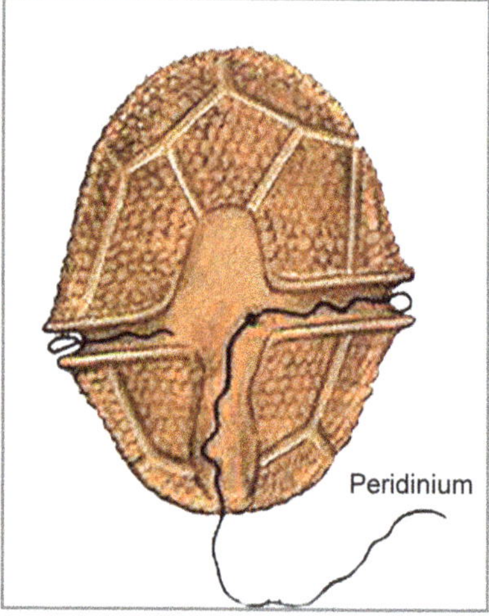

1. **Describe the above pictures and what is the relation with the history of this patient?**
2. **What is your diagnosis?**
3. **Which poison is responsible here and how does it enter into the human body?**
4. **What is the mechanism of its action?**
5. **Which systems are involved by this toxin?**
6. **How can you diagnose this toxin?**
7. **What is the specific treatment?**

Answers

1. This is the picture of tropical fish known as coral reef fish and second one is the picture of dinoflagellates.
2. Diagnosis is sea nonbacterial food-induced food poisoning, the toxin being ciguatera.
3. Poison responsible is ciguatera toxin which is produced by dinoflagellates like *Gambierdiscus toxicus*. It is transferred through the food web as algae which is consumed by herbivorous fish which in turn is consumed by carnivorous fish. When human being will consume this fish, this toxin enters into the human being.
4. This ciguatera toxin activates voltage-gated sodium channels which present in the cell membrane leading to increased permeability to sodium ion thereby depolarizing the nerve cells and resulting in different spectrum of neurologic manifestations.
5. Following systems are involved by this toxin:
   a. Neurological system:
      - Extreme circumoral paresthesia
      - Myalgia
      - Arthralgia
      - Dysesthesia
      - Headache
      - Vertigo
      - Weakness
   b. Gastrointestinal system:
      - Abdominal pain
      - Vomiting
      - Diarrhea
      - Nausea
   c. Cardiovascular system:
      - Bradycardia
      - Arrhythmia
      - Hypertension
   d. Neuropsychiatry:
      - Hallucination
      - Depression
      - Memory concentration problem
      - Giddiness
6. Diagnosis mainly clinical but confirmation can be done by detection of toxin in the contaminated fish.

7. Treatment:
   a. Intravenous mannitol has to be given at a rate of 0.5–1 g/kg of body weight over half an hour and should be given within 48–72 hours of ingestion of the fish. It acts by:
      - Reduction of cerebral edema
      - Scavenging the free radicals which are generated by this toxin

   - Reduction of its action at the sodium/potassium channels
   b. To prevent the hypovolemic shock, a large amount of isotonic fluids is administered.
   c. If required, intravenous pressor agents can be given to increase the pressure after administration of the intravenous fluid.

CASE 30

A 19-year-old male habitual intaker of outside food came to the outpatient department with abdominal pain with fever and bloody diarrhea alternating with constipation. On examination, there is tachycardia and tender left colonic area. His following findings are:

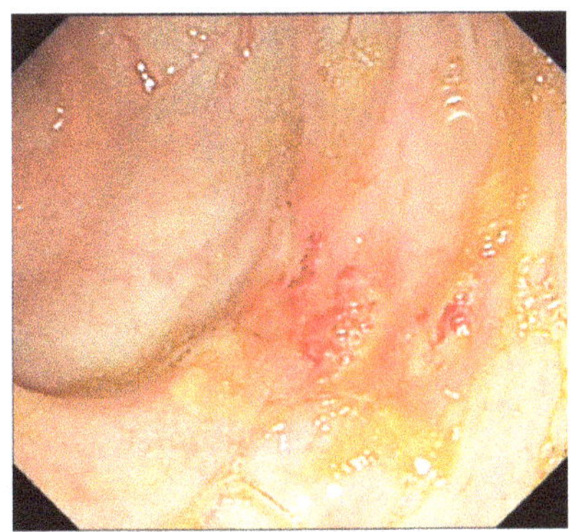 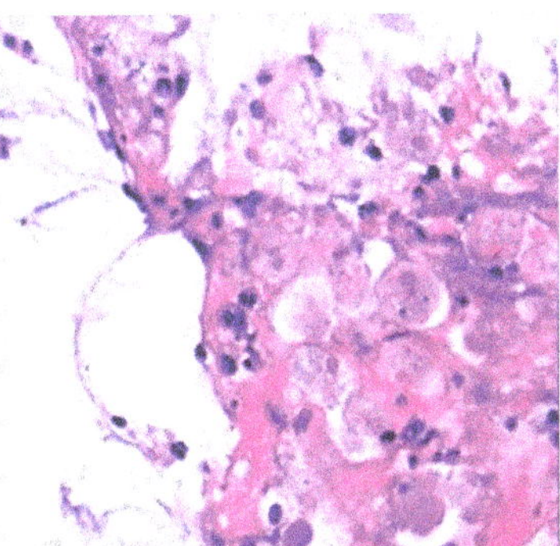 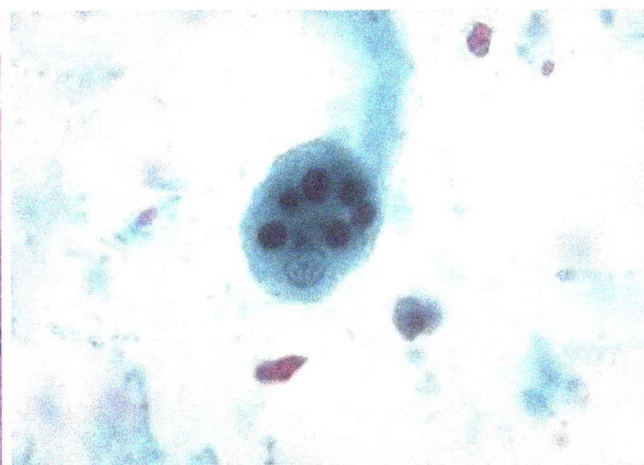

1. **Describe the above pictures.**
2. **What is your diagnosis?**
3. **What are the complications?**

Answers

1. Description of the above pictures:
   a. Colonoscopic features are multiple irregular erosions which are covered with bloody exudates in the cecum.
   b. Histological features are:
      - The presence of superficial ulcers located in the lamina propria
      - Presence of the inflammatory exudates on the surface of the mucosa
      - Exudates is composed of fibrin, inflammatory cells, and necrotic tissue.

2. The diagnosis is amebic ulcer producing acute amebic colitis.

3. Complications of amebic colitis:
   a. Fulminant amebic colitis
   b. Toxic megacolon
   c. Ameboma
   d. Rectovaginal fistula
   e. Perforation of the bowel
   f. Stricture formation
   g. Peritonitis
   h. Gastrointestinal bleeding
   i. Intussusception

CASE 31

A 30-year-old male has been admitted with bloody diarrhea, pain in the right lower quadrant a week after consumption of meat in a hotel.

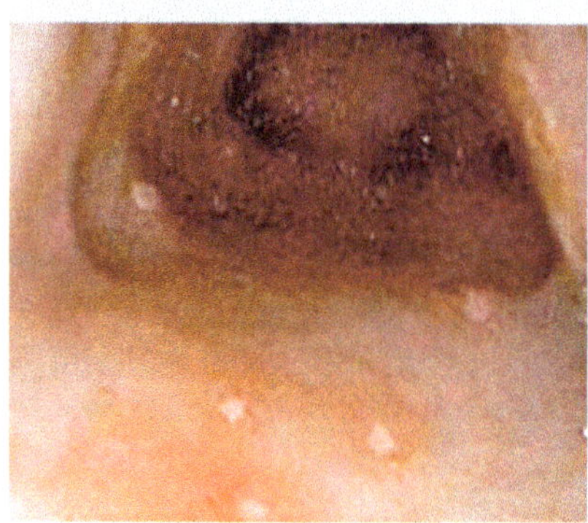 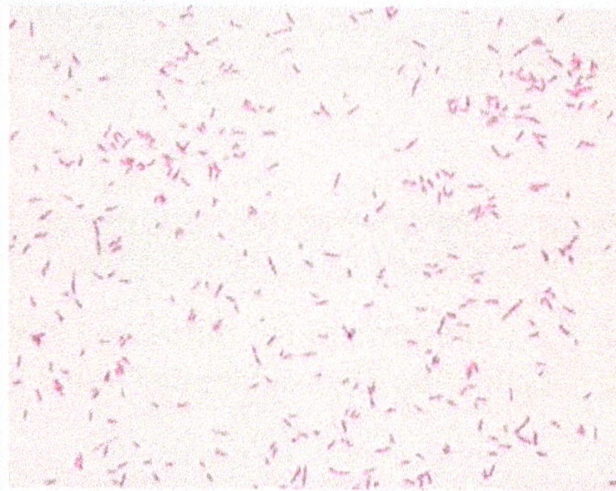 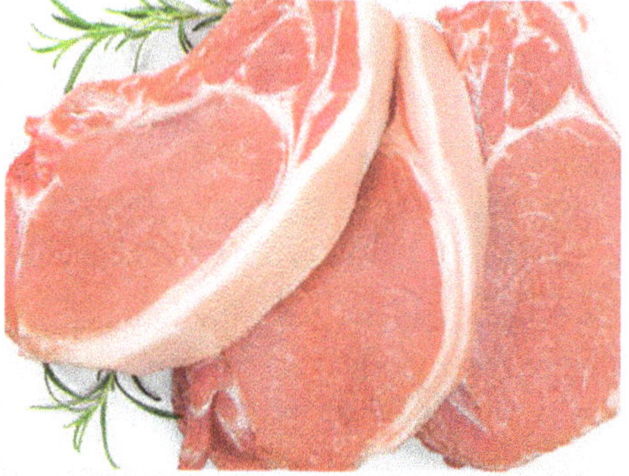

1. **Describe the pictures demonstrated above.**
2. **What is your diagnosis?**
3. **What is the pathogenesis of this disease?**
4. **What are the complications?**
5. **How can you treat the disease?**

Answers

1. Description of the above pictures:
   a. Colonoscopy demonstrates multiple discrete superficial ulcers having bloody exudates seen in the cecal area.
   b. Microscopical picture demonstrates gram-negative bacilli
   c. Third picture demonstrates the flesh of the pork that has been eaten by the patient.
2. The diagnosis is Yersinia enterocolitis.
3. Pathogen enters the small intestine passing through the stomach to localize into the lymphoid tissue as well as mesenteric lymph nodes. In the intestine, they will colonize into the Peyer's patches from where they will spread.
   a. These bacteria produce urease enzyme that will breakdown into ammonia that protects these bacteria from the harsh acidic environment in the stomach cavity.
   b. These bacteria also produce attachment invasion focus and YadA that will:
      - Confer resistance against the complement-mediated opsonization
      - Prevent phagocytosis
   c. These bacteria also contain Yops or *Yersinia* outer membrane proteins that will block the secretion of tumor necrosis factor-α (TNF-α) and interleukin-8 thereby arresting phagocytosis.
   d. Some strains also produce yersiniabactin that will bind with iron in a depleted state thereby allowing the bacteria to thrive and grow. These bacteria will utilize the siderophore of other organism to chelate iron.
4. Complications are:
   a. Gastrointestinal complications:
      - Peritonitis
      - Bowel perforation
      - Diffuse ulcerative ileitis and colitis
      - Intussusception
      - Paralytic ileus
      - Toxic megacolon
      - Cholangitis
      - Mesenteric venous thrombosis
      - Small bowel necrosis
   b. Extraintestinal complications:
      - Hepatic abscess
      - Splenic abscess
      - Renal abscess
      - Lung abscess
      - Septicemia
      - Osteomyelitis
      - Endocarditis
      - Myocarditis

- • Suppurative lymphadenitis
- • Glomerulonephritis
- • Hepatic failure
- • Mycotic aneurysm
5. Treatment:
    a. Drug of choice is:
        - • Trimethoprim-sulfamethoxazole
        - • Aminoglycosides
    b. Other drugs are:
        - • Tetracycline
        - • Quinolones
        - • Cephalosporin
    c. Proper hydration
    d. Nutritional support

CASE 32

A 30-year-old nondiabetic male presented in the casualty department with sudden distention of the abdomen along with pain having prior history of bloody dysentery with mucopurulent stool and tenesmus but without any features of dehydration following intake of outside food.

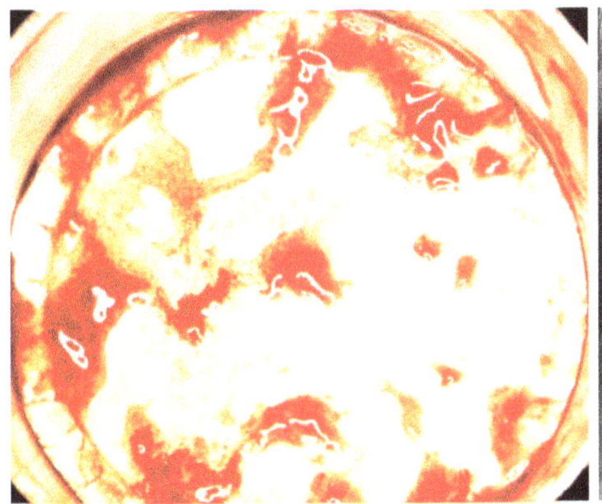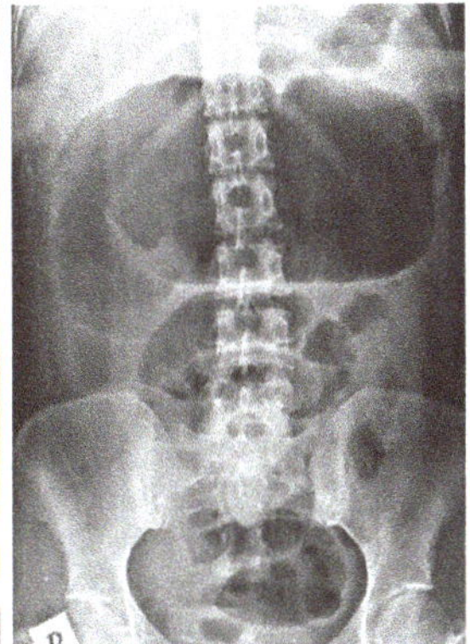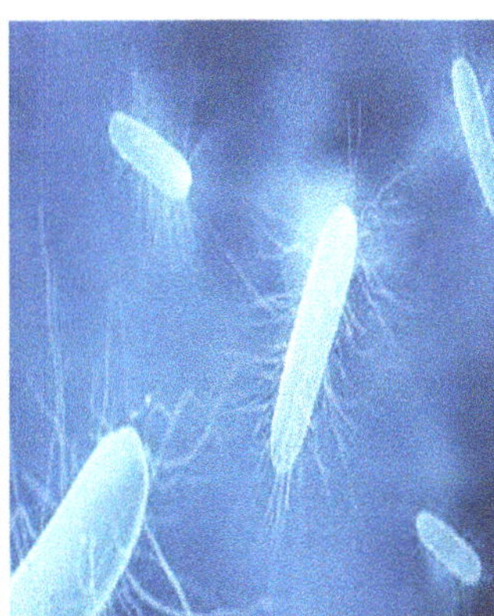

1. **What are the findings?**
2. **What is your diagnosis?**
3. **What are the predisposing factors of the second picture?**
4. **Which species have common genomic sequences of these bacteria?**
5. **What are the major genomic signatures of these bacteria?**
6. **Which age is very vulnerable to complication?**
7. **What are the risk factors in clinically severe cases?**
8. **Name two major complications of this disease.**
9. **What is the "gold standard" method for the diagnosis of this disease?**
10. **What is the major difficulty in this process and how can you overcome it?**

Answers

1. Description of the above pictures:
    a. First picture demonstrates stool with mucus and bright red blood in a pot.
    b. Abdominal X-ray demonstrates:
        - • Greatest distention of the ascending and descending colon along with dilatation of the transverse colon
        - • Loss of haustral pattern
    c. Third picture demonstrates presence of gram-negative bacilli

2. The diagnosis is *Shigella* dysentery with complication like toxic megacolon.

3. Predisposing factors of toxic megacolon are:
    a. Hypokalemia
    b. Use of opioids
    c. Anticholinergic drugs
    d. Loperamide
    e. Psyllium seeds
    f. Antidepressants

4. Following bacteria have common genetic variations:
    a. *E. coli* K-12

b. *Shigella flexneri* 2a
c. *Shigella sonnei*
d. *Shigella dysenteriae* type 1
e. *Shigella boydii*

5. Three moajor genomic signatures are:
   a. 215 kb virulence plasmid carrying most of the genes which is required for the invasive capacity.
   b. Absence of alteration of genetic sequences encoding the products like lysine hydroxylase.
   c. Presence of a gene that encodes the cytotoxin Shiga toxin in *S. dysenteriae*

6. Extremes of age like children of <5 years old and elderly patients are vulnerable to complications.

7. Risk factors for clinically severe cases:
   a. Nonbloody diarrhea
   b. Moderate-to-severe dehydration
   c. Bacteremia in HIV patients and severely malnourished patients
   d. Absence of fever
   e. Abdominal tenderness
   f. Rectal prolapse

8. Two major complications of this disease are:
   a. Toxic megacolon
   b. Hemolytic uremic syndrome

9. Gold standard methods of diagnosis are isolation and identification of the bacteria from the fecal material.

10. In absence of any nearby laboratory facility, the bacteria will be diagnosed as these are very fragile due to rapid change in temperature and pH. It can be overcome by carrying these materials in the buffered glycerol saline or Cary-Blair medium as these are the holding medium.

CASE 33

A 35-year-old HIV-infected woman presented in emergency department with recurrent seizures and headache with signs of cerebellar involvement following an episode of fever, headache, and diarrhea 2 days after intake of underprocessed foods of animal and hot dogs. On examination, there is tachycardia, mild neck rigidity, and altered mental status. Her cerebrospinal fluid (CSF) demonstrated white blood cell count of 3,200/cc with modest neutrophilic predominance, low glucose, and Gram stain demonstrated the following feature and MRI brain showed also following features:

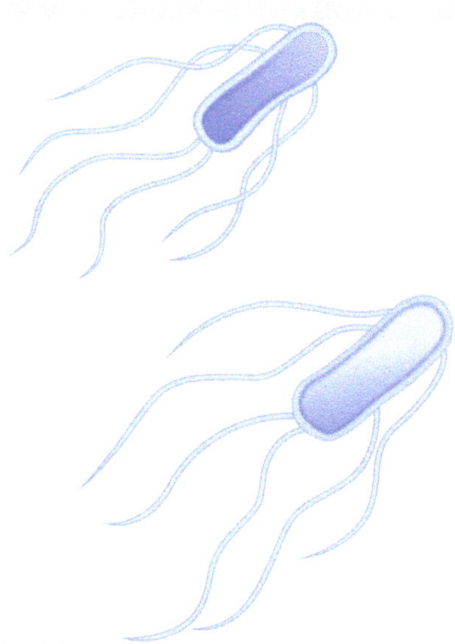

1. **What are your findings?**
2. **What is your diagnosis?**
3. **What are the serotypes in this organism, and human beings are susceptible to which serotypes?**
4. **Which group of patients are at high risk?**
5. **What are the common complications occurring in pregnant women?**
6. **What is granulomatosis infantiseptica?**

Answers

1. The picture demonstrated short gram-positive anaerobic motile bacilli.
2. Patient is suffering from listeriosis.
3. Serotypes are based on the somatic as well as flagellar antigens. Human beings are susceptible to:
   a. Serotype 1/2a
   b. Serotype 1/2b
   c. Serotype 4b
4. Following groups of patients are at high risk:
   a. Older adults—these patients are at increasing risk in each decade over 59 years of age.
   b. Patients with impaired cellular immunity
   c. Patients with hematologic malignancy
   d. Bone marrow transplants
   e. Receipt of glucocorticoids or immunosuppressive drugs
5. Following complications occur in pregnant women:
   a. Fetal loss
   b. Premature birth
   c. Abnormal delivery at term like increased heart rate or meconium staining of the amniotic fluid
6. Granulomatosis infantiseptica is characterized by disseminated microabscesses as well as granuloma present in the skin, spleen, and liver as a result of severe uterine infection from *Listeria monocytogenes*. In this condition, the infant may be stillborn or die soon after birth.

CASE 34

A 28-year-old man, villager of Bihar, came to the outpatient department with recurrent nonbloody diarrhea with abdominal cramping and arthralgia. On examination, patient is anemic and has tender periumbilical region. His endoscopy followed by chromoendoscopy was done and biopsy was taken from the duodenal wall.

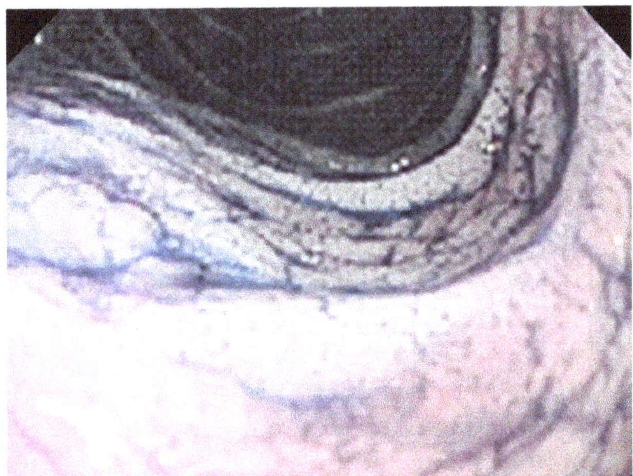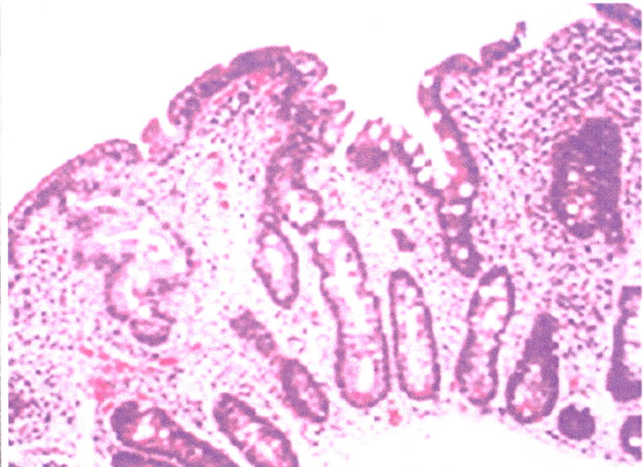

Serum demonstrated vitamin D3 is 9 IU, serum iron is 15 mg/cc, and serum calcium is 8 mg/cc.

Left hand picture demonstrated conventional EGD + chromoendoscopy (0.5% indigo carmine) demonstrates atrophic foci and mosaic patterns. Right hand picture demonstrated slide stained with HE (40x): duodenal mucosa with poorly distinguishable villi, crypt hyperplasia and lymphocytosis.

1. **Describe the above pictures.**
2. **What is your diagnosis?**
3. **What human leukocyte antigen (HLA) alleles whose absence excludes this disease?**
4. **What are the serological investigations to be done and which antigen is responsible?**
5. **What is the mechanism of diarrhea?**
6. **What are the other associated diseases occurring in this disease?**

Answers

1. Description of the above pictures:
   a. Endoscopy along with chromoendoscopy demonstrated atrophic foci and mosaic pattern of mucosa.
   b. Histology from the duodenal mucosa demonstrated:
      - Poorly distinguishable villi, i.e. blunting of the villi
      - Cryptic hyperplasia
      - Lymphocytosis
2. The diagnosis is adult celiac disease.
3. Absence of the following alleles excludes the celiac disease:
   a. HLA-DQ2
   b. HLA-DQ8
4. The antibodies are:
   a. Tissue transaminase antibody IgA
   b. Antiendomysial antibody IgG
   c. Deamidated antigliadin antibody IgG
   d. In case of IgA deficient patient, antigliadin antibodies IgG and tissue transglutaminase IgG antibodies
5. Mechanism of diarrhea:
   a. Steatorrhea due to villus atrophy in the proximal part of the small intestine
   b. Lactase deficiency
   c. Cryptic hyperplasia leading to secretary diarrhea
   d. Hypersecretion of the fluid from the cryptic epithelium
6. Associated diseases are:
   a. Type 1 diabetes mellitus
   b. Autoimmune thyroid disease
   c. Dermatitis herpetiformis
   d. Down syndrome
   e. Turner syndrome

CASE 35

A 60-year-old nondiabetic, nonsmoker male started hematemesis 2 hours ago while he was working at computer. He vomited nearly 2 cups of bright red blood and passed black tarry stool twice. He has been on NSAID to get relief of pain from osteoarthritis. He has a habit of taking eight beers daily. On examination, he had orthostatic hypertension, tachycardia, SpO_2 94% at room air. Abdomen is tender and soft, splenic tip is palpable, and free fluid is present. Rectal examination demonstrated maroon-colored stool. Laboratory examination revealed WBC count of 7,200/cc, hemoglobin of 9 g/dL, platelet count of 100,000/cc, and liver and renal function tests were normal.

1. **What are the differential diagnoses with pathologic factors?**
2. **Describe Rockall score.**
3. **What are the endoscopic predictors of rebleeding?**
4. **Which medications should be given to this patient for acute treatment prior to endoscopy?**
5. **What are the endoscopic methods of treatment of upper gastrointestinal bleeding?**

Answers

1. Differential diagnoses are:
   a. Peptic ulcer disease:
      - NSAIDs
      - *Helicobacter pylori* infection
      - Cushing ulcer
      - Curling ulcer
   b. Erosive esophagitis:
      - Gastroesophageal reflux disease
      - Alcohol
      - NSAIDs
      - Radiation
      - Infection
   c. Esophageal varices:
      - Chronic liver disease
      - Splenic vein thrombosis
   d. Gastric varices:
      - Chronic liver disease
      - Splenic vein thrombosis
   e. Mallory–Weiss syndrome:
      - Retching
      - Coughing
      - Heavy ingestion of alcohol
   f. Vascular malformation:
      - Angiodysplasia
      - Dieulafoy's lesion
      - Portal hypertensive gastropathy
      - Gastric antral vascular ectasia (GAVE)
      - Rendu–Osler–Weber disease

g. Neoplasm:
  - Smoking
  - Family history of gastric cancer
  - *Helicobacter pylori* infection

2. Rockall score:

Variable	Score 0	Score 1	Score 2	Score 3
Age	<60 years	60–90 years	>80 years	Renal failure Or Liver failure
Shock		Pulse is >100 beats/min Systolic blood pressure of >100 mm Hg.	Pulse is >100 beats/min Systolic blood pressure of <100 mm Hg.	
Comorbidity				
Diagnosis	Mallory–Weiss tear	Rest of the differential diagnoses	Malignancy	
Stigmata of recent hemorrhage	None		Blood Visible vessels	

3. Following are the endoscopic score of rebleeding:

Endoscopic findings	Risk of rebleeding	Treatment
Arterial spurting	90%	Proton pump inhibitor + Endoscopic hemostasis
Nonbleeding visible vessel	50%	Proton pump inhibitor + Endoscopic hemostasis

Continued

Continued

Endoscopic findings	Risk of rebleeding	Treatment
Adherent clot	25–30%	Proton pump inhibitor ± Endoscopic hemostasis
Oozing without visible vessels	10–20%	Proton pump inhibitor ± Endoscopic hemostasis
Pigmented clot	7–10%	Proton pump inhibitor
Clean-based ulcer	3–5%	Proton pump inhibitor

4. Patient should be resuscitated with intravenous fluid through the large-bore intravenous lines with continuous administration of PPI in case of peptic ulcer and in case of suspected varices intravenous octreotide.

5. Following are the methods of endoscopic treatment of upper gastrointestinal bleeding:
   a. In case esophageal varices:
      - Sclerotherapy
      - Band ligation
   b. Gastric varices: Intravariceal glue
   c. Peptic ulcer bleeding can be treated by:
      - Bipolar cautery
      - Heater probe cautery
      - Argon plasma coagulation
      - Endoscopic clip
      - Injection therapy

CASE 36

A 27-year-old man went to casualty department with several episodes of bleeding per rectum following cramping abdominal pain on the day of completing marathon race which ceased automatically. His blood pressure was 95/50 mm Hg with tachycardia. Laboratory results demonstrated hemoglobin level of 15 g/dL and other tests are normal.

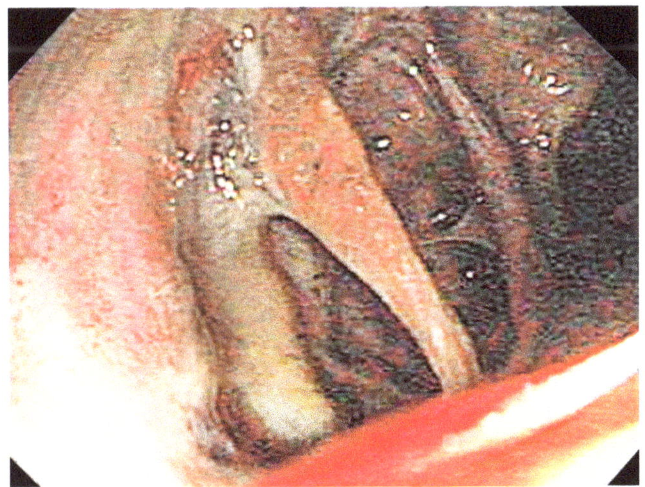

1. **What is your diagnosis and why?**
2. **Which areas are the most vulnerable points of ischemia in acute cases?**
3. **What are the protective factors for preventing this disease?**
4. **What should be the radiological investigation in this case?**
5. **What are the typical features of acute disease?**
6. **How can you treat this case?**

Answers

1. This patient developed acute cramping abdominal pain and bleeding per rectum following marathon race. So, in this case, there may be severe dehydration leading to severe vascular insufficiency. There may be associated vasoconstriction in the mesenteric vessels. So, the diagnosis is acute vascular insufficiency of the mesenteric vessels.

2. Intestine is supplied by celiac artery, superior mesenteric artery, and inferior mesenteric arteries with extensive collateralization within these vessels and major arcades. Within the colon, collateral vessels meet in the two areas:
   a. At the splenic flexure
   b. Descending or sigmoid colon

   So, these areas are vulnerable to decrease in the blood flow leading to acute ischemia. Hence, these points are known as Griffith's point and Sudeck's point respectively.

3. Protective factors to prevent acute intestinal ischemia are:
   a. Abundant collateralization
   b. Autoregulation of blood flow
   c. Increased extraction of oxygen from the blood

4. Following radiological investigations should be done to detect the acute intestinal ischemia:
   a. Duplex ultrasound has high sensitivity and high specificity. It can demonstrate high peak velocity of flow in the superior mesenteric artery which indicates severe bowel ischemia.
   b. Magnetic resonance angiography

5. Following are the acute features of the disease:
   a. Nausea
   b. Vomiting
   c. Cramping abdominal pain
   d. Recurrent urge to defecate
   e. Bleeding per rectum
   f. Normal common imaging studies

6. Since this case is acute and if not properly and timely treated, it may lead to cardiovascular collapse. Methods of treatment include:
   a. Moist oxygen administration
   b. Hemodynamic stability
   c. Correction of electrolyte abnormalities
   d. Administration of blood and blood products
   e. Avoidance of vasopressors
   f. Administration of broad-spectrum antibiotics with administration of probiotics and prebiotics

CASE 37

A 24-year-old man has been admitted with 6–8 eight episodes of diarrhea occasionally mixed with stool, low-grade fever, and cramping abdominal pain for the last 6 months with history of tenesmus. He lost nearly 8 kg weight within this period. On physical examination, blood pressure is 120/85 mm Hg, pulse rate 80 beats/minute, and temperature 100°F. Laboratory results demonstrated hemoglobin of 7 g%, mean corpuscular volume (MCV) of 65 fl, WBC of 14,000/cc, and rest of the laboratory tests were normal. His endoscopic feature was as given below:

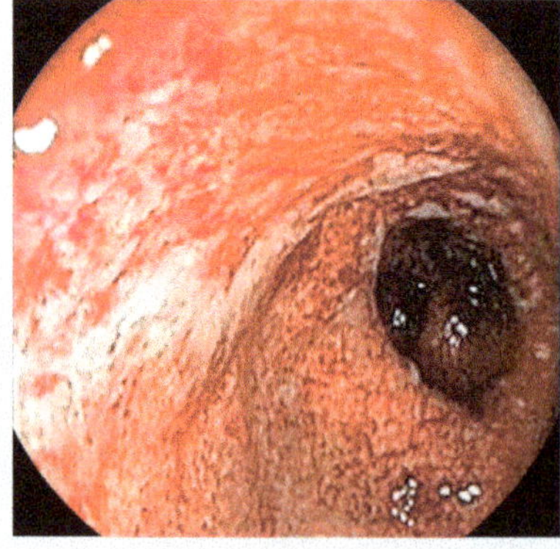
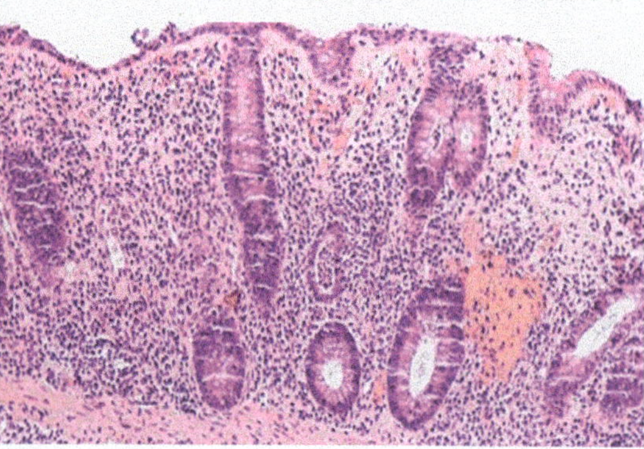

1. **What are the features in the colonoscopy?**
2. **What are the histologic features in the picture?**
3. **What is your diagnosis?**
4. **From the history can you guess the extent of colonic involvement?**
5. **What are the specific tests in the stool that should be used in this disease?**

Answers

1. Features in the above colonoscopy are:
   a. Marked erythema involving whole colonic mucosa.
   b. Mucosal friability
   c. Intervening mucosa is not normal.
   d. Presence of exudation on the surface of the mucosa
2. Histologic features in the above picture are:
   a. Inflammation is limited to mucosa and submucosa.
   b. Distorted cryptic architecture of the colonic mucosa
   c. Crypts are bifid and numbers are decreased.
   d. Gap inbetween the crypts and muscularis mucosae is increased.
   e. Congestion of the mucosal vessels
   f. Mucosal edema
   g. Infiltration with the inflammatory cells and focal hemorrhage
3. The diagnosis is acute extensive ulcerative colitis.
4. This is extensive and severe ulcerative colitis because:
   a. Whole colon is involved.
   b. Stool is liquid in nature and mixed with blood, whereas in case of proctitis only the stool may not be hard having streak of blood on its surface.
   c. Cramping abdominal pain which is not usually present.
   d. Presence of tenesmus suggests involvement of rectum
5. Following tests should be performed in the stool:
   a. Intestinal inflammation can be detected by fecal lactoferrin present in the activated neutrophil.
   b. Fecal calprotectin present in the monocytes and neutrophil correlates with:
      - Histological inflammation
      - Predict the relapse
      - Detect pouchitis

CASE 38

A 52-year-old man has been admitted with recurrent bloody diarrhea for >5 years and a dermatological manifestation on the feet for >6 years. As the patient has been suffering from depression and taking antidepressive, but suddenly developed acute distention of the abdomen along with increasing pain all over the abdomen.

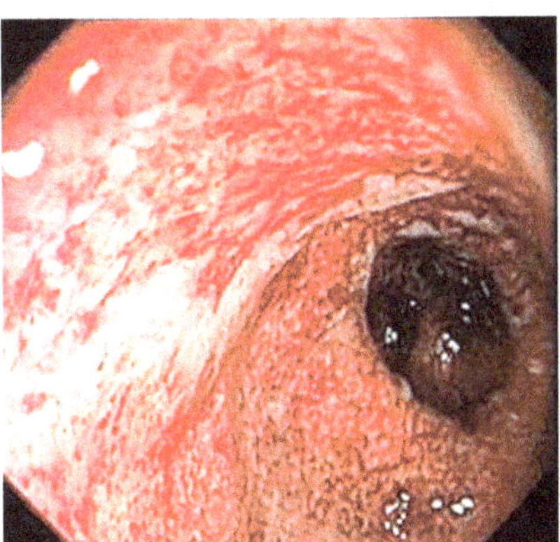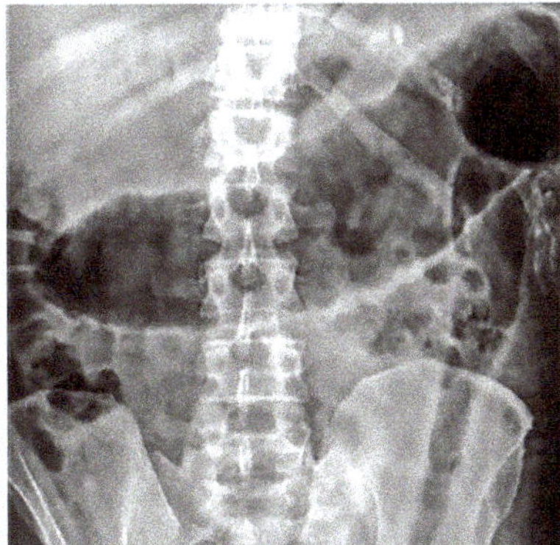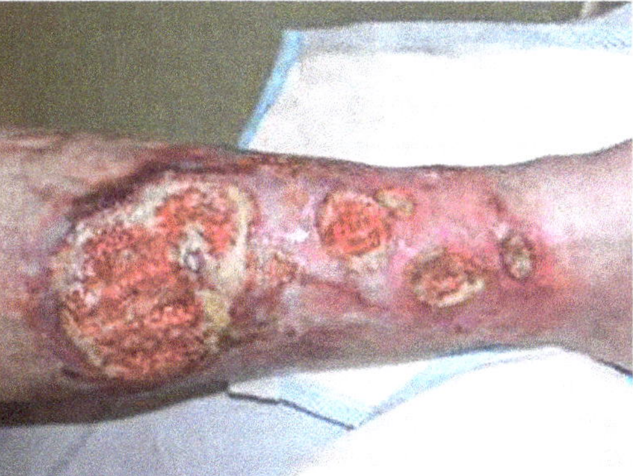

1. **Describe the above pictures.**
2. **What is your diagnosis?**
3. **Name 9 complications of this disease.**

Answers

1. Description of the above pictures:
   a. Features in the above colonoscopy are:
      - Marked erythema involving whole colonic mucosa
      - Mucosal friability
      - Intervening mucosa is not normal.
      - Presence of exudation on the surface of the mucosa
   b. Straight X-ray of abdomen demonstrates:
      - Dilated transverse colon of >10 cm in diameter
      - Surface border is shaggy.
      - Loss of haustra pattern
      - Presence of thumbprinting
   c. Dermatological feature includes:
      - There is presence of multiple ulcers on the shin bone.
      - Superior edge of the proximal ulcer has characteristic purple edge.
2. The diagnosis is ulcerative colitis with toxic mega-colon and extraintestinal manifestation in the form of pyoderma gangrenosum.
3. Extraintestinal manifestations of the ulcerative colitis:
   a. Rheumatologic disorders:
      - Peripheral arthritis
      - Sacroiliitis
      - Ankylosing spondylitis
   b. Metabolic bone disorders:
      - Osteoporosis
      - Osteonecrosis
   c. Dermatological disorders:
      - Erythema nodosum
      - Pyoderma gangrenosum
      - Psoriasis
      - Pyoderma vegetans
      - Sweet syndrome
      - Aphthous stomatitis
   d. Ocular disorders:
      - Uveitis
      - Episcleritis
   e. Hepatobiliary disorders:
      - Fatty liver
      - Cholelithiasis
      - Primary sclerosing cholangitis
   f. Urologic: Nephrolithiasis
   g. Hematological: Thromboembolic disorders
   h. Cardiorespiratory diseases:
      - Endocarditis
      - Myocarditis
      - Pleuropericarditis
      - Interstitial lung disease
   i. Others:
      - Pancreatitis
      - Systemic amyloidosis

CASE 39

A 64-year-old man came to outpatient department with progressive dysphagia to solid and assessed according to the WHO performance status I. Upper endoscopy demonstrates probably malignant tumor seen within the lower esophageal mucosa 22 cm distant from esophagus. Computerized tomography of the chest demonstrated the presence of 4 cm tumor localized in the upper thoracic esophagus without any evidence of distant metastasis.

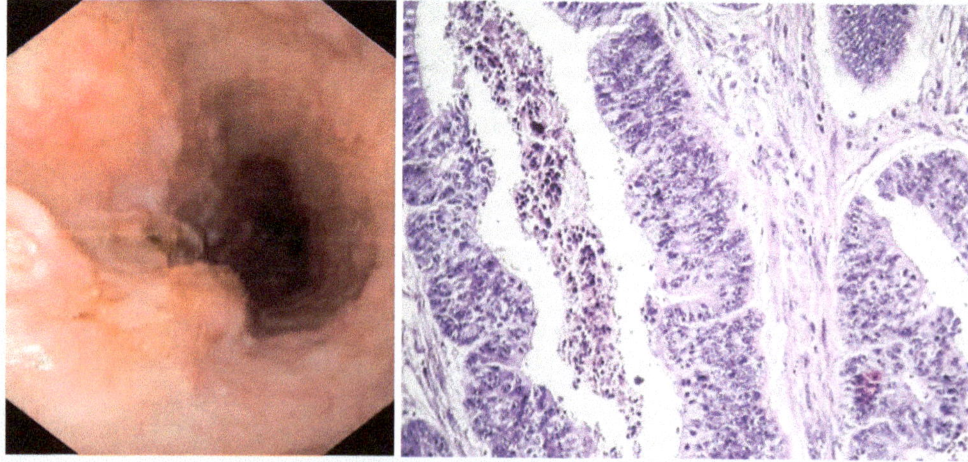

1. **What are the investigations that should be done in this patient and show the reasons?**
2. **Mention the staging of esophageal cancer.**
3. **How can you classify esophageal cancer histologically?**

Answers

1. Following investigations should be done:
   a. PET-CT: It is recommended in case of resectable esophageal cancer to exclude any distant metastasis.
   b. Endoscopic ultrasonography of the esophagus to stage the tumor, hence it is recommended.
   c. Since the tumor is present above the level of carina, i.e., <25 cm from carina. Tracheobronchoscopy is recommended for excluding tracheal invasion according to the European Society for Medical Oncology.
2. Staging of esophageal carcinoma:
   TNM classification of esophageal cancer:

T-status	
Tis	High-grade dysplasia
T1	Invasion of lamina propria, muscularis mucosae, or submucosa
T2	Invasion of muscularis propria
T3	Invasion to adventitia

Continued

Continued

T-status	
T4a	Invasion to resectable adjacent structure (pleura, pericardium, and diaphragm)
T4b	Invasion to unresectable adjacent structure (aorta, trachea, and vertebral body)
N-status	
N0	No regional lymph node metastasis
N1	1–2 positive regional lymph node
N2	3–6 positive regional lymph node
N3	7 or more positive regional lymph node
M-status	
M0	No distant metastasis
M1	Distant metastasis

3. Histological classification:

G1	Well differentiated
G2	Moderately differentiated
G3	Poorly differentiated
G4	Undifferentiated

CASE 40

A 72-year-old smoker with mild chronic obstructive pulmonary disease (COPD) on inhaler presented with progressive dysphagia. Upper gastrointestinal endoscopy demonstrated 40 mm carcinoma at 36 cm from the incisor tooth but not bordering the gastroesophageal (GE) junction. Endoscopic ultrasound demonstrated the invasion of the tumor to lamina propria, but not to submucosa. There was no lymphadenopathy. Whole body PET-CT demonstrated absence of lymphadenopathy and distant metastasis.

1. **What is the staging of esophageal cancer?**
2. **Describe the T-status in tumor staging.**
3. **Which treatment is suitable in this case?**
4. **What do you mean by limited esophageal cancer?**
5. **Is there any role of radiofrequency ablation in this disease?**

Answers

1. As this cancer invades lamina propria, there is absence of lymphadenopathy or distant metastases, the stage of esophageal cancer is T1a, N0, and M0.
2. Tumor staging:
   a. T1: Tumor invades to lamina propria or submucosa
   b. T1a: Tumor invades mucosa, submucosa, or lamina propria
   c. T1b: Tumor invades submucosa
   d. T2: Tumor invades muscularis mucosae
3. As there is no distant metastasis or lymphadenopathy, endoscopic submucosal or endoscopic mucosal resection of the tumor is the method of treatment.

4. Limited esophageal cancer can be defined as the invasion of the tumor restricted up to muscularis propria in absence of distant metastases or any lymphadenopathy.

5. As this tumor is resectable and no evidence of spread, radiofrequency ablation has no role in this disease.

CASE 41

A 72-year-old patient presented with a stent within the esophagus to relieve from dysphagia as he was diagnosed as suffering from metastatic adenocarcinoma of esophagus. But, he requested the doctor to resect the tumor as he had been suffering from retrosternal pain.

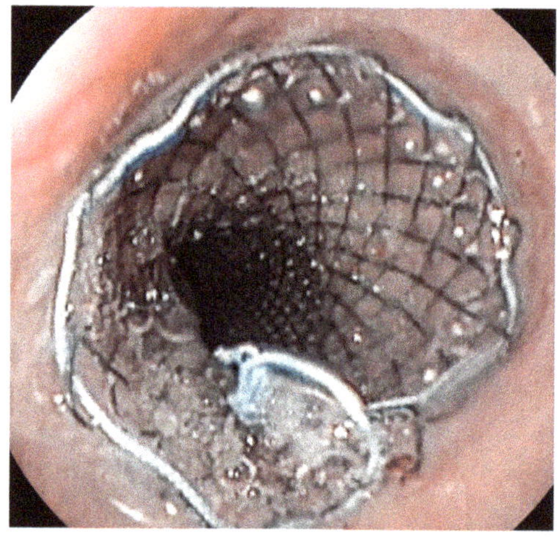

1. **Which stent is demonstrated here?**
2. **What are the modalities of therapy that are effective here?**

Answers

1. The stent here is self-expandable metal stent which is introduced in the esophageal cavity.
2. The proper therapy to be given here is the combination of:
   a. Self-expandable metallic stent: It is introduced into the esophagus to relieve dysphagia; but, it may produce chest discomfort.
   b. Brachytherapy: It is a type of intraluminal radiotherapy in which radioactive source will be placed within the esophageal cavity thereby delivering the proper dose of radiation minimizing the adverse side effects; as a result dysphagia can be relieved further.
   c. Chemotherapy: It is given as palliative therapy in this case having good performance status, but it has little role in squamous cell carcinoma of esophagus.

CASE 42

A 45-year-old man having chronic cough, hoarseness of voice underwent upper gastrointestinal endoscopy which demonstrated salmon-colored patch at the upper end of esophagus 16 cm from the incisors. ENT checkup demonstrated inflamed laryngeal fold.

1. **What is cervical inlet patch?**
2. **How is it formed?**
3. **What are the treatment protocols in this patient?**
4. **Is there any chance of malignancy in this area?**

Answers

1. Cervical inlet patch is a congenital condition where the heterotopic gastric mucosa is formed in the upper esophagus.
2. As a result of incomplete embryonic transformation of the esophageal mucosa from columnar to squamous epithelium. Mainly fundic mucosa is seen histologically which leads to increased production of acids resulting spectrum of symptoms.
3. Therapies are:
   a. Proton pump inhibitors
   b. Different endoscopic approaches:
      - Argon plasma coagulation
      - Endoscopic resection of the heterotopic mucosa
      - Radiofrequency ablation
4. Yes, there is chance of squamous cell carcinoma at this area.

CASE 43

A 65-year-old man underwent reviewed upper gastrointestinal endoscopy for surveillance of Barrett's esophagus.

1. **Histologically which mucosa supports Barrett's esophagus without dysplasia?**
2. **After 1 year, surveillance endoscopy demonstrated evidence of intestinal metaplasia without dysplasia histologically. When should the next surveillance endoscopy be done?**
3. **After 3 years, repeat endoscopy demonstrated low-grade dysplasia in the two out of four sections. How can it be managed?**
4. **After 6 months, again surveillance endoscopy was done and there was evidence of high-grade dysplasia. What should be the next approach?**

Answers

1. Histologically, metaplastic columnar epithelial cells of intestine are confirmed 1 cm above the gastroesophageal junction. The pathognomonic of Barrett's esophagus is multilayered epithelium and diagnosis is confirmed by the islands of squamous epithelium.
2. In case of nondysplastic Barrett's esophagus, progression to malignancy is 0.3% yearly, but it is much more in case of any grade of dysplasia. Repeat surveillance depends upon the length of Barrett's esophagus. Repeat endoscopy is done if the length is >3 cm and if it is <3 cm repeat surveillance endoscopy should be done within 3–5 years.
3. Radiofrequency ablative therapy should be offered. In case of visible dysplastic lesion, it can be removed by endoscopic mucosal resection.
4. Endoscopic resection of the dysplastic mucosa should be staged for planning the next therapy. Other methods like "cap and snare" or band ligation can be done to resect the visible lesions. As all the visible lesions are resected then radiofrequency ablation should be done in the residual Barrett's epithelium.

CASE 44

A 60-year-old male presented with 3 years history of progressive dysphagia to both solid and liquid and retrosternal discomfort. As his upper gastrointestinal endoscopy was normal, high-resolution manometry of esophagus was performed. It showed:

Integrated relaxation pressure of 30 mm Hg (normal is <15 mm Hg) and distal contractile integral (DCI) is 90 (normal being 450–8,000). Since DCI is >450, distal latency is not necessary.

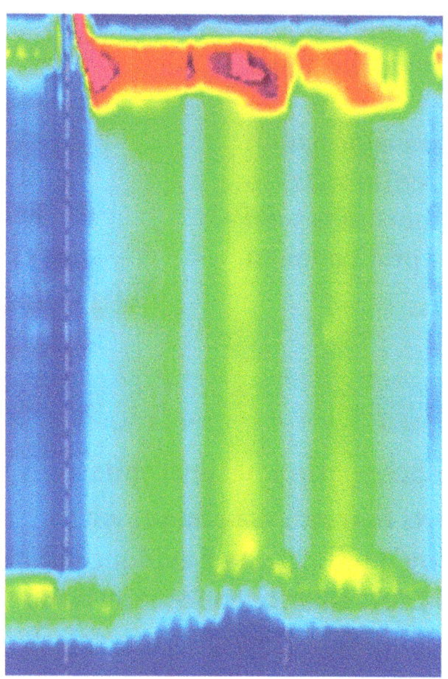

1. **What is your diagnosis?**
2. **What does "abnormally elevated integral relaxation pressure" indicate?**
3. **What are the cardinal features in this disease?**
4. **Classify this disease.**
5. **Why it is not pseudoachalasia?**

Answers

1. The diagnosis is type II achalasia cardia.
2. Abnormally increased integral relaxation pressure indicates failure of relaxation of lower esophageal sphincter.
3. The cardinal features of this disease are:
   a. Loss of normal peristalsis
   b. Elevated pressure of the lower esophageal sphincter
4. Classification of achalasia:

Subtypes of achalasia	Distinguishing features
Classical achalasia	Esophageal pressure is <30 mm Hg (dark blue)
	No panesophageal pressure

Continued

Continued

Subtypes of achalasia	Distinguishing features
Type II (with esophageal compression) achalasia	Panesophageal pressurization is >20% swallows (green color)
Type III achalasia (spastic)	>20% of swallows with premature contraction along with distal contractile integral of >450

5. Pseudoachalasia is less likely because of the following reasons:
   a. Long duration of symptoms
   b. Age is <50 years.
   c. Normal endoscopic appearances
   d. Normal integrated relaxation pressure

CASE 45

A 40-year-old psychiatric patient was admitted in the hospital within 5 hours of ingestion of cylindrical battery, two coins, and scalpel blade.

How can you retrieve the foreign body?

Answer

Foreign body can be retrieved by:

a. Within 2–6 hours, endoscopy should be done to retrieve sharp object and battery.

b. Within 24 hours, urgent endoscopy should be done in case of ingestion of risky object in the stomach.

c. Overtube which should be used in case of sharp object ingested because that may damage the esophageal mucosa during retrieval.

CASE 46

A 30-year-old man came to outpatient department with flatulent dyspepsia refractory to omeprazole and metronidazole. Upper gastrointestinal endoscopy was performed while he is on medication and it demonstrated multiple duodenal ulcers in the duodenal bulb and *H. pylori* test was negative. Serum gastrin is 88 pmol/L, C-reactive protein (CRP) is 8 mg/dL, and hemoglobin is 13 g%.

1. **What are the differential diagnoses?**
2. **Which is the most likely diagnosis?**
3. **Is there any association of negative urease test with PPI?**
4. **What are the features of Zollinger–Ellison (ZE) syndrome?**
5. **What are the infections in HIV disease producing refractory ulcers?**

Answers

1. Following are the differential diagnoses:
   a. *Helicobacter pylori* infection
   b. Peptic ulcer disease
   c. ZE syndrome
   d. HIV infection leading to secondary infection producing gastritis
   e. Crohn's ulcer
2. The most likely diagnosis is *H. pylori*-related duodenal ulcer.
3. Proton pump inhibitor compromises the urease test leading to negative urease test. So in spite of *H. pylori* infection, urease test will be negative. Hence, this PPI should be stopped at least for 2 weeks prior to this test.
4. This is not a case of ZE syndrome as the classical features of this syndrome are:
   a. Diarrhea
   b. Ulcer should be present in the second part of the duodenum.
   c. Severe ulceration which is resistant to PPI.
   d. Absence of intake of NSAIDs intake
   e. Large gastric folds
   f. Fasting gastrin level is >1,000 pg/mL.
5. Following infections leading to production of ulcers refractory to treatment:
   a. *Cytomegalovirus*
   b. Herpes simplex virus

CASE 47

A 40-year-old smoker obese male came in outpatient department with flatulent dyspepsia in spite of two courses of anti-*H. pylori* treatment.

1. **What are the factors producing resistance to the treatment?**
2. **What are the factors responsible for treatment failure?**
3. **What are the virulence factors present in *H. pylori*?**
4. **In case of high metabolic index, which is responsible for treatment failure?**
5. **Which host genetic factor is responsible for treatment success?**

Answers

1. Following factors are responsible for resistance to the treatment:
   a. Primary treatment failure occurring in 20% of patients.
   b. Smokers
   c. High basal metabolic index
2. Following factors responsible for treatment failure:
   a. Host genetic factor
   b. *Helicobacter pylori* virulence factor
   c. Antimicrobial resistance
   d. Compliance with therapy
   e. Duration of therapy
3. Two factors are present in *H. pylori*:
   a. CagA protein
   b. VacA toxin
4. In case of high metabolic index, reduced bioavailability is responsible for treatment failure.
5. Interleukin-1β-511 T/T genotype and failure with C/C and C/T genotypes.

CASE 48

A 65-year-old nonsmoker male having Billroth I gastrectomy 19 years ago came to gastroenterology clinic with severe weakness and on examination he was found to be anemic.

1. **What are the causes of this anemia in this patient?**
2. **How do the above deficiencies occur?**
3. **What are the types of operation that should be done in ulcers in different sites?**

Answers

1. Following are the causes of anemia:
   a. Iron
   b. Vitamin B_{12} deficiency
   c. Folic acid deficiency
2. Following are the causes of the above deficiencies:
   a. In case of postgastrectomy, ferric iron cannot be converted to ferrous form prior to its absorption from the duodenum.
   b. Vitamin deficiency occurs because of loss of intrinsic factor which is secreted by the parietal cells in the stomach.
   c. Folate deficiency occurs secondary to vitamin B_{12} deficiency which is required for conversion of methyltetrahydrofolic acid to tetrahydrofolic acid.
3. For duodenal ulcer Billroth II gastrectomy and for gastric ulcer Billroth II gastrectomy are of choice.

CASE 49

A 65-year-old man suffered from epigastric discomfort in spite of taking daily rabeprazole for nearly 10 years. He underwent gastroscopy which demonstrated mild erythema in the body; from there endoscopic biopsy was taken which demonstrated:

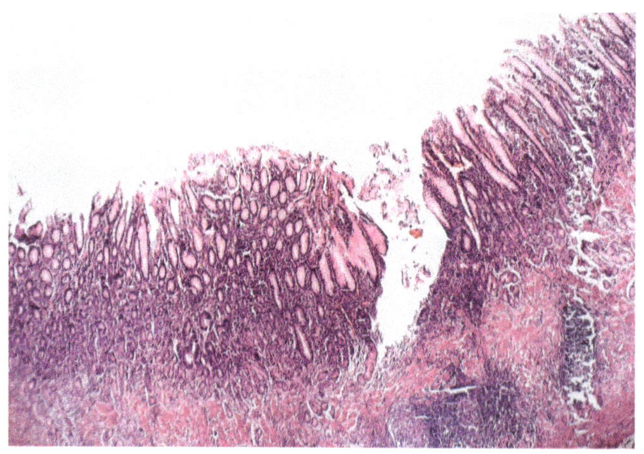

1.   **What is seen in the above histologic picture?**
2.   **Based on this histologic feature, what should be the interval of doing surveillance endoscopy?**
3.   **What are the high-risk features that are responsible for developing gastric carcinoma?**
4.   **Why is surveillance endoscopy done on this patient?**

Answers

1.   Histological features demonstrate:
     a.   Almost complete absence of specialized gastric glands
     b.   Extensive intestinal metaplasia
     c.   Focal pyloric metaplasia
     d.   Absence of *H. pylori*
2.   At least every 3 years surveillance of upper gastro-intestinal endoscopy is required.
3.   Following are the high-risk features for developing gastric carcinoma:
     a.   High-risk ethnicity
     b.   Family history of gastric carcinoma
     c.   Residence of high-risk areas
     d.   Presence of dysplasia in biopsy
     e.   Presence of extensive intestinal metaplasia in the biopsy
     f.   Operative link on gastric assessment stage III and IV
4.   For the following reasons, surveillance endoscopy is done:
     a.   Presence of intestinal metaplasia in case of chronic atrophic gastritis will lead to development of dysplasia and intestinal type adenocarcinoma.
     b.   For adequate grading and staging, four nontargeted biopsies from four quadrants.
     c.   Additional targeted biopsies are also taken

CASE 50

A 45-year-old nonsmoker male came to gastroenterology clinic with upper abdominal discomfort in spite of taking low-dose omeprazole for 6 months. He underwent gastroscopy which demonstrated three polyps in the fundic region, >1.5 cm in diameter. Targeted biopsies were taken.

1.   **What should be the next step?**
2.   **What are the types of gastric epithelial polyp?**
3.   **Write the characteristics of the fundal polyp.**
4.   **What is the relation of PPI with fundal polyp?**
5.   **Which epithelial polyp is likely to develop malignancy and what are its characteristics?**

Answers

1.   Endoscopy should be repeated for excision of the polyps because the size of the polyps is >1.5 cm.
2.   There are three types of gastric epithelial polyps:
     a.   Fundic gland polyp
     b.   Hyperplastic polyp
     c.   Adenomatous polyp
3.   Characteristics of the fundic gland polyp:
     a.   It is present in the fundal or upper gastric body mucosa.
     b.   It has no cancerous risk unless it is associated with familial adenomatous polyposis.
     c.   If its size is >1 cm, there is chance of dysplasia.
     d.   It is not associated with *H. pylori* infection.
4.   Fundic gland polyp is associated with long-term use of PPI and this polyp regresses when the PPI will be stopped.
5.   Adenomatous poly is likely to develop malignancy. Its characteristics are:
     a.   It is present in the antral mucosa and incisura.
     b.   It is single in number.
     c.   It is pinkish in color.
     d.   It is sessile or pedunculated.

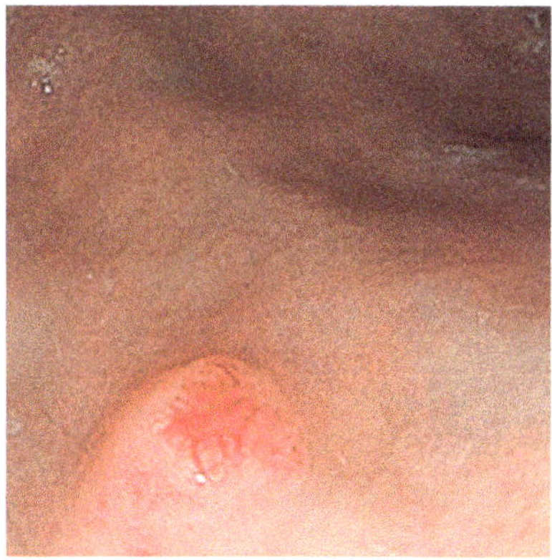

CASE 51

A 60-year-old male underwent upper gastrointestinal endoscopy as he complained of upper abdominal pain. It demonstrated:

Biopsy was taken that showed:

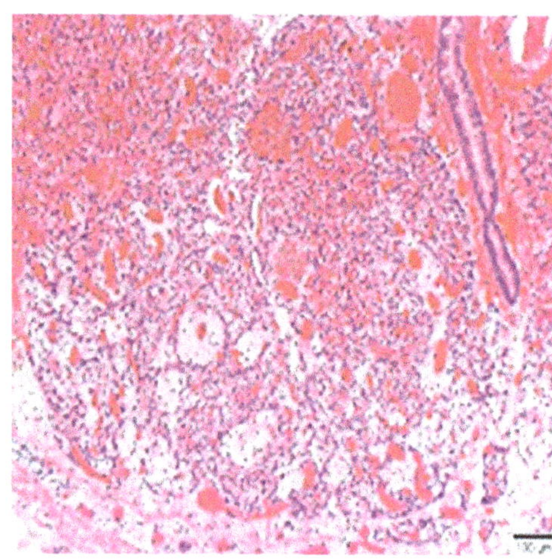

Laboratory results demonstrated hemoglobin level of 10 g/dL, serum ferritin of 10 ng/dL, 8% transferrin saturation, and serum vitamin B_{12} of 90 ng/L and positive anti-intrinsic factor antibodies. CT scan of abdomen is normal.

1. **What is the finding in the endoscopy?**
2. **What are the histological features?**
3. **What is your likely diagnosis?**
4. **What are the characteristics of this disease?**
5. **What are other features associated with this disease?**
6. **What are the different types of this disease?**

Answers

1. Endoscopic picture demonstrated presence of red-colored smooth surfaced lesion of nearly 5 mm in diameter seen on the lateral curvature of the stomach.
2. Histological features demonstrate:
   a. Sheets of cribriform islands as well as glandular structure
   b. Tumor cells are uniform with small amount eosinophilic cytoplasm
3. The diagnosis is type 1 neuroendocrine tumor.
4. Characteristics of this type 1 neuroendocrine tumor are:
   a. Small reddish nodule; may be multiple
   b. Increased serum gastrin level
   c. There is presence of enterochromaffin like cells.
   d. No progression to metastasis.
   e. Ki-67 index: It is ≤3%.
5. Associated features with this tumor are:
   a. Chronic atrophic gastritis
   b. Vitamin B_{12} deficiency
6. There are three types of tumor:
   a. Type 1 neuroendocrine tumor
   b. Type 2 neuroendocrine tumor
   c. Type 3 neuroendocrine tumor

CASE 52

A 59-year-old male with history of postprandial epigastric discomfort underwent upper gastrointestinal endoscopy which demonstrated round smooth-surfaced lesion without any sign of erosive areas seen in the fundal mucosa in retroflexed view. Biopsy was taken from that lesion for immunohistochemistry that demonstrated positivity for CD117.

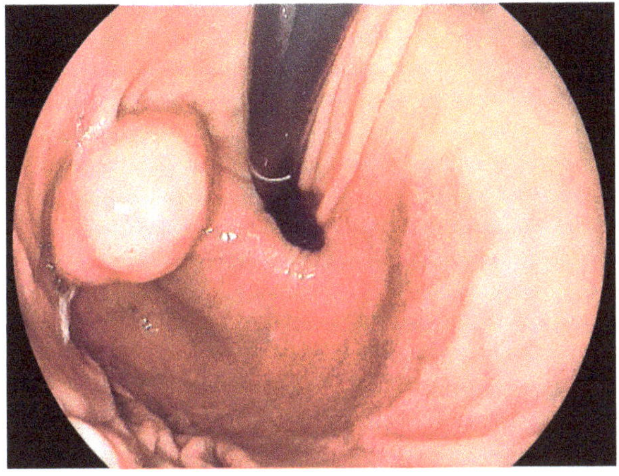

1. **What is your diagnosis?**
2. **What is the next step in the diagnosis of this disease?**
3. **What are the positive markers for this lesion?**
4. **What are the uses of enterography in this lesion?**
5. **What are the types of this lesion according to the risk?**

Answers

1. It is a case of gastrointestinal stromal tumor.
2. Next step in the diagnosis is CT scan of abdomen.
3. Positive markers for this tumor are:
    a. CD117
    b. CD34
    c. DOG-1
4. Enterography can assess the following:
    a. Location of the tumor
    b. Diagnosis staging
    c. Invasion to nearby structure
    d. Perforation of the stomach
    e. Metastasis to other organs
5. According to the risk, there are three types of tumor:
    a. Low-risk tumor: It can be resected laparo-scopically.
    b. High-risk metastatic tumor: It can be resected along with administration of 400 mg imatinib daily.
    c. Unresectable tumor: It can be resectable with neoadjuvant imatinib.

CASE 53

A 72-year-old man underwent upper gastrointestinal endoscopy that demonstrated a lesion in the antrum.

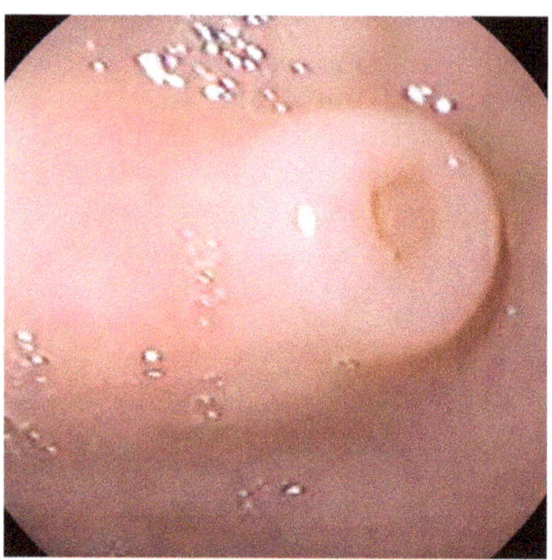

1. **Describe the lesion.**
2. **What is your diagnosis?**
3. **What is the usual site of lesion?**
4. **What should be the next investigation in this case and how does it look like?**
5. **What are the complications?**

Answers

1. There is a round smooth-surfaced submucosal lesion with central umbilication having diameter of <2 cm in seen in the antral mucosa.
2. The diagnosis is pancreatic rest present in the gastric antrum.
3. Pancreatic rest is usually present in the gastric antrum or anywhere in the foregut as well as midgut.
4. Next investigation should be endoscopic ultrasound which can effectively diagnose and can differentiate from gastrointestinal stromal tumor. It will demonstrate as either hypoechoic or intermediate echoic heterogeneous lesion having indistinct border.
5. Complications of this pancreatic rest are:
   a. Ulceration
   b. Gastric outlet obstruction
   c. Rarely malignancy

CASE 54

A 28-year-old nonsmoker man with history of abdominal pain, diarrhea in spite of intake of long-standing rabeprazole and anti-*H. pylori* treatment, nonintake of NSAIDs, and family history of pancreatic tumor in his father underwent gastroscopy that revealed:

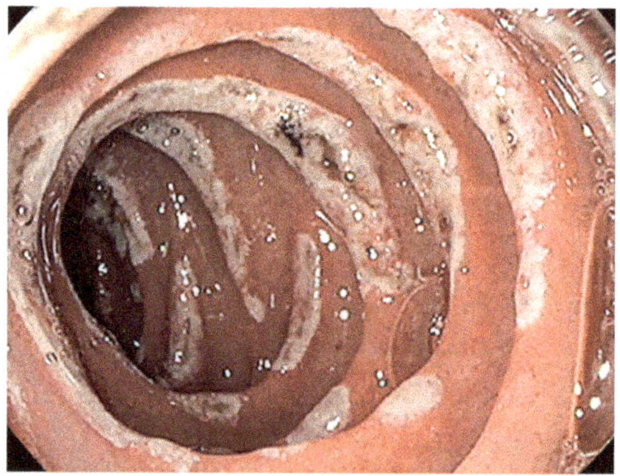

1. **What is the endoscopic finding?**
2. **What is your suspected diagnosis?**
3. **Which test is essential for confirming the diagnosis?**
4. **What is the pathophysiology for diarrhea and ulcers?**
5. **What are the laboratory tests that should be performed in this case and why?**
6. **Which special test should be performed to diagnose this disease?**

Answers

1. Gastroscopy demonstrated multiple superficial ulcers seen involving the second and third part of the duodenum.
2. The suspected diagnosis is ZE syndrome.
3. Serum level of gastrin should be measured, and it should be >1,000 pg/mL.
4. Gastrinoma is the functional endocrine tumor releasing large amount of gastric acid leading to formation of multiple duodenal ulcers. Diarrhea occurs due to hypersecretion of acids leading to development of malabsorption.
5. Following tests should be performed to diagnose it as a part of multiple endocrine neoplasia type 1 (MEN1):
    a. Serum calcium
    b. Serum parathyroid hormone
    c. Serum prolactin
6. Secretin stimulation test: Secretin usually suppresses the release of gastrin from the G cells. But, failure of suppression of gastrin level to <200 pg/mL following administration of secretin is the diagnostic of gastrinoma.

CASE 55

A 69-year-old female has been diagnosed as T2N adenocarcinoma of stomach. Now, she asked the doctor about the risk of cancer in her son in future.

1. **What will doctor answer to the patient?**
2. **What are the other risk factors for gastric carcinoma?**
3. **What is the treatment option in this patient?**

Answers

1. As male has threefold increased risk of developing gastric cancer. Hence, her son is prone to develop gastric cancer in future.
2. Other risk factors are:
    a. Age: There is an increased risk of this cancer with advancing age.
    b. Family history: There is increased incidence of this cancer in the first-degree relatives.
    c. Infection with *H. pylori*: There is increased incidence of noncardiac gastric carcinoma with this infection.
    d. Tobacco smoking
3. This patient is in stage IIB gastric carcinoma. So, the treatment options are:
    a. Radical gastrectomy
    b. If there is gap of at least 5 cm between the upper margin of the tumor and the gastroesophageal junction, in that case subtotal gastrectomy is indicated.
    c. Otherwise total gastrectomy along with pre-operative chemotherapy are indicated.

CASE 56

A 55-year-old woman with history of GERD on omeprazole therapy suffered from abdominal distention, intermittent vomiting, and >4 kg weight loss. On examination, there is succussion splash and distention of abdomen. Her gastroscopic finding and magnetic resonance enterography are normal. Thyroid function test, fasting glucose, and creatinine are normal.

1. **What is your probable diagnosis?**
2. **Which test confirms the diagnosis?**
3. **What are the most common causes of gastroparesis?**
4. **How can wireless capsule motility study diagnose the gastric emptying?**

Answers

1. As the patient has been suffering from delayed gastric emptying without any mechanical obstruction, hence the patient has gastroparesis.
2. Gastric emptying scintigraphy of solid-phase meal at 4 hours should be done to confirm the diagnosis.
3. The most common cases of gastroparesis are:
   a. Diabetes mellitus
   b. Postgastric surgery
   c. Idiopathic
4. Wireless capsule motility study measures temperature, pressure, and pH when it traverses through the gastrointestinal tract. There is sudden increase in pH when it passes from the stomach into the duodenal cavity.

CASE 57

A 54-year-old man with history of celiac disease on gluten-free diet has undergone upper gastrointestinal endoscopy due to upper abdominal pain. Endoscopic biopsy was taken.

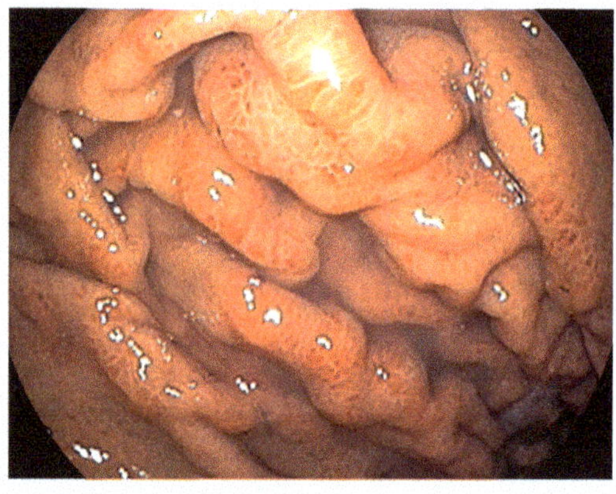
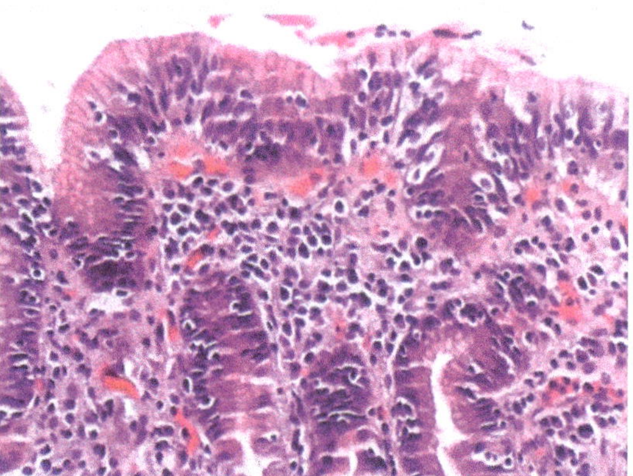

1. **Describe the above pictures.**
2. **What is your diagnosis?**
3. **What are the associated diseases?**

Answers

1. Description of the above pictures:
   a. Endoscopic pictures demonstrated:
      - Erosions
      - Nodularity
      - Mucosal elevations
      - Tiny ulcerations.
   b. Histological pictures demonstrate:
      - Increased intraepithelial lymphocytes—this is defined as >25 intraepithelial lymphocytes per 100 gastric surface and foveolar epithelial cells.
      - Most of the lymphocytes are small having halo appearance.
      - Proliferation of the epithelial cells
      - Hyperplasia of the foveolar epithelial cells
      - Immunohistochemistry may demonstrate $CD3^+$ and $CD8^+$ T lymphocytes.
2. The diagnosis is lymphocytic gastritis.
3. Following conditions are associated with lymphocytic gastritis:
   a. Infections:
      - *Helicobacter pylori* infection
      - HIV infection

b. Autoimmune etiologies:
  - Celiac disease
  - Crohn's disease
  - Lymphocytic enterocolitis

c. Neoplasia:
  - Lymphoma
  - Carcinoma

d. Medication: Ticlopidine

CASE 58

A 50-year-old man presented with abdominal pain, nausea, and vomiting in the clinic. On examination, there was pedal edema. Endoscopy done and biopsy was taken from the suspected region.

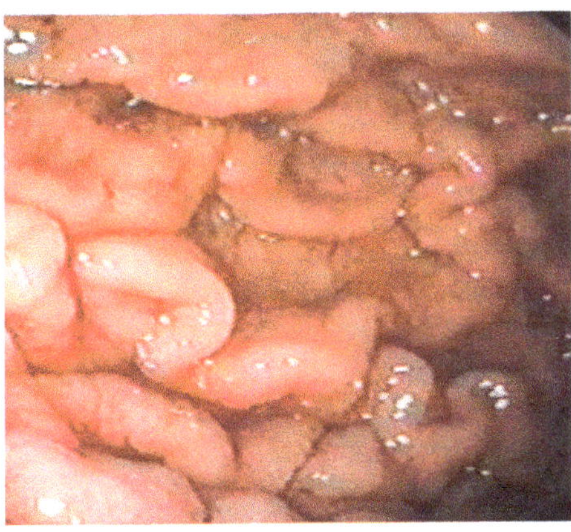 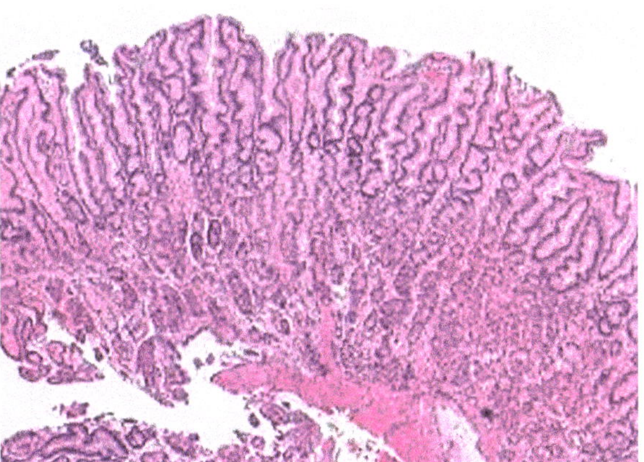

1. **Describe the above pictures.**
2. **What is your diagnosis?**
3. **Why is there pedal edema?**
4. **What are the diseases commonly associated?**
5. **What is the increased risk in this condition?**
6. **What is the intragastric pH in this disease?**

Answers

1. Description of the above pictures:
    a. Endoscopic picture demonstrates thickening giant gastric folds in the fundus and upper gastric body with antral sparing.
    b. Histological picture demonstrates:
      - Foveolar hyperplasia with corkscrew appearance
      - Cystically dilated deep glands
      - Preservation of linear architecture
      - Increased mucus
      - Atrophy of the oxyntic glands
2. Diagnosis is Menetrier's disease.
3. Pedal edema is due to hypoalbuminemia.
4. Following diseases are commonly associated:
    a. *Helicobacter pylori* infection
    b. *Cytomegalovirus* infection
    c. Inflammatory bowel disease
    d. Ankylosing spondylitis
5. There is an increased risk of gastric carcinoma.
6. Intragastric pH will be high due to decreased acid production and atrophy of the oxyntic glands.

CASE 59

A 65-year-old male came to outpatient department with weakness and dyspnea on exertion. On examination, the patient was anemic. His gastroscopy was done which demonstrated:

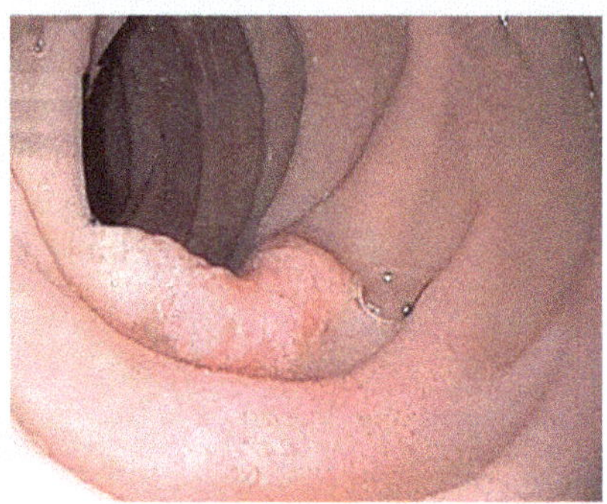 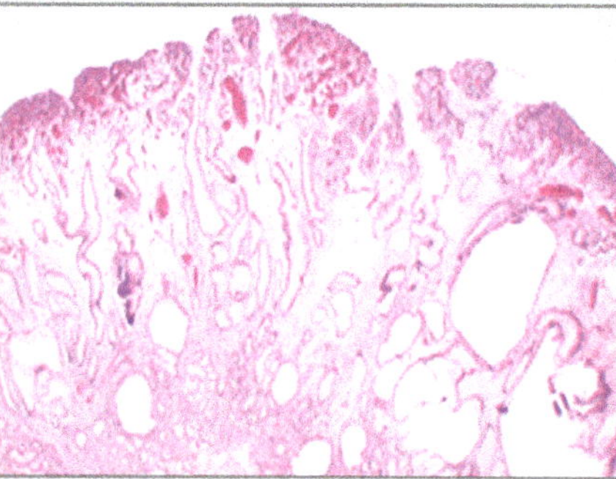 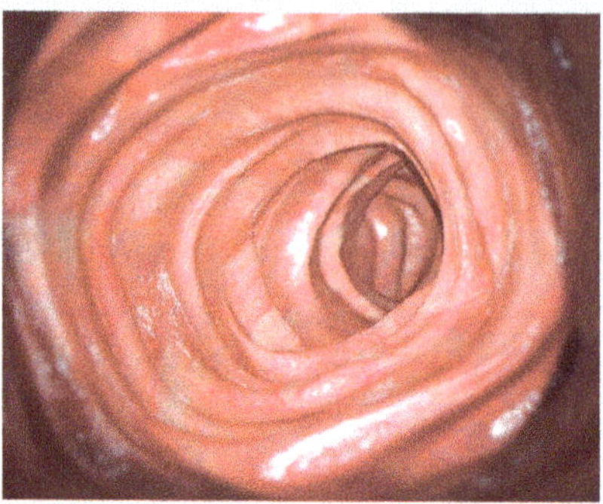

1.   **Describe the endoscopic and histopathologic features.**
2.   **What is your diagnosis?**
3.   **What are the characteristics in this disease?**
4.   **What are the surgical methods required in this disease for resection of the lesion?**

Answers

1.   Description of the pictures:
     a.   Endoscopy demonstrates mass lesion seen in the second part of the duodenum.
     b.   Histologic picture demonstrates:
          •   Presence of small tubular gland lined by eosinophilic absorptive epithelium containing pseudostratified and hyperchromatic nuclei
          •   Absence of dysplasia
     c.   Colonoscopy is normal up to cecum.
2.   Diagnosis is duodenal adenoma in the second part of the duodenum.
3.   Most of the duodenal adenomas are present in the distal part of the duodenum. There is 85% chance of transformation to malignancy. Hence, surgical resection of the adenoma is mandatory. Again, high-grade dysplastic lesion and large nonampullary sporadic duodenal adenoma of ≥20 mm in diameter are highly prone to develop adenocarcinoma. Hence, submucosal resection is necessary.
4.   Options of surgical resection include:
     a.   Laparoscopic-assisted endoluminal surgery
     b.   Laparoscopic excision of the polyp
     c.   Duodenectomy
     d.   Pancreaticoduodenectomy

CASE 60

A 69-year-old poor rickshaw driver has a history of pancreatic cancer developed gradually increasing postprandial abdominal distention and vomiting and anorexia. CT scan was done in this patient which revealed:

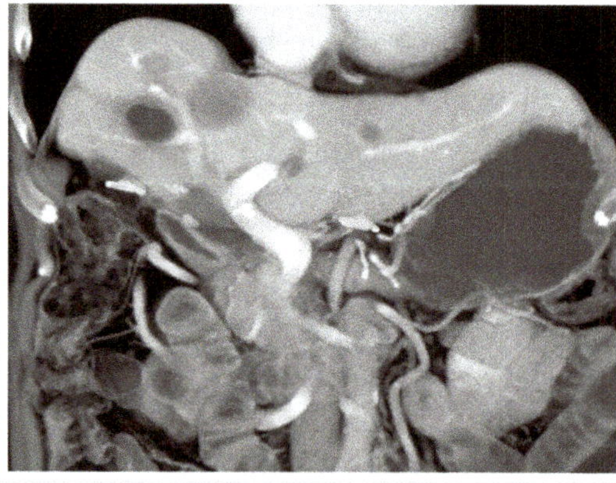

1. **Describe the CT scan of the abdomen in the above picture.**
2. **What is the immediate treatment?**
3. **What are the treatment options?**

Answers

1. CT scan demonstrates distended stomach due to gastric outlet obstruction as a result of local infiltration as well as extrinsic compression of the pancreatic cancer.
2. Immediate treatment is the decompression of the stomach by large-bore nasogastric tube.
3. Management includes:
   a. Opium analgesia
   b. Decompression of the stomach by nasogastric tube
   c. Endoscopic or fluoroscopic placement of the stent across the stricture area
   d. In case of incomplete obstruction, nasojejunal feeding tube should be inserted for providing nutrition to the patient.
   e. Surgical option is bypassing the stricture area along with gastrojejunostomy.

CASE 61

A 35-year-old female with no comorbidities came to emergency department with shortness of breath. Emergency computerized tomography pulmonary angiogram was performed which denied pulmonary embolism but detected calcification on the wall of the gallbladder with multiple calculi within the cavity were found. Her liver function test demonstrated serum bilirubin 1.2 mg/dL, alkaline phosphatase (ALP) level 122 U/L, and serum glutamic pyruvic transaminase (SGPT) 18 U/L.

1. **What is the importance of calcification in the wall of the gallbladder?**
2. **What should be the next step in this case?**

Answers

1. There is spotty calcification on the wall of the gallbladder which may lead to gallbladder carcinoma in future as compared to homogeneous calcification. This type of gallbladder is known as porcelain gallbladder. This type of gallbladder is associated with gallbladder stone.
2. As there is chance of cancer of the gallbladder in future, cholecystectomy is the choice.

CASE 62

A 38-year-old female developed abdominal pain 12 hours after the laparoscopic cholecystectomy for acute cholecystitis. There was a presence of bile in the surgical drain. Urgent CT scan of abdomen was done which demonstrated collection in the abdomen. An urgent endoscopic retrograde cholangiopancreatography (ERCP) was done which demonstrated:

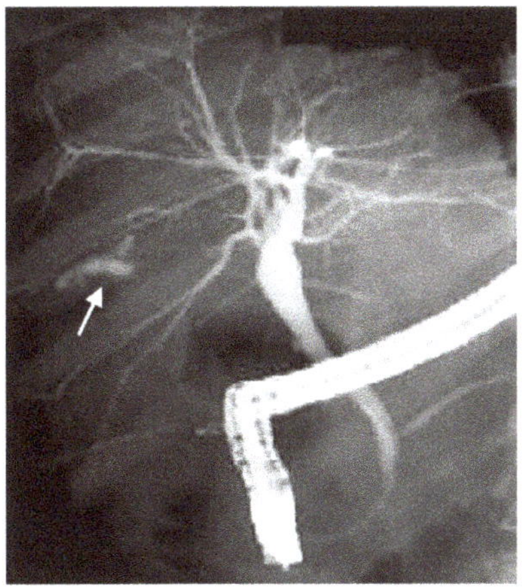

1. **What does the ERCP describe?**
2. **What is your diagnosis?**
3. **What are the common sites of leakage of bile postcholecystectomy?**
4. **What is the most common picture in this case?**
5. **What should be the method of treatment and why?**

Answers

1. ERCP demonstrates leakage of bile from the duct of Luschka and absence of the filling defect in the biliary tree.
2. The diagnosis is postcholecystectomy biliary leak from the duct of Luschka.
3. Following are the sites of leakage postcholecystectomy:
   a. Cystic duct stump
   b. Duct of Luschka
   c. Common bile duct (CBD)
   d. Common hepatic duct
   e. Gallbladder
4. Most common clinical picture is abdominal pain along with percutaneous leakage of biliary fluid from the wound site or from the drain.
5. Endoscopic approach to produce low pressure flow direction of the bile for draining the bile away from the site of leak thereby allowing the epithelium to regenerate and seal, the method being endoscopic sphincterotomy and/or endoscopic stenting of the biliary tree.

CASE 63

A 75-year-old male with past history of insertion of drug-eluting coronary stent as he suffered from acute myocardial infarction 6 months ago and on clopidogrel and aspirin and bisoprolol was admitted with acute right upper abdominal pain and jaundice with sepsis. His blood level demonstrated bilirubin of 12 mg/dL, ALP of 328 U/L, alanine aminotransferase (ALT) of 38 U/L, INR of 1.3, total count of 14,500/cc, platelet count of 170,000/cc, and CRP of 82 mg/L. His abdominal ultrasonography followed by magnetic resonance cholangiopancreatography (MRCP) demonstrated as below:

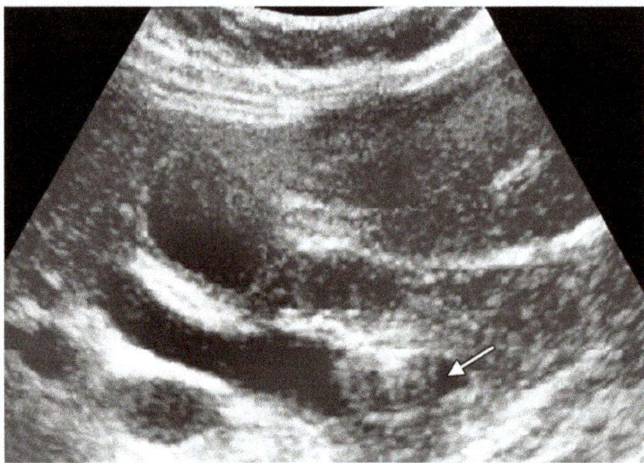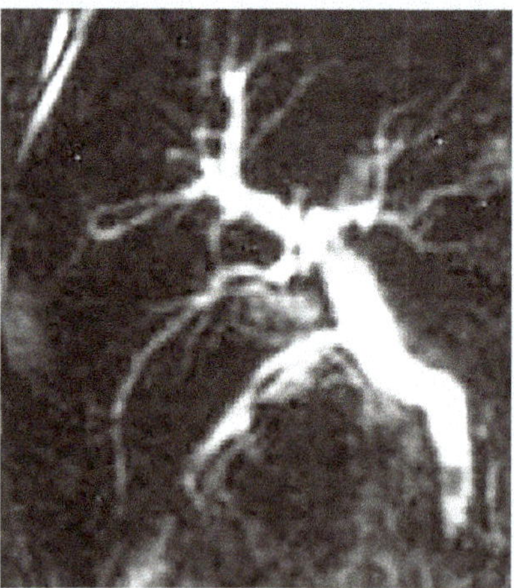

1. **Describe the above pictures?**
2. **What is your diagnosis?**
3. **What should be the method of treatment in this patient?**

Answers

1. Description of the above images:
   a. Ultrasonography of the abdomen demonstrated presence of large stone in the distal part of common bile duct.
   b. MRCP demonstrated presence of a large stone in the distal part of the common bile duct.
2. The diagnosis is stone in the common bile duct leading to sepsis in a case of patient having drug eluting coronary artery stent from acute myocardial infarction.
3. As the patient is on clopidogrel and aspirin, no percutaneous procedure is advisable. So, following procedures can be accepted:
   a. ERCP for biliary stenting without sphincterotomy
   b. In case of large common bile duct, stone should be broken by extracorporeal lithotripsy to break the stone followed by ERCP to extract the fragments of stones by small sphincterotomy.
   c. After consultation with the cardiologists regarding the temporary safe, discontinuation of the aspirin and clopidogrel prior to the interventional procedure.

CASE 64

A 25-year-old male presented with no comorbidities after returning from the Kashmir tour developed sudden spasmodic right upper abdominal pain. His urgent ultrasound of the abdomen demonstrated as below:

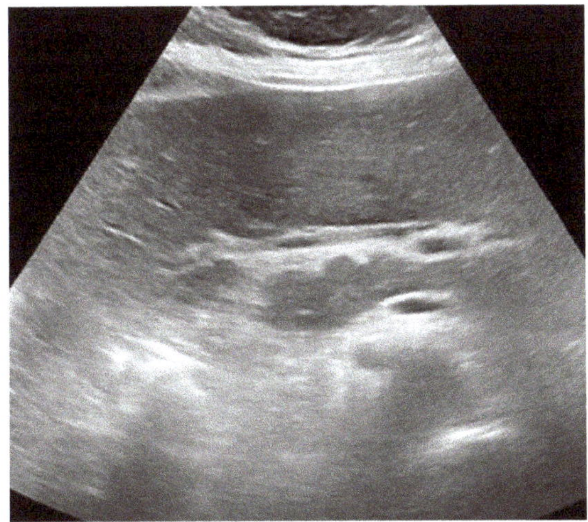

1. **What is seen in the above picture?**
2. **What is your diagnosis?**
3. **What are the clinical features of the different systems involvement?**
4. **Why is there acute abdominal pain in case of biliary ascariasis?**
5. **What are the other flukes that enter in the distal part of the ducts?**

Answers

1. Distal common bile duct containing multiple hypoechoic tubular structures having well-defined echogenic wall seen in the common bile duct.
2. The diagnosis is ascariasis in the common bile duct.
3. Following are the features of involvement of the different organs:
   a. Gastrointestinal system: Intestinal obstruction, peritonitis, and pancreatitis
   b. Lungs: Asthma and pneumonia
   c. Common bile duct and pancreatic duct: Cholangitis, acute pancreatitis, and cholecystitis hepatolithiasis.
4. Slow writhing movement of the ascaris during entry into the common duct through the ampulla of Vater leading to sphincter spasm resulting in acute abdominal pain.

5. Following flukes enter into the distal biliary canaliculi like small- and medium-sized ducts and beyond the spatial resolution of the USG:

   a. *Fasciola hepatica*
   b. *Clonorchis sinensis*
   c. *Opisthorchis viverrini*

CASE 65

A 29-year-old male came to gastroenterology clinic with recurrent history of right upper quadrant pain for 6 years in spite to cholecystectomy done 3 years before and three episodes of cholangitis for which ERCP was performed in each episode with common bile duct clearance for calculi. Blood report demonstrated serum bilirubin 2.5 mg/dL, ALP 240 U/L, ALT 72 U/L, hemoglobin 12.5 g/dL, total count 10,500/cc, and platelet count 210,000/cc.

USG of abdomen demonstrated the following.

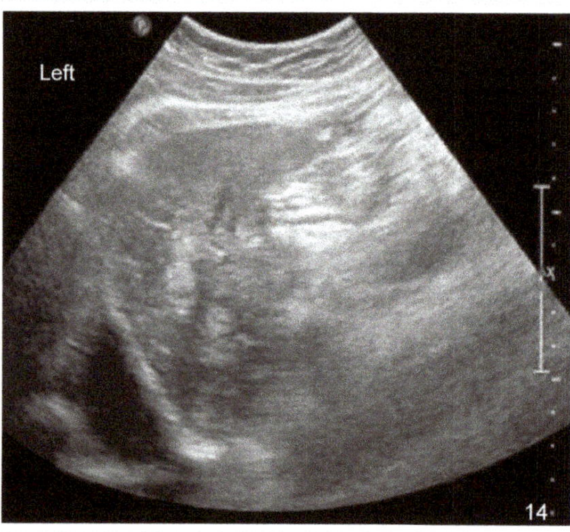

Genetic analysis demonstrated homozygous mutation (c.139C>T) in *ABCB4* gene.

1. **What is being demonstrated in the ultrasonography of abdomen?**
2. **What is your diagnosis?**
3. **What are the other characteristics in this disease?**
4. **What is the treatment for this disease?**
5. **What is the rare complication in this disease?**

Answers

1. Ultrasonography of abdomen demonstrated multiple foci of intrahepatic microlithiasis in both the lobes in the liver.
2. It is a genetic disease due to mutation of the *ABCB4* gene leading to development of low phospholipid-associated microlithiasis.
3. Following are the characteristics in this disease:
   a. It occurs in patients <40 years of age
   b. Intrahepatic cholelithiasis
   c. Intrahepatic bile duct stones
   d. Gallbladder cholesterol stones
   e. Recurrent biliary symptoms despite of cholecystectomy
4. Treatment is ursodeoxycholic acid (UDCA). Dose is 15 mg/kg/day to dissolute the stones.
5. Rare complication in this disease is primary biliary cirrhosis.

CASE 66

A 35-year-old woman presented with history of primary sclerosing cholangitis, fever with chill and rigor, worsening of serum biochemistry in the form of jaundice. MRCP was done which demonstrated:

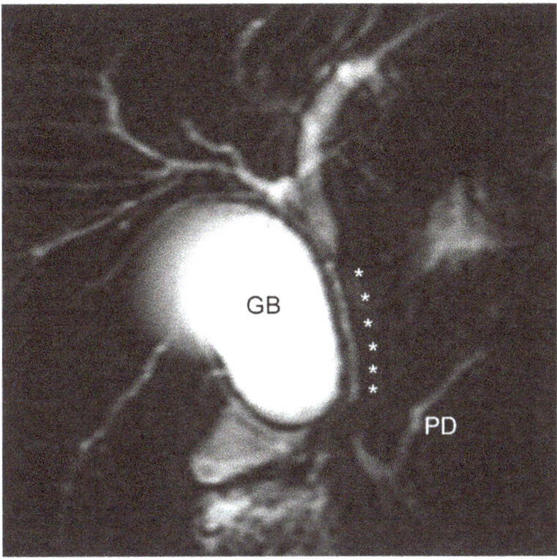

1. **What has been demonstrated in the above MRCP?**
2. **What do you define dominant stricture in case of primary biliary cirrhosis?**
3. **What is the importance of dominant stricture?**
4. **What are the indications of taking ductal sampling during ERCP in this case?**
5. **Why are antibiotics prescribed in this case prior to ERCP?**

Answers

1. MRCP demonstrated dominant stricture involving whole common bile duct and distal common hepatic duct. There is dilatation of intrahepatic duct, gallbladder, and pancreatic duct.
2. In primary biliary cirrhosis, dominant stricture can be defined as follows:
   a. Extrahepatic stenosis of ≤1.5 mm in diameter in the common bile duct
   b. ≤1 mm in the main hepatic duct within 2 cm of hilum
3. Importance of dominant stricture:
   a. It is associated with increased risk of cholangio-carcinoma and mortality.
   b. It is associated with polymorphism of CD14. It is a key mediator of immune system.
4. Indications of ductal sampling during ERCP in this case:
   a. Worsening of symptoms of obstruction like jaundice, pruritus, and cholangitis.
   b. Rapid increase in the ALP and ALT levels
   c. Progression of the existing stricture that can be identified in MRCP.
5. Antibiotics should be prescribed prior to ERCP because there is a chance of incomplete biliary drainage and cholangitis.

CASE 67

A 70-year-old man has been admitted with progressively increasing jaundice with progressive weight loss. His MRCP demonstrated the following:

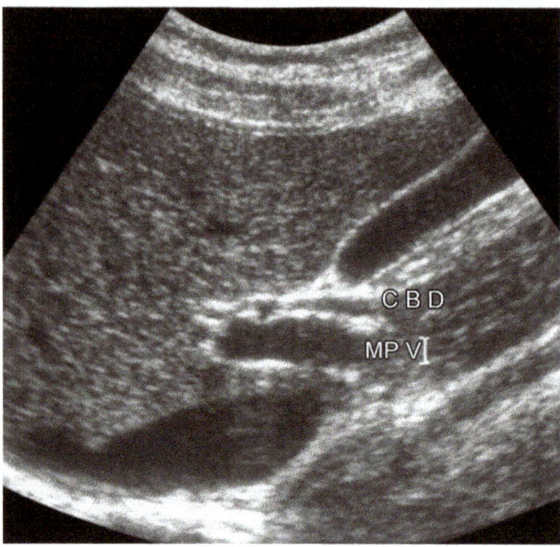

1. **What has been demonstrated in MRCP?**
2. **What is the probable diagnosis?**
3. **What are the areas in the ducts involved in this case?**
4. **What are the epidemiologic risk factors in this case?**

Answers

1. MRCP demonstrated that there is suspicious stricture in the mid part of common bile duct with dilatation of proximal common bile duct and intrahepatic biliary canaliculi.
2. Probable diagnosis is cholangiocarcinoma.
3. Following areas are involved in this case:
   a. Intrahepatic ducts
   b. Perihilar ducts
   c. Distal biliary tree
4. Following are the risk factors in cholangiocarcinoma:
   a. Primary sclerosing cholangitis
   b. Age: Age-related incidence is increased in Hispanic as well as Asian populations whereas lowest incidence in case of non-Hispanic black and white populations.
   c. Geographical variations: In South-East Asia, there is increased risk due to infection with hepatobiliary flukes like *Opisthorchis viverrini* as well as *Clonorchis sinensis* leading to chronic biliary inflammation resulting cholangiocarcinoma.
   d. *Fasciola hepatica* in Asia and Africa
   e. Hepatolithiasis is the most common cause if intrahepatic cholangiocarcinoma in Asia.
   f. Choledochal cyst like Caroli's disease characterized by multiple segmental dilatations involving intrahepatic bile ducts
   g. Congenital hepatic fibrosis

CASE 68

A 60-year-old male suffering from hepatocellular carcinoma secondary to the hepatitis C virus (HCV)-positive cirrhosis underwent liver transplantation 4 months ago presented with progressive jaundice in the hepatology clinic. Operation: Modified piggyback operation with common hepatic artery to common hepatic artery and common blie duct to common bile duct anastomosis.

On investigation, his serum bilirubin was 9 mg/dL, ALP 100 U/L, ALT 502 U/L, CRP 7 mg/L, and albumin 3.5 g/dL. Tacrolimus level 8 ng/mL and blood culture being negative.

Magnetic resonance cholangiopancreatography demonstrated diffuse irregularity and dilated intrahepatic biliary radicles. There is also anastomosis between nondilated common hepatic duct with dilated native common bile duct.

1. **What is the cause of jaundice?**
2. **How can you diagnose nonanastomotic biliary stricture?**
3. **What are the causes of anastomotic stricture?**
4. **How is anastomotic stricture being treated?**
5. **What are the causes of nonanastomotic stricture?**
6. **What is ischemic cholangiopathy?**
7. **What are the risk factors of ischemic cholangiopathy?**

Answers

1. Progressively increasing jaundice due to:
   a. Anastomotic biliary stricture at the site of bile duct anastomosis in case of choledochocholedochostomy or choledochojejunostomy
   b. Nonanastomotic biliary stricture
2. Nonanastomotic stricture can be diagnosed by triple phase CT scan or ultrasound Doppler study for excluding hepatic artery thrombosis or hepatic artery stenosis because biliary tree is supplied from hepatic artery exclusively.
3. Causes of anastomotic stricture are:
   a. Small caliber bile duct
   b. Donor-recipient bile duct size mismatch
   c. Anastomotic site tension
   d. Excessive use of electrocautery to control bleeding
4. Anastomotic stricture can be treated by stenting or dilatation during ERCP.
5. Causes of nonanastomotic stricture are:
   a. Hepatic artery thrombosis
   b. Hepatic artery stenosis
   c. Ischemic cholangiopathy
6. Ischemic cholangiopathy is characterized by nonischemic stricture in presence of patent hepatic artery leading to progressive biliary stasis or recurrent biliary sepsis occurring within 12 months of liver transplant.
7. Following are the risk factors of ischemic cholangiopathy:
   a. Prolonged ischemia time
   b. *Cytomegalovirus* infection
   c. Donation after circulatory death

CASE 69

A 40-year-old man presented in the hepatology clinic with recurrent cholangitis. Ultrasound demonstrated dilated common bile duct. Endoscopic cholangiopancreatography demonstrated dilated common bile duct without any evidence of stone. MRCP was done which demonstrated:

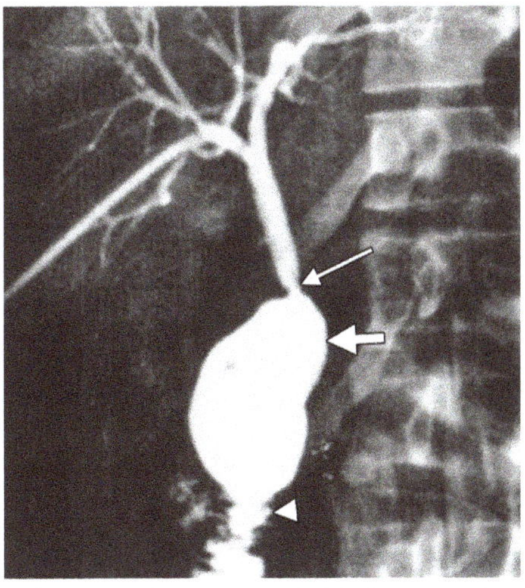

1. **What are the findings in the MRCP?**
2. **What is your diagnosis?**
3. **What are the risks in this case?**
4. **What are the types of this disease?**
5. **What is the epidemiology of this disease?**

Answers

1. MRCP demonstrated spindle-shaped dilatation along the length of the common bile duct.
2. The diagnosis is choledochal cyst type 1.
3. Following are the risks in case of choledochal cyst:
   a. Stone formation
   b. Ductal stricture
   c. Pancreatitis
   d. Cholangiocarcinoma
4. There are five types of choledochal cyst:
   a. Type I: There is dilatation of common bile duct. It may be cystic (A), focal (B), or fusiform (C).
   b. Type II: This can be described as diverticulum of common bile duct.
   c. Type III: It is known as choledochocele representing dilatation of distal common bile duct.
   d. Type IV: It is characterized by dilatation of intrahepatic and extrahepatic biliary tree (A) or only extrahepatic duct (B).
   e. Type V: It is also known as Caroli's disease consisting of multiple intrahepatic dilatations.
5. Epidemiology of choledochal cyst: It is characterized by the congenital dilatation of common bile duct commonly present in the infancy with jaundice and biliary colic. Female-to-male ratio is 4:1.

CASE 70

A 28-year-old asymptomatic man addicted to one recreational drug presented in the hepatology clinic with following types of liver function test:

Serum bilirubin 8 mg/dL, alkaline liver function test 350 U/L, and ALT 52 U/L. MRCP demonstrated the following:

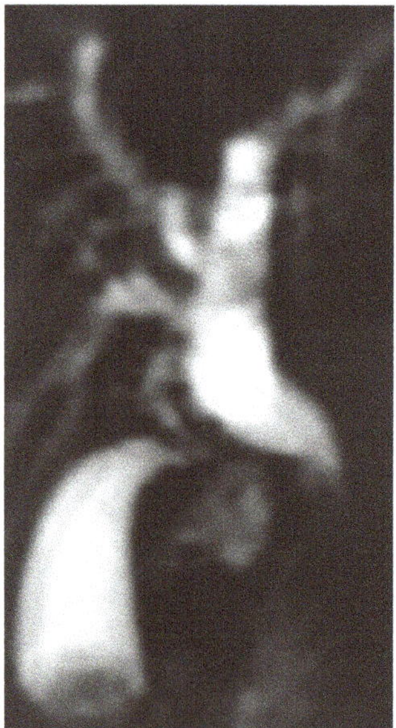

1. **What does the MRCP demonstrate?**
2. **What is your most probable diagnosis?**
3. **What is the pathophysiology behind this drug producing this disease?**
4. **What are the cholangiographic presentations in this case?**
5. **What is the risk with the use of methadone use?**

Answers

1. MRCP demonstrates extrahepatic dilatation of common bile duct with distal tapering.
2. Most probable diagnosis is ketamine abuse.
3. This drug produces biliary cholangiopathy through the chronic stimulation of the N-methyl-D-aspartic acid receptor present in the biliary smooth muscles leading to production of inflammation and fibrosis resulting in stricture as well as dilatation ultimately. As the disease is chronic, hence repeated exposure leads to result abnormal liver function test.

4. Following are the cholangiographic patterns of presentation:
   a. Diffuse extrahepatic dilatation
   b. Fusiform extrahepatic dilatation with distal tapering
   c. Intrahepatic dilatation
   d. Beading of the intrahepatic duct with normal extrahepatic duct
5. Methadone use is associated with:
   a. Dysfunction of sphincter of Oddi
   b. Dilatation of common bile duct
   c. Dilatation of pancreatic duct

CASE 71

A 49-year-old Nigerian came to the United States of America and developed severe cough with expectoration and fever. He was admitted in emergency department and subsequently diagnosed as pneumococcal pneumonia. His serology demonstrated as positive for HIV, CD4$^+$ count showed 10 cell/μL, platelet count of 110,000/cc, and white blood cell count of 5,500/cc. Liver function test demonstrated ALP of 400/IU, bilirubin of 9 mg/cc, and ALT level of 90 U/L. His MRCP was done and it demonstrated:

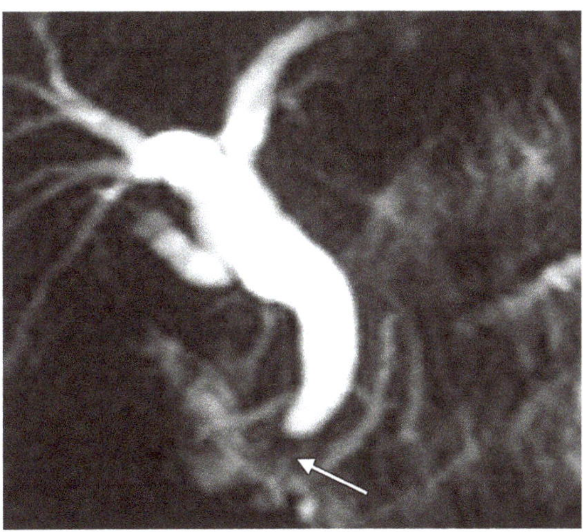

1. **What is the finding in MRCP?**
2. **What is your likely diagnosis?**
3. **What are the types of hepatobiliary diseases in this HIV infection?**
4. **What is the description of this disease?**
5. **What are the common infecting organisms associated with this disease?**

Answers

1. MRCP demonstrated that there is feature of dilatation of common bile duct with smooth tapering along with multiple dilatations and narrowing of the intrahepatic bile ducts.
2. The diagnosis is hepatobiliary cholangiopathy as a result of colonization with *Cryptosporidium parvum*.

3. There are following types of hepatobiliary diseases in HIV infection. These are:
   a. Diseases associated with immunosuppression leading to:
      - AIDS cholangiopathy
      - Acalculous cholecystitis

- AIDS-related neoplasm like Kaposi's sarcoma and non-Hodgkin lymphoma
- Vanishing bile duct syndrome
  b. Highly active antiretroviral therapy (HAART) leading to drug-induced hepatotoxicity
  c. Worsening coinfection with hepatitis B or C virus leading to progression of the fibrosis.
  d. Nonalcoholic fatty liver disease (NAFLD)
  e. Nodular regenerative hyperplasia
4. AIDS cholangiopathy is a syndrome of biliary obstruction due to infection leading to bile duct stricture associated with advanced immunosuppression occurring in patients with poor access to AIDS medication or noncompliance to the medication.
5. Following organisms are associated with this disease:
  a. *Cryptosporidium parvum*
  b. *Cytomegalovirus*
  c. Microsporidium
  d. *Giardia*
  e. *Histoplasma*
  f. *Mycobacterium avium* complex

CASE 72

A 40-year-old type I diabetic nonalcoholic patient came to outpatient department with acute abdominal pain radiating to back. On examination, epigastric region is tender. On investigation, serum amylase was 1,250 U/L, serum lipase of 2,300 U/L, ALT of 167 U/L, ALP of 180 U/L, and triglyceride of 797 mg/dL.

1. **What is your likely diagnosis?**
2. **What is the etiology in this case and why?**
3. **Why not triglyceride is the etiology?**
4. **What are the dermatological signs in this disease?**
5. **What are the phases in this disease and in which phase this patient resides?**

Answers

1. The diagnosis is acute pancreatitis.
2. The etiology is gallstone-induced pancreatitis because more than three times elevation of ALT level above normal is of >95% predictive value in diagnosing gallstone as the cause.
3. Triglyceride level should be nearly 1,000 mg/dL to diagnose this as a cause of acute pancreatitis.
4. Pancreatic necrotic tissue will track along the falciform ligament as well as into retroperitoneal area leading to development of ecchymoses in the:
  a. Periumbilical region—Cullen's sign
  b. In the flank—Grey Turner sign
5. There are two phases of acute pancreatitis:
  a. Early phase lasting for 1 week being mediated by systemic inflammatory response and there is an increased risk of extrapancreatic organ failure.
  b. Late phase occurring in case of moderate-to-severe type of acute pancreatitis. Here, there is an increased risk of:
  - Local complications
  - Infections
  - Different organ failure

This patient is in the early phase of acute pancreatitis.

CASE 73

A 50-year-old hypertensive, nondiabetic, dyslipidemic female having history of intake of red wine daily for >5 years with occasional binge drinking has been admitted with sharp upper abdominal pain radiating to back and anorexia and nausea. She has a family history of hypertension and diabetes in her father, but her two sons are healthy. She was a smoker but quit 4 years ago. Two days prior to this episode, she took five glasses of wine. On examination, she has tachycardia, blood pressure, respiration normal, afebrile, and no stigmata of liver disease. On abdominal examination, epigastric region is tender, bowel sound is normal, and no hepatosplenomegaly.

Laboratory test demonstrated there is leukocytosis, AST level is 120 U/L but ALT level 40 I/U, ALP 80 I/U, and bilirubin level 1 mg/dL.

1. **What is the likely diagnosis?**
2. **What should be the next investigations?**
3. **After proper diagnosis, how can you assess the disease severity?**
4. **What is the definition of severity of acute pancreatitis?**
5. **What is CT severity score and what are the limitations?**

Answers

1. The likely diagnosis is acute pancreatitis.
2. Next investigation for confirming the diagnosis is estimation of serum amylase and lipase.
3. Following are the different scores for assessing the severity of the acute pancreatitis:
   a. BISAP scoring system:
      - Blood urea nitrogen >25 mg/dL
      - Impaired mental status—Glasgow Coma Scale of <15
      - SIRS—it can be defined as presence of two or more of the following:
        ○ Temperature of >38°C or <36°C
        ○ Respiratory rate of >20 breaths/minute or $PaCO_2$ of <32 mm Hg
        ○ Pulse rate of >90 beats/minute
        ○ White blood cell count of either <400/cc or >12,000/cc
      - Age > 60 years
      - Presence of pleural effusion as detected on imaging
   b. Ranson criteria:
      - At the time of admission:
        ○ Age > 55 years
        ○ White blood cell count > 16,000/cc
        ○ Blood glucose > 200 mg/dL
        ○ Lactate dehydrogenase > 350 U/L
        ○ AST > 250 U/L.
      - After 48 hours of admission:
        ○ Hematocrit—fall by >10%
        ○ Blood urea nitrogen—increase by >5 mg/dL
        ○ Serum calcium < 8 mg/dL
        ○ pO_2 < 60 mm Hg
        ○ Base deficit of >4 mEq/L
        ○ Fluid sequestration of >6,000 mL
4. There are three types of severity in acute pancreatitis:
   a. Mild acute pancreatitis:
      - Absence of organ failure
      - Absence of local and/or systemic complications
      - Rare mortality
   b. Moderately severe pancreatitis:
      - Presence of transient organ failure of <48 hours
      - Presence of local systemic complications of <48 hours
   c. Severe pancreatitis:
      - Presence and persistent organ failure of >48 hours
      - Single organ failure
      - Multiple organ failure
      - Mortality is extremely high.
5. CT severity score in acute pancreatitis is:

   Balthazar score:
   a. A: Normal pancreas—0
   b. B: Enlargement of pancreas—1
   c. C: Inflammatory changes in the pancreas and peripancreatic fat—2
   d. D: Ill-defined peripancreatic fluid collection—3
   e. E: Two or more poorly defined peripancreatic fluid collection—4

   Pancreatic necrosis:
   a. None: 0
   b. ≤30%: 2
   c. >30–50%: 4
   d. >50%: 6

CASE 74

A 36-year-old nondiabetic, nonhypertensive, nonsmoker, and normolipidemic patient developed acute abdominal pain. Patient has been suffering from ileocecal Crohn's disease and started 250 mg azathioprine once daily. MRCP demonstrated normal common bile duct, normal intrahepatic biliary structure, and no gallstone. There is no family history.

1. **What is your likely diagnosis?**
2. **In this patient, what are the possible etiologies for this diagnosis?**
3. **What are the risk factors associated with it?**
4. **Which is the possible treatment?**
5. **Is there any chance of recurrence of this condition?**

Answers

1. The most likely diagnosis is acute pancreatitis.
2. Following are the possible etiologies:
   a. Here the most likely cause is azathioprine administration.
   b. Other drug-induced cause is 5-aminosalicylate and metronidazole
   c. As there is increased prevalence of gallstones in Crohn's disease, choledocholithiasis may be the cause.
   d. Autoimmune causes:
      - Autoimmune pancreatitis
      - Primary sclerosing cholangitis
3. Following are the risk factors associated with this disease:
   a. Female sex
   b. Cigarette smoking
   c. Exposure to glucocorticoids
   d. Certain human leukocyte antigen polymorphism
4. Possible treatment here is the removal of the azathioprine administration.
5. Yes, there should be recurrence after reintroduction of azathioprine.

CASE 75

A 45-year-old woman postcholecystectomy developed gallstone-induced cholangitis. So, after proper treatment of the infection, ERCP was arranged to take out the residual gallstones present in the common bile duct with sphincterotomy for ductal clearance. But within 1 day after the procedure, the patient developed acute abdominal pain and was admitted in ICU.

1. **What is the possible diagnosis?**
2. **What are the risk factors for the development of this disease?**
3. **What are the drugs that should be recommended prior to this procedure?**

Answers

1. Patient developed post-ERCP pancreatitis.
2. Risk factors for this disease are:
   a. Patient-related factors:
      - Female gender
      - Functional biliary sphincter disorder like sphincter of Oddi dysfunction
      - Previous history of pancreatitis
   b. Procedure-related risk factors:
      - Repeated and prolonged attempt for cannulation
      - Passage of pancreatic guidewire
      - Injection of large amount of dye into the pancreatic duct
3. Per rectal diclofenac or oral indomethacin should be administered either prior to or postprocedure.

CASE 76

A 67-year-old male has been admitted with severe epigastric pain radiating to back. On examination, there is severe epigastric tenderness. Blood report demonstrated hemoglobin of 12 mg/dL, total count of WBC 15,000/cc, platelet count of 200,000/cc, electrolytes and renal function test normal, but ALP was 198 U/L, serum ALT 70 U/L, serum amylase 1010 U/L, and lipase 892 U/L.

1. **What is your diagnosis?**
2. **What investigation should be the first choice?**

3. **When is CT scan required and how can you grade the severity?**
4. **Which urinary tests should be done to diagnose acute pancreatitis?**
5. **Is there any importance of interleukins in case of acute pancreatitis?**
6. **What are the serum markers elevated in case of acute pancreatitis?**

Answers

1. The definite diagnosis is acute pancreatitis.
2. The prime and foremost investigation that should be done in this case is abdominal ultrasound because this can detect the gallstones as an underlying etiology.
3. CT scan is needed which is required for diagnosing pancreatic necrosis and extrapancreatic inflammation. Contrast-enhanced CT scan is required as it can distinguish between the edematous pancreas and necrotizing pancreatitis. CT severity score in case of acute pancreatitis:
   a. Point (A):
      - Normal pancreas: 0
      - Pancreatic enlargement: 1
      - Pancreatic or peripancreatic fat inflammation: 2
      - Single peripancreatic fluid collection: 3
      - More than two fluid collections and/or retroperitoneal air: 4
   b. Point (B):
      - No pancreatic necrosis: 0
      - Up to 30% of the gland: 2
      - 30–50% of the gland: 4
      - >50% of the gland: 6
   CT severity index: A + B
   a. Mild pancreatitis: 0–2
   b. Moderate pancreatitis: 3–6
   c. Severe pancreatitis: 7–10
4. Following tests in urine should be done to diagnose acute pancreatitis:
   a. Trypsinogen activation peptide
   b. Anionic pepsinogen
5. Following interleukins are important in the first few hours of acute pancreatitis:
   a. Interleukin-1
   b. Interleukin-6
   c. Interleukin-8
6. Following serum markers are elevated in case of acute pancreatitis:
   a. Procalcitonin
   b. Polymorphonuclear elastase
   c. Pancreatic-associated protein
   d. Amylase
   e. Lipase
   f. Glucose
   g. Calcium
   h. Procarboxypeptidase B
   i. Carboxypeptidase B activation peptide
   j. Trypsinogen-2
   k. Phospholipase A2
   l. Amyloid protein A
   m. Substance P
   n. Antithrombin III
   o. Platelet-activating factor
   p. IL-1, IL-6, and IL-8

CASE 77

A 50-year-old man was admitted with acute abdominal pain after excessive alcohol consumption. He was diagnosed alcohol-induced acute pancreatitis. On examination, there was tachycardia, blood pressure of 90/50 mm Hg, respiratory rate of 24 breaths/minute, SpO_2 of 93%, hemoglobin of 13 g/dL, total count of WBC 15,000/cc, and platelet count of 300,000/cc.

1. **Which fluid is required for resuscitation and why?**
2. **What are the immediate results of fluid resuscitation?**
3. **If hypotension persists in spite of adequate resuscitation of fluid, what are the steps?**
4. **At what rate the fluid can be given?**
5. **Why is hydroxyethyl starch not given?**
6. **What should be the proper strategy of nutrition?**
7. **What are the factors in acute pancreatitis that should prevent enteral nutrition as it is impossible?**
8. **In case of severe acute pancreatitis, what are the criteria for starting the oral feeding?**

Answers

1. Ringer lactate is the fluid of choice for resuscitation, because it reduces the incidence of SIRS as compared to administration of normal saline.
2. Successful fluid resuscitation will result in:
   a. Warm peripheries
   b. Good pulse volume
   c. Normalization of arterial blood pressure
   d. Good urine output
   e. Improved mixed venous oxygen tension
3. If the patient is still hypotensive in spite of adequate fluid resuscitation, following steps are taken:
   a. Dopamine should be given at a rate of 10–15 mL/kg/minute as slow intravenous infusion
   b. In case associated vasoconstriction, dobutamine is preferred choice.
4. Ringer lactate should be given at a rate of 5–10 mL/kg/hour as it will help in:
   a. Diminished need for mechanical ventilation
   b. Abdominal compartment syndrome
   c. Sepsis leading to increased mortality
5. Hydroxyethyl starch is not given because it will produce renal failure.
6. Following should be nutritional strategies:
   a. In case of mild-to-moderate pancreatitis, oral feeding should be started as soon as possible. If the patient is intolerant to oral feeding, enteral tube feeding should be started within 2–3 days of admission to prevent sepsis.
   b. In case of severe pancreatitis with presence of SIRS, enteral tube either via nasogastric or nasojejunal tube feeding should be started as it will reduce:
      • Systemic infection
      • Multiorgan failure
      • Need for surgical intervention
   c. In severe pancreatitis when there is reduced gastric emptying, nasojejunal tube is of choice.
   d. If the patient fails to fulfil the nutrition through oral or nasogastric tube, parenteral nutrition is of choice. In this case, the main choice is L-glutamine as it will reduce the incidence of sepsis leading to mortality.
7. Following factors in acute pancreatitis make impossible for enteral nutrition:
   a. Vomiting
   b. Abdominal distention
   c. Paralytic ileus
   d. Peritonitis
   e. Severe sepsis
8. Following are the criteria to start the oral feeding in acute pancreatitis:
   a. Absence of abdominal pain
   b. Reduction of lipase and amylase to normal levels
   c. Absence of complications like pancreatic fistulas
   d. Resolution of paralytic ileus as detected by appearance of bowel sounds

CASE 78

A 45-year-old man presented with persisting abdominal pain even after 4 months of gallstone-induced acute pancreatitis. MRCP of the abdomen demonstrated:

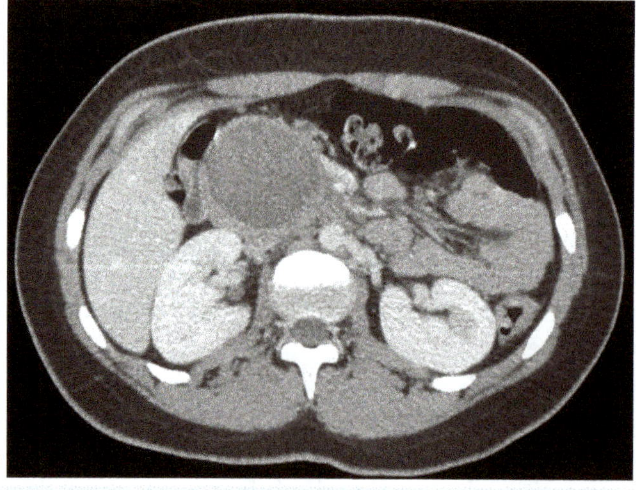

1.   **What is the feature in MRCP?**
2.   **What is the incidence of this finding in acute pancreatitis?**
3.   **What are the characteristic features of this disease?**
4.   **What are the fate of this pseudocyst?**
5.   **What are the treatment modalities in this case?**

Answers

1.   Feature in MRCP is pancreatic pseudocyst.
2.   There is 10–20% incidence in case of acute pancreatitis.
3.   Following are the characteristic features in this disease:
     a.   It is characterized by encapsulated collection of the fluids having well-defined inflammatory wall.
     b.   It usually occurs within 4 weeks of interstitial edematous pancreatitis.
     c.   It will mature >4 weeks of acute pancreatitis.
4.   Following are the fate of pseudocyst:
     a.   Complete resolution in 70% cases
     b.   Biliary obstruction
     c.   Gastric outlet obstruction: Bleeding in the pseudocyst
     d.   Infection
5.   Endoscopic or surgical or endosonographic cystogastrostomy

CASE 79

A 45-year-old man has come to gastroenterology clinic with recurrent abdominal pain over 6 months. So, MRCP of abdomen was done. It demonstrated:

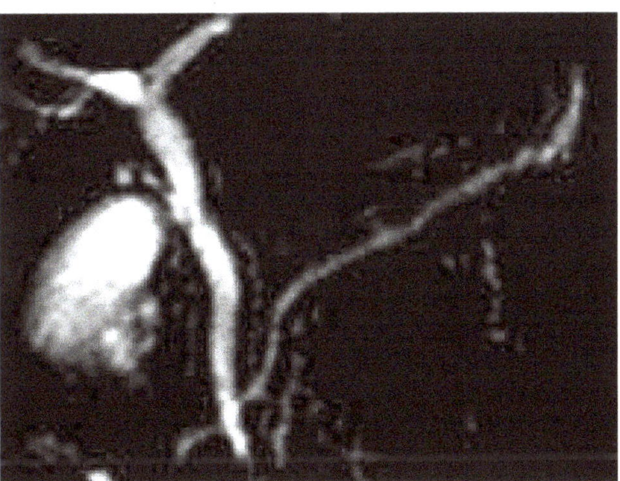

1.   **What is the finding in MRCP?**
2.   **What is your diagnosis?**
3.   **How is this formed?**
4.   **Why is there recurrent pain in this disease?**

Answers

1. MRCP demonstrated pancreatic divisum with normal biliary tree.
2. The diagnosis is pancreatic divisum.
3. This will result from the failure of fusion of ventral and dorsal pancreatic duct during gestation resulting in separation of two ductal systems without any connection in-between them.
   a. One is dorsal pancreatic duct or duct of Santorini which enters into the minor papilla directly.
   b. Other is ventral pancreatic duct or duct of Wirsung which enters into the major papilla.
4. Recurrent pain is due to incomplete drainage through the minor papilla.

CASE 80

A 70-year-old chronic heavy smoker came to outpatient department with 4 months history of weight loss along with pale semisolid malodorous stool. He had a history of intake of 26 units of alcohol weekly. Fecal elastase level is <40 ng/mL and serum amylase is normal.

1. **What is your most likely diagnosis?**
2. **What is the cause of malabsorption?**
3. **What are the risk factors of this disease?**
4. **In case of heavy alcohol intake, what are the proposed factors responsible for development of chronic pancreatitis?**
5. **In case of pancreatic duct obstruction, what are the causes of chronic pancreatitis?**
6. **If this occurs at a young age, what is the cause behind it?**
7. **Is there any risk of cancer in this disease?**

Answers

1. The most likely diagnosis is chronic pancreatitis.
2. Malabsorption occurs as a result of destruction of >90% of exocrine cells of pancreas.
3. Following are the risk factors in this disease:
   a. Heavy alcohol intake—history of alcohol intake of >150 g/day for at least 5–10 years
   b. Tobacco—it will lead to rapid development of pancreatic calcification.
   c. Obstruction of pancreatic duct
   d. Tropical pancreatitis
   e. Hereditary causes
   f. Autoimmune causes
   g. Metabolic factors
4. In case of heavy alcohol intake, following factors are responsible for development of chronic pancreatitis:
   a. Genetic variation which involves polymorphism of proteins which is involved in the cellular antioxidant defense of alcohol metabolism.
   b. Consumption of high-protein diet
   c. Consumption of high-fat diet
   d. Hyperlipidemia
   e. Exposure to bacterial endotoxin
   f. Smoking
5. Causes of pancreatic duct obstruction are:
   a. Pancreatic tumor
   b. Ductal tumor
   c. Ampullary tumor
   d. Benign ductal stricture
   e. Pancreatic divisum with stenosis of minor papilla
6. If it occurs in the young, it is mostly due to hereditary pancreatitis. The causes are:
   a. *Protease serine 1* gene: It is autosomal dominant. This gene encodes trypsinogen. Mutation of this gene leads to autoactivation of trypsin within the pancreas resulting in activation of zymogen to active form. It will autodigest the pancreatic tissue.
   b. Other mutations are *SPINK1* gene.
   c. Cystic fibrosis transmembrane conductance regulator gene
7. In case of hereditary chronic pancreatitis, there is chance of pancreatic cancer.

CASE 81

A 60-year-old heavy smoker came to the outpatient department with foul smelling semisolid stool and weight loss for the last 8 months. His fecal elastase level is <50 ng/mL. MRCP of abdomen done which is shown below:

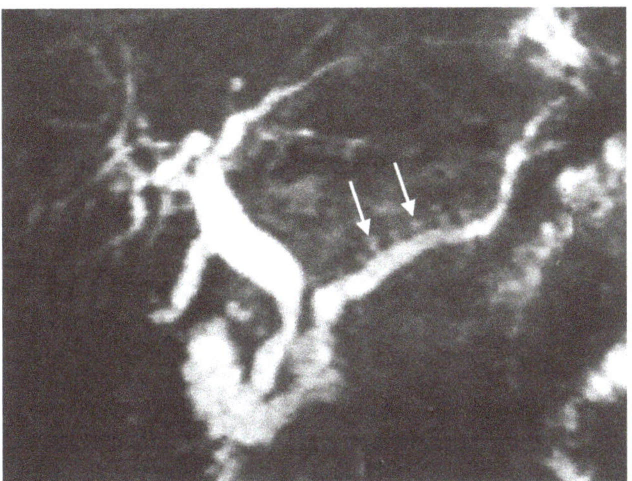

1. **What is the feature in MRCP?**
2. **What is the most likely diagnosis?**
3. **What is the cause of steatorrhea?**
4. **Is there any chance of vitamin deficiency in chronic pancreatitis?**
5. **What are the causes of pancreatic exocrine insufficiency?**
6. **What are the tests for pancreatic insufficiency?**

Answers

1. There is evidence of alternate cystic dilatation and constriction in the length of pancreatic duct.
2. The most likely diagnosis is chronic pancreatitis.
3. Steatorrhea is due to pancreatic exocrine insufficiency of >90%.
4. There is increased risk of deficiency of fat-soluble vitamins like A, D, E, and K.
5. Following are the causes of exocrine insufficiency:
   a. Cystic fibrosis
   b. Chronic pancreatitis
   c. Pancreatic neoplasm
   d. Postpancreatic resection
   e. Acute necrotizing pancreatitis
   f. Celiac disease: In this case, the causes are villus atrophy and impaired production of cholecystokinin and pancreozymin.
6. Following are the tests for pancreatic exocrine efficiency:
   a. Coefficient of fat absorption
   b. Measurement of feces over 3 days after fat-controlled diet
   c. Breath test with ^{13}C-labeled triglyceride breath test
   d. Estimation of pancreatic secretion volume with secretin-MRCP
   e. Direct sampling of duodenal content to estimate pancreatic secretion after secretin administration—bicarbonate level of <80 mEq/L is diagnostic.

CASE 82

A 45-year-old heavy smoker and chronic alcoholic patient came to outpatient department with chronic abdominal pain. MRCP demonstrated:

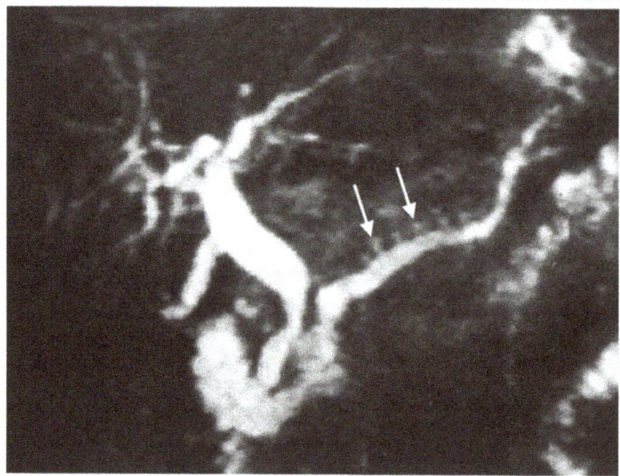

1. **What is demonstrated in MRCP?**
2. **What is the likely diagnosis?**
3. **What can be demonstrated in the CT scan of abdomen in this disease?**
4. **What may be the finding in the ERCP?**
5. **What are the causes of pancreatic pain?**
6. **How can the pancreatic pain be managed?**

Answers

1. MRCP demonstrated alternate constriction and dilatation in the whole length of pancreatic duct looking like "chain of lake" appearance.
2. The most likely diagnosis is chronic pancreatitis.
3. Following features are seen in the CT scan in abdomen:
   a. Calcification
   b. Ductal stones
   c. Abnormal size of the pancreas
   d. Dilated pancreatic duct
   e. Pseudocyst
4. Features in the ERCP are:
   a. Stone in the pancreatic duct
   b. Normal diameter of main pancreatic duct up to 3 mm
   c. Irregularities of the main pancreatic duct and also its side branches
5. Following are the causes of pancreatic pain:
   a. Structural pathology:
      - Pseudocyst
      - Duodenal obstruction
      - Common bile duct pathology
   b. Ductal lesions:
      - Stricture
      - Calculi
   c. Neurogenic pain
6. Pancreatic pain can be relieved by the following ways:
   a. Cessation of alcohol
   b. Cessation of smoking
   c. Pharmacological routes like:
      - Opioid administration
      - Tramadol: It is preferred over morphine because of its fewer gastrointestinal side effect.
      - Gabapentin
      - Antidepressant
      - Anxiolytics
   d. Blocking of the celiac axis

CASE 83

A 57-year-old male has been admitted with painless jaundice, pruritus, deep yellow-colored urine, and progressive weight loss. He has a history of allergy, nasal congestion, and eczema.

Blood report demonstrated raised IgG4. CT scan of the abdomen demonstrated bulky pancreatic head. Pancreatic duct is irregular with distal obstruction of common bile duct and bilateral enlarged kidneys and localized lymphadenopathy.

1. **What is your likely diagnosis?**
2. **What are the features of this disease?**
3. **What are the other conditions where IgG4 may be elevated?**
4. **Wat are the typical features of this disease?**
5. **What is the main therapy in this disease?**

Answers

1. The most likely diagnosis is type 1 autoimmune pancreatitis in case of IgG4-related diseases.
2. This disease is fibroinflammatory mass-like lesion involving different organs in the body mainly in male with history of atopy.
3. In the following conditions IgG4 may be elevated:
   a. Malignancy
   b. Many inflammatory conditions
   c. 5% healthy individuals
4. Following features can be seen in the pancreas in this disease:
   a. Diffuse sausage-shaped pancreas
   b. In half of the patients discrete mass in the pancreatic head
5. The main drug in this disease is prednisolone as this disease is steroid responsive. Rituximab can be given in case of relapse or side effects of steroid.

CASE 84

A 40-year-old man was admitted in the emergency with recurrent episodic upper abdominal pain, postprandial vomiting, and progressive weight loos. On examination, epigastric region is tender. Blood examination demonstrated leukocytosis, ALT 55 IU/L, ALP 122 IU/L, bilirubin 1.5 mg/dL, and amylase 188 IU/L. CA 19-9 and IgG4 are within normal limits.

CT scan of abdomen demonstrated that second portion of the duodenum is abnormally enhanced with focal thickening of the wall and pancreatic head is enlarged.

Endoscopy and histology from this part demonstrated:

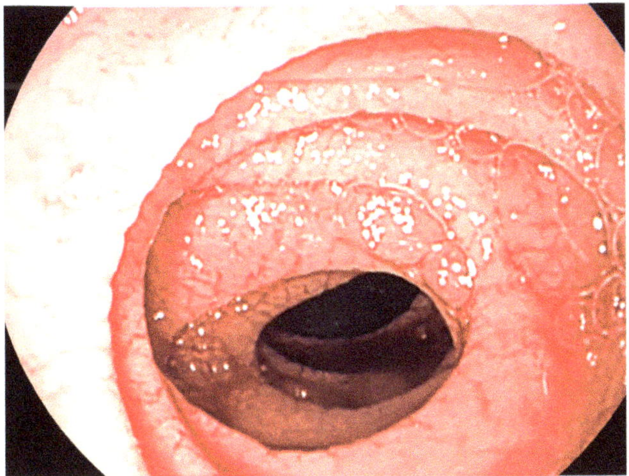
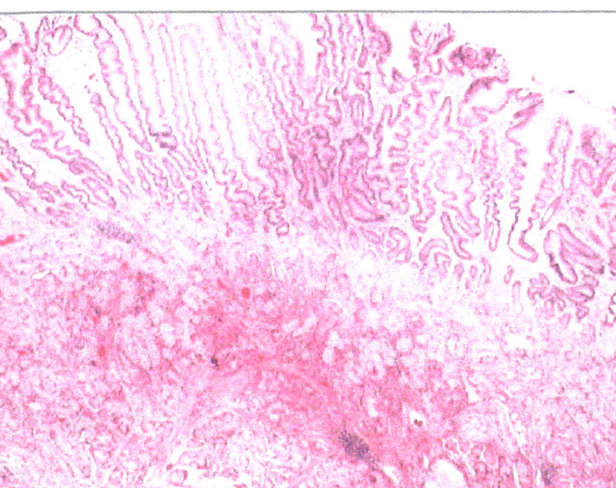

1. **What are the findings in the above pictures?**
2. **What is your most likely diagnosis?**
3. **What are the common characteristics of this disease?**
4. **What are the typical histological pictures in this disease?**
5. **What is the treatment of choice in this disease?**

Answers

1. Description of the above pictures:
    a. Endoscopic picture demonstrated stenosis with edematous wall in the first and second part of the duodenum.
    b. Histology from the duodenal second part demonstrated hyperplasia of the Brunner's gland with evidence of multiple spindle cells.
2. It is paraduodenal pancreatitis or groove pancreatitis—an uncommon variety of segmental pancreatitis.
3. Following are the characteristics of this disease:
    a. It affects groove in-between the duodenal wall and pancreatic head and common bile duct. Sometimes, this disease surrounds the minor ampulla and accessary duct.
    b. It will affect the males of 40–50 years of age.
    c. There may be a history of abuse of alcohol.
    d. Blood biochemical and serological pictures are similar to described above.
4. Typical histological pictures:
    a. Duodenal wall cysts
    b. Hyperplasia of Brunner's gland
    c. Dilatation of Santorini's duct
    d. Protein plaques in the pancreatic duct
5. Treatment of choice is pancreatoduodenectomy.

CASE 85

An 85-year-old nonalcoholic hypertensive and nondiabetic patient has been admitted in gastroenterology unit with painless progressively increasing jaundice, deep yellow-colored urine, and clay-colored stool. On USG, there is enlarged pancreatic head, dilatation of common bile duct, and intrahepatic biliary canaliculi. On examination, only there is jaundice. Blood biochemistry showed bilirubin 15.7 mg/dL, ALT 100 mg/dL, ALP 580 IU/L, and CA 19.9 857 U/mL. PET scan demonstrated:

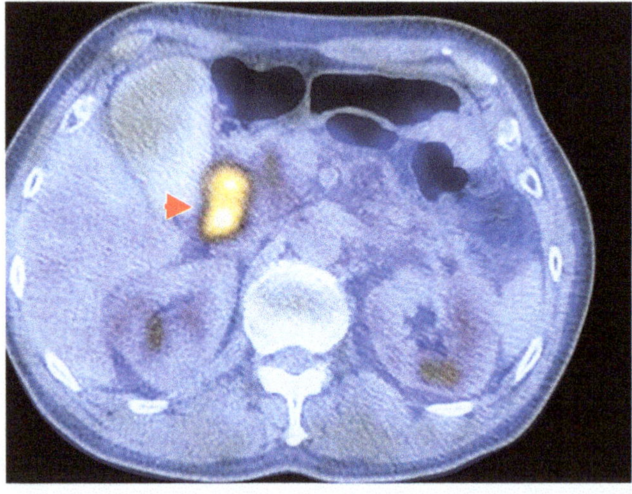
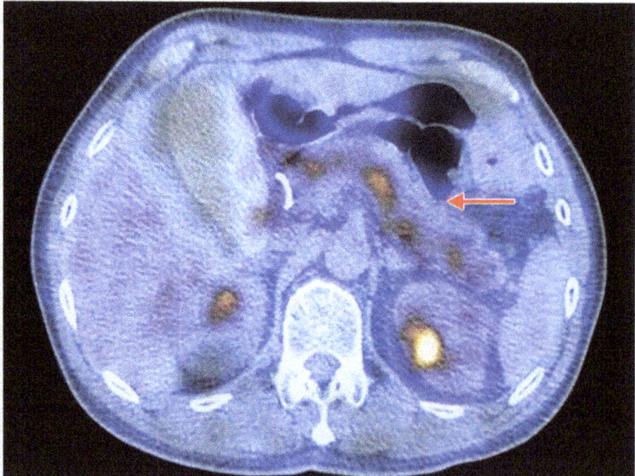

1. **What is the PET-CT demonstrated above?**
2. **What is your diagnosis?**
3. **What are the family history-related risk factors for this disease?**
4. **What is CA 19-9?**

5. With which blood group is this antigen related?
6. Which Lewis blood group does not contain this CA 19-9?
7. What are the causes where CA 19-9 is elevated?
8. Does this antigen have any prognostic value?
9. Describe the stage of this disease.

Answers

1. PET-CT demonstrated intense hypermetabolic areas in the pancreatic head and tail and focally in the peripancreatic area. There is absence of extrapancreatic lesion.
2. The diagnosis is pancreatic cancer without any extrapancreatic spread.
3. Family-related risk factors are:
   a. Hereditary pancreatitis: It is an autosomal dominant disease.
   b. Pancreatic cancer—7% chance of getting cancer in the first-degree relatives
4. CA 19-9 carbohydrate antigen sialyl Lewis A. It is 86% sensitive and 87% specific for pancreatic cancer.
5. CA 19-9 is related to blood group Lewis antigen. Patient containing Le (α-β+) or Le (α+β-) blood group will express CA 19-9.
6. Lewis blood group Le (α-β-) does not contain this antigen.
7. Any cause of having cholestasis may increase the level of this antigen.
8. After resection of the pancreatic tumor if the level of this antigen does not normalize, it is prognostically poor as any level of ≥500 U/mL is associated with poor prognosis after surgery.

9. TNM staging system:
   a. T1S: Carcinoma in situ
   b. T1: Tumor limited to pancreas, <2 cm in greatest dimension
   c. T2: Tumor limited to pancreas, >2 cm in dimension
   d. Tumor extends into any of the following:
      - Duodenum
      - Bile duct
      - Peripancreatic tissue
   e. Tumor extends into any of the following:
      - Stomach
      - Spleen
      - Colon
      - Adjacent large vessels
   f. N0: No lymph node involvement
   g. N1: Regional lymph node involvement
   h. M0: No distant metastasis
   i. M1: Distant metastasis

Stage I: T1–T2, N0, M0
Stage II: T3 N0, M0
Stage III: T3 N0 M0–T3, N1, M0
Stage IVA: Any T, any N, M0
Stage IVB: Any T, any N, M1

CASE 86

A 28-year-old man has been admitted with severe diarrhea and stool culture detected enteropathogenic *E. coli*. Oral rehydration therapy has been started.

1. Which receptor is involved in oral rehydration therapy and why?
2. What do you mean by transporter?
3. Gastrointestinal infection affects which receptors?
4. Which substances should be added in the novel oral rehydration therapy?
5. In this infection, ORS is helpful or not?
6. What are the other receptors that are present in the colon involved in the electrolytes secretion or absorption?

Answers

1. Sodium–glucose cotransporter 1 (SGLT1) is responsible for sodium and water absorption coupled with glucose, in infectious diarrhea these receptors are preserved.
2. Transporter is the transmembrane protein which mediates ion and other solute transport.
3. Gastrointestinal infections affect both secretory and/or absorptive receptors.
4. In the novel oral rehydration therapy:
   a. Starch should be added as it will help in the absorption of sodium in the colon by providing short-chain fatty acids.
   b. Zinc should be added as it works by alteration of chloride homeostasis
5. In this, enteropathogenic *E. coli* activity of the SGLT1 is inhibited. As a result, the patient is less responsive to oral rehydration therapy.
6. Other receptors in the intestines:
   a. In the distal colon which helps in absorption of sodium will be decreased in infection with murine *Salmonella*.
   b. NKCC1: It is present on the basolateral wall of the colon and supplies chloride ion for secretion. Expression of this transporter will be increased in *Salmonella* and *E. coli* infections.
   c. Cystic fibrosis transmembrane conductance regulator (CFTR) receptors present in the apical surface of the intestinal epithelial cells and are responsible for efflux of sodium.
   d. GLUT1: It is responsible for glucose transport. It has no role in the ORS absorption.

CASE 87

A 40-year-old man has been admitted with a 6-month history of severe diarrhea with abdominal bloating sensation in spite of fasting. On examination, the patient was dehydrated and flushed. Blood tests demonstrated serum potassium 1.9 mEq/L, sodium 145 mEq/L, creatinine 1.5 mg/L, and urea 160 mg/dL. Fecal osmotic gap is <50 mOsm/kg.

1. **What is your likely diagnosis and why?**
2. **What are the classical pictures of this disease?**
3. **What is the classical history of this disease?**
4. **How is the diarrhea produced?**
5. **What is the main pathophysiology in this disease?**
6. **How is this disease confirmed?**
7. **What are the images required for this disease?**
8. **What are the management strategies in this case?**

Answers

1. The diagnosis is VIPoma because the classical pictures of this disease are:
   a. Secretory diarrhea
   b. Hypokalemia
   c. Dehydration
2. The classical pictures of the disease are:
   a. Secretary diarrhea of >3 L/day in spite of prolonged fasting
   b. Hypokalemia having level of <3 mEq/L
   c. Hyperglycemia
   d. Hypercalcemia
   e. Hypochlorhydria
   f. Signs of dehydration
   g. Facial flushing
3. This is neuroendocrine non-β islet cell tumor originating from pancreas in 90% of cases, more in women having age in-between 30 and 50 years.
4. Vasoactive intestinal polypeptide stimulates secretion of fluid and electrolytes from the intestinal epithelium and cholangiocytes in the bile duct.
5. This tumor stimulates intestinal cyclic adenosine monophosphate and gastric acid. It will also promote:
   a. Vasodilatation
   b. Glycogenolysis
   c. Lipolysis
   d. Bone resorption
6. Disease is confirmed by measuring the serum level of vasoactive intestinal polypeptide.
7. Following imaging studies are done for diagnosis of this disease:
   a. Contrast-enhanced CT scan of abdomen for localization of the disease
   b. MRI in case of indeterminate lesion or to detect metastases

c. Somatostatin receptor angiography by using radiolabeled octreotide or lanreotide to detect occult metastases within or outside the abdomen

d. Endoscopic ultrasound to detect accurate extent of the disease

8. Following are the management schedule:

a. Management of the fluid and electrolytes

b. Inhibition of secretion of octreotide or lanreotide

c. Glucocorticoid, if the patient is refractory to somatostatin analog

d. Interferon-α, in case of nonresponder to somatostatin analog and glucocorticoid

e. Complete surgical resection in the form of distal pancreatectomy to dissect primary tumor

f. Treatment of the metastatic areas

CASE 88

A 38-year-old man came to outpatient department with long-lasting diarrhea and wants to know regarding the gut hormones.

What are the gut hormones? Mention their names with its site of production.

Answer

Name	Site of production	Stimulation	Action
Glucagon-like peptide 1	L cell of small intestine	Ingested carbohydrate	• Inhibits gastric emptying glucagon release • Appetite • Stimulates glucose-dependent release of insulin
Glucagon-like peptide 2	L cells in the small intestine	Ingested carbohydrate	• Inhibits gastric emptying • Gastric acid production • Stimulates growth of small bowel mucosa • Increases mesenteric blood flow
Cholecystokinin	I cells in the small intestine	Ingested food and protein	• Stimulates contraction of gallbladder • Delays gastric emptying
Gastrin	G cells in the stomach	• High pH • High-grade gastric distention • Histamine • Amino acid • Acetylcholine	• Stimulates production of gastric acid • Gastric hypertrophy
Somatostatin	D cells in the stomach, small intestine, and pancreas	• Gastrin • Gastric acid • VIP • Low-grade gastric distention • Acetylcholine	• Inhibits production of gut hormones • Production of gastrin • Reduces pancreaticobiliary secretion • Reduces gastrointestinal motility • Contraction of gallbladder

CASE 89

A 40-year-old obese doctor came to obesity clinic. On examination, his body mass index (BMI) is 35 kg/m^2. He wanted to know about the obesity from you. What is your opinion regarding leptin?

1. **What is leptin?**
2. **Where is it found?**
3. **What is the function of this hormone?**
4. **In obese patient, what is the condition of leptin?**

Answers

1. Leptin, a satiety hormone of LEP gene in obese patient. It will be increased in response to eating.
2. It is found
   a. In the fat cells
   b. In the placenta
   c. In the breast milk
3. It produces a signal to the brain in response to increased fat mass leading to increased level in the serum. It will reduce the food intake through:
   a. Decreased expression of neuropeptide Y in hypothalamus
   b. Increased transcription of pro-opiomelanocortin as well as α-melanocyte-stimulating hormone
4. Following are the conditions of leptin in obese man:
   a. In case of mutation or abnormalities of leptin gene leading to complete deficiency of leptin and it is associated with hyperphagia resulting in obesity.
   b. Resistance to supraphysiological dose of leptin in case of obesity in spite of increased concentration of leptin.

CASE 90

A 49-year-old obese man presented with BMI level of 40 kg/m^2 prior to bariatric surgery. He has given his consent to the research study regarding ghrelin.

1. **What is ghrelin?**
2. **From where is it secreted?**
3. **When is it secreted and decreased?**
4. **What is the function of ghrelin?**
5. **What is the relation of ghrelin with obesity?**
6. **What will be the fate of ghrelin after gastric bypass surgery?**

Answers

1. Ghrelin is a satiety hormone.
2. It is secreted from the:
   a. Oxyntic glands in the fundus
   b. Duodenum
   c. Pancreas
   d. Pituitary gland
   e. Kidney
3. It is secreted in response to fasting having a surge before meals during cephalic phase and falls in response to carbohydrate food as compared to protein or fat.
4. Ghrelin:
   a. Increases the gastric emptying
   b. Increases the secretion of growth hormone from the pituitary gland affecting the bone metabolism
5. There is an inverse relationship between the serum level of ghrelin and obesity. So, in case of obesity, postprandial level of ghrelin will be impaired.
6. After gastric bypass surgery like sleeve gastrectomy:
   a. Serum ghrelin level will be lowered.
   b. There is no premeal surge of ghrelin.

   As a result, there will be an improved balance of energy after bariatric surgery.

CASE 91

A 7-year-old boy has been admitted with abdominal pain with distention, nausea, and progressive weight loss. His upper and lower gastrointestinal endoscopy and abdominal sonography were normal. His blood biochemistry and stool examination were within normal limit.

1. **What is the next investigation should be done?**
2. **What is the aim of that investigation?**
3. **What are the other methods of investigation that can be done and what is the difference from the previous one?**

Answers

1. Catheter-based manometry using multiple pressure sensors most accurately measure the small bowel contractility pattern in the form of amplitude and propagation. In this method, sensor is placed in the duodenum or proximal jejunum to measure the physiology of the whole small bowel.

2. The above method will provide the information regarding the neuropathic versus myopathic pattern.

3. Following are the methods that are used for intestinal motility:

   a. Wireless motility capsules will provide information regarding the amplitude of contraction at a given point in the small bowel but cannot provide the information regarding the propagation of contractions. It can provide information regarding propagation through the pylorus and ileocecal valve thereby small propagation can be calculated.

   b. Small bowel scintigraphy can accurately measure the transit but is lacking in standardization.

   c. Lactulose hydrogen breath test can provide information regarding the small bowel transit.

CASE 92

A 30-year-old single mother has been admitted with history of intermittent abdominal pain with alternate constipation and diarrhea for the last 20 years. She had no history of vomiting, weight loss, unremarkable past medical or surgical or drug history. Physical examination is normal. Routine laboratory tests including complete blood count, blood glucose, and metabolic panel are all normal. Upper and lower gastrointestinal endoscopy and small bowel enteroscopy were normal.

1. **What is your diagnosis?**
2. **How can you classify the diagnosis?**
3. **Define criteria of your diagnosis?**
4. **What are the types of stool in this disease usually?**
5. **What are the other symptoms unrelated to intestine?**
6. **What are the risk factors here for this diagnosis?**
7. **What are the conservative treatments for this disease?**

Answers

1. The most likely diagnosis is IBS.

2. Classification of IBS:

   a. IBS-C: Constipation with abnormal movement of the bowel (Bristol stool scale type 1 and 2 in >25% and type 6 and 7 in <25% of bowel movements)

   b. IBS-D: Diarrhea due to abnormal bowel movement (Bristol stool scale type 6 and 7 in >25% and type 1 and 2 in <25% of bowel movements)

   c. IBS-M: Alternate constipation and diarrhea (Bristol stool scale 1 and 2 in >25% and type 6 and 7 in >25% of bowel movement)

   d. Unclassified IBS: It will meet the diagnostic criteria for IBS but cannot be categorized to any of the previous subtypes.

3. Rome criteria IV:

   At least 1 day per week of recurrent abdominal pain or discomfort associated with two or more of the following criteria with symptom onset for at least 3 months:

   a. Related to defecation which is either increasing or improving pain.

   b. Associated with change in the frequency of stool

   c. Associated with change in the form of stool

4. Types of stool has been classified according to the Bristol stool scale:

   a. Type 1: Separate hard lump like nuts

   b. Type 2: Sausage-shaped but lumpy

   c. Type 3: Like sausage but there are cracks on the surface

   d. Type 4: Like sausage or snake, smooth and soft

   e. Type 5: Soft blobs with clear-cut edges

   f. Type 6: Fluffy pieces with ragged edges and a mushy stool

   g. Type 7: Watery, no solid pieces, entirely liquid

5. Following symptoms unrelated to intestine:

   a. Migrain headache

   b. Fibromyalgia

   c. Sleep disturbances

   d. Anxiety

   e. Depression

   f. Chronic pelvic pain

6. Risk factors for the diagnosis: Since the patient is single mother. So, anxiety or depression is the risk factor here.
7. There are different types of treatment in different types of IBS:

Constipation–predominant IBS	
Psyllium husk	3.4 g twice daily after meals
Magnesium hydroxide	2–4 tablespoonful daily
Lactulose	10–20 g twice daily
Polyethylene glycol	17 g to be dissolved in one glass of water and to be taken once or twice daily
Tegaserod	6 mg twice daily
Cisapride	5–10 mg before meals
Lubiprostone	8 µg twice daily after meals
Linaclotide	290 µg once daily
Plecanatide	3 mg once daily

Continued

Continued

Diarrhea–predominant IBS	
Loperamide	2–4 mg once daily
Diphenoxylate	1 tablet 3–4 times daily
Alosetron	1 mg twice daily
Cholestyramine	4 g with each meal
Eluxadoline	100 mg twice daily
For abdominal pain	
Smooth muscle relaxants like mebeverine hydrochloride, dicyclomine, and hyoscine	1–3 times daily before meals
Tricyclic antidepressants (amitriptyline and clomipramine)	10–50 mg at night
Serotonin reuptake inhibitors (fluoxetine, sertraline, and escitalopram)	10–15 mg once daily

CASE 93

A 46-year-old man suffering from functional abdominal pain has been nonresponsive to antispasmodic, antidepressants, and hypnotics.

1. **What should be prescribed in this patient?**
2. **What are the general measures for management of functional abdominal pain?**
3. **What are the sites of dysfunction of brain–gut axis?**
4. **What is the stepwise management of functional abdominal pain?**
5. **Which drug should be avoided in this type of pain?**

Answers

1. Gabapentin
2. Following are the general measures of functional abdominal pain:
   a. Validation of symptoms
   b. Education of underlying condition
   c. Setting of achievable goals
3. Dysfunction of the brain–gut axis occurs at the following levels:
   a. Peripheral sensitization in case of postinfectious IBS
   b. Central sensitization at spinal dorsal horn
   c. Descending modulation of pain pathways from the brain
4. Stepwise management of functional abdominal pain:
   a. First line of management: Low-dose amitriptyline at night
   b. Second line of management: Serotonin nonadrenergic reuptake inhibitors such as duloxetine and venlafaxine
   c. Psychological therapies:
      - Cognitive behavioral therapy
      - Relaxation therapy
      - Hypnotherapy
      - Stress management
   d. Gabapentin and pregabalin act in the pain-signaling axis in the central nervous system
5. Opioids should be avoided in functional abdominal pain as there is risk of:
   a. Hyperalgesia
   b. Narcotic bowel syndrome
   c. Psychological dependence

CASE 94

You have been directed to give advice to a group of patients with celiac disease. What will be your advice regarding the gluten-free drink?

1. **What are the drinks not gluten free?**
2. **Which drinks are gluten free?**
3. **Which grains are to be avoided?**
4. **In the gluten-free diet, what is the amount of gluten present?**

Answers

1. Following drinks are not gluten free:
   a. Barley water
   b. Squash
   c. Malted milk drink
   d. Beers
   e. Ales
   f. Lagers
   g. Stouts
2. Following drinks are gluten free:
   a. Wine
   b. Spirits
   c. Sherry
   d. Cider
   e. Port
3. Following grains are avoided:
   a. Bulgur wheat
   b. Semolina
   c. Spelt
   d. Wheat
   e. Rye
4. In the gluten-free diet, 20 parts per million or fewer gluten is present.

CASE 95

A 28-year-old patient diagnosed with celiac disease 14 years back has come to gastroenterology clinic with persistent abdominal pain, alteration of bowel habit, and bloating. His had histology of the duodenal mucosa 12 years back. He has no nutritional deficiency. His recent histology from the duodenal mucosa has been demonstrated as below:

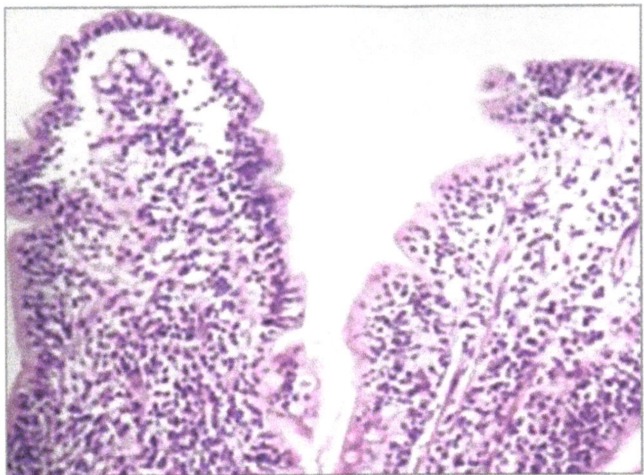
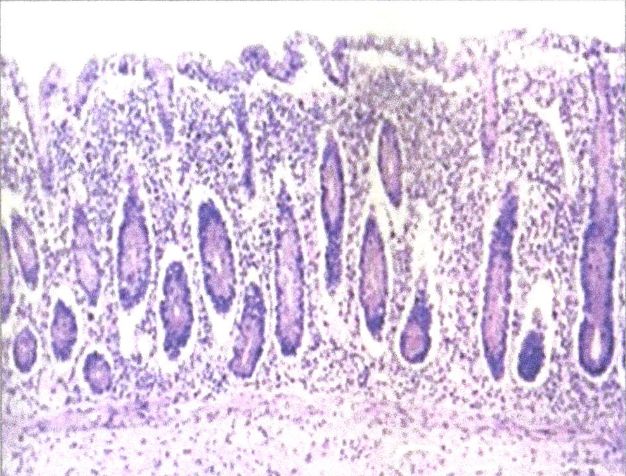

1. **Describe the above histology from the duodenal mucosa.**
2. **Describe this histological classification.**
3. **Is the histology improved with gluten-free diet?**
4. **What is your diagnosis and why?**

Answers

1. Two histology from the duodenal mucosa demonstrated:
   a. Left one demonstrated total villus atrophy
   b. Right one demonstrated intraepithelial lymphocytosis and absence of villus atrophy
2. Histological classifications (Marsh classification) from the duodenal mucosa:

Classifi-cation	Description	Intraepithe-lial lympho-cytosis	Hyper-plasia of crypt	Villus atrophy
Marsh 0	Normal	No	No	No
Marsh 1	Intraepithelial lymphocytosis	Yes	No	No
Marsh 2	Intraepithelial lymphocytosis and cryptic hyperplasia	Yes	Yes	No

Continued

Continued

Classifi-cation	Description	Intraepithe-lial lympho-cytosis	Hyper-plasia of crypt	Villus atrophy
Marsh 3A	Partial villus atrophy	Yes	Yes	Yes (partial)
Marsh 3B	Subtotal villus atrophy	Yes	Yes	Yes (subtotal)
Marsh 3C	Total villus atrophy	Yes	Yes	Yes (total)

3. Yes, after 6–12 months intake of gluten-free diet, histological changes improve, but intraepithelial lymphocytosis will be present.
4. It is a postceliac disease IBS as there is vitamin deficiency, resolution of villus atrophy in presence of bowel habit alteration and persistent bloating.

CASE 96

A 30-year-old man with celiac disease complained in the medicine outpatient department with backache and bone pain. X-ray of the pelvis demonstrated as below:

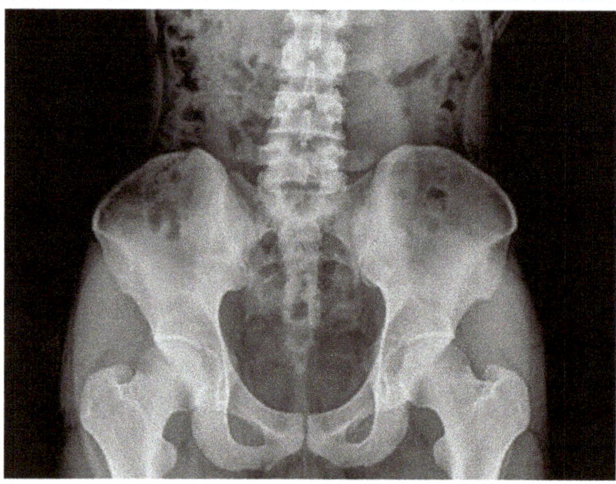

1. **What is demonstrated in the straight X-ray of pelvis?**
2. **What is the metabolic panel that should be investigated in this disease?**
3. **What is the screening method that should be done in this disease?**

Answers

1. X-ray of the pelvis demonstrated evidence of osteoporosis.
2. Following metabolic panel should be investigated:
   a. Serum ionic calcium
   b. Vitamin D
   c. Serum ALP
3. Screening method:
   a. In case of osteopenia and osteoporosis, DEXA scan should be done every 2–3 years.
   b. In case of normal bone density, DEXA should be done every 5 years.

CASE 97

A 55-year-old female having history of parathyroidectomy and resection of the pituitary microadenoma developed abdominal pain with bloating and vomiting and diarrhea. She has also a history of wheezing and facial flushing. Her upper and lower gastrointestinal endoscopy were normal. CT enterography demonstrated presence of mass in the mid ileal region. There are also some lesions in the liver.

1. **What is your diagnosis?**
2. **What are the features of this disease?**
3. **What is the cause of facial flushing?**
4. **What are the other features of that disease that also cause facial flushing?**
5. **What investigation should be of choice to confirm that specific cause?**
6. **What restriction should be maintained to prevent the false positivity of that test?**
7. **What are the specific markers of this tumor?**

Answers

1. The diagnosis is MEN1.
2. The following features of this tumor are:
   a. Parathyroid tumor
   b. Pancreatic tumor
   c. Anterior pituitary tumor
3. The cause of facial flushing is a carcinoid tumor.
4. Other features of this carcinoid tumor are:
   a. Wheezing
   b. Facial flushing
   c. Diarrhea
5. The investigation to confirm the diagnosis of carcinoid tumor is 24 hours urinary excretion of 5-HIAA to measure the end product of serotonin metabolism.
6. Patient should avoid following serotonin/tryptophan-rich food to prevent false positivity of the test:
   a. Kiwi fruit
   b. Pineapple
   c. Walnuts
   d. Aubergine
7. Following are the specific markers of this MEN type 1:
   a. Chromogranin A
   b. Chromogranin B
   c. Chromogranin C

CASE 98

A 50-year-old chronic alcoholic patient taking 160 units of alcohol weekly has been admitted in the emergency department with severe diarrhea passing 6–8 times daily. He has disorientation. On examination, mental test score is 4/10. Neurological examination is normal other than disorientation and no nystagmus or ophthalmoplegia. Skin lesion demonstrated the following:

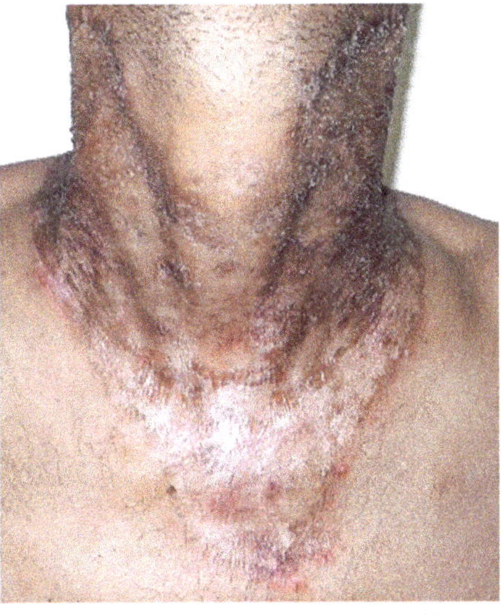

1. **What is the lesion seen in the above picture?**
2. **What is your diagnosis?**
3. **What are the features of your diagnosis?**
4. **Why is it uncommon in well-developed countries?**
5. **What is the cause of this disease in this patient?**

Answers

1. There is evidence of photosensitive erythematous rash in the neck in the "V"-shaped distribution.
2. The most likely diagnosis is niacin deficiency.
3. Following are the features in favor of the diagnosis:
   a. Dermatitis
   b. Dementia
   c. Diarrhea
   d. If untreated death
4. It is not an endemic disease because in the developed countries the patient takes meat, mushrooms, fish, peanut and yeast, and fortified cereals.
5. This is common in alcoholic because the patient will suffer from nutritional deficiency or malnutrition.

CASE 99

A 42-year-old patient having history of alcoholic excess as well as spondylitis came to outpatient department with loose stool and abdominal bloating. He has been taking long-term trimethoprim to correct recurrent urinary tract infection. Blood test demonstrated hemoglobin 10 g/dL and MCV 110 fl. Folate is low. Ferritin and vitamin B_{12} are normal.

1. **What is the cause of folate deficiency in this patient and why?**
2. **What are the other causes of folate deficiency?**
3. **In what form is folate reabsorbed in the intestine?**
4. **Which is the rate-limiting enzyme for folate metabolism?**
5. **How can you differentiate it from celiac disease?**

Answers

1. The cause of folate deficiency is longtime administration of trimethoprim because this drug will inhibit the dihydrofolate reductase, which will reduce the monoglutamate form absorbed from the intestine to dihydrofolate and then to tetrahydrofolate leading to folate deficiency.
2. Other causes of folate deficiency are:
   a. Dietary deficiency in the context of excess alcohol
   b. Increased folate utilization:
      - Pregnancy
      - Lactation
      - Chronic hemolytic anemia
   c. Malabsorption through the small intestine:
      - Celiac disease
      - Crohn's disease involving small bowel
   d. Medication:
      - Trimethoprim
      - Methotrexate
3. Folate is absorbed in the monoglutamate form from the jejunum.
4. Rate-limiting enzyme is dihydrofolate reductase.
5. In celiac disease, there is associated vitamin B_{12} deficiency as well as iron-deficiency anemia with low ferritin and high CRP. So here isolated folate deficiency is not possible in celiac disease.

CASE 100

A 56-year-old type 2 diabetic female with ischemic heart disease has come to gastroenterology clinic with tingling sensation in the lower limbs and weight loss. She is taking medications such as metformin, aspirin, and PPI. Her blood test demonstrated 9.5 g/dL hemoglobin, MCV 110 fl, folate level 2.6 µg/L, vitamin B_{12} 120 ng/L, and anti-intrinsic factor antibodies are negative.

1. **What is your impression from the above case?**
2. **What is your diagnosis?**
3. **What are the neurological manifestations in this disease?**
4. **What is the cause of peripheral tingling of the lower limbs?**
5. **What is the total stored content of this substance?**
6. **What is the mechanism of deficiency in this case?**

Answers

1. Above history demonstrates:
   a. Low vitamin B_{12}
   b. Low hemoglobin
   c. High MCV
   d. Peripheral tingling involving the lower limb
   e. Absence of the intrinsic factor antibodies in the circulation
   f. Patient is on metformin for diabetes, aspirin for ischemic heart disease, and PPI for gastric mucosal protection.
2. The most likely diagnosis is megaloblastic anemia with peripheral neuropathy due to long-term metformin and PPI intake.
3. Neurological manifestations in case of vitamin B_{12} deficiency are:
   a. Peripheral neuropathy
   b. Subacute combined degeneration of the spinal cord

4. S-adenosyl methionine is required for methyl donor in the synthesis of polyamine as well as transmethylation reaction which is responsible for myelin synthesis and maintenance. So, deficiency of S-adenosylmethionine leads to abnormal methylation of the phospholipid like phosphatidylcholine resulting in abnormal neuronal conduction which ultimately leads to myelopathy and encephalopathy.

   Another active form of cobalamin, adenosylcobalamin, acts as mitochondrial cofactor in the conversion of L-methylmalonyl-CoA to succinyl-CoA. So in case of vitamin B_{12} deficiency, there is increased amount of L-methylmalonyl-CoA which ultimately forms methylmalonic acid which is responsible for abnormal myelination leading to defective neural transmission.
5. Total stored content of vitamin B_{12} is 2–4 mg.
6. Metformin results in deficiency by altering the calcium homeostasis. PPI produces this deficiency through the gastric acid hyposecretion.

CASE 101

A 78-year-old alcoholic poor man has come to outpatient department with pain and swelling in the right knee without any history of trauma not under any medication. On examination, the following lesions are seen. His hematological test demonstrates low ferritin. Coagulation profiles and urinalysis are normal.

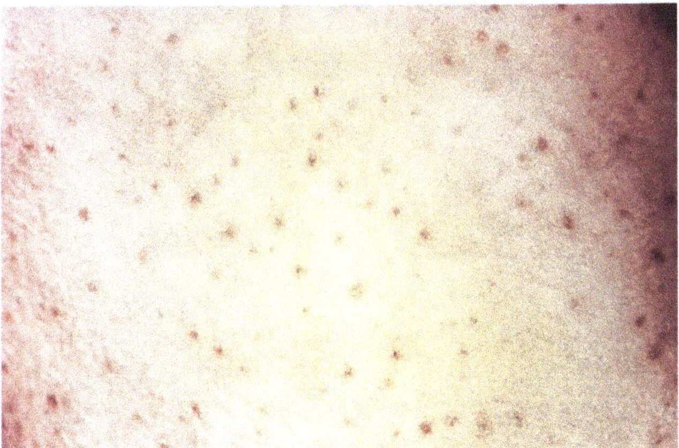
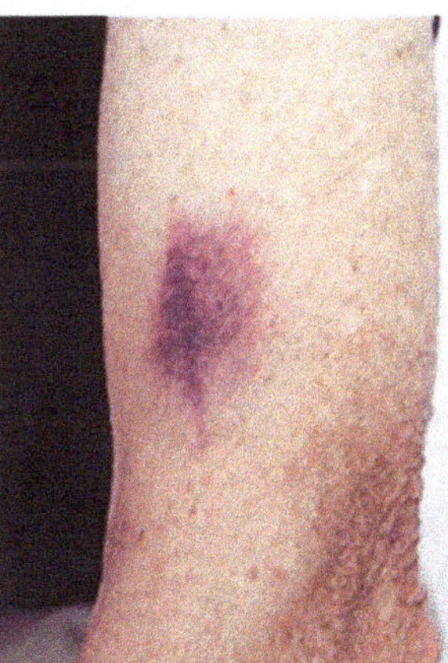
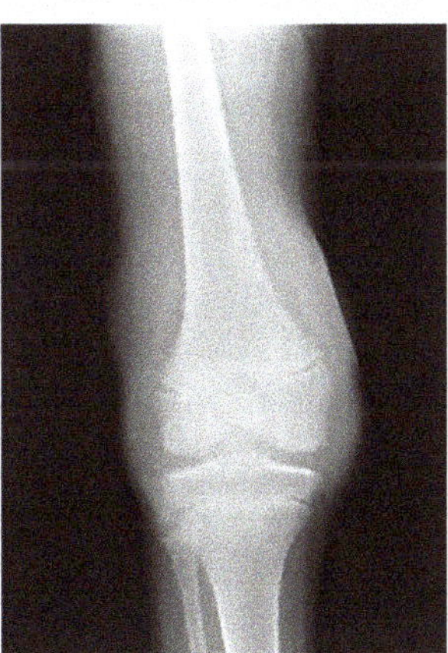

1. **Describe the above pictures.**
2. **What is your likely diagnosis and why?**
3. **What is the pathophysiology behind the above pictures?**
4. **Name the good sources of this nutrient.**
5. **What are the classical signs of this micronutrient?**
6. **What is the mainstay of the diagnosis of this micronutrient?**

Answers

1. The above pictures demonstrated:
   a. Perifollicular hemorrhage
   b. Ecchymoses
   c. Straight X-ray demonstrating the swelling of the joint probably blood
2. The most likely diagnosis is scurvy due to deficiency of vitamin C because of defective collagen synthesis and decreased ferritic because of decreased absorption of iron.
3. The main pathophysiology behind the picture is:
   a. Defective collagen synthesis due to deficient cross-linking in the connective tissue
   b. Defective absorption of iron from the small intestine

4. Good sources of this micronutrient are:
   a. Fruits
   b. Green vegetables
   c. Potatoes
   d. Tomatoes
5. Classical signs of the deficiency of this micronutrient are:
   a. Petechiae
   b. Ecchymoses
   c. Perifollicular hemorrhages
   d. Hemorrhage in the gums
   e. Hemorrhage in the joints
6. Mainstay of the diagnosis is plasma and leukocyte level of vitamin C.

CASE 102

A 35-year-old woman, resident of rural China, has been admitted in cardiac emergency ward with exertional breathlessness and oliguria just after her arrival in India. On examination, there were evidences of congestive cardiac failure, with bilateral basal decreased breath sounds and fine crepitations. According to her family member, there were recent changes in the mood in that patient. Hematological tests and blood biochemistry were normal. Echocardiography demonstrated global reduced systolic function along with left ventricular dyskinesia. Her chest X-ray demonstrated a blunted bilateral costophrenic angle. Her thyroid function test demonstrated thyroid-stimulating hormone (TSH) is high and low T4 and T3.

1. **What is your diagnosis?**
2. **What are the differential diagnoses in this condition?**
3. **What is the probable cause and why?**
4. **What is the pathophysiology behind this condition?**

Answers

1. It is a case of dilated cardiomyopathy which is characterized by cardiomyopathy in a woman of childbearing age.
2. The differential diagnoses are
   a. Selenium deficiency
   b. Thiamine deficiency
3. Selenium deficiency is the most likely cause because in this there is change in mood of that patient and thyroid function was abnormal. In thiamine deficiency, there is no change in mood and thyroid function test is also normal.

4. In the human being, selenium is the important component of:
   a. Selenoprotein
   b. Glutathione peroxidase:
      - Cytosolic glutathione peroxidase prevents the cardiomyocytes from the oxidant damage which will be catebolized by selenoproteins to get maximum effect.
      - It will reduce the production of inflammatory cytokines.
   c. Iodothyronine deiodinase 2—it will convert thyroxine to its more active form triiodothyronine.

So, deficiency of selenium will lead to development of dilated cardiomyopathy and decreased production of thyroid hormone.

d. It also takes part in the cell-mediated immunity and function of natural killer cells.

In severe selenium deficiency, there are changes in the mood and dysfunction of the skeletal muscles.

CASE 103

A 2-year-old child came to outpatient department with abdominal pain, cramping, and diarrhea which worsened after taking milk and ultimately diagnosed as a case of lactose intolerance.

1. **What do you mean by lactase activity?**
2. **What is the most common cause of lactase deficiency in adult?**
3. **Which gene is responsible for this genetic disease?**
4. **Which test can be done in this disease to diagnose?**
5. **What are the cases where this test will be negative?**

Answers

1. Lactase is a disaccharidase enzyme that breaks down the disaccharide into glucose and galactose which will be absorbed readily from the intestinal wall mucosa through active transport by SGLT1 and glucose transporter 2 (GLUT2). Undigested lactose will be acted upon by intestinal bacteria to form methane, hydrogen ion, carbon dioxide, and short-chain fatty acids.

2. In adult, common cause of lactase deficiency is lactase nonpersistence which is a primary genetic disease.

3. Lactase gene presents on the chromosome number 2. If two wild type genes are present in one person, then this person can be considered to have lactase nonpersistence.

4. Lactose-hydrogen breath test: It will measure the hydrogen gas in the expired breath in response to oral lactose load.

5. In following cases, hydrogen breath test will be negative:

   a. Hydrogen nonproducer leading to false negativity
   b. Altered anatomy of the bowel
   c. Small intestinal bacterial overgrowth
   d. Rapid gastrointestinal transit leading to false positivity

CASE 104

A 45-year-old female suffering from progressive systemic sclerosis came to outpatient department with abdominal flatulence, abdominal cramping, and nonbloody stool. Her hematological blood test demonstrated hemoglobin 10 g/dL, MCV 112 fl, folate level 19 μg/L. Colonoscopy and upper gastrointestinal endoscopy were normal, but duodenal mucosal histology only demonstrated intraepithelial lymphocytosis but absence of chronic inflammatory cell in the lamina propria.

1. **What is your most likely diagnosis and why?**
2. **What should be the mode of treatment?**
3. **What are the drugs to be avoided in this case?**
4. **Why is it a case of celiac disease?**
5. **Why is there anemia?**

Answers

1. The most likely diagnosis is small bowel bacterial overgrowth in a case of female with progressive systemic sclerosis. It occurs due to decreased intestinal motility leading to stasis of the bowel content resulting in increased growth of the bacteria.
2. Line of treatment is administration of the antibiotics to address the bacterial overgrowth:
   a. Metronidazole
   b. Co-amoxiclav
   c. Rifaximin
   d. Norfloxacin
   e. Cotrimoxazole
   f. Ciprofloxacin
3. Following drugs should be avoided as they will further decrease the intestinal motility:
   a. Anticholinergics
   b. Opioids
4. It is not a case of celiac disease because in case of duodenal mucosal histology there should be atrophy of the villus and presence of lymphocytes in the lamina propria.
5. As there is increased intestinal bacterial overgrowth, it will hamper the absorption of vitamin B_{12} from the terminal ileum leading to macrocytic anemia.

CASE 105

A 60-year-old male having previous history of ileocecal resection to treat Crohn's disease came to gastroenterology clinic with complaint of nonbloody diarrhea. He has no history of weight loss, anorexia, abdominal pain, fever, and no extraintestinal manifestation. His complete blood count, vitamin B_{12}, and folate level as well as CRP were also within normal limit.

1. **What is the most likely diagnosis?**
2. **Why do you have this diagnosis?**
3. **What are the other causes of bile acid malabsorption?**
4. **How can it be diagnosed?**
5. **Which drug is used in this case?**

Answers

1. The most likely diagnosis is bile acid malabsorption leading to nonbloody diarrhea in a case of ileocecal resection in patient with Crohn's disease.
2. As bile acid is absorbed from the distal ileum, resection of >100 cm of distal ileum will hamper the absorption of the bile acids leading to its entry into the colon resulting in diarrhea.
3. Following are the other causes of bile acid malabsorption:
   a. Primary disease of the terminal ileum
   b. HIV infection
   c. Defect in the synthesis of the bile acids
   d. Defect in the transport of bile acids
4. Bile acid malabsorption can be diagnosed by measurement of 7-day retention of orally administered selenium labeled bile acid.
   a. Retention of 10–15% suggests mild bile acid malabsorption
   b. 5–10% retention suggests moderate bile acid malabsorption
   c. <5% retention suggests severe bile acid malabsorption
5. In this case, bile acid sequestrant cholestyramine is used in this bile acid malabsorption-related diarrhea.

CASE 106

A 35-year-old man presented in outpatient department with joint pain, weakness, and cramping abdominal pain on omeprazole. On examination, patient is anemic. Hematological test demonstrated evidence of iron-deficiency anemia. On further enquiry, he confessed occasional intake of over-the-counter medication. Upper gastrointestinal endoscopy demonstrated multiple superficial duodenal ulcers. MR enterography demonstrated presence of a stricture in the small intestine. Serum gastrin level was normal. Liver function test demonstrated bilirubin, serum glutamic-oxaloacetic transaminase (SGOT), SGPT, and ALP level were normal but serum albumin level is 1.8 g/dL.

1. **What is the most likely diagnosis?**
2. **What are the points in favor of this diagnosis?**
3. **What are the structures affected by NSAIDs?**
4. **Why there is abdominal pain?**
5. **How can you diagnose the etiology?**
6. **How it can be treated?**

Answers

1. The most likely diagnosis is NSAID-induced enteropathy.
2. The tetrad of this diagnosis is:
   a. Iron-deficiency anemia
   b. Small bowel ulceration
   c. Abdominal pain
   d. Hypoalbuminemia due to protein losing enteropathy
3. Following structures are affected by NSAIDs:
   a. Stomach
   b. Duodenum
   c. Jejunum
   d. Ileum
   e. Colon
4. Cramping abdominal pain in this patient is due to partial obstruction of the small intestine due to production of diaphragm like fibrotic stricture.
5. NSAID as an etiology can be diagnosed by:
   a. History of over-the-counter medication
   b. Serum or urinary content of NSAIDs
6. This patient can be treated by:
   a. Withdrawal of the NSAIDs can resolve the intestinal ulceration.
   b. Treatment of anemia
   c. Duodenal ulcers can be treated by PPIs.
   d. Intestinal stricture can be treated by endoscopic dilatation of the intestine or stricturoplasty.

CASE 107

A 40-year-old man with history of Crohn's colitis has been admitted in the hospital with severe exacerbation of this disease which required administration of the hydrocortisone intravenously.

1. **Which is responsible for this exacerbation of inflammation in Crohn's colitis as compared to ulcerative colitis?**
2. **What are the key components of intestinal homeostasis?**
3. **Which cytokines are produced in large amount in Crohn's disease?**
4. **Which cytokine is produced in increased amount in inflammatory bowel disease mucosa?**
5. **What is the function of Th17 cytokine?**

Answers

1. Cytokine driven by dysregulated immune response to microbial and environmental antigen are responsible for cellular interactions in the intestine both in healthy state and in disease.
2. Following factors governed by cytokine network are responsible for maintaining the intestinal homeostasis:
   a. Epithelial barrier function
   b. Host defense pathways
   c. Immune regulation
   d. Tissue repair
   Disruption of this network will lead to inflammation and inflammatory bowel disease subsequently.
3. After being exposed to foreign antigen, $CD4^+$ cells will be activated and differentiate into Th1, Th2, or Th17 cells. Th1 cells produce following cytokines like:
   a. IL-2: It is produced in Crohn's disease in large amount by mucosal T cells indicating significant response.
   b. IL-6
   c. Interferon-γ: It is also produced in increased amount but not in ulcerative colitis. It will induce the production of IL-12 and IL-18.
   d. Tumor necrosis factor-α
4. IL-6 is produced in increased amount in mucosa in case of inflammatory bowel disease which in turn induces:
   a. Activation of immune cells

b. Inhibition of apoptosis: Induction of Th17 cell differentiation

5. Function of Th17:
    a. It produces multiple cytokines like:
        - IL-21
        - IL-22
        - IL-23
    b. It will induce the proinflammatory cytokines through the stimulation of Th1 cells.

CASE 108

A 37-year-old pregnant woman having 15 years history of ileocolic Crohn's disease went to antenatal clinic. Neither she has a family history of Crohn's disease nor her husband.

1. **What are the risk factors of her child having Crohn's disease?**
2. **What are the evidences that prove the genetic susceptibility of the child to develop Crohn's disease?**

Answers

1. Following are the risk factors for developing this disease in the child:
    a. If the first-degree relative is affected.
    b. Genetic susceptibility is greater in Crohn's disease.
    c. If one parent is affected, 9% chance of developing this disease in Crohn's disease.
2. Following are the evidences of genetic susceptibility to this disease:
    a. According to extensive genome-wide association studies, 240 genes are associated with inflammatory bowel disease.
    b. According to the above studies, *ATG16L1* and *IRGM* genes are associated with Crohn's disease and involved in autophagy.
    c. Nucleotide-binding oligomerization domain containing protein-2 is associated with fibrostenosing variety of Crohn's disease. These genes are prevalent in European or Ashkenazi Jewish descent.
    d. *HLA* genes are implicated in the susceptibility as well as severity of Crohn's disease and ulcerative colitis.
    e. Genetic factors are more common if the disease is early in onset.

CASE 109

A 29-year-old nonsmoker man has been admitted with acute exacerbation of ulcerative colitis for which he required infliximab after being nonresponder to intravenous steroid.

1. **What do you mean by acute severe ulcerative colitis?**
2. **What the other causes have to be excluded in this case and how?**
3. **What should be the next step of treatment?**
4. **What is the dose in acute severe ulcerative colitis?**
5. **What are the indications of colectomy?**
6. **What are the types of colectomy usually performed?**

Answers

1. Acute severe ulcerative colitis can be defined as daily six or more bowel movements along with at least any one sign of toxicity:
    a. Tachycardia
    b. Fever
    c. Anemia with hemoglobin level of 10.5 g/dL
    d. Raised inflammatory marker, i.e., erythrocyte sedimentation rate (ESR)—30 mm/1st hour
2. Following causes have to be excluded:
    a. *Clostridium difficile*
    b. *Cytomegalovirus* infection—it should be done by sigmoidoscopy with minimal inflation and taking the biopsy for:
        - Immunohistochemistry staining
        - Rapid viral culture method
        - PCR-based assay
3. One-third of these patients require colectomy

4. In case of acute severe ulcerative colitis:
   a. Single-dose infliximab at 5 mg/kg is the rescue therapy in this patient.
   b. Accelerated dose of infliximab of >5 mg/kg is not more effective as compared to single-dose therapy.
5. Following are the indications of colectomy:
   a. Failure of treatment with glucocorticoids despite other medical therapy
   b. Complications of severe attack
   c. Severe attack which fails to respond to medical intervention
   d. Dysplasia
   e. Carcinoma
   f. Chronic continuous use of the drugs hampering the quality of life
6. Following types of colectomy are performed:
   a. Subtotal colectomy with ileostomy
   b. Proctocolectomy with Brooke ileostomy
   c. Colectomy with ileorectal anastomosis
   d. Proctocolectomy with ileal pouch-anal anastomosis

CASE 110

A 25-year-old man came to the gastroenterology clinic with history of passage of blood and mucus with stool 6–8 times daily along with abdominal pain. He also suffered from recurrent mouth ulcers and has a family history of ankylosing spondylitis. On examination, he has tachycardia, aphthous ulcers in the mouth, and tender right iliac fossa. His leg reveals:

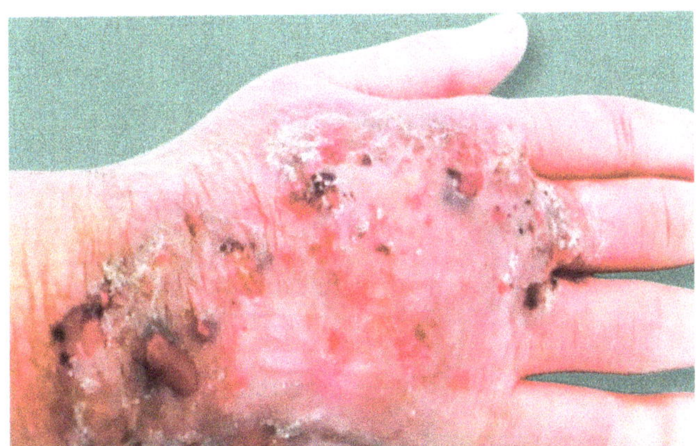

1. **What does the above picture show here?**
2. **What is your diagnosis and why?**
3. **What should be the important investigation that should be done here?**
4. **What should be the findings in the colonoscopy in this disease?**
5. **How can you assess the severity of the disease endoscopically?**

Answers

1. Presence of multiple pustules which are broken down to ulcer having violaceous border or edges with considerable necrosis diagnostic of pyoderma gangrenosum.
2. Diagnosis is acute ulcerative colitis because of the following reasons:
   a. Extraintestinal manifestation like aphthous ulcers in the mouth
   b. Pyoderma gangrenosum
   c. Passage of blood and mucus with stool
3. Important and basic examinations to be done here are:
   a. Stool culture for:
      - *Clostridium difficile*
      - *Escherichia coli* O157:H7
      - *Salmonella*
      - *Shigella*
      - *Yersinia*
      - *Campylobacter*

b. Straight X-ray of abdomen findings:
  - Edematous and irregular margin of the colon
  - Thickening of the wall of the colon
  - Dilated colonic segments in case of toxic megacolon
4. Findings in the colonoscopy are:
   a. Superficial erosions with loss of vascularity and hyperemic mucosa—earliest sign
   b. Granular, friable, and ulcerated lesion with presence of pseudopolyp
   c. No intervening mucosa is normal without any skip areas.

5.

Ulcerative colitis endoscopic index of severity score	Mayo score	Endoscopic features
0	0	Normal
1–3	1	• Erythema • Decreased vascular pattern • Mild friability
4–6	2	• Marked erythema • Absent vascular pattern • Friability • Erosions
7–8	3	• Spontaneous bleeding • Ulcerations

CASE 111

A 35-year-old male presented with periumbilical pain and passage of blood and mucus with stool for 20 days. His colonoscopic findings are the following:

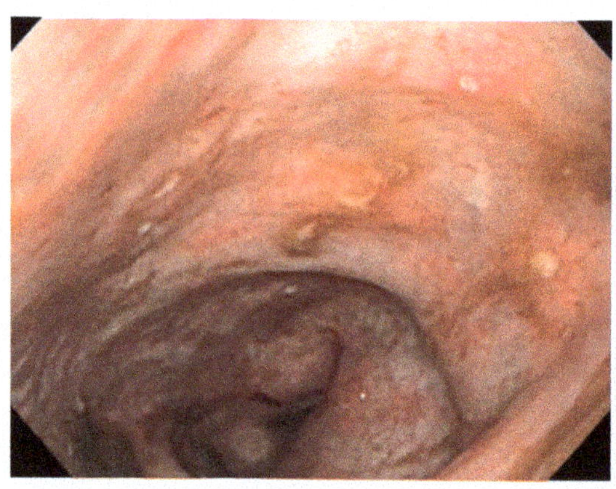
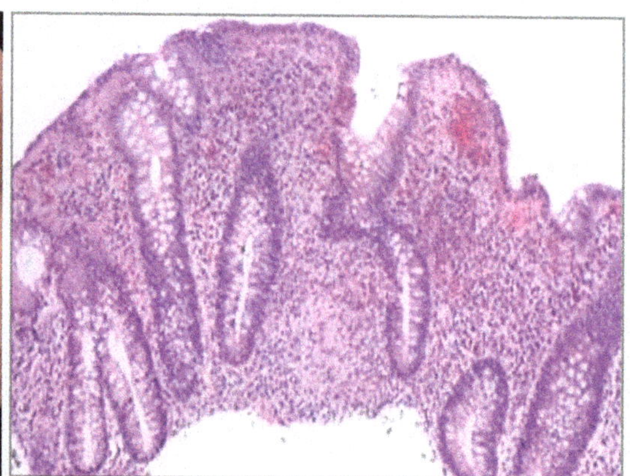

1. **What are the colonoscopy findings?**
2. **What are the biopsy features in this patient?**
3. **What is your diagnosis?**
4. **Which of the Montreal classification stage is consistent with this patient?**
5. **What are the genetic factors associated with this disease?**
6. **What are the environmental factors associated with this disease?**
7. **What are the immunological factors responsible for this disease?**

Answers

1. Colonoscopy demonstrated in the cecum:
   a. Presence of aphthous ulcer
   b. Cobblestoning appearances of the mucosa
   c. Serpiginous ulcer
   d. Stricture in the terminal ileum

2. Biopsy picture demonstrated the following:
   a. Focal inflammatory infiltrates around the crypts
   b. Ulceration of the superficial mucosa
   c. Invasion of the inflammatory cells into the deeper layer of the mucosa
   d. Presence of noncaseating granuloma

3. Diagnosis is Crohn's disease involving the ascending colon and the terminal ileum leading to formation of stricture at the ileocecal junction.
4. The revised Montreal classification stage of Crohn's disease is:
   a. Age at diagnosis (A)
      - A1: 16 years or younger
      - A2: 17–40 years
      - A3: >40 years
   b. Location (L):
      - L1: Terminal ileum
      - L2: Colon
      - L3: Ileocolon
      - L4: Upper gastrointestinal tract (modifier)
   c. Behavior (B): Perianal disease modifier (B):
      - B1: Nonstricturing, nonpenetrating
      - B2: Stricturing
      - B3: Penetrating
      - B4: Stricturing + Perianal
      - B5: Penetrating + Perianal
   In this patient, the stage is A2, L3, and B2.
5. Following genetic factors are associated with Crohn's disease:
   a. First-degree relative of this patient is 20-fold increased risk of developing this disease.
   b. 25% patients with Crohn's disease have family history of inflammatory bowel disease.
   c. Mutation of the following genes involved in the presentation of bacterial antigen as well as innate immune response will lead to development of Crohn's disease:
      - Autophagy-related 16-like 1, i.e., ATG16L1—it may be protective or increased risk for Crohn's disease based on the single nucleotide polymorphism.
      - Nucleotide-binding oligomerization domain containing 2, i.e., NOD2 which is also known as caspase recruitment domain family member 15, i.e., CARD15—here three mutations in the leucine-rich repeats, is associated with increased risk of developing Crohn's disease.

- Immunity-related GTPase, i.e., IRGM is associated with increased risk of Crohn's disease.
- Interleukin-23 receptor, i.e., IL-23R is associated with increased risk of developing Crohn's disease.

6. Following environmental factors are associated with Crohn's disease:
   a. Social class:
      - Upper middle class—increased risk
      - Male bricklayers, security personnel, women involved in the cleaning or maintenance business—lower risk
   b. Smoking—increased
   c. Breastfeeding—protective.
   d. NSAIDs—potential precipitants of this disease
7. Immunological factors and microbial factors:
   a. Loss of barrier in-between the luminal contents and the mucosal epithelium—increase in incidence of inflammation
   b. Intestinal microbes
   c. Depletion of as well as lowered diversity of the members of mucosa associated phyla Firmicutes and Bacteroides is associated with this disease which is known as dysbiosis.
   d. Prominent infiltration of the innate immune cells in the lamina propria:
      - Polymorphonuclear leukocytes
      - Macrophages
      - Dendritic cells
      - Natural killer cells
   e. Adaptive immune cells in the lamina propria:
      - B cells
      - T cells
   f. Elevation of the cytokines and chemokines:
      - Tumor necrosis factor-α
      - Interleukin-1β
      - Interferon-γ
      - Interleukin-23
      - Th17 pathway

CASE 112

A 25-year-old male came to gastroenterology clinic with 20 days history of passage of mucus and blood with stool along with abdominal pain, fever, and backache. His colonoscopy along with biopsy was performed which demonstrated:

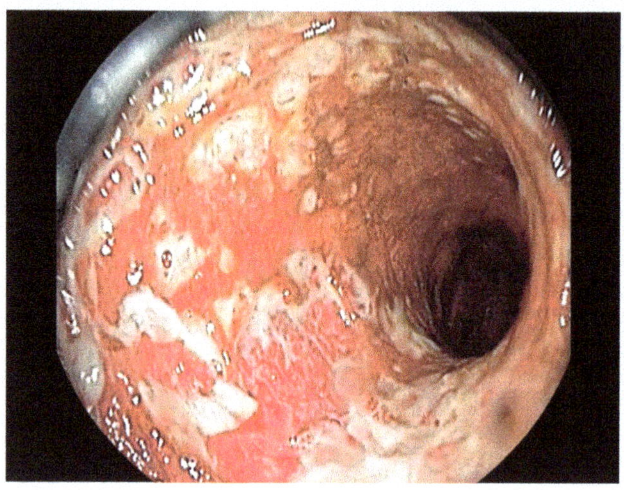
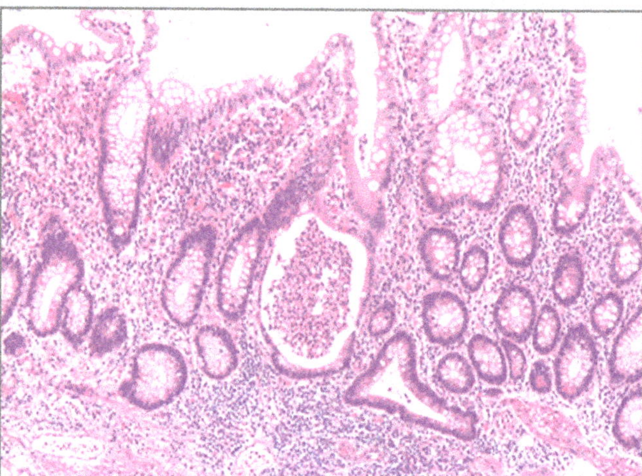

1.   **What are the colonoscopic features in this disease?**
2.   **What are the biopsy features in this picture?**
3.   **What is your diagnosis?**
4.   **What is the main differential diagnosis in this history?**
5.   **How can you differentiate between the two?**
6.   **Is it chronic or active disease and why?**
7.   **What do you mean by quiescent disease?**

Answers

1.   Colonoscopic features:
     a.   Granularity and friability of the colonic mucosa
     b.   No intervening normal mucosa
     c.   Severe hyperemic mucosa with pseudomembrane formation
     d.   Loss of normal vascularity
2.   Histological features in this picture are:
     a.   Expansion of the lamina propria by lympho-plasmocytes infiltration
     b.   Presence of basal lymphoid cellular aggregates
     c.   Distortion of the cryptic architecture
     d.   Cryptic abscess
3.   Diagnosis is acute exacerbation of chronic ulcerative colitis.
4.   Main differential diagnoses are:
     a.   Infective colitis
     b.   Crohn's colitis

5.   Basal plasmacytic infiltration in-between the cryptic bases and the muscularis mucosae is the diagnostic of ulcerative colitis. Absence of granuloma formation excludes Crohn's disease.
6.   This is an acute exacerbation of chronic ulcerative colitis. This is not a case of acute ulcerative colitis because following features are not present:
     a.   Invasion of cryptic epithelium by polymorphonuclear leukocytes leading to cryptitis
     b.   Accumulation of neutrophils within the lumen producing cryptic abscess
7.   Quiescent disease is characterized by absence of neutrophils in the mucosa in presence of chronic mucosal injury:
     a.   Cryptic distortion
     b.   Atrophy of the mucosa
     c.   Paneth cell metaplasia

CASE 113

A 45-year-old female with history of Crohn's disease came to gastroenterology clinic with rectal discharge along with perianal pain and also pain during defecation. Laboratory investigations demonstrated hemoglobin 11.5 g/dL, white blood cell count 12,000/cc, and CEP 70 mg/L.

1. **What is the most likely diagnosis?**
2. **What should be the useful investigation for this diagnosis?**
3. **What other investigation can be performed for diagnosis?**
4. **How can you manage this case?**
5. **Classify this disease.**
6. **How can you treat these fistulae?**

Answers

1. The most likely diagnosis is perianal fistula. It may be associated with perianal abscess as there is associated perianal pain.
2. Contrast-enhanced MRI should be the investigation of choice to diagnose perianal fistulizing Crohn's disease.
3. Endoscopic anorectal ultrasound can also be done provided there is no rectal stenosis.
4. Following is the process of management of perianal fistulae:
   a. Classification of the perianal fistulae
   b. Definite mapping of the fistulae.
   c. Which organ has been affected—it should be determined.
   d. Concurrent disease should be ascertained.
   e. Exclusion of sepsis
   f. Assessment of the general condition of the patient including the morbidities
5. Park classification of perianal fistula:
   a. Intersphincteric anal fistula
   b. Trans-sphincteric anal fistula
   c. Suprasphincteric anal fistula
   d. Extrasphincteric anal fistula

Another classification of perianal fistula:
   a. Simple fistula:
      • Superficial perianal fistula
      • Superficial anovaginal fistula
      • Intersphincteric perianal fistula
      • Intersphincteric anovaginal fistula
   b. Complex fistula:
      • Trans-sphincteric perianal fistula
      • Suprasphincteric perianal fistula
      • Extrasphincteric perianal fistula
      • Enterocutaneous fistula
      • Enteroenteric fistula
      • Enterovesical fistula
      • Rectovaginal fistula
6. Treatment of fistulae:
   a. Simple fistulae in case of Crohn's disease if asymptomatic do not require treatment usually.
   b. Simple fistulae in case of Crohn's disease if symptomatic should be treated by Seton placement along with broad-spectrum antibiotics like metronidazole with or without ciprofloxacin.
   c. Complex perianal fistulae in Crohn's disease should be treated by infliximab or adalimumab along with adequate surgical drainage as these drugs induce and maintain the closure of the fistulae.

CASE 114

A 25-year-old female student with past history of suspected IBS came to gastroenterology clinic with periumbilical pain with weight loss of >4 kg in 2 months but absence of loose motion. Her hemoglobin was 11 g/dL and albumin level 3.4 g/dL.

1. **Which investigation should be done for the diagnosis?**
2. **Which is the investigation of choice in the diagnosis of small bowel pathology?**
3. **What imaging studies should be done in Crohn's disease?**

Answers

1. Ileocolonoscopy should be the first choice as it can directly visualize the mucosa of colon or ileum along with histopathological correlation.
2. Capsule endoscopy should be the investigation of choice in the diagnosis of small bowel Crohn's disease when ileoscopy is unsuccessful.
3. Radiological investigations for the diagnosis of Crohn's disease are:
   a. Small bowel follow-through: It can detect:
      - Stricture or
      - Fistula
      - Cobblestoning pattern, i.e., mucosal edema alternating with ulcerations
   b. Computerized tomography: It can detect:
      - Perforation of intestine
      - Abscesses
      - Fistula
   c. MR enterography: It can detect:
      - Assesses the inflammation in the bowel wall
      - Submucosal inflammation followed by fibrosis
      - Different complications like fistula, perforation, or abscess
      - Small bowel ulceration, stricture, and fistula

      It should be considered in case of woman of childbearing age because the other imaging should not be done.

CASE 115

A 29-year-old female smoker with family history of inflammatory bowel disease came to gastroenterology clinic with 4 months history of periumbilical pain and 4 kg weight loss. On examination, her periumbilical region was tender. Investigation demonstrated hemoglobin level 11 g/dL and albumin 2.3 g/dL. Her abdominal ultrasound was done.

1. **What are the features that can be found in ultrasonography?**
2. **What are the markers of inflammation and what do these indicate?**
3. **What is the advantage of measuring fecal calprotectin level?**
4. **Which serological markers are seen in the serum in this patient?**

Answers

1. Ultrasonographic features in Crohn's disease are:
   a. Mural changes:
      - Thickening of the bowel wall with increased vascularization
      - Stratification of bowel wall is lost.
      - Altered echogenicity of the bowel wall
      - Increased color Doppler signal
      - Lack of peristalsis
      - Prominent submucosal layer
   b. Extramural changes:
      - Mesentery becomes hyperechoic and thickened.
      - Mesentery becomes vascular.
      - Mesenteric nodes become enlarged.
      - Hypertrophy of the mesenteric fat
   c. Complications of Crohn's disease:
      - Fistula
      - Abscesses
      - Stricture
2. Markers of inflammation are:
   a. C-reactive protein
   b. ESR

   Elevation of these markers:
   a. Correlate with clinical, endoscopic, and radiological measures of the existing disease activity
   b. Predict the relapse
   c. Identify the patient who is the person for colectomy because this patient suffers from severe ulcerative colitis.
3. Fecal calprotectin level in Crohn's disease:
   a. >250 µg/g of stool correlates with:
      - Presence of large ulcerations
      - Mucosal healing
   b. >203 µg/g of stool—it will predict the recurrence in postoperative cases of Crohn's disease.
4. Following serological markers are present in the serum of Crohn's disease:
   a. Perinuclear antineutrophil cytoplasmic antibodies (pANCAs)—present in 20% of patient
   b. Anti-saccharomyces cerevisiae antibodies (ASCAs)
   c. Anti-Bir1—it is associated with penetrating small bowel Crohn's disease and fibrostenosing Crohn's disease.
   d. Anti-OmpC

CASE 116

A 30-year-old man was on infliximab 5 mg/kg intravenously 8 weekly, azathioprine 50 mg orally, and 2.4 g mesalazine for acute severe ulcerative colitis for 6 months and was on complete resolution. But after that patient again started semisolid stool mixed with occasional blood four times daily. On investigation, trough level of infliximab was 2.7 µg/mL with undetectable antibodies to infliximab. Fecal calprotectin level was increased up to 850 µg/g of stool.

1. **What should be the next step?**
2. **What should be the recurrence of the disease?**
3. **How the relapse should be treated?**
4. **In what condition, the drug should be changed and why?**
5. **If trough level is normal and antibodies are also detected, in that case what should be the treatment option?**

Answers

1. Next step should be:
   a. Colonoscopy
   b. Fecal calprotectin
   c. CRP level
   d. Imaging studies
2. Here, the trough level of infliximab is low and the antibodies are absent. So, here the dose of the infliximab is inadequate leading to relapse of the disease.
3. So, here the dose of the drug has to be increased.
4. If the antibodies can be detected, in that case the loss of response should be due to immunogenicity to infliximab. In that case, the drug has to be changed to alternative anti-TNF agent or immunomodulator has to be added.
5. If the trough level of the drug is normal and antibodies are absent, in that case inflammation may not be triggered by TNF-mediated pathways, in that case also drug having different mechanism of action should be given for the disease control.

CASE 117

A 75 year-old-man presented with steroid-dependent left-sided ulcerative colitis. You want to start azathioprine. Patient will ask you about this drug.

1. **What is the risk of using this drug?**
2. **Which drug will increase the risk further?**
3. **How does this drug act?**
4. **What is the indication of starting this drug?**
5. **What are pathways of metabolism of this drug?**

Answers

1. This drug is associated with increased risk of lymphoma mainly in elderly.
2. It is an immunomodulator. It is prodrug so this has to be metabolized to 6-thioguanine to exert its effect and it takes at least 3 months to demonstrate its effect.
3. Addition of infliximab will enhance the risk of lymphoma further.
4. Requirement of more than two courses of oral corticosteroids within the span of 12 months
5. Azathioprine will be metabolized to mercaptopurine which in turn is metabolized to following three compounds:
   a. 6-mercaptopurine (inactive form) catabolized by thiopurine methyltransferase (TPMT)
   b. Thiourate (inactive form) catalyzed by xanthine oxidase
   c. 6-thioguanine nucleotide (active form) catalyzed by hypoxanthine-guanine phosphoribosyl transferase.

CASE 118

A 75-year-old morbidly obese woman having history of chronic obstructive sleep apnea and past history of heart failure has been admitted with severe bloody diarrhea of >15 times per day along with abdominal pain. She has a history of NYHA IV heart failure. On examination, her pulse rate was 95 beats/minute and blood pressure was 130/70 mm Hg. Immediately intravenous steroid was started. After the third day of administration, the number of stool was reduced to 3 times/day, pulse rate became 72 beats/minute, temperature was normal, and blood pressure was 120/80 mm Hg.

On the third day, investigation demonstrated hemoglobin level 9.5 g/dL with white blood cell count of 10,000/cc, platelet count of 500,000/cc, but CRP was raised to 50 mg/L.

1. **What is Oxford day 3 criteria?**
2. **Does this patient meet the criteria? If yes, what should be the next step?**
3. **Define acute severe ulcerative colitis.**
4. **What should be the rescue therapy of choice?**
5. **Which is the best combination in this patient?**

Answers

1. Oxford day 3 criteria:
   a. Frequency of stool is ≥9/day
      Or,
   b. CRP is ≥45 mg/L and frequency of stool is 3–8/day.
2. This patient meets the criteria. So in this patient, continuation of steroid therapy is not helpful rather patient should undergo colectomy. Otherwise second-line rescue therapy can be started with the following drugs:
   a. Cyclosporine
   b. Infliximab
3. Acute severe ulcerative colitis can be defined by Truelove and Witts criteria:
   a. Frequency of stool ≥6 times/day plus any one of the following:
      - Tachycardia having >90 beats/minute
      - Temperature of >37.8°C
      - Hemoglobin < 10.8 g/dL
      - Raised ESR or CRP of >30
4. Choice of rescue therapy:
   a. Following are the factors in favor of infliximab:
      - Hypocholesterolemia of <3 mmol/L or hypomagnesemia of <0.5 mmol/L—increased risk of neurotoxicity with this drug
      - Epilepsy
      - Hyperkalemia or hypertension
      - Renal impairment/hepatic impairment
   b. Following are the factors in favor of infliximab:
      - Azathioprine-Inactive in patient
      - Shorter half-life—if more likely to need colectomy
      - History of tuberculosis, hepatitis B, multiple sclerosis of NYHA III or IV heart failure
5. Infliximab is relatively contraindicated in this patient as this patient has a history of NYHA IV heart failure. So, cyclosporine along with thiopurine or vedolizumab as these drugs can be given in elderly.

CASE 119

A 30-year-old man presented with tenesmus, lower abdominal pain, and bloody diarrhea two times per day. Left-sided colonoscopy and histopathology was performed which demonstrated as below:

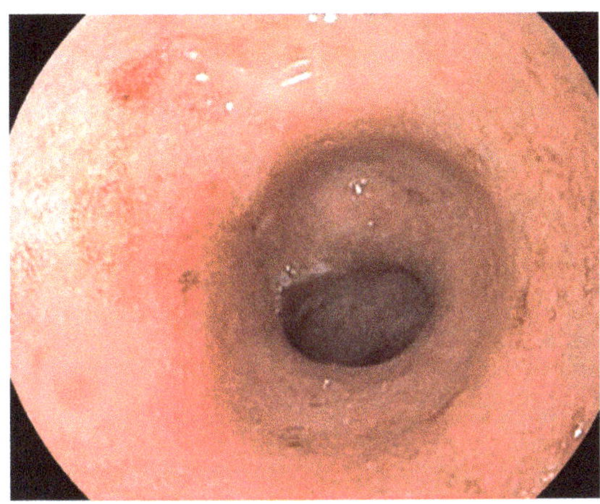 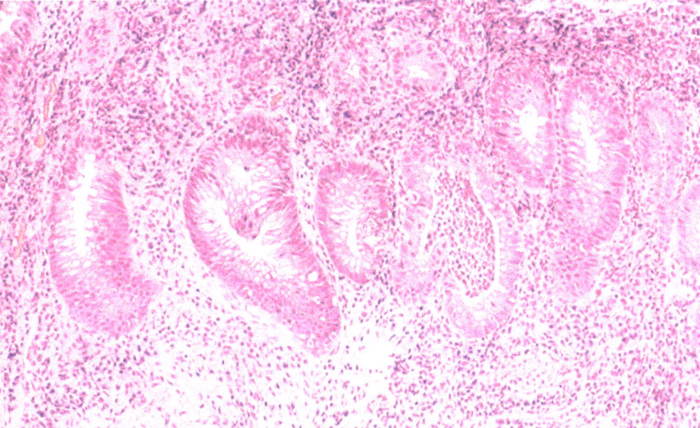

1. **Describe the above pictures.**
2. **What is your diagnosis?**
3. **What is the line of treatment?**
4. **What are the drawbacks in the treatment of above patient?**
5. **What should be the line of treatment in refractory cases?**

Answers

1. Description of colonoscopy—this lesion has been extended to 15 cm from the anus:
   a. Mucosa is granular.
   b. Loss of vascularity
   c. Presence of superficial ulcerations

   Description of histopathology:
   a. Presence of cryptitis
   b. Mucosal expansion by full-thickness lympho-plasmacytosis leading to cryptic dilatation and distortion
   c. Cryptic abscess
   d. Absence of dysplasia
2. Diagnosis is ulcerative proctitis.
3. Treatment to be given is:
   a. Up to 10 cm from the anus, mesalazine suppositories are effective in 90% cases as compared to oral preparation.
   b. Beyond 10 cm from the anus, mesalazine liquid enema is preferred up to splenic flexure.
4. Drawbacks in above treatment:
   a. Acceptability to suppositories or enema
   b. Retention discomfort
   c. Prolonged bed rest
   d. Difficulties in the self-administration
5. In refractory proctitis:
   a. Oral corticosteroids
   b. Immunosuppressive therapies
   c. With or without biological therapies

CASE 120

A 40-year-old woman has undergone proctocolectomy with ileal pouch-anal anastomosis as he was diagnosed inflammatory bowel disease and was refractory to medical therapy. But 7 months later, the patient came to outpatient department with nondiarrhea, tenesmus, and lower abdominal pain. Pouchoscopy was done which demonstrated:

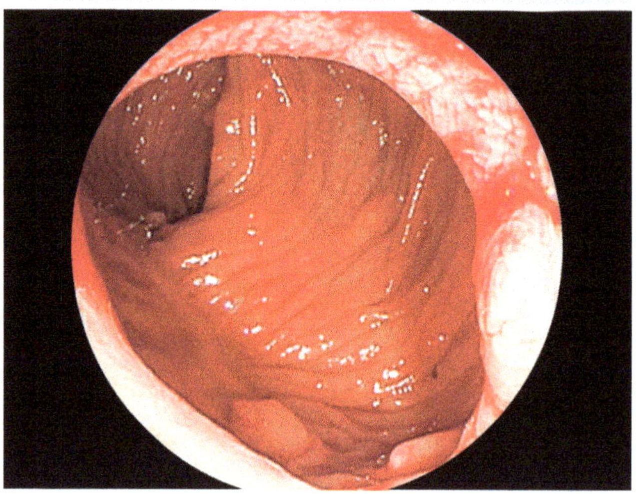

1. **Describe the picture of pouchoscopy.**
2. **What is your diagnosis?**
3. **What are the classical symptoms of pouchitis?**
4. **What are the classical endoscopic features in case of pouchitis?**
5. **What are the future complications of pouchitis?**
6. **What should be the treatment in this case?**

Answers

1. Pouchoscopy demonstrates:
   a. Hyperemic mucosa
   b. Presence of aphthous ulcers
   c. Presence of erosions
   d. Mucosal exudates
2. The diagnosis is pouchitis.
3. Classical pictures of pouchitis are:
   a. Abdominal cramping
   b. Fecal frequency
   c. Tenesmus
   d. Fecal urgency
   e. Pelvic discomfort
4. Classical endoscopic pictures are:
   a. Patchy mucosal erythema
   b. Mucosal friability
   c. Loss of vascular pattern
   d. Mucosal hemorrhage and erosions
5. Following are the complications of pouchitis:
   a. Chronic pouchitis
   b. Peripouch sepsis
   c. Pouch intussusception
   d. Pouch volvulus
   e. Irritable pouch syndrome
6. Treatment of acute pouchitis is short course of antibiotic therapy with probiotic VSL#3 as it will prevent relapse.

CASE 121

A 40-year-old man having 7 years history of ileocecal Crohn's disease has come to gastroenterology clinic with cramping abdominal pain with nausea, weight loos, and vomiting. Colonoscopy was advised and it showed below. CT enterography demonstrated 7 cm long stricture in the terminal ileum involving ileocecal valve along with dilatation of the proximal small bowel.

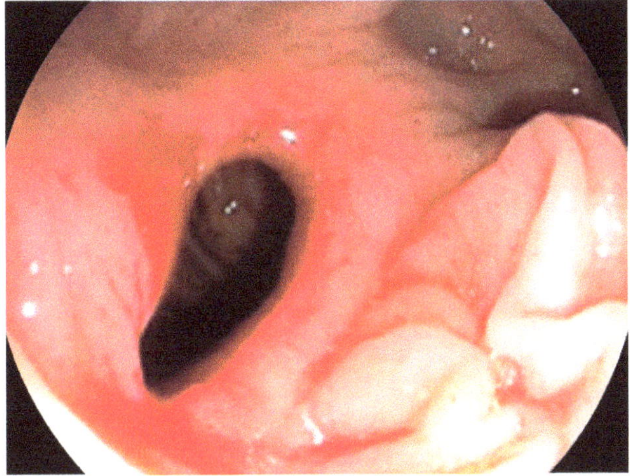

1. **What is the colonoscopic features here?**
2. **What is your diagnosis?**
3. **How can you treat this patient?**
4. **If the patient is malnourished, what should be the line of treatment?**

Answers

1. Colonoscopy demonstrates:
   a. Evidence of narrowing and deformity at the ileocecal junction through which the scope cannot be negotiated into ileal cavity.
   b. Absence of ulcer or erosion in the cecal mucosa
   c. Loss of normal vascularity in the cecal mucosa
2. Diagnosis is stricture at the ileocecal junction without any evidence of active Crohn's disease.
3. Following are the line of treatment:
   a. If the length of the stricture is <5 cm, endoscopic dilatation with or without stenting.
   b. If the length of the stricture is >5 cm, then ileocecal resection is the method of choice.
4. If the patient is malnourished, there should be various types of postoperative complications. To avoid this, two-stage procedure is done:
   a. Resection of the diseased segment with formation of stoma
   b. Delayed restoration of the continuity

CASE 122

A 32-year-old man has been admitted with abdominal pain, bloody diarrhea, and nausea. Colonoscopy demonstrated acute severe ulcerative colitis and being treated with intravenous hydrocortisone. But on the fourth day, patient developed acute abdominal pain and examination showed tachycardia and diffuse rebound tenderness of the abdomen.

His hematological and biochemical investigation demonstrated hemoglobin 8 g/dL, sodium 145 mmol/L, potassium 2.1 mmol/L, magnesium 0.45 mmol/L, and albumin 2.1 g/L.

Straight X-ray abdomen demonstrated:

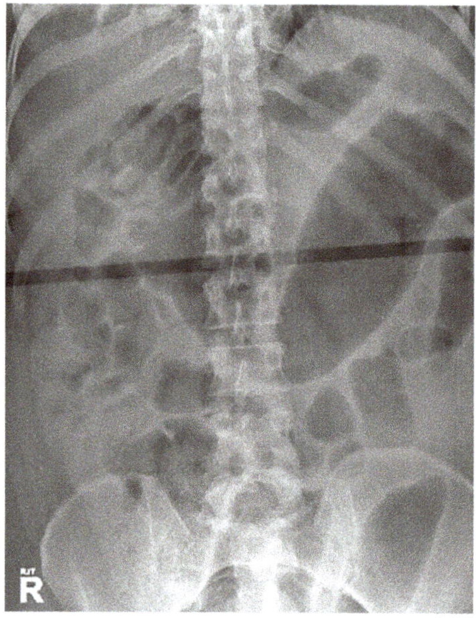

1. **What has been demonstrated in the above straight X-ray of abdomen?**
2. **What is the cause of it?**
3. **What are the causes of this disease?**
4. **What are the risk factors in this disease?**
5. **What is the pathogenesis of this disease?**
6. **What is the definition of this disease?**
7. **What are the criteria of toxic megacolon?**
8. **What is the medical management of this disease?**
9. **What is the surgical management in this disease?**
10. **What are the complications of this disease?**

Answers

1. Straight X-ray demonstrated dilatation of descending colon and transverse colon in case of acute severe ulcerative colitis.
2. The cause is hypomagnesemia leading to wasting of potassium through the secretion of potassium leading to development of toxic megacolon.
3. Causes of toxic megacolon:
   a. Inflammatory:
      - Ulcerative colitis
      - Crohn's disease
   b. Infectious causes:
      - *Salmonella*
      - *Shigella*
      - Campylobacter colitis
      - *Clostridium difficile*
      - *Entamoeba histolytica*
      - *Cytomegalovirus*
      - Enterohemorrhagic or enteroinvasive *E. coli*
   c. Ischemia
4. Risk factors associated with this disease are:
   a. Hypomagnesemia
   b. Hypokalemia
   c. Medications:
      - Opioid
      - Antimotility agents
      - Antidepressants
   d. Barium enema
   e. Colonoscopy

5. Pathogenesis in this disease:

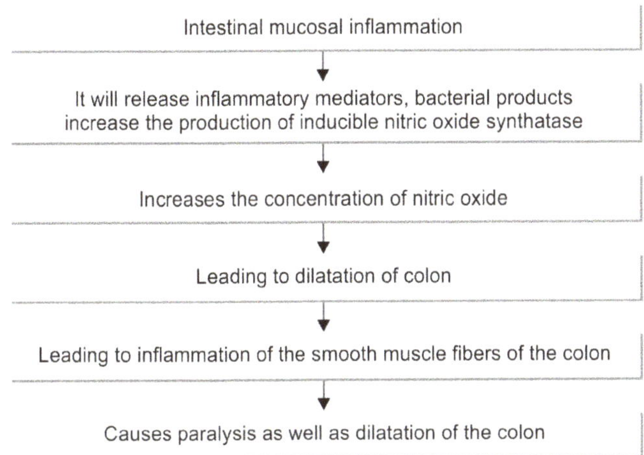

6. Definition of the disease: Toxic megacolon can be defined as total or nonobstructive dilatation of the colon, i.e., diameter of the colon of >5.5 cm or cecum of >9 cm.

7. Criteria of toxic megacolon:
    a. Radiological evidence of dilatation of the colon of >6 cm.
    b. At least any three of the following:
        - Fever of >38°C
        - Heart rate of >120 beats/minute
        - Anemia
        - Neutrophilic leukocytosis of >10,500/cc

c. At least any one of the following:
    - Altered sensorium
    - Dehydration
    - Electrolyte disturbances
    - Hypotension

8. Medical management of this disease:
    a. Intravenous fluid for adequate dehydration
    b. Use of antibiotics such as metronidazole and vancomycin
    c. In case of *Cytomegalovirus*, ganciclovir should be given.
    d. In case of *Clostridium difficile*, vancomycin or fidaxomicin should be given.
    e. In case ulcerative colitis, hydrocortisone 100 mg over 6 hours or methylprednisolone 60 mg daily for 5 days
    f. Insertion of nasogastric tube to decompress the stomach

9. Surgical management of this disease:
    a. Subtotal colectomy with ileostomy with either Hartmann pouch, sigmoidostomy, or rectostomy

10. Complications of toxic megacolon:
    a. Perforation of bowel
    b. Peritonitis
    c. Abscess
    d. Abdominal compartment syndrome

CASE 123

A 45-year-old man with history of inflammatory bowel disease came to department of dermatology with the following dermatological manifestations:

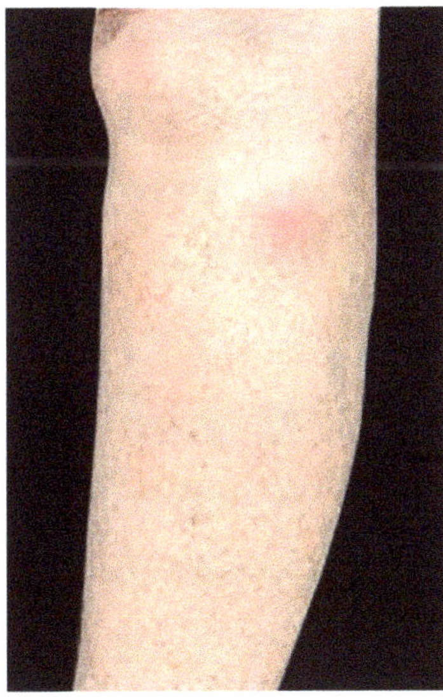

1. **Describe the lesion.**
2. **What is your diagnosis?**
3. **What are the causes of this lesion?**
4. **What is the main pathophysiology behind it?**

Answers

1. These are erythematous deep firm, solid nodules, which are painful in palpation and present on the extensor aspect of the leg.
2. Diagnosis is erythema nodosum.
3. Causes of this lesion are:

   Infectious causes:
   - Tuberculosis
   - Leprosy
   - *Mycoplasma* pneumonia
   - Leptospirosis
   - Psittacosis
   - *Chlamydia trachomatis*
   - Cat scratch disease

   a. Viral disease:
   - Infectious mononucleosis
   - Hepatitis B and C virus
   - Epstein–Barr virus
   - Herpes simplex virus
   - HIV virus

   b. Fungal disease:
   - Histoplasmosis
   - Blastomycosis
   - Coccidioidomycosis

   c. Parasitic:
   - Amebiasis
   - Giardiasis

   Noninfectious causes:

   a. Drugs:
   - Antibiotics
   - Sulfonamides
   - Miscellaneous causes:
     - Bromide
     - Iodide
     - OCP

   b. Malignancy:
   - Leukemia
   - Lymphoma
   - Occult malignancies

   c. Inflammatory bowel disease:

   d. Miscellaneous causes:
   - Whipple's disease
   - Behcet disease
   - Pregnancy

4. Pathophysiology in this disease: It occurs due to type IV hypersensitivity to many antigens. Antigen-antibody complexes in the venules of the subcutaneous fat leading to production of oxygen-free radicals, formation of TNF-α, and granuloma.

CASE 124

A 30-year-old hypertensive woman with history of quiescent Crohn's disease came to the emergency department with fever, headache, arthralgia, and mouth ulcers following influenza vaccination. On examination, there was raised temperature, and multiple erythematous tender papules on her neck as well as at the site of immunization.

Laboratory investigation demonstrated CRP 70 mg/L and there was leukocytosis.

1. **What is your diagnosis?**
2. **What are the characteristics of this disease?**
3. **What are the causes of this disease?**
4. **What are the genetic factors involved in this disease?**
5. **What are the clinical diagnostic criteria?**
6. **How can you treat this disease?**

Answers

1. The diagnosis is acute febrile neutrophilic dermatosis or Sweet syndrome described by Robert Sweet.
2. Following are the characteristics in this disease:
   a. Sudden-onset, tender erythematous nodules or plaques
   b. Fever
   c. Arthralgia
   d. Headache
   e. Ocular inflammation
   f. Oral or genital lesions rarely
3. Following are the causes of this disease:
   a. Several malignancies:
      - Acute myeloid leukemia (AML)
      - Chronic myeloid leukemia (CML)
      - Multiple myeloma
      - Myelodysplastic syndrome
      - Monoclonal gammopathy
      - Lymphoma
      - Solid tumors rarely
   b. Inflammatory causes:
      - Inflammatory bowel disease
      - Systemic lupus erythematosus (SLE)
      - Rheumatoid arthritis
      - Sjögren syndrome
      - Dermatomyositis
      - Behcet disease
      - Hashimoto thyroiditis
   c. Postinfectious syndrome
   d. Drugs:
      - Antibiotics
      - Antihypertensives
      - Immunosuppressives
      - Antiepileptics
      - Anticancer drugs
      - Antipsychotics
      - Antithyroid drugs
4. Following genetic factors involved in this disease:
   a. *HLA-B54* in Japanese population
   b. Mutation in *MEFV* in Mediterranean population
   c. Chromosome 3q abnormalities
5. Following are the clinical diagnostic criteria:
   a. Sudden onset of appearance of tender, plaques, or nodules
   b. Neutrophilic infiltration in the dermis in absence of vasculitis

   For diagnostic confirmation, following are the criteria:
   a. Temperature of >38°C
   b. Preceded by upper respiratory or gastrointestinal infection, presence of malignancy, pregnancy, or inflammatory disorders
   c. Polymorphonuclear leukocytosis
   d. Elevated inflammatory markers
   e. Positive response to corticosteroids
6. This disease can be treated by:
   a. 2–4 weeks tapering course of steroids
   b. Injection of intralesional steroids
   c. Administration of topical steroids

CASE 125

A 22-year-old boy with childhood history of Crohn's disease came to emergency department with history of painless congestion in the eye in absence of change in the vision.

1. **What is your diagnosis?**
2. **What are the ocular features in Crohn's disease?**
3. **What are the risk factors for ocular involvement?**
4. **How can you treat this case?**

Answers

1. Since the patient has a history of inflammatory bowel disease, congestion in the eye in absence of pain, or loss of vision, the diagnosis is episcleritis.
2. Other ocular features in this disease are:
   a. Scleritis: It is characterized by inflammation of scleral vessels leading to pain and visual disturbances worsening at night.
   b. Uveitis: It is characterized by inflammation of the middle layer of the eye as well as choroid. There are two subtypes:
      - Anterior uveitis: Involvement of iris with or without ciliary body.
      - Posterior uveitis: Involvement of choroid and retina or in-between ciliary body and retina.

3. Following are the risk factors for episcleritis:
   a. Female sex
   b. Presence of arthropathy in case of Crohn's disease

4. Episcleritis can be treated by topical steroids and analgesics.

CASE 126

A 30-year-old man having history of Crohn's disease came to the clinic with loose motions 2–3 times per day with pain in the right iliac fossa and extreme fatigue. Laboratory investigation demonstrated hemoglobin 10 g/dL, MCV 75 fl, ferritin 88 µg/L, serum iron 9 µmol/L, and CRP 20 mg/L.

1. **What is your diagnosis?**
2. **What should be the level in ferritin deficiency anemia?**
3. **What are the recommendations in the treatment of iron-deficiency anemia?**

Answers

1. The diagnosis is iron-deficiency anemia in case of inflammatory bowel disease.
2. Ferritin level in case of iron-deficiency anemia:
   a. In absence of inflammation, it should be <30 µg/L.
   b. In presence of inflammation, it should be <100 µg/L.
3. Intravenous iron should be considered in case of the following:
   a. Clinically active disease
   b. Intolerance to oral iron
   c. Level of hemoglobin is <10 g/dL.
   d. If the patient requires erythropoiesis-stimulating agents

CASE 127

A 50-year-old man with history of pancolitis for 14 years and was on 4 g mesalazine as maintenance therapy. His paternal uncle and his son developed colonic carcinoma. About 3 years ago colonoscopy was performed and it demonstrated normal findings but biopsy taken from the colonic mucosa demonstrated microscopic inflammation having Nancy histological index grade III.

1. **When should the surveillance colonoscopy be done?**
2. **What are the risk factors of developing colonic carcinoma in patient with ulcerative colitis?**

Answers

1. Surveillance colonoscopy:
   a. According to British Society of Gastroenterology, surveillance colonoscopy should be done after 10 years of the disease onset who is under remission. Two to four biopsies should be taken at random fashion at every 10 cm within the colon as well as rectum.
   b. In case of extensive colitis, annual surveillance colonoscopy should be performed every year as there is chance of colonic carcinoma which increases to 8–16% in 20 and 30 years, respectively.

2. Following are the risk factors for developing colonic carcinoma in patient with ulcerative colitis:
   a. Ulcerative colitis with evidence of dysplasia in colonic biopsies
   b. Duration of the disease
   c. Extensive colitis
   d. Family history of colonic carcinoma
   e. Evidence of primary sclerosing cholangitis in patient with ulcerative colitis—it is five times more common.
   f. Young disease of onset
   g. Male sex

CASE 128

A 25-year-old woman having history of intake of azathioprine for treating ulcerative colitis suddenly has been diagnosed as pregnant and is of 10 weeks of gestation. Now, she has the following questions regarding the different medications.

1. **What is the fear in woman regarding the adverse effect in the fetus?**
2. **What is the effect of azathioprine in fetus?**
3. **Is there any effect of thiopurine in breastfeeding?**
4. **What about 5-aminosalicylic acid in pregnancy?**

Answers

1. The young woman has a fear of developing developmental defect to the fetus if she will be on the medication as she thinks that the drug will cross through the placenta.
2. Azathioprine or its metabolite can cross the placenta, but according to different meta-analyses, there is no increased risk of adverse outcome on pregnancy if she is on this drug.
3. After intake of this drug, it will be secreted for 4 hours in breast milk. Hence, expression of the breast milk for that time period is advisable.
4. As sulfasalazine is associated with the folate malabsorption, hence high dose of folic acid should be given during pregnancy to prevent any adverse effect.

CASE 129

A 30-year-old woman previously treated with infliximab for treating pancolitis that was diagnosed 1 year ago and she has been under remission for last 7 months. Now, she wants to start family. So, colonoscopy demonstrated absence of macroscopic as well as microscopic features of colitis.

1. **In case of active disease, why is it advised not to take pregnancy?**
2. **What is the effect of infliximab in the treatment of this disease in case of pregnancy?**
3. **If infliximab is continued throughout the third trimester, what advice should be given regarding the baby's vaccination schedule?**

Answers

1. In case of active disease, pregnancy should be prohibited until the remission of the disease because this inflammatory bowel disease is associated with low birth weight and preterm baby.

   Again, there is chance of flare of this disease and this should be treated actively and aggressively with any drug except methotrexate.
2. Infliximab should be given in the pregnant woman with active disease. It will cross the placenta and will be detectable for 2–7 months in the baby after discontinuation of this drug. Hence, this drug should be discontinued after 24–26th week unless the disease activity dictates the continuation of the drugs.
3. If the drug is continued throughout the third trimester, the live vaccination should be avoided for at least 6 months after birth.

CASE 130

A 70-year-old woman received four cycles of immunotherapy for treating metastatic melanoma starting 49 days ago. She was also on methotrexate along with folic acid for treating rheumatoid arthritis. Now, she complained of nonbloody loose motion with abdominal discomfort. Colonoscopy demonstrated following features:

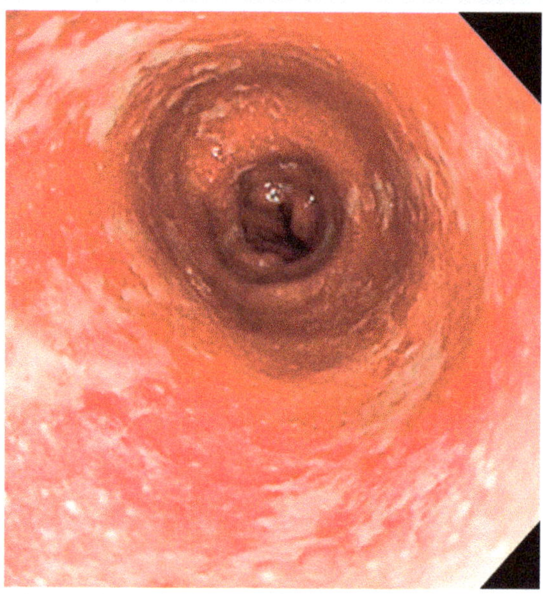

1. **Describe the above picture.**
2. **What is your diagnosis?**
3. **What is the mechanism of diarrhea?**
4. **Which drugs should be used in this case?**
5. **In this case if there is predominance of nausea or vomiting, what may be the cause?**
6. **Mention the treatment in this case.**

Answers

1. Colonoscopic picture in the rectum demonstrates:
   a. Patchy colitis
   b. Loss of the vascular pattern
   c. Presence of small superficial ulcers
2. Diagnosis is immunotherapy-mediated colitis.
3. Immunotherapy produces diarrhea by inhibiting the checkpoint of the immune system. Gastrointestinal immune-related side effects are mainly responsible for diarrhea.
4. Checkpoint inhibitors are used in the treatment of this disease as well as lung cancer.
5. The cause may be due to immunotherapy-related gastritis.
6. In this case, oral steroid at a dose of 1 mg/kg/day should be given for 3–5 days. In that case, infliximab at a dose of 5 mg/kg/day can be considered.

CASE 131

A 45-year-old male with history of hypertension and atrial fibrillation was taking telmisartan and bisoprolol respectively and pain killer for osteoarthritis. He developed lower respiration tract infection for which he did a course of amoxicillin 2 weeks ago. Now, he came to emergency department with left-sided abdominal pain with loose stool with bleeding per rectum for 1 day. On examination, blood pressure is 80/50 mm Hg and pulse is irregularly irregular with rate of 110 beats/minute. Laboratory investigation demonstrated hemoglobin 12 g/dL, CRP 12 mg/L, serum lactate 4 mmol/L, and total leukocyte count 15,500/cc. Endoscopy at the splenic flexure demonstrated:

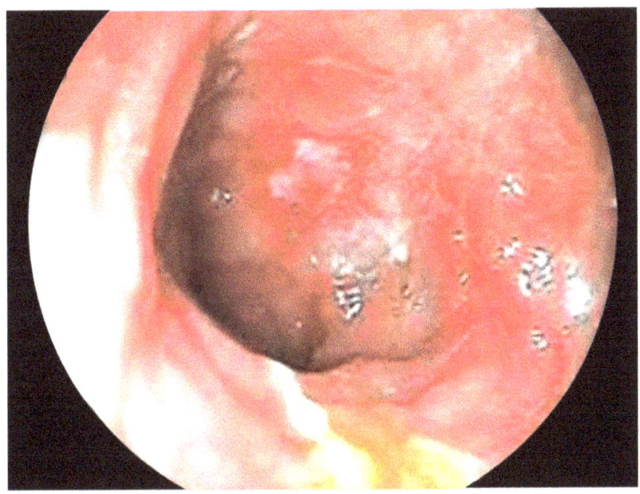

1. **Describe the colonoscopic picture.**
2. **What is your diagnosis and give your reasons?**
3. **Why is splenic flexure involved?**
4. **Why is it not a case of antibiotic-associated diarrhea?**
5. **What are the causes of this disease?**
6. **What are the risk factors that cannot be resolved with conservative treatment?**
7. **Why was serum lactate raised?**

Answers

1. Colonoscopic features are the following:
    a. Friable and edematous mucosa
    b. Petechial hemorrhages
    c. Fragile mucosa
    d. Segmental erythema
    e. Longitudinal ulceration
2. Diagnosis is ischemic colitis. Points in favor are:
    a. Endoscopic appearances in the mucosa
    b. Low blood pressure
    c. Presence of atrial fibrillation
    d. History of hypertension
3. Superior mesenteric artery supplies the small intestine from the duodenum to mid-transverse colon and rest of the colon up to superior aspect of rectum is supplied by inferior mesenteric artery. Collateral flow is maintained by the marginal artery of Drummond running parallel to the colon and also through the arc of Riolan. This marginal artery runs also along the splenic flexure. It is absent in the 5% of the population. So, ischemic injury occurs in the following watershed areas of the colon:
    a. Griffith point in the splenic flexure
    b. Sudeck point in the sigmoid colon
4. It is not a case of pseudomembranous colitis, because:
    a. Absence of pseudomembrane
    b. There is a gap of >14 days between the onset of diarrhea and last dose of antibiotics.
5. Causes of ischemic colitis are:
    a. Physiological:
        • Heart failure
        • Atherosclerosis
        • Systemic inflammatory response syndrome
        • Concurrent malignancy

b. Pharmacological:
- Sex hormones
- Chemotherapy
- Cardiac glycosides
- Diuretics
- Interferon
- Vasopressin
- Statin

c. Repair of abdominal aortic aneurysm
d. Bowel preparation in colonoscopy

6. Following factors associated with severity cannot be resolved by conservative treatment:
   a. Male sex
   b. Right-sided colitis
   c. Lack of rectal bleeding
   d. Renal dysfunction
   e. Colonic stricture
   f. Peritonitis

7. Serum lactate was raised due to hypoperfusion leading to systemic dysfunction.

CASE 132

A 50-year-old male underwent loop ileostomy as he suffered from refractory Crohn's disease and has no symptom and any therapy for last 4 years, then suddenly developed rectal bleeding, discharge of mucus, and tenesmus. So, the ileoscopy was performed which was normal macroscopically. So diagnosis was "diversion colitis".

1. **When can diversion colitis occur?**
2. **What is the main cause of diversion colitis and why?**
3. **How can you treat this patient?**

Answers

1. Diversion colitis can occur within a few months to at least 3 years after the loop ileostomy.
2. Diversion colitis can occur due to deficiency of short-chain fatty acids because their deficiency leads to ischemia to the colorectal mucosa.

   Carbohydrate in the colon is metabolized into short-chain fatty acids by colonic bacteria like butyric acid and it:
   a. Provides nutrition to the colonic mucosa
   b. Acts as oxidative substrate to the colonocytes
   c. Also relaxes the vascular smooth muscles

3. The treatment is:
   a. Enema of short-chain fatty acids
   b. Corticosteroid enema can be given.
   c. Mesalazine enema can be given.
   d. Definite surgical treatment is restoration of continuity as well as fecal stream.

CASE 133

A 60-year-old woman having history of depression for which she is on sertraline presented in the clinic with loose stool for last 15 years. Her all the laboratory tests including anti-tTG antibody IgA and fecal elastase were within normal limit. Colonoscopy was also normal.

1. **What is the most likely diagnosis?**
2. **What are the types of this disease?**
3. **What are the provocating factors in this disease?**
4. **Is there any contribution to this disease?**
5. **Which is the diagnostic of the disease?**
6. **What are the histologic features in this disease?**
7. **How can you manage this patient?**

Answers

1. The most likely diagnosis is microscopic colitis which is based on the history of long-time intake of antipsychotic drug along with all the negative investigations and colonoscopy findings.

2. There are two types of microscopic colitis:
   a. Collagenous colitis
   b. Lymphocytic colitis

3. Following are the provocating factors for developing this colitis:
   a. Proton pump inhibitors
   b. Selective serotonin reuptake inhibitors
   c. Thyroid dysfunction
   d. Celiac disease
   e. NSAIDs
   f. Statins
   g. Smoking
4. Following genes are associated with the disease:
   a. *HLA-DQ2*
   b. *HLA-DQ1*
   c. *HLA-DQ3*
   d. *HLA DR3-DQ2*
5. Histology from the pancolonic mucosa mostly from the right-sided colonic mucosa is the diagnosis of this disease.

6. Following are the histologic findings:
   a. In case of collagenous colitis:
      - Cryptic architecture will be intact.
      - Increase in colonic mucosal subepithelial collagen layer
      - >10 μm thick made of collagen type I and III rather than collagen type IV
   b. In case of lymphocytic colitis:
      - Increased number of intraepithelial lymphocytes
      - Subepithelial collagen layer will be absent.
      - Presence of >20 lymphocytes per 100 epithelial cells
7. Management of this disease:
   a. Removal of offensive medication
   b. In case of mild symptom, antidiarrheal agent

CASE 134

A 75-year-old diabetic man came to gastroenterology clinic with history of severe cramping, abdominal pain, and severe loose motion for the last 2 days just after completion of clindamycin course for treating osteomyelitis in the right fifth metatarsal bone. Colonoscopy was done and it showed the following:

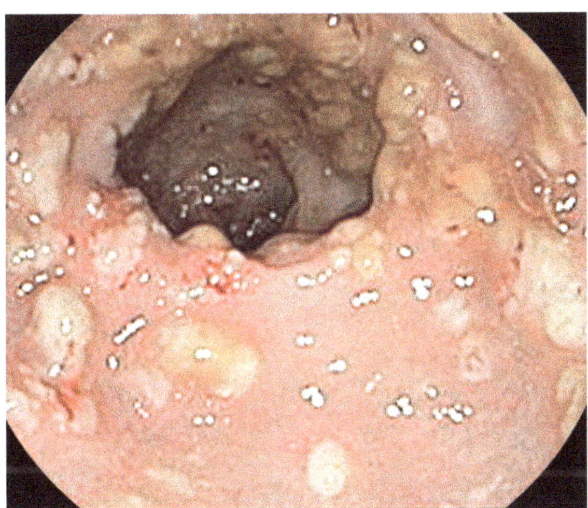

1. **Describe the above picture.**
2. **What is your most likely diagnosis?**
3. **Which organism is responsible for this disease?**
4. **What is the route of transmission?**
5. **What is the pathophysiologic mechanism in this disease?**
6. **What is the screening test to be done in this disease?**
7. **What are the further tests done to confirm the diagnosis?**
8. **What are the complications in this disease?**

Answers

1. The above picture demonstrates raised occasionally hemorrhagic nodules or plaques covering the mucosa.
2. The most likely diagnosis is pseudomembranous colitis.
3. *Clostridium difficile*, gram-positive bacillus, is responsible for this disease following a course of antibiotic.
4. This organism is transmitted through the fecal-oral route.
5. This organism produces two types of toxins:
   a. Toxin A (enterotoxin)
   b. Toxin B (cytotoxin)
   These toxins:
   a. Produce colonic inflammation
   b. Disrupt the colonic cell cytoskeleton
   c. Cellular death
6. There are two screening tests:
   a. Glutamate dehydrogenase antigen testing: Glutamate dehydrogenase is produced by both toxin- and nontoxin-producing bacteria. This antigen testing can confirm whether the organism colonizes the colonic mucosa or not. This is rapid screening test with sensitivity of >96%.
   b. Nucleic acid amplification test
7. Following tests should be performed to confirm the diagnosis:
   a. Testing of cytotoxin:
      - Cell culture cytotoxicity assay: Highly sensitive, but expensive as well as time-consuming.
      - Enzyme immunoassay: It can detect both the toxins and it is an easy test. But false-negative test rate is high.
      - Polymerase chain reaction
   b. Anaerobic fecal culture: This test is not routinely used.
8. Following are the complications:
   a. Toxic megacolon
   b. Bowel perforation
   c. Sepsis

CASE 135

A 25-year-old Indian female swimmer went to North America for swimming competition. After returning from there, she suddenly noticed some dermatological features on the back. Her hematological tests demonstrated eosinophil count 1.6×10^9/L and fecal microscopy and culture were negative.

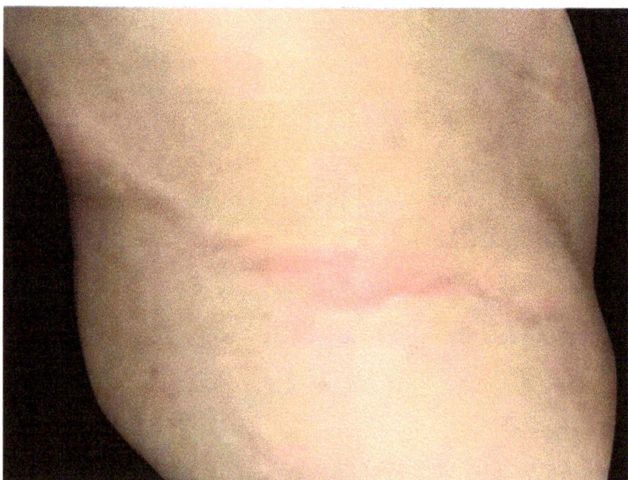

1. **Describe the above picture.**
2. **What is the most likely diagnosis?**
3. **What is the characteristic of the rash?**
4. **How can the infection be transmitted?**
5. **What are the features of chronic infection?**
6. **What is the complication in this disease?**
7. **What is the definite treatment in this disease?**

Answers

1. The lesion can be described as raised serpiginous wheal developed in the back of the trunk.

2. The most likely diagnosis is cutaneous larva currens caused by *Strongyloides stercoralis*. The diagnosis is based on the specific lesion, the patient's return from North America, and peripheral eosinophilia.

3. Rash can be described as creeping eruption due to migration of larvae subcutaneously. Rash can be described as transient wheal develops on the trunk of the body

4. This is an autoinfection transmitted through the gastrointestinal tract. It infects the human being through the contact with the soil containing larvae.

5. Chronic infection is characterized by intermittent diarrhea, abdominal pain, and loss of weight, dry cough, and wheeze if the larvae will migrate into the lungs.

6. Rare complication is hyperinfection syndrome occurring in the immunosuppressed patients when chronically infected which is characterized by:
   a. Bloody diarrhea
   b. Perforation of the bowel
   c. Gram-negative septicemia
   d. Pulmonary exudates
   e. Meningoencephalitis

7. The treatment is ivermectin.

CASE 136

A 45-year-old corporate worker came to emergency department with 8 days history of fever and abdominal pain with bloody diarrhea following a dinner from a hotel taking meat stew. On examination, there was raised temperature and tender periumbilical. Laboratory examination demonstrated white blood count 16,000/cc and CRP 20 mg/L. Other parameters were normal.

1. **What is your most likely diagnosis and why?**
2. **What are the risk factors for this infection?**
3. **What are the late complications in this disease?**
4. **What is the specific treatment for this disease?**
5. **Name one preventive strategy for *Campylobacter jejuni* infection.**

Answers

1. The most likely diagnosis is acute invasive diarrhea due to infection with *Campylobacter jejuni* based on the following findings:
   a. Intake of poultry meat
   b. Incubation period of 3–7 days

2. Following are the risk factors for *Campylobacter jejuni* gastroenteritis:
   a. Age-group:
      - <5 years
      - Between 20 and 29 years
   b. Male sex
   c. Consumption of:
      - Raw or undercooked poultry or other meat
      - Unpasteurized milk and dairy products
      - Untreated water
   d. Contact with firm animals

3. Late complications in this disease:
   a. Reactive arthritis
   b. Guillain–Barré syndrome

4. Specific drugs in this disease are:
   a. Azithromycin
   b. Erythromycin

5. The preventive strategies "farm-to-fork" for controlling the *Campylobacter jejuni* infection. The description of this strategy:
   a. Farm:
      - Ensuring animal health through the preventive medicine
      - Ensuring the biosecurity
         ○ Appropriate ventilation
         ○ Appropriate cleaning
         ○ Safe handling of the manure
         ○ Elimination of still water
   b. Regarding slaughterhouse and processing of the meat:
      - Sanitation and good hygiene maintenance
      - Use of hazard analysis and critical control points
      - Separation of the uncontaminated from the contaminated meat and animals
   c. Kitchen:
      - Refrigeration of the meat and poultry
      - Cross-contamination should be avoided.
      - Poultry cooking in 74°C and meat cooking in 71°C
   d. In case of individual, proper handwashing

CASE 137

A 35-year-old African man presented in the emergency department with 2 weeks history of fever along with loose motion up to 18–22 times daily. On examination, temperature was increased. Laboratory examination revealed white blood count 800/cc, hemoglobin 9 g/dL, CRP 88 mg/L, and CD4+ count 40/cc. HIV serology was positive. Sigmoidoscopy demonstrated:

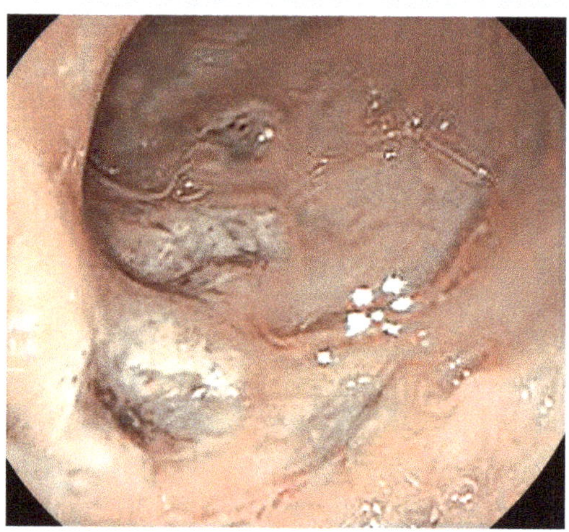

1.   **Describe the above colonoscopy picture.**
2.   **What is the most likely diagnosis?**
3.   **What are the risk factors in this disease?**
4.   **What are the indications of colonoscopy in this patient?**
5.   **What are the complications in this disease?**
6.   **How can you treat this patient?**

Answers

1.   Colonoscopic picture of left colon demonstrates:
     a.   Mucosal erythema
     b.   Loss of normal vascular pattern
     c.   Punched-out ulcer which is well defined.
2.   The most likely diagnosis is Cytomegalovirus colitis in patient with immunodeficiency.
3.   Following are the risk factors in this disease:
     •   Immunodeficiency syndrome
     •   Corticosteroid therapy
     •   Hematological malignancy
     •   Patient on hemodialysis
     •   Cancer therapy
     •   Immunocompetent persons
4.   Indications of therapy in this patient are:
     a.   Reactivation of *Cytomegalovirus* leads to Cytomegalovirus colitis and evidences of high-grade density of this virus on histopathological examination
     b.   In case of corticosteroid refractory- or steroid-dependent patient in spite of low density of *Cytomegalovirus*
     c.   Evidence of large punched-out ulcer in the left colon

5.   Following are the complications in this disease:
     a.   Chronic inflammation
     b.   Perforation of the large bowel
     c.   Toxic megacolon
     d.   Formation of pseudomembrane
     e.   Ischemic colitis
     f.   Severe hemorrhage
6.   This patient can be treated by:
     a.   Intravenous ganciclovir should be given as first line of treatment and this can be changed to oral valganciclovir in outpatient department and should be continued for 3–6 weeks.
     b.   Foscarnet can be given as second line of therapy in case of resistance to ganciclovir or toxicity of ganciclovir as it has following side effects:
         •   Renal impairment
         •   Seizures
     c.   If the patient has associated with *Cytomegalovirus* retinitis, 2 weeks of treatment of *Cytomegalovirus* is required prior to commencement of ART because there is chance of increasing intraocular inflammation as a result of immune reconstitution syndrome.

CASE 138

A 45-year-old male with history of acromegaly for >15 years underwent colonoscopy and a hyperplastic polyp was found and excised endoscopically.

1. **What is your next advice?**
2. **What are the indications of colonoscopy in this patient?**

Answers

1. Colonoscopic surveillance is required every 3 years.
2. Following are the indications for colonoscopic screening in this patient:
   a. This patient is at risk of developing colonic adenocarcinoma.
   b. Screening for colonoscopy is required after the age of 40 years.
   c. If in the first screening adenomatous polyp was found and level of insulin, like growth factor is above the maximum of the age corrected normal 3 yearly screening is required.
   d. If first screening colonoscopy demonstrated hyperplastic polyp or serum insulin-like growth factor is normal, then screening is required at every 5–10 years' interval.
   e. As most of the polyps are present on the right side of the colon, hence colonoscopy rather than sigmoidoscopy may be required.

CASE 139

A 35-year-old woman came to the gastroenterology clinic with chronic diarrhea and was advised colonoscopy which demonstrated multiple polyps in the ascending, transverse, and descending colon. On enquiry, there was family history of colonic cancer in her grandmother and surgery of the polyp in her maternal uncle. Other family blood-related relatives are normal and healthy.

1. **What is the likely diagnosis?**
2. **Is it an inherited disease, if so, which is responsible for this disease and how?**
3. **In this disease, what percentage will have chance of carrier, how many suffer and how many are not at all affected?**
4. **Maximum how many polyps may be present in this disease?**
5. **What is the chance of developing colonic carcinoma in these patients?**
6. **Is there any other cancer present in these patients?**
7. **Is there any chance of upper gastrointestinal cancer?**
8. **How can you manage this case?**

Answers

1. The most likely diagnosis is MUTYH-associated polyposis.
2. As it is an autosomal recessive disease, and the gene responsible for this disease is *MUTYH* gene, hence mutation of each copy of gene from both parents will lead to development of this polyposis. In that case parents are known as carriers.
3. As it is autosomal recessive, there is 1 in 4 children will be affected phenotypically, 2 in 4 children will be carrier containing one mutant gene only, and 1 in 4 children will be completely normal.
4. Nearly 100–1,000 polyps are present in these patients.
5. In these homozygous patients, there is 100% chance of developing carcinoma in colon at 60 years of age.
6. There is chance of developing breast cancer in female having biallelic mutation in the carriers.
7. Yes, there is a chance of duodenal cancer in 4% cases.
8. Management of the case:
   a. In patients having biallelic carriers of *MUTYH* gene, surveillance colonoscopy should be started at 18–20 years then at yearly basis.
   b. Upper gastrointestinal endoscopy should be started at 35 years of age.
   c. Prophylactic colectomy should be considered depending on the:
      - Number of polyps
      - Degree of dysplasia
   d. Screening of the breast should be done at regular intervals.

CASE 140

A 45-year-old woman having past history of operation of breast cancer came to outpatient department with central abdominal pain. On examination, there was evidence of the following:

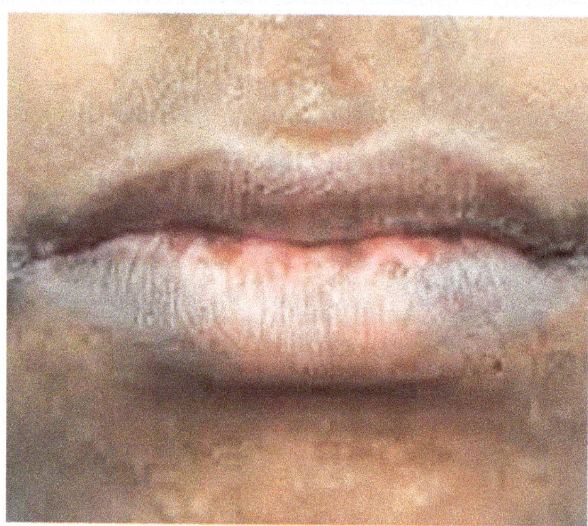

1. **What has been described in the above picture?**
2. **What is the most likely diagnosis?**
3. **What is the risk of this disease?**
4. **What are the diagnostic criteria in this patient?**
5. **How can you manage this patient?**
6. **What are the possible complications in these patients?**

Answers

1. There is evidence of perioral pigmentation.
2. The most likely diagnosis is Peutz–Jeghers (PJ) syndrome based on the history of perioral pigmentation along with central abdominal pain.
3. There is an increased risk of breast cancer, stomach cancer, colon cancer, and pancreatic cancer.
4. Diagnostic criteria of PJ syndrome: This is based on any one of the following:
   a. Presence of ≥2 histologically confirmed PJ polyps
   b. Any number of PJ polyps in a patient having family history of PJ syndrome in close relatives.
   c. Evidence of characteristic perioral mucocutaneous pigmentation in a patient having family history of PJ syndrome in close relatives.
   d. Presence of any number of PJ polyps having characteristics of mucocutaneous pigmentation.
   e. A pathogenic variant in STK11

5. Following are the methods of management:
   a. Surveillance gastroscopy, colonoscopy, and video endoscopy should be started at 8 years of age and then small bowel surveillance should be done 3 yearly.
   b. In case of normal findings in baseline gastroscopy or colonoscopy, the next surveillance can be deferred up to 18 years of age.
   c. In case of presence of polyp in baseline gastroscopy or colonoscopy, the next surveillance endoscopy should be repeated 3 yearly.
   d. In case of symptomatic patient, investigation should be started earliest.
   e. Elective polypectomy should be done to prevent complications.
6. Two possible complications occur in this patient:
   a. Intussusception
   b. Gastrointestinal bleeding

CASE 141

The patient has been suffering from constipation for years and ultimately diagnosed as dyssynergic defecation problem.

1. **What is the therapy which is based on instrument in this case?**
2. **What are the other methods of therapy?**
3. **In refractory cases, what should be the modality of treatment?**

Answers

1. Biofeedback therapy: It is an instrument-based therapy where the instrument is used to record the bodily activities of the patient which in turn provides feedback to the different sensory stimuli in the body like visual, auditory as well as visual stimuli. It is used to rehabilitate anorectal function. It requires active engagement, motivation, and preserved cognition of the patient.
2. Other modalities of therapy are:
    a. Constipating medications should be avoided.
    b. Timed toilet training
    c. Exercise
    d. Laxative use
    e. Myectomy of the anal sphincter
    f. Botulinum toxin can be injected at the anal sphincter for paralyzing the anal sphincter and spasm.
3. In refractory cases of constipation, following surgery can be considered:
    a. Colectomy
    b. Ileostomy
    c. Ileorectal anastomosis

CASE 142

A 50-year-old woman previously diagnosed as a case of IBS came to gastroenterology clinic with history of accidental leakage and soiling of the garment with stool for last 1 year. She was chronic smoker for the last 20 years and history of vaginal delivery following episiotomy at 25 years of age. She is overweight. On rectal examination, there was decreased anal muscular tone.

1. **What is your diagnosis?**
2. **What are the strongest risk factors for this disease?**
3. **What are the other risk factors in this disease?**
4. **How can you treat the patient?**

Answers

1. The most likely diagnosis is fecal incontinence.
2. The strongest risk factors are:
    a. Irritable bowel syndrome
    b. Prior cholecystectomy
    c. Diarrhea
3. Other less common risk factors are:
    a. Current smoking
    b. Obesity
    c. Urinary stress incontinence
    d. Rectocele
4. Following are the baseline assessments in this case:
    a. Proper medical and obstetric history
    b. Enquire regarding the bowel habit of the patient
    c. Fecal load or treatable causes of diarrhea should be considered.
    d. Red flag sign for gastrointestinal cancer should be considered.
    e. Searching for any evidence of disc prolapse or cauda equina syndrome
    f. Rectal examination should be done to detect:
        - Rectal prolapse
        - Third-degree hemorrhoids
        - Injury to anal sphincter and any trauma in the anus
        - Assessment of cognition of the patient

CASE 143

A 54-year-old man came to gastroenterology clinic with abdominal bloating. Since the last few years, he has been on laxative to prevent constipation. Colonoscopy was performed and it demonstrated:

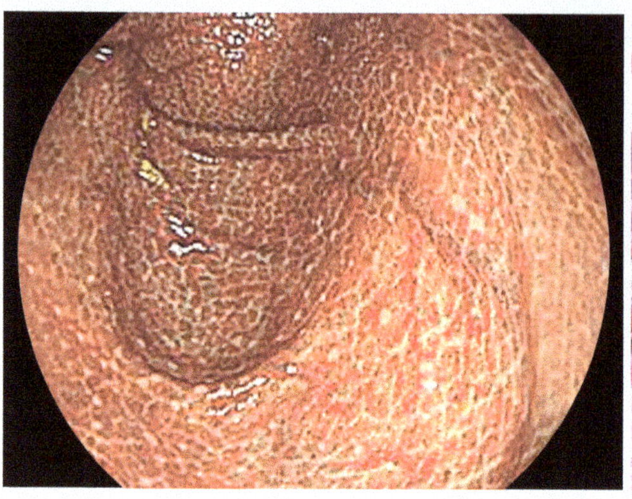 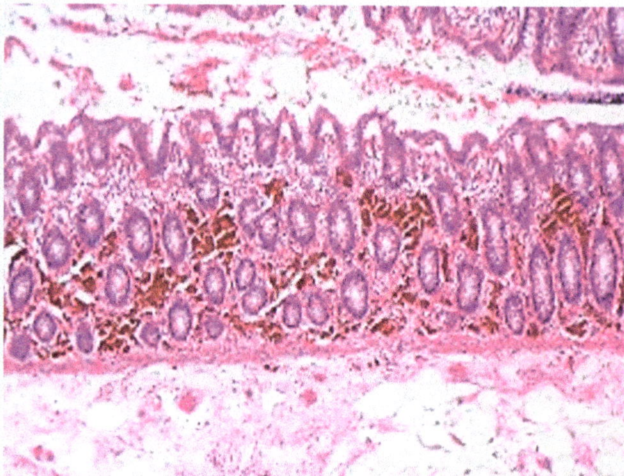

1. **What has been demonstrated in the above pictures?**
2. **What is your diagnosis?**
3. **What is the most common cause of this condition?**
4. **Describe the pathophysiology of this condition.**
5. **Which part of the colon is mostly involved and why?**
6. **How does this laxative work within the bowel?**
7. **What is brown bowel syndrome?**

Answers

1. The above pictures demonstrated:
   a. Colonoscopic picture demonstrated heavily pigmented mucosa looking like skin of the leopard.
   b. Histologic picture demonstrated pigment-laden macrophages seen by periodic acid–Schiff stain.
2. The most likely diagnosis is melanosis coli.
3. Most common cause is chronic use of laxatives containing senna.
4. Anthraquinone present in the laxatives after intake travels down the intestinal tract in inactive form until it will reach into the large intestine where it will be converted to active form. This active form will damage the cells in the wall of the colon leading to cellular apoptosis. After the cellular death, they will create dark pigment which is nothing but macrophages containing lipofuscin pigment within the lamina propria. This is visible under the colonoscopy.

5. It mostly involves proximal colon as compared to distal colon and this is due to distribution of the macrophages within the colonic wall.
6. Anthraquinone laxative works in the following ways:
   a. It will stimulate active transport of chloride ion into the gut lumen leading to development of osmotic gradient resulting in pulling of water within the lumen of the gut.
   b. It will prevent reabsorption of water, potassium, and sodium by inhibiting the Na-K-ATPase present on the enterocytes leading to excretion into feces.
   c. It increases the peristalsis of the intestinal wall by stimulating local prostaglandin.
7. Brown bowel syndrome is characterized by brown discoloration of the colon due to deposition of lipofuscin in the tunica muscularis rather than colonic mucosa.

CASE 144

A 55-year-old nondiabetic woman with history of chronic constipation for the last 18 years passing stool every 4–5 days came to clinic with abdominal bloating and flatulence. Her thyroid, liver, and renal function tests were normal. She was not taking any antipsychotic drug or sedatives. She has not been suffering from any neurological disorders. She underwent slow transit study of the bowel.

1. **What is this method of study?**
2. **What are the types of functional constipation?**
3. **Describe Rome IV criteria for IBS.**
4. **What are the causes of secondary constipation?**
5. **Why constipation is more common in elderly?**
6. **Why constipation is more common in the last month of pregnancy?**
7. **What are the patterns of dyssynergic defecation in anorectal manometry?**

Answers

1. This test measures the colonic transit time study after taking a capsule containing 24 radiopaque markers. In this method, one capsule will be ingested on the day 1. On the day 6, straight X-ray of abdomen will be taken.
   a. In case of normal colonic transit, <5 markers will remain in the colon.
   b. In case of delayed colonic transit, ≥6 markers will remain scattered throughout the colon.
   c. In case of dyssynergic defecation, ≥6 markers are present in the rectosigmoid colon, but in the rest of the colon there is normal transit of markers.
2. There are three types of functional or primary constipation:
   a. Slow transit constipation which is characterized by prolonged delay in the transit time of stool throughout the colon.
   b. Dyssynergic defecation or pelvic floor dyssynergia: It is characterized by difficulty or inability to expel the stool from the anorectum.
   c. Irritable bowel syndrome with predominant constipation: This is characterized by symptoms of constipation with abdominal pain or discomfort.
3. Rome IV criteria for IBS:
   Recurrent abdominal pain on average at least one day or week in the past 3 months associated with two or more of the following:
   a. Related to defecation and/or
   b. Associated with change in frequency of stool and/or
   c. Associated with a change in form of stool

4. Causes of secondary constipation are:
   a. Pathology in the colon:
      - Stricture
      - Anal fissure
      - Cancer
      - Proctitis
      - Rectocele
      - Intestinal pseudo-obstruction
      - Megacolon
      - Diverticulosis
   b. Neurological disorders:
      - Parkinsonism
      - Lesions in the spinal cord
      - Multiple sclerosis
      - Stroke
      - Spina bifida
   c. Metabolic disorders:
      - Hypothyroidism
      - Hypercalcemia
      - Diabetes mellitus
   d. Psychotic disorders:
      - Depression
      - Anxiety
      - Various eating disorders
   e. Drugs like opioids
   f. Western diet
5. Constipation is more common in elderly because of the following reasons:
   a. Lack of normal bowel movement during aging
   b. Lack of proper diet
   c. Lack of adequate fluid intake
   d. Lack of adequate physical activity

e. Use of different drugs

f. Illness

g. Loose fitting dentures or loss of tooth leading to difficulty in chewing

h. Intake of low-fiber diet because of difficulty in chewing

i. Presence of rectocele

j. Pelvic floor dyssynergia

6. It is more common in third trimester of pregnancy because of:

   a. Significant increase in sex hormones

   b. Decreased movement of the intestine

   c. Delayed emptying of the intestine because of mechanical pressure by the gravid uterus

7. There are four patterns in dyssynergic defecation in anorectal manometry:

   a. Pattern 1:
      - Paradoxical increase in pressure
      - Elevated intrarectal pressure of ≥45 mm Hg

   b. Pattern 2:
      - Inability to produce enough expulsive forces
      - Without increasing intrarectal pressure
      - Along with paradoxical increase in the intra-anal pressure

   c. Pattern 3:
      - Enough expulsive forces
      - Incomplete decrease in intra-anal pressure of <20% of baseline normal

   d. Pattern 4:
      - Inability to produce sufficient expulsive forces
      - Without increase in the intrarectal pressure
      - No inadequate reduction in residual intra-anal pressure or absence of intra-anal pressure

CASE 145

A 70-year-old man with alcoholic cirrhosis came to hepatic clinic, where triphasic CT scan was performed and it demonstrated a mass of 4×4 cm present in the right lobe of the liver which enhanced vividly in the arterial phase and hypoattenuated in the portal venous phase and there is no distant metastasis. Patient was advised to do transarterial chemoembolization (TACE).

1. **Which artery is required for the TACE?**
2. **What is Barcelona clinic liver cancer (BCLC) staging system in hepatocellular carcinoma?**
3. **What is TACE?**
4. **In which stage of liver cancer, TACE is considered as first line of therapy?**
5. **Hepatic artery supplies in which segment of the liver?**
6. **What are the complications of TACE?**

Answers

1. Hepatic artery is selected. As hepatic artery is the branch of celiac artery, hence the procedure should be started through the celiac artery.

2. BCLC staging of the hepatocellular cancer: Five stages—

   a. Stage 0 (very early stage):
      - Size of the tumor is <2 cm.
      - Feeling well (performance status 0)
      - Liver working normally (Child–Pugh A)

   b. Stage A (early stage):
      - Single tumor of any size or up to three tumors, all are <3 cm.
      - Feeling well (performance status 0)
      - Liver functioning well (Child–Pugh A or B)

   c. Stage B (intermediate stage):
      - Many tumors in the liver
      - Patient feeling well (performance status 0)
      - Liver working well (Child–Pugh A or B)

d.   Stage C (advanced stage):
   - Spreading of cancer into the blood vessels, lymph nodes, or other body organs
   - Patient feeling less well or less active (performance status 1 or 2)
   - Liver still working well (Child–Pugh A or B)

e.   Stage D:
   - Severe liver damage (Child–Pugh C)
   - Patient needs the help of others to look after him (performance status 3 or 4)

3.   Transcatheter arterial chemoembolization (TACE) is rapid injection of the viscous emulsion of chemoembolic drugs into the blood vessels which is supplied to the tumor through the right or left hepatic artery depending upon the involved side.

4.   BCLC stage 2 is considered as first line of therapy in this case.

5.   Hepatic artery supplies:
   a.   Right hepatic artery supplies I, V, VI, VII, and VIII segments of the liver
   b.   Left hepatic artery supplies II, III, and IV segments of the liver

6.   Post-TACE complications:
   a.   Fever
   b.   Self-limiting nausea
   c.   Abdominal pain
   d.   Transient liver decompensation
   e.   Rarely irreversible hepatic failure

CASE 146

A 45-year-old man with history of cirrhosis came to gastroenterology clinic with jaundice and gradual abdominal distention. He was advised transjugular liver biopsy and measurement of portal pressure.

1.   How can you calculate hepatic venous pressure gradient (HVPG)?

2.   How HVPG can be graded?

3.   What are the complications of portal hypertension?

Answers

1.   HVPG = Wedged hepatic venous pressure (WHVP) – Free hepatic venous pressure (FHVP). Median of three readings can be taken.

2.   HVPG can be graded as follows:
   a.   Normal: 1–5 mm Hg
   b.   Preclinical sinusoidal hypertension: 6–98 mm Hg.
   c.   Clinical sinusoidal portal hypertension: It is $\geq$10 mm Hg. It is a risk factor for hepatic decompensation within 3 months of resection of liver in case of hepatocellular carcinoma.
   d.   Elevation of $\geq$12 mm Hg—associated with ascites and variceal bleeding

3.   Complications of portal hypertension:
   a.   Consumptive coagulopathy leading to thrombo-cytopenia
   b.   Venous collaterals on the abdominal wall
   c.   Ascites
   d.   Spontaneous bacterial peritonitis
   e.   Hepatic hydrothorax
   f.   Hepatorenal syndrome
   g.   Hepatic encephalopathy
   h.   Hepatopulmonary syndrome
   i.   Portopulmonary hypertension
   j.   Cirrhotic cardiomyopathy
   k.   Chronic bleeding from portal hypertensive gastropathy leading to iron-deficiency anemia
   l.   Bleeding from the varices

CASE 147

A 65-year-old male has been admitted with decompensated alcoholic cirrhosis for measurement of HVPG and liver biopsy. Reading demonstrated as:

Free hepatic venous pressure (FHVP) 12/12/12 mm Hg and wedged hepatic venous pressure (WHVP) 30/30/30 mm Hg. Liver biopsy demonstrated:

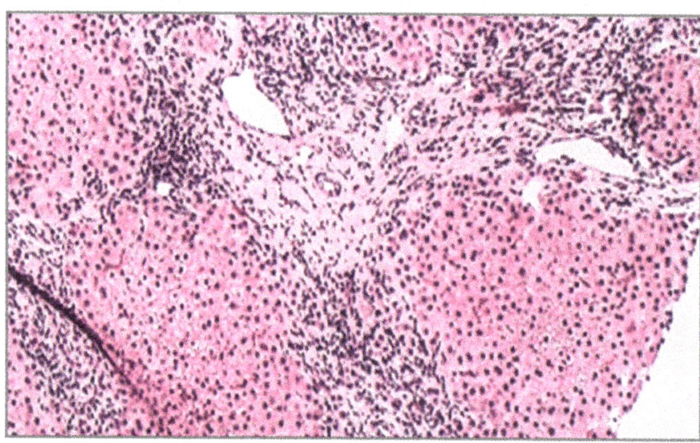

1. **What is the histological feature in the above histology?**
2. **What is the amount of HVPV?**
3. **What is your likely diagnosis?**

Answers

1. The histology of the liver demonstrated the following:
   a. Absence and paucity of bile ducts
   b. Infiltration with focal chronic inflammatory cells in the periportal area

2. HVPG = 30 – 12 = 18 mm Hg
3. The most likely diagnosis is severe portal hypertension in a case of primary biliary cirrhosis.

CASE 148

A 60-year-old obese patient with a history of nonalcoholic cirrhosis has been admitted in ICU with variceal bleeding. On admission, HVPV was measured. Then the patient was treated with 40 mg of propranolol orally thrice daily for 5 days. Then again HVPG was measured.

On admission: FHVP = 15/16/16 and WHVP = 40/40/40

After propranolol therapy: FHVP = 14/14/14 and WHVP = 35/35/35

1. **What is the change in the HVPG in the above case?**
2. **What is your interpretation?**

Answers

1. In the first case: HVPG = 24 mm Hg; in the second case: HVPG = 21 mm Hg. So, difference is 3 mm Hg.

2. Significant improvement in the HVPG after treatment with propranolol is considered when the reduction of HVPG is at least 12 mm Hg or 20% reduction from the baseline.

CASE 149

A 65-year-old cirrhotic male admitted with abdominal distention. His HVPG was measured. His CT scan of abdomen was demonstrated:

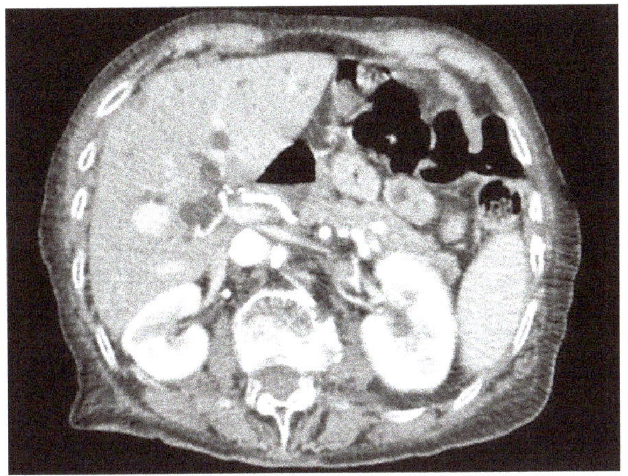

1. **What does the above CT scan abdomen picture demonstrate here?**
2. **What is the HVPG?**
3. **What is your interpretation?**

Answers

1. Above CT scan abdomen picture demonstrated that there are multiple shunts in-between the hepatic veins in the liver.

2. Here, FHVP = 15/15/15 mm Hg and WHVP = 18/18/18 mm Hg. So, HVPG = 3 mm Hg.

3. Wedged hepatic portal gradient is abnormally low which may be due to shunt in-between the hepatic veins.

CASE 150

A 50-year-old woman came to gastroenterology clinic with right-sided upper abdominal pain. Ultrasonography of the abdomen demonstrated a hemangioma in the right lobe of the liver. CT scan of the abdomen demonstrated:

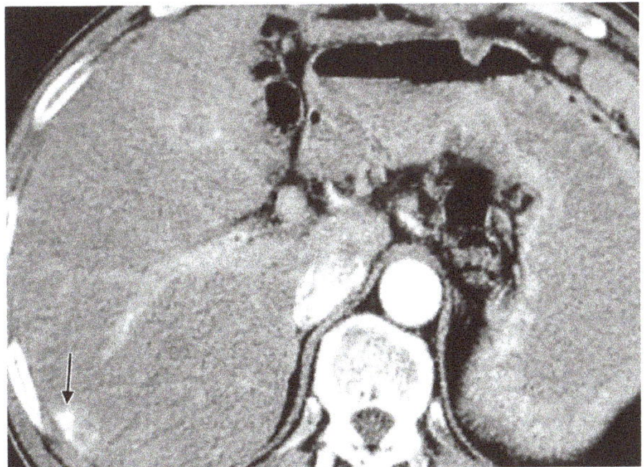

His FHVP = 15 and WHVP = 25 mm Hg

1. **What is your CT scan finding?**
2. **What is HVPG?**
3. **What is your interpretation?**
4. **What is your treatment?**

Answers

1. CT scan of the abdomen demonstrated arterioportal communication seen during arterial phase and a rare cause of portal hypertension.

2. HVPG = 10 mm Hg

3. It interprets as a case of portal hypertension.

4. This case can be treated by coil embolization of arterioportal shunt.

CASE 151

A 56-year-old type 2 diabetic patient suffering from nonalcoholic steatotic hepatitis with cirrhosis having no feature of decompensation. Gastroscopy demonstrated the following features:

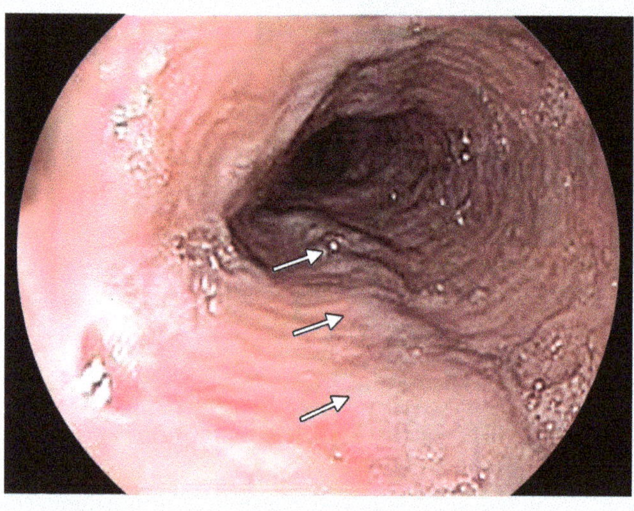 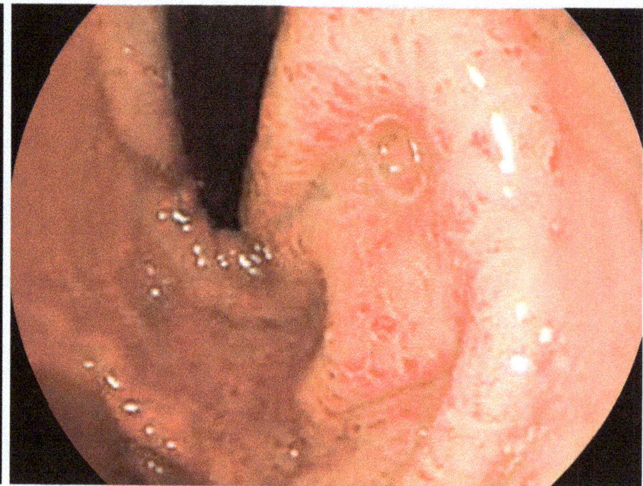

1. **What are the findings in the above pictures?**
2. **When the repeat gastroscopy should be done?**
3. **How is portal vein formed?**
4. **What are the effects of portal hypertension?**
5. **How do the esophageal varices develop?**
6. **How do gastric varices develop?**
7. **What are the sites where varices can develop?**
8. **Which patient should avoid gastroscopy?**

Answers

1. Gastroscopy demonstrated the following:
   a. Two columns of early esophageal varices in the lower third of esophagus.
   b. There is evidence of early portal gastropathy characterized by multiple submucosal ecchymoses with congested fundal mucosa.
2. The repeat gastroscopy should be done at the end of 1 year because of the following reasons:
   a. Early esophageal varices that are collapsed easily on insufflation.
   b. There are no high-risk stigmata in gastroscopy.
   c. There is no feature of decompression.
3. Portal vein is formed by confluence of superior mesenteric vein and the splenic vein behind the pancreas and responsible for the 70% of blood supply to the liver bed. The branches are:
   a. Cystic vein
   b. Left gastric vein
   c. Right gastric vein
4. Following are the effects of portal hypertension:
   a. Dilatation of the portal venous tributaries leads to development of varices that may bleed easily.
   b. Different collaterals connect the portal and the systemic vein resulting in shunt which will predispose to hepatic encephalopathy.
5. Dilatation of the anterior as well as posterior tributaries of left gastric vein leading to production of esophageal varices

6. Gastric varices develop from:
    a. Left gastric veins
    b. Gastric vein
    c. Gastroepiploic veins
7. Other varices are:
    a. In the rectum: From superior hemorrhoidal vein
    b. Retroperitoneum:
        • Gonadal vein
        • Lumbar vein
        • Paraduodenal vein

c. Around the surgical stoma as a result of communication between the relocated mesenteric veins and cutaneous veins

8. Following patients should avoid gastroscopy:
    a. If patient having liver stiffness, measurement of <15 kPa and platelet count >150,000/cc can avoid gastroscopy.
    b. If HVPG is <10 mm Hg, gastroscopy can be avoided.

CASE 152

A 45-year-old patient with cirrhosis underwent screening gastrointestinal endoscopy. It demonstrated the following finding:

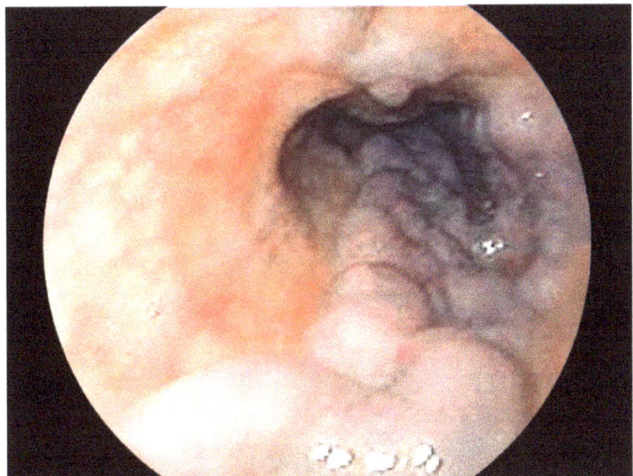

1. **What is the finding in the above picture?**
2. **What is the cause for developing the above features?**
3. **What are pathophysiologies for developing the above feature?**
4. **What are the risk factors for variceal bleeding?**
5. **What are the complications of variceal bleeding?**
6. **How can you manage the active bleeding?**
7. **What precaution should be taken during administration of terlipressin?**

Answers

1. The above picture demonstrated evidence of gastroesophageal varices.
2. Portal hypertension is responsible for developing gastroesophageal varices.
3. Following are the pathophysiologies of portal hypertension which in turn produces gastroesophageal varices:
    a. Increased resistance to portal blood flow at the level hepatic sinusoids—it is caused by:
        • Intrahepatic vasoconstriction due to:
            ○ Decreased production of nitric oxide
            ○ Increased release of angiotensinogen, endothelin-1, and eicosanoids
        • Remodeling of sinusoids leading to disruption of blood flow
    b. Increased portal blood flow resulting from hyperdynamic circulation due to dilatation of splanchnic blood flow through the following mediators:
        • Nitric oxide
        • Prostacyclin
        • Tumor necrosis factor

4. Following are the risk factors for variceal bleeding:
   a. Size of the varices: As the size is gradually increasing in size, there is risk of bleeding.
   b. Advanced Child–Pugh classification leading to increased risk of variceal hemorrhage
   c. Presence of red color sign in the varices during gastroscopy
   d. Active consumption of alcohol
5. Complications of the variceal bleeding are:
   a. Aspiration
   b. Hepatic encephalopathy
   c. Multiorgan failure
   d. Perforation of esophagus
   e. Death
6. Following are the treatments of active bleeding:
   a. Hemodynamic resuscitation
   b. Intravenous access for administration of fluid, blood, and drugs
   c. Overtransfusion should not be done as it increases the risk of portal pressure and rebleeding risk.
   d. Coagulopathy should be started as it increases the bleeding risk.
   e. Sedation and nephrotoxic drugs should be avoided.
   f. Intravenous octreotide at a dose of 50 µg bolus followed by intravenous transfusion to decrease the portal pressure
   g. Intravenous terlipressin should be given 2 mg 4 hourly for 2–3 days followed by 1 mg 4 hourly.
   h. 250 mg erythromycin should be given intravenously 30 minutes to 2 hours prior to endoscopy.
   i. Band ligation of the variceal bleeding as compared to sclerotherapy
   j. If the endoscopic treatment fails, self-expandable metal stent or peroral placement of Sengstaken–Blakemore tube for at least 24–48 hours
   k. As there is chance of secondary bacterial infection, antibiotics like norfloxacin or ceftriaxone should be given for a week.
7. During administration of terlipressin and serum sodium estimation should be done as this drug produces hyponatremia by reducing the solute-free water through the kidney by activation of vasopressin 2 receptor activation.

CASE 153

A 45-year-old nondiabetic patient from Bangladesh came to gastroenterology clinic with progressively increasing distention of the abdomen. His blood report demonstrated hemoglobin 12.5 g/dL, platelet count 155,000/cc, white blood cell count 9,000/cc, bilirubin 3.2 mg/dL, serum enzyme level normal, serum albumin 3.3 g/dL, ascitic fluid albumin 1.2 g/dL, and ascitic fluid cell count 150/cc.

1. **What type of ascites and why?**
2. **What are the three main causes of ascites?**
3. **What are the other causes of ascites?**
4. **How can you differentiate whether the ascites is due to heart failure or due to cirrhosis?**
5. **Is there any importance of measuring the serum level of CA-125 in ascites?**
6. **What are the features of chylous ascites?**
7. **What are the complications related to paracentesis?**

Answers

1. It is transudative ascites because the serum-ascites albumin gradient (SAAG) is 3.3/1.2, i.e., >1.1
2. Three main causes of transudative ascites are:
   a. Cirrhosis
   b. Congestive cardiac failure
   c. Budd–Chiari syndrome
3. Other causes of ascites are:
   a. Transudative ascites:
      - Massive hepatic metastasis
      - Pericarditis
      - Idiopathic portal fibrosis
      - Portal vein thrombosis
   b. Exudative ascites:
      - Tuberculosis
      - Malignant peritonitis
      - Pancreatitis
      - Subacute bacterial peritonitis
      - Peritoneal carcinomatosis

4. Ascitic fluid albumin estimation can differentiate heart from cirrhosis:
    a. In case of heart failure, ascitic fluid is >2.5 g/dL because compliant hepatic sinusoids will allow protein-rich fluid to leak into the abdominal cavity leading to increase in ascitic fluid albumin.
    b. Whereas, in case of cirrhosis, vascular permeability will be restricted by the fibrous tissue leading to maintaining the ascitic fluid protein level to <2.5 g/dL.
5. As CA-125 is secreted by healthy mesothelial cells and ovarian tumor cells, this level can be increased in both males and females in ascites of any cause.
6. Chylous ascites produces following features:
    a. Diarrhea
    b. Steatorrhea
    c. Malnutrition
    d. Edema
    e. Nausea
    f. Enlarged lymph nodes
    g. Fever
    h. Night sweats
7. Following are the paracentesis-related complications:
    a. Infection
    b. Bleeding
    c. Perforation of bowel
    d. Electrolyte imbalance
    e. Kidney injury
    f. Leakage of ascitic fluid through the abdominal wall

CASE 154

A 55-year-old patient with alcoholic cirrhosis has been admitted with inversion of sleep rhythm and behavioral changes following constipation of some days. He left alcohol for 8 months. He was on diuretics, propranolol, and lactulose. On examination, his blood pressure was 90/60 mm Hg, pulse rate 120 beats/minute, spider nevi in the chest, presence of ascites, and no neurological deficit.

On investigation, his hemoglobin was 9 g/dL, platelet count 70,000/cc, bilirubin 2.3 mg/dL, normal level of enzyme, urea 60 mg/dL, creatinine 1.6, and sodium 122 mEq/L. Serology was negative.

1. **What is your most likely diagnosis?**
2. **How can you classify this disease?**
3. **What are the tests to be done to detect minimal changes in this disease?**
4. **What are the mimics of hepatic encephalopathy?**

Answers

1. The most likely diagnosis is grade II episodic type C hepatic encephalopathy being precipitated by constipation in a case of decompensated alcohol-related cirrhosis.
2. Classification of the disease:
    a. According to etiology:
        - Type A: Hepatic encephalopathy associated with acute liver failure (ALF)
        - Type B: In case of predominant portosystemic shunting without liver disease associated with hepatic encephalopathy
        - Type C: Hepatic encephalopathy associated with cirrhosis of liver
    b. According to clinical severity:
        - Covert hepatic encephalopathy: Minimal hepatic encephalopathy + West Haven grade I
        - Overt hepatic encephalopathy: It includes West Haven grade II to IV hepatic encephalopathy
    c. According to the time course:
        - Episodic hepatic encephalopathy: Difference in-between the episodes is ≥6 months with intervening periods without neurological symptoms. It is further subdivided into:
            - Precipitated hepatic encephalopathy
            - Spontaneous hepatic encephalopathy
            - Recurrent hepatic encephalopathy: Evidence of two episodes within 6 months
        - Minimal hepatic encephalopathy
        - Persistent hepatic encephalopathy: It is characterized by presence of alteration in the behavior present persistently with intermittent relapses of overt hepatic encephalopathy. It is further subdivided into the following:

- ○ Mild hepatic encephalopathy
- ○ Severe hepatic encephalopathy
- ○ Treatment-dependent hepatic encephalopathy
3. Following tests are done to detect the minimal hepatic encephalopathy:
   a. International Society for Hepatic Encephalopathy recommends following psychometric hepatic encephalopathy score for the diagnosis of minimal hepatic encephalopathy:
      - Number connection test A: Here, randomly distributed numbers have to be joined serially as quickly as possible.
      - Number connection test B: Here, randomly distributed numbers as well as letters have to be joined in alternating series as quickly as possible, i.e., 1-A-2-B-3-C like this.
      - Line copying test: Here, a given line has to be traced as quickly as possible.
   - Digit symbol test: Here, a sheet is given to the patient where each digit from 1 to 9 is assigned a symbol. Patient has to write down the symbol under each digit within a given a time.
   - Mosaic test: Here, the cubes having various designs on each face have to be placed within a given time in such a way that upper faces will form a particular design.
4. Following are the mimics of hepatic encephalopathy:
   a. Dyselectrolytemia
   b. Encephalitis
   c. Myxedema coma
   d. Sepsis-induced encephalopathy
   e. Cerebrovascular accidents
   f. Alcohol intoxication
   g. Wernicke's encephalopathy
   h. Withdrawal of alcohol
   i. Delirium tremens

CASE 155

A 55-year-old patient with alcoholic cirrhosis has been admitted with inversion of sleep rhythm and behavioral changes following constipation of some days. He left alcohol for 8 months. He was on diuretics, propranolol, and lactulose. On examination, his blood pressure was 90/60 mm Hg, pulse rate 120 beats/minute, spider nevi in the chest, presence of ascites, and no neurological deficit.

On investigation, his hemoglobin was 9 g/dL, platelet count 70,000/cc, bilirubin 2.3 mg/dL, normal level of enzyme, urea 60 mg/dL, creatinine 1.6, and sodium 122 mEq/L. Serology was negative.

1. **What is your most likely diagnosis?**
2. **What is the West Haven classification along with the stages?**
3. **What are the effects of ammonia once it will cross the blood–brain barrier?**
4. **What are the factors affecting the ammonia level?**
5. **What are the factors precipitating hepatic encephalopathy?**
6. **Mention the strategies in the management of hepatic encephalopathy?**
7. **What is the mechanism of action of lactulose?**

Answers

1. The most likely diagnosis is grade II episodic type C hepatic encephalopathy being precipitated by constipation in a case of decompensated alcohol-related cirrhosis.
2. West Haven classification of hepatic encephalopathy with stages:
   a. Grade 0: No obvious changes, but it consists of potentially underlying mild disease—minimal hepatic encephalopathy.
   b. Grade 1:
      - Minimal lack of awareness
      - Euphoria or anxiety
      - Shortened attention span
      - Altered sleep rhythm
      - Impaired performance of calculations
   c. Grade 2:
      - Lethargy or apathy
      - Minimal disorientation for time or place
      - Subtle personality changes
      - Inappropriate behavior
      - Dyspraxia
      - Persistence of asterixis
   d. Grade 3:
      - Somnolence progressing toward stupor but responsive to verbal stimuli

- Confusion
- Gross disorientation
- Bizarre behavior
    e. Grade 4: Coma
3. Following are the neurotoxic effects of ammonia once it will cross the blood–brain barrier:
    a. Alteration in the molecular transport such as electrolytes, amino acids, and water in the astrocytes and neurons
    b. Increased synthesis of glutamines from glutamates by astrocytes
    c. Inhibition of generation of excitatory and inhibitory postsynaptic potentials
    d. Impaired metabolism of amino acids
    e. Increased activity of γ-aminobutyric acid (GABA) leading to impaired utilization of energy
4. Following factors affect the ammonia level:
    a. High-dietary protein intake
    b. Gastrointestinal bleeding
    c. Prolonged fasting due to:
        - Breakdown of the muscles
        - Intense physical activity
    d. Presence of renal dysfunction
    e. Post-transjugular intrahepatic portosystemic shunt (post-TIPSS)
5. Following factors precipitate hepatic encephalo-pathy:
    a. Gastrointestinal bleeding
    b. Infections
    c. Trauma
    d. Dehydration
    e. Uremia
    f. Constipation
    g. Excessive protein in the diet
    h. Hyperkalemia
    i. Hyponatremia
    j. Sedatives or tranquilizers
    k. Diuretic therapy
6. Following are the strategies in the management of hepatic encephalopathy:
    a. Covert hepatic encephalopathy: Therapy with lactulose or lactitol
    b. Acute episode of hepatic encephalopathy:
        - First choice is lactulose by either retention enema or orally depending upon the consciousness of the patient.
        - If the patient is not responding to lactulose, intravenous L-ornithine-L-aspartate should be an alternative.
        - In case of intolerance to lactulose, polyethylene glycol can be given.
    c. Prevention of recurrence:
        - Lactulose should be recommended.
        - Rifaximin should be given as an add-on therapy to lactulose.
7. Mechanism of action of lactulose:
    a. It inhibits the production of ammonia by following processes:
        - Conversion of lactulose to lactic acid and acetic acid leading to acidification in the gut lumen. As a result ammonia is converted to ammonium which is impermeable to mucous membrane of the gastrointestinal tract. So, it leads to reduction in the concentration of ammonia in the circulation.
        - It inhibits the ammonia-forming bacteria and increases the production of nonam-monia forming lactobacilli.
        - It acts as cathartic thereby reducing the load in the gut bacteria.

CASE 156

A 55-year-old man has been admitted with alcoholic cirrhosis with oliguria and diarrhea for 2 days. His laboratory investigation demonstrated blood urea 178 mg/dL and serum creatinine 3.2 mg/dL. Liver function test demonstrated within normal limit.

1. **What is your most likely diagnosis?**
2. **What is the differential diagnosis?**
3. **How can you differentiate these two diagnoses?**

Answers

1. The most likely diagnosis is prerenal acute kidney injury in a case of alcoholic cirrhosis.
2. The differential diagnosis is hepatorenal syndrome–acute kidney injury.
3. Following are the points in favor of acute tubular necrosis—acute tubular injury:
   a. Acute kidney injury is caused by either ischemic injury or nephrotoxic damage of renal tubular cells resulting in formation of "muddy brown" cast which can be demonstrated in the urine microscopy.
   b. Impairment of reabsorption of sodium and urea leading to increased excretion of free sodium to >2–3%.
   c. Neutrophil gelatinase-associated lipocalin will be elevated.

Following are the points in favor of hepatorenal syndrome–acute kidney injury:
   a. Integrity of the tubular epithelium will be intact.
   b. Free excretion of sodium and urea will be low.
   c. Neutrophil gelatinase-associated lipocalin will be normal.

CASE 157

A 48-year-old hypertensive married IT professional having sedentary lifestyle consuming 80 g of alcohol on the weekend attended liver clinic for raised liver enzymes. She has no history of drug intake. She has a family history of coronary artery disease. On examination, her BMI was 33.02 g/m², waist circumference 90 cm, blood pressure 140/90 mm Hg, pulse rate 90 beats/minute, and hepatomegaly. USG demonstrated liver size of 12.2 cm with increased echo, spleen size 8 cm, portal vein 9.5 cm, and no ascites. Her blood test demonstrated hemoglobin of 13.2 g/dL, platelet count of 150,000/cc, total count of WBC 8,000/cc, total bilirubin of 2 mg/dL, ALT of 100 IU/L, AST of 95 IU/L, ALP of 108 IU/L, INR of 1.15, albumin level of 3.8 g/dL, serology negative triglyceride 300 of mg/dL, LDL of 98 IU/L, renal function test normal, and HbA1c of 6.7.

Transient elastography demonstrated 8.2 kPa and controlled attenuated parameter of 329.

1. **What type of injury occurred in this patient?**
2. **What is the normal range for ALT and AST?**
3. **What histories are required to be elicited while evaluating cases of raised liver enzymes?**
4. **What patterns of elevation of hepatic enzymes occurring in different types of hepatitis?**
5. **Why AST level is higher than ALT in case of alcoholic hepatitis?**
6. **If ALP is raised, what tests should be done to detect the involvement of liver?**
7. **What are the causes of increased or decreased ALP?**

Answers

1. In the above blood picture, liver enzymes are elevated indicative of hepatocellular injury as in this injury there is disproportionate elevation of the ALT and AST as compared to ALP. On the other hand, ALP is disproportionately elevated as compared to AST or ALT. Here, R ratio should be evaluated to delineate the cause of injury.

   $$R = \dfrac{\text{ALT/upper limit of normal}}{\text{AP/upper limit of normal}}$$

   a. In case of hepatocellular injury, ALT is more than two times of upper level of normal and R = ≥5
   b. In case of cholestatic liver injury, ALP is more than two times of upper level of normal and R = ≤2.
   c. In case of mixed hepatic injury, ALT and AP both are two times upper limit of normal or 5 > R > 2.

2. Classically normal range of ALT is 5–35. According to recent guideline in case of male and female, normal ALT levels are 29–33 IU/L and 19–25 IU/L, respectively.

3. Following histories are required to be elicited for diagnosing elevated enzymes of the liver:
   a. History of arthritis and skin rash indicates autoimmune diseases
   b. History of anorexia, generalized weakness, and low-grade fever suggests viral hepatitis
   c. History of weight loss, anorexia, and generalized weakness suggests hepatocellular carcinoma

d. History of itching, dark urine, and clay-colored stool suggests congestive phase of viral hepatitis and any type of cholestasis

e. History of tattooing, illicit drug use, needle pricks, blood transfusion, and renal failure in dialysis suggests hepatitis C virus pathology

f. History of blood transfusion, sharing of unsterilized shaver, and sexual promiscuity suggests viral B pathology

g. History of drug intake to detect drug-induced liver injury

h. History of any extrahepatic disorder such as cardiac and thyroid disorders

i. History of inflammatory bowel disease as it may lead to extraintestinal manifestations of liver injury

j. History of any chronic morbidity such as diabetes mellitus, obesity, hypertension, hyperuricemia, and dyslipidemia

k. Family history of hepatocellular failure or death due to liver disease

4. Following are the patterns of transaminases in different types of liver involvement:

a. AST is greater than ALT: It occurs in—
- Alcoholic hepatitis
- Cirrhosis of any etiology
- Ischemic hepatitis
- Congestive hepatopathy
- Acute Budd–Chiari syndrome
- Total parenteral nutrition

b. ALT is greater than AST: It occurs in—
- Nonalcoholic steatohepatitis
- Acute and chronic viral hepatitis
- Drug-induced liver injury
- Autoimmune hepatitis (AIH)
- Metabolic liver disorders
- Sepsis-induced liver dysfunction

c. Nonhepatic causes of elevated liver enzymes:
- Rhabdomyolysis
- Cardiac injury
- Thyroid disorders
- Strenuous exercise
- Adrenal insufficiency
- Hemolysis

- Macro-ASTemia: It is characterized by formation of complexes by AST and immunoglobulins which lead to its reduced clearance.

5. Following are the causes of elevated AST as compared to AST in alcoholic hepatitis:

a. Due to damage of the mitochondria in the hepatocytes, there is elevation of AST.

b. ALT is very sensitive to pyridoxine which occurs in alcoholic patient.

So, the ratio becomes AST: ALT is 5:1. But AST level is never >400 U/L.

6. As the origin of ALP is from bone, intestine, placenta, kidney, and liver, in case of liver injury, serum γ-glutamyl transpeptidase level should also be elevated which will not be elevated in other involvement of other organs.

7. Causes of elevated or lowering of ALP:

a. Hepatic causes of:
- Intrahepatic or extrahepatic or both types of cholestasis.
- Infiltrative disorders:
  - Granulomatous diseases such as tuberculosis and sarcoidosis
  - Amyloid disease
  - Lymphoma
  - Fungal infections
  - Cancers
- Liver abscesses
- Ductopenia
- Vanishing bile duct syndrome
- Benign intrahepatic cholestasis in pregnancy

b. Nonhepatic causes of raised ALP:
- Cardiac failure
- Hemophagocytic lymphohistiocytosis
- Thyroid disorders
- Bone diseases

c. Causes of low ALP:
- Hypothyroidism
- Wilson's disease
- Hemolysis
- Congenital hypophosphatasia
- Aceruloplasminemia

CASE 158

A 24-year-old male has been admitted in emergency with history of low-grade fever for 5 days associated with nausea, malaise, yellowish discoloration of eyes for 3 days, drowsiness, and irrelevant talk for 1 day. He has no history of blood transfusion, tattooing, illicit drug use, intake of alcohol, and no such history in his family members and in the surrounding community. On examination, he is deeply icteric and there is flapping tremor.

His blood picture demonstrated hemoglobin level of 12 g%, platelet count of 150,000/cc, total WBC count of 15,000/cc, total bilirubin of 10 g/dL out of which 8 g/dL was direct bilirubin. ALT and AST were 1,400 and 801 IU/L, respectively, ALP 101 of IU/L, albumin of 3.5 g/dL, and INR of 2.2, and viral serology all are negative except hepatitis E virus (HEV) immunoglobulin M (IgM) which was positive. Procalcitonin was 1.5, serum sodium 124 mEq/L, and potassium 4.4 mEq/L, and renal function test was normal.

1. **What is your diagnosis?**
2. **How can you differentiate it from acute liver injury?**
3. **What are the common liver diseases producing this condition?**
4. **How can you classify this disease?**

Answers

1. Acute hepatocellular failure in a case of HEV-positive acute hepatitis
2. In case of acute liver injury, there is dysfunction of liver as well as coagulopathy like INR of >1.5, but there is no evidence of alteration of consciousness. But in case of ALF, there should be jaundice along with INR of ≥1.5 associated with any degree of encephalopathy but there is no preexisting liver disease.
3. Following common diseases produce this condition:
   a. Drug-induced liver injury
   b. Overdose of acetaminophen
   c. Autoimmune hepatitis
   d. Ischemic hepatitis
   e. Budd–Chiari syndrome
   f. Acute fatty liver in pregnancy
   g. Infection with hepatotropic viruses such as HAV, HEV, and HBV.
4. Acute liver failure according to the duration of jaundice:
   a. Hyperacute ALF: Up to 7 days
   b. Acute ALF: 7–28 days
   c. Subacute ALF: 28 days to 26 weeks

CASE 159

A 24-year-old male has been admitted in emergency with history of low-grade fever for 5 days associated with nausea, malaise, yellowish discoloration of eyes for 3 days, drowsiness, and irrelevant talk for 1 day. He has no history of blood transfusion, tattooing, illicit drug use, intake of alcohol, and no such history in his family members and in the surrounding community. On examination, he is deeply icteric and there is flapping tremor.

1. **What is your diagnosis?**
2. **Describe the King's college criteria in this disease.**
3. **How can ALFED model predict the outcome in ALF?**
4. **What are the clinical prognostic indicators in this disease?**
5. **What are the other scoring systems required in case of ALF for hepatic transplantation?**
6. **What is the role of optic nerve sheath diameter in this disease?**
7. **What is the role of plasmapheresis in ALF?**

Answers

1. Acute liver failure in a case of HEV-positive acute hepatitis

2. King's college criteria for emergency liver transplantation:
   a. Paracetamol and Hyperacute etiologies:
      - Arterial pH <7.3 after resuscitation.
      - Lactate level >3 mmol/L
      - Any three of the following:
         ○ INR > 6.5
         ○ Hepatic encephalopathy grade III
         ○ Serum creatinine > 300 µmol/L
   b. Nonparacetamol etiologies:
      - INR > 6.5
      - Any three of the following:
         ○ Indeterminate etiology
         ○ Age < 10 or > 40 years
         ○ Jaundice to encephalopathy >7 days
         ○ Bilirubin > 300 µmol/L
         ○ INR > 3.5

3. ALFED (acute liver failure early dynamic model) score:

Variable over 3 days	Scores assigned
Hepatic encephalopathy, persistent, or progressed to grade >2	2
INR, persistent, or prolonged to level ≥5	1
Arterial ammonia, persistent, or increased to level ≥123 µmol/L	2
Serum bilirubin, persistent, or increased to level ≥15 mg/dL	1

   Risk stratification based on ALFED model:
   a. 0 to 1: Low risk, expected mortality 2.6%
   b. 2 to 3: Moderate risk, expected mortality 19%
   c. 4 to 6: High risk, expected mortality 88%.

4. Clinical prognostic indicators in this disease:
   a. Age ≥ 50 years
   b. Jaundice encephalopathy interval >7 days
   c. At presentation, grade 3 to 4 encephalopathy
   d. Presence of cerebral edema
   e. Prothrombin time ≥ 35 seconds
   f. Creatinine ≥ 1.5 mg/dL

   According to this indicator, 3 to 6 should be considered optimum for differentiating between survivors and nonsurvivors.

5. Other scoring system required for ALF:
   a. Clichy criteria or Beaujon-Paul Brousse criteria: It can identify the patients for emergency transplantation of liver:
      - Hepatic encephalopathy stage ≥ 3
      - Level of factor V < 20% or < 30% based on the age
   b. Model for end-stage liver disease (MELD) score: It is used for listing the patients for liver transplantation or outcome after performing TIPSS. If this score is >33, prognosis is poor and he or she will require urgent liver transplantation.
   c. Acute liver failure study group index (ALFSG Index): It can predict transplant-free survival. It is based on the following criteria:
      - Grade of hepatic encephalopathy
      - Etiology of liver failure
      - Level of bilirubin
      - INR
      - Requirement of vasopressor

6. Optic nerve sheath is continuous with the dura mater of the brain. Subarachnoid space in the brain is continuous with that in the optic nerve sheath. So, it can reflect in the change in pressure of CSF within the subarachnoid space in the brain. This optic sheath diameter can be measured by ultrasonography. There is a linear correlation between intracranial pressure and optic nerve sheath diameter. The cutoff value is >5.2 mm of sheath when intracranial pressure is >20 mm Hg.

7. Plasmapheresis:
   a. Acts as bridge to transplant of liver
   b. Helps to select the modality when transplant will be the only option.

CASE 160

A 40-year-old male came to liver clinic with 1 week history of malaise, low-grade fever, yellowish discoloration of urine, and conjunctiva. He has family history of hepatitis B virus-induced jaundice 2 months ago. He has no history of intravenous drug use, blood transfusion, and tattooing. On examination, there was jaundice and tender hepatomegaly. On ultrasonography, liver is 11.5 cm in length having regular margin and smooth surface, spleen is 9 cm in length and diameter of the portal vein is 9 cm and absence of pleural fluid.

1. **What is your likely diagnosis?**
2. **What are the signs of hepatocellular failure in the hand?**
3. **When this disease is known as chronic hepatitis?**
4. **Mention the classical stages of chronic infection.**
5. **According to American Association for the Study of Liver Disease (AASLD) guideline, what are the cutoff values of upper limit of ALT?**
6. **What is the screening recommended for hepatitis B virus infection?**
7. **If the patient is hepatitis B surface antigen (HBsAg) negative, anti-HBs negative, but anti-HBc positive, what will be the implication?**

Answers

1. The most likely diagnosis is hepatitis B virus-induced hepatitis.
2. Following are the signs of hepatocellular failure in the hand:
   a. Jaundice
   b. Flapping tremor
   c. White nails
   d. Palmar erythema
   e. Dupuytren's contracture
3. If the HBsAg is positive for at least 6 months, this disease is known as chronic hepatitis B infection.
4. Following are the stages of chronic HBV infection:

Phase	ALT	HBV DNA	HBeAg	Liver biopsy
Immune tolerant	Normal usually	Increased	Positive	Minimal inflammation
Immune active	Increased	Increased	Positive	Moderate inflammation
Immune control (inactive chronic hepatitis B)	Normal	Undetectable or Low	Positive	Minimal necro-inflammation
Immune reactivation	Increased	Increased	Positive	Moderate-to-severe inflammation or fibrosis

The above stages have been modified by European Association for the Study of the Liver (EASL) guidelines in 2017 as follows:

Phase	ALT	HBV DNA	HBeAg	Liver biopsy
HBeAg positive Chronic infection	Normal usually	$>10^7$	Positive	Minimal inflammation

Continued

Continued

Phase	ALT	HBV DNA	HBeAg	Liver biopsy
HBeAg positive Chronic hepatitis	Increased	10^4 to 10^7	Positive	Moderate inflammation
HBeAg negative Chronic infection	Normal	<2,000	Negative	None
HBeAg negative Chronic hepatitis	Increased	>2,000	Negative	Moderate-to-severe inflammation or fibrosis

5. According to AASLD guideline, the upper limit of normal ALT value is 29–33 U/L for males and 19–25 U/L for females.
6. Following are the recommended strategies for HBV screening of HBV:
   a. Promiscuity between men
   b. Intravenous drug use
   c. Patient under hemodialysis
   d. People living with HIV patients
   e. Regular blood donors
   f. Chronic hepatitis C patients
   g. Patients under immunosuppressive therapies
   h. Homosexuality or heterosexuality with HIV patients
   i. Incarcerated patients
   j. Pregnant women
   k. Infants born to HIV-infected mother
   l. Traveling to countries having high prevalence of HBV infection.
7. The following scenarios are there:
   a. This patient had previous exposure to HBV infection.

b. Recovered already from acute HBV infection in the early life and anti-HBs titer is going down to low level of titer or at undetectable level.

c. Chronic infection for decades followed by clearance of HBsAg

d. Patient is in the window phase of acute infection with HBV.

e. Mutation of HBsAg leading to false-negative HBsAg

CASE 161

1. **What do the above pictures demonstrate?**
2. **What is the end point of therapy in HBV infection in chronic HBV patient?**
3. **What are the recommendations of HBV therapy according to AASLD and EASL?**
4. **In case of acute HBV infection, what are the recommendations of therapies?**
5. **What are the recommendations in case of pregnant patient?**
6. **What are the drug options in the treatment of chronic HBV infection?**

Answers

1. The above pictures are the drugs used in treatment of HBV infection in patient infected with HBV.

2. The goals of therapies are the following:

   a. To prevent the progression of the disease as the cirrhosis once sets in, within 5 years, decompensation rate will be 20% and risk of developing hepatocellular carcinoma will be 2–5%.

   b. Elimination of integrated DNA or closed covalent circular DNA (cccDNA). But it is very difficult to achieve.

   c. Loss of HBsAg: It is commonly used parameter. But, this may be present if the cell wall may be present in the blood in spite of clearing of virus.

   d. The most monitorable parameter is HBV DNA suppression to very low or undetectable level.

   e. Normalization of ALT

3. Recommendations of HBV therapy according to AASLD and EASL guidelines are:

Characteristics	AASLD (2018)	EASL (2017)
HBeAg positive	• HBV DNA > 20,000 IU/L • ALT more than two times of upper limit of normal	• HBV DNA > 2,000 IU/L • ALT level more than upper limit of normal • And/or at least moderate necroinflammation/fibrosis
HBeAg negative	• HBV DNA > 2,000 IU/L • ALT level more than two times upper limit of normal	• HBV DNA > 2,000 IU/L • ALT level more than upper limit of normal • And/or at least moderate necroinflammation/fibrosis
Compensated cirrhosis	Adult with compensated cirrhosis even in presence of virus level of <2,000 IU/L should be given.	Any detectable HBV DNA regardless of ALT level
Decompensated cirrhosis	All patients	Any detectable HBV DNA regardless of ALT level plus assessment of liver transplant

Continued

Continued

Characteristics	AASLD (2018)	EASL (2017)
Additional patients who may require therapies	• Adults > 40 years of age • Normal ALT level • HBV DNA ≥ 1,000,000 IU/L with significant necroinflammation or fibrosis • Family history of cirrhosis or hepatocellular carcinoma • Extrahepatic manifestations	• Patients with HBV DNA of >20,000 IU/L and ALT of more than two times upper limit of normal regardless the degree of fibrosis • Family history of cirrhosis or hepatocellular carcinoma

4. 90–95% of acute HBV infection will clear virus spontaneously.

   According to EASL guideline, following patients should be treated:

   a. Acute hepatitis B having INR of >1.5

      Or,

   b. Protracted course having marked jaundice of >4 weeks.

   According to AASLD guidelines:

   Acute liver failure or protracted severe course having:

   • Total bilirubin of >3 mg/dL or direct bilirubin > 1.5 mg/dL

   • INR of >1.5

   • Encephalopathy

   • Ascites

5. The recommendations in case of pregnant patients are:

   a. All the patients with chronic hepatitis B-positive liver disease should be delivered in the institution.

   b. All the newborn should be given immunoglobulin and vaccines just after delivery.

   c. In patients with high level of HBV DNA and HBeAg, positive treatment should be started according to the following guidelines:

   • According to AASLD guidelines if HBV DNA is > 200,000 IU/L, tenofovir disoproxil fumarate (TDF) should be started at 28 weeks of pregnancy.

   • According to EASL guidelines, TDF should be started at 24–28 weeks of pregnancy and it should be continued up to 12 weeks after the delivery if:

     ○ HBV DNA level > 200,000 IU/L

        Or,

     ○ HBsAg levels is 4 log10 IU/mL

     ○ Evidence of fibrosis or cirrhosis

6. Following are the drug options for chronic hepatitis B infection:

   a. Nucleotide analogs having low barrier of resistance:

   • Lamivudine

   • Adefovir dipivoxil

   • Telbivudine

   b. Pegylated interferon-α

   c. Nucleotide with high barrier of resistance:

   • Entecavir

   • Tenofovir disoproxil fumarate

   • Tenofovir alafenamide (TAF)

CASE 162

A 40-year-old patient having history of HBsAg positivity has been taking antiviral therapy for 2 years and HBV DNA level was undetectable. Patient suddenly developed progressively increasing jaundice and HBV DNA level was increased to >1,000 IU/L.

1. **What is your diagnosis?**
2. **How can you define this disease?**
3. **How can you differentiate acute HBV infection from HBV reactivation?**
4. **How can you differentiate it from acute B virus flare?**
5. **What are the conditions where entecavir TAF is preferred over TDF?**
6. **How can you define cure in HBV infection?**
7. **What are the newer biomarkers for HBV infection?**

Answers

1. This is a case of reactivation of hepatitis B virus under continuous treatment with antiviral therapy.
2. This reactivation of HBV can be defined in patients who are HBsAg-positive as follows:
   a. ≥2 log increase in the HBV DNA level as compared to its baseline level
   b. HBV DNA level is ≥3 log or 1,000 IU/mL in a patient who had previous level undetected.
   c. HBV A level ≥ 4 log, i.e., 10,000 IU/L who had previous level undetected.

   If the patient is anti-HBc positive, reactivation can be defined as follows:
   a. Detectable HBV DNA
   b. Reappearance of HBsAg in the blood
3. Difference between the acute HBV infection and reactivation of chronic HBV infection:

Characteristics	Reactivation of chronic HBV infection	Acute hepatitis B virus infection
History	Past history in case of the affected patients Family history of chronic HBV hepatitis	Recent exposure to HBV infection
Lever enzymes	High	High
Jaundice	Present	Present
Prodrome	May be present	May be present
IgM anti-HBc	Low, i.e., <1:1,000	High, i.e., >1:1,000
HBV DNA level	>1,000 copies/mL	<1,000 copies/mL
In follow-up	Persistence of HBsAg after 6 months	95% patients clear the virus from the circulation
Histology	Presence or absence of chronicity	No evidence of chronicity

4. In case of acute HBV flare ALT level is ≥3 times normal above the baseline level and >100 IU/L.
5. In the following conditions, entecavir/TAF is preferred over TDF:
   a. Age > 60 years. But, TAF will not require dose adjustment if the age is >12 years and body weight is >35 kg along with estimated creatinine clearance of >15 mL/min or <15 mL/min and under dialysis.
   b. Presence of bone disease like osteoporosis
   c. History of fragile fracture
   d. Chronic use of steroid or other drugs that produce osteopenia
   e. Renal dysfunction:
      - Effective GFR of <60 mL/min/1.73 m^2
         - Entecavir dose should be adjusted if eGFR value is <50 mL/min.
      - Phosphate level < 2.5 mg/dL
      - Albumin 30 mg/24 hours or moderate dipstick proteinuria
      - Patient under hemodialysis
6. There are various types of cure in HBV infection under treatment:
   a. Sterilizing cure:
      - cccDNA is not detected but there is no active transcription.
      - Integrated DNA is not detected.
   b. Idealistic functional cure:
      - cccDNA is detected without no active transcription.
      - Presence or absence of integrated DNA
   c. Realistic functional cure:
      - cccDNA is detected without any active transcription.
      - Integrated DNA is detected.
   d. Attainable partial functional cure:
      - cccDNA is detected with low level of active transcription.
      - Integrated DNA is detected.
7. There are two new biomarkers developed for HBV infection. These are:
   a. Serum HBV RNA: It is a mixture of:
      - Intact pregenomic and subgenomic, spliced RNA
      - Poly A free RNA species

   (It will correlate to pgRNA which is the direct measure of transcriptional activity of cccDNA, also to intrahepatic content of pgRNA and cccDNA).

   Limitation of this RNA:
      - Avoidance of cross-detection to cross detect HBV DNA
      - Characterization of HBV RNA whether it is pgRNA, total RNA, spliced RNA, or truncated RNA.)
   b. HBcrAg: It can measure the combined antigenic component of:
      - Denatured HBeAg
      - HBV core antigen
      - Truncated incompletely processed core or precore protein

It measures:

- Intrahepatic cccDNA and its transcription activity.
- If HBV DNA is undetectable, its presence indicates continued transcription from cccDNA.
- It can predict the incidence of relapse after stopping the treatment.

- It can predict the relapse in case of continued treatment and to diagnose whether it is treatment-induced or spontaneous.
- To detect the strategies of newer targeting therapies targeting cccDNA

Its limitation: It requires improvement for monitoring the response in patients who are on antiviral therapy.)

  c. Quantitative anti-HBc antibody

  d. Level of serum interferon-inducible protein-10

CASE 163

A 55-year-old male having no history of comorbidities has been admitted in the liver clinic with gradual painless generalized abdominal distention and swelling of the legs for 1 month. He had no history of dyspnea, orthopnea, periorbital swelling, fever, hematemesis or melena or alteration of sleep pattern or jaundice, no sexual promiscuity or high-risk behavior, but there is history of blood transfusion 25 years back. On examination, only there was pallor, spider nevi in the front upper chest, palpable spleen, and moderate ascites. On blood examination, his hemoglobin was 8.5 g/dL, platelet count 90,000/cc, total leukocyte count 6,000/cc, serum bilirubin 2 mg/dL, AST 100 IU/L, ALT 50 IU/L, ALP 125 IU/L, albumin 3 g/dL, and INR 1.5. Serology showing anti-HCV positive, and electrolytes and renal function tests are within normal limit. So quantitative HCV RNA was done and it was 9×10^6/L.

Abdominal ultrasound demonstrated the following:

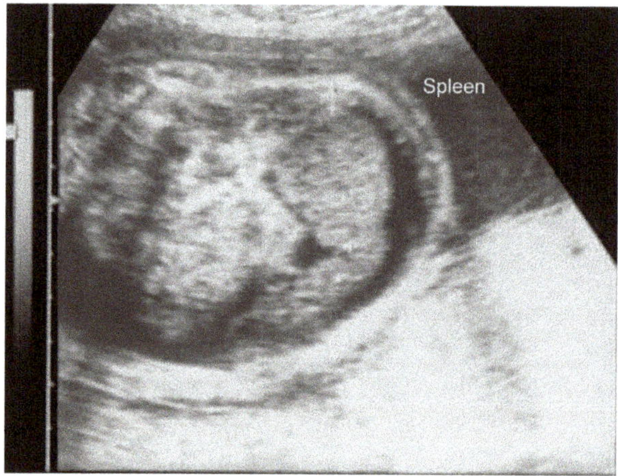

1. **What is present in the above picture?**
2. **What is your most likely diagnosis?**
3. **What factors enhancing the disease progression to fibrosis?**
4. **With which there is no association of disease progression to fibrosis?**
5. **Which groups of population require continuous screening of this disease?**
6. **How can you evaluate this disease?**
7. **Is genotype necessary during HCV therapy?**

Answers

1. Ultrasound of the abdomen demonstrated enlarged spleen and moderate ascites.
2. This is a case of hepatitis C virus-related decompensated cirrhosis with evidence of hypersplenism.

3. Following are the factors enhancing the disease progression toward fibrosis:
   a. Established risk factors:
      - Host related:
        - Old age
        - Duration of infection

- ○ Obese patient
- ○ Hepatic steatosis
- ○ Severe necroinflammation:
  - – Insulin resistance
  - – White race
- ○ Immunosuppression
- • Viral factors:
  - ○ HCV coinfection with genotype 3
  - ○ Coinfection with HIV
- • Environmental factors:
  - ○ Consumption of alcohol
  - ○ Smoking
  - ○ Use of marijuana
- b. Possible association:
  - • Male sex
  - • Increased content of iron in the liver
4. There is no association of viral load with disease progression to fibrosis.
5. Following groups of population require continuous screening for HCV infection:
   a. High-risk exposure:
      - • Patients are on maintenance hemodialysis.
      - • Children born to HCV-positive mother
      - • Exposure of the health worker to:
        - ○ Needlestick injury
        - ○ Mucosal injury to HCV-positive blood
   b. High-risk behavior:
      - • Intravenous drug abuse
      - • High-risk sexual behavior:
        - ○ Multiple sexual partner
        - ○ Male homosexuals
   c. Other:
      - • Persistently raised ALT and AST

- • Coinfection with:
  - ○ Hepatitis B virus
  - ○ HIV
6. Evaluation of a patient with hepatitis C virus infection:
   a. Primary diagnosis—anti-HCV positive
   b. Virological assessment:
      - • Quantitative estimation of HCV RNA
      - • In case of selected patient, HCV genotype
      - • In case of selected patient, resistance-associated substitution (RAS) of the drugs
   c. Assessment of severity of liver disease:
      - • Noninvasive measurement of fibrosis:
        - ○ Blood: Aspartate aminotransferase to platelet ratio index (APRI)
        - ○ Radiological: FIB-4, transient elastography
      - • Ancillary tests like:
        - ○ USG/CT scan
        - ○ α-fetoprotein to exclude hepatocellular carcinoma
   d. Evaluation of comorbidities:
      - • Renal function test
      - • Test for HBsAg
      - • ELISA test for HIV
      - • Pregnancy test during childbearing age
7. As the pangenotype drug is available, HCV genotyping is not essential, but in the following selected cases, genotyping of HCV is essential:
   a. In case cirrhosis, selection of the cost-effective therapies
   b. For determination of relapse versus reinfection
   c. As there is a worse prognosis in case of genotype 3, so for prediction of prognosis is essential.

CASE 164

A 55-year-old male having no history of comorbidities has been admitted in the liver clinic with gradual painless generalized abdominal distention and swelling of the legs for 1 month. He had no history of dyspnea, orthopnea, periorbital swelling, fever, hematemesis or melena or alteration of sleep pattern or jaundice, no sexual promiscuity or high-risk behavior, but there is history of blood transfusion 25 years back. On examination, only there was pallor, spider nevi in the front upper chest, palpable spleen, and moderate ascites. On blood examination, his hemoglobin was 8.5 g/dL, platelet count 90,000/cc, total leukocyte count 6,000/cc, serum bilirubin 2 mg/dL, AST 100 IU/L, ALT 50 IU/L, ALP 125 IU/L, albumin 3 g/dL, and INR 1.5. Serology showing anti-HCV positive, electrolytes and renal function tests are within normal limit. So quantitative HCV RNA was done, and it was 9×10^6/L. Patient told the doctor to start antiviral therapy.

Abdominal ultrasound demonstrated the following:

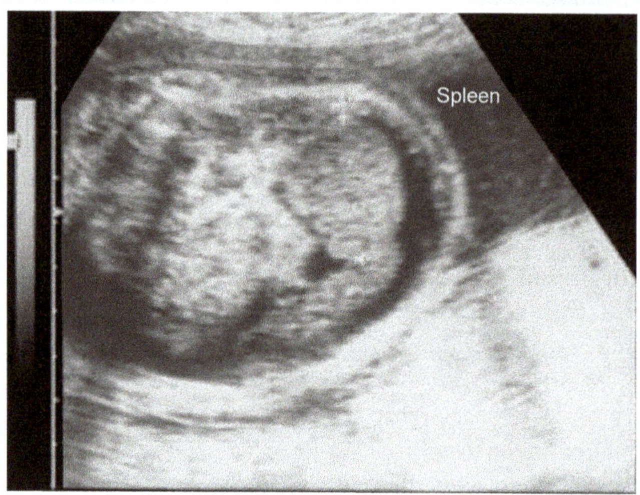

1.   **What is your diagnosis?**
2.   **Prior to commencement of therapy, what cautions do you want to take regarding medicine?**
3.   **How will you manage the patient with cirrhosis by antiviral therapy?**
4.   **How should you monitor during ribavirin therapy?**
5.   **What do you know regarding the role of RAS testing in this disease management?**
6.   **What is occult HCV infection?**

Answers

1.   This is a case of HCV-infected decompensated cirrhosis with evidence of hypersplenism.
2.   Following precautions should be taken prior to commencement of antiviral therapy:
     a.   Use of CYP enzyme inducer such as phenytoin, carbamazepine, and phenobarbital are contra-indicated as these drugs will reduce the concentration of the antiviral drugs.
     b.   Use of NS3-4A protease inhibitor such as grazoprevir, glecaprevir, and voxilaprevir are contraindicated in case of Child–Pugh B or C decompensated cirrhosis or prior history of decompensation, because there is chance of higher concentration of protease inhibitors leading to increased chance of toxicity.
3.   Management of the patient with cirrhosis by antiviral therapy:
     a.   Confirmation of the diagnosis: Baseline investigations such as APRI, transient elastography, or FIB-4
     b.   In case of noncirrhotic patient:
          • Sofosbuvir (400 mg) + daclatasvir (60 mg) × 12 weeks.

• HCV RNA level should be checked after 12 weeks of treatment completion to get sustained virological response.
• If HCV RNA is not detected, there is sustained virological response.

c.   Compensated Child–Pugh A cirrhosis:
     • Sofosbuvir 400 mg + velpatasvir 100 mg for 12 weeks
     • HCV RNA level should be checked after 12 weeks of treatment completion to get sustained virological response.
     • If HCV RNA is not detected, there is sustained virological response.
     • If HCV RNA is detected, patient should be referred to higher center.
d.   Decompensated Child–Pugh B or C cirrhosis:
     • Sofosbuvir 400 mg + velpatasvir 100 mg + ribavirin 600–1,200 mg for 12 weeks
     • In case of intolerance to ribavirin, then sofosbuvir 400 mg + velpatasvir 100 mg for 24 weeks

AASLD 2019 treatment for HCV-induced cirrhosis:
• HCV-positive noncirrhotic patients:

- o Following patients are noneligible in these criteria:
  - – Prior treatment
  - – eGFR is <30 mL/min/m^2
  - – Coinfection with HBV or HIV
  - – Ongoing pregnancy
  - – Known or suspected hepatocellular carcinoma
  - – Prior transplantation of liver
- o Pretreatment assessment:
  - – Clinical signs of cirrhosis like nodularity of liver with or without splenomegaly
  - – Laboratory testing prior to treatment
  - – Assessment of cirrhosis by noninvasive and laboratory testing:
    - ▪ FIB-4 score of >3.25
    - ▪ Transient elastography score of >12.5 kPa
  - – Noninvasive serological test if the value above the proprietary cutoff for cirrhosis
  - – Assessment of drug-to-drug interactions
- o Recommended treatment:
  - – Glecaprevir 300 mg + pibrentasvir 120 mg for 8 weeks
  - – Sofosbuvir 400 mg + velpatasvir 100 mg for 12 weeks
- For chronic HCV compensated cirrhosis:
  - o Pretreatment assessment:
    - – Clinical signs of cirrhosis like nodularity of liver with or without splenomegaly
    - – Laboratory testing prior to treatment
    - – Assessment of cirrhosis by non-invasive and laboratory testing:
      - ▪ FIB-4 score of >3.25
      - ▪ Transient elastography score of >2.5 kPa
    - – Noninvasive serological test if the value above the proprietary cutoff for cirrhosis
    - – Assessment of drug-to-drug interactions
  - o Recommended regimens:
    - – For genotype 1 to 6: 300 mg glecaprevir or 120 mg pibrentasvir after meals orally for 8 weeks
    - – For genotype 1, 2, 4, 5, and 6: 400 mg sofosbuvir or 100 mg velpatasvir orally daily for 12 weeks.

4. Following are the processes of monitoring of the patients during ribavirin therapy:
   a. As ribavirin may cause hemolysis leading to produce symptomatic anemia, hemoglobin measurement is advisable at 0, 2, 4, 6, 8, 10, and 12 weeks:
      - If the hemoglobin level is below 10 g/dL, dose of the ribavirin therapy should be reduced to 600 mg.
      - If the hemoglobin level is below 8 g/dL, ribavirin should be temporarily discontinued.
      - If the patient is a known case of ischemic heart disease, weekly monitoring of hemoglobin is advisable. If the hemoglobin level will be reduced by >2 g/dL within a short interval as compared to the baseline level ribavirin therapy should be discontinued.
   b. Ribavirin also produces:
      - Rash
      - Shortness of breath
      - Sore throat
      - Glossitis
   c. As this drug is known teratogenic, every woman under this treatment should be advised to use effective contraception during the therapy with this drug and 6 months post-therapy.

5. The RAS test is indicated in the following situations based on the type of regimen:
   a. Sofosbuvir/velpatasvir and sofosbuvir/daclatasvir: In case of genotype 3, NS5A RAS Y93H is recommended. If positive, ribavirin or voxilaprevir, but it is not recommended in case of decompensated cirrhosis.
   b. Elbasvir or grazoprevir: If RAS is positive in case of HCV genotype 3, alternate regimen should be advised.
   c. Sofosbuvir or ledipasvir: If RAS is positive in case of genotype 1a, alternate regimen should be advised.

6. Occult HCV infection is characterized by presence of HCV DNA in the hepatocytes as well as in the mononuclear cells in the peripheral blood in spite of undetectable HCV RNA in the serum. It has following two types of profiles:
   a. During evaluation of liver disease patient is:
      - Serum HCV RNA is negative.

- Anti-HCV antibody is negative.
- Liver tissue HCV RNA is positive.

b. In patient with spontaneous clearance of or posttreatment clearance of HCV RNA where:

- Serum HCV RNA is negative.
- Anti-HCV antibody is negative.
- Liver tissue HCV RNA is positive.

CASE 165

A 55-year-old male having no history of comorbidities has been admitted in the liver clinic with gradual painless generalized abdominal distention and swelling of the legs for 1 month. He had no history of dyspnea, orthopnea, periorbital swelling, fever, hematemesis or melena or alteration of sleep pattern or jaundice, no sexual promiscuity or high-risk behavior, but there is history of blood transfusion 25 years back. On examination, only there was pallor, spider nevi in the front upper chest, palpable spleen, and moderate ascites. On blood examination, his hemoglobin was 8.5 g/dL, platelet count 90,000/cc, total leukocyte count 6,000/cc, serum bilirubin 2 mg/dL, AST 100 IU/L, ALT 50 IU/L, ALP 125 IU/L, albumin 3 g/dL, and INR 1.5. Serology showing anti-HCV positive, electrolytes and renal function tests are within normal limit. So quantitative HCV RNA was done and it was 9×10^6/L. Patient told the doctor to start antiviral therapy. Patient will undergo transplantation of liver.

Abdominal ultrasound demonstrated the following:

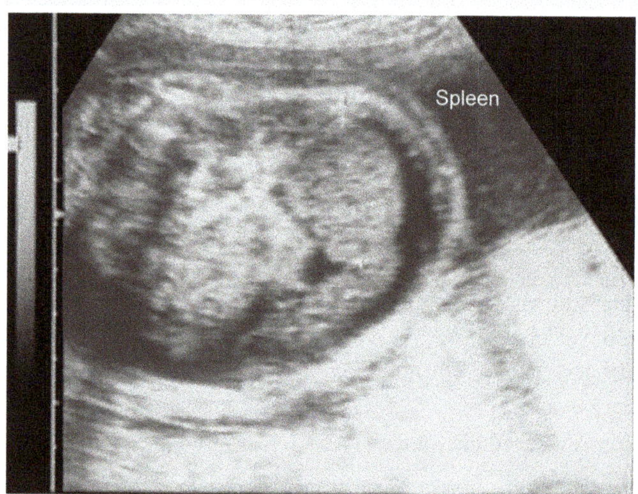

1. **What is your diagnosis?**
2. **What is the optimum time of starting the HCV therapy?**
3. **What is the recommended regimen in case of post-transplant patient?**

Answers

1. This is a case of decompensated cirrhosis with evidence of hypersplenism.
2. Optimum timing of commencement of therapy:
   a. Immediately after liver transplant, when postoperative issues will be resolved.
   b. Before development of significant liver disease
   c. When the immunosuppression level will be achieved.
   d. There is no ongoing episode of acute rejection.

3. According to AASLD recommendation in case of posttreatment:
   a. 400 mg glecaprevir + 120 mg pibrentasvir orally daily for 12 weeks
   b. 400 mg sofosbuvir + 100 mg velpatasvir orally daily for 12 weeks
   c. In case of genotype 1, 4, 5, and 6, 400 mg sofosbuvir + 90 mg ledipasvir orally daily for 12 weeks

CASE 166

A 29-year-old female having no history of comorbidities came to antenatal clinic for initial checkup. On enquiry, she has a history of blood transfusion 25 years back. On examination, only there was pallor, spider nevi in the front upper chest, palpable spleen, and moderate ascites. On blood examination, his hemoglobin was 11.5 g/dL, platelet count 190,000/cc, total leukocyte count 9,000/cc, serum bilirubin 1.2 mg/dL, AST 45 IU/L, ALT 50 IU/L, ALP 108 IU/L, albumin 3 g/dL, and INR 1.1. Serology showing anti-HCV positive, electrolytes and renal function tests are within normal limit. So, quantitative HCV RNA was done and it was 9×10^6/L. Patient told the doctor that she was very anxious for her HCV positivity.

Abdominal ultrasound demonstrated the following:

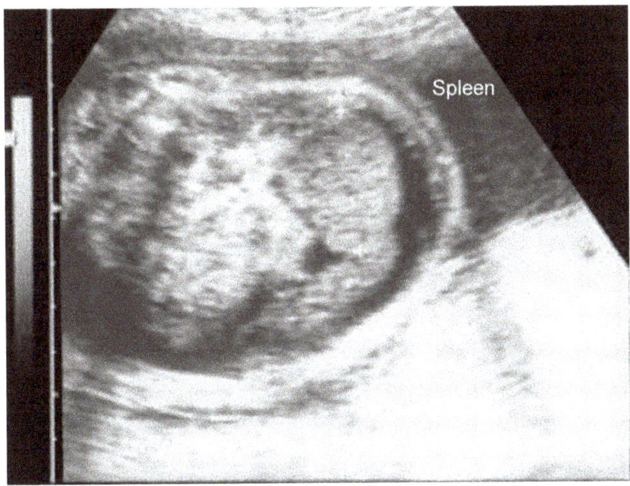

1. **What should be advice of the doctor to the pregnant lady?**
2. **What should be the advice for the child after birth?**

Answers

1. Strategies of treatment with HCV therapy in pregnant lady:
    a. Treatment during pregnancy is not recommended.
    b. During delivery of the baby, invasive procedures like instrument-assisted delivery and fetal scalp monitoring should be avoided.
    c. After delivery of the baby, breastfeeding should be continued except in case of cracked nipple. Again, in 10–25% cases there will be spontaneous clearing of the virus in the postpartum period. So, one should wait at least for 9–12 months in the postpartum period prior to initiation of the antiviral therapy.
2. Advice for the child got birth from HCV-positive lady:
    a. Child should be evaluated at 18 months for anti-HCV antibody. If this is positive, HCV RNA should be done in 3 years.
    b. Treatment should be started at ≥3 years of age. But treatment should be started earlier if following manifestations may occur:
        - Advanced liver fibrosis
        - Any one extrahepatic manifestations:
            ○ Cryoglobulinemia
            ○ Rash
            ○ Glomerulonephritis
    c. As per the recommendations of AASLD:
        - If the age is 3–11 years and HCV genotype is 2 and 3: If the weight is <47 kg, dose of ribavirin is 15 mg/kg of body weight.
        - If the age is >3 years and patient is genotype 1, 4, 5, or 6 positive:
            ○ Dose of sofosbuvir:
                - If the body weight is <17 kg: 150 mg for 12 weeks
                - If the body weight is 17–35 kg: 200 mg for 12 weeks
                - If the body weight is >35 kg: 400 mg for 12 weeks

- ○ Dose of ledipasvir:
  - – If the body weight is <17 kg: 33.75 mg for 12 weeks
  - – If the body weight is 17–35 kg: 45 mg for 12 weeks
  - – If the body weight is >35 kg: 90 mg for 12 weeks
- ○ If the age is >12 years or weight is >45 kg: Glecaprevir or pibrentasvir for 8 weeks.

CASE 167

A 31-year-old male with end-stage renal failure was on maintenance hemodialysis for the last 5 years. But, suddenly he was found to be HCV positive. Immediately, the patient was asked to undergo HCV RNA and liver function test and HCV RNA showed 230,000 IU/mL. Liver function test was normal except that ALT is 58 IU/L and AST 48 IU/L.

1. **What is your diagnosis?**
2. **What is the plan of HCV therapy in this patient?**

Answers

1. This patient suffering from end-stage renal failure in a case of chronic kidney disease has been recently cross-infected with HCV virus through the hemodialysis procedure.
2. Plan of HCV therapy in this patient:
   a. If the patient is willing to do renal transplant, complete cure of HCV is required as it will reduce the all-cause mortality.
   b. Complete cure of HCV will lead to better graft survival after living donor transplantation.
   c. In case of advanced fibrosis or compensated cirrhosis, after complete cure of HCV liver transplantation can be avoided.
   d. Drug of choice should be sofosbuvir with daclatasvir or ledipasvir.
   e. In these drugs, no dose reduction is required.

CASE 168

A 45-year-old man who is already HIV positive and under retroviral therapy recently developed deranged liver function. While checking the viral serology, he was found to be HCV positive.

What is the drug combination that should be given with dose adjustment?

Answers

- Reduced dose of daclatasvir with boosted protease inhibitor like ritonavir or atazanavir with dose reduction to 30 mg/day
- Reduced dose of daclatasvir along with increasing the dose of efavirenz, etravirine, or nevirapine to 90 mg/day
- If eGFR is <60 mL/min/1.73 m^2, fixed dose of sofosbuvir-velpatasvir and sofosbuvir-ledipasvir should be avoided. Alternatively, TAF should be started.
- Ribavirin should be avoided when stavudine, zidovudine, or didanosine are used as retroviral therapy because there is risk of:
  - ○ Acute pancreatitis
  - ○ Worsening of anemia
- If the patient is newly diagnosed HIV, in that case CD4 count will be low. So, there is a chance of false negativity of HCV. In that case, quantitative estimation of HCV RNA should be done.

CASE 169

A 45-year-old hypertensive, type 2 diabetic nonalcoholic male having sedentary lifestyle and mixed diet has come to medical clinic with elevated liver enzymes during his routine checkup. On examination, his BMI was 32 kg/m^2 and waist circumference of 94 cm, blood pressure of 150/90 mm Hg, pulse rate of 80 beats/minute, and regular. Per abdomen examination is nonsignificant. Echocardiographic picture demonstrated:

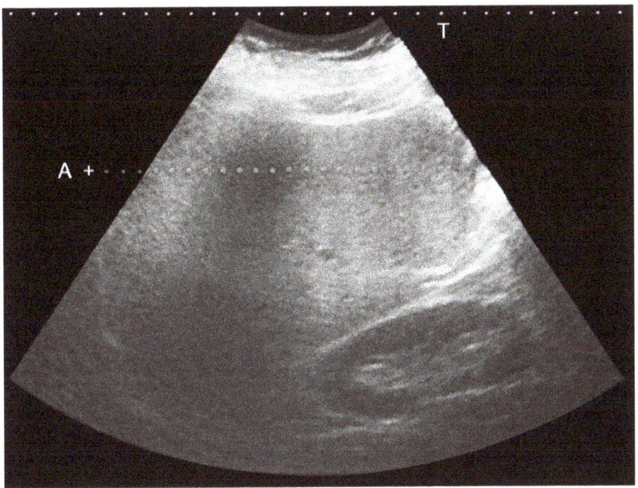

1. **What is your likely diagnosis?**
2. **How can you diagnose it?**
3. **Define this disease.**
4. **What are the risk factors in this disease?**
5. **What are the mechanisms involved in the evolution of the disease?**
6. **What are the noninvasive measurements to be done in this disease?**
7. **What is the risk of hepatocellular carcinoma in this disease?**
8. **What is MAFLD?**

Answers

1. This is a case of NAFLD.
2. Following two characteristics are required for the diagnosis of NAFLD:
    a. Presence of fat in the liver demonstrated either by ultrasonography or MRI or by histology.
    b. Exclusion of other causes of fat accumulation in the liver like use of medicine that is responsible for hepatic steatosis or any hereditary disorder responsible for fat accumulation.
3. Nonalcoholic fatty liver disease is present in two forms:
    a. Nonalcoholic fatty liver disease: It is characterized by steatotic changes of >5% without any evidence of hepatocellular injury.
    b. Nonalcoholic steatohepatitis: It is characterized by nonalcoholic fatty liver along with inflammation within the liver with or without hepatic fibrosis.
4. Following are the risk factors for this disease:
    a. Established risk factors:
        - Obesity
        - Type 2 diabetes mellitus
        - Dyslipidemia
        - Hypertension
        - Age
        - Sex
        - Ethnicity
    b. Evolving risk factors:
        - Obstructive sleep apnea
        - Psoriasis
        - Endocrinopathies
        - Colorectal cancer
        - Polycystic ovarian disease (PCOD)
        - Osteoporosis

5. Following mechanisms are involved in the development of NAFLD:
   a. Increased entry of fatty acids from adipocytes to liver cells
   b. Increased uptake of free fatty acids by the hepatocytes from the circulation
   c. Stimulation of hepatic lipogenesis mediated by:
      - Insulin
      - Glucose
      - Endoplasmic reticulum stress mediated
   d. Endoplasmic reticulum stress-mediated inhibition of export of lipid from the liver
6. Noninvasive tests for assessing the case:

Serum-based test	Components
Aspartate aminotransferase to platelet ratio index	• Aspartate aminotransferase • Platelet count
Nonalcoholic fatty liver disease fibrosis score	• Age • Body mass index • Hyperglycemia • Platelet count • Albumin • AST/ALT ratio
Fibrosis-4	• Age • AST • Platelet count • ALT
Enhanced liver fibrosis test	• Age • Hyaluronic acid • Tissue inhibitors metalloproteinase-1 • Procollagen-III, N-terminal propeptide

7. Nonalcoholic fatty liver disease is the fastest evolving cause of hepatocellular carcinoma having range of 0.5–2.6% in the NAFLD-induced cirrhosis. Following are the risk factors associated with cirrhosis:
   a. Male gender
   b. Light drinker
   c. High fibrosis-4 index
8. "MAFLD" denotes "metabolic dysfunction-associated fatty liver disease". Proposed criteria for MAFLD are based on:
   a. Evidence of hepatic steatosis on histology
   b. Imaging
   c. Serum biomarkers

Along with one of the following three criteria:
   - Overweight/obesity
   - Presence of type 2 diabetes mellitus
   - Metabolic dysregulation: It can be defined as presence of any two of the following criteria:
      ○ Waist circumference of ≥102/88 cm in case of Caucasian men or women, respectively or ≥90/80 cm in Asian men or women, respectively.
      ○ Blood pressure of ≥130/80 mm Hg or on specific antihypertensive drugs
      ○ Serum triglyceride of ≥150 mg/dL or on specific drugs
      ○ Presence of prediabetes (fasting plasma glucose level of 100–125 mg/dL or 2 hours postprandial plasma glucose level of 140–199 mg/dL or HbA1c level of 5.7–6.4%.
      ○ Presence of plasma HDL-cholesterol of <40 mg/dL in case of men or <50 mg/dL in case of women or on the treatment with specific drug
      ○ Homeostasis model assessment (HOMA)—insulin resistance score of ≥2.5
      ○ Plasma high-sensitivity CRP (hs-CRP) level of >2 mg/dL.

CASE 170

A 45-year-old corporate worker having history of intake of 40–70 g/day whiskey 6 days per weeks with increase at the weekend for last 2 months due to stress on the job. He had no history of blood transfusion, over-the-counter drug intake, tattooing, and unsafe needle practices. On examination, he has tachycardia, jaundice, spider angioma, palmar erythema, hepatomegaly, and no ascites.

Laboratory details are: total leukocyte count is 12,500/cc, bilirubin 9 mg/dL, AST 150 IU/L, ALT 70 IU/L, ALP 95 IU/L, and INR 1.7. Serology for all hepatitis viruses and ANA are negative. Serum electrolytes and renal markers are normal.

Echocardiography and histology of liver demonstrated:

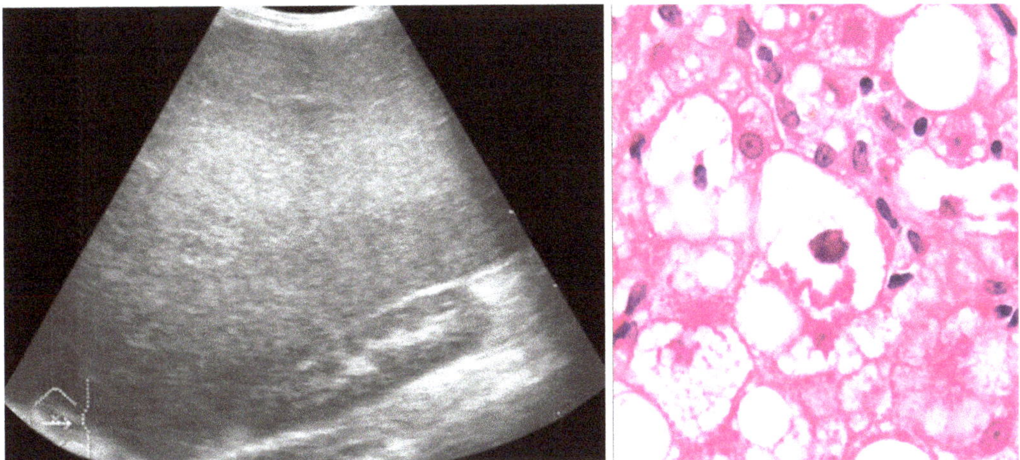

1.   **What is the feature demonstrated in the ultrasonography and histology of liver?**
2.   **In which other diseases may this body be found?**
3.   **What is your diagnosis?**
4.   **What are the diagnostic criteria in this disease?**
5.   **What percentage of patients will develop cirrhosis?**
6.   **What are the peripheral features suggestive of alcoholic cirrhosis?**
7.   **What are the features of severe alcoholic hepatitis?**

Answers

1.   Demonstration of the above pictures:
     a.   Ultrasonography of abdomen demonstrated hepatomegaly.
     b.   Histology of liver demonstrated Mallory–Denk body—it is cytoplasmic hyaline inclusion bodies found in the hepatocytes.
2.   In the following cases, this histological picture may be found:
     a.   Nonalcoholic fatty liver disease
     b.   Primary biliary cirrhosis
     c.   Hepatocellular carcinoma
     d.   Chronic cholestasis
     e.   Focal nodular hyperplasia
     f.   Patient on glucocorticoid therapy
     g.   Intestinal bypass surgery for obesity
     h.   Weber–Christian disease
     i.   Von Gierke disease
     j.   Indian childhood cirrhosis
3.   The diagnosis is alcoholic liver disease.
4.   Following are the criteria for the diagnosis of this case:

Minimum criteria for the diagnosis	Possible alcoholic hepatitis
Serum bilirubin > 3 mg/dL	Does no meet the minimum criteria Or, Has potential confounders
Consumption of more than three standard drinks, i.e., 40 g/day for female and four drinks, i.e., 50–60 g/day for >6 months	Inconsistent history of alcohol
<2 months from the last drink to the development of jaundice	Atypical laboratory studies: • AST <50 IU/L • AST/ALT > 400 IU/L • AST to ALT ratio > 1.5
AST > 50 IU/L but AST and ALT are both <400 IU/L	History of recent hemorrhagic or septic shock
AST/ALT ratio > 1.5	Positive immune markers: • ANA > 1:160 • Antismooth muscle cell antibody 1:80
	Possibility of DILI
	Liver biopsy should be done to confirm the diagnosis.

Continued

Continued

Minimum criteria for the diagnosis	Possible alcoholic hepatitis
Probable alcoholic hepatitis	Definite alcoholic hepatitis
It will meet the minimum criteria for alcoholic hepatitis without confounding factors	• Clinical alcoholic hepatitis • Biopsy proven alcoholic hepatitis
It will meet the minimum criteria for alcoholic hepatitis without confounding factors	
Negative immune markers: ANA < 1:160 ASMA < 1:80	
Absence of: Sepsis Shock Use of cocaine	
Drug use at risk of DILI within 1 month Liver biopsy is mandatory for the diagnosis.	

5. If the patients continue taking at least 50 g of alcohol daily for >5 years continuously, 10–20% of them develop alcoholic cirrhosis
6. Peripheral features of alcoholic cirrhosis:
   a. Parotid enlargement
   b. Palmar erythema
   c. Dupuytren's contracture
7. Following are the features of severe alcoholic hepatitis:
   a. Presence of ascites
   b. Bleeding from the varices
   c. Cutaneous markers of coagulation failure
   d. Hepatic encephalopathy
   e. Acute kidney injury

CASE 171

A 45-year-old corporate worker having history of intake of 40–70 g/day whiskey 6 days per week with increase at the weekend for the last 2 months due to stress on the job. He had no history of blood transfusion, over-the-counter drug intake, tattooing, and unsafe needle practices. On examination, he has tachycardia, jaundice, spider angioma, palmar erythema, hepatomegaly, and no ascites.

Laboratory details are: total leukocyte count is 12,500/cc, bilirubin 9 mg/dL, AST 150 IU/L, ALT 70 IU/L, ALP 95 IU/L, and INR 1.7. Serology for all hepatitis viruses and ANA are negative. Serum electrolytes and renal markers are normal.

Echocardiography and histology of liver demonstrated:

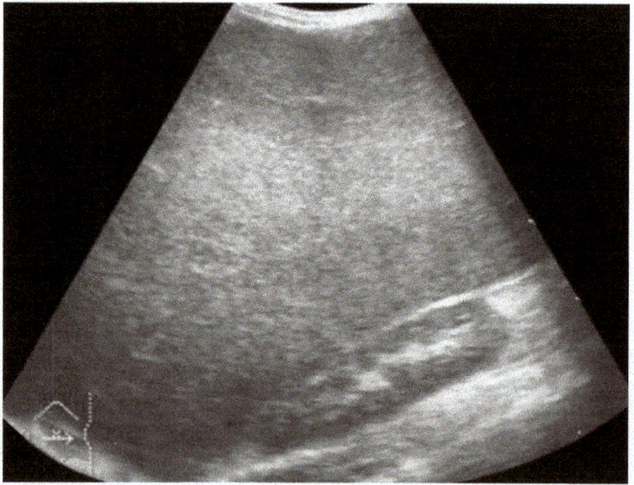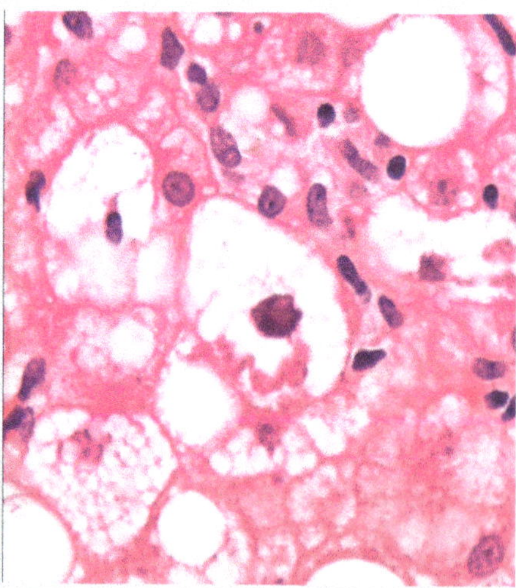

1. **What is the feature demonstrated in the ultrasonography and histology of liver?**
2. **What are the classical histological features in alcoholic hepatitis?**
3. **What is the score for histology of alcoholic hepatitis?**
4. **What are the clinical scores for assessing the severity of the patient?**

Answers

1. Demonstration of the above pictures:
   a. Ultrasonography of abdomen demonstrated hepatomegaly.
   b. Histology of liver demonstrated Mallory–Denk body—it is cytoplasmic hyaline inclusion bodies found in the hepatocytes.
2. Classical histological features of alcoholic hepatitis are:
   a. Alcoholic steatohepatitis—it is characterized by:
      - Macrovascular steatosis
      - Lobular neutrophilic infiltrate
      - Mallory–Denk bodies
      - Satellitosis
      - Megamitochondria
      - Zone 3 perivenular injury
      - Infiltration with polymorphonuclear cells
      - Chicken wire fibrosis
   b. Fibrosis
   c. Cirrhosis
3. There are three stages of severity, i.e., (1) mild, (2) moderate, and (3) severe. According to four histologic components, these are:
   a. Stage of fibrosis

   b. Bilirubinostasis
   c. Megamitochondria
   d. Polymorphonuclear cellular infiltration
4. Following are the clinical scores for assessing the severity in this patient:

Severity score of alcoholic hepatitis	Formula	Cutoff for the severe alcoholic hepatitis
Maddrey discriminant function	4.6 × [Patient's prothrombin time – control prothrombin time] + total bilirubin in mg/dL	≥32
MELD	Total bilirubin International normalized ratio Creatinine	≥20
Glasgow alcoholic hepatitis score	Age White blood cell count Urea Bilirubin	≥9
ABIC	Age Bilirubin International normalized ratio Creatinine	More than 9

CASE 172

A 50-year-old chronic alcoholic patient came with right upper abdominal pain and weight loss. On examination, there was tender hepatomegaly and his peripheral features were as demonstrated below. His viral serology was negative, ANA was negative, INR was 1.2, and liver function test demonstrated ALT 122 IU/L and AST/ALT ratio was 1.9. Echocardiography demonstrated liver span of 18 cm.

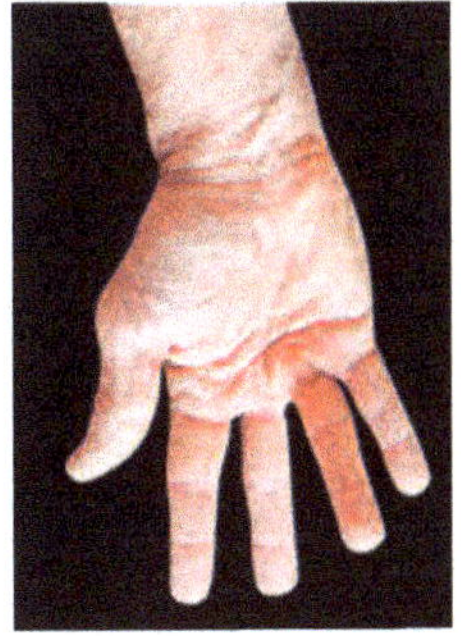
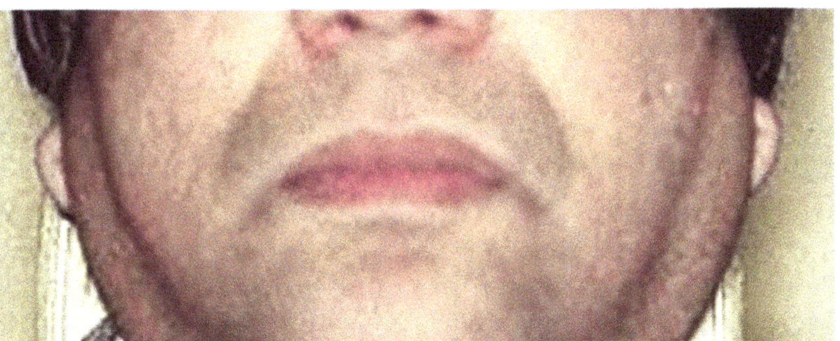

1. **What do the above pictures demonstrate?**
2. **What is your diagnosis?**
3. **Provide the criteria as per the National Institute on Alcohol Abuse and Alcoholism.**
4. **Describe the pathophysiology of alcoholic liver injury.**
5. **What are the management options in this disease?**
6. **What are the specific measures to be given to this patient?**

Answers

1. The above pictures demonstrated:
   a. Palmar erythema
   b. Dupuytren's contracture
2. Patient has been suffering from alcoholic hepatitis.
3. Criteria as per the National Institute on Alcohol Abuse and Alcoholism are the following:
   a. Onset of jaundice within 60 days of heavy alcohol consumption of >50 g daily for minimum 6 months.
   b. Serum bilirubin of >3 mg/dL
   c. Elevation of AST to 50–400 IU/L
   d. AST/SALT ratio of >1.5
   e. There is no other cause of hepatitis.
4. Pathophysiology of alcoholic hepatitis:
   a. Alcohol in the hepatocyte undergoes oxidative metabolic pathway leading to production of reduced ratio of NAD to NADH, as a result there is inhibition of oxidation of triglyceride and fatty acids thereby aggravating lipogenesis.
   b. Translocation of endotoxin from intestine to hepatocytes in the form of lipopolysaccharides where in the Kupffer cells it will bind to toll-like receptor 4 and CD14 to release large amount of reactive oxygen species which in turn release the following factors which will accumulate in the neutrophils and macrophages leading to development of clinical features of alcoholic liver disease:
      - Cytokines
      - Tumor necrosis factor-α
      - Interleukin-8
      - Monocyte chemotactic protein-1
      - Platelet-derived growth factor
5. Management options for this disease:
   a. Abstinence of alcohol with follow-up clinical assessment:
   b. Nutritional support
   c. Administration of thiamine
   d. Supplementation of zinc
   e. Search for any infection
6. Specific treatment:
   a. Corticosteroid—oral prednisolone 40 mg daily for 28 days, it is preferred as compared to prednisone as will not require metabolism in the liver to get its effect. If the patient is unable to take this drug orally, methylprednisolone is the drug of choice. If the Lille score is >0.45 even after 4 weeks of drug therapy, steroid should be discontinued. If the Lille score is <0.45, in that case steroid should be continued for another 3–4 weeks.
   b. In case of nonresponder to steroid, pentoxifylline should be given at a dose of 400 orally thrice daily for 28 days.
   c. Fecal microbiota transplantation has shown potential benefit.
   d. Administration of granulocyte colony-stimulating factor
   e. Amoxicillin–clavulanic acid
   f. Metadoxine
   g. Interleukin-22
   h. Anakinra—interleukin-1 receptor antagonist
   i. Obeticholic acid
   j. Molecular adsorbent recycling system

CASE 173

A 35-year-old chronic alcoholic patient having recent history of binge drinking of alcohol has come to emergency department progressively increasing yellowish discoloration of urine and conjunctiva for 25 days along with progressively increasing abdominal distention for 12 days and disorientation for 2 days prior to admission. No history of bleeding from any sites, no sensorial alteration, or decreased urine output. On examination, there was deep jaundice, tachycardia, pitting pedal edema, bilateral enlargement of parotid gland, and enlarged nontender liver having irregular surface and gross ascites. Ultrasonography demonstrated coarse echogenic liver, splenomegaly, and ascites with diameter of portal vein of 14 mm.

Ascitic fluid examination demonstrated cell count of 200/cc having neutrophil 65%, protein 1.8 g/dL, and SAAG 1.4. Laboratory examination demonstrated negative for hepatitis viral serology, bilirubin 12 mg/dL with ALT 77 IU/L, AST 65 IU/L, ALP 90 IU/L, INR 1.9, sodium 128 IU/L, urea 60 mg/dL, and creatinine 1.2 mg/dL.

1. **What is your diagnosis and why?**
2. **What are the other nomenclature systems of this disease?**
3. **What are the differences between acutely decompensated cirrhosis and this patient?**
4. **What are the proposed subtypes of acutely decompensated cirrhosis?**
5. **What are the scoring systems used for stratifying the prognosis of this patient?**
6. **Mention the pathophysiological concept of this disease which is different from decompensated cirrhosis.**
7. **What are the emerging therapies in this patient?**

Answers

1. The diagnosis is acute on chronic liver failure (ACLF) because of the following points:
   a. History of significant alcohol intake
   b. Progressively increasing yellowish discoloration within a span of 4 weeks
   c. History of disorientation for 2 days
2. Following are the different nomenclature systems:
   a. According to Asian-Pacific Association for the Study of the Liver (APASL) in 2014, "acute hepatic insult" is characterized by:
      - Serum bilirubin of ≥5 mg/dL
      - Coagulopathy with INR of ≥1.5 with prothrombin level <40%
      - Evidence of ascites with or without encephalopathy
      - Previous diagnosis of liver disease or undiagnosed liver disease
      - Associated with high 28 days mortality
   b. According to EASL:
      - The prerequisite is underlying cirrhosis.
      - Scoring system according to different organ failures:
        ○ Total bilirubin is >12 mg/dL indicating liver failure.
        ○ Serum creatinine is >2 mg/dL or requirement of renal replacement therapy (RRT) indicating renal failure.
        ○ West Haven hepatic encephalopathy grade 3 or 4 indicating cerebral failure
        ○ INR of >1.5 or platelet count of <20,000/cc indicating coagulation failure
        ○ Requirement of vasopressin indicating circulatory failure
        ○ PaO_2/FiO_2 ratio of <200 or SpO_2/FiO_2 ratio of <214

   ACLF can be classified based on organ failure:
   - ACLF-1: Single organ failure
   - ACLF-2: Patient with two organ failure
   - ACLF-3: Patient with three or more organ failure

   c. According to the World Gastroenterology Organization (WGO):
      - Type A (noncirrhotic): In patient with existing chronic liver disease, there is sudden flare of the baseline investigations.
      - Type B (compensated cirrhosis): These patients will experience decompensation following acute insult.
      - Type C (decompensated cirrhosis): These patients will already in a stage of decompensation experience worsening of decompensation.

3. Difference between the acute decompensation of cirrhosis and acute on chronic liver failure:

Parameters	Acute decompensation of cirrhosis	Acute on chronic liver failure
Presentation	Usually subsequent presentation or as index case	Index always
Organ involvement	Hepatic or extrahepatic organs	Always hepatic
Duration between insult and presentation	Up to 12 weeks	Within 4 weeks
Preexisting cirrhosis	Always present	May or may not be present
28 days mortality	Low	Always high
Systemic inflammation	Moderate inflammation	High-grade inflammation
Presence of decompensation	Presence or absence of decompensation	Always absent

4. Following are the subtypes of acutely decompensated cirrhosis:
   a. Pre-ACLF: This case will evolve into ACLF within 90 days with high systemic inflammation as well as mortality.
   b. Unstable decompensated cirrhosis: There are complications of severe portal hypertension leading to frequent hospitalization which is not due to ACLF.
   c. Stable decompensated cirrhosis
5. Following are the scoring systems for stratifying the prognosis in this patient:
   a. Patient satisfying the definition of APASL regarding ACLF
   b. The North American Consortium for the study of End-stage Liver Disease (NACSELD) score
   c. MELD score
   d. Acute Physiology and Chronic Health Evaluation (APACHE) score
   e. Simple organ failure count (SOFC) score
6. Following are the pathophysiological concepts of this patient which are different from decompensated cirrhosis:
   a. A state of exaggerated immune response
   b. State of immune dysregulation
   c. State of immune dysfunction
7. Following are the emerging therapies in this patient:
   a. Plasmapheresis
   b. Extracorporeal liver support system
   c. Transplantation of fecal microbiota
   d. Administration of granulocyte colony-stimulating factor

CASE 174

A 58-year-old patient with known history of decompensated alcoholic cirrhosis in the form of diuretic responsive ascites has been admitted with progressive abdominal distention with diffuse pain all over the abdomen in spite of no recent history of fever, nausea, vomiting, or oliguria. Also, he has no history of any operative interventions. On examination, he has the following peripheral features along with grade II ascites. Hematological reports demonstrated hemoglobin 8.5 g/dL, platelet count 100,000/cc, total bilirubin 3.5 mg/dL, AST 60 IU/L, ALT 48 IU/L, and INR 1.4. Viral serology, urea and creatinine, and electrolytes were normal. Ascitic fluid analysis demonstrated total cell count of 600/cc with neutrophilic predominance and SAAG 1.5.

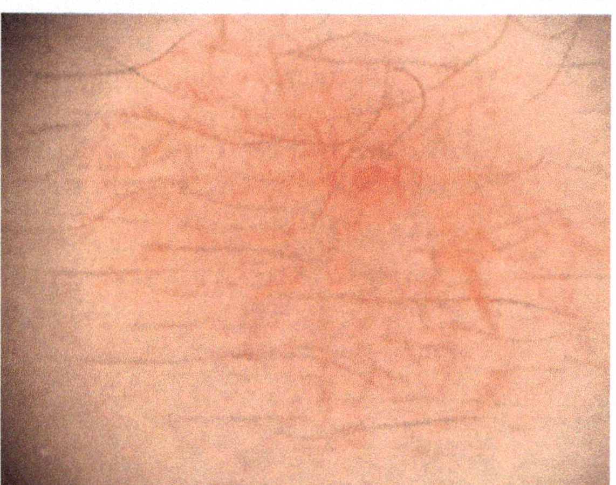
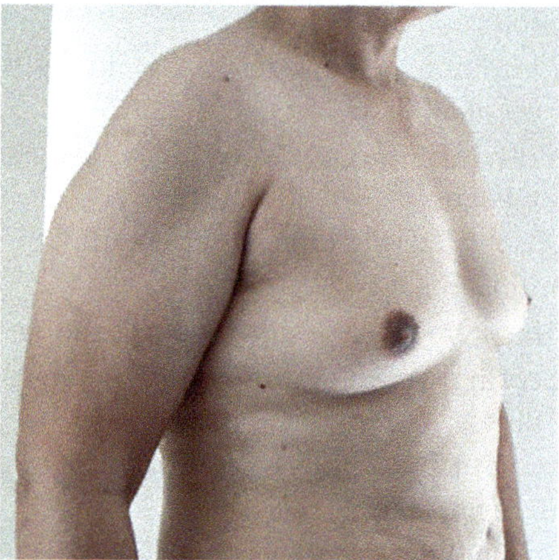

1. **Describe the above pictures.**
2. **How can you grade the feature in the right-hand side picture?**
3. **What is uncomplicated ascites?**
4. **How can you grade the ascites?**
5. **What do you mean by SAAG and what is the importance of SAAG?**
6. **Enumerate the cause of ascites based on SAAG.**

Answers

1. The above pictures demonstrate:
   a. Spider angioma which can be described as presence of central arteriole from which spreading of capillaries and their branches as legs of spider. If the central arteriole is compressed with pinhead, all the capillaries will be blanched.
   b. Gynecomastia which can be described as enlargement of breast tissue in men having no lobules.

2. Depending upon the enlargement of breast, it can be classified as three types:
   a. Grade I: There is small enlargement without any skin excess.
   b. Grade IIa: Here, there is moderate enlargement of breast tissue without any skin excess.
   c. Grade IIb: Here, there is moderate enlargement of breast tissue with extra skin.
   d. Grade III: There is marked enlargement of breast tissue along with extra skin.

3. Uncomplicated ascites has absence of any of the following features:
   a. Infected ascites
   b. Refractory ascites
   c. Ascites associated with features of hepatorenal syndrome

4. Gradation of ascites:
   a. Grade 1: Ascites can be detected only by ultrasonography of abdomen. It is mild ascites.
   b. Grade 2: In this type, there is moderate symmetrical distention of the abdomen. It is moderate.
   c. Grade 3: In this type, there is marked abdominal distention, which is also known as gross ascites.

5. SAAG can be described as serum-ascites albumin gradient. Value of SAAG is ≥1.1, which is responsible for transudative ascites and SAAG of <1.1, which is responsible for exudative ascites.

6. Based on value of SAAG, ascites can be classified as:
   a. Causes of SAAG of ≥1.1:
      - Heart failure
      - Portal hypertension
      - Hypothyroidism
      - Hepatic venous outflow tract obstruction
   b. Causes of SAAG of <1.1:
      - Tubercular ascites
      - Subacute bacterial peritonitis
      - Malignant ascites
      - Pancreatic ascites
      - Nephrotic syndrome

CASE 175

A 58-year-old patient with known history of decompensated alcoholic cirrhosis in the form of diuretic responsive ascites has been admitted with progressive abdominal distention with diffuse pain all over the abdomen in spite of no recent history of fever, nausea, vomiting, or oliguria. Also, he has no history of any operative interventions. On examination, he has the following peripheral features along with grade II ascites. Hematological reports demonstrated hemoglobin 8.5 g/dL, platelet count 100,000/cc, total bilirubin 3.5 mg/dL, AST 60 IU/L, ALT 48 IU/L, and INR 1.4. Viral serology, urea and creatinine, and electrolytes were normal. Ascitic fluid analysis demonstrated total cell count of 500/cc with neutrophilic predominance and SAAG 1.5.

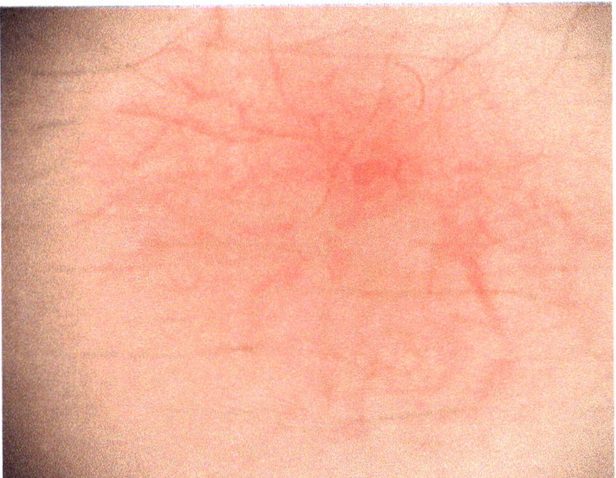
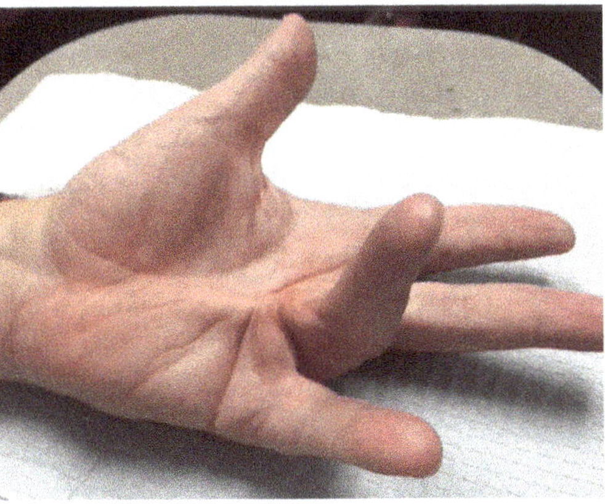

1. **Describe the above pictures.**
2. **What is site of tapping of ascitic fluid and why?**
3. **What should be the algorithm of treatment of uncomplicated ascites?**
4. **When should diuretic be stopped in this case?**
5. **How can you estimate the sodium balance in case of ascites?**

Answers

1. Description of the above pictures:
   a. Spider angioma which can be described as presence of central arteriole from which spreading of capillaries and their branches as legs of spider. If the central arteriole is compressed with pinhead, all the capillaries will be blanched.
   b. Dupuytren's contracture: It is characterized by thickening as well as tightening of the connective tissue affecting the fascia of the palm leading to contracture of the ring and third fingers mostly.

2. Site of tapping of ascites should be in the lower left quadrant for the following reasons:
   a. This area is thinner.
   b. This area has comparatively greater fluid pocket.

   Right lower quadrant should be avoided because of the following reasons:
   a. Wall is thicker as compared to left lower quadrant wall.
   b. There is risk of distention of cecum if the patient is on laxatives.

   Site should be 15 cm lateral to umbilicus to avoid injury to liver and spleen.

   Tapping should not be done around the umbilicus because superior and inferior epigastric arteries run lateral to umbilicus and way toward midinguinal point and there is chance of injury to these arteries.

3. Treatment algorithm of uncomplicated ascites:
   a. Restriction of sodium intake to 4.6–6.9 g/day along with complete avoidance of salt in the prepared meals
   b. Potassium-sparing diuretics like spironolactone should be started with 100 mg daily with gradually increasing the dose every third day to maximum of 400 mg daily so as to monitor the loss of weight to at least 2 kg per week.
   c. If the patient does not lose weight >2 kg per week or there is hyperkalemia, loop diuretic like furosemide 40 mg/day up to maximum 160 mg daily.
   d. In case of patient with grade 3 ascites, combination of furosemide and spironolactone should be given.
   e. If the patient develops painful gynecomastia, amiloride should be started.
   f. If a low response to furosemide, then torsemide can be given.
   g. Target of weight loss with diuretics:
      - In patient without edema, weight loss should be at least 0.5 kg/day.
      - In patient with edema, weight loss should be at least 1 kg/day.
   h. After resolution of ascites, dose of the diuretic should be reduced to the lowest effective dose.

4. Diuretic should be stopped in the following conditions:
   a. If sodium level is <125 mmol/L.
   b. Stage 1A renal injury
   c. Evidence of hepatic encephalopathy
   d. Progressively increasing muscle cramps
   e. In case of serum potassium:
      - If it is <3 mmol/L, furosemide should be stopped.
      - If it is >6 mmol/L, spironolactone should be stopped.

5. Net sodium in the blood = Total intake of sodium – Net loss of sodium from the blood through insensible loss.

   78 mmol/day = (88 – 10) mmol/day, assuming there is no renal loss of sodium.

   So, weight in the form of fluid to be gained every day = Gain in sodium/Sodium concentration in the ascitic fluid.

   Now, serum sodium = accumulation of sodium in ascitic fluid = 135 mmol/L

   So, daily gain in weight = 78/135 = 0.58 kg

   So, weekly accumulation of fluid = 0.58 × 7 = 4.06 L

   In case of large volume paracentesis, 6–8 L of fluid is taken out. One has to wait for another 2 weeks at least for reaccumulation of ascitic fluid.

CASE 176

A 58-year-old patient with known history of decompensated alcoholic cirrhosis in the form of diuretic responsive ascites has been admitted with progressive abdominal distention with diffuse pain all over the abdomen in spite of no recent history of fever, nausea, vomiting, or oliguria. Also, he has no history of any operative interventions. On examination, he has following peripheral features along with grade III ascites. Hematological reports demonstrated hemoglobin 8.5 g/dL, platelet count 100,000/cc, total bilirubin 3.5 mg/dL, AST 60 IU/L, ALT 48 IU/L, and INR 1.4. Viral serology, urea and creatinine, and electrolytes were normal. Ascitic fluid analysis demonstrated total cell count of 200/cc with lymphocytic predominance and SAAG 1.5.

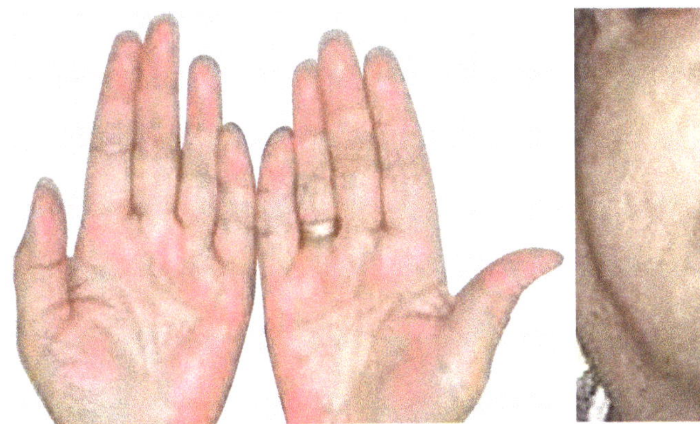 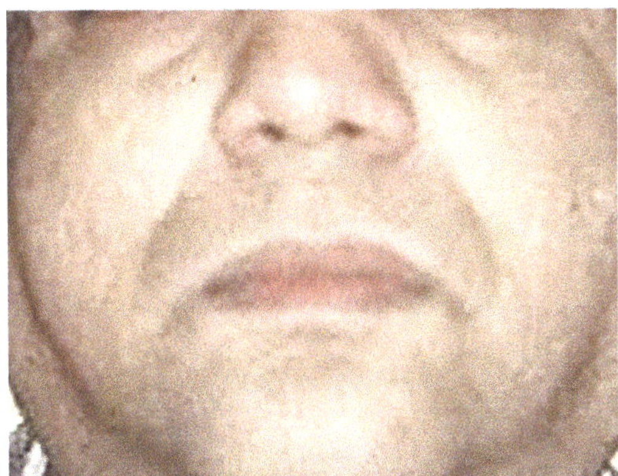

1. **Describe the above pictures.**
2. **What is your diagnosis?**
3. **Why is there abdominal pain?**
4. **What is large volume paracentesis and its indications?**
5. **How circulatory imbalance will occur after large volume paracentesis?**
6. **How this paracentesis-induced circularoty dysfunction can be prevented?**

Answers

1. Description of the above pictures:
   a. There is evidence of hyperemia in the thenar and hypothenar eminences.
   b. There is evidence of bilateral painless swelling of the parotid gland.
2. The diagnosis is decompensated alcoholic cirrhosis with evidences of hepatocellular failure.
3. Abdominal pain may be due to:
   a. Huge abdominal distention leading to tightness in the abdomen
   b. Compartment syndrome
   c. Increased abdominal pressure leading to stretching of the abdominal muscles
4. Large volume paracentesis can be defined as drainage of ≥5 L of ascitic fluid in a single sitting in grade III ascites.

   Indications of large volume paracentesis:
   a. To give relief from respiratory distress in case of tense ascites
   b. To prevent abdominal pain from:
      - Tense ascites
      - Increased intra-abdominal pressure
      - Compartment syndrome
   c. To prevent impending rupture of umbilical hernia
5. Paracentesis-induced circulatory dysfunction is a vasomotor phenomenon characterized as >50% increased plasma renin activity from the pretreatment level to >4 ng/mL/hour on the fourth day of paracentesis resulting in renal failure, hyponatremia, hepatic encephalopathy, and lastly decreased overall survival due to:
   a. Aggravated arteriolar vasodilatation
   b. Sudden decrease in high intra-abdominal pressure
6. Paracentesis-induced circulatory dysfunction can be prevented by:
   a. Infusion of 6–8 g of 20% salt poor albumin per liter drainage of ascitic fluid during large volume paracentesis

CASE 177

A 58-year-old patient with known history of decompensated alcoholic cirrhosis in the form of diuretic responsive ascites has been admitted with progressive abdominal distention with diffuse pain all over the abdomen in spite of no recent history of fever, nausea, vomiting, or oliguria. Also, he has no history of any operative interventions. On examination, he has the following peripheral features along with grade III ascites. Hematological reports demonstrated hemoglobin 8.5 g/dL, platelet count 100,000/cc, total bilirubin 3.5 mg/dL, AST 60 IU/L, ALT 48 IU/L, and INR 1.4. Viral serology, urea and creatinine, and electrolytes were normal. Ascitic fluid analysis demonstrated total cell count of 200/cc with lymphocytic predominance and SAAG 1.5.

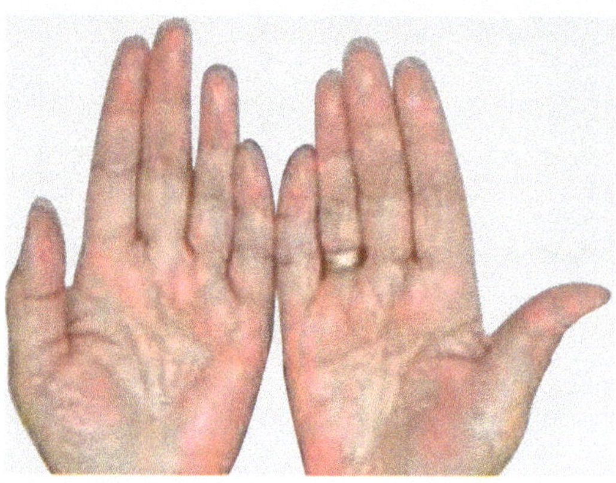 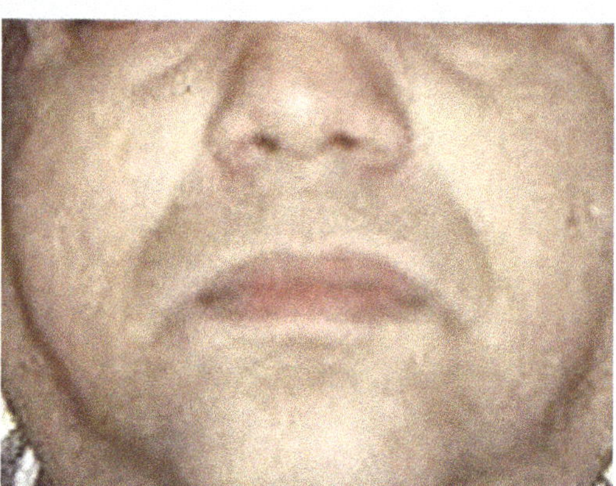

1. **Describe the above pictures.**
2. **What is your diagnosis?**
3. **Define refractory ascites.**
4. **Classify refractory ascites.**
5. **What are the defining criteria for refractory ascites?**

Answers

1. Description of the above pictures:
    a. There is evidence of hyperemia in the thenner and hypothenner eminences.
    b. There is evidence of bilateral painless swelling of the parotid gland.
2. The diagnosis is decompensated alcoholic cirrhosis with evidences of hepatocellular failure.
3. Refractory ascites can be defined as presence of free fluid in the abdomen that cannot be mobilized or its early recurrence cannot be prevented by medical intervention.
4. There are two types of refractory ascites:
    a. Diuretic resistant: This can be described as:
        - Lack of response to diuretic therapy
        - Lack of response to sodium restriction
    b. Diuretic intractable ascites: It can be described as development of diuretic-induced complications precluding the use of effective dose of diuretics.
5. Following are the defining criteria for refractory ascites:
    a. According to duration of treatment:
        - Intensive diuretic therapy—400 mg spirono-lactone daily plus 160 mg furosemide daily for 1 week who is on salt restrict diet with <90 mmol daily.
    b. Lack of response:
        - Mean loss of weight of <0.8 kg in 4 days
        - Urinary output of sodium is less than the sodium intake.
    c. Recurrence of ascites early: It can be defined as reappearance of grade 2 to 3 ascites within 4 weeks of initial mobilization.
    d. Diuretic-induced complications like:
        - Development of hepatic encephalopathy in absence of other precipitating factors
        - Renal impairment in the form of decrease in serum sodium to >10 mmol/L to <125 mmol/L
        - Changes in the serum potassium to <3 mmol/L or >6 mmol/L
        - Incapacitating cramps in the muscles

CASE 178

A 58-year-old patient with known history of decompensated alcoholic cirrhosis in the form of diuretic responsive ascites has been admitted with progressive abdominal distention with diffuse pain all over the abdomen, fever, nausea, and occasional vomiting. Also, he has no history of any operative interventions. On examination, he has the following peripheral features along with grade III ascites. Hematological reports demonstrated hemoglobin 8.5 g/dL, platelet count 100,000/cc, total bilirubin 3.5 mg/dL, AST 60 IU/L, ALT 48 IU/L, and INR 1.4. Viral serology, urea and creatinine, and electrolytes were normal. Ascitic fluid analysis demonstrated total cell count of 500/cc with neutrophilic predominance and SAAG 1.0.

1. **What is your diagnosis?**
2. **What are the criteria of your diagnosis?**
3. **What are the etiologies of this case?**
4. **What are the risk factors of your diagnosis?**
5. **Why anaerobic infection is not common in ascitic fluid?**
6. **What are the subtypes of your diagnosis?**
7. **What is the pathophysiology of your diagnosis?**
8. **What are the criteria of this disease due to secondary cause?**

Answers

1. The most likely diagnosis is subacute bacterial peritonitis.
2. Criteria for the diagnosis are:
   a. Underlying evidence of long-standing cirrhosis
   b. Polymorphonuclear leukocytes of >250/cc
   c. Exclusion other causes of secondary bacterial peritonitis
3. Following are the etiologies for the diagnosis:
   a. Gram-negative aerobic organisms: *Klebsiella pneumoniae*
   b. Grame-positive aerobic organism:
      - *Streptococcus pneumoniae*
      - *Streptococcus viridans*
4. Following are the risk factors of the diagnosis:
   a. Decompensated cirrhosis
   b. Past history of subacute bacterial peritonitis (SBP): In these patients, following features may indicate the predictors of future SBP:
      - Child–Turcotte–Pugh (CTP) score of ≥9
      - Bilirubin of ≥3 mg/dL
      - Serum creatinine of ≥1.2 mg/dL and blood urea nitrogen of ≥25 mg/dL
      - Serum sodium level of ≤130 mEq/L
      - Ascitic fluid total protein level <1.5 g/dL
   c. Low complement levels
   d. Reduced protein synthesis in the liver
   e. Along with:
      - Prolonged prothrombin time
      - Protein level in the ascitic fluid <1 g/dL

- Long-term proton pump therapy promoting bacterial growth in the gut and its translocation

5. Since there is high oxygen tension in the ascitic fluid, anaerobic organism is less common in this fluid.
6. Subtypes of subacute bacterial peritonitis are:
   a. Culture-negative SBP or culture negative neutrocytic ascites: It is characterized by neutrophil count in the ascitic fluid of >250/cc in absence of positive blood culture.
   b. Bacterascites:
      - Monomicrobial nonneutrocytic bacterascites: It is characterized by count of neutrophil <250/cc in the ascitic fluid and fluid culture demonstrated single bacterial organism.
      - Polymicrobial nonneutrocytic bacterascites: It is characterized by count of polymorphonuclear neutrophil <250/cc and demonstration of multiple organisms in the ascitic fluid on culture. Causative factors being:
         ○ Perforation of gut
         ○ After paracentesis
7. Pathophysiology of this SBP:
   a. Increased intestinal permeability
   b. Concomitant intestinal bacterial overgrowth

After translocation, these bacteria will go to regional mesenteric lymph nodes. From here:
   a. The bacteria will enter the systemic circulation then to ascitic fluid.

b. Rupture of the involved mesenteric node in the setting of increased portal pressure leading to dissemination in the fluid

8. Criteria for the secondary cause leading to peritonitis:

a. Glucose level <50 mg/dL
b. Concentration of protein >10 g/L
c. Level of lactate dehydrogenase in the ascitic fluid is more than that in the serum.

CASE 179

A 45-year-old chronic alcoholic man came to gastroenterology clinic with progressively increasing swelling with diffuse abdominal pain, fever, and oliguria for the last 15 days. He has no history of vomiting or facial puffiness. There is no surgical intervention.

On examination, no pedal edema, blood pressure 105/60 mm Hg, pulse rate 110 beats/minute, regular and grade III ascites, and urine output was 350 mL in the last 1 day. Examination of ascitic fluid demonstrated total count of 600/mL, with 85% neutrophil, protein 1.9 and SAAG of 1.5, and sugar 70 mg/dL.

Laboratory investigation demonstrated hemoglobin level 8 g/dL, total count 15,000/cc, platelet count 125,000/cc, bilirubin level 4 mg/dL, AST and ALT slightly above normal, serum albumin 2.9 g/dL, INR 1.6, serology negative, serum sodium 124 mEq/L, potassium 4.2 mEq/L, urea 65, and creatinine 2.2 mg/dL.

1. **What is your most likely diagnosis?**
2. **What are the criteria according to Acute Kidney Injury Network (AKIN) criteria for acute kidney involvement?**
3. **Mention the stage of acute kidney involvement.**
4. **Mention the causes of acute kidney involvement in cirrhosis.**
5. **What are the findings in the urine analysis in case of acute kidney involvement in cirrhosis?**
6. **Mention the differentiating points between the intrinsic renal disease and prerenal failure.**

Answers

1. The most likely diagnosis is decompensated alcoholic cirrhosis complicated by spontaneous bacterial peritonitis and acute kidney injury.

2. According to Acute Kidney Injury Network criteria for acute kidney injury reduction kidney function within 48 hours and it can be manifested by either:

   a. Rise in serum creatinine by >0.3 mg/dL within 48 hours
   b. Rise in serum creatinine by ≥50% from the baseline or by a factor 1.5 from the baseline.
   c. Decrease in the documented urine output, i.e., <0.5 mL/kg of body weight/hour for >6 hours.

3. Staging of acute kidney injury:

Stage of acute kidney injury	Serum creatinine criteria	Urine output criteria
I	Increase in serum creatinine by ≥0.3 mg/dL Or, Increase in serum creatinine by 1.5–1.9 times from the baseline	Urine output <0.5 mL/kg/hour for 6–12 hours

Continued

Continued

Stage of acute kidney injury	Serum creatinine criteria	Urine output criteria
II	Increase in serum creatinine by 2.0–2.9 times from the baseline	Urine output <0.5 mL/kg/hour for ≥12 hours
III	Increase in serum creatinine by ≥3.0 times from the baseline Or Serum creatinine ≥4.0 mg/dL Or Renal replacement therapy Or In patients of <18 years, decrease in estimated glomerular filtration rate to <35 mL/min/1.73 m^2	Urine output <0.3 mL/kg/hour for ≥24 hours or anuria for ≥12 hours

4. Causes of acute kidney injury in cirrhosis are:
   a. Prerenal causes:
      - Depletion of volume:
         ○ Gastrointestinal bleeding

- ○ Gastrointestinal fluid loss
- ○ Use of diuretics
- ○ Sepsis
- Effective perfusion will be decreased:
  - ○ Hepatorenal syndrome
  - ○ Cardiorenal syndrome
  - ○ Use of NSAIDs and COX-2 inhibitors
  - ○ Use of radiological contrast
  b. Intrinsic renal injury:
  - Acute tubular necrosis:
    - ○ Ischemia
    - ○ Sepsis
    - ○ Toxins
    - ○ Drugs
    - ○ Radiological contrast media
  - Glomerular diseases
  - Interstitial kidney disease
  c. Postrenal cause: Obstructive uropathy

5. Following are the findings in the urine analysis in acute kidney injury in cirrhosis:

Indicators	Pathologies
Pigmented granular cast	Toxic acute tubular injury
	Ischemic acute tubular injury
Red blood cell cast	Glomerulonephritis
Significant proteinuria	Glomerulonephritis

6. Following are the differences between prerenal disease and intrinsic renal disease:

Parameters	Prerenal injury to kidney	Intrinsic renal disease
Urine microscopy	No casts	Granular cast
		RBC cast
Osmolality of urine	>500 mOsmol/kg	<350 mOsmol/kg
Urinary sodium	<10 mEq/L	>20 mEq/L

CASE 180

A 45-year-old chronic alcoholic man came to gastroenterology clinic with progressively increasing swelling and oliguria for the last 110 days. He has no history of vomiting or facial puffiness and no surgical intervention.

On examination, presence of pedal edema, blood pressure 105/60 mm Hg, pulse rate 110 beats/minute, regular, grade III ascites, and urine output was 350 mL in the last 1 day. Examination of ascitic fluid demonstrated total count of WBC 300/mL, with 60% neutrophil, protein 1.9, and SAAG of 0.9.

Laboratory investigation demonstrated hemoglobin level 9 g/dL, total count 9,000/cc, platelet count 125,000/cc, bilirubin level 4 mg/dL, AST and ALT slightly above normal, serum albumin 2.9 g/dL, INR 1.6, serology negative, serum sodium 124 mEq/L, potassium 4.2 mEq/L, urea 165, and creatinine 3.2 mg/dL.

1. **What is your most likely diagnosis?**
2. **What are the types of this syndrome?**
3. **Mention the biomarkers that differentiate this syndrome from acute kidney injury?**
4. **What are the vasoconstrictors used in this syndrome with mechanism of actions.**
5. **What are the predictors of response to terlipressin therapy?**
6. **In case of nonresponder to terlipressin, what should be the next step of management?**

Answers

1. The most likely diagnosis is hepatorenal syndrome in a case of decompensated alcoholic cirrhosis.
2. New definition of hepatorenal syndrome:

Hepatorenal syndrome + Acute kidney injury	Increase in serum creatinine of ≥0.3 mg/dL within 48 hours
	And/or
	Urine output of ≤0.5 mL/kg of body weight in ≥6 hours
	Or
	Increase in serum creatinine of ≥50% from the baseline (lowest available in last 3 months)

Continued

Continued

Hepatorenal syndrome in nonacute kidney injury	
Hepatorenal syndrome in acute kidney disease	Effective glomerular filtration rate <60 mL/min/1.73 m² for <3 months in absence of structural causes
	Increase in serum creatinine <50% from the baseline (lowest available in last 3 months)
Hepatorenal syndrome in chronic kidney disease	Effective glomerular filtration rate <60 mL/min/1.73 m² for ≥3 months in absence of structural causes

3. Following are the potential biomarkers that can differentiate hepatorenal syndrome from acute tubular necrosis:

a. Urinary neutrophil gelatinase-associated lipocalin (uNGAL): The cutoff value is 220 μg/g of creatinine in 88% of patients with hepatorenal syndrome with acute kidney injury. The value is below this level.

b. Fractional excretion of urinary sodium (FeNa): The cutoff value of <0.2% can differentiate hepatorenal syndrome from acute kidney injury.

c. Cystatin C

d. Interleukin-18

e. Kidney injury molecule-1

f. Liver-type fatty acid-binding protein

4. Following are the vasoconstrictors used in this syndrome:

Vasocons-trictors	Mechanism of action	Dosage
Terlipressin	• It is vasopressin analog • It acts on the V1 receptors present on the vascular smooth muscles • It exerts its maximum effect on the mesenteric as well as cutaneous circulation	In can be given at a dose of 0.5 mg intravenously 4–6 hourly In case of nonresponse, it can be increased up to 1 mg 4–6 hourly
Noradrena-line	• It is α- and β-adrenergic agonist • It acts as potent vasoconstrictor • It increases the cardiac output • It has limited effect on splanchnic circulation	It should be given as 0.5–3 mg/hour with a target of maintaining mean arterial pressure of ≥10 mm Hg

Continued

Continued

Vasocons-trictors	Mechanism of action	Dosage
Octreotide	• It will inhibit glucagon and other vasodilatory molecule release • It acts as vasoconstrictor of systemic as well as splanchnic circulation • It acts as vasoconstrictor of portosystemic collaterals	It is given as intravenous infusion as 50 μg as bolus dose which is followed by 50 μg/hour as continuous intravenous infusion
Midodrine	It is α-1 agonist leading to vasoconstriction of systemic and splanchnic circulation	It can be given as 7.5 mg thrice daily and can be increased up to 15 mg thrice daily with a target of mean arterial pressure of ≥10 mm Hg

5. Following are the predictors of response to terlipressin therapy:

a. Baseline bilirubin <10 mg/dL

b. Early increase in mean arterial pressure of 5 mm Hg at day 3

6. In case of nonresponder to terlipressin, following management should be commenced:

a. Medical therapy in the form of sequential administration of noradrenaline along with terlipressin

b. Surgical therapies:
   • Transjugular intrahepatic portosystemic shunt
   • Renal replacement therapy

CASE 181

A 70-year-old man with alcoholic cirrhosis came to hepatic clinic, where triphasic CT scan was performed and it demonstrated a mass of 4 × 4 cm present in the right lobe of the liver which enhanced vividly in the arterial phase and hypoattenuated in the portal venous phase and there is no distant metastasis. Patient was advised to do TACE.

1. **What are the causes of irregular surface of the liver?**

2. **What are the factors responsible for protection from the hepatocellular carcinoma?**

3. **What are the complications in this disease?**

Answers

1. Following are the causes of the irregular surface of the liver:
   a. Micronodular or macronodular cirrhosis
   b. Hepatocellular carcinoma
   c. Hepatic abscess
   d. Secondaries in the liver
   e. Multiple hepatic cysts

2. Following factors protect the liver from developing hepatocellular carcinoma:
   a. Coffee intake
   b. Statin in case of diabetes

3. Complications of hepatocellular carcinoma are:
   a. Portal hypertension
   b. Hepatic venous thrombosis
   c. Hepatocellular failure
   d. Spreading to other organs

CASE 182

A 45-year-old chronic alcoholic patient taking 140 g daily for >8 years but having no other comorbidities came to emergency department with alteration of consciousness following massive bout of vomiting of blood. On examination, patient was icteric, blood pressure 90/50 mm Hg, pulse rate 132 beats/minute, regular, pedal edema, peripheral features of alcoholic liver disease like palmar erythema, bilateral enlargement of parotid gland, liver three-finger firm, nontender and sharp margin, surface irregular, and spleen three finger.

On laboratory investigation, hemoglobin 9.5 mg/dL, platelet count 120,000/cc, leukocyte count 15,000/cc, total bilirubin 6.5 mg/dL, SGOT 156 IU/L but SGPT normal, hepatitis viral serology is negative, urea 80 mg/dL, creatinine 1.4 mg/dL, and serum sodium 128. Hepatic venous pressure gradient was >10 mm Hg.

His upper gastrointestinal endoscopy was done which demonstrated:

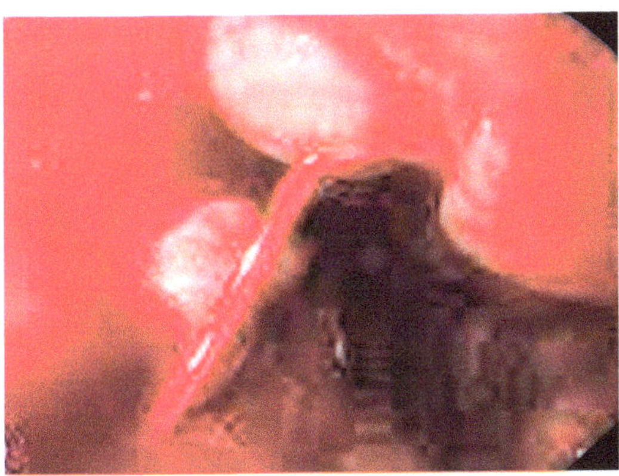
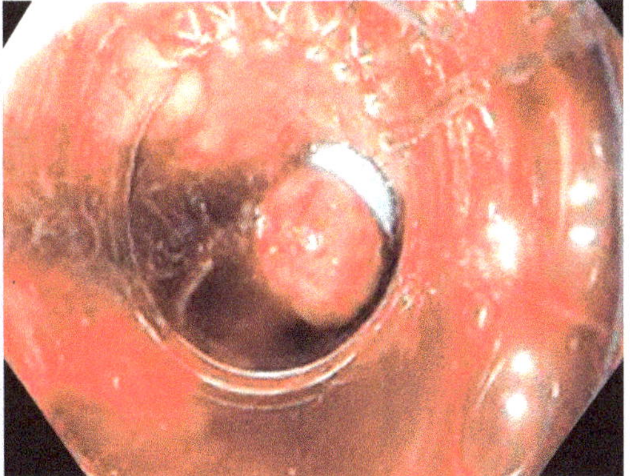

1. **Describe the above endoscopic pictures.**
2. **What is your diagnosis?**
3. **What are the points in favor of your diagnosis?**
4. **In this case, what are the risk factors of poor outcome?**
5. **What are the factors responsible for an excellent outcome in this patient?**
6. **What are the prognostic significances based on HVPG in this patient?**
7. **What are the vasoactive treatments in case of variceal hemorrhage?**
8. **What are the indicators of failure to control the variceal bleeding?**
9. **Is there any role of prophylaxis with antibiotics in this case?**
10. **What antibiotic is of choice in this case and why?**
11. **What are the factors that decide the timing of endoscopic treatment?**
12. **What is the primary prophylaxis to prevent this bleeding?**
13. **What is the mechanism of action of the drugs used in this disease?**
14. **What are noncirrhotic portal hypertension?**
15. **How can you differentiate this case from noncirrhotic portal hypertension?**

Answers

1. There are two pictures of endoscopy:
   a. First endoscopic picture demonstrated evidence of bleeding esophageal varices.
   b. Second endoscopic picture demonstrated banding done in the bleeding varix.
2. The most likely diagnosis is bleeding esophageal varices in a case of decompensated alcoholic cirrhosis with clinically significant portal hypertension leading to features of hemorrhagic shock.
3. Points in favor of this diagnosis are:
   a. History of alcohol intake for long duration
   b. History of jaundice
   c. History of hematemesis
   d. Presence of stigmata of cirrhosis
   e. Presence of hepatosplenomegaly
   f. Pitting edema
4. Following are the risk factors of poor outcome:
   a. Hepatic venous portal gradient of >20 mm Hg has five times increased risk of poor outcome.
   b. Child–Pugh having hepatic portal venous gradient of >20 mm Hg.
   c. Previous history of acute variceal bleeding but not receiving any portal pressure reducing agent
   d. Presence of ascites
   e. Presence of hepatic encephalopathy
5. Following factors are responsible for excellent outcome in this patient:
   a. Hepatic portal venous gradient of <10 mm Hg
   b. Absence of ascites
   c. Absence of hepatic encephalopathy
   d. Child–Pugh score of 1
   e. No previous history of variceal bleeding
6. Prognostic significance in the patient with cirrhosis based on HVPG:
   a. ≤5 mm Hg: Noncirrhotic portal hypertension
   b. >5 but <10 mm Hg: Portal hypertension
   c. >10 but <12 mm Hg: Clinically significant portal hypertension but predictive of decompensation
   d. >12 but <16 mm Hg: Variceal hemorrhage
   e. >16 but <20 mm Hg: Variceal rebleeding
   f. >20 but <30 mm Hg: It is very much difficult to control hemorrhage. So, there is increased mortality.
   g. >30 mm Hg: Spontaneous bacterial peritonitis
7. Following are the vasoactive therapies in this patient:
   a. Terlipressin:
      - 1–2 mg every 4 hourly till the control of bleeding

- Then 1 mg every 4 hourly as maintenance.
- Caution:
  ○ Arrhythmias
  ○ Tissue ischemia
  ○ Potential development of hyponatremia
   b. Somatostatin:
      - Bolus dose is 250 mg intravenously.
      - Followed by continuous infusion of 250–500 μg hourly
   c. Octreotide:
      - Initial bolus dose is 50 μg.
      - Followed by continuous infusion of 50 μg hourly
8. Following are the indicators of failure to control the bleeding:
   a. Fresh hematemesis
   b. Nasogastric aspiration of ≥100 mL of blood ≥2 hours after the start of a specific treatment with the drug or after therapeutic endoscopy
   c. Development of hypovolemic shock
   d. Drop of hemoglobin level 3 g/dL from the baseline within 24 hours in absence of any transfusion
   e. Drop of hematocrit of 9% within 24 hours in absence of any transfusion
9. Antibiotic prophylaxis is given to:
   a. Reduce the mortality
   b. Reduce the incidence of infection
   c. Reduce the early bleeding
   d. Reduce the total hospital stay
10. Ceftriaxone is the antibiotic of choice because:
    a. If the patient is on quinolone prophylaxis
    b. Advanced cirrhosis: Any two or more of the following:
       - Ascites
       - Hepatic encephalopathy
       - Severe malnutrition
       - Serum bilirubin level is >3 mg/dL.
    c. High prevalence of documented resistance to quinolone
11. Following are the factors upon which the treatment will depend:
    a. Vital signs of the patient
    b. Amount of hemorrhage
    c. Presence or absence of active bleeding—this can be judged from:
       - Color of the blood
       - Amount and frequency of vomiting

Endoscopy should be performed without delay if:
- The color of the blood is bright red.
- Presence of hematochezia
- Unstable vital signs

Endoscopy can be delayed if the following features are seen:
- Stable vital signs
- Vomiting of black-colored blood with food
- Absence of hematemesis or hematochezia within last 12 hours

12. Primary prophylaxis of prevention of variceal bleeding:
    a. For medium to large varices irrespective of Child–Pugh score
    b. Small high-risk varices with red wale sign
    c. Small varices with Child–Pugh class C

Following drugs are given as prophylaxis:
    a. Propranolol at a dose of 20–40 mg daily
    b. Carvedilol at a dose of 6.25 mg daily

13. Mechanism of action:
    a. Propranolol by blocking following receptors:
        - $\beta1$ receptor—decreases the cardiac output
        - $\beta2$ receptor—reduction of the splanchnic blood flow
    b. Carvedilol by following mechanism:
        - $\beta1$—it decreases the cardiac output
        - $\beta2$—reduction in the splanchnic blood flow
        - $\alpha1$ and production of nitric oxide—it will decrease the intrahepatic resistance as well as produces systemic and intrahepatic vasodilatation.

14. Noncirrhotic portal hypertension can be defined as presence of portal hypertension in absence of cirrhosis of liver but presence of acquired hepatic periportal fibrosis.

15. Differentiation of noncirrhotic portal hypertension from cirrhotic portal hypertension:

Cirrhotic portal hypertension	Noncirrhotic portal hypertension
Onset is insidious	Onset is acute or sudden
Presence of ascites	Absence of ascites
Recurrence of hematemesis is uncommon	Common recurrence of hematemesis
Anemia is moderate	Anemia will be severe
Pedal edema	Absence of edema
Hepatic encephalopathy is common	Hepatic encephalopathy is not common
Biopsy demonstrated cirrhosis	Biopsy demonstrated portal fibrosis

CASE 183

A 45-year-old chronic alcoholic patient taking 140 g daily for >8 years but having no other comorbidities came to emergency department with alteration of consciousness following massive bout of vomiting of blood. On examination, patient was icteric, blood pressure 90/50 mm Hg, pulse rate 132 beats/minute, regular, pedal edema, peripheral features of alcoholic liver disease like palmar erythema, bilateral enlargement of parotid gland, liver three finger firm, nontender and sharp margin, surface irregular, and spleen three finger.

On laboratory investigation, hemoglobin 9.5 mg/dL, platelet count 120,000/cc, leukocyte count 15,000/cc, total bilirubin 6.5 mg/dL, SGOT 156 IU/L but SGPT normal, hepatitis viral serology is negative, urea 80 mg/dL, creatinine 1.4 mg/dL, and serum sodium 128. Hepatic venous pressure gradient was >10 mm Hg.

His upper gastrointestinal endoscopy was done which demonstrated:

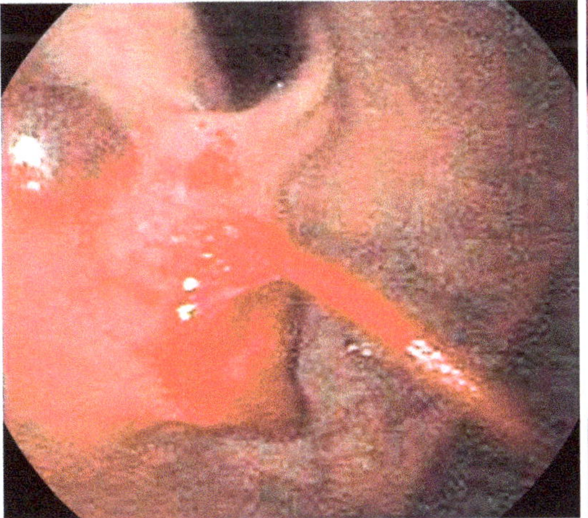
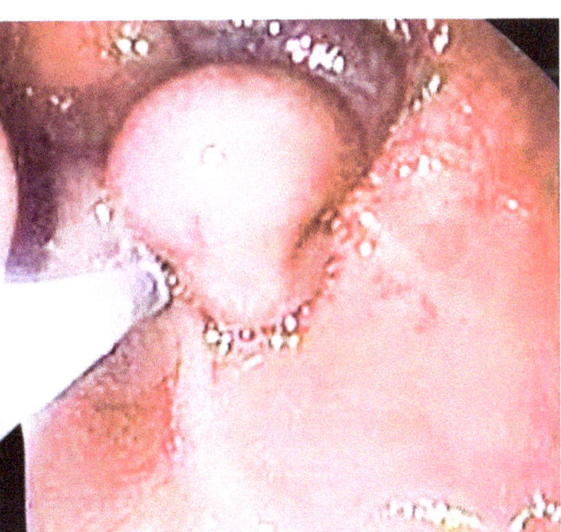

1. **What is the above findings in the upper gastrointestinal endoscopy?**
2. **What is your diagnosis?**
3. **Classify the picture demonstrated above.**
4. **What should be the treatment in this case?**
5. **How can you prevent the rebleeding rate?**
6. **What are the signs of hepatocellular failure?**
7. **What are the causes of upper gastrointestinal bleeding?**
8. **What are the complications of cirrhosis?**
9. **What are the five causes of death in cirrhosis?**

Answers

1. The above pictures of upper gastrointestinal endoscopy demonstrated:
   a. Bleeding esophageal varices
   b. Banding of the gastric varices
2. The most likely diagnosis is bleeding gastric varices in a case of decompensated alcoholic cirrhosis with clinically significant portal hypertension leading to features of hemorrhagic shock.
3. Classification of the gastric varices:
   a. GOV1: Esophageal varices extending below the gastric cardia into the lesser curvature
   b. GOV2: Esophageal varices extending below the gastric cardia into fundus
   c. IGV1: It is characterized by isolated varices in the fundus.
   d. IGV2: Isolated varices anywhere in the stomach like antrum, body, or pylorus.
4. Types of treatment in case of gastric varices:
   a. In GOV1 or IGV1 band ligation
   b. In GOV2 and IGV2 combination therapy with banding
   Endoscopic sclerotherapy with cyanoacrylate glue or alcohol should not be given in GOV1 and IGV1 because:
   a. Success rate is low.
   b. High rebleeding rate
   But in case of GOV2, endoscopic obturation should be the choice.
5. Gastric variceal bleeding can be prevented by:
   a. Repeated session of injection of cyanoacrylate glue
   b. Administration of nonselective β-blockers
   c. TIPSS
   d. Balloon-occluded retrograde transvenous obliteration (BRTO)
6. Following are the signs of hepatocellular failure:
   a. Presence of jaundice
   b. Circulatory changes:
      • Palmar erythema
      • Spider angioma
      • Cyanosis because of arteriovenous shunting in the lung
      • Clubbing
   c. Endocrinal changes:
      • Libido
      • Loss of axillary and pubic hair
      • Gynecomastia
      • Testicular atrophy
      • Impotence in males
      • Breast atrophy
      • Irregular menses and amenorrhea in females
   d. Hemorrhagic manifestations:
      • Bruises
      • Epistaxis
      • Menorrhagia
   e. Others:
      • White nails
      • Diffuse pigmentation
      • Dupuytren's contracture
      • Parotid enlargement
7. Following are the causes of upper gastrointestinal bleeding:
   a. Esophageal varices
   b. Gastric varices
   c. Portal congestive gastropathy
   d. Gastroduodenal ulceration
   e. Mallory–Weiss tear
8. Following are the complications of cirrhosis:
   a. Portal hypertension
   b. Hepatocellular failure
   c. Hepatic encephalopathy
   d. Spontaneous bacterial peritonitis
   e. Increased incidence of peptic ulcer

f. Hepatocellular carcinoma

g. Anemia

h. Hepatopulmonary syndrome

i. Hepatorenal syndrome

j. Hypoproteinemia

k. Tendency for hemorrhage

9.
a. Hepatocellular failure

b. Severe gastrointestinal bleeding

c. Primary liver cancer

d. Infections

e. Hepatic encephalopathy

CASE 184

A 28-year-old hypothyroid female on 50 µg levothyroxine has been admitted with yellowish discoloration of conjunctiva and urine for 15 days. On enquiry, she admitted the history of recurrent self-limiting jaundice in the last 2 years. She had neither significant family or drug history nor any surgical history. On examination, she was mildly anemic and icteric, normal BMI, per abdomen liver, and spleen is not palpable. Laboratory investigation demonstrated hemoglobin 9.5 g/dL, platelet count 150,000/cc, and white blood cell count 10,000/cc. Total bilirubin 5 mg/dL with ALT, AST, and ALP were 350, 510, and 102, respectively. Her viral serology was negative. Renal function and electrolyte test were normal, but ANA was strongly positive.

1. **What is your diagnosis?**
2. **What are points in favor of your diagnosis?**
3. **What are the recent diagnostic scoring systems for diagnosis of this patient?**
4. **What are the limitations in this scoring systems?**
5. **What are the classical clinical presentations in this disease?**
6. **What are the extrahepatic diseases to be enquired in this disease?**
7. **Is there any hereditary role in this case?**
8. **What are the causes of jaundice of >6 months?**

Answers

1. The most probable diagnosis is chronic AIH.
2. Following are the points in favor of AIH:
   a. Young female
   b. Background of autoimmune disease like thyroid disorder
   c. History of recurrent jaundice
   d. Positive autoimmune serology
   e. Raised transaminases
3. Revised International Autoimmune Hepatitis Group scoring system in 1999:

Criteria	Score	Criteria	Score
Female	+2	HLA-DRB1*03 positive Or DRB1*04 positive	+2
ALP:AST or ALT ratio: >3 <1.5	 −2 +2	Alcohol use <25 g/day >60 g/day	 +2 −2

Continued

Continued

Criteria	Score	Criteria	Score
ANA/SMA Or LKM >1:80 1:80 >1:40 1:40 AMA positive	 +3 +2 +1 0 −4	Liver biopsy Interface hepatitis Plasmacytoid infiltrate Hepatic rosettes No specific feature Biliary changes Fat, granuloma, and others	 +3 +1 +1 −5 −3 −3
Gamma globulin levels: More than two upper levels of normal 1.5–2 upper level of normal 1–1.4 upper level of normal	−4 +3 +2 +1	Concurrent immune disease (thyroiditis, colitis, etc.)	+2
Viral marker Positive Negative	 −3 +3	Other liver-related markers (anti-SLA and anti-actin)	+2

Continued

Continued

Criteria	Score	Criteria	Score
Hepatotoxic drugs TACE (Transarterial chemoembolization) No	−4 +1	Response to treatment Complete response Relapse	+2 +3
Pretreatment scores: • Definite diagnosis: >15 • Probable diagnosis <15 Posttreatment score: • Definite diagnosis: >17 • Probable diagnosis: 12–17			

4. Following are the limitations in the above scoring system:
   a. Lack of validation for the specific groups like acute severe AIH and AIH presenting with acute liver failure.
   b. The scoring system relies on immunofluorescence than ELISA for serological markers.
   c. Unproven efficacy in the following settings:
      • Overlap syndrome
      • Concomitant NAFLD
      • Post-liver transplant AIH
5. Following are the classical clinical presentations of AIH:
   a. Asymptomatic AIH:
      • It occurs in 25–35% of patients
      • Within the period of 32 months 25–75% patients develop symptoms
      • Its histology similar to that of symptomatic patients
   b. Chronic hepatitis:
      • It occurs in one-third of the patients
      • Most common are fatigue, arthralgia, menorrhea, or malaise but most common being easy fatigability
      • In certain cases, jaundice may be present.
   c. Cirrhosis: It can present in 25% patients.
   d. Acute severe AIH or AIH with ALF:
      • Asymptomatic AIH in patients with no previous history of chronic liver disease:
         ○ Jaundice
         ○ INR is >1.5 but <2.
         ○ Absence of encephalopathy
      • Autoimmune hepatitis with ALF in patients with previous history of chronic liver disease:
         ○ Jaundice

         ○ INR is >2.
         ○ Absence of encephalopathy
   • Acute presentation—it can be characterized by presentation within 30 days from onset.
   • ANA is absent or becomes weakly positive in 29–30% of patients.
   • IgG levels normal in 25–39% of patients
   • Following are the features in the AIH-ALF histology:
      ○ Central perivenulitis
      ○ Plasma cells enriched inflammatory infiltrate
      ○ Massive hepatic necrosis
      ○ In 32% cases, presence of lymphoid follicles
6. Following are the extrahepatic features in AIH:
   a. Presence of concurrent extrahepatic diseases in 14–44% of patients
      • More common in women
      • Positive family history
      • HLA-DRB1*04:01
   b. Most common is autoimmune thyroid disease.
   c. Other diseases are:
      • Type 1 diabetes mellitus
      • Ulcerative colitis
      • Pernicious anemia
      • Rheumatoid arthritis
      • Different autoimmune dermatological disorders:
         ○ Alopecia areata
         ○ Urticaria
         ○ Vitiligo
         ○ Leukocytoclastic vasculitis
7. Role of heredity:
   a. In case of young patient, positive for HLA-B8 and HLA-DR3
   b. In case of old patient, HLA-DRY
8. Causes of jaundice of >6 months:
   a. Cholestatic viral hepatitis
   b. Chronic AIH
   c. Chronic hepatitis
   d. Cirrhosis of liver
   e. Malignancy of liver
   f. Alcoholic hepatitis
   g. Drug-induced hepatitis
   h. Wilson's disease
   i. Primary biliary cirrhosis
   j. Obstructive cirrhosis due to extrahepatic biliary tract obstruction
   k. Congenital hyperbilirubinemia

CASE 185

A 28-year-old hypothyroid female on 50 µg levothyroxine has been admitted with yellowish discoloration of conjunctiva and urine for 15 days. On enquiry, she had the history of recurrent self-limiting jaundice in the last 2 years. She had neither significant family or drug history nor any surgical history. On examination, she was mildly anemic and icteric, normal BMI, per abdomen liver, and spleen are not palpable. Laboratory investigation demonstrated hemoglobin 9.5 g/dL, platelet count 150,000/cc, and white blood cell count 10,000/cc. Total bilirubin 5 mg/dL with ALT, AST, and ALP were 350, 510, and 102, respectively. Her viral serology was negative. Renal function and electrolytes test were normal, but ANA was strongly positive.

1. **What is your diagnosis?**
2. **What are the histological features in this case?**
3. **Name the drugs that can produce this type of liver injury.**
4. **How can you differentiate this disease from drug-induced liver injury?**
5. **What are the indications of treatment according to 2010 AASLD guideline?**
6. **What are the first-line therapies in this case?**
7. **What are the criteria of response to treatment according to AASLD 2019 guideline?**
8. **What you have to check prior to administration of azathioprine?**
9. **What are the second-line treatments in this disease?**

Answers

1. The most likely diagnosis is AIH.
2. Following are the cardinal features in this disease:
   a. Interface hepatitis—it is the hallmark for this diagnosis.
   b. Panacinar hepatitis
   c. Plasma cell infiltration
   d. The early severe case of the histological stage is centrilobular zonal necrosis. It may coexist with interface hepatitis.
   e. Emperipolesis
   f. Hepatic rosettes
   g. In some cases, IgG4 positivity may be present.
3. Following drugs are responsible for similar type of liver injury:
   a. Minocycline
   b. Infliximab
   c. Nitrofurantoin
   d. Methyldopa
   e. Statins
   f. Propylthiouracil
   g. Isoniazid
   h. Diclofenac
   i. Adalimumab
   j. Immune cytokine checkpoint inhibitors
4. Following are the differentiating points that can differentiate this disease from drug-induced liver injury:
   a. Drug-induced injury is always acute onset but AIH is chronic onset.
   b. Temporal association implicates drug-induced liver injury
   c. Hypersensitivity features such as rash, peripheral eosinophilia, and presence of eosinophils in urine are present in drug-induced liver injury.
   d. Presence of other types of autoimmune disorders are more common in AIH.
   e. Though prednisolone is the drug of choice in both the cases but relapse is more common in AIH.
   f. Histological features of fibrosis are common in AIH.
5. Absolute indications of treatment of AIH according to AASLD 2019 guidelines:
   a. AST is >10 times upper limit of normal
   b. AST is more than five times of upper limit of normal and γ-globulin level is more than two times of upper limit of normal.
   c. Bridging or multiacinar necrosis on histology
   d. Evidence of incapacitating symptoms
6. First-line therapies in this disease are:
   a. Prednisolone 40–60 mg daily or 20–40 mg daily in combination with azathioprine
   b. Azathioprine 50–150 mg daily or 1–2 mg/kg of body weight daily.
7. Following are the criteria of response to treatment according to AASLD 2019 guideline:
   a. Biochemical remission: It is characterized by normalization of serum AST and ALT and IgG levels. But, level of IgG may be permanently elevated once the is developed.

b. Histological remission: It is characterized by absence of any inflammation in the liver post-treatment.

c. Incomplete response: It is characterized by improvement in the histological as well as laboratory findings but not enough to satisfy the criteria of remission.

d. Relapse: It is characterized by exacerbation of the disease activity after the induction of remission or after withdrawal of the drug.

e. Treatment failure: It is characterized as despite of the standard therapy there is worsening of the laboratory as well as histological findings.

f. Intolerance to treatment: It is characterized by inability to continue the maintenance therapy due to appearance of drug-related side effects.

8. Following are the checkpoints prior to azathioprine administration:

a. TPMT activity

b. Vaccination hepatitis A virus and B virus

c. If the patient is HBsAg negative but anti-HBc positive, he or she should be assessed periodically for the reactivation of hepatitis B virus when the patient is on standard dose of steroid combined with azathioprine.

d. If the patient is on high dose of steroid or B-cell depleting drug, he should be treated with hepatitis B virus therapy.

e. Following should be monitored:
- Vitamin D status
- Bone mineral density
- Features of metabolic syndrome

9. Following are the second-line drugs in this disease:

a. Mycophenolate mofetil

b. Cyclosporine

c. Calcineurin inhibitor

d. 6-mercaptopurine

e. Biologics:
- Infliximab
- Rituximab

CASE 186

A 50-year-old nondiabetic, nonhypertensive female came to gastroenterology clinic with yellowish discoloration of the conjunctiva, progressively increasing pruritus, weight loss, fatigue, and chills. Patient had no history of abdominal pain, fever, no intake of medication, no history of recent medication, tattooing, abnormal sexual behavior, blood transfusion, or substance abuse. On examination, there was jaundice, and scratch mark all over the body. Abdominal examination demonstrated evidence of firm nontender liver, sharp margin, splenomegaly, and no free fluid in the abdomen.

Laboratory examination demonstrated hemoglobin 9.5 g/dL, platelet count 8,500/cc, total bilirubin 4.2 mg/dL with direct fraction 3.2 g/dL, AST 98 IU/L, ALT 59 IU/L, alkaline phosphatase 486 IU/L, and viral serology and antinuclear factor negative but antimitochondrial antibody (AMA) positive.

1. **What is the most likely diagnosis?**
2. **How can you identify the types in this case?**
3. **What are the epidemiological characteristics in this disease?**
4. **What is the natural history of this disease?**
5. **What are the specific antibodies for this disease?**
6. **What is the cause of pruritus and how can you treat pruritus in this case?**
7. **What is the cause of osteoporosis in this disease and how can you treat osteoporosis?**

Answers

1. The most probable diagnosis is primary biliary cholangitis associated with cirrhosis.

2. Cholestasis results from either formation of bile or impairment of bile flow through the biliary canaliculi. So, there are two types of stasis:

a. Intrahepatic biliary stasis

b. Extrahepatic cholestasis

First step in the diagnosis of cholestasis is increased level of serum ALP. But, this enzyme is elevated due to many causes; however, an associated raised level of γ-glutamyl transpeptidase will support the diagnosis of cholestasis.

Second step is the proper clinical positive and negative family history.

Third step is performing the ultrasound of the abdomen to differentiate between intrahepatic and extrahepatic cholestasis.

Fourth step is to perform:

a. MRCP

b. EUS

c. Antimitochondrial antibody

d. Biopsy of liver

e. ERCP

3. Following are the epidemiological characteristics in this disease:

a. This disease occurs in middle-aged female with female-to-male ratio of 10:1.

b. Peak incidence is in the fifth decade.

c. Highest prevalence of this disease occurs in Spain, Canada, Scandinavian countries, and UK.

4. Natural history of this disease:

a. Preclinical or silent phase: Here, the patient is positive for AMA but biochemically silent.

b. Asymptomatic phase: Here, the patient is AMA positive associated with biochemical abnormalities. This phase may be prolonged up to 20 years, but on an average, 30% patients remain symptomatic up to 5 years.

c. Symptomatic phase: In this phase, the patient may present with pruritus, abdominal pain, jaundice, and hepatomegaly. Subsequently, patient develops evidence of portal hypertension and lately ascites in 20% of cases and 10–15% patients develop varices.

d. Stage of liver failure: In this phase, the jaundice becomes progressive.

5. Following are the antibodies specific for this disease:

a. Antimitochondrial antibodies against different mitochondrial antigens.

   • AMA PDH-E2 is directed against E2 component of mitochondrial ketoacid dehydrogenase complexes.

   • Other AMAs are clinically relevant, these are anti-M4, anti-M8, and anti-M9.

   • This antibody can be determined by immunofluorescence and ELISA.

b. Antinuclear antibodies:

   • It is positive in 30–50% cases.

   • By immunofluorescence, following types of ANA are highly specific for this disease:

      I. Multiple nuclear ANA

      II. Rim ANA pattern

c. Anti-Kelch-12

d. Anti-hexokinase-1

e. Anti-glycoprotein 210 antibodies correlate with the disease progression toward hepatic failure

f. Anti-P62 antibodies correlate with the disease progression toward hepatic failure

g. Anticentromere antibodies correlate with portal hypertension

h. Anti-np62 antibody

i. Anti-sp100 antibody

6. Following factors are responsible for pruritus in this disease:

a. Bile acid retention

b. Increased opioidergic tone

c. Autotoxin activity

Treatment:

a. First line of therapy is administration of cholestyramine.

b. Second line of therapy is rifampicin 150–300 mg daily.

c. Opioid antagonists

d. Antihistaminics

e. Sertraline

f. Plasmapheresis

g. In case of refractory pruritus, the option is liver transplantation.

7. Following are the risk factors for osteoporosis:

a. Advanced age

b. Lower BMI

c. High histological stage of this disease

d. Severe cholestasis

Mechanism of osteoporosis: Bilirubin inhibits osteoblastic activity leading to interfere with bone formation

Treatment:

a. Supplementation of vitamin D and calcium, when the femur score is <1.5.

b. Bisphosphonates should be administered in patients with advanced risk of fracture.

CASE 187

A 50-year-old nondiabetic, nonhypertensive female came to gastroenterology clinic with yellowish discoloration of the conjunctiva, progressively increasing pruritus, weight loss, fatigue, and chills. Patient had no history of abdominal pain, fever, no intake of medication, no history of recent medication, tattooing, abnormal sexual behavior, blood transfusion, or substance abuse. On examination, there was jaundice, and scratch mark all over the body. Abdominal examination demonstrated evidence of firm nontender liver, sharp margin, splenomegaly, and no free fluid in the abdomen.

Ultrasonography demonstrated the following features:

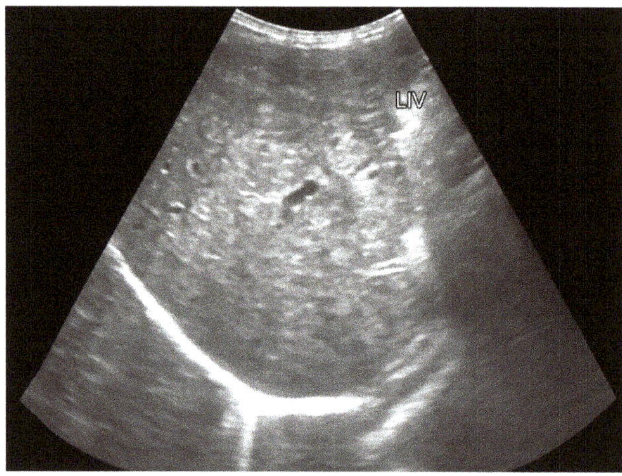

Laboratory examination demonstrated hemoglobin 9.5 g/dL, platelet count 8,500/cc, total bilirubin 4.2 mg/dL with direct fraction 3.2 g/dL, AST 98 IU/L, ALT 59 IU/L, alkaline phosphatase 486 IU/L, and viral serology and antinuclear factor negative but AMA positive. Liver biopsy demonstrated:

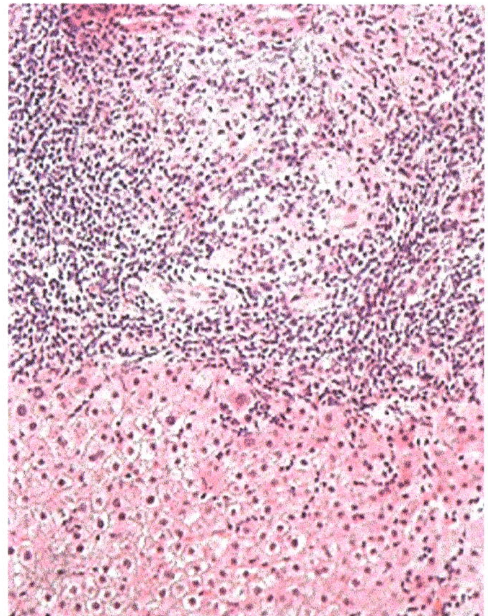

1. **What do the above two pictures demonstrate?**
2. **What is your most likely diagnosis?**
3. **What are the indications of liver biopsy?**
4. **What is the staging system of this disease according to histology?**
5. **What is the use of UDCA in this disease?**
6. **What are the criteria for the response to UDCA?**

Answers

1. The above ultrasonographic picture demonstrates narrowing and obliteration of the intrahepatic biliary canaliculi along with increased echogenicity.

   Histologic picture demonstrates:
   a. Inflammation of the bile ducts
   b. Periductal epithelioid granuloma
   c. Proliferation of bile ductules
   d. Fibrosis

2. The most likely diagnosis is primary biliary cholangitis leading to cirrhosis.

3. Indications of liver biopsy:
   a. Presence of low titer AMA or negative
   b. History of intake of hepatotoxic drugs
   c. Prominent features of hepatitis in the form of elevation of transaminases
   d. If there is suspicion of concurrent pathology.
   e. Overlapping of this disease with AIH

4. Ludwig staging system of primary biliary cholangitis according to liver biopsy:
   a. Stage 1—portal stage: Characterized by:
      - Bile duct abnormalities
      - Portal inflammation
   b. Stage 2—periportal stage: This stage is characterized by periportal fibrosis with or without periportal inflammation or prominent portal tract with seemingly intact newly formed limiting plates.
   c. Stage 3 or septal stage: This stage is characterized by septal fibrosis with active inflammatory paucicellular septa or both the features are present.
   d. Stage 4 or cirrhosis: In this stage, nodules along with various degrees of inflammation should be present.

5. UDCA acts by following mechanisms in this disease:
   a. Increase in the hydrophilic bile acid profile
   b. Stimulation of bile secretion
   c. Immunomodulatory action
   d. Protection against cytokine-related injury

6. Following are the criteria of response to UDCA in this disease:
   a. Mayo criteria: Alkaline phosphatase is less than two times of upper limit of normal.
   b. Paris I criteria:
      - Serum ALP is less than three times of upper limit of normal.
      - Serum AST is less than two times of upper limit of normal.
      - Serum bilirubin is less than 1 mg/dL.
   c. Paris II criteria:
      - Serum ALP is less than 1.5 times of upper limit of normal.
      - Serum AST is less than 1.5 times of upper limit of normal.
      - Serum bilirubin is less than 1 mg/dL.
   d. Spanish criteria: Reduction of serum ALP is 40% of baseline or to the normal value.
   e. Rotterdam criteria: Normalization of the bilirubin level and/or albumin, ALP, and platelets.

CASE 188

A 40-year-old man presented in the emergency department with fever with chill, progressively yellowish discoloration of urine and conjunctiva associated with itching, clay-colored stool for 25 days, and pain in the right upper abdomen for 7 days. He has long-standing history of 3–5 times per day blood-mixed loose stool for the last 3 years for which he was treated by metronidazole and other antibiotics in the primary health center. He had past history of intermittent jaundice for the last 1 year that had been treated with intravenous medication. He has no history of addiction to alcohol, tattooing, joint pain and skin rash, medication, and surgical or endoscopic history.

On examination, there was jaundice, scratch marks all over the body, shiny nails, and BMI 22 kg/m^2. Vitals are normal. Liver was enlarged 4 cm below the right midclavicular line and nontender. Spleen and gallbladder were not palpable.

Laboratory investigations demonstrated bilirubin 14 mg/dL with direct fraction of 11 mg/dL. AST, ALT, and ALP were 110, 140, and 410 IU/L, respectively. Serology, ANA, ASMA, and AMA were negative.

USG and MRCP demonstrated the following.

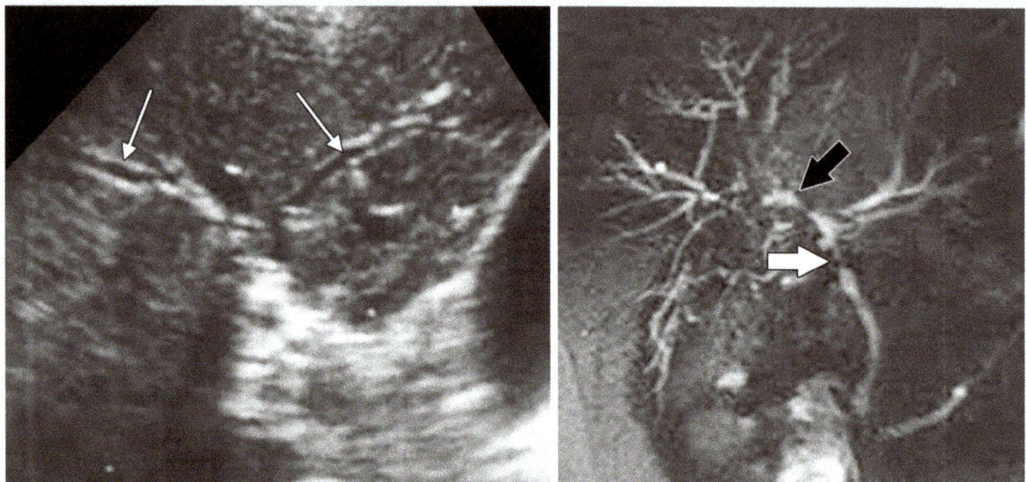

1. **What has been described in the above pictures?**
2. **What is the most probable diagnosis?**
3. **What are the points in favor of this diagnosis?**
4. **ERCP was done and it was found normal. What is the next diagnostic investigation in this case?**
5. **Describe Amsterdam classification in respect of cholangiographic changes in this disease?**
6. **Is there any role of autoantibodies in this disease?**
7. **What are the modes of presentation in this disease?**

Answers

1. Description of the above pictures:
   a. Ultrasonography of the abdomen demonstrated:
      - Thickening and dilatation of the intrahepatic biliary canaliculi
      - Moderately thickened gallbladder wall
   b. NRCP picture demonstrated:
      - Multifocal stricture in the intrahepatic and extrahepatic bile ducts leading to beaded appearance of the biliary canaliculi
      - Upstream intrahepatic bile duct stricture extending to the liver periphery
2. The most likely diagnosis is primary sclerosing cholangitis. It is the extraintestinal manifestation of inflammatory bowel disease.
3. Following points are in favor of this diagnosis:
   a. History suggestive of cholestatic jaundice
   b. Raised ALP, i.e., R ratio of <2
   c. Mixed cholestatic hepatitis, i.e. R ratio in between 2 and 5
   d. MRCP suggestive of multifocal biliary stricture with beaded appearance of intrahepatic canaliculi

   e. History of long-standing recurrent bloody diarrhea
4. If ERCP is normal, liver biopsy should be done and following features are the characteristic of this disease:
   a. Proliferation of the bile duct
   b. Periductal inflammation
   c. Periductal fibrosis looking like "onion skin" lesion.
   d. Obliteration of the bile duct
5. Amsterdam classification of primary sclerosing cholangitis in respect to cholangiographic changes:

Type	Intrahepatic features	Extrahepatic features
0	Normal	Normal
I	Multifocal changes in the contour of the bile duct, minimum dilatation	Slight irregularities in the caliber of the duct There is absence of stricture
II	There are multifocal strictures along with sac-like dilatation and reduced ductal arborization.	Evidence of segmental stricture

Continued

Continued

Type	Intrahepatic features	Extrahepatic features
III	With adequate filling pressure, central branches of the bile ducts are opacified. Severe narrowing with pruning is present.	Entire length of the common bile duct demonstrates strictures.
IV		Duct contour is extremely irregular. There is diverticulum like outpouchings.

6. Following autoantibodies may be present in this disease but their values are uncertain:
   a. Antineutrophil cytoplasmic antibody in 50–85% of cases
   b. In 70% cases, antinuclear antibody
   c. In 15% cases, anti-smooth muscle antibody
   d. In 30% cases, antiendothelial cell antibody
   e. In 50% cases, anticardiolipin antibody
   f. In 10% cases, thyroperoxidase
   g. In 4% cases, thyroglobulin
   h. In 15% cases, rheumatoid factor

7. Following are the modes of presentation in this case:
   a. Asymptomatic patients with abnormal liver function test
   b. Patient has positive family history of inflammatory bowel disease having cholestatic feature in the liver function test
   c. Presence of jaundice with pruritus
   d. Evidence of hepatic failure leading to deepening of jaundice
   e. Decompensated chronic liver disease leading to formation of ascites and/or varices
   f. Evidence of cholangiocarcinoma

CASE 189

A 40-year-old man presented in the emergency department with fever with chill, progressively yellowish discoloration of urine and conjunctiva associated with itching, clay-colored stool for 25 days, and pain in the right upper abdomen for 7 days. He has long-standing history of 3–5 times per day blood mixed with loose stool for last 3 years for which he was treated by metronidazole and other antibiotics in the primary health center. He had past history of intermittent jaundice for last 1 year that had been treated with intravenous medication. He has no history of addiction to alcohol, tattooing, joint pain and skin rash, medication, and surgical or endoscopic history.

On examination, there was jaundice, scratch marks all over the body, shiny nails, and BMI 22 kg/m^2. Vitals are normal. Liver was enlarged 4 cm below the right midclavicular line and nontender. Spleen and gallbladder were not palpable.

Laboratory investigations demonstrated bilirubin 14 mg/dL with direct fraction of 11 mg/dL. AST, ALT, and ALP were 110, 140, and 410 IU/L, respectively. Serology, ANA, ASMA, and AMA were negative.

USG and MRCP demonstrated the following. Colonoscopy was also performed.

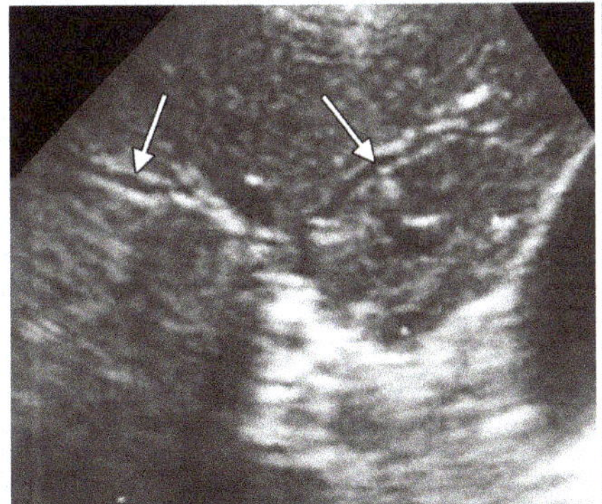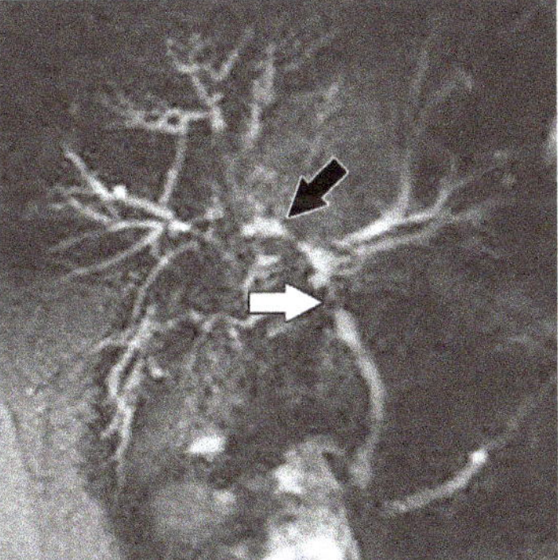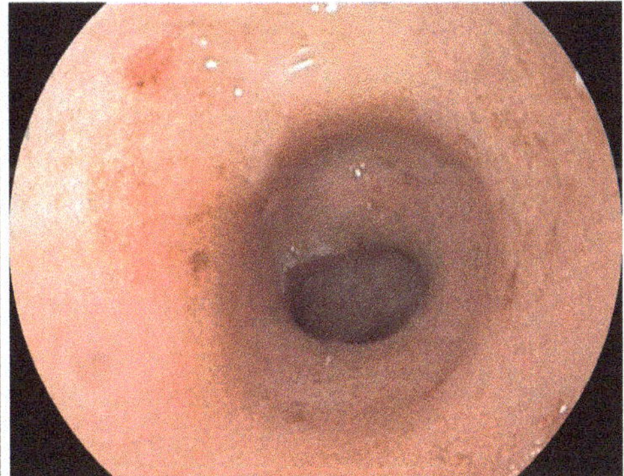

1. **What has been described in the above pictures?**
2. **What is the most probable diagnosis?**
3. **What are the variants of this disease?**
4. **What are the various prognostic indices seen in this disease?**
5. **What are the four different scores in this disease?**
6. **What is the dominant stricture in this disease?**
7. **How dominant stricture can be managed?**
8. **What are the classical features in this case?**

Answers

1. Description of the above pictures:
   a. Ultrasonography of the abdomen demonstrated:
      - Thickening and dilatation of the intrahepatic biliary canaliculi
      - Moderately thickened gallbladder wall.
   b. NRCP picture demonstrated:
      - Multifocal stricture in the intrahepatic and extrahepatic bile ducts leading to beaded appearance of the biliary canaliculi
      - Upstream intrahepatic bile duct stricture extending to the liver periphery
   c. Colonoscopic picture demonstrates:
      - Multiple superficial ulcers
      - Loss of vascular architecture in the colonic mucosa
      - Mucosa appears granular
      - Presence of mucous on the colonic wall
2. The most likely diagnosis is primary sclerosing cholangitis. It is the extraintestinal manifestation of inflammatory bowel disease.
3. Following are the variants in this disease:
   a. Classic primary sclerosing cholangitis involving both the intrahepatic and extrahepatic ducts.
   b. Small duct primary sclerosing cholangitis
   c. Primary sclerosing cholangitis–AIH overlap—it occurs in nearly 10% of cases
   d. Noninflammatory bowel disease—primary sclerosing cholangitis
   e. Autoimmune sclerosing cholangitis in pediatric age-group
4. Following are the prognostic indicators in this disease:
   a. Age: As the age increases prognosis becomes poor.
   b. Albumin: There is an inverse relation between serum albumin and prognosis.
   c. Alkaline phosphatase: Its increasing level is associated with poor prognosis.
   d. Small duct involvement: This type of involvement is associated with good prognosis as compared to large duct involvement.
   e. Serum bilirubin: Persistently raised bilirubin level for more than 3 months is associated with poor prognosis.
   f. Enhanced liver fibrosis (ELF) test: It is a strong predictor of the prognosis in this disease.
   g. Level of IgG4: Its high level is associated with shortened liver transplant-free survival.
   h. Histological stage: It follows Ludwig or Ishak or Nakanuma score.
   i. Spleen size in ultrasound: Its size of more than 12 cm is associated with poor prognosis.
5. Following are the clinical scores in this disease:
   a. Mayo score involving age, bilirubin, hemoglobin, histological stage, and inflammatory bowel disease
   b. King's college score involving age, histological stage, hepatomegaly, ALP, histological stage, and splenomegaly
   c. Multicenter model involving age, serum bilirubin, and splenomegaly
   d. Scandinavian model involving age, serum bilirubin, and histological stage
6. Dominant stricture in ERCP can be defined as:
   a. Stenosis of the common bile duct ≤1.5 mm in diameter
      And/or
   b. Hepatic duct diameter of ≤1 mm within 2 m of the main hepatic confluence
7. Endoscopic management of dominant stricture is dilatation along with concomitant ductal sampling by brush cytology and/or endobiliary biopsy of the stricture with/without stenting to improve the survival in this patient.
8. Following are the classical features in primary sclerosing cholangitis:
   a. Extensive colitis with pancolitis

b. Rectal sparing
c. More common is backwash ileitis.
d. Disease activity is milder.
e. There is high risk of colorectal cancer.

f. There is a high risk of postproctocolectomy pouchitis.
g. There is a higher chance of peristomal varices in patients with ileostomy.

CASE 190

A 38-year-old obese woman on oral contraceptive pill having no other comorbidities came to gastroenterology clinic for routine checkup because of vague abdominal pain. She was advised whole abdomen ultrasonography which demonstrated well-demarcated mass size being 7 cm diameter in the liver with early enhancement in the arterial phase and isoattenuation during the portal venous phase. MRI of liver also demonstrated early enhancement with gadolinium.

1. **What is the most likely diagnosis?**
2. **What are the risk factors in this disease?**
3. **What are the different subtypes of this mass?**
4. **What are the prognostic factors in this mass?**
5. **What are the complications in this disease?**
6. **What are the different treatments in this disease?**
7. **What are the macroscopic features in this disease?**

Answers

1. The most likely diagnosis is hepatocellular adenoma.
2. Following are the risk factors in hepatocellular adenoma:
    a. Oral contraceptive pills
    b. Anabolic steroid
    c. Metabolic syndrome
    d. Noncontraceptive estrogen supplements
    e. Obesity
3. Following are the different subtypes of hepatocellular adenoma:
    a. HNF1A-mutated hepatocellular adenoma
    b. β-catenin-mutated hepatocellular adenoma
    c. Inflammatory hepatocellular adenoma
    d. Sonic hedgehog hepatocellular adenoma
4. Following are the prognostic factors in hepatocellular adenoma:
    a. Men
    b. Larger tumors
    c. β-catenin-mutated hepatocellular adenoma
5. Complications of this adenoma are:
    a. Hemorrhage
    b. Malignant transformation
6. Following are the treatments of hepatocellular adenoma:
    a. In case of female:
        - Weight reduction
        - Stopping the oral contraceptive pills
        - Follow-up MRI surveillance after 6 months
    b. In case of male: Surgical resection as there is chance of malignant transformation
7. Following are the macroscopic features of resected hepatocellular adenoma:
    a. Majority and well circumscribed
    b. The mass is uncapsulated or pseudocapsulated
    c. Its color is light as compared to surrounding liver.
    d. Presence of foci of necrosis, hemorrhage, and bile staining
    e. Lack of significant fibrosis and nodularity

CASE 191

A 60-year-old nonalcoholic, type 2 diabetic, hypertensive, and dyslipidemic patient had been suffering from NAFLD. After few years due to some upper abdominal discomfort, he was advised ultrasonography and demonstrated two masses of about 3.5 cm and 3.2 cm, normal portal vein, and no ascites. So, triphasic CT scan was advised which demonstrated two irregular nodular lesions in VII segment showing arterial enhancement followed by delayed phase washout.

1. **What is the most probable diagnosis?**
2. **What are the points in favor of this diagnosis?**
3. **What is staging system in this disease?**
4. **What is LI-RADS?**
5. **Name three classification systems in this disease?**
6. **What are the common clinical presentations in this disease?**
7. **What are the paraneoplastic manifestations in this disease?**
8. **What are the sites of extrahepatic metastasis?**
9. **What are the percutaneous strategies in this disease?**
10. **What are the limitations of percutaneous therapies?**
11. **What are the transarterial therapies in this disease?**
12. **What are the indications and complications of TACE and transarterial radioembolization (TARE)?**
13. **What are the emerging therapies in this disease?**

Answers

1. The most probable diagnosis is hepatocellular carcinoma.
2. Following are the points in favor of this diagnosis:
   a. Presence of metabolic syndrome
   b. Presence of NAFLD
   c. Biochemical evidence of cirrhosis
   d. Imaging evidence of cirrhosis
   e. Presence of space-occupying lesion having arterial enhancement and delayed phase washout.
3. Barcelona Clinic Liver Cancer System (BCLC system) in hepatocellular carcinoma:

BCLC stage	Character of tumor	Extrahepatic spread	Estimated survival
0 (very early)	Single nodule of <2 cm	Nil	
A (early)	Single or 2–3 nodule of ≤3 cm	Nil	>5 years
B (intermediate)	Multinodular	Nil	2 years
C (advanced)	Extrahepatic spread	Portal vein or extrahepatic spread	8–13 years
D (terminal)	End-stage liver function	Incurable and widespread disease	3 months

4. LI-RADS, i.e., Liver Imaging Reporting and Data System: It is a classification system. It can estimate the likelihood of hepatocellular carcinoma in the high-risk patients, and it is validated in case of cirrhosis. By this criteria, lesion can be classified into following categories:
   a. LR-1: Definitely benign
   b. LR-2: Probably benign
   c. LR-3: Immediate probability of malignancy
   d. LR-4: Probably hepatocellular carcinoma
   e. LR-5: Definite hepatocellular carcinoma
5. Following three classification systems of hepatocellular carcinoma:

Classification system	Features
Alberta classification system	• Transarterial radioembolization α-fetoprotein in algorithm should be included • It provides for transplant beyond Milan criteria • Sorafenib restricted to Child–Pugh class A only
Hong Kong liver cancer system	• Predominantly derived from HBV-HCC • Five stages I to V • Early tumor: Single nodule ≤ 5 cm or ≤3 tumor nodule • Aggressive surgical resection
Cancer of the Liver Italian Program	• Prognostic scoring system • Includes α-fetoprotein-based stratification along with cutoff at the level of 400 ng/dL

6. Following are the common clinical presentations in hepatocellular carcinoma:
   a. Asymptomatic patient
   b. Constitutional symptoms

c. Pyrexia of unknown origin

d. Abdominal mass

e. Decompensation of cirrhosis

f. Jaundice

Following are the signs:

a. Hepatomegaly

b. Splenomegaly

c. Ascites

d. Fever

e. Wasting

f. Hepatic bruit

g. Jaundice

7. Paraneoplastic manifestations in the hepatocellular carcinoma are:

a. Carcinoid syndrome

b. Hypertension

c. Hypercalcemia

d. Neuropathy

e. Hypoglycemia

f. Hypertrophic osteoarthropathy

g. Polymyositis

h. Polycythemia

i. Thrombophlebitis migrans

j. Watery diarrhea syndrome

8. Following are the sites of extrahepatic metastasis from common to rare sites:

a. Lung

b. Lymph node

c. Bone

d. Adrenal gland

e. Peritoneum

9. Following are the percutaneous strategies in the treatment of hepatocellular carcinoma:

a. Percutaneous ethanol injection

b. Radiofrequency ablation

c. Microwave ablation

d. Cryoablation

e. Irreversible electroporation

10. Following are the limitations of percutaneous therapies:

a. Radiofrequency ablation: Limitations:
   - Thermal injury to adjacent structures
   - Heat effect near the major vessels

b. Microwave ablation: Limitation—heat sink effect

c. Cryoablation: Limitation—cryoshock

d. Irreversible electroporation: Limitation—general anesthesia is required.

11. Following are the transarterial therapies in the hepatocellular carcinoma:

a. Transarterial embolization

b. Transarterial chemoembolization

c. Transarterial radioembolization with yttrium-90 microspheres

12. Indications of TACE are:

a. BCLC-B stage of hepatocellular carcinoma

Complications of TACE are:

a. Postembolization syndrome

b. Decompensation and hepatic failure

c. Abscesses

d. Gastrointestinal ulceration

Indications of TARE are:

a. Advanced and unresectable hepatocellular carcinoma

b. Acts as bridge to liver transplant

Complications of TARE are:

a. Liver failure

b. Radiation-induced liver disease

c. Biliary complication

d. Gastrointestinal complication

e. Postembolization syndrome

f. Radiation pneumonitis

13. Following are the emerging therapies in hepatocellular carcinoma:

a. Immune checkpoint inhibitors along with locoregional therapy: Nivolumab + TACE

b. Immune checkpoint inhibitors along with tyrosine kinase inhibitors: Lenvatinib + pembrolizumab

CASE 192

A 40-year-old male came to hepatology clinic with pain in the right upper abdomen for the last 2 months, progressively increasing abdominal distention for 20 days, and yellowish discoloration of the eyes for 10 days. He had past history of pain in the same area for the last 3 years but recovered after taking treatment but no previous history of altered consciousness, bleeding from any sites, or jaundice. On examination, there was jaundice, mild pallor, pedal edema, hepatosplenomegaly, and ascites with protruding umbilicus. Laboratory investigation, his hemoglobin was 9 g/dL, platelet count 80,000/cc, total bilirubin 5 mg/dL, ALT 190 IU/L, ALP 150 IU/L, viral serology negative, serum electrolytes and renal function test negative, and JAK2 negative.

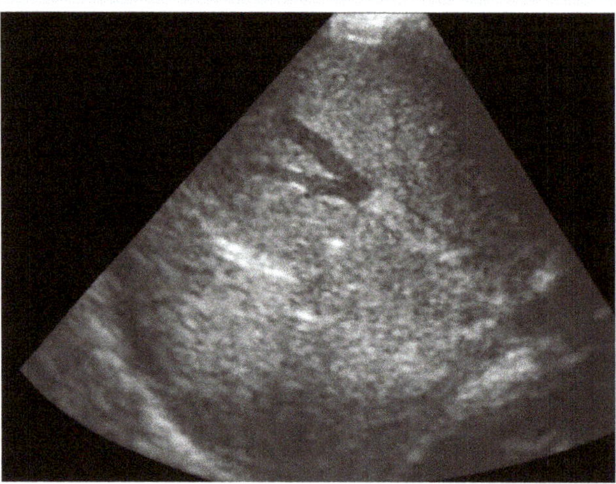

1. **What does the above picture demonstrate?**
2. **What is your diagnosis?**
3. **Define this disease.**
4. **What are the clinical variants in this disease?**
5. **What is the pathophysiology in this disease?**
6. **What are the predisposing factors in this disease?**
7. **What are the types of congenital membrane produced in this disease?**
8. **What are the pathogeneses of ascites in this disease?**
9. **What are the factors associated with a good prognosis in this disease?**
10. **What do you mean by prognostic index in this disease?**
11. **What are the complications in this disease?**

Answers

1. The above picture demonstrates thrombosis of hepatic vein with patent right and left hepatic veins.
2. The diagnosis is Budd–Chiari syndrome.
3. This disease can be defined as thrombotic or non-thrombotic obstruction of the hepatic venous outflow anywhere from the hepatic venules to the junction of the inferior vena cava leading to development of ascites, hepatomegaly, and abdominal pain.
4. There are three clinical variants in this disease:
   a. Acute and subacute form: It is characterized by:
      - Rapidly developing abdominal pain
      - Jaundice
      - Ascites
      - Hepatomegaly
      - Renal failure
   b. Chronic form: It is characterized by:
      - Progressive ascites
      - Absence of jaundice
      - In 50% cases, renal impairment
   c. Fulminant form: It is characterized by:
      - Uncommon presentation
      - Features of fulminant failure
      - Ascites
      - Tender hepatomegaly
      - Jaundice
      - Renal failure

5. Pathophysiology in this disease:
   a. Congestion of the hepatic parenchyma due to poor hepatic venous outflow resulting from blocked hepatic veins, intrahepatic inferior vena caval obstruction or combination of two. Presentation of the disease depends upon the location, extent, and acuity of obstruction. Progressive and differential occlusion of the hepatic veins results in alternative drainage areas in the congested hepatic parenchyma into the adjacent venous territories leading to development of the subcapsular as well as intraparenchymal collaterals.
   b. Caudate lobe is hypertrophied because this lobe has independent drainage into the inferior vena cava.
   c. Part of the hepatic parenchyma that can manage to drain through the developed collaterals becomes hypertrophied leading to heterogeneous parenchymal as well as vascular distribution.
   d. Hypertrophied caudate lobe compresses the inferior vena cava leading to further compromisation of the venous outflow.
   e. Hepatic parenchymal congestion leads to:
      - Cellular necrosis
      - Sinusoidal capillarization
      - Epithelial dysfunction
      - Activation of stellate cells
      - Progressive fibrosis of the hepatic parenchyma

6. Following are the predisposing factors in this disease:
   a. Hematologic disorders:
      - Paroxysmal nocturnal hemoglobinuria (PNH)
      - Polycythemia rubra vera
      - Myeloproliferative syndrome
      - Antiphospholipid syndrome
      - Essential thrombocytosis
   b. Inherited thrombotic diathesis:
      - Protein S deficiency
      - Protein C deficiency
      - Antithrombin III deficiency
      - Factor V Leiden deficiency
   c. Chronic infection:
      - Aspergillosis
      - Hydatid cyst
      - Syphilis
      - Tuberculosis
   d. Chronic inflammatory disease:
      - Inflammatory bowel disease
      - SLE
      - Sjögren's syndrome
      - Sarcoidosis
   e. Tumors:
      - Hepatocellular carcinoma
      - Adrenal carcinoma
      - Renal cell carcinoma
      - Right atrial myxoma
   f. Congenital membranous obstruction

7. There are three types of congenital membranous obstruction:
   a. Type I: Here, membrane is present in the inferior vena cava or in the atrium
   b. Type II: There is absence of a segment of the inferior vena cava
   c. Type III: In this type, inferior vena cava cannot be filled, and collaterals have been developed.

8. There are two stages in the development of the ascites in this disease:
   a. In early stage due to hepatic venous outflow tract obstruction, there is increase in the hydrostatic pressure leading to exudation of the fluid rich in protein through the fenestration of the sinusoid into the interstitium. Usually, these protein-rich fluids are absorbed by the lymphatic channels but as the disease progresses, the exudate will overwhelm the absorptive capacity of the lymphatics leading to development of high protein ascites.
   b. In the late or advanced stage, there is increased deposition of the type IV collagen within the perisinusoidal space leading to capillarization of the sinusoids, as a result the protein will restricted into the sinusoidal spaces. So, now only protein-poor fluid will enter into the interstitium leading to formation of low protein ascites.

9. Following factors are associated with good prognosis in this disease:
   a. Younger age at the time of diagnosis
   b. Low Child–Pugh score
   c. Absence of ascites
   d. Easily controlled ascites
   e. Low serum creatinine level

10. Prognostic index in the disease:

    (Ascites score × 0.75) + (Pugh score × 0.28) + (age × 0.037) + (creatinine level × 0.0036)

    Score if <5.4, it is associated with good prognosis.

11. Complications in this disease are:
    a. Hepatic encephalopathy
    b. Variceal hemorrhage
    c. Hepatorenal syndrome
    d. Portal hypertension
    e. Complications associated with hepatic decompensation
    f. Complications associated with hypercoagulable states

CASE 193

This is a picture of 28-year-old male having cavernous transformed portal vein having unknown etiology. Magnetic resonance cholangiography and portography demonstrates:

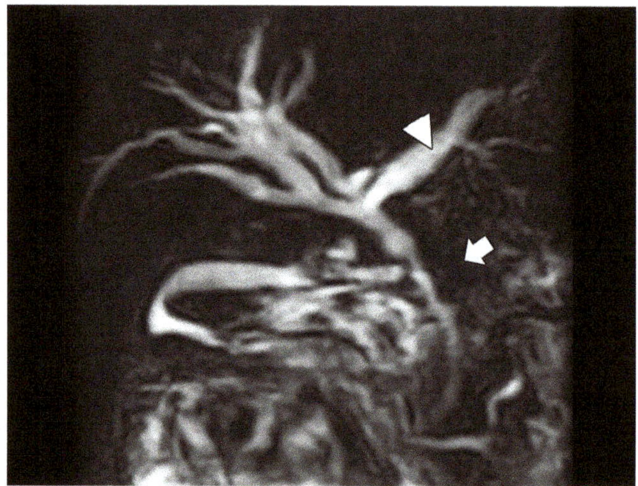

1. **Describe the above picture.**
2. **What is your most likely diagnosis?**
3. **Mention the criteria for making this diagnosis.**
4. **What are the cholangiographic abnormalities seen in this disease?**
5. **What are the venous plexuses surrounding the biliary tract?**
6. **What are the diagnostic modalities in this disease?**
7. **What are the different types of classification of this disease?**

Answers

1. Description of the above picture:
    a. Dilatation of the extrahepatic and intrahepatic bile duct
    b. Extrinsic impression and irregular contour
2. The most likely diagnosis is portal cavernoma cholangiopathy
3. Following are the criteria for making this diagnosis:
    a. Presence of portal cavernoma
    b. Typical cholangiographic changes evidenced on ERCP or MRCP
    c. Absence of other causes of the biliary changes
4. Following are the cholangiographic abnormalities seen in this disease:
    a. Extrinsic impression or indentations
    b. Shallow impression or indentations
    c. Irregular ductal contour
    d. Filling defects
    e. Stricture
    f. Angulation of bile duct
    g. Dilatation of the upstream
    h. Ectasia
5. Two venous plexuses are responsible for the drainage of the biliary tract:
    a. Fine reticular epicholedochal venous plexus of Saint is present on the bile duct wall
    b. Venous plexus of Petren into which the above blood drains
6. Following are the diagnostic modalities in this disease:
    a. Ultrasonography with color Doppler study

b. MRCP with MR portography:
- Comprehensive noninvasive techniques
- It can delineate accurately biliary changes.
- It can demonstrate the relationship between biliary changes and collaterals.
- It can ascertain suitable vein.
- It can distinguish between the bile duct varices and CBD.

c. Endoscopic ultrasound can delineate following types of choledochal collaterals:
- Paracholedochal collaterals: These are present at a distance from fibromuscular layer.
- Pericholedochal collaterals: It is characterized by large varices of >1 mm which present outside and adjacent to the fibromuscular layer.
- Epicholedochal collaterals: Varices of <1 mm in size lying outside and adjacent to the fibromuscular layer
- Intracholedochal collaterals:
  ○ Varices at <1 mm distant from the stent or stone
  ○ Varices with wall of common bile duct on both the sides

d. ERCP: It is the gold standard method for diagnosis in this disease.

e. IDUS and cholangiography

7. There are two classifications in this disease:

a. Chandra classification:
- Type I: Extrahepatic ducts are involved only.
- Type II: Intrahepatic ducts are involved only.
- Type IIIa: There are extrahepatic duct along with involvement of unilateral intrahepatic bile duct.
- Type IIIb: There are extrahepatic duct along with involvement of unilateral intrahepatic bile duct.

b. Liver in Progression (LIP) classification:
- Grade I: There are irregularities or angulations of the biliary tree.
- Grade II: There are indentations or strictures without upstream dilatation of the biliary tree.
- Grade III: Presence of strictures with upstream dilatation of the biliary tree

CASE 194

A 24-year-old man having history of AIDS with CD4 count 10 came to emergency department with sudden right upper abdominal pain, nausea, and vomiting for 2 days. MRCP was advised. It demonstrated the following:

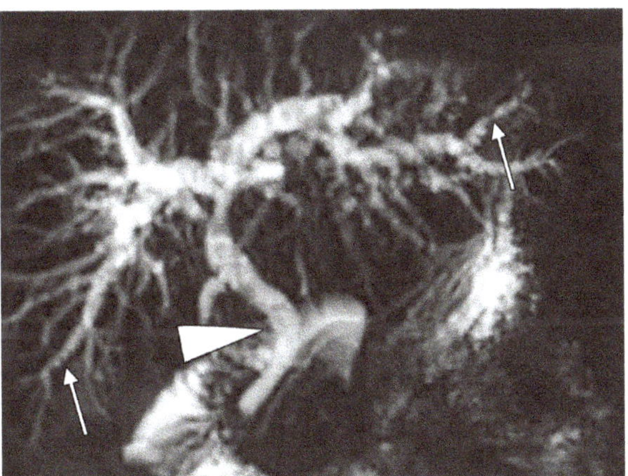

1. **Describe the above picture.**
2. **What is your diagnosis?**
3. **What are the etiologies in this disease?**
4. **What is the risk factor?**
5. **How can you diagnose it?**
6. **How can you treat this disease?**

Answers

1. The above picture demonstrates:
   a. Multiple strictures involving the peripheral intrahepatic ducts
   b. Intrahepatic and extrahepatic bile ducts are diffusely dilated with abrupt narrowing near the ampulla.
2. The most likely diagnosis is AIDS cholangiopathy.
3. Following are the etiologies in this disease:
   a. *Cryptosporidium parvum:* It is the most common pathogen.
   b. *Cytomegalovirus*
   c. Microsporidia
4. Risk factor: CD4 count is <20.
5. Following are the methods of diagnosis:
   a. MRCP or ERCP:
      - Papillary stenosis—most common finding
      - Papillary stenosis in one-third of cases—there is combination of intrahepatic dilatation as well as multifocal intrahepatic biliary strictures having alternating normal segments or saccular dilatation.
      - In 20% cases, there is characteristic beaded appearance.
6. Following are the methods of treatment:
   a. Symptomatic treatment by:
      - Opioids
      - Neural plexus blockers
   b. Treatment of opportunistic infection
   c. Ursodeoxycholic acid for improving abdominal pain as well as normalization of liver status
   d. Restoration of immune function with HAART therapy
   e. Endoscopic sphincterotomy

CASE 195

A 55-year-old type 2 diabetic and hypertensive male on metformin and amlodipine taking <0 units of alcohol weekly came to medicine clinic for routine health checkup. Physical examination is normal except basal metabolic index of 32 kg/m^2.

Laboratory investigation demonstrated routine blood tests were normal. Liver function test demonstrated bilirubin 0.5 mg/dL, ALT 120 IU/L, AST 45 IU/L, ALP 85 IU/L, albumin 3.8 g/mL, and INR 1.

1. **What are the differential diagnoses?**
2. **What are the structures in the human body where AST and ALT are found?**
3. **What is the importance of the ratio of AST to ALT?**
4. **What are the causes of elevated ALT?**
5. **What are the causes of raised ALP?**
6. **What are the additional tests to be done in this case?**
7. **What invasive as well as noninvasive investigations should be done that can help and manage this disease subsequently?**

Answers

1. Following are the differential diagnoses:
   a. Alcoholic liver disease
   b. Nonalcoholic fatty liver disease
   c. Autoimmune hepatitis
   d. Chronic hepatitis B
   e. Chronic hepatitis C
   f. Hemochromatosis
2. Following are the structures in the human body produce AST and ALT:
   a. For ALT: Cytosol in the hepatocyte
   b. For AST:
      - Liver
      - Cardiac muscle
      - Skeletal muscle
      - Kidney
      - Brain
      - Pancreas
3. Importance of AST-to-ALT ratio:
   a. AST-to-ALT ratio of >2: Alcoholic liver disease
   b. AST-to-ALT ratio of ≥0.8 suggests NAFLD
4. Following are the causes of elevated ALT:
   a. Elevation of <100 IU/L:
      - Nonalcoholic fatty liver disease
      - Chronic hepatitis B
      - Chronic hepatitis C

- Celiac disease
- Hemochromatosis
- Nonhepatic causes:
  - Hemolysis
  - Strenuous exercise
  - Thyroid disease
  - Myopathy

b. Moderately elevated AST (between 100 and 350 IU/L):
- Alcoholic hepatitis
- Autoimmune hepatitis
- Wilson disease
- Budd–Chiari syndrome
- Acute biliary obstruction
- All the causes of above responsible for elevation of <100 IU/L

c. Major elevation of >1,000 IU/L:
- Acute viral hepatitis
- Paracetamol poisoning
- Autoimmune hepatitis
- Ischemic hepatitis
- Budd–Chiari syndrome

5. Following are the causes of ALP:
a. Elevation of less than three times upper limit of normal:
- Hepatitis
- Cirrhosis
- Infiltrative disease in the liver

- Sepsis
- Congestive cardiac failure

b. Elevation of more than three times upper limit of normal:
- Biliary obstruction by:
  - Stone
  - Pancreatic carcinoma
  - Cholangiocarcinoma
- Primary sclerosing cholangitis
- Sepsis
- Metastases in the liver
- Hepatocellular carcinoma
- Sarcoidosis
- Amyloidosis
- Liver injury due to cholestatic drugs

6. Additional tests, i.e., transient elastography should be done to diagnose hepatic fibrosis.
7. Following noninvasive tests should be done:
a. Serological markers:
- Direct markers:
  - Procollagen type III amino-terminal peptide
  - Serum hyaluronic acid
- Indirect markers:
  - AST-to-platelet ratio index
  - FIB-4 score
  - NAFLD fibrosis score

b. Radiological markers—transient elastography
Invasive test for the diagnosis is liver biopsy.

CASE 196

A 50-year-old man has been admitted in the emergency department with severe repeated bouts of hematemesis and melena for 2 days. On examination, patient was pale, pulse rate 120 beats/minute, blood pressure 90/60 mm Hg, and respiratory rate 28 breaths/minute. Following features are also present:

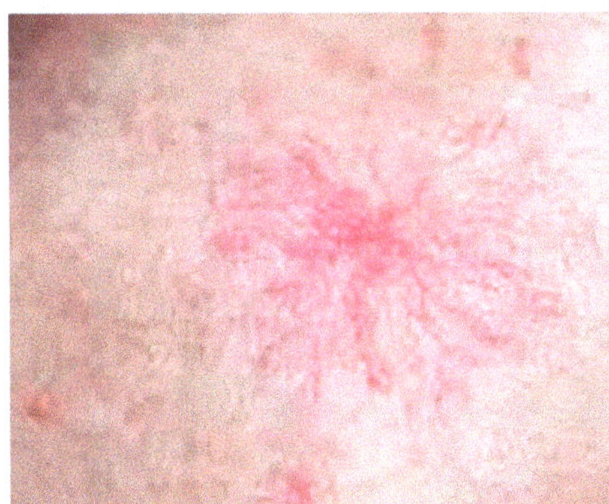
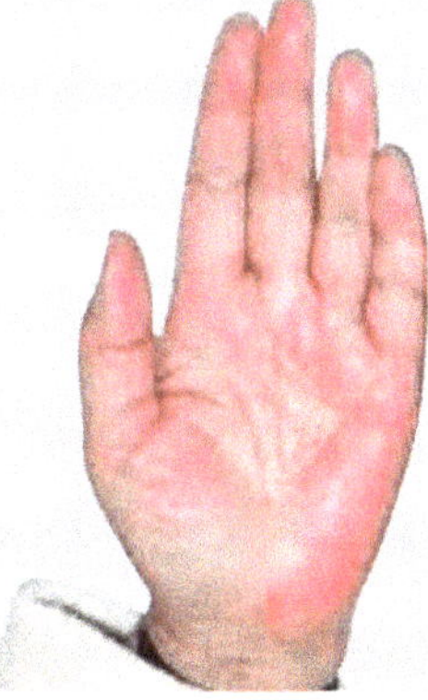

Laboratory investigation demonstrated hemoglobin 5 g/dL, bilirubin 1.8 mg/dL, ALT 78 IU/L, and creatinine 0.78 mg/dL. Abdominal ultrasonography and endoscopy demonstrated:

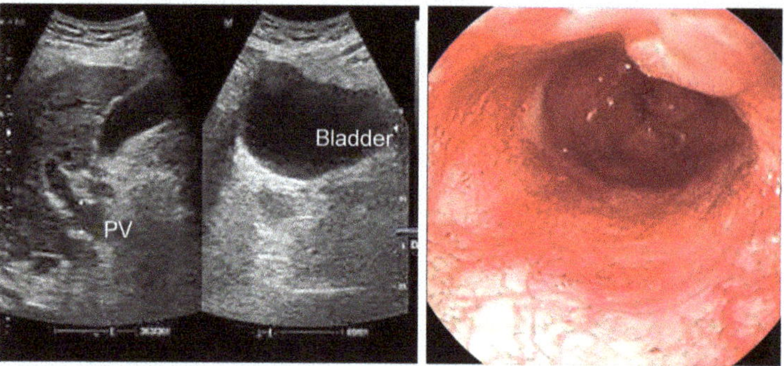

1. **What do the above pictures demonstrate?**
2. **What is the most likely diagnosis?**
3. **What is the normal pressure gradient across the sinusoid?**
4. **What is the definition and classification of portal hypertension?**
5. **How can you classify varices?**
6. **What are the high-risk signs for bleeding in the varices?**

Answers

1. The above pictures demonstrate:
   a. Spider nevi
   b. Palmar erythema
   c. Ultrasonography demonstrated hepatospleno-megaly
   d. Endoscopy demonstrated bleeding varices.
2. The most likely diagnosis is bleeding varices from portal hypertension in a case of cirrhosis.
3. Normal pressure across the sinusoids is 3 mm Hg which allows flow of blood from portal vein to hepatic venous system.
4. Portal hypertension can be defined as the increase in pressure in the portal vein is more than 6 mm Hg. Portal hypertension is significant when the portal pressure is >10 mm Hg.

   Classification of the portal hypertension:
   a. Presinusoidal portal hypertension:
      - Extrahepatic:
        ○ Portal venous thrombosis
        ○ Splenic vein thrombosis
        ○ Extrinsic portal vein compression
      - Intrahepatic:
        ○ Idiopathic portal hypertension
        ○ Sarcoidosis
        ○ Schistosomiasis
        ○ Primary biliary cirrhosis
   b. Sinusoidal portal hypertension:
      - Cirrhosis
      - Acute alcoholic hepatitis
   c. Postsinusoidal portal hypertension:
      - Budd–Chiari syndrome
      - Obstruction of the inferior vena cava
      - Constrictive pericarditis
      - Veno-occlusive disease
5. There are two types of grading system:
   a. Size of the varices:
      - Large >5 mm in diameter
      - Small <5 mm in diameter
   b. According to grade:
      - Grade I: Straight and small varices which can be depressed by the insufflation.
      - Grade II: Presence of tortuous varices occupying less than half of the esophageal lumen
      - Grade III: Presence of large varices occupying more than half of the esophageal lumen
6. Following are the high-risk signs on the varices seen through the endoscopy:
   a. Red wheals
   b. Cherry red spot
   c. Hemostatic spots

CASE 197

A 60-year-old man has been admitted with confusion and agitation with history of inversion of sleep rhythm for the last 4 days following 6 days of constipation. He had neither past history nor family history of viral hepatitis. On examination, there was mild jaundice, moderate ascites, hepatomegaly, and flapping tremor.

Blood investigation demonstrated bilirubin 3.51 mg/dL, AST 120 IU/L, ALT 55 IU/L, platelet count 60,000/cc, and creatinine 1.45 mg/dL.

1. **What is your most likely diagnosis?**
2. **Define this disease.**
3. **What is the first feature in this disease and how can it be diagnosed?**
4. **What are the psychometric tests for diagnosing this type of disease?**
5. **What is the pathophysiology in this disease?**

Answers

1. The most likely diagnosis is hepatic encephalopathy, the precipitating factor being constipation.
2. The hepatic encephalopathy characterized by spectrum of neuropsychiatric abnormalities ranging from subtle psychomotor changes to confusion and coma occurring in a case of impaired liver function test with or without portosystemic shunting.
3. First feature in this disease is psychomotor slowing and it can be detected by psychometric testing.
4. Following are the psychiatric tests:
   a. Psychometric hepatic encephalopathy score:
   b. Stroop test
   c. Critical flicker frequency
   d. Continuous reaction time
   e. SCAN test
   f. Inhibitory control test
5. Pathophysiology in this disease:
   a. Due to portosystemic shunting, ammonia and other toxic product bypass the liver to enter into the systemic circulation to enter brain leading to development of cerebral edema and dysfunction of astrocytes.
   b. Depletion of muscle volume produces sarcopenia leading to hepatic encephalopathy as muscles are the important organ for the detoxification of ammonia.
   c. Hyponatremia increases the cerebral edema and astrocyte dysfunction.
   d. Inflammatory response syndrome due to infection leads to development of hepatic encephalopathy.
   e. Gut dysbiosis and small bowel bacterial overgrowth are also responsible for encephalopathy.

CASE 198

A 60-year-old woman has been admitted with yellowish discoloration of urine following heavy intake of alcohol for the last 10 days. She had recurrent past history of admission for alcohol intoxication. On examination, she was deeply jaundiced and had moderate ascites.

1. **What is your most likely diagnosis?**
2. **Is there any relation of alcohol intake with alcoholic hepatitis?**
3. **What is the pathophysiology in this disease?**
4. **How can you assess the severity of this disease?**

Answers

1. The most likely diagnosis is alcoholic hepatitis.
2. Risk of cirrhosis can be determined by volume of alcohol and strength of alcohol. This risk increases with intake of alcohol >30 g/day, and the highest risk being >100 g/day.
3. Pathophysiology in this disease:
   a. In the liver, alcohol is metabolized to acetaldehyde by alcohol dehydrogenase which in turn converted into acetate by the enzyme in the mitochondrial acetaldehyde dehydrogenase. In the process of conversion, alcohol dehydrogenase reduces NAD

to NADH leading to increased accumulation of NADH which inhibits neoglucogenesis and oxidation of fatty acid resulting in fatty infiltration in the liver.

b. Alcohol is metabolized by P450 cytochrome 2E1 pathway leading to free oxidation radicals' generation through the oxidation of NADPH to NADP and this is upgraded in case of chronic alcohol use.

c. In case of chronic alcohol use, hepatic macrophages are activated leading to production of TNF-α and reactive oxygen species.

d. There is depletion of antioxidants like vitamin E as well as glutathione resulting in apoptosis leading to hepatic necrosis.

e. Free oxygen species induces peroxidation of the lipid.

4. Following are the methods of assessing the severity of this disease:

a. Maddrey discriminant function: 4.6 × (PT in seconds – Control PT in seconds) + (Serum bilirubin in μmol/L)
   - If the value is ≥32, there is high short-term mortality and there is benefit from steroid administration.
   - If the value is <32, there is low short-term mortality but do not benefit from steroid administration.

b. Glasgow alcoholic hepatitis score: It includes following variables such as age, serum bilirubin, urea, prothrombin time, and WBC count.

c. Model for end-stage liver disease (MELD) score: It is based on the variables such as serum bilirubin, creatinine, and INR. The score is ranges from 6 to 40.

CASE 199

A 60-year-old type II diabetic, obese hypertensive smoker over 20 years came for routine checkup and found ALT 66 IU/L, other component of liver function test, renal function test, hematological test, and HbA1c 8.5%. He has no history of alcohol intake and no past history of viral hepatitis. Ultrasonographic features are normal:

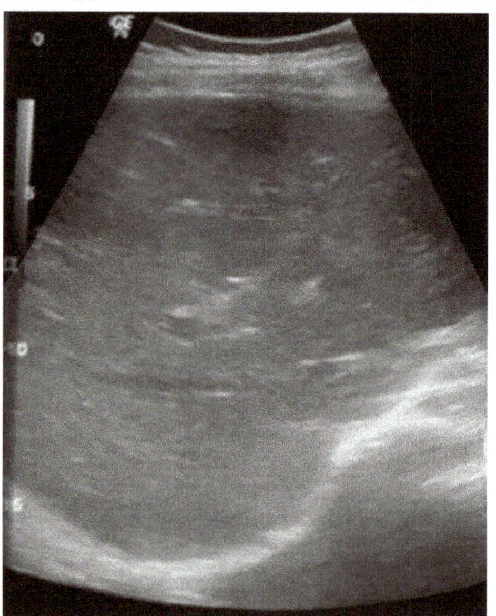

1. **What does the above picture demonstrate?**
2. **What is the most likely diagnosis and on what factors?**
3. **What is the significance of a high NAFLD fibrosis score?**
4. **What are the processes of investigation?**
5. **What is the approach to manage this case?**

Answers

1. The above picture demonstrated fat infiltration with hyperechoic areas in the liver.
2. The patient has:
   a. Elevated ALT, echogenic
   b. Infiltration in the liver
   c. Metabolic risk factors:
      - Type II diabetes
      - Hypertension
      - Obesity
   d. Absence of alcohol intake
   e. Absence of viral serology
   Hence, the diagnosis is NAFLD.
3. NFS helps to identify the patient with NAFLD. If it is associated with liver biochemistry, albumin and thrombocytopenia is indicative of cirrhosis.
   a. Low NFS has high negative predictive value for advanced hepatic fibrosis.
   b. Intermediate or high NFS value has low positive predictive value. In this case, further investigations are required.
4. Next, noninvasive investigation is transient elastography for measuring the liver stiffness and correlating with the clinical findings. If there is discordance between these two in that case liver biopsy is the ultimate choice.
5. Following are the approaches to management:
   a. Lifestyle modification:
      - Weight loss
      - Exercise
      - Cessation of smoking
   b. Treatment of metabolic syndrome:
      - Statins
      - Metformin
      - GLP-1 agonists
      - Thiazolidinediones
   c. Vitamin E
   d. Obeticholic acid

CASE 200

A 2-year-old child having history of inflammatory bowel disease on 5-aminosalicylic acid with colonoscopy surveillance came to gastroenterology clinic with progressively increasing discoloration of urine conjunctiva and itching.

1. **What is your most likely diagnosis?**
2. **What is the investigation to confirm the diagnosis?**
3. **What are the classical features in the histological picture in this disease?**
4. **What are the histological stages in this disease?**

Answers

1. The most likely diagnosis is primary sclerosing cholangitis.
2. MRCP is the diagnosis as it demonstrates:
   a. Multifocal strictures in the bile duct
   b. Segmental dilatations
3. Most important classical features in this disease are:
   a. Periductal concentric fibrosis surrounding interlobular and septal bile ducts—it is known as onion skin fibrosis.
   b. Concentric fibrosis along with obliteration of the small ducts—it is known as obliterative fibrous cholangitis. It is the diagnosis.
4. Ludwig described the following four histological stages:
   a. Stage 1: Portal inflammation
      - Mild inflammation confined to the portal tracts.
      - Minimal fibrosis.
   b. Stage 2: Periportal fibrosis
      - Extension of inflammation and fibrosis beyond the portal tracts.
      - Early signs of periportal fibrosis without significant architectural distortion.
   c. Stage 3: Bridging fibrosis
      - Bridging of fibrosis between portal tracts or from portal tracts to central veins.
      - Progressive architectural distortion.
   d. Stage 4: Cirrhosis
      - Extensive fibrosis and nodule formation.
      - Complete architectural distortion of the liver (cirrhosis).

CASE 201

A 30-year-old 36th weeks gravid female suddenly developed abdominal pain, nausea, and vomiting. Laboratory investigation demonstrated bilirubin 5 mg/dL, AST 1,405 IU/L, INR 1.9, white blood cell count 17,000/cc, platelet count 78,000/cc, and blood sugar 52 mg/dL.

1. **What are the differential diagnoses?**
2. **How can you differentiate the above causes?**
3. **What is the most likely diagnosis?**
4. **What are the criteria of fatty liver of pregnancy?**
5. **What is the cause of hypotension and agitation in this case?**
6. **Why may the ALP be elevated in the normal pregnancy?**
7. **What is the level of α-fetoprotein in normal physiological pregnancy?**

Answers

1. Differential diagnoses are:
   a. Hyperemesis gravidarum
   b. Intrahepatic cholestasis in pregnancy
   c. Hypertension-related liver diseases
   d. Preeclampsia/eclampsia
   e. HELLP (Hemolysis, Elevated Liver enzymes, and Low Platelets) syndrome
   f. Infarction in the liver

2. Above causes can be differentiated by the following means:
   a. Hyperemesis gravidarum:
      - It occurs before 9th week of pregnancy
      - It is more common in case of multiple or molar pregnancy.
      - In 50% cases, ALT is elevated to 2–5 times the normal.
      - Normal bilirubin level
   b. Intrahepatic cholestasis of pregnancy:
      - It occurs in third trimester
      - Presence of pruritus on the palms and soles without rash and can be relieved within 6 weeks of pregnancy.
      - Increased level of serum bile acids >11 µmol/L
      - 1.5–8 times increase in ALT above normal
      - Normal bilirubin level
      - Antimitochondrial antibody, viral serology, and anti-smooth muscle cell antibody are negative.
   c. Preeclampsia/eclampsia:
      - It occurs after 20 weeks of gestation
      - Presence of hypertension
      - Presence of proteinuria of >300 mg/day
      - Seizure: It will appear in case of eclampsia.
      - Visual disturbances
      - Peripheral edema
   d. HELLP syndrome:
      - It occurs between 28th and 36th week of pregnancy
      - Bleeding tendency
      - Raised ALT but normal bilirubin level
      - Risk factors:
         o Previous history of preeclampsia/eclampsia
         o HELLP syndrome
         o Multiparity
         o Diabetes
         o Obesity
         o Chronic hypertension
         o Molar pregnancy
   e. Acute fatty liver of pregnancy:
      - It appears after 36 weeks of pregnancy but always before delivery
      - In severe cases, severe vomiting or encephalopathy
      - Abnormal liver function test:
         o Hyperbilirubinemia
         o Severely elevated ALT
         o Acute renal dysfunction
         o Leukocytosis
         o Thrombocytopenia

3. The most likely diagnosis is acute fatty liver of pregnancy.

4. The criteria of fatty liver of pregnancy: Six or more features in absence of other etiologies:
   a. Vomiting
   b. Pain abdomen
   c. Polydipsia/polyuria

d. Encephalopathy
e. Raised bilirubin > 0.82 mg/dL
f. Hypoglycemia of <2 mg/dL
g. Leukocytosis of >11,000/cc
h. Uric acid level > 5.72 mg/dL
i. Ammonia level > 42 IU/L
j. Ascites or hyperechoic liver in ultrasound
k. Creatinine level > 1.7 mg/dL
l. Coagulopathy: Prothrombin time > 14 seconds or activated partial thromboplastin time of >34 seconds
m. On biopsy, there is microvascular stasis.

5. The hypotension may be due to:
   a. Hypoglycemia
   b. Encephalopathy
   c. Hepatic rupture
6. ALP level will be elevated in normal pregnancy because it will be produced from placenta as well as fetus during bone development. But to exclude the biliary part of ALP, serum γ-glutamyl transpeptidase should be measured.
7. α-fetoprotein is increased in pregnancy because it is produced by the fetus.

CASE 202

A 45-year-old man came to outpatient department with oval painless swelling in the right groin which according to him increases in size during straining and decreases in lying down position. On examination, there was evidence of something coming out through the superficial inguinal ring but deep inguinal ring was intact.

1. **What is the most likely diagnosis?**
2. **Classify this disease.**
3. **How can you differentiate these diseases?**
4. **What are the age incidences in this disease?**
5. **Why is it more common in males?**
6. **Why does it occur in adult age?**
7. **What are the coverings of the structure coming out through the ring?**
8. **What are the boundaries of the inguinal canal?**
9. **What are the contents of the spermatic cord?**
10. **Describe the boundaries of Hesselbach's triangle.**

Answers

1. The most likely diagnosis is direct inguinal hernia.
2. There are two types of hernia:
   a. Direct inguinal hernia: It is characterized by protrusion of contents of the abdomen through the weak area of the anterior abdominal wall through its posterior wall due to weakness of the muscles of the abdominal wall.
   b. Indirect inguinal hernia: It is a defect present since birth in the lower abdominal wall. The inguinal canal usually closes in the developing fetus before birth. But in some cases, both the opening remains open after birth and abdominal contents will protrude through the canal leading to development of indirect inguinal hernia.

3. Following are the differentiating points:

Direct hernia	Indirect hernia
Acquired	Congenital
Sac enters into the inguinal canal through the posterior wall	The contents come through the deep inguinal ring into the inguinal canal
Less common	More common
It occurs as a result of weakness on the anterior abdominal wall	There is persistence of the processus vaginalis.
It occurs in elderly	It occurs in infant
Neck of the hernial sac is present medial to inferior epigastric artery.	Neck of the hernial sac is present lateral to inferior epigastric artery.

4. Age incidences:
   a. Direct inguinal hernia is more common in elderly between 70 and 80 years of age.
   b. Indirect inguinal hernia is common in infants as it is a developmental defect.
5. It is more common in males because in males inguinal canal is large.
6. Anterior abdominal wall muscles are supplied by:
   a. Inferior intercostal nerves
   b. Iliohypogastric nerve
   c. Ilioinguinal nerve
   Injury to these nerves during abdominal surgery will lead to weakness of the anterior abdominal muscles resulting in the chance of development of direct inguinal hernia.
7. Covering structures of the inguinal hernia are:
   a. Transversalis fascia forms the posterior wall of the contents in the inguinal ring in direct inguinal hernia
   b. Processus vaginalis is the covering of the content that protrudes through the deep ring into the inguinal canal and exits through the external inguinal ring.
8. Boundaries of the inguinal canal are:
   a. Anterior wall is composed of:
      - Aponeurosis of the external oblique muscle which is strengthened by the internal oblique muscle laterally.
   b. Posterior wall known as floor which is formed by:
      - Transversalis fascia
      - Conjoint tendon
      - Deep inguinal ring
   c. Roof or superficial wall is formed by:
      - Medial crus of the aponeurosis of external oblique muscle
      - Musculoaponeurotic arches of internal oblique muscles
      - Transverse abdominal muscles
      - Transversalis fascia
   d. Inferior wall is formed by:
      - Inguinal ligament
      - Reinforced medially by lacunar ligament
      - Reinforced laterally by iliopubic tract
9. Contents of the spermatic cord are:
   a. Ductus deferens
   b. Artery of the ductus deferens
   c. Testicular artery
   d. Cremasteric artery
   e. Pampiniform plexus of veins
   f. Genital branch of the genitofemoral nerve
   g. Lymphatics
   h. Sympathetic and parasympathetic nerves
10. Boundaries of the Hesselbach's triangle:
    a. Medially the lateral border of the rectus abdominis muscle
    b. Laterally by inferior epigastric vessels
    c. Inferiorly inguinal ligament

CASE 203

A 25-year-old man having past history of hematemesis came to emergency department with acute abdominal pain. She had past history of similar pain abdomen. She used to take tea or coffee. He was advised upper gastrointestinal endoscopy which demonstrated:

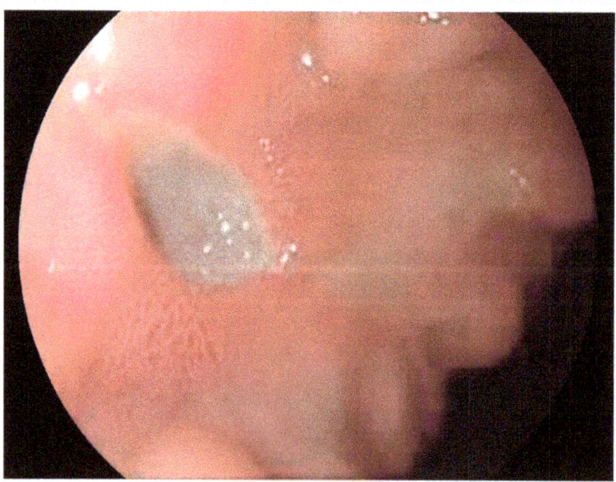

1. **What is your diagnosis?**
2. **In which area of the stomach, there is an increased incidence of ulcer?**
3. **What type of congenital abnormality in the ileum may develop peptic ulcer?**
4. **What is the cause of epigastric pain?**
5. **What are the anatomical relations of stomach?**
6. **What is the blood supply of the stomach?**

Answers

1. The endoscopic picture demonstrated punched-out ulcer on the lesser curvature of stomach.
2. The lesser curvature of stomach in-between the fundus and antrum is the area of ulcer.
3. Meckel's diverticulum is the area of congenital abnormality of the gut which may secrete acid that may be responsible for development of ulcer in future.
4. Pain from the stomach carries this sensation through the splanchnic nerve to reach T7 and T8 spinal segments. Again the epigastric region is supplied by T7 and T8 segments of the spinal cord. Hence, the stomach pain is referred to this epigastric region.
5. Anatomical relations of the stomach:
   a. Anteriorly:
      - Left lobe of the liver
      - Diaphragm
      - Anterior abdominal wall
   b. Posteriorly:
      - Omental bursa
      - Pancreas
      - Left kidney
      - Adrenal gland
      - Spleen
      - Splenic artery
   c. Superiorly:
      - Esophagus
      - Diaphragm
   d. Inferiorly and laterally: Transverse mesocolon
6. Blood supply of the stomach: Blood supply of the stomach originates from the abdominal aorta—
   a. It is provided by the two anastomotic systems:
      - Anastomosis along the lesser curvature: Union of the—
        ○ Right gastric artery originating from common hepatic artery
        ○ Left gastric arteries originating from celiac trunk
      - Anastomosis along the greater curvature: Union of the—
        ○ Right gastroomental artery originating from gastroduodenal artery
        ○ Left gastroomental artery originating from splenic artery
   b. Direct branches:
      - Short and posterior gastric arteries from the splenic artery supply the fundus and upper part of the body.
      - Gastroduodenal artery originating from the common hepatic artery supplies the pylorus of the stomach.

CASE 204

A 6-month-old baby was taken to the emergency ward with history of the severe projectile vomiting along with poor gain in weight. On examination, there was a palpable mass in the epigastrium. Ultrasonography demonstrated:

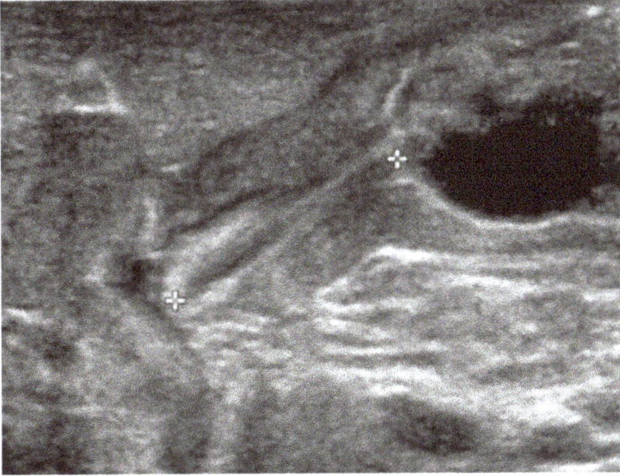

1. **What has been described in the above picture?**
2. **What is your most likely diagnosis?**
3. **What is the cause of projectile vomiting?**
4. **Is it a congenital abnormality?**
5. **Why is it more common in males?**

Answers

1. Ultrasonographic picture demonstrated thickened pyloric part of the stomach.
2. The most likely diagnosis is hypertrophic pyloric stenosis.
3. As with the contraction of the stomach, the food cannot enter into the small intestine, the chyme automatically will move upward to exit out in projectile nature.
4. It is not present during birth but will develop later.
5. The hormone testosterone induces hypertrophy of the pyloric muscles. Hence, it is five times more common in males.

CASE 205

A 45-year-old chronic alcoholic for 15 years having past history of hematemesis has been admitted with progressively increasing distention of abdomen and upper abdominal pain. On examination, his blood pressure 130/80 mm Hg, pulse rate 100 beats/minute, ascites, and hepatosplenomegaly. Endoscopy demonstrated the following:

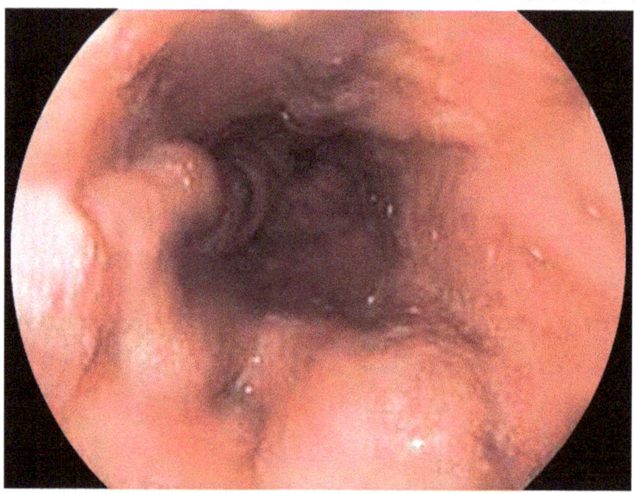

1. **What is the finding in the upper gastrointestinal endoscopy?**
2. **What is your diagnosis?**
3. **What is the anatomical basis of hematemesis?**
4. **What is the basis of ascites?**
5. **Enumerate the different sites of portocaval anastomosis.**

Answers

1. Endoscopy demonstrated two grade II and two grade I esophageal varices.
2. The diagnosis is portal hypertension in a case of alcoholic cirrhosis.
3. Following are the anatomical basis of hematemesis:
   a. Fibrosis around the portal blood vessels leading to increased portal venous pressure leading to reversal of flow of blood from the portal to systemic circulation resulting in varicosity of the esophageal veins (systemic circulation) at the lower end of esophagus.
4. Increased pressure of the fibrous tissue surrounding the portal vessels leading to increase in the pressure within the superior mesenteric vein and splenic vein. As a result, fluid will come out of the capillaries leading to accumulation of the fluid into the peritoneal cavity.

5. Following are the different sites of portocaval anastomosis:

Sites	Portal veins	Systemic veins
Lower esophagus	Left gastric veins	Lower branches of esophageal veins
Upper part of anal canal	Superior rectal veins	Middle and inferior rectal veins
Umbilicus	Paraumbilical veins	Epigastric veins
Area of liver	Intraparenchymal branches of right branch of portal vein	Retroperitoneal veins
Hepatic and splenic flexures	Omental and colonic veins	Retroperitoneal veins
Hepatic and splenic	Ductus venosus	Inferior vena cava

CASE 206

A 48-year-old woman came to outpatient department with history of fatigue, amenorrhea, yellowish discoloration of the conjunctiva, and increased pigmentation all over the body but not anemic. On examination, there was jaundice and palmar erythema. Abdominal examination demonstrated there was hepatomegaly and presence of ascites. Her complete blood count demonstrated hemoglobin was 15 g/dL, bilirubin was 4.5 mg/dL, and AST and ALT levels were 67 and 100 IU/L, respectively.

1. **What is the most likely diagnosis?**
2. **What are the points in favor of this diagnosis?**
3. **Define this disease.**
4. **What are the types of this disease?**
5. **What are the organs involved in the disease from deposition of iron?**
6. **What is the total body iron store and what is the amount in this disease?**
7. **Is there any genetic relation with this disease?**
8. **In this disease, why iron is absorbed in a large amount?**
9. **What is the cardiac manifestation in this disease?**
10. **Why should this disease be early detected?**
11. **Name five most common causes of hyperpigmentation.**
12. **What is the line of investigation in this case?**
13. **What is the most common cause of death in this disease?**
14. **What will be the effect of intake of shellfish in this patient?**
15. **What are the causes of iron overload leading to hemochromatosis?**
16. **What are the complications in this disease?**

Answers

1. The most likely diagnosis is hemochromatosis.
2. Following are the points in favor of this diagnosis:
   a. Age is >30 years.
   b. Presence of generalized hyperpigmentation
   c. Presence of hepatomegaly
   d. Jaundice
   e. Ascites
3. Hemochromatosis is an autosomal recessive disorder characterized by increased absorption of iron and its subsequent deposition into the liver, skin, and other organs in the body resulting from the mutation of gene encoding the protein involved in the metabolism of iron.
4. Following are the types of hemochromatosis:
   a. Type I or HFE-related hereditary hemochromatosis: It is autosomal recessive disease.
   b. Type 2a or due to mutation of *hemojuvelin* gene or type 2b or mutation of *hepcidin* gene-related hemochromatosis—autosomal recessive disease. Age of onset is 15–20 years.
   c. Type 3 or mutation of transferrin receptor 2 gene-related hemochromatosis: It is autosomal recessive and present in white as well as nonwhite subjects. Age of onset is 30–40 years.
   d. Type 4 or mutation of *ferroportin* gene-related hemochromatosis: It is autosomal dominant. Age of onset is 10–80 years.
5. Following organs are involved in this disease:
   a. Liver
   b. Skin
   c. Pancreas
   d. Joints
   e. Testes
   f. Pituitary
   g. Abdomen
   h. Kidneys
6. Total body iron is 4 g and it should be increased to 10 g.
7. Four genetic mutations are involved in this primary hemochromatosis in 90% cases:
   a. Mutation in the chromosome number 6.
   b. *HJV*
   c. *HAMP*
   d. *TIR1*

   In 10% severe hemochromatosis, there is no such mutation.

8. Iron is absorbed from the duodenal mucosa by the duodenal metal transporter-1 which is also known as NRAMP2. In this disease, there is increased expression of this transporter leading to iron overloading.
9. Cardiac manifestation in this disease is due to deposition of iron in the cardiac muscle fibers resulting in dilated cardiomyopathy as well as conduction system further resulting in different types of arrhythmias.
10. Early detection of this disease is beneficial as it will:
    a. Do early venesection in patient in absence of diabetes mellitus or cirrhosis to prevent progression of this disease
    b. Prevent hepatocellular carcinoma
11. Five causes of hyperpigmentation are:
    a. Primary biliary cirrhosis
    b. Pellagra
    c. Uremia
    d. Hemochromatosis
    e. Addison's disease
12. Following investigations should be done in this case:
    a. Increased level of serum ferritin
    b. Increased saturation of transferrin as normal value will exclude this disease.
    c. Measurement of iron store in the liver tissue
    d. Noninvasive method of measuring the iron store in the liver
    e. Hereditary hemochromatosis gene
13. Most common cause of death in this disease is hepatocellular carcinoma.
14. There is increased risk of sepsis if this patient with genetic hemochromatosis will take the shellfish due to *Vibrio vulnificus*.
15. Following are the causes of iron overload leading to hemochromatosis:
    a. Massive intake of iron orally
    b. Increased absorption of iron in spite of normal intake of iron
    c. Massive transfusion of red blood cells
16. Following are the complications in this disease:
    a. Diabetes mellitus
    b. Hepatocellular carcinoma
    c. Congestive cardiac failure
    d. Hypogonadism
    e. Osteoporosis increased risk of infection with:
       - *Yersinia enterocolitica*
       - *Listeria monocytogenes*
       - *Vibrio vulnificus*

CASE 207

A 28-year-old man came to outpatient department with abnormal dancing movement. On examination, there is hepatosplenomegaly and anemia. Psychiatric examination demonstrated behavioral as well as emotional changes. Eye examination demonstrated the following features:

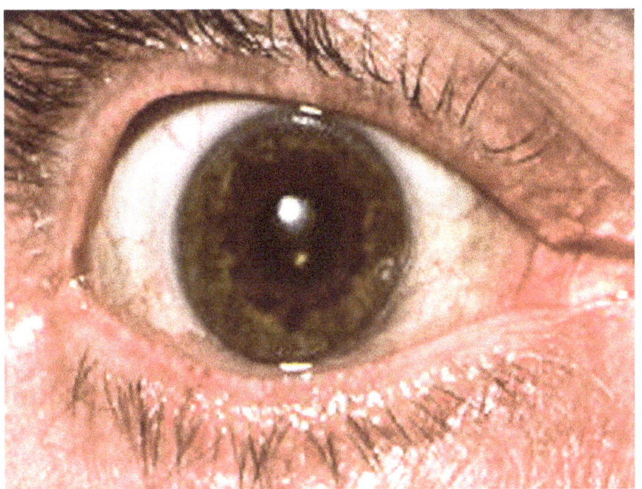

1.   **What is demonstrated in the above picture?**
2.   **Where is this feature found in this patient?**
3.   **What is your most likely diagnosis?**
4.   **What are the neurological manifestations present in this disease?**
5.   **What is the genetic defect in this disease?**
6.   **What are the common causes of this eye finding?**
7.   **What are the most common neurological features found in this disease?**
8.   **What are the pathophysiologies behind this disease?**
9.   **What are biochemical features found in this disease?**
10.   **Mention three renal manifestations in this disease.**
11.   **How can you confirm this disease?**
12.   **Mention the six radiological features in this disease.**

Answers

1.   Slit lamp examination demonstrated fine granular pigmented deposits in the Descemet membrane of the cornea in the ring form. It is most marked at the superior and inferior poles of cornea.
2.   Kayser–Fleischer (K-F) ring is found in patients with Wilson disease demonstrating neuropsychiatric manifestation but not with hepatic manifestation.
3.   This patient has been suffering from Wilson's disease.
4.   The neurological manifestations are:
     a.   Tremor of Parkinsonism
     b.   Involuntary or dancing movements—chorea
     c.   Ataxia
     d.   Dystonic spasm
     e.   Dysarthria
     f.   Incoordination
     g.   Rigidity
5.   This is autosomal recessive disease. Defect being located in the chromosome number 13 affecting mutation of adenosine triphosphatase 7B protein, i.e., Wilson's disease protein which is responsible for transport of copper. It may be related with family history of consanguinity. Another common mutation is substitution of HIO69Q. It is present in one-third of the patients.
6.   Common causes of the above eye features are:
     a.   Wilson's disease
     b.   Primary biliary cirrhosis
     c.   Cryptogenic cirrhosis

    d.   Chronic active hepatitis

    e.   Cirrhosis

    f.   Long-standing intrahepatic cholestasis

7. Most common neurologic features in this disease are difficulty in speaking and difficulty in writing in the school.

8. Following are the pathophysiologies in this disease:

   a. Excessive absorption of copper from the intestine

   b. Decrease in the clearance or excretion of copper by the liver

   c. Increased deposition of the copper in the following tissues:
      - Liver
      - Cornea
      - Brain
      - Kidneys

9. Following biochemical changes occur in this disease:

   a. Low level of ceruloplasmin

   b. Serum copper may be normal, high, or low.

   c. Excretion of the copper through the urine will be increased.

10. Following three renal manifestations are present in this disease:

    a. Aminoaciduria

    b. Renal tubular acidosis

    c. Renal calculi

11. Diagnosis can be confirmed by any one of the following:

    a. K-F ring and serum ceruloplasmin level is <20 mg/L

    b. Serum ceruloplasmin < 200 mg/L and copper content in the liver biopsy is >250 mg/g of dry liver tissue.

    c. Urinary copper level > 40 µg/day and <100 µg/day and low level of ceruloplasmin

12. Following six radiological features are present in this disease:

    a. Evidence of osteopenia in hands and feet.

    b. Arthropathy

    c. Articular abnormalities in the knee, wrist, foot, hip, shoulder, and elbow:
       - Fragmentation of subchondral bone
       - Cyst formation

    d. Osteomalacia and rickets

    e. Periosteal bone formation

    f. Chondrocalcinosis

CASE 208

A 45-year-old woman has been admitted with acute abdominal pain radiating to right side of her back at the lower end of scapula after having heavy meal and vomiting.

1. **What is the most likely diagnosis?**
2. **Why there is abdominal pain and vomiting following heavy meal?**
3. **Why the pain has been referred to the right scapula?**
4. **If the gallbladder is inflamed, where the pain will be referred and why?**

Answers

1. This is a case of cholelithiasis.

2. As the food reaches the duodenal cavity, cholecystokinin will be released leading to contraction of the gallbladder. Since the stone is present in the gallbladder, the stone will be squeezed into cystic duct resulting in abdominal pain.

3. Visceral pain from the gall passes along the splanchnic nerves to the T7 and T8 spinal root. Infrascapular region is supplied by the T7 and T8. Hence, this has been referred to as the infrascapular region.

4. In case of acute cholecystitis, inflammation of the gallbladder irritates C3 and C4 segments of phrenic nerve. Again, right shoulder region is supplied by the same spinal segments. Hence, the pain of acute cholecystitis is referred to right shoulder.

CASE 209

A 60-year-old man admitted with painless bleeding per rectum just after defecation and it was in the form of drop of blood splashing in the pan. During proctoscopy, following features are found:

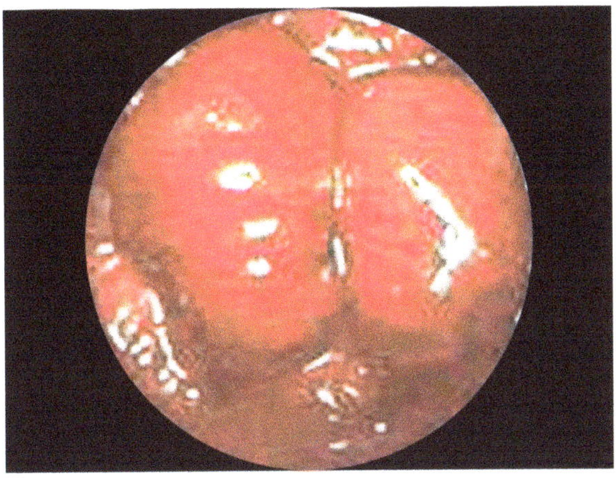

1. **What is the feature seen in the proctoscopy?**
2. **What is your diagnosis?**
3. **What is this?**
4. **Why is the bleeding painless here?**
5. **Describe the anatomical basis of this feature.**
6. **What are the causes of this disease?**
7. **Classify this disease.**
8. **Why is the other one painful?**
9. **What is the embryological relevance of pectinate line?**

Answers

1. The above feature demonstrated the evidence of internal hemorrhoids.
2. Patient has been suffering from internal hemorrhoids.
3. Internal hemorrhoid is characterized by dilatation of superior or internal rectal venous plexus leading to appearance of radicle of superior rectal veins at 3, 7, and 9 o' clock positions.
4. Internal hemorrhoids are present above the pectinate line. The mucous membrane above the pectinate line is supplied by the autonomic nerve plexus; hence, the bleeding is painless. But pain may occur due to stretching of the anus.
5. Following are the anatomical bases of internal hemorrhoids:
   a. In case of constipation and hard stool, it gives pressure upon the venous radicle leading to pooling of blood in these venous radicles having poor venous return leading to development of varices.
   b. In case of patient with chronic obstructive lung disease, the increased abdominal pressure may aggravate this condition.
   c. In case of advanced age, supporting tissue of anal cushion will degenerate leading to prolapse of the mucosal venous radicles.
6. Following are the causes of internal hemorrhoids:
   a. Constipation
   b. Straining during defecation and coughing
   c. Obesity
   d. Pregnancy
7. Hemorrhoids can be classified into two types:
   a. Internal hemorrhoids
   b. External hemorrhoids
8. External hemorrhoids occur below the pectinate line due to dilatation of the inferior rectal veins. Area below the pectinate line is supplied by sensory nerves; hence, external hemorrhoids are painful.
9. Pectinate line which is also known as dentate line is the area of portosystemic communication. Area above this line originates from endoderm and area below this line originates from ectoderm.

CHAPTER 6

Geriatric Medicine

CASE 1

An 80-year-old hypertensive on medication, diet-controlled diabetic male having past history of upper respiratory tract infection and frontal sinusitis treated with antibiotic has been admitted with headache for 5 days and confusion for 1 day and two seizures in 6 hours.

On examination, patient was confused, temperature 101°F, pulse rate 102 beats/min, regular, and blood pressure 150/90 mm Hg. All the systemic examination was normal except there was right-sided extensor plantar response.

Laboratory investigation demonstrated hemoglobin was 15 g/dL, white blood cell count 26,000/cc, erythrocyte sedimentation rate (ESR) 78 mm/1st hour, urea 62 mg/dL, and creatinine 1.1 mg/dL. Liver function test and serum electrolytes were normal.

1. **What is the most likely diagnosis?**
2. **What are the points in favor of your diagnosis?**
3. **What are the other differential diagnoses?**
4. **What is the investigation that confirms the diagnosis?**
5. **Can skull X-ray help in the diagnosis?**
6. **What is the cause of the increased serum urea?**
7. **What are the diseases will spread to develop this disease?**

Answers

1. The most likely diagnosis is cerebral abscess.
2. Points in favor of this diagnosis are:
   a. Delirium
   b. Headache
   c. Fever
   d. Past history of sinusitis and upper respiratory tract infection
   e. Leukocytosis
3. Other differential diagnoses are:
   a. Cerebral tumor
   b. Bacterial sinusitis
4. CT scan is the investigation which will confirm the diagnosis because of the following reasons:
   a. It will demonstrate a mass lesion. After injection of the contrast, it will demonstrate ring enhancement. It is due to surrounding cerebral edema.
   b. It will provide the proper view of the air sinuses.
5. Skull X-ray will demonstrate mucosal edema in the different sinuses but cannot help to differentiate the diagnosis.
6. Serum urea was raised in this patient for the following reasons:
   a. Patient was febrile leading to evaporation of fluid from the body.
   b. Patient was confused as a result he did not take fluid to replenish.
   c. Hypercatabolism leading to increased nitrogen turnover
7. Following infections spread through the hematogenous route:
   a. Sinusitis
   b. Lung abscess
   c. Bronchiectasis
   d. Penetrating head trauma
   e. Middle ear infection
   f. Skin and subcutaneous sepsis
   g. Infection in the intracerebral venous sinuses

CASE 2

A 78-year-old hypertensive male admitted in the medicine department with left-sided hemiparesis and in eye examination following were found:

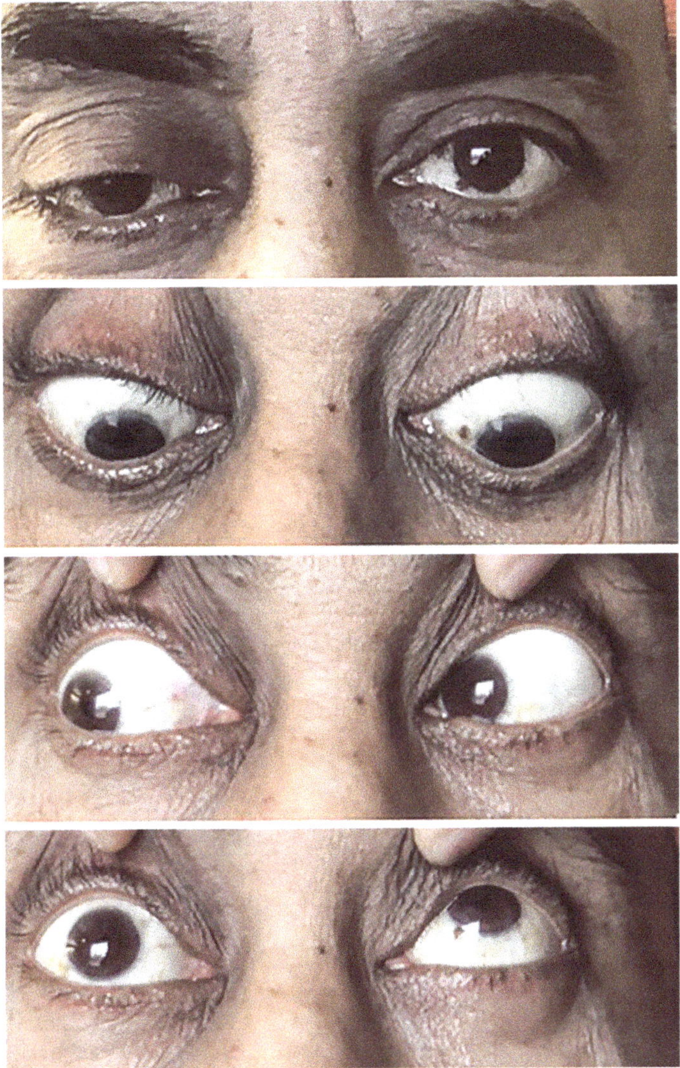

1. **What is your diagnosis regarding the eye examination?**
2. **What is your syndromic diagnosis?**
3. **What are the eye muscles involved in this case?**
4. **What is the site of lesion in this case?**
5. **What are the causes of this disease?**
6. **Whether pupil is involved in this disease?**
7. **What may be the associated abnormalities in this disease?**
8. **What may be the complications in this disease?**

Answers

1. The eye examination revealed:
   a. Right-sided ptosis
   b. Normal infraduction
   c. Normal abduction of right lateral rectus and normal adduction of left medial rectus
   d. Impaired supraduction of the right eye on upward gaze
2. The syndromic diagnosis is Weber syndrome.
3. Following are the eye muscles involved in this case:
   a. Medial rectus
   b. Superior rectus
   c. Inferior rectus
   d. Inferior oblique
4. Site of lesion is:
   a. Oculomotor fascicles in the interpeduncular cisterns
   b. Cerebral peduncle
5. Causes of the lesion in the decreasing order of frequency:
   a. Cardioembolism
   b. Thrombosis
   c. Large artery-to-artery embolism
   d. Intrinsic perforator branch disease leading to lacunar infarct
6. If upper and middle midbrain are involved, the pupil will be unresponsive and dilated. But, if the lower midbrain is involved, the pupil will be spared.
7. Following may be the associated abnormalities:
   a. Involvement of the red nucleus leading to ataxia
   b. Involvement of the substantia nigra leading to development of parkinsonism
8. Following are the complications in this disease:
   a. Massive posterior circulation infarction
   b. Tonsillar herniation
   c. Evolving hydrocephalus
   d. Secondary complications like:
      - Aspiration pneumonia
      - Contracture
      - Bedsores
      - Deep vein thrombosis
      - Pulmonary embolism
      - Urinary tract infection

CASE 3

An 82-year-old man having history of osteoarthritis of both knee and ischemic heart disease came to medical clinic with history of five falls within a span of 2 months which was according to the patient due to loss of balance. He had no history of unconsciousness and vertigo.

On examination, there was orthostatic hypotension, pulse demonstrated atrial fibrillation, mini-mental scale examination was 26/30, and muscle power 4/5. There was cataract in both the eyes.

1. **What types of intervention is required to reduce the incidence of frequent fall?**
2. **Why digoxin cannot be used in this case?**
3. **Administration of which drug can reduce the frequent falls?**
4. **How the balance is maintained in the elderly patient?**
5. **What are the complications of falls?**
6. **How can you prevent fall?**

Answers

1. Following types of interventions can reduce the frequent falls:
   a. Active and passive physiotherapy can reduce the weakness, muscle strengthening, training of the gait, and balance of the lower limb.
   b. Patient may get benefit from changes in the pain reduction medication. But number of medications should be reduced as intake of more than four medications may lead to frequent fall.
   c. Intake of sedative drugs may lead to frequent falls.
2. Digoxin can control the ventricular rate in patient with atrial fibrillation but cannot cardiovert the patient to maintain sinus rhythm. Since this patient's heart rate is within control, hence this drug cannot be used in this patient.
3. Warfarin should be used in this patient to prevent further falls.
4. Balance of the human body is maintained through the composite action during standing and motion:
   a. Sensory input from the following system:
      - Vision
      - Vestibular system
      - Proprioceptive system

b. Processing of the sensory input in the central nervous system

c. Effector system through the musculoskeletal organ

5. Complication of falls:
   a. Injuries:
      - Subdural hematoma
      - Injury to the brain
      - Painful soft-tissue injury
      - Fractures of:
        ○ Hip
        ○ Femur
        ○ Humerus
        ○ Ribs
        ○ Wrist
   b. Hospitalization:
      - Consequences of immobilization:
        ○ Deconditioning
        ○ Deep vein thrombosis
      - Risk of:
        ○ Hospital-acquired infection
        ○ Iatrogenic illness
      - Disability:
        ○ Physical injury
        ○ Psychological
      - Death
6. By following methods one can prevent falls:
   a. Environmental hazards management
   b. Training of sensory balance
   c. Physical therapy
   d. High-intensity resistance strength training
   e. Multifactorial intervention program
   f. Effective hip protector use

CASE 4

An 81-year-old hypertensive female patient having chronic obstructive lung disease and osteoarthritis leading to fractured hip treated by screw came to medicine department with dizziness but no loss of consciousness. On examination, she has frailty.

1. **Is dual-energy X-ray absorptiometry (DEXA) required in this case?**
2. **Who should be treated for osteoporosis?**
3. **Who are at risk of fracture?**
4. **What is measured in DEXA?**
5. **What are the drugs used in osteoporosis?**

Answers

1. It can diagnose osteoporosis. As she had history of fracture, it is not necessary and appropriate in considering his age and frailty. Again osteoarthritis will interfere with the result.
2. According to Royal College of Physicians (RCP) who had history of fracture and osteopenic should be treated for osteoporosis.
3. Following are at risk of fracture:
   a. Advanced age
   b. Female sex
   c. Prior history of fracture
   d. Smoker
   e. Corticosteroid use
   f. Low body mass index
   g. Alcohol intake
   h. Secondary osteoporosis
4. DEXA measures T-scores and Z-scores.
   a. The T-scores measure the differences between bone mineral density and mean value of bone mineral density in the young adult. These are measured in standard deviations.
      - Osteopenia is diagnosed in the scores are between negative 1 and negative 2.5.
      - Osteoporosis can be diagnosed in the score is below negative 2.5.
   b. The Z-score is the number of deviations below or above the age-matched bone mineral density. Secondary osteoporosis can be diagnosed if the score is less than negative 1.5.
5. Following drugs are used in case of osteoporosis:
   a. Bisphosphonates:
      - Alendronate: It will reduce the incidence of fracture of hip, spine, and wrist.

- Risedronate: It will reduce the vertebral as well as nonvertebral fracture by 40% over 3 years.
- Intravenous zoledronic acid: It will reduce 70% spine fracture and 40% hip fracture over 3 years.

b. Other drugs:
- Estrogen-only replacement
- Salmon calcitonin
- Conjugated estrogen-progestin hormone replacement
- Raloxifene: It is estrogen receptors modulators. It reduces resorption of osteoclast.
- Teriparatide: It is recombinant parathormone which stimulates osteoblast to produce bone.
- Denosumab—RANKL inhibitors: It is monoclonal Ig2 that will inhibit receptor activator of nuclear factor kappa-B ligand (RANKL) thereby inhibiting binding with RANK.

CASE 5

A 79-year-old man came to medicine clinic with his wife as he has been suffering from swaying and difficulty in initiation of movements and also incontinence of urine. His CT scan demonstrated:

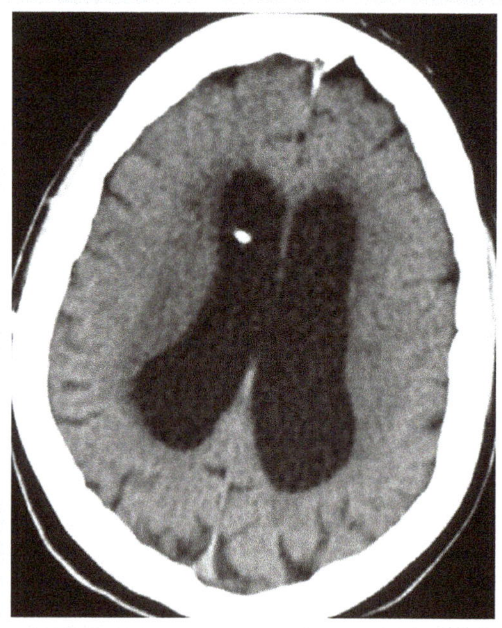

1. **What is the finding in the CT scan of brain?**
2. **What is your diagnosis?**
3. **What is the pathophysiology of idiopathic hydrocephalus?**
4. **What are the criteria in this diagnosis?**
5. **What are the causes of abnormal gait?**
6. **What are the causes of dementia?**
7. **What are the causes of urinary incontinence?**
8. **What are the typical features of gait in this disease?**
9. **What are the features in MRI of brain suggestive of this diagnosis?**
10. **What are the favorable outcomes after surgery?**
11. **What are the unfavorable outcomes after surgery?**

Answers

1. CT scan of brain demonstrated huge dilatation of lateral ventricles.
2. This is a case of normal pressure hydrocephalus (NPH).
3. The pathophysiology of idiopathic hydrocephalus:
    a. Increased pulse pressure in cerebrospinal fluid
    b. Increased flow of cerebrospinal fluid through the aqueduct
    c. Reduced compliance of the subarachnoid space
    d. Reduction of cerebral blood flow
    e. Reduced reabsorption of cerebrospinal fluid into the venous system due to increased vascular resistance
    f. Reabsorption of the cerebrospinal fluid through the transependymal flow rather than through pacchionian granulations
    g. Altered expression of tumor necrosis factor-α and transforming growth factor-β
    h. Failure of drainage of vasoactive metabolites
    i. Loss of Windkessel effect in the basal arteries in the skull
4. The clinical criteria for the diagnosis are:
    a. Gait apraxia
    b. Urinary incontinence
    c. Dementia
5. Causes of abnormal gait are:
    a. Increased intracranial pressure produces compression as well as stretching of the fibers of the corticospinal tract in the corona radiata supplying the lower limbs.
    b. Periventricular white matter and prefrontal regions are poorly perfused.
    c. Structures in the brain stem like pedunculo-pontine nucleus are compressed.
6. The causes of dementia are:
    a. Due to enlargement of the ventricles, cortex is pushed against the inner table of calvarium leading to shearing forces resulting in dementia.
7. Causes of urinary incontinence are:
    a. In the early stage, periventricular sacral fibers of the corticospinal tract are stretched leading to loss of voluntary control of bladder contraction.
    b. In the later stage, dementia may lead to incontinence.
8. Typical features of gait in this disease are:
    a. External rotation of the foot
    b. Poor clearance of foot like shuffling, festination, or tripping
    c. Notable difficulty in turning of the body in its long axis
    d. Failure of the initiation of gait
9. Following are the features in brain MRI suggesting this diagnosis:
    a. Evans index: It is frontal horn ratio which is characterized by maximal width of frontal horn of the ventricle divided by transverse inner diameter of the skull. If the ratio is >0.3, it suggests significant ventricular enlargement.
    b. Callosal angle should be in-between 40° and 90° in this disease.
    c. Size of the temporal horn: There is disproportionate widening of the ventricles as compared to cerebral sulci.
    d. Normal size of the fourth ventricle in the face of enlarged third and lateral ventricle is suggestive of NPH.
    e. Dilated Sylvian fissure
    f. Coronal section at the level of posterior commissure demonstrates narrow subarachnoid space surrounding the outer surface of the brain and narrow medial cistern
    g. There is bulging of the roof of the lateral ventricles
    h. Study of cerebrospinal fluid demonstrates >24.5 mL/min in this disease
10. Following are the favorable outcomes after surgery:
    a. Lack of lesion in the white matter in MRI brain
    b. Aqueductal stroke volume is >42 µL.
    c. There is resistance to outflow of cerebrospinal fluid is >18 mm Hg.
    d. B-wave is longer than 50% of intracranial pressure during monitoring time.
11. Following are the unfavorable outcomes after surgery:
    a. Severe dementia
    b. When the presenting feature is dementia.
    c. Either misdiagnosis or delayed recognition
    d. MRI features demonstrating lesion in the white matter

CASE 6

An 80-year-old male smoker admitted with history of progressively increasing cough with expectoration of greenish sputum and breathlessness for 7 days and fall while standing from sitting position 3 days ago and few episodes of confusion in last 2 days. After admission, he suddenly experienced sharp knife-like pain in the central part of the chest which was aggravated during deep inspiration as well as coughing.

On examination, there were crackles in both lung bases and respiratory rate 26 beats/min. During treatment, patient suddenly developed worsening of respiratory distress and blood pressure 90/60 mm Hg.

Laboratory examination demonstrated neutrophilic leukocytosis. Chest X-ray demonstrated:

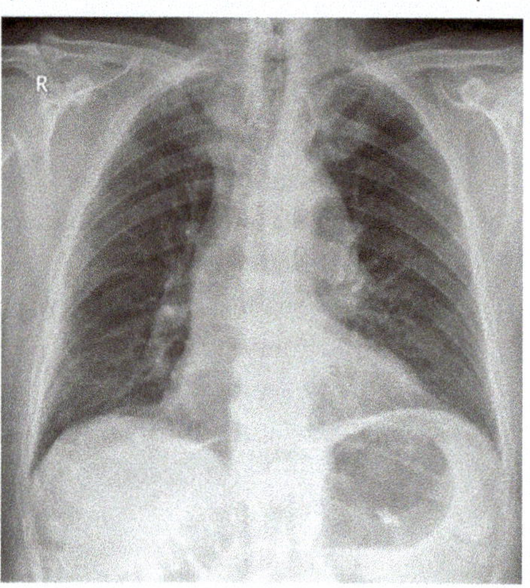
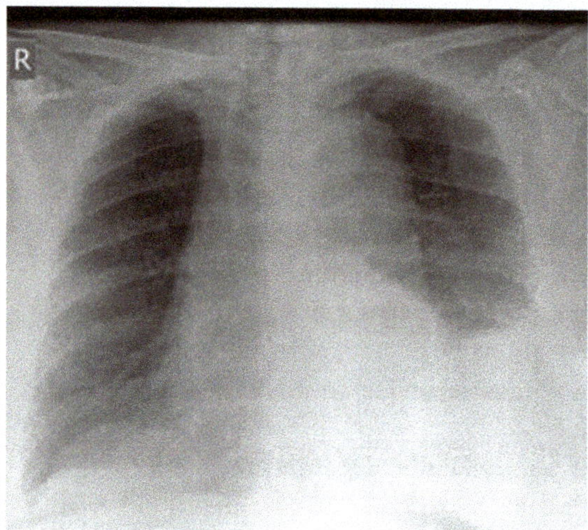

1. **What is shown in the left-sided chest X-ray?**
2. **What is your diagnosis and why?**
3. **What are the other causes of hypotension to be excluded?**
4. **What is demonstrated in the right chest X-ray?**
5. **What are the fallacies of chest ultrasound?**
6. **What should be the next investigation of choice to detect the underlying pathology?**
7. **What is your most likely diagnosis?**
8. **What is the pathogenesis in this disease?**
9. **What are the radiological features suggestive of the disease?**
10. **What are the factors in favor of good outcome in this patients after surgery?**

Answers

1. The chest X-ray demonstrated:
   a. Unfolding of the thoracic aorta—which is due to degenerative changes in the wall of the aorta.
   b. Slightly coarsening of the bronchovascular markings
   c. Early inflammatory shadow at the left lung base
   d. Normal cardiothoracic ratio

2. The working diagnosis is sepsis because of the following points:
   a. Neutrophilic leukocytosis
   b. High ESR
   c. Lower respiratory tract infection
   d. Low blood pressure

3. The other causes responsible for hypotension to be excluded:
   a. No hypoxia
   b. No evidence of dehydration
   c. No physical signs or radiological evidence of heart failure
   d. No evidence in the clinical history or clinical signs leading to sympathetic neuropathy resulting in hypotension

4. Right-sided chest X-ray demonstrated:
   a. Left-sided pleural effusion
   b. Expansion of the intrathoracic aorta

5. The fallacies of the chest ultrasound are the following:
   a. Confirm the presence of pleural fluid and guide sampling

b. Do not provide any information regarding heart and great vessels

6. Next investigation of choice is CT scan of thorax which can demonstrate:
   a. Abnormal dilatation of the aorta
   b. Some leakage of fluid into the pleural cavity
   c. Presence of mass lesion eroding from the aorta

7. The most likely diagnosis is mycotic aneurysm affecting thoracic aorta.

8. Pathogenesis of mycotic aneurysm:
   a. Bacteremia: It is commonly in older people affecting preexisting atherosclerosis or aneurysm.
   b. Local injury or bacterial inoculation resulting from:
      - Intravenous drug use
      - Trauma
      - Iatrogenic causes, i.e., percutaneous intervention
   c. Local spread from vertebral osteomyelitis or intra-abdominal sepsis
   d. Septic emboli from infective endocarditis associated with emboli in vasa vasorum

9. Following radiological features are suggestive of this disease:
   a. Saccular and lobulated contours
   b. Inflammation of the soft-tissue surrounding the vessel wall
   c. Collection of fluid in the perianeurysmal area
   d. Intramural collection of air around the blood vessels

10. Factors in favor of good outcome in this patients after surgery are:
    a. Preceding good functional status
    b. Lack of copathologies
    c. Normal renal function
    d. Normal left ventricular function
    e. Preservation of aortic valve

CASE 7

An 82-year-old man having history of recurrent falls came to emergency department with left-sided chest pain. Chest X-ray demonstrated:

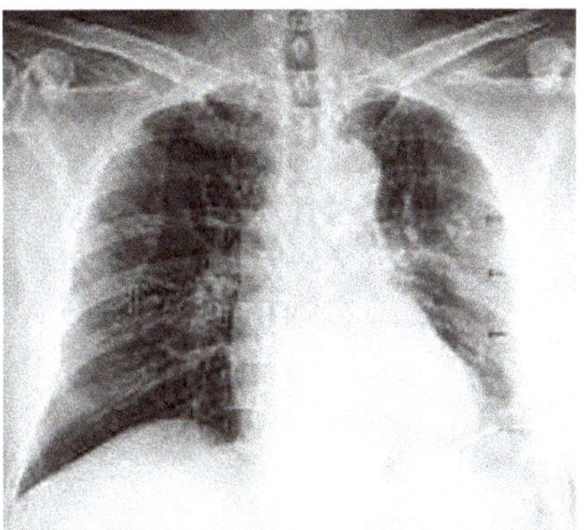

After admission patient developed progressively increasing breathlessness and saturation of 84% in room air. Percussion of right side of the chest revealed stony dull sound and auscultation demonstrated absent breath sound. Chest X-ray demonstrated:

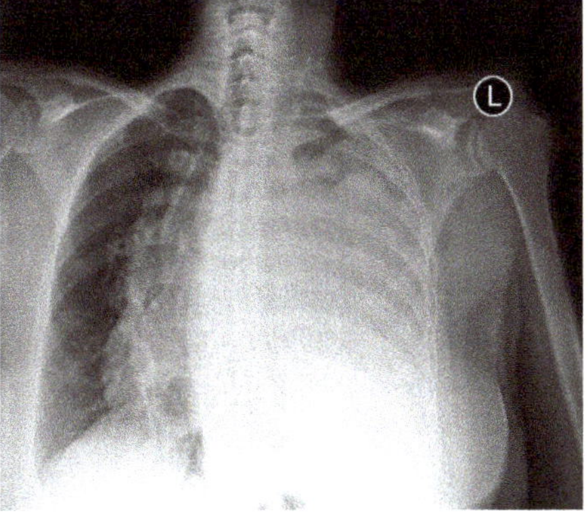

1. **What are demonstrated in the above chest X-ray?**
2. **What is the cause of this picture demonstrated above?**
3. **Is there any relation if rib fracture with mortality?**
4. **What are the ribs that are associated with fracture?**
5. **What are the causes of spontaneous rib fracture?**

Answers

1. First X-ray of chest demonstrated multiple fractures of 4th, 5th, and 6th rib of left side. Second X-ray of chest demonstrated massive right-sided pleural effusion.
2. The cause of this left-sided pleural effusion due to fractured rib and the fluid is bloody effusion.
3. Relation of rib fracture with mortality:
   a. Single rib fracture is associated with 5% mortality.
   b. Seven or more rib fractures are associated with 13–69% mortality.
4. Relation of rib with fracture:
   a. 1st, 2nd, and 3rd ribs are hardest to break.
   b. 4th to 10th ribs are very vulnerable to fracture.
   c. 11th and 12th ribs are mobile and very difficult to break.
5. Causes of rib fracture:
   a. Osteoporosis
   b. Rib metastasis
   c. Hyperparathyroidism

CASE 8

An 81-year-old man having history of several falls and unsteadiness of gait but no headache came to neurology department with loss of balance during walking which disappeared while sitting position.

On examination, features of osteoarthritis like Heberden's node in his hands. He had history of immature cataract and some degree of sensorineural hearing loss. He had no postural hypotension, neurological signs, and all other systemic examinations were normal. CT scan demonstrated:

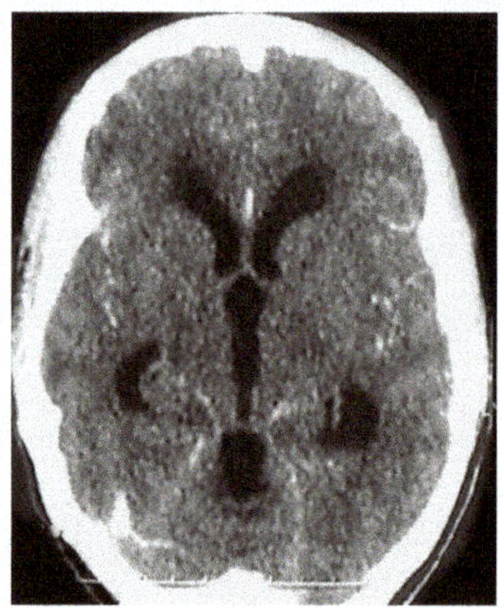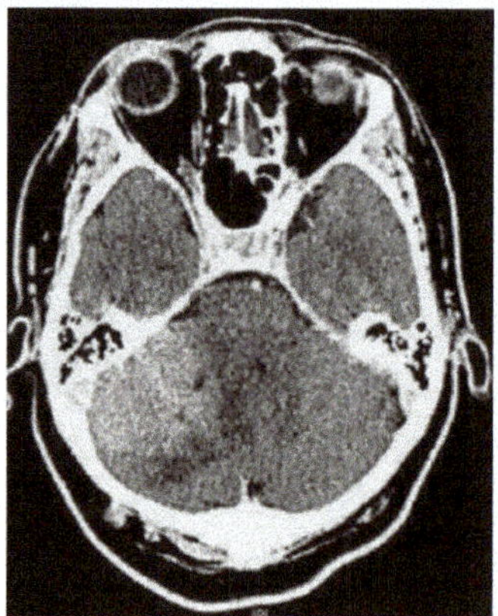

1. **What are the features demonstrated in above CT scan of brain?**
2. **What are the causes of disequilibrium?**
3. **How can you differentiate vertigo from disequilibrium?**
4. **What is your diagnosis?**
5. **What are the types of lesion seen in this area?**
6. **What are the differentiating features in schwannoma from meningioma?**
7. **What are the complications following surgery of the tumor?**

Answers

1. There is dilatation of both lateral ventricles, i.e., third and fourth ventricles. With cerebral atrophy related to age in the first CT scan of brain.

   In the second CT scan of brain demonstrated: extra-axial enhancing mass involving the right cerebellopontine angle overlying the cerebellar hemisphere producing mass effect leading to compression of the fourth ventricle.

2. Cases of disequilibrium:
   a. Visual impairment
   b. Drug intoxication
   c. Hearing loss
   d. Psychological issue

3. Vertigo can be defined as sensation of rotation of self or surroundings in relation to the patient which may be due to vestibular, central or vestibular, or central nervous system disorders.

4. The patient has been suffering from cerebellopontine angle tumor.

5. Following lesions are seen in this area:
   a. Schwannoma: This lesion involves 5th, 7th, 9th, 10th, and occasionally 11th cranial nerves.
   b. Meningioma: It arises from the dura of the petrous part of temporal bone from the proliferation of arachnoidal meningothelial cells.
   c. Epidermoid tumor arises during neural tube closure from congenital misdisplacement of ectodermal cells
   d. Arachnoid cyst: It results from splitting of embryonic arachnoid membrane filled up with cerebrospinal fluid.

6. Differentiating features in meningioma from schwannoma are the following:
   a. Hyperdense appearances in noncontrast CT scan of brain
   b. Lack of erosion in the internal auditory canal
   c. Broad dural attachment
   d. Cleft of cerebrospinal fluid in-between the brain parenchyma and tumor
   e. Thickening of the dura around the tumor known as dural tail sign
   f. Hyperostosis
   g. Ice cream cone shape
   h. Presence of calcification

7. Complications following surgery:
   a. Headache
   b. Hemorrhage
   c. Stroke
   d. Vascular injury
   e. Infection
   f. Injury to the cranial nerve
   g. Nerve dysfunction

CASE 9

An 88-year-old man having history of hypertension on thiazide and telmisartan came to medicine outpatient department (OPD) with anorexia, fever with intermittent chills, and pain in the front left lower chest. He was given antidiabetic, antipyretic, and proton pump inhibitors. His serum sodium was 130 mEq/L. His plasma and urine osmolality were 292 mOsmol/kg and 630 mOsmol/kg, respectively.

After 3 days, he suddenly watched the following:

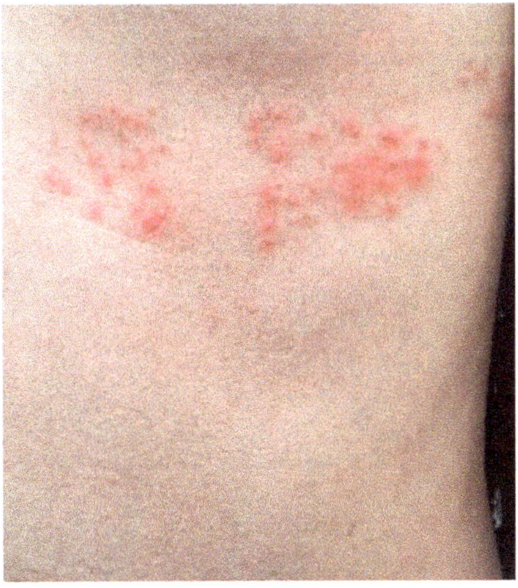

1. **What is shown in the above picture?**
2. **What is your diagnosis?**
3. **How can you manage this patient?**
4. **What is the cause of hyponatremia?**
5. **What are the differential diagnoses in this case?**
6. **What is the pathophysiology of this disease?**
7. **What are the complications in this disease?**

Answers

1. The above picture demonstrated papulovesicular eruptions having erythematous base seen in the lower right and left part of the chest along the specific dermatome.
2. The patient has been suffering from herpes zoster.
3. Following drugs are used:
   a. Acyclovir should be administered five times daily for 8 days.
   b. Topical capsaicin can be administered to decrease the incidence of postherpetic neuralgia. But it should not be given during the acute attack.
   c. Gabapentin can be given to decrease the incidence of postherpetic neuralgia. But, it should not be given during the acute attack.
4. Hyponatremia is mostly due to chronic intake of thiazide. This is not due to SIADH as the urine and serum osmolality both were normal.
5. As the patient is very aged, this disease may be due to suppressed cell-mediated immunity. In this patient, there is anorexia, weight loss, night sweat, and high ESR are all predisposing factors which include:
   a. Multiple myeloma
   b. Lymphoma
   c. Carcinoma
   d. Chronic infection
6. Dormant herpes zoster virus present in the dorsal nerve root being escape from the control of T lymphocytes replicate, then migrate down the axon of that nerve root and reach the specific dermatome.
7. Following are the complications of this disease:
   a. Postherpetic neuralgia
   b. Blindness due to conjunctivitis
   c. Herpes panophthalmitis
   d. Eight cranial nerve involvement leading to deafness
   e. Disseminated herpes zoster infection leading to:
      - Pneumonitis
      - Encephalitis
      - Meningitis

CASE 10

An 80-year-old hypertensive diabetic male came to eye department with recurrent sudden development of loss of vision in the inferior quadrant. His blood pressure was 170/90 mm Hg, pulse rate 90 beats/min, regular, and other systemic examination was normal. There was no carotid bruit heard. Funduscopic examination demonstrated:

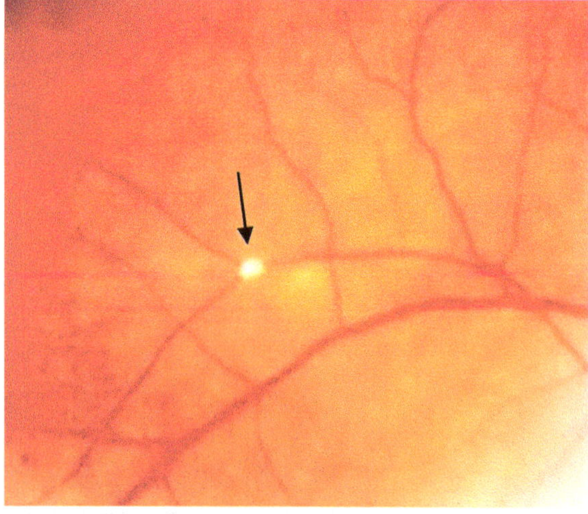

1. **What is demonstrated in the fundoscopy?**
2. **What is the next investigation to be done in this case?**
3. **What are the possible risk factors for this eye finding?**

Answers

1. Fundoscopy demonstrated presence of cholesterol emboli in the superior temporal branch of the left retinal artery. There is no evidence of retinal detachment, no evidence of diabetic retinopathy, and cupping.
2. Carotid Doppler study is required to detect the stenosis of the carotid artery which may require surgery for correction if the stenosis is >75% in this artery.
3. Following are the probable risk factors:
   a. Smoking
   b. History of coronary artery bypass graft
   c. Older age
   d. Hypertension
   e. High systolic blood pressure
   f. Male sex
   g. Coronary artery disease
   h. Total cholesterol

CASE 11

An 82-year-old diabetic man was admitted with sudden onset of left-sided hemiparesis. CT scan of brain demonstrated evolving infarction on the left cerebral hemisphere in the territory of middle cerebral artery. Laboratory investigation demonstrated complete blood count, liver function and renal function tests, clotting screens, and ECG were within the normal limit.

1. **How the patient should be managed?**
2. **What are the inclusion criteria in this patient?**
3. **Name seven exclusion criteria in this case?**

Answers

1. As usual if the patient presents within 3 hours of the incidence, the treatment of choice is thrombolysis. But as this patient is >80 years old and diabetic, the incidence of complication following thrombolysis was very high. Hence, here the treatment of choice is 300 mg aspirin immediately followed by administration of daily dose of 75 mg orally.
2. The inclusion criteria in this patient are:
   a. Age 18–80 years
   b. Clear time of onset
   c. Clinical signs of definite stroke
   d. Within 3 hours of incidence
   e. National Institutes of Health Stroke Scale (NIHSS) score of >4 but <25
3. Following seven exclusion criteria of thrombolysis are:
   a. Rapidly improving symptoms or minor stroke symptoms
   b. History of trauma or stroke within 3 months
   c. History of hemorrhage from different sites within 3 weeks
   d. History of major surgery—obstetric delivery within 2 weeks
   e. High premorbid dependency
   f. Known clotting disorders
   g. Incidence of seizures at the onset of stroke

CASE 12

A 78-year-old diabetic and hypertensive male after being discharged from the hospital being recovered through open abdominal surgery from subacute intestinal obstruction readmitted in the medical unit with the complaint of severe mid-dorsal back pain.

On examination, blood pressure was 155/95 mm Hg, pulse rate 90 beats/min, and temperature 102°F. All other systemic examinations were normal. There was one scar seen during abdominal examination.

Laboratory examination demonstrated mild neutrophilic leukocytosis, high ESR, and low albumin. ECG was normal and presence of osteophytes on the dorsal spine.

1. **What are the differential diagnoses in this case?**
2. **What are the points in favor of sepsis in this patient?**
3. **Which investigation is specific in this case?**
4. **Why isotope bone scan is not the choice in this case?**
5. **Why CT scan of bone is not of the choice in this patient?**
6. **What is the most likely diagnosis?**
7. **What are the other differential diagnoses and how can you exclude these diagnoses?**
8. **How can you define this disease?**
9. **What are the risk factors in this disease?**

Answers

1. The differential diagnoses are:
   a. Acute pain in the bone by:
      - Fracture
      - Malignancy
      - Infection
   b. Soft-tissue pain from the supporting structure due to:
      - Infection
      - Malignancy
      - Trauma
      - Noninfective inflammatory conditions
   c. Paraspinal masses
   d. Prolapsed intervertebral disk due to:
      - Direct pressure on the ligamentous structures
      - Impingement on the spinal cord
      - Impingement on the nerve root
2. Following are the points in favor of sepsis in this patient:
   a. High ESR
   b. Recent abdominal surgery
   c. Recent insertion of intravenous catheter
3. MRI of spine is the investigation of choice because it will demonstrate:
   a. The inflammation in the paraspinal inflammation
   b. The inflammation in the intervertebral disk
   c. The inflammation in the bone
4. Isotope bone scan is not the choice of investigation as it will demonstrate the abnormal uptake in the bone in case of infection or fracture or malignant condition in the bone but it cannot delineate the soft-tissue inflammation.

5. CT scan of spine can detect the most of the pathologies but it is less sensitive than MRI in detecting active inflammation if there is no overt destruction of the bone.
6. The most likely diagnosis is septic diskitis.
7. The other differential diagnoses are:
   a. Prolapse of the intervertebral disk but it usually occurs in lumbar or sacral vertebrae.
   b. Osteoporotic collapse of the vertebrae: It is excruciatingly painful and plain X-ray demonstrates minimal changes.
   c. Crush fracture: Normal alkaline phosphatase produces the injury to the bone less likely.
   d. Metastatic bone disease: Onset of pain is gradual not all on a sudden. Alkaline phosphatase is expected to be high. Plain X-ray can demonstrate abnormal picture in the bone.
   e. Acute osteomyelitis: It may be the closet to this diagnosis, and in some cases septic diskitis may be associated with underlying osteomyelitis.
8. Septic diskitis can be defined as inflammation of the intervertebral disk extending into discovertebral junction, into epidural space, posterior vertebral elements as well as paraspinal soft tissues.
9. Following are the risk factors in this disease:
   a. Different invasive procedures
   b. Resection of rectal cancer
   c. Carcinomas
   d. Diabetes mellitus
   e. Bacterial endocarditis
   f. Septicemia following urinary tract infection

CASE 13

An 88-year-old man was admitted with fracture at the neck of the femur and operative fixation was performed as emergency. During hospital day, he developed severe hospital-acquired pneumonia and was under ventilator. After discharging from hospital, he was unable to walk because he was too weak to walk.

On examination, his vitals were normal. All the systemic examinations were normal except the quadriceps muscles were wasted due to long-term bedridden.

Laboratory examination demonstrated albumin level was 2.2 mg/dL, alkaline phosphatase was 300 IU/L, and rest of the other parameters were within normal limit.

1. **What is the most important underlying cause of this severe weakness in this patient?**
2. **Define this disease.**
3. **What are the factors contributing to sarcopenia?**
4. **How can you assess this disease?**
5. **How can you confirm this disease?**
6. **What are the physical performances to detect this disease?**
7. **What are the complications in this disease?**
8. **What are the histopathological changes occurring in the muscle fibers?**
9. **How can you treat the patient?**

Answers

1. This patient has been suffering from sarcopenia.
2. Sarcopenia can be defined as reduction of the muscle mass below 2 standard deviation below the mean for young healthy reference group affecting the elderly as well as sedentary populations.
3. Following are the factors contribute to sarcopenia:
   a. Decrease in size and number of the type II muscle fibers
   b. Inactivity
   c. Insulin resistance
   d. Obesity
   e. Reduced concentration of growth factor and androgen in the serum
   f. Inadequate intake of protein
   g. Blunted synthesis of muscle protein in response to protein meals or resistance exercise
   h. Chronic disease:
      - Chronic obstructive pulmonary disease
      - Chronic kidney disease
      - Diabetes mellitus
      - Cancer
      - HIV
   i. Physical inactivity
4. Sarcopenia can be assessed by:
   a. Handgrip test
   b. Chair stand test

5. Confirmation of sarcopenia:
   a. Quantification of:
      - Total body skeletal muscle mass (SMM)
      - Appendicular skeletal muscle mass (ASM)
      - Cross-sectional area of a skeletal muscle
      - Correlation of height, weight, or BMI
6. Following performances are done to detect the sarcopenia:
   a. Gait speed test
   b. Short physical performance battery: It consists of the following tests:
      - Chair stand test
      - Standing balance
      - Walking speed

      Minimal and maximal achieving score are 0 and 12 respectively.
   c. Timed-up and go test
   d. The 400-m walk test
7. Following are the complications in this disease:
   a. It is associated with increased mortality in patients with:
      - End-stage renal disease (ESRD)
      - Pancreatic cancer
      - Chronic heart failure
   b. Sarcopenia associated with dose-related toxicities who are taking chemotherapy in patients with:
      - Hepatocellular carcinoma
      - Renal cell carcinoma
      - Breast cancer

c. It is associated with increased incidence of postoperative complications in patients with:
- Undergoing general surgical procedure
- Liver transplantation
- Colorectal surgery

8. Following are the histopathological changes in the muscle fibers:
   a. Reduced number of muscle fibers
   b. Decrease in the diameter of the muscle fibers
   c. Dysfunction of mitochondria
   d. Density of the mitochondria are diminished
   e. Accumulation of inclusion bodies in the myocytes

f. Accumulation of fat with age because adipose tissue within the lean body mass

9. This patient can be treated by following means:
   a. Exercise treatment
   - Aerobic and load-bearing exercise
   - Galvanic stimulation to the muscle fibers can cause muscle contraction.
   - Massage will improve the sense of well-being leading to decrease in the muscle tension.
   - If the patient is protein and potassium depleted, additional protein and potassium supplementation should be given.

CASE 14

An 82-year-old male presented with acute severe sudden abdominal pain during resection of submucosal resection of the submucosal polyp followed by collapse state in the emergency department.

On examination, pulse rate 112 beats/min and blood pressure 80/50 mm Hg. Abdominal examination revealed cardboard tenderness and peristaltic sound nearly nil. X-ray demonstrated:

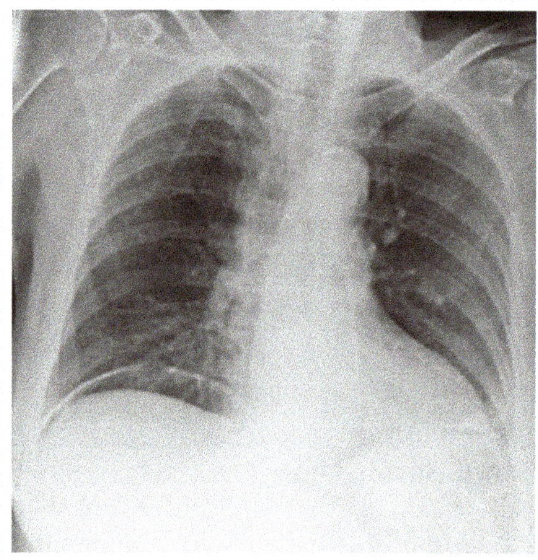

1. **What does the above picture demonstrate?**
2. **What is your diagnosis?**
3. **What are the endoscopy-related gases under diaphragm?**
4. **What are the CT findings in the gastric perforation?**
5. **What are the surgical repairs in this patient taken?**
6. **What are the complications of the gastric perforation?**
7. **Who are at increased risk of perforation?**

Answers

1. The above picture demonstrated gas under the light crus of diaphragm.
2. The diagnosis is gas under the diaphragm from perforation of hollow viscus.

3. Following are the endoscopy-related gastric perforation:
   a. Polypectomy
   b. Endoscopic mucosal resection
   c. Dilatation of anatomic stricture

   d. Scope of barotrauma

   e. Medications

   f. Caustic injuries

4. CT scan of abdomen in case of gastric perforation:
   a. Mesenteric air
   b. Discontinuity of the hollow viscus wall
   c. Extraluminal enteric contrast
   d. Free abdominal fluid
   e. Mesenteric hematoma
   f. Thickening of the bowel wall
   g. Extravasation of the intravenous contrast

5. Following surgical operations can be taken in this patient:
   a. Primary repair where the defect can be primarily closed suture.
   b. Graham patch repair where the defect is plugged with the well-visualized omental pedicle.
   c. Modified Graham patch repair where there is primary closure of the defect followed by flap application.
   d. Wedge resection where perforated area should be resected from the healthy tissue if it is on the greater curvature of the stomach and distant from either gastroesophageal junction or pyloric orifice.

6. Following are the risks of this disease:
   a. Infection of the wound
   b. Sepsis
   c. Malnutrition
   d. Delirium
   e. Multiorgan failure
   f. Obstruction of the bowel and adhesion

7. Following patients are at increased risk of this disease:
   a. Advanced disease
   b. Dementia
   c. Sepsis
   d. Hypoxia
   e. Electrolyte abnormalities
   f. Metabolic abnormalities
   g. Intraoperative complications

CASE 15

An 83-year-old woman with history of constipation came to emergency department with acute pain abdomen, vomiting, and distention. Urgent straight X-ray was taken instantaneously which was:

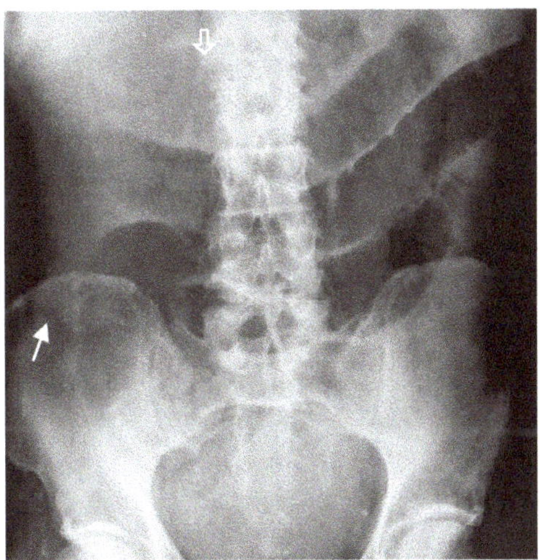

1. **What does the above picture demonstrate?**
2. **What is your diagnosis?**
3. **Where are the common sites of the disease?**
4. **What is the epidemiological incidence of this disease?**
5. **Which patients are most likely involved in this disease?**
6. **What is the direction of rotation in case different parts of intestine?**
7. **What are the complications in this disease?**
8. **What are the complications of surgery?**

Answers

1. The straight X-ray demonstrated dilatation of the small and large bowel loops. There is fluid seen in the right colon and gas fluid transverse colon.

2. In the face of constipation with a sudden history of acute abdominal pain, the diagnosis is that vomiting may lead to volvulus.

3. In case of elderly, sigmoid colon is the most common site of volvulus formation followed by cecum, splenic flexure, and transverse colon.

4. Epidemiological correlation:
   a. This disease is extremely common in younger subject developing countries, but in the developed countries affecting the elderly and frail female.
   b. Constipation is responsible for this disease in Western countries whereas high fiber diet is responsible in African population.

5. Following patients are most likely to be involved by this disorder:
   a. Neuropsychiatric disorder
   b. Multiple sclerosis
   c. Parkinson's disease
   d. Bedridden patients in the nursing home
   e. Duchenne type of muscular dystrophy
   f. Visceral myopathy
   g. Chagas disease

6. Sigmoid colon becomes loaded with fecal matter and susceptible to torsion in the counterclockwise direction. Due to repeated torsion, mesentery becomes shortened due to chronic inflammation.

   Cecal volvulus is either organoaxial (like cecocolic or true cecal) or, mesentricoaxial like cecal bascule.

   Ascending colon and ileum will twist on each other in the clockwise direction.

7. Complications of this disease are:
   a. Gangrene
   b. Bowel strangulation
   c. Perforation
   d. Peritonitis

8. Complications of the surgery in this disease are:
   a. Recurrence
   b. Anastomotic leak
   c. Wound infection
   d. Sepsis
   e. Pelvic abscess
   f. Fecal fistula
   g. Complications of ileostomy and colostomy

CASE 16

A 79-year-old male came to gastroenterology clinic with anorexia and dyspepsia. Upper gastrointestinal endoscopy was advised but the patient refused it. But, this patient agreed to perform barium meal of the stomach which demonstrated:

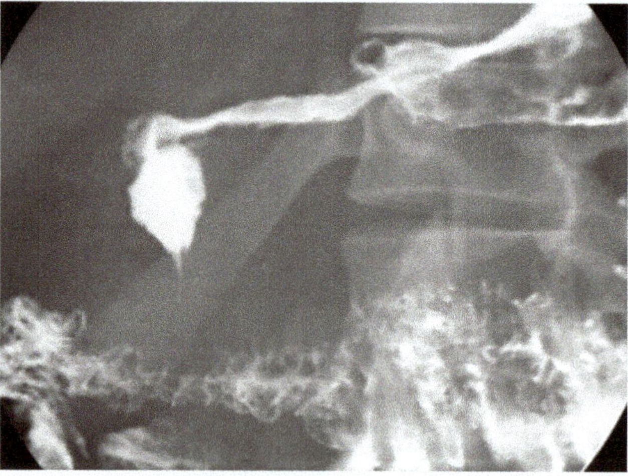

1. What has been demonstrated in the above picture?
2. What is your diagnosis?
3. What are the genes associated with this disease?
4. What are the cancers associated with this disease?
5. What are the differential diagnoses in this case?

Answers

1. Barium meal study of the stomach demonstrated luminal annular narrowing along the long segment which extends upto pyloric channel.

2. The diagnosis is linitis plastica. It is a phenotype of gastric carcinoma, also known as signet cell carcinoma or Scirrhous carcinoma.

3. Following genes are associated with linitis plastica:
   a. E-cadherin—mutation of its germine gene leads to occurrence of this disease
   b. Human epidermoid growth factor 2 gene—its upregulation or its increased expression

4. Breast cancer, colonic cancer, and ovarian cancer are associated with this linitis plastica.

5. Following are the differential diagnoses and process of exclusion:
   a. Atrophic gastritis: It presents with dyspepsia and decreased distensibility due to mucosal destruction and loss of mucosal folds.
   b. Hypertrophic gastritis due to *Helicobacter pylori*: There is mucosal fold hypertrophy but intact distensibility.
   c. Corrosive gastritis: Proper history of acid intake along with feature of corrosive gastritis.
   d. Watermelon stomach with loss of distensibility: Here, there will be features of hepatic decompensation and features of portal hypertension.

CASE 17

An 85-year-old hypertensive female having history of stroke for the past 5 years came to emergency department with history of drowsiness. Immediate urine dipstick test demonstrated positive for blood, protein, leukocytes, and nitrites. On examination, his vitals were normal.

Laboratory examination demonstrated total leukocyte count 18,000/cc and raised ESR. He was prescribed amoxicillin for 7 days. But after 7 days, he developed bloody diarrhea with lower abdominal pain and blood pressure 90/50 mm Hg, pulse rate 110 beats/min, and temperature 101°F. Colonoscopy demonstrated:

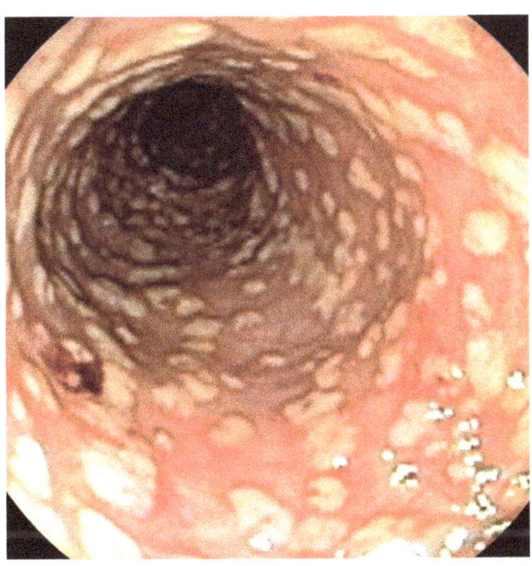

1. **What does the above picture demonstrate?**
2. **What is your diagnosis?**
3. **What are the points in favor of your diagnosis?**
4. **What are the other differential diagnoses and how can you exclude these diagnoses?**
5. **What is the difference in the incidence of females with positive urine analysis with or without long-term catheter?**
6. **What is the pathophysiology of this infection?**
7. **What is the common algorithm to detect the *Clostridium* infection in the stool?**
8. **What are the criteria of severe *Clostridium difficile* colitis?**
9. **What are the complications in this disease?**

Answers

1. The above colonoscopy picture diagnosis demonstrates raised yellowing, occasionally hemorrhagic nodules which conglomerate to produce pseudomembranes.
2. The specific diagnosis is pseudomembranous colitis.
3. Following are the points in favor of your diagnosis:
   a. Fever
   b. Severe diarrhea
   c. Relatively mild abdominal pain
   d. Preceding course of antibiotics
4. The other differential diagnoses are:
   a. Ischemic colitis:
      - Much more severe abdominal pain
      - Blood staining with stool
   b. Antibiotic-associated diarrhea:
      - Absence of fever
      - Diarrhea is not severe.
   c. Norovirus infection:
      - Absence of blood in the stool
      - Abdominal pain is not severe.
      - Stool test to detect the presence of *C. difficile* toxin in the stool.
5. The difference in the incidence of females with positive urine analysis with or without long-term catheter:
   a. In absence of catheter, 50% females demonstrate >100,000 bacteria and >10 white blood cells per high power field (HPF) in urine.
   b. In presence of long-term catheter, 80% females demonstrate >100,000 bacteria and >10 white blood cells per HPF in urine.
6. Pathophysiology of this infection: *C. difficile* produces colitis through the production of exotoxin A and B which lead to generation of inflammation in the colonic mucosa, disruption of colonic cytoskeleton and ultimately cellular death. Pseudomembranes is developed due to hyperstimulation of the body's immune system by these toxins thereby drawing the neutrophils to invade the colonic mucosa.
7. Common algorithm to detect glutamate dehydrogenase antigen in the stool by enzyme immunoassay, if positive, then *Clostridium* toxin A and B have to be detected.
8. Criteria of severe *C. difficile* colitis are:
   a. Leukemoid reaction of >35,000/cc
   b. Hypotension
   c. Admission to intensive care units
   d. Elevated serum lactate
   e. Evidence of end organ damage
9. Following are the complications in this disease:
   a. Perforation of colon
   b. Toxic megacolon
   c. Sepsis

CASE 18

An 80-year-old male on wheel chair as a consequence of paraparesis due to lesion in the dorsal spine level fell down on the floor and became bedridden. Within 2 months, he developed pressure sores in the sacral region. This bed sores were dressed properly but its ulcer base was not healed. The patient suddenly developed low-grade fever, anorexia, and increasing pain in the bed sore. After 2 days during dressing the wound, he noticed whitish granular materials coming from the base of the wound.

Laboratory investigation demonstrated neutrophilic leukocytosis, raised ESR, and C-reactive protein (CRP) of 102, and protein electrophoresis demonstrated polyclonal gammopathy.

1. **What is the most likely diagnosis?**
2. **What are the points in favor of your diagnosis?**
3. **Whether straight X-ray of the sacrum is useful or not?**
4. **What should be the specific investigation to be done here?**
5. **Which type of dressing is the best process in this case?**
6. **Why other dressing is not done here?**

Answers

1. The most likely diagnosis is osteomyelitis.
2. Points in favor of this diagnosis are:
   a. Low-grade fever
   b. Neutrophilic leukocytosis
   c. High ESR
   d. High CRP
   e. Polyclonal rise in the immunoglobulins
   f. Delayed healing of the pressure sores
   g. Appearance of the granular materials from the base of the ulcers
3. Straight X-ray of the sacrum can detect the presence of osteomyelitis in advanced case but it cannot detect the extent of osteomyelitis.
4. MRI of the sacrum and pelvis is the best option in this case.
5. Nonadherent deep wound dressing is the best option in this case.
6. Vacuum-assisted dressing can speed up the wound healing in case of proper debridement and appearance of sufficient granulation tissue, but in case of osteomyelitis, this dressing is contraindicated. Occlusion with larval debridement should be done in case of difficult removal of the necrotic tissue. But, this type of dressing should not be done in case of underlying bone infection.

CASE 19

An 80-year-old patient having past history of prostatectomy, hypertension on diuretics came to medical clinic with history of frequent falls and deterioration of memory.

On examination, all the vitals were normal, Mini-Mental State Examination (MMSE) score was 17/30, and AMTS score was 5/10. All the systemic examinations were normal except there was dyspraxia, poor balance and brisk deep tendon reflexes, plantar reflexes flexor, and absence of primitive reflexes.

Cerebrospinal fluid (CSF) features demonstrated opening pressure normal. Protein, chloride, sugar, and WBC were normal. ECG and chest X-ray were normal. CT brain revealed age-related cerebral atrophy. EEG demonstrated as given below:

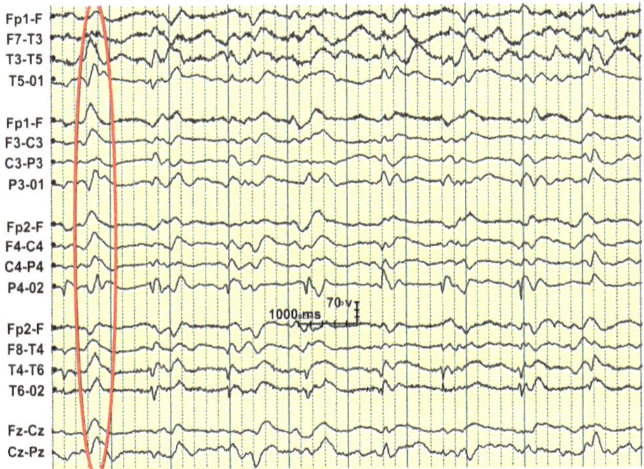

1. **What is the EEG feature?**
2. **What is the most likely diagnosis?**
3. **What are the points in favor of your diagnosis?**
4. **Why it is not NPH?**
5. **Define this disease.**
6. **What are the types of this disease?**
7. **What are the biomarkers in this disease?**

Answers

1. EEG demonstrated bilateral synchronous periodic epileptiform discharges in typical repetitive pattern.
2. The most likely diagnosis is Creutzfeldt–Jakob disease.
3. Points in favor of this diagnosis:
   a. Subacute onset
   b. Mixed cognitive disorders and motor signs
   c. Myoclonic jerk
   d. Specific EEG abnormality
4. This is not a case of NPH because there is absence of:
   a. Gait disorder
   b. Urinary incontinence
   c. Disproportionate enlargement of the ventricles
5. Creutzfeldt–Jakob disease is rare group of fatal transmissible spongiform encephalopathies caused by prion proteins.
6. Following are the types of this disease:
   a. Sporadic type:
      - It is the most common type.
      - It occurs in 85% of cases
      - It occurs spontaneously
      - Age of onset is 55–75 years having median age of 68 years and mean age of 61 years.
      - 90% patient will die within 1 year.
      - Mean duration of survival is 4–8 months.
   b. Familial disease:
      - It occurs in 10% of cases
      - It is the second most common type.
      - There is family history.
      - Genetic mutation test is positive.
      - There is autosomal mutation in *PRNP* gene that encodes prion proteins.
   c. Acquired disease:
      - It is <1% of cases.
      - Mean age is 29 years.
      - Transmission from human or animal to human being.
      - In MRI, there is pulvinar sign.
   d. Bovine spongiform encephalopathy or "mad cow" disease
7. The biomarkers in this disease CSF biomarkers are:
   a. 14-3-3 proteins
   b. Total tau protein
   c. Neuron-specific enolase

CASE 20

An 85-year-old hypertensive man having history of peripheral vascular disease on antihypertensive medication such as lisinopril, calcium channel blockers, and diuretics came to medical clinic with history of falls twice while rising from the chair.

On examination, patient is slightly drowsy, lethargic, disorientated, vitals normal, feet cool, absent pulse in the artery dorsalis pedis in both the feet but both the femoral and popliteal pulses were present. Respiratory system revealed basal crackles in the both bases, and neurological system normal.

Laboratory investigation demonstrated serum urea 110 mg/dL, creatinine 6.2 mg/dL, potassium 6 mmol/L, bicarbonate 14 mmol/L, pH 7.37, PO_2 9.8 kPa, PCO_2 4.1 kPa, and liver function test normal. Chest X-ray demonstrated slight hyperinflation of the chest. 8 weeks earlier serum urea was 35 mg/dL and creatinine was 1.8 mg/dL. Urine was positive for protein.

1. **What is the most likely cause of renal failure?**
2. **Why it is not due to abdominal aortic dissection?**
3. **Is the patient suffering from ESRD?**
4. **What is the most important step in the treatment of this patient?**
5. **What is the cause of falls in this patient?**

Answers

1. The most likely diagnosis is renal arteriosclerosis.
2. This case is not due to abdominal aortic dissection because:
   a. It is usually more catastrophic.
   b. Patient will be anuric.
   c. There will be no time to become acidotic metabolically and no chance of adequate compensation.
3. This patient has not been suffering from ESRD because patient was nearly completely normal 8 weeks ago and his renal function test was normal.
4. Most important step in this case is omission of lisinopril as there will be improvement of the renal function after discontinuation of this drug. Because this drug will reduce the renal plasma flow as well as glomerular filtration rate if the renal artery is normal.
5. As this patient gave history of falls while rising from the chair, he should be suffering from orthostatic hypertension and can be detected by measuring the blood pressure in lying down and also in standing position. Fall also may be due to the antihypertensive drugs.

CASE 21

An 84-year-old diabetic on diabetic diet, hypertensive on thiazide, atorvastatin, and aspirin female came to medical clinic with sudden pain in the left foot and pain in the left index finger.

On examination, all the vitals were normal, plantar fascia was tender, patient's proximal interphalangeal (PIP) joints of left index finger swollen, and tender. All other systems were normal.

Laboratory investigation demonstrated serum glutamic pyruvic transaminase (SGPT) 55 IU/L and white blood cell 5,700/cc.

1. **Mention the differential diagnoses.**
2. **What is the most likely diagnosis?**
3. **Is there any relation of this disease with the drugs the patient taking?**
4. **What causes raised SGPT to slightly upper level of normal?**
5. **Mention the risk factors in this disease in this patient.**
6. **What are the complex interactions in the pathophysiology of gout?**

Answers

1. The differential diagnoses are:
   a. Gout: It occurs due to deposition of uric acid crystals in the PIP joints of left index finger.
   b. Trauma: Here, there is no history of trauma and the female is compos mentis.
   c. Pseudogout: It usually involves large joints like knee and wrist. It does not involve plantar fascia.
   d. HLA-B positive enthesitis: It involves plantar fascia. It is a chronic condition and peak incidence in case of younger people.
   e. Sepsis
   f. Rheumatoid arthritis
   g. Systemic lupus erythematosus (SLE)
   h. Seronegative arthropathy
   i. Postinfective arthropathies
2. The most likely diagnosis is gouty arthritis.
3. The patient is taking thiazide and low-dose aspirin. Both the drugs will reduce the clearance of the uric acid leading to formation of overt gout.
4. The following causes raised SGPT to slightly upper level of normal:
   a. Low-dose aspirin
   b. Statin
   c. Fatty infiltration in the liver
5. Following are the risk factors involved in this disease:
   a. Hypertension
   b. Obesity
   c. Diabetes mellitus
   d. Cardiovascular disease
   e. Medications like thiazide and aspirin
   f. Elderly
6. Following are the complex interactions in the pathophysiology of gout:
   a. Genetic, metabolic as well as other factors will lead to hyperuricemia.
   b. Physiologic, metabolic, and other factors are responsible for formation of monosodium urate monohydrate crystals.
   c. Soluble cellular and innate immune response leading to formation of crystal formation and initiation of inflammatory response.

d. Immune mechanism will lead to resolution of this crystal-induced inflammation.

e. Chronic inflammation, immune cell effects, and effect of crystals on the chondrocytes and osteoblast and osteoclast lead to bony erosion, injury to joint, and tophi formation.

CASE 22

An 85-year-old hypertensive, type II diabetic female having history of mastectomy for treating breast carcinoma and ischemic heart disease was brought to emergency department with head injury following crushing head against the concrete wall.

On examination, blood pressure was 175/100 mm Hg, pulse rate 96 beats/min, irregular, respiratory rate 16 breaths/min with normal breathing pattern, Glasgow Coma scale (GCS) 7/15, and body temperature 94°F. Systemic examinations were normal. Head examination demonstrated laceration in the area of the posterolateral part of the skull.

Laboratory investigation demonstrated total white blood cell count 12,000/cc, hemoglobin 12 mg/dL, electrolytes normal, urea 55 mg/dL, creatinine 1.1 mg/dL, and plasma glucose 296 mg/dL.

1. **Which factors are associated with poor prognosis in this patient?**
2. **What should be the next line of investigation?**
3. **What is the most immediate management in this patient?**
4. **How cold temperature of the body is treated in this patient?**
5. **If the CT scan of brain is normal, what is your diagnosis?**
6. **Which type of head injury is common in this old age?**
7. **Which patient is prognostically better?**

Answers

1. Following factors are associated with the prognosis in this patient:
   a. Glasgow Coma score is associated with the poor prognosis in this patient Low:
   b. Uncontrolled hypertension not responding to the treatment
   c. Diabetic vascular disease not responding to the treatment
   d. New onset atrial fibrillation is also poor prognostic factor because it is associated with:
      • Myocardial infarction
      • Sepsis
      • Pulmonary embolism
2. CT scan of the head should be done in this case to detect intracerebral hemorrhage or any brain contusion.
3. Since the GCS is 7/15, patient requires immediate intubation to prevent aspiration of gastric content and pharyngeal content because the patient may lose gag reflex.
4. To treat the cold body temperature, patient should be covered with blanket with regular measurement of body temperature at hourly interval since the normalization of the temperature.
5. The most probable diagnosis is cerebral concussion. This is not a case of metabolic or respiratory acidosis because the respiratory rate was 16 breaths/min which is very unusual.
6. In the old age, dura mater is adherent firmly with the skull leading to rare incidence of extradural hemorrhage, whereas cerebral atrophy as a consequence of aging of dementia leads to increased venous wall fragility that bridge the subdural space resulting in the increased risk of cerebral hematoma.
7. Following patients are prognostically better:
   a. Good preinjury functional score
   b. Few comorbidities
   c. Absence of dementia
   d. Good renal function

CASE 23

An 80-year-old nondiabetic, nonhypertensive female came to medicine OPD with history of severe tingling of the both lower leg and for that she was sleepless at night and moved to-and-fro to get relief from that leg pain.

Laboratory investigation demonstrated hemoglobin level 8 g/dL, mean corpuscular volume (MCV) 68 fL, and total iron-binding capacity (TIBC) high. Thyroid, renal, and liver function tests were normal.

1. **What is the most likely diagnosis?**
2. **What is the definition of this disease?**
3. **What are the types of the disease?**
4. **What are the medications associated with this disease?**
5. **In which stage of pregnancy it is very common?**
6. **If this disease is under control, what are the signs in favor of the re-emergence or augmentation of this disease?**
7. **What are the nonpharmacological management in this patient?**
8. **What are the drugs can be administered in this disease?**

Answers

1. This feature is consistent with restless leg syndrome.
2. This disease is characterized by irreversible desire to move the legs to get relief from the tingling symptoms.
3. This disease is classified into following types:
   a. Primary or idiopathic
   b. Secondary type:
      - Iron deficiency
      - Diabetes mellitus
      - Chronic renal disease
      - Folate deficiency
      - Magnesium deficiency
      - Peripheral neuropathy
      - Venous insufficiency
      - Celiac disease
      - Amyloidosis
      - Fibromyalgia
4. Following medications are associated with this disease:
   a. Anticonvulsants like phenytoin
   b. Antidepressant like amitriptyline
   c. β-blockers
   d. Histamine-2 antagonists
   e. Lithium
   f. Neuroleptics
   g. Withdrawal from the vasodilators or sedatives
5. During the third stage of pregnancy, this disease is very common.
6. If the disease is under control, following criteria should be met to diagnose the presence of this disease:
   a. Symptoms occur early in the evening
   b. Symptoms are very intense in the morning.
   c. Symptoms will extend to the upper part of the body.
7. Following are the nonpharmacological management in this disease:
   a. Exercise
   b. Sleep hygiene
   c. Massage of the limbs
   d. Hot and cold baths
   e. Electrical stimulation of the feet
   f. Elimination of caffeine in the diet during bedtime
8. Following drugs can be given in this disease:
   a. Pregabalin: This drug is effective up to 1 year.
   b. Ropinirole, pramipexole, and rotigotine: These drugs are effective up to 6 months.
   c. Gabapentin for 1 year
   d. Levodopa for 1 year

CASE 24

An 85-year-old hypertensive female was brought to emergency department with history of progressively increasing drowsiness following fall in her house.

On examination, she was drowsy, afebrile, pulse rate 94 beats/min, regular, blood pressure 160/90 mm Hg, respiratory rate 16 breaths/min, and GCS 12/15. CNS examination revealed right-sided plantar extensor. CT scan of brain demonstrated:

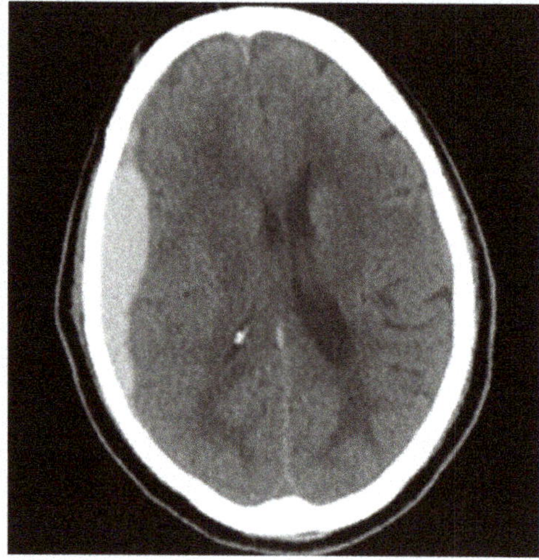

1.   **What is demonstrated in the CT scan of brain?**
2.   **How can you differentiate this disease from subdural hematoma?**
3.   **What are the causes of this disease?**
4.   **How can you classify this disease?**
5.   **How radiologists estimate the amount of hemorrhage in the brain?**
6.   **In which case surgery is required?**

Answers

1.   The above CT scan of brain demonstrated hyperdense shadow seen left side in-between skull and dura mater
2.   Differences between extradural and subdural hematoma:

Extradural hematoma	Subdural hematoma
Biconvex or lenticular shaped	Diffuse or concave shaped
Temporal or temporoparietal region	Entire surface may be involved
Middle meningeal artery is involved.	Tearing of the bridging veins
Classically there is lucid interval	There is underlying brain damage
Outcome depends upon the status of the patient prior to surgery	Prognosis is worse as compared to extradural hematoma

3.   The causes of extradural hematoma:
     a.   Traumatic
     b.   Nontraumatic:
          - Infective
          - Coagulopathy
          - Hemorrhagic
          - Vascular malformation

4.   Classification of extradural hematoma according to radiologic progression:
     a.   Type 1: Acute—it occurs on 1st day associated with "swirl" of the unclotted blood.
     b.   Type 2: Subacute—it occurs between 2nd and 4th day; it is usually solid.
     c.   Type 3: Chronic—it occurs between 7th and 20th day; it is mixed or lucent appearance along with contrast enhancement.

5.   Estimation of amount of blood in the brain in case of hemorrhage:
     a.   Maximum diameter of hemorrhage on the CT slice with largest area of hemorrhage
     b.   Maximum diameter 90° to "a" on the same slice of CT scan
     c.   The number of CT slices with hemorrhage multiplied by the thickness of slice in centimeters

     So the calculation is abc/2.

6.   In following cases, surgery is required:
     a.   Acute extradural hemorrhage
     b.   Hematoma of >30 mL regardless of GCS score.
     c.   GCS of <9 with pupillary abnormalities like anisocoria

CASE 25

A 78-year-old man was taken to physician by his wife because her sleep was disturbed by the frequent episodes of thrashing to her face in most of the nights for last 1 year leading to development of bruises. During this attack, she faced difficulty in awakening him from the sleep. Her husband also told about his vivid dreams during sleep.

On examination, all the vitals were normal. All the systemic examinations were normal; only there was evidence of injury as a consequence of hitting his head against bed.

All the laboratory examinations were normal.

1. **What is the most likely diagnosis?**
2. **How can you define this disease?**
3. **Why it is not nocturnal epilepsy?**
4. **Why it is not a case of restless leg syndrome?**
5. **Why it is not a case of hypnagogic myoclonus?**
6. **What are the systems involved in this disorder?**
7. **What is the line of treatment in this disorder?**
8. **How can you follow-up this patient?**

Answers:

1. The most likely diagnosis is rapid eye movement (REM) sleep behavior disorder.
2. The disease can be defined as violent movements of all the limbs with vocalizations while the patient is dreaming during the phase of REM phase of sleep cycle occurring mostly in male as compared to female with male-to-female ratio of 9:1.
3. Nocturnal epilepsy is not the case because:
   a. The description is typical like that of REM sleep disorder.
   b. Absence of features of generalized epilepsy like tongue biting and incontinence
4. This is not a case of restless leg syndrome because:
   a. Patient is always awake.
   b. There is unusual sensation in the lower limb.
   c. There is irreversible urge to move the legs to get relief from tension.
5. Hypnagogic myoclonus is not a case because:
   a. It occurs in all ages
   b. It occurs in an individual as he or she is drifting into sleep initially.
   c. There are evidences of one or two muscular jerks that may be associated with sensation of falling.
   d. During this time, the patient will awake transiently then fall into sleep.
6. Two systems are involved in this disorder:
   a. Generation of muscle atonia due to active inhibition of neurons in the medulla
   b. Suppression of motor skeletal activity that involves the input from forebrain
7. The first line of treatment in this disorder is 0.5–1 mg clonazepam at night orally.

   Patient with extrapyramidal disorder like Parkinson's disease, Lewy body disease as well as progressive supranuclear palsy will respond to L-dopa or pramipexole.
8. If this patient is a part of Lewy body dementia, follow-up is required to find any sign of:
   a. Parkinsonism
   b. Progressive supranuclear palsy
   c. Multisystem atrophy
   d. Cognitive decline

CASE 26

An 80-year-old man having past history of poor stream of urine was brought to emergency department in drowsy state following several attacks of shivering and hematuria.

On examination, temperature was 101°F, blood pressure 150/90 mm Hg, and pulse rate 112 beats/min. Abdominal examination revealed tender renal angle. Per rectal examination demonstrated large and firm prostate.

Laboratory investigation demonstrated leukocytes 20,000/cc, ESR 34 mm/1st hour, urea 120 mg/dL, and creatinine 4 mg/dL.

1. **What is the most likely diagnosis and why?**
2. **What is the most useful diagnostic test in this case?**
3. **Is prostate-specific antigen (PSA) reliable in this case?**
4. **Is cystoscopy is useful in this case?**

Answers

1. The most likely diagnosis is urinary tract infection. Points in favor of this diagnosis are:
   a. Presented with fever with chill and rigor
   b. High neutrophilic leukocytosis
   c. Feature of obstruction in the lower urinary tract
   d. Renal angle tenderness
   e. Raised ESR due to acute phase response
2. Collection of urine through the catheter is the diagnosis of choice if the patient is unable to pass urine due to prostatic hypertrophy. This urine is sent for microbiological diagnosis.
3. PSA is not reliable in this case because PSA can be very high in case of urinary sepsis.
4. Cystoscopy is not usually done until.
   - Sepsis is controlled.
   - Obstruction will be relieved.

CASE 27

An 87-year-old man came to emergency department with drowsy state. Medical student calls for hypodermoclysis to manage the patient.

1. **What is the procedure he wants to learn?**
2. **What is hypodermoclysis?**
3. **What are the indications of hypodermoclysis?**
4. **What are the contraindications of hypodermoclysis?**

Answers

1. He wants to learn how to set up a subcutaneous infusion
2. Hypodermoclysis is a process of infusion of fluids subcutaneously to hydrate easily in mild to moderately dehydrated adult patients.
3. Indications of hypodermoclysis:
   a. For prevention and treatment of mild to moderately dehydrated patients due to:
      - Poor oral intake
      - Diarrhea
      - Use of diuretics
      - Dysphagia
      - Drowsiness
      - Confusion
      - Difficult to feed enterally or parenterally
   b. In the terminal phase of life:
      - Request of the patient
      - To administer opioid or other analgesics
      - To reduce the symptoms of dry mouth, confusion, or constipation
4. Contraindications of hypodermoclysis:
   a. In case of fluid overload
   b. In bleeding disorders
   c. Shock
   d. Circulatory failure
   e. Severe dehydration

CASE 28

An 82-year-old woman having past history of total hip replacement 8 years ago came to emergency department with history of headache, exertional dyspnea, increased tiredness, and low back pain.

On examination, patient was pale. Vitals were normal. All the systems were normal, except the spine revealed tenderness at L2 level and few areas in the skull tender.

Laboratory investigation demonstrated hemoglobin 8.3 g/dL, white blood cell count 4,000/cc, and platelet count 110,000/cc, ESR 100 mm/1st hour, urea 177 mg/dL, creatinine 3.8 mg/dL, alkaline phosphatase 250 U/L, and blood viscosity 1.92 mPa/s. X-ray of skull demonstrated:

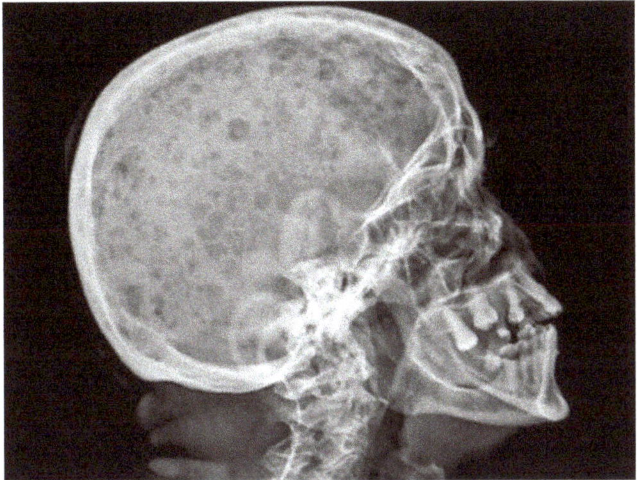

1. **What is the finding in the above X-ray?**
2. **What is the most likely diagnosis?**
3. **What is the result of hypercalcemia ion in this patient?**
4. **What is the effect of renal failure?**
5. **What is the cause of anemia in this patient?**
6. **What is the result of bony lesions in this patient?**
7. **What is the National Comprehensive Cancer Network guideline regarding the laboratory studies in this disease?**
8. **What are the differential diagnoses in this case?**
9. **What are the complication in this disease?**

Answers

1. The above lateral view of the skull of X-ray demonstrated multiple punched-out appearances in the skull.
2. The most likely diagnosis is multiple myeloma.
3. Hypercalcemia will lead to:
   a. Increased thirst and urination
   b. Bone pain
   c. Abdominal pain
   d. Nausea and vomiting
   e. Mental status
4. Renal failure results:
   a. Edema
   b. Acidosis
   c. Electrolyte disturbances
5. Anemia results from:
   a. Replacement of the bone marrow by the plasma cells
   b. Decreased formation of erythropoietin

6. Bony lesion results:
   a. Pathological fracture
   b. Vertebral collapse
   c. Reduced height
   d. Compression of the spinal cord
   e. Radicular pain
   f. Kyphosis
7. National Comprehensive Cancer Network guideline regarding the laboratory studies in this disease are as follows:
   a. Complete blood count, differential count, and platelet count
   b. Blood urea nitrogen, creatinine, electrolyte, albumin, and calcium
   c. Serum lactate dehydrogenase and $\beta 2$ microglobulin
   d. Serum immunoglobulin, serum protein electrophoresis, and serum immunofixation electrophoresis

e. 24 hours proteinuria, urine protein electrophoresis, and urine immunofixation electrophoresis
f. Assay of serum free light chain
g. Whole body low-dose CT scan
h. Aspiration and biopsy of bone marrow and/or flow cytometry including cytogenetics
i. Fluorescence in situ hybridization (FISH) of plasma cells

8. Following are the differential diagnoses and they can be excluded by following:
   a. Monoclonal gammopathy of undetermined significance:
      - Serum monoclonal protein of <3 g/dL
      - Clonal bone marrow cells <10%
      - No evidence of end organ damage
   b. Smoldering multiple myeloma:
      - Serum monoclonal protein of ≥3 g/dL
      - Clonal bone marrow cells between 10 and 59%
      - No evidence of end organ damage
   c. Solitary plasmacytoma:
      - Normal bone marrow
      - Solitary lesions made up of clonal plasma cells
      - No end organ damage
      - Negative image outside of the single lesions
   d. Waldenstrom macroglobulinemia:
      - Lymphoplasmacytic lymphoma that can be noted in the bone marrow
      - M protein is IgM. It is unusual in multiple myeloma
      - Presence of MYD88L265P
      - Following symptoms occur:
        - Peripheral neuropathy
        - Lymphadenopathy
        - Anemia
        - Hepatosplenomegaly

9. Complications in this disease are:
   a. Common complications:
      - Hypercalcemia
      - Renal insufficiency
      - Infection
      - Skeletal lesions
      - Anemia
   b. Less common complications:
      - Venous thromboembolism
      - Hyperviscosity syndrome

CASE 29

An 80-year-old female having past history of rheumatoid arthritis leading to gross deformity of the small joints of hands and feet on methotrexate weekly and daily folic acid and replacement of the deformed stenosed mitral valve by Austin Moore prosthesis came to medical outdoor with an ulcer on the leg.

On examination, her vitals were normal. All the peripheral pulses were palpable. Cardiological examination revealed prosthetic first heart sound and second heart sound normal. No splenomegaly on examination of abdomen. Musculoskeletal examination demonstrated deformed PIP joints of hand and effusion of the right knee joint.

Laboratory examination revealed total white blood cell count 5,000/cc, hemoglobin 11 g/dL, double-stranded deoxyribonucleic acid (DSDNA) positive, antinuclear antibody (ANA) positive, and CRP 50 mg/L. Leg ulcer demonstrated:

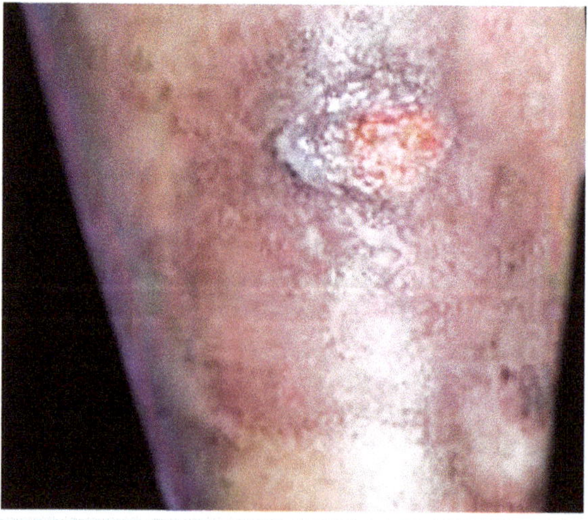

1. **What is the ulcer seen in the leg?**
2. **Why it is not a case of venous insufficiency?**
3. **Why it is not a case of cellulitis?**
4. **Why it is not thromboembolic disease?**
5. **Mention the diagnostic criteria in this disease.**
6. **What are the syndromes associated with this ulcer?**
7. **What are the drugs used in this disease?**

Answers

1. This ulcer has slightly scalloped edge with deep basal slough and inflamed rim surrounding the ulcer. So, this is case of pyoderma gangrenosum.
2. As there is no history of venous insufficiency and the mode of onset is not slow, hence, it does not support the venous insufficiency.
3. This ulcer is not accompanied by:
   a. Extensive area of cutaneous erythema
   b. Fever
   c. High white blood cell count
4. It is not a sequela of thromboembolic disease because all the peripheral pulses are palpable and extremities are warm.
5. Diagnostic criteria in this disease are:
   a. Major criteria:
      - Rapid progression of a painful necrolytic cutaneous ulcer with irregular violaceous as well as undetermined border
      - Other causes of cutaneous ulceration have been excluded.
   b. Minor criteria:
      - History suggestive of pathology or cribriform scarring
      - Systemic diseases associated with pyoderma gangrenosum
      - Histopathology demonstrated:
         ○ Sterile dermal neutrophilia
         ○ Mixed inflammation
         ○ Lymphocytic vasculitis
      - Response to treatment with steroids

   Two major and any two minor criteria can confirm the diagnosis.
6. Following syndromes are associated with this ulcer, i.e., pyoderma gangrenosum:
   a. PAPA syndrome: It includes pyoderma gangrenosum, acne, pyogenic sterile arthritis.
   b. PASH syndrome: It includes pyoderma gangrenosum, acne, and hidradenitis suppurativa.
7. Following drugs are used in this case:
   a. Systemic corticosteroids
   b. Azathioprine
   c. Anti-TNF-α drugs:
      - Etanercept
      - Adalimumab
   d. Anti-interleukin-12/23 inhibitor: Ustekinumab
   e. Interleukin-1β monoclonal antibody: Canakinumab
   f. Anti-interleukin-6 monoclonal antibody: Tocilizumab

CASE 30

A 78-year-old female came to medicine outdoor with palpitation, weakness, vertigo, and tinnitus. On examination, there was pallor and pulse rate 110 beats/min.

Laboratory examination demonstrated hemoglobin 6 g/dL and stool for occult blood test positive. The colonoscopy was advised and demonstrated:

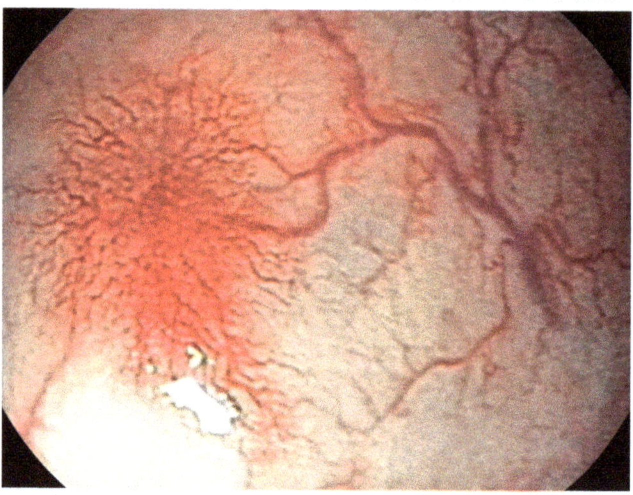

1. **What is the finding in the colonoscopy?**
2. **What is this disease?**
3. **How it is formed?**
4. **How it can be diagnosed radiologically?**
5. **What are the endoscopic therapies in this disease?**

Answers

1. The colonoscopy demonstrated dilated blood vessels in the mucous membrane in the colon.
2. This disease is characterized by stretching as well as dilatation of the blood vessels leading to loss of blood in the wall of colon. It may also present in the stomach.
3. It is formed as a result of rhythmic contraction of the colon leading to stretching of the wall of the blood vessels resulting in formation of the arteriovenous malformation, which ultimately form angiodysplasia.
4. Radionuclide scanning can detect bleeding up to 0.1–0.5 mL/min. There are two types of scanning:
   a. Tc-99m pertechnetate autologous red blood cell
   b. Technetium sulfur colloid
5. Following are the endoscopic therapies in this disease:
   a. Argon plasma coagulation ablation
   b. Electrocoagulation
   c. Endoscopic clip and band ligation
   d. Injection sclerotherapy

CASE 31

An 80-year-old man having no family history of tremor came to medical outdoor with difficulty in the movement of his right shoulder without any relief and writing difficulty.

On examination, the face is masked face, slowness in movement, and cogwheel rigidity. He was taking 125 mg Madopar thrice daily, but after taking drugs the patient developed involuntary movement involving face and hands.

1. **Why it is not benign or thyrotoxic tremor?**
2. **Why it is not cerebellar tremor?**
3. **Why the shoulder pain will occur?**

4. **What are the risk factors of shoulder stiffness?**
5. **What are the conditions mimicking shoulder pain?**
6. **What is the staging of shoulder pain?**
7. **What are the complications in this joint disease?**
8. **What are the best options of treatment in this patient?**
9. **What are the types of drug-induced abnormal movement of upper limbs and face?**
10. **Describe UK Parkinson's disease Brain Bank criteria.**

Answers

1. This patient developed tremor of right hand whereas thyrotoxic tremor or benign tremor is always bilateral tremor.
2. It is not cerebellar tremor because it is not associated with vertigo.
3. Parkinson's disease is associated with frozen shoulder.
4. Following are the risk factors of frozen shoulder:
    a. Diabetes
    b. Thyroid cause
    c. Surgery to shoulder
    d. Trauma to shoulder
    e. Open heart surgery
    f. Menopause
    g. Cervical disease in the neck
5. Following conditions mimicking frozen shoulder pain:
    a. Poststroke subluxations of shoulder
    b. Subacromial pathology
    c. Rotator cuff tendinopathy
    d. Referred pain like Pancoast tumor
6. Staging of frozen shoulder:
    a. Stage 1: Freezing in 2–9 months—early stage. This is painful phase which will be worse at night with gradual restriction of movement at the glenohumeral joint.
    b. Stage 2: Frozen in 4–12 months. There is stiffness with persisted restriction of the movement and less pain in the glenohumeral joint.
    c. Stage 3: Thawing in 12–42 months. This is recovery phase when there is gradual return of motion around the joint.
7. The complications of this frozen shoulder:
    a. Residual pain
    b. Residual stiffness
    c. Fracture of humerus
    d. Rupture of the tendon of biceps during manipulation of shoulder

8. Treatment should be delayed until there is functional impairment and the drug of choice is levodopa along with peripheral decarboxylase inhibitor. Contralateral thalamotomy should be done in patient whose tremor is refractory to drug therapy.
9. There are three types of drug-induced dyskinesia:
    a. Beginning-of-dose dyskinesia: If the patient starts high dose too frequently.
    b. Peak-dose dyskinesia: It occurs when the blood level of this drug is highest.
    c. Off-period dyskinesia: This movement occurs when the plasma level of this drug will be lowest.
10. UK Parkinson's disease criteria for Parkinson's disease:
    a. Bradykinesia plus any one of the following:
        - Rigidity
        - Resting tremor
        - Disordered posture, balance, and gait
    b. None of the following:
        - Recent exposure to neuroleptic, toxin, or drug
        - Past history of oculogyric crisis or encephalitis
        - Stepwise strong progression
        - Cerebellar signs or pyramidal signs
        - Severe autonomic failure
        - Supranuclear paralysis of downward gaze
        - Cerebellar or frontal lobe tumors
        - Communicating hydrocephalus
    c. Clinical signs that can differentiate idiopathic parkinsonism from parkinsonian disorders:
        - Asymmetric onset of parkinsonism
        - Good response to levodopa and development of dyskinesia
        - Oculomotor and pyramidal signs are absent.
        - Early memory disturbances are absent. Hallucination and confusional episodes are unrelated to treatment.
        - Early postural disability and falls

CASE 32

A 75-year-old having history of carcinoma of rectum with metastasis into the liver already admitted in the ward suddenly developed massive bleeding per rectum.

On examination, patient became collapsed, pulse thread, and blood pressure 80/50 mm Hg.

1. **What is your next action for the patient?**
2. **The patient died in spite of the treatment. What will be the next course of action?**
3. **Name seven points when coroner should be informed in case of death of the patient.**

Answers

1. As this is the terminal illness, so attempting to recover the patient from this symptom is not justified and it will not be successful, because this bleeding is of arterial origin. So, the aim should be to sedate the patient by administering intravenous midazolam to relieve from distress in the last moment of life.

2. This patient should not require to refer to coroner court as the cause of the hemorrhage is from rectal cancer. It should be the duty of the doctor to attend the patient during his last illness and to issue the certificate of death. The death certificate should not be issued by the doctor who is not present during the last illness. In case of any doubt in the issuing death certificate, in that case he or she can discuss with the coroner's office.

3. Following are the seven circumstances when coroner should be informed:
   a. Unknown cause of death
   b. Patient was admitted in dead condition or died within 24 hours of admission.
   c. If death occurs within 24 hours of operation or after administration of anesthetic drugs.
   d. If the attending doctor has not seen him or her within 14 hours of death.
   e. Traumatic death or alleged traumatic death
   f. Suicide or suspected suicide
   g. Death from criminal action or in suspicious circumstances.

CASE 33

An 80-year-old nonsmoker, nondiabetic, and nonhypertensive man with prior history of recurrent urinary tract infection relieved by proper culture-specific antibiotics came to medical outdoor with complaint of dorsal back pain not responding to paracetamol, weight loss, anorexia, and occasional hematuria for last 2 months.

On examination, there was pallor, pulse rate 102 beats/min, regular, blood pressure 135/80 mm Hg, afebrile, respiratory rate 16 breaths/min, and no lymphadenopathy. All the systemic examinations were normal except there was tenderness in the sacral and D6 region.

Laboratory investigation revealed hemoglobin 9 g/dL, total white blood cell count 6,500/cc, urea 95 mg/dL, creatinine 1.5 mg/dL, alkaline phosphatase 220 IU/L, and corrected calcium 13.5 mg/dL. Straight X-ray of the spine demonstrated:

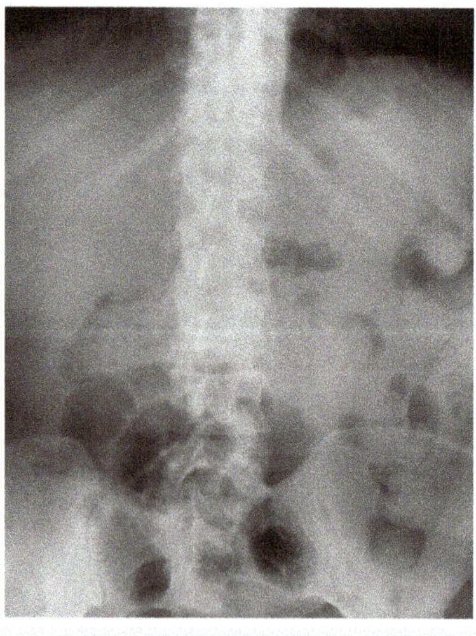

1. **What is shown in the above X-ray?**
2. **What is the most likely diagnosis?**
3. **Why alkaline phosphatase has been increased?**
4. **Is there are requirement of estimation of serum aluminum?**
5. **Why the serum levels of urea and creatinine have been raised?**
6. **Is there any chance of cure of hypercalcemia in this case by calcitonin?**
7. **Why there is anemia in this case?**
8. **What is Gleason's pattern of this disease?**

Answers

1. The above straight X-ray of the spine demonstrated extensive sclerosis of the spine.
2. This patient has been suffering from carcinoma prostate as he has:
   a. Dysuria
   b. Hematuria
   c. Extensive sclerosis of the vertebrae
3. Alkaline phosphatase has been increased here as it has been released from the vertebrae and there is significant dysfunction in the liver function test.
4. If there is any suspicion of drinking the water contaminated with aluminum, in that case serum aluminum is required.
5. As the patient has been suffering from anorexia, hence he was reluctant to drink. So, obviously this patient has been suffering from prerenal azotemia thereby serum urea and creatinine have been raised. Again hypercalcemia exacerbates the dehydration.
6. Calcitonin can be given in this case, but the dose of calcitonin that is required to reduce the serum level of calcium in this hypercalcemia due to malignancy. It may lead to undesirable side effects. Hence, there is reason to start this drug in this case.
7. Here, there is anemia in this case due to following causes:
   a. Direct suppression of the bone marrow by the malignant deposits
   b. Indirect suppression of the bone marrow in the context of extensive malignancy
8. Gleason's pattern of prostate cancer:
   a. Grade 1: Small and uniform glands
   b. Grade 2: Presence of more stroma between the glands
   c. Grade 3: Distinctly infiltrative margins
   d. Grade 4: Irregular masses of neoplastic glands
   e. Grade 5: Only occasional gland formation

CASE 34

A 75-year-old hypertensive male was found on the floor by his son and was taken to emergency department.

In the emergency department during examination, he was found conscious, pulse rate 100 beats/min, and blood pressure 150/95 mm Hg. Neurological examination demonstrated left-sided hemiparesis along with left-sided homonymous hemianopia. CT scan of brain demonstrated:

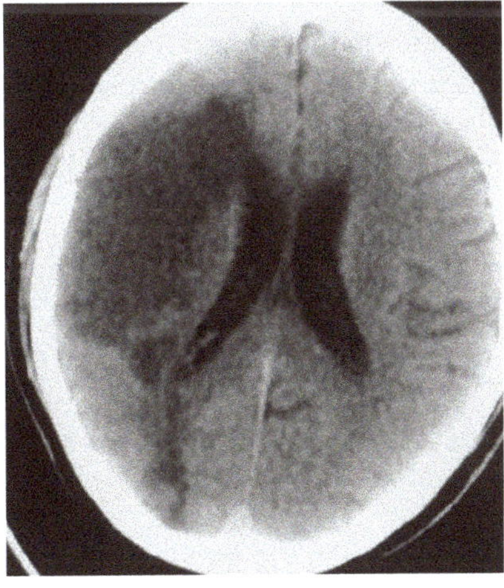

1. **What is demonstrated in the above CT scan of brain?**
2. **What is your diagnosis?**
3. **How can you classify this disease?**

Answers

1. Above CT scan brain demonstrated hypodense lesion in the left cerebral hemisphere in the middle cerebral artery territory with shifting of the midline to the left with perilesional edema.
2. This patient has been suffering from right-sided hemiparesis due to left cerebral infarction in the left middle cerebral artery territory.
3. Classification of stroke according to Bamford:

Type of infarct	Diagnosis
Cerebral infarction	If a CT scan performed within 28 days of symptom, onset shows an area of low attenuation, no relevant abnormality, or an area of irregular high attenuation within a larger area of low attenuation (i.e., an area of hemorrhagic infarction) or, If a necropsy examination shows an area of cerebral infarction (pale or hemorrhagic) in a region compatible with the clinical signs and symptoms
Lacunarinfarct (LACI)	One of the four classic clinical lacunar syndromes. Patients with faciobrachial or brachiocrural deficits are included, but more restricted deficits are not

Continued

Continued

Type of infarct	Diagnosis
Total anterior circulation infarct (TACI)	Combination of new higher cerebral dysfunction (e.g., dysphasia, dyscalculia, and visuospatial disorders), homonymous visual field defect, and ipsilateral motor and/or sensory deficit of at least two areas of the face, arm, and leg. If the conscious level is impaired and formal testing of higher cerebral function or the visual fields is not possible, a deficit is assumed
Partial anterior circulation infarct (PACI)	Only two of the three components of the TACI syndrome, with higher dysfunction alone, or with a motor/sensory deficit more restricted than those classified as LACI (e.g., confined to one limb, or to the face and hand but not the whole arm)
Posterior circulation infarct (POCI)	Any of the following: ipsilateral cranial nerve palsy with contralateral motor and/or sensory deficit, bilateral motor and/or sensory deficit, disorder of conjugate eye movement, cerebellar dysfunction without ipsilateral long-tract deficit (i.e., ataxic hemiparesis), or isolated homonymous visual field defect

(OCSP: Oxfordshire Community Stroke Project)

CASE 35

An 85-year-old hypertensive on digoxin and aspirin, smoker having 40 packs-year came to medical outdoor with complaint of severe pain in the feet and inability to walk.

On examination, pulse rate was 70 beats/min, irregularly irregular, blood pressure 160/90 mm Hg. Cardiovascular and respiratory examinations were normal. Abdominal examination revealed an expansile mass. All the peripheral pulses were normal. Arterial brachio-pedal index in the left was 0.92 and 0.95 on the right.

Laboratory investigation demonstrated total white blood cell count of 11,000/cc, eosinophil count 1,100/cc, ESR 70 mm/1st hour, urea 95 mg/dL, and D-dimer 0.8 mg/L.

Abdominal ultrasound demonstrated the evidence of infra-renal abdominal aortic aneurysm.

Left feet demonstrated:

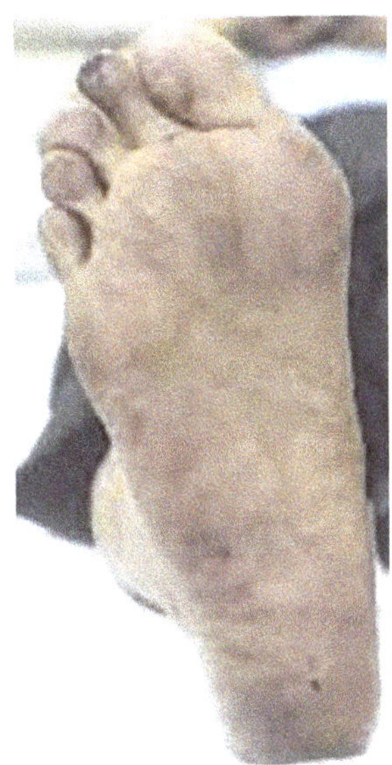

1. **What is shown in the figure?**
2. **What is your diagnosis with points in favor of this diagnosis?**
3. **What are the risk factors in this disease?**
4. **What is the definite diagnosis in this disease?**
5. **What is the pathophysiology of this disease?**
6. **What is the prognosis in this disease?**
7. **What are the dermatological manifestations in this disease?**

Answers

1. There is evidence of gangrene of the right second toe.
2. The diagnosis is cholesterol crystal embolism. Points in favor of this diagnosis are:
   a. Sudden onset of obstruction of the small vessels
   b. Presence of peripheral pulses
3. Following are the risk factors in this disease:
   a. Male sex
   b. Hypertension
   c. Diabetes mellitus
   d. Peripheral vascular disease
   e. Atherosclerosis of the ascending aorta
   f. Advanced age
   g. Renal failure
   h. Patient undergoing interventional vascular procedure
   i. Cardiovascular surgery
4. The diagnosis is confirmed by biopsy of the arterioles which demonstrate:
   a. Presence of cholesterol crystals spaces because the crystals will be dissolved at the time of preparation.
   b. Presence of spindle-shaped cleft surrounded by hyperplastic intimal tissue as well as giant cells.

5. Pathophysiology of this disease:

Spontaneous, traumatic or iatrogenic rupture of the plaques in the aorta or its branches
↓
Plaque containing cholesterol, fibrin-calcified debris, and platelet will lodge into medium and small size arteries
↓
Mechanical occlusion of these arteries
↓
Inflammation due to deposition of the foreign body, recruitment of leukocytes, and activation of compliment
↓
End organ damage

6. The prognosis in this disease is very poor, but it will depend upon the sites of plaques whether it is above or below the origin of renal artery.
   a. If it is above the origin of renal artery, there will be invariably renal failure leading to high mortality.
   b. If it is below the origin of renal artery, the prognosis is better. There may be gangrene of the toe.
   c. But overall prognosis is bad because once plaque rupture, there is chance of further rupture of the plaque.

7. Following are the dermatological manifestations in this disease:
   a. Retiform purpura
   b. Blue or purple toe
   c. Ulcers
   d. Gangrene
   e. Livedo reticularis
   f. Small nail bed infarct
   g. Pain in the foot and toe

CASE 36

A 75-year-old diabetic woman long-term resident of Africa came to medical outdoor with chief complaint of foul-smelling stool floating in the pan, weight loss, and postprandial abdominal pain for several months.

Laboratory investigation demonstrated hemoglobin 9 g/dL, MCV 105 fL, leukocyte count 10,000/cc, and lipase 150 IU/L. Plain straight X-ray of abdomen demonstrated:

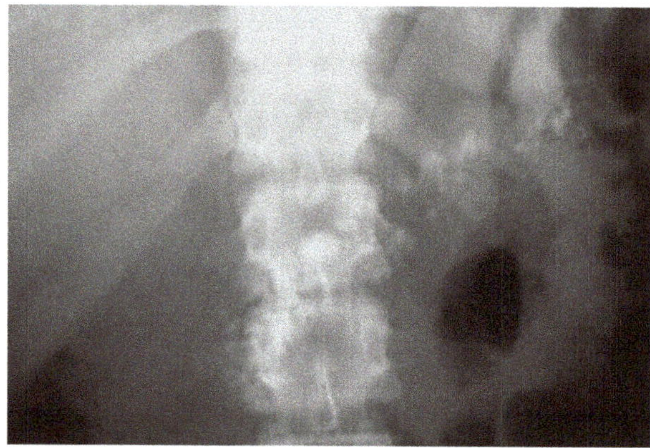

1. **What has been demonstrated in the above picture?**
2. **What is your diagnosis?**
3. **What is the most common cause of this disease?**
4. **What is the pathophysiology regarding this disease?**
5. **What is the current guideline regarding the diagnosis of chronic pancreatitis?**

Answers

1. Straight X-ray of abdomen demonstrated presence of calcifications throughout the region of pancreas.
2. The diagnosis is chronic calcific pancreatitis.
3. The most common cause of chronic pancreatitis is alcohol consumption. Alcohol increases protein secretion from the acinar cells to make the fluid more viscus which may lead to ductal obstruction resulting in acinar fibrosis followed by atrophy.
4. There are several theories in the development of chronic pancreatitis.
   a. According to one theory, failure of increased secretion of bicarbonate in response to increased secretion of proteins from the acini. These abundant proteins ultimately combine to block the pancreatic duct.
   b. Activation of the intraparenchymal enzymes within pancreatic gland
   c. Diminished ability of the pancreatic cells to respond to calcium signaling leading to alteration of feedback mechanism resulting in promotion of another cycle and thereby cellular death.
5. Current guideline to assess the pancreas:
   a. CT scan of abdomen is the ideal test for assessing the morphology of the pancreas.
   b. CT scan of abdomen is done to exclude the other pathologies.
   c. When CT scan is abnormal, magnetic resonance cholangiopancreatography (MRCP) should be done.
   d. Secretion stimulated MRCP should be done to detect any subtle changes in the pancreatic duct and can help in assessing of the ductal compliance as well as exocrine function.
   e. Endoscopic ultrasound should be done to assess the ductal and parenchymal changes in early course.

CASE 37

A 90-year-old completely housebound female having past history of fall leading to fracture of the right femur came to medical outdoor with complaint of decreased mobility and generalized body aches. She used to live alone.

On examination, the vitals were normal, abdomen, and central nervous system normal. Chest wall was tender. There was weakness of the proximal muscles of upper limb but not tender. The patient was given steroid but without any relief.

Laboratory investigation demonstrated ESR 34 mm/1st hour, urea 78 mg/dL, creatinine 4 mg/dL, corrected calcium 1.7 mg/dL, and alkaline phosphatase 250 U/L.

1. **What are the differential diagnoses?**
2. **How can you exclude all the differential diagnoses to come into conclusion?**
3. **What is the treatment in this patient?**
4. **What are the newly proposed criteria in the diagnosis of this disease?**

Answers

1. The differential diagnoses are:
   a. Osteomalacia
   b. Polymyalgia rheumatic
   c. Polymyositis
   d. Multiple myeloma
2. The process of exclusion:
   a. Osteomalacia:
      - Elderly female
      - Frail and housebound state
      - Low corrected calcium in the blood
      - Muscles are weak but not tender
      - High serum alkaline phosphatase
   b. Polymyalgia rheumatic—it is not the diagnosis because:
      - ESR is not high.
      - Failure to respond to corticosteroids
      - Serum alkaline phosphatase should not be very high.
      - Corrected calcium should not be very high.
   c. Polymyositis is not the diagnosis because:
      - Muscle is not tender.
      - High ESR is absent.
      - Creatine phosphokinase (CPK) level is not increased.
   d. Multiple myeloma is not the diagnosis because:
      - ESR is not high.
      - Serum corrected calcium is low.
3. The treatment is vitamin D3 60 k once weekly for 12 weeks followed by calcium vitamin D3 combination. If the patient has malabsorption syndrome or chronic liver disease or hypoparathyroidism, higher dose of vitamin D is required to maintain normocalcemia.
4. Newly proposed criteria in absence of liver and kidney diseases:
   a. Elevated parathormone level
   b. Elevated level of alkaline phosphatase
   c. Low level of urinary calcium
   d. Low intake of calcium of <300 mg daily or low calcidiol level of <30 nmol/L

CHAPTER 7

Hemato-Oncology

A 70-year-old male admitted in the medicine department with nocturia, polyuria, and abdominal pain. On examination, there was anemia and a nodule on the abdomen. His laboratory investigations demonstrated hemoglobin 7.5 g/dL, platelet count 100,000/cc, white blood cell 5,000/cc, creatinine 10 mg/dL, calcium 14.5 mg/dL, total protein 12 g/dL, and uric acid 7 mg/dL. Bone marrow demonstrated:

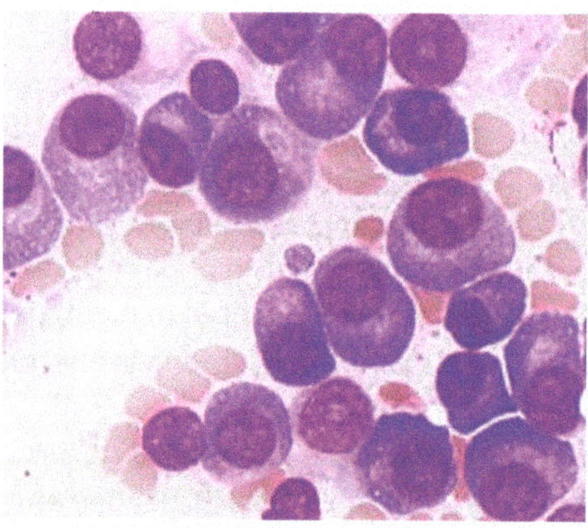 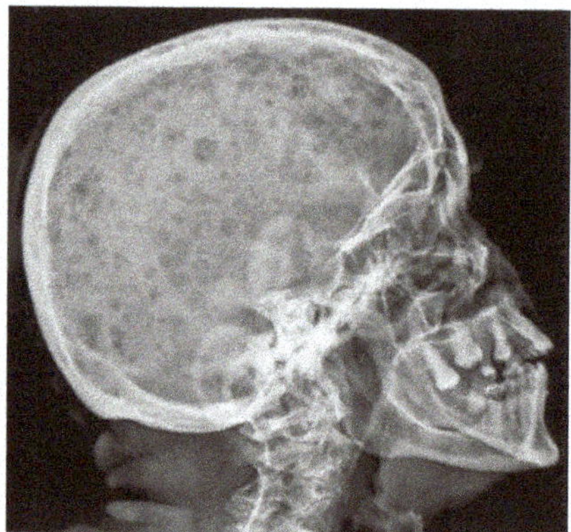

1. What has been shown in the above pictures?
2. What does the blood picture demonstrate?
3. What is your diagnosis?
4. What is the cause of the nodule in the patient's body?
5. Define the pentad in this disease?
6. What is the demographic incidence in this disease?
7. What are the predisposing factors in this disease?
8. What are the different criteria in this disease?
9. What are the causes of anemia in this disease?
10. What are the common organisms responsible for recurrent infection in this disease?
11. What are the causes of increased bleeding tendency in this disease?
12. What are the causes of renal failure in this disease?
13. What are the different types of cells found in this disease?
14. In the bone marrow trephine biopsy, what are the patterns of this abnormal cells found?
15. What are the panels used for detecting these abnormal cells clone in the flow cytometry?
16. What are the prognostic factors that lower survival in this disease?

17. **What are the diseases in which the plasma cells rich inflammatory infiltrate seen?**
18. **What are International Staging System Criteria in this disease?**
19. **Mention the causes of death in this disease.**
20. **What are the conditions when should we think of this disease?**
21. **What are the tests for Bence Jones protein in urine?**
22. **What are the value of free light chain in this disease?**
23. **What Hevylite assay?**
24. **What are the importance of cytogenetics in this disease?**

Answers

1. The above pictures demonstrate:
   a. In the bone marrow: Sheets of plasma cells which looks like normal plasma cells having eccentric nucleus containing "spoke wheel"-like chromatin and deeply basophilic cytoplasm and perinuclear halo.
   b. Multiple punched-out lesion throughout the skull indicating lytic lesions.
2. Blood picture demonstrates:
   a. Anemia
   b. Thrombocytopenia
   c. High creatinine indicating renal failure
   d. Hypercalcemia
   e. High protein
3. This patient has been suffering from multiple myeloma.
4. The nodule is developed as a result of plasma cells infiltration.
5. Following are the pentad of multiple myeloma:
   a. Presence of monoclonal protein in the serum and/or urine
   b. Anemia
   c. Hypercalcemia
   d. Lytic lesions in the bone and/or bone pain
   e. Renal failure
6. Following are the demographic incidences in this disease:
   a. Age: This disease occurs in middle-aged or elderly patients.
   b. Sex: Males are more commonly affected as compared to females.
   c. Race: This disease is more common African-American as compared to Caucasians.
   d. Familial: This disease is more common in person having incidence of this disease in the first-degree relatives.

7. Predisposing factors are the following:
   a. Radiation exposure:
      - It is more common in Japanese atomic bomb survivors.
      - It is two times more common in radiologists as compared to physicians.
      - Persons with diagnostic or therapeutic X-ray exposures.
   b. Exposures to:
      - Herbicides
      - Pesticides
      - Metal industries
   c. Chronic stimulation with antigen in the immune system in:
      - Various infections
      - Inflammations
      - Connective tissue disorders
   d. Viral infections:
      - HIV
      - Hepatitis C
      - Herpes virus 8
8. Different criteria in this spectrum of this disease are the following:
   a. Monoclonal gammopathy of undetermined significance:
      - Myeloma protein: <3 g/dL
      - Bone marrow: Monoclonal plasmacytosis <10%
      - No evidence of other B cell malignancy
      - Absence of myeloma-related end organ disease
   b. Smoldering multiple myeloma:
      - Clonal plasmacytosis: >10% but <60%
      - Absence of disease-related symptoms in the host:
        ○ Absence of anemia
        ○ Absence of hypercalcemia

- ○ No bone disease
- ○ Absence of renal insufficiency
  - c. Symptomatic multiple myeloma:
    - Myeloma protein in the serum protein and/or urine
    - Plasmacytoma
    - Hypercalcemia
    - Anemia
    - Lytic bone lesion
    - Hyperviscosity
    - Amyloidosis
    - Infections

9. Following are the causes of anemia in this disease:
   a. Normal hematopoietic cells will be replaced by the plasma cells.
   b. Overactive cytokines like interleukin-1 and tumor necrosis factor-α inhibit erythropoiesis
   c. Bleeding
   d. Kidney damage leading to decreased production of erythropoietin
   e. Increased apoptosis of the erythropoietic cells by the FAS ligand

10. Following common organisms are responsible for the infections in this patient:
    a. *Staphylococcus aureus*
    b. *Streptococcus pneumoniae*
    c. *Haemophilus influenzae*
    d. Gram-negative *Escherichia coli*

11. Following are the causes of increased bleeding tendency in this disease:
    a. Infiltration of the bone marrow by the plasma cells
    b. Uremia
    c. Hyperviscosity
    d. Abnormal protein

12. Following are the causes of renal failure in this disease:
    a. Deposition of Bence Jones protein in the glomerular basement membrane as well as tubular basement membrane
    b. Hypercalcemia leads to nephrocalcinosis
    c. Dehydration
    d. Hyperuricemia
    e. AL type amyloid deposits
    f. Filtration of light chain protein through the glomerulus
    g. Acute or chronic pyelonephritis
    h. Use of nephrotoxic drugs
    i. Infiltration of myeloma cells in streaks or nodules

13. Following are the different types of cells found in this disease:
    a. Flame cells seen commonly in immunoglobulin A (IgA) myeloma
    b. Mott cells or Morula cells in grape-like accmulation
    c. Russel bodies: It is found in the form of cherry red refractile round bodies made of synthesized immunoglobulins.
    d. Dutcher bodies can be found after periodic acid–Schiff (PAS) staining.
    e. Gaucher-like cells
    f. Presence of crystalline rods in the cytoplasm

14. Following pattern of plasma cells are found in the bone marrow trephine biopsy:
    a. Nodular or broadband type
    b. Diffuse fully packed marrow which will replace the normal hematopoietic cells.
    c. Presence of interstitial with or without paratrabecular seams of the plasma cells

15. Following are the panels used for detecting these abnormal cells clone in the flow cytometry:
    a. CD19
    b. CD45
    c. CD38
    d. CD138
    e. CD56
    f. Cytoplasmic κ and λ

16. Following are the prognstic factors that lower survival in this disease:
    a. β_2 microglobulin level >5.5 mg/L due to increased burden of tumor
    b. Increased secretion of λ light chain
    c. Elevated level of lactate dehydrogenase
    d. High level of C-reactive protein (CRP)
    e. Serum albumin level of <3.5 g/dL
    f. Plasmablastic morphology
    g. Plasma cells labeling index is >1%.
    h. High degree of plasma cell infiltration in the bone marrow
    i. Increased number of cytogenic anormalities, e.g., t(4:14), t(14;16), t(14,20), etc.
    j. CD28, CD44 positive, and CD56.

17. Following are the diseases in which reactive plasma cells rich inflammatory infiltrate seen:
    a. Chronic osteomyelitis
    b. Cholesteatoma
    c. Nasal polyp

18. International staging system criteria:
    a. Stage I:
        - β_2 microglobulin <3.5 mg/L
        - Serum albumin level of ≥3.5 g/dL
    b. Stage II:
        - Neither stage I and stage III. Two criteria for stage II:
            i. Serum β_2 microglobulin <3.5 mg/L but serum albumin <3.5 g/L
                Or,
            ii. Serum β_2 microglobulin 3.5–5.5 mg/L irrespective of serum albumin
    c. Stage III: Serum β_2 microglobulin >5.5 mg/L
19. Causes of death in this disease are the following:
    a. Recurrent bacterial or fungal infections
    b. Renal failure
    c. Acute leukemia
    d. Myelodysplastic syndrome
    e. Hemorrhage
20. In case of following symptoms, one should think of multiple myeloma in a patient:
    a. History of backache with signs of paraplegia
    b. Anemia of obscure reason
    c. Pathological fracture
    d. Unexplained bone pain
    e. Involvement of multiple vertebrae
    f. Features of chronic renal disease
    g. Unexplained high erythrocyte sedimentation rate (ESR)
    h. Presence of Bence Jones protein in the urine
21. If the urine of the patient is allowed to heat to 55–60°C, there is evidence of cloudy precipitate, but if the temperature of the urine is increased to 90°C. The precipitate will disappear. This test is very sensitive because only 0.3 mg/mL of this potein can be detected.
22. The normal value of free κ is 3.3–19.4 mg/L and free λ level is 5.7–26.3 mg/L and normal ratio of κ/λ is 0.26–1.65.
23. Hevylite assay can measure the intact immunoglobulin, i.e., serum heave plus isotype light chain as well as concentration of each subtype of immunoglobulin, i.e., IgGκ, IgGλ, IgAκ, IgAλ, IgMκ, and IgMλ.
24. Importance of cytogenetics in this disease are:
    a. The most common translocation in the chromosome is in the heavy chain locus on the chromosome number 14q32. It is found in the 55% of cases.
    b. In 50% cases, there is partial deletion of chromosome 13 and it has adverse prognosis.
    c. The patient with t(4;14) and t(14;16) has worst prognosis.

CASE 2

A 45-year-old man came to medical clinic with abdominal pain and loose motion for 6–8 times/day along with rectal bleeding for 3 months. Patient is pale and generalized abdominal tenderness.

Hematological report demonstrated hemoglobin 8 g/dL, mean corpuscular volume (MCV) 105 fL, and platelet count 100,000/cc. His colonoscopy demonstrated:

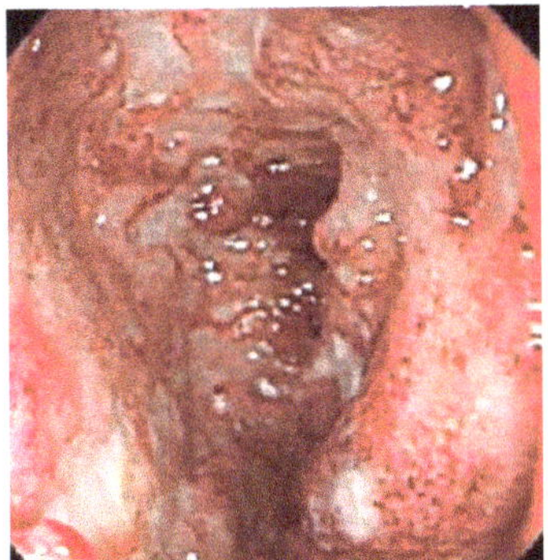
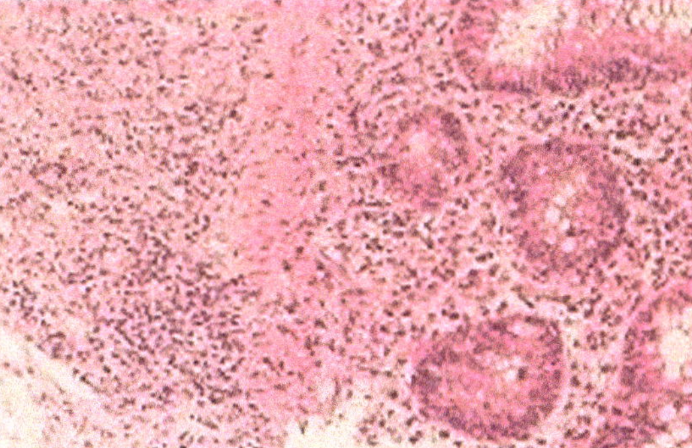
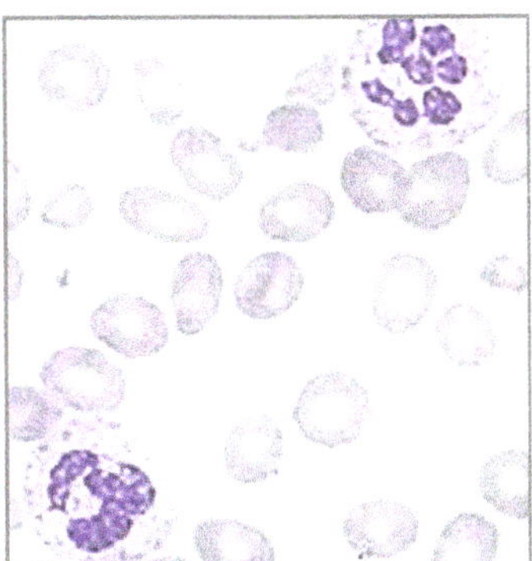

1. **What is shown in the colonoscopy?**
2. **What is the histologic feature in the biopsy specimen from ulcers in the colon?**
3. **Describe the peripheral blood picture in this patient?**
4. **What is your diagnosis?**
5. **How can you classify macrocytosis?**
6. **How can you define this disease?**
7. **What is the significance of transcobalamin in relation to this vitamin?**
8. **What are the intestinal causes of this disease?**
9. **What are the drugs producing this disease?**
10. **Which step in the biochemical reaction is interrupted by this vitamin deficiency?**
11. **What is methyl trap hypothesis and how can it be aggravated?**
12. **Which characteristic feature in the peripheral blood is suggestive of this vitamin deficiency?**
13. **What are the neurological manifestations in this vitamin deficiency and how it can be aggravated?**
14. **What are the features of peripheral blood picture other than macrocytosis?**
15. **How can this vitamin assayed in the serum?**
16. **Which is the early marker of this vitamin deficiency in the serum?**
17. **Which is the very sensitive marker that can be measured both in the serum and urine?**
18. **What are the conditions where homocysteine level will be increased in serum?**
19. **What are the hematological responses to therapy following this vitamin administration?**
20. **Which defect will not return to normal inspite of vitamin B12 therapy?**

Answers

1. Colonoscopy demonstrates deep ulcers with cobble-stoning appearances with narrowing of the lumen in the ascending colon.
2. Histology from the area of ulcer demonstrates infiltration of the inflammatory cells in the lamina propriya and the submucosa along with the presence of cryptic abscesses.
3. Peripheral blood picture demonstrates ovalomacrocytosis of the red blood cells and hypersegmented neutrophils.
4. This patient has been suffering from megaloblastic anemia in case of Crohn's disease.
5. Macrocytosis of the red blood cells can be subdivided into two types:
   i. Megaloblastic, where there is presence of both macrocytes and macro-ovalocytes:
      - Vitamin B12 deficiency
      - Folate deficiency
      - Cytotoxic drugs interfering with the synthesis of neucleic acids
      - Drugs interfering with the metabolism of folate:
        ○ Methotrexate
        ○ Primidone
        ○ Phenobarbitone
        ○ Phenytoin
      - Type I and II dyserythropoietic anemia
      - Erythroleukemia
      - Myelodysplastic syndrome
   ii. Nonmegaloblastic, i.e., round ovalocytes:
      - Hemolytic anemia
      - Hemorrhagic anemia
      - Liver disease
      - Aplastic anemia
      - Hypothyroidism
      - Alcohol toxicity
6. Megaloblastic anemia can be defined as macrocytic normochromic peripheral blood picture with megaloblastic bone marrow due to the defective DNA synthesis resulting from vitamin B12 deficiency.
7. Transcobalamin I (haptocorrin) derived from granulocytes binds firmly with cobalamin and release it slowly to the tissues. Transcobalamin II (holotranscobalamin) being synthesized in the liver less firmly bound to cobalamin thereby will release this into the tissue.
8. Intestinal causes of vitamin B12 deficiency:
   a. Tropical sprue
   b. Celiac disease

c. Ileal resection

d. Crohn's disease

e. Bacterial overgrowth:
- Diverticulitis
- Blind loop syndrome

f. Low pH in the intestine: Zollinger–Ellison syndrome

9. Following drugs interfere with the absorption of cobalamin:

a. Colchicine

b. Alcohol

c. Metformin

d. Neomycin

e. Para-aminosalicylic acid

10. During the formation of methionine from homocysteine by methionine synthetase using cobalamin where methyltetrahydrofolate acts as methyl group donor and tetrahydrofolate is formed. This tetrahydrofolate is converted into 5,10-methylenetetrahydrofolate which in turn converts deoxyuridine monophosphate to deoxythymidine monophosphate for DNA synthesis and 5,10-methylenetetrahydrofolate itself will be converted to dihydrofolate. Deficiency of cobalamin inactivate the methionine synthatase resulting in accumulation of the methyltetrahydrofolate as it will not be converted into tetrahydrofolate, thereby folate will be unavailable for the synthesis of DNA.

11. During the formation of methionine from homocysteine by methionine synthetase using cobalamin where methyltetrahydrofolate acts as methyl group donor and tetrahydrofolate is formed. This tetrahydrofolate is converted into 5,10-methylenetetrahydrofolate which in turn converts deoxyuridine monophosphate to deoxythymidine monophosphate for DNA synthesis and 5,10-methylenetetrahydrofolate itself will be converted to dihydrofolate. Deficiency of cobalamin inactivate the methionine synthatase resulting in accumulation of the methyltetrahydrofolate as it will not be converted into tetrahydrofolate, thereby folate will be unavailable for the synthesis of DNA. This is known as methyl trap hypothesis.

    S-adenosyl methionine inhibits synthesis of methyltetrahydrofolate, so the deficiency of S-adenosyl methionine leads to increased synthesis of methyltetrahydrofolate thereby aggavating the methyl trap.

12. Peripheral blood picture demonstrates:

a. Macrocytes

b. Anisocytosis

c. Giant hypersegmented neutrophil having five or more lobes in >5% neutrophils—it is earliest sign of megaloblastic anemia.

13. Neurological manifestations in this disease are the following:

a. Subacute combined degeneration of the spinal cord involving:
- Posterior column leading to loss of joint sense, vibration sense, and ataxia
- Lateral column leading to development of spastic paraplegia

b. Features of peripheral neuropathy characterized by:
- Pain and needles in the distal extremities
- Cold extremities
- Numbness in the gloves and stocking distribution

14. Features other than macrocytes seen in the peripheral blood picture are the following:

a. Basophilic stippling

b. Multiple Howell–Jolly bodies

c. Cabot's ring

d. Sieve-like appearance of megaloblast due to presence of open fine chromatin

15. Vitamin B12 can be assayed in the serum by the following methods:

a. Microbiological assay

b. Radioactive B12 assay
- Radioisotopes dilution method
- Radioimmunoassay

c. Competitive protein binding assay with:
- Chemiluminescence system
- Fluorescence detection system

16. Serum holotranscobalamin II which is the active fraction of plasma cobalamin is more specific and early marker of vitamin B12 deficiency.

17. As vitamin B12 deficiency decreases the conversion of methylmalonate to succinate, hence there is increased level of methylmalonic acid in the serm and urine.

18. In the following conditions, there is increased level of plasma homocysteine:

a. Vitamin B12 deficiency

b. Folate deficiency

c. Renal failure

    d. Hypothyroidism

    e. Genetic polymorphism

19. Following are the hematological responses during therapy:

    a. On the third day to fourth day, there will be reticulocytosis with peak on seventh day.

    b. Normoblastic erythropoiesis by 24–48 hours

    c. White blood cell count and platelet count will come to normal level within a week.

    d. By 12th to 14th day hypersegmented neutrophil will disappear.

    e. Within 48 hours serum iron level comes to normal.

    f. Within 1–2 weeks serum lactate dehydrogenase comes to normal

    g. Within few days serum level of methylmalonic acid and homocysteine will come to normal.

    h. Neurological manifestations will return to normal gradually

20. Only atrophic changes in the stomach mucosa will not return to normal, hence chance of gastric cancer will remain.

CASE 3

A 45-year-old man came to medical clinic with abdominal pain for 3 months. Patient is pale and generalized abdominal tenderness.

Hematological report demonstrated hemoglobin 8 g/dL, MCV 105 fL, and platelet count 100,000/cc. Upper gastrointestinal endoscopy demonstrated as below. Peripheral blood picture also showed as below:

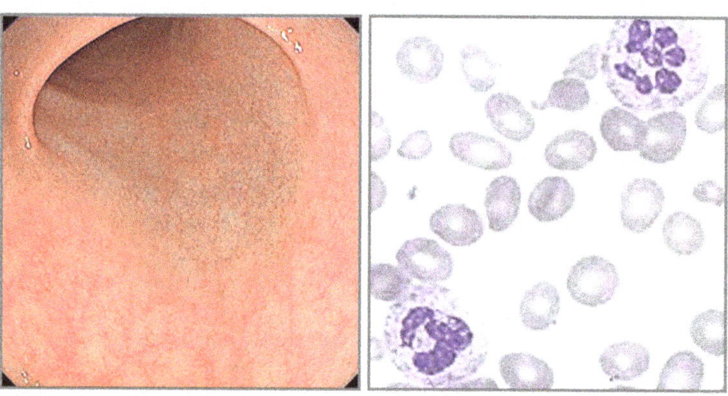

1. **What is shown in the above pictures?**
2. **What is your diagnosis?**
3. **What are the demographic characteristics of this disease?**
4. **What is the main pathology in this disease?**
5. **What are the other diseases associated with this condition?**
6. **What are the organ changes seen in this disease?**
7. **What are the autoantibodies specific for this disease?**
8. **Which specific test can differentiate the etiologies of the vitamin deficiency?**

Answers

1. The above pictures show:

    a. Endoscopy of stomach demonstrates atrophic shining mucosa with increased vascularity suggestive of chronic atrophic gastritis

    b. Peripheral blood picture demonstrates ovalo-macrocytosis of the red blood cells and hyper-segmented neutrophils

2. The definite diagnosis is pernicious anemia leading to megaloblastic anemia.

3. Following are the demographic characteristics of this disease:

    a. It is seen in Scandinavian and European countries.

    b. It occurs in fifth decade of life

    c. It is more common in females.

4. Pathophysiology of this disease:

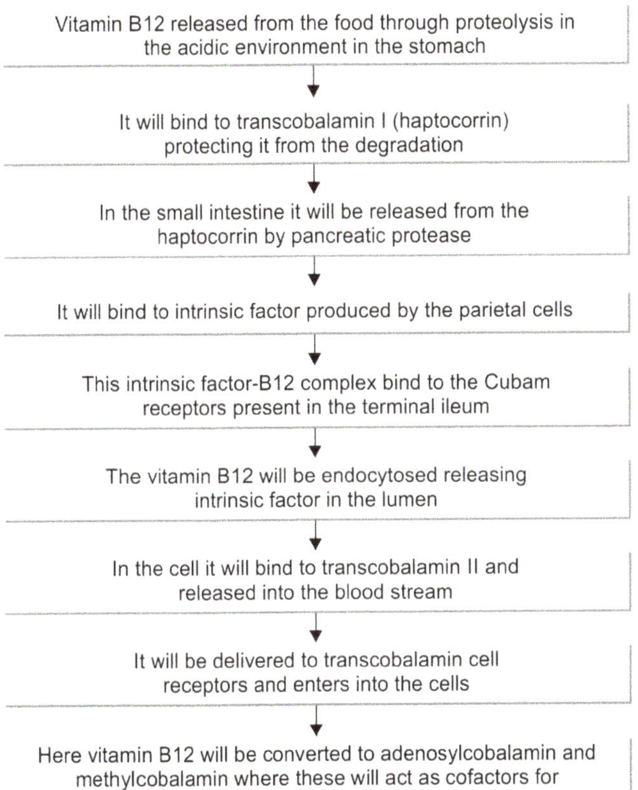

5. Following are the diseases associated with this condition:
   a. Type 1 diabetes mellitus
   b. Autoimmune thyroid disease
   c. Vitiligo
   d. Hypoadrenalism
   e. Myasthenia gravis
6. Following are the organ changes in this disease:
   a. Shiny, glazed, and beefy tongue indicating atrophic glossitis
   b. Atrophic gastritis
   c. Subacute combined degeneration of the spinal cord
7. Following are the autoantibodies specific for the pernicious anemia:
   a. Type 1 blocking antibodies interfering with the binding of intrinsic factor with the vitamin B12. It is present both in gastric juice and plasma.
   b. Type II blocking antibodies which attach with:
      • Intrinsic factor
      • Vitamin B12—intrinsic factor complex
   c. Parietal canalicular antibodies—it is related to gastric mucosa.
8. Schilling test: It can differentiate the etiology which may be intrinsic factor deficiency or intestinal malabsorption.
   a. After administration of radioactive vitamin B12 if the 24 hours urinary excretion of less than the administered dose, it is due to deficiency of intrinsic factor.
   b. If the test is repeated with high amount of intrinsic factors, and the amount to be excreted in 24 hours is less than 1% of administered dose, it may be due to ileal lesion.

CASE 4

A 40-year-aged female came to medical clinic with history of fatigability, weakness, pallor and bruising, and spiking fever. Complete blood count demonstrated hemoglobin 7.8 g/dL and total white blood cell count 38,500/cc. Bone marrow picture demonstrated:

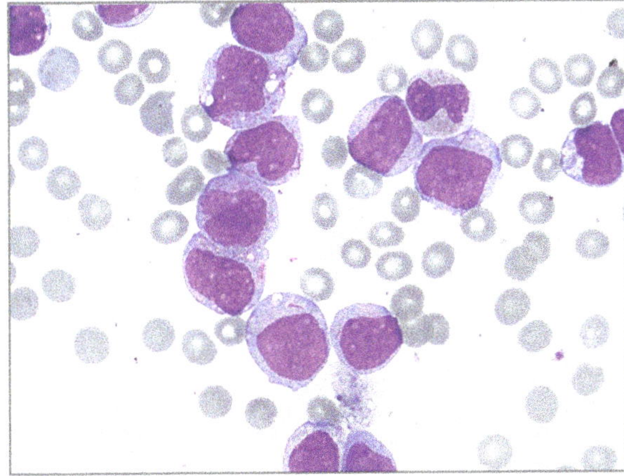
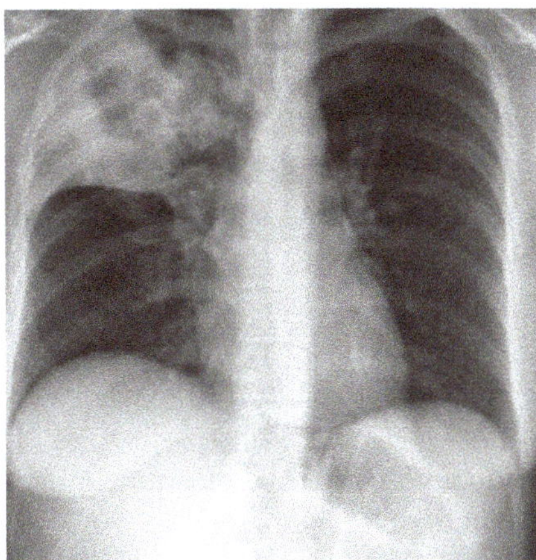

1. What has been shown in the bone marrow biopsy?
2. What is shown in the chest X-ray?
3. What is the definite diagnosis?
4. What is the most likely cause of fever?
5. What are the types of maturation occurring in this disease?
6. What are the hereditary risk factors for developing this disease?
7. Classify this disease.
8. What is the significance of cytochemistry in this disease?
9. What is the significance of myeloperoxidase in these cells?
10. What is the significance of esterase in this disease?
11. Describe the characteristic feature of chloroma?
12. Why coagulation tests are done in this disease?
13. Which serum enzyme is specifically elevated?
14. What are the clinical prognostic factors in this disease?
15. How can you treat this disease?
16. What are the criteria for complete remission?
17. What are the principles of therapy in this disease?
18. What do you mean by minimal residual disease?

Answers

1. Bone marrow picture demonstrates primitive leukemic cells having Auer rods—diagnostic of acute leukemia.
2. Anteroposterior (AP) view of chest X-ray demonstrates pneumonic consolidation involving right upper zone with central cavitation suggestive of staphylococcal pneumonia.
3. This patient has been suffering from acute myeloid leukemia.
4. The most likely cause of fever in this case is due to pneumonic consolidation.
5. There are two types of mutations seen in this disease:
   a. Mutations involving ability of the hematopoietic cells to proliferate like BCR-ABL and FLT3.
   b. Mutations preventing the maturation of the hematopoietic cells like PML-RARA, RUNX1, RUNX1T1, and MLL.
6. Following are the hereditary risk factors for developing acute leukemia:
   a. Down syndrome
   b. Bloom syndrome
   c. Fanconi syndrome
7. According to World Health Organization (WHO) classification in 2016:
   a. Acute myeloid leukemia with recurrent genetic abnormalities
   b. Acute myeloid leukemia with myelodysplasia-related changes
   c. Therapy-related acute myeloid leukemia
   d. Acute myeloid leukemia not otherwise categorized
   e. Myeloid sarcoma
   f. Myeloid proliferations related to Down syndrome
   g. Blastic plasmacytoid dendritic cell neoplasm
   h. Acute leukemia of ambiguous lineage

   According to FRENCH, AMERICAN, and BRITISH classification (FAB classification):
   a. M0: Acute myeloid leukemia with minimal differentiation
   b. M1: Acute myeloid leukemia without maturation
   c. M2: Acute myeloid leukemia with maturation
   d. M3: Acute promyelocytic leukemia
   e. M4: Acute myelomonocytic leukemia
   f. M5:
      • Acute monoblastic leukemia—M5a
      • Acute monocytic leukemia—M5b
   g. M6: Acute erythroid leukemia
   h. M7: Acute megakaryocytic leukemia
8. Significance of cytochemistry in this disease: Various lipids, enzymes, and different substances present in the cytoplasm of the hematopoietic cells for:
   a. Differentiation lymphoblasts from myeloblasts
   b. Differentiation of different subtypes of acute myeloid leukemia
   c. Detection of the enzyme deficiencies in the myeloid cells

9. Significance of myeloperoxidase in this disease: This enzyme is present in the primary granules in the neutrophil which is cyanide resistant and eosinophilic granules which is cyanide sensitive. It is absent in the primitive myeloblasts but as the cells become mature toward the stage of promyelocyte the myeloperoxidase become positive.

10. Significance of esterases in this disease: There are two groups of leukocyte esterases:
    a. Specific esterase stained specifically with naphthol AS-D chloroacetate
    b. Nonspecific esterase stained α-naphthyl acetate esterase

11. Characteristic features of chloroma are the following:
    a. The name appears from its green appearance due to myeloperoxidase. It may occur:
        - At the time of diagnosis
        - It may occur prior to diagnosis of acute myeloid leukemia
        - It will represent acute blastic transformation of myelodysplastic syndrome or chronic myeloid leukemia.
        - It occurs as an extramedullary relapse in the treated cases of acute myeloid leukemia.

12. Following coagulation tests should be performed in this disease:
    a. Prothrombin time
    b. Activated partial thromboplastin time
    c. D-dimer
    d. Fibrinogen level

13. Serum lactate dehydrogenase and serum lysozyme will be raised in M4 and M5 varieties of acute myeloid leukemia.

14. Following are the prognostic factors in this disease:
    a. Age
    b. Acute myeloid leukemia arising from myelodysplastic syndrome
    c. Treatment-related acute myeloid leukemia
    d. Performance status
    e. Extramedullary disease
    f. Comorbidities

15. Treatment in this condition:
    a. Combination of 100–200 mg/m^2 cytarabine intravenous infusion for 7 days along with 3 days of 60–90 mg/m^2 daunorubicin or idarubicin as induction therapy. But, addition of etoposide along with the above induction therapy can improve the survival.
    b. For preventing relapse high-dose cytarabine with or without allogenic hematopoietic stem cell transplantation
    c. Maintenance therapy includes:
        - Immunotherapy
        - Demethylating agents
        - Targeted therapy
    d. Consolidation therapy includes 2–3 mg/m^2 twice daily on day 1, 3, and 5.

16. Following are the criteria for complete remission:
    a. <5% of blast cells in normocellular bone marrow
    b. Return of peripheral blood count to normal:
        - Neutrophil >1,500/cc
        - Platelet >100,000/cc
        - Hemoglobin level >10 g/dL
    c. Disappearance of signs and symptoms

17. Principles of therapy in acute myeloid leukemia are:
    a. In case of t(8;21), induction therapy followed by consolidation therapy
    b. In case of t(15;17), all-trans retinoic acid (ATRA) and induction therapy which are followed by consolidation therapy.
    c. In case of inv(16) or t(16;16)
    d. Unfavorable cytogenic abnormalities: Aggressive therapies and hematopoietic stem cell transplantation in the first remission.

18. Minimal residual disease is a type of disease which cannot be detected by conventional light microscopy of the blood as well as bone marrow postremission induction chemotherapy. It can be diagnosed by various modern technique by following criteria:
    a. 1 blast cell in 20 normal cells for morphology
    b. 1 in 10^2 for cytogenetics
    c. 1 in 10^4 to 10^5 for flow cytometry
    d. 1 in 10^6 for polymerase chain reaction

CASE 5

A 45-year-old male presented in the medical clinic with history of fatigue, weakness, recurrent infections, and bleeding from the nose and severe swelling with pain in the calf muscles. On examination, there is pallor, and the calf demonstrated as below. Peripheral blood picture demonstrated as below:

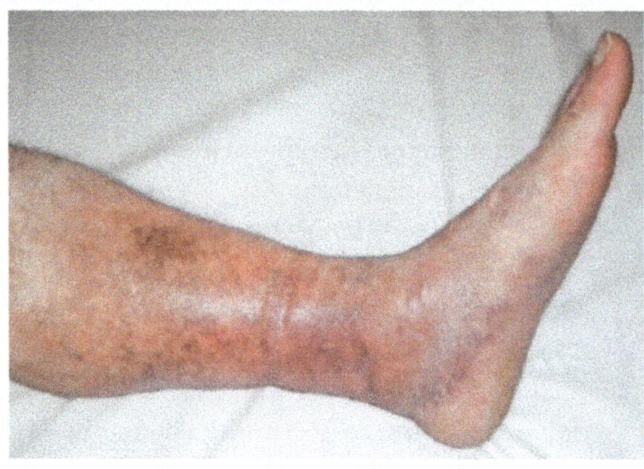 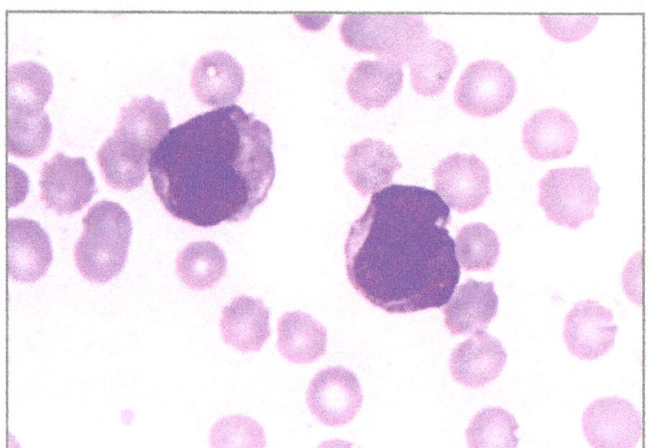

1. **What is shown in the above pictures?**
2. **What is your diagnosis?**
3. **What is the specific immunohistochemical feature in this disease?**
4. **What is the genetic basis of this disease?**
5. **What are the other cytogenic abnormalities found in this disease?**
6. **What are the risk factors in this disease?**
7. **What is the pathophysiology in this disease?**
8. **What is the typical description of the cell in this disease?**
9. **What is the coagulation workup to be done in this disease?**
10. **How can this specific type be classified?**
11. **How can you treat this disease?**
12. **What are the supportive therapies given to this patient?**
13. **What are the drug-induced toxicities in this patient?**
14. **What are the complications possible in this case?**

Answers

1. Above pictures demonstrate:
   a. Diffusely erythematous swelling of the left calf muscle suggestive of deep venous thrombosis
   b. Peripheral blood picture demonstrates promyelocyte with Auer rods
2. This patient has been suffering from acute promyelocytic leukemia.
3. These promyelocytic cells are:
   a. Negative for HLA-DR and CD34
   b. Positive for CD33 and CD13

4. In 95% of cases, there is balanced translocation between 15 and 17.
5. Other cytogenetic abnormalities are the following:
   a. t(5;17)(q35;q21) fuse RARα with nucleophosmin
   b. t(11;17)(q23,q21) fuse RARα with promyelocytic leukemia zinc finger
   c. t(11;17)(q13;q21) fuse RARα with nuclear mitotic apparatus
   d. t(17,17)(11;q21) fuse RARα with *STAT5b* genes
6. Following are the risk factors:
   a. Chemotherapy
   b. Ionizing radiation

c. Industrial solvents

d. Other toxic agents

7. Pathophysiology in this disease:

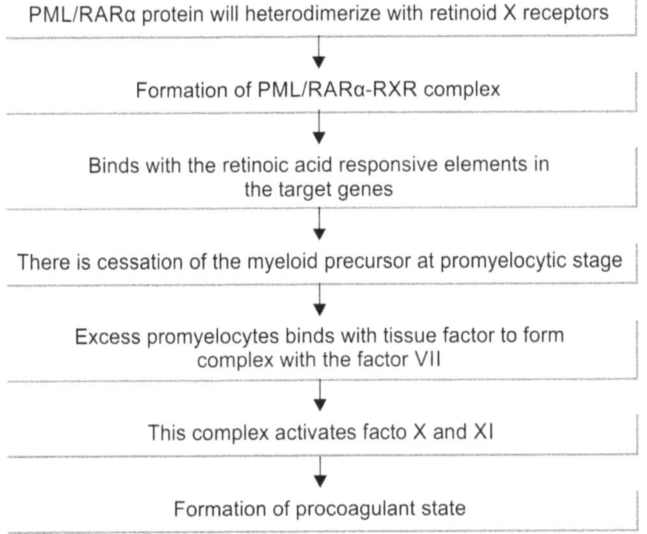

8. The typical description of the promyelocytic cell:

a. The nuclei in the promyelocytic cell are increased, bilobed, folded, kidney-shaped, or dumbbell shaped.

b. High nucleus-cytoplasmic ratio

c. Fine chromatin

d. Prominent nucleoli

e. Violet granules in the cytoplasm

f. Intense myeloperoxidase activity

g. In the microgranular variant less prominent Auer rods and pellets

9. Following coagulopathy workup should be done in this disease:

a. Platelet count

b. Prothrombin time

c. Activated partial thromboplastin time

d. D-dimer

e. Fibrin split products

f. Fibrinogen estimation

10. Acute promyelocytic leukemia can be classified into following types:

a. Low risk: White blood cell ≤ 10,000/cc and platelet count ≥ 40,000/cc

b. Intermediate risk: White blood cell ≤ 10,000/cc and platelet count ≤ 40,000/cc

c. High risk: White blood cell > 10,000/cc

11. All-trans retinoic acid is the mainstay of treatment and it should be started even before the cytogenic

confirmation. The cure rate can be increased by administering this drug along with anthracycline derivatives.

- Arsenic trioxide by dissociating the PML/RARα-RXR complex from the target gene increases the differentiation of the malignant cells clone. ATRA along with arsenic trioxide should be used for induction and consolidation in case of low and intermediate risk PML patients.

- ATRA along with arsenic oxide with gemtuzumab ozogamicin should be used in case of high-risk patient in absence of cardiac dysfunction. Maintenance therapy is not required for those patients who already received induction and consolidation treatment.

12. Following supportive therapies are required:

a. In patients with history of coagulopathy should be treated to maintain fibrinogen level >150 mg/mL with administration of cryoprecipitate and fresh frozen plasma.

b. Platelet should be maintained above 50,000/cc by platelet transfusion.

c. In case of granulocytopenia with fever, empirical antibiotic should be administered to treat gram-negative bacteria.

d. In case of suspected catheter-related infection vancomycin should be given.

e. If the fever persists for >5 days even after commencement of antibiotic therapy, antifungal drug should be started.

13. Following are the retinoic acid derivatives induced toxicities may occur in this patient is benign intracranial hypertension which is characterized by:

a. Headache

b. Increased intracranial pressure

c. Papilledema

d. Improves with lumbar puncture

14. Possible complications in this case are the following:

a. Differentiation syndrome or cytokine release syndrome after commencement of differentiating agent and it is characterized by the following features:

- Fever

- Peripheral edema

- Pulmonary edema

- Hypoxemia

- Pleural or pericardial effusion

- Multiorgan dysfunction

- White blood cell count of >10,000/cc

This can be treated urgently by intravenous dexamethasone 10 mg twice daily.

b. Hyperleukocytosis due to administration of the differentiating agents resulting in rapid differen-

tiation of the immature promyelocytes. It is treated by systemic steroids.

c. ECG monitoring for measuring QT interval in case of arsenic trioxide therapy.

CASE 6

A 55-year-old female came to surgical clinic with a breast mass along with the pain in the bone. Blood biochemistry demonstrated hypercalcemia. The picture of breast mass, picture of peripheral blood, and bone marrow aspirates under microscope:

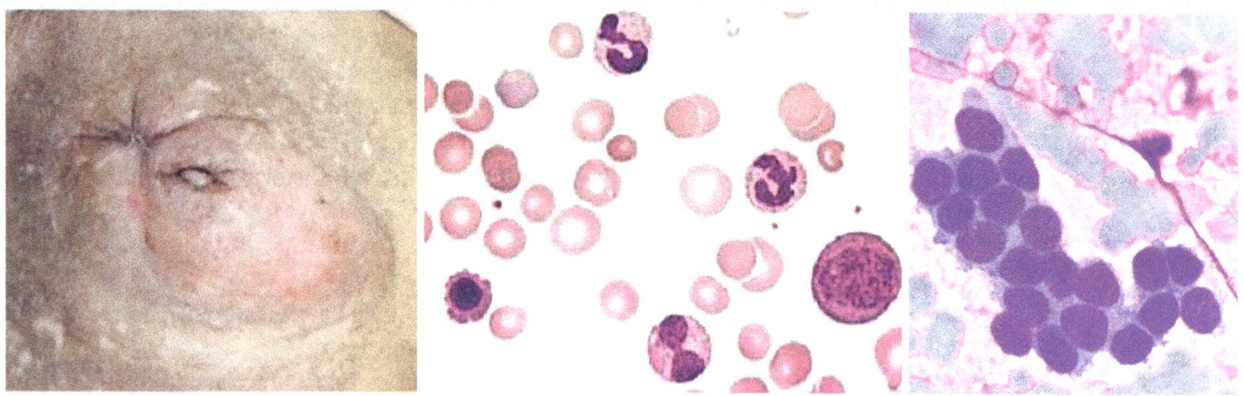

1. **What are the pictures described above?**
2. **What are the causes of bone pain?**
3. **What is your diagnosis?**
4. **Which can confirm the infiltration of the marrow?**
5. **What is the importance of immunohistochemistry in this disease?**
6. **What are the risk factors for this disease?**
7. **What is the age-wise incidence rate in this disease?**
8. **Which gene is involved in this disease?**
9. **How can you divide this disease histologically?**
10. **What further tests should be done in this case?**
11. **What are the basic principles of treatment in this disease?**
12. **What is the role of radiotherapy in this disease?**
13. **How can you stage this disease and in which stage this case will fall?**
14. **What are the complications of this disease based on different types of treatment?**
15. **How can you follow-up this patient?**

Answers

1. Description of the above pictures:
   a. There is fungating mass involving the left breast. Tumor is looking like peau d'orange in appearance.
   b. Peripheral blood picture demonstrates immature myeloid cells along with erythroblast in the peripheral blood.
   c. Bone marrow aspirates showed solid nests of tumor cells containing hyperchromatic nuclei.
2. Bone pain is due to infiltration of the bone marrow with tumor cells.
3. This patient has been suffering from stage four breast carcinoma having secondaries in the bone marrow.
4. Trephine biopsy can confirm the diagnosis of bone marrow infiltration.

5. Immunohistochemistry is useful for confirmation of the origin of the infiltrating cells, i.e., epithelial cells are positive for cytokeratin.
6. Risk factors for this disease are the following:
   a. Age: Advanced age
   b. Sex: Females are most commonly involved.
   c. Personal history of breast cancer: History of cancer in one breast will increase the likelihood of development of cancer in other breast.
   d. Histologic risk factor: Lobular carcinoma in situ and proliferative changes with atypia are the important category of risk factors for breast cancer.
   e. Family history of breast cancer: First-degree relative for breast cancer has two-to threefold increased incidence of breast cancer.
   f. Genes: *BRCA1* and *BRCA2* are the two genes increase the incidence of breast cancer.
   g. Reproductive risk factor: Lifetime exposure to estrogen increases the incidence of breast cancer which include:
      - Onset of menarche before the 12 years of age
      - History of child birth after the age of 30 years
      - Nuliparity
      - History of menopause after the age of 55 years
   h. Exogenous hormonal use increases the incidence of breast cancer like:
      - Use of contraception in case of premenopausal women
      - Hormone replacement therapy in case of postmenopausal women
7. Age-wise incidence of breast cancer:
   a. At the age of 20–24 years: Incidence is 1.5/100,000 population
   b. At 70–79 years of age: Incidence is 421.3/100,000 population
8. *BRCA1* and *BRCA2* genes are involved in this disease.
9. In relation of basement membrane, breast cancer is divided into two forms:
   i. Invasive form
   ii. Noninvasive form
   Noninvasive form again can be subdivided into:
   a. Lobular carcinoma in situ
   b. Ductal carcinoma in situ: It can be subdivided into four types:
      i. Papillary
      ii. Cribriform
      iii. Solid
      iv. Comedo
10. Following tests should be done in this case:
    a. Mammography: It is the most common modality of investigation but it is not sensitive in case of young woman
    b. Ultrasonography: It should be used for assessing the consistency and size of the breast mass.
    c. Magnetic resonance imaging: It is used in case of:
       - Occult lesion
       - Suspected bilateral multifocal malignancy
       - Response to neoadjuvant chemotherapy
       - Bone scan can confirm the secondary deposits
11. Following are the basic principles of treatment of this disease:
    a. To reduce the local recurrences
    b. To reduce the risk of metastatic spread
12. Significance of radiotherapy in this disease:
    a. It reduces the recurrences of cancer by 50% at 10 years
    b. It reduces the cancer-related death by 20% if done after breast conservative surgery
    c. It is not required for female of >70 years old who is lymph node negative but hormone receptor positive.
    d. It is beneficial in case of:
       - Tumor of >5 cm larger in diameter
       - Tumor invading the chest wall and skin having positive lymph nodes
       - Advanced cases with metastasis in the central nervous system or bone
13. Staging of breast cancer according to American Joint Committee:
    a. Primary tumor:
       - Tis: Carcinoma in situ, Pagets, or no tumor
       - T1: <2 cm
         - T1a: 0.1–0.5 cm
         - T1b: 0.5–1 cm
         - T1c: 1–2 cm
       - T2: 2–5 cm
       - T3: Larger than 5 cm
       - T4:
         - T4a: Chest wall involvement
         - T4b: Involvement of skin
         - T4c: Involvement of skin and chest wall
         - T4d: Inflammatory carcinoma
    b. Regional lymph node involvement:
       - N1: Mobile ipsilateral axillary lymph nodes
       - N2: Fixed/mobile matted ipsilateral axillary lymph nodes

- N3:
  - N3a: Ipsilateral infraclavicular lymph nodes
  - N3b: Ipsilateral internal mammary lymph nodes
  - N3c: Ipsilateral supraclavicular lymph nodes
  c. Distant metastases:
  - M1: Distant metastases:
    - Stage 0: Tis
    - Stage 1: T1N0
    - Stage 2: T2N0, T3N0, T0N1, T1N1, and T2N1
    - Stage 3: Skin and rib involvement, matted lymph nodes
    - Stage 4: T3N1, T0N2, T1N2, T2N2, T3N2, Any T, N3T4, and any N
    - Stage 5: M1

This patient has been suffering from stage 5 disease.

14. Complications are the following:
  a. Surgery-related complications:
  - Infection
  - Bleeding
  - Pain
  - Permanent scarring
  - Cosmetic issues
  - Altered sensation in the chest area
  b. Chemotherapy-related complications:
  - Nausea, vomiting, and diarrhea
  - Loss of memory
  - Loss of hair
  - Vaginal dryness
  - Neuropathy
  - Menopausal symptoms
  c. Complications related to hormonal therapy:
  - Hot flushes
  - Fatigue
  - Nausea
  - Vaginal dryness
  - Impotence in male with breast cancer
  d. Radiotherapy-related complications:
  - Pain
  - Skin changes
  - Nausea
  - Hair loss
  - Neuropathy

15. Follow-up of this patient:
  a. Patient should be followed up for cancer recurrences and spread.
  b. Yearly or biannual follow-up by mammography of the treated as well as other unaffected breast
  c. In case of any suspicion, the patient should report the clinic.

CASE 7

A 7-year-old boy following an episode of fever for 4 days came to the medical clinic with history of the skin lesions like below. His blood count demonstrated hemoglobin 12 g/dL, white blood count 9,000/cc, platelet count 90,000/cc, international normalized ratio (INR) 1.1, activated partial thromboplastin time (APTT) normal, and fibrinogen normal. Serum urea and creatinine were 27 mg/dL and 0.9 mg/dL, respectively.

His peripheral blood picture demonstrated as below:

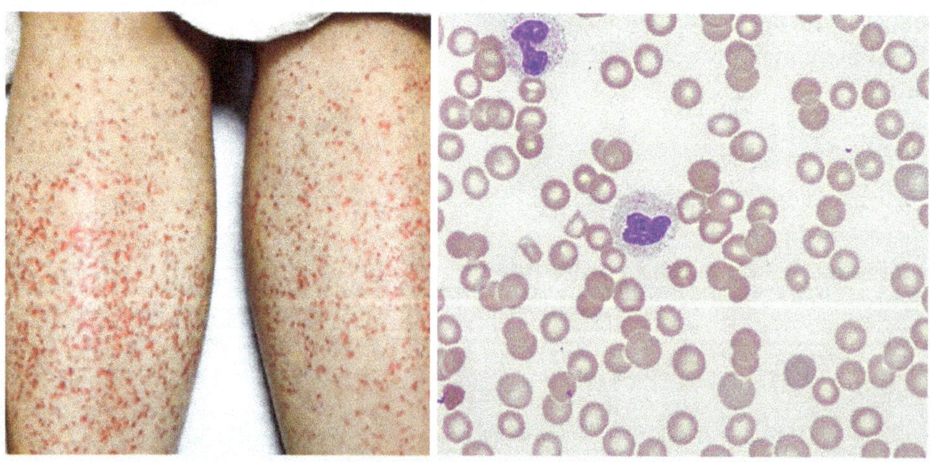

1. Interpret the peripheral blood picture?
2. Interpret the above blood report.
3. Describe the picture of the patient.
4. What is your diagnosis?
5. When do you suspect the hematological malignancy?
6. What should be the picture of bone marrow in this case?
7. What should be the clinical form of this disease according to the International Working group?
8. Name seven drugs responsible for this disease?
9. How can you classify this disease and which form of disease is preponderant in female and why?
10. What is the characteristics of the gestational variety of this disease and why?
11. In what semester neonatal variety of this disease occurs in pregnant woman?
12. What are the risks in the pregnant patient with this disease?
13. What is the mechanism of this disease induced by this drugs?
14. What is the pathophysiology of this disease occurring in the childhood?
15. What are the tests should be done in this case and why?
16. What are the indications of active therapy in this disease and what are the conditions where no therapy should be done?
17. What is the treatment of choice in severe cases?
18. What is the risk of administering steroids in pregnant patient?
19. What is the choice of operation in this case and when?
20. In neonatal case, which treatment is preferred and why?
21. When the platelet will rise in untreated case of neonates and why?
22. What is the risk of administering rituximab in this case?
23. What is the advantages and disadvantages of administration of anti-D globulin in this patient?
24. What are the mechanisms of actions of the following drugs in this case:
    a. Fostamatinib
    b. Efgartigimod and rozanolixizumab
    c. Sutimlimab
    d. Rilzabrutinib
25. What is the rationale of using thrombopoietin and what is its disadvantages?
26. What are the causes of consumptive thrombocytopenia?
27. What are the causes of this disease due to decreased production of platelets?

Answers

1. Peripheral blood picture demonstrates few clumps of platelets in the field with variation in the size of the platelets.
2. Above blood report demonstrates:
    a. Low platelet count
    b. Absence of red blood cell fragmentation and polychromasia
    c. INR, APTT, and fibrinogen are normal which will exclude disseminated intravascular coagulation.
    d. Urea and creatinine are within normal limit which excludes hemolytic-uremic syndrome (HUS).
3. Picture of the patient demonstrates feature of purpura in the both lower limbs.
4. This patient has been suffering from immune thrombocytopenic purpura (ITP).
5. When the thrombocytopenia cannot improve spontaneously over the few days course and prior to treatment of immune thrombocytopenia.
6. Following should be the picture in the bone marrow in this disease:
    a. Increased size of megakaryocytes
    b. Number of megakaryocytes are normal or increased.
    c. Immature form of megakaryocytes, i.e., smooth forms containing single nuclei and scanty cytoplasm.
    d. Because of accelerated destruction of platelets, the platelet will be in the younger form.

7. According to the International Working group, following are the clinical phases of this disease:
   a. Newly diagnosed ITP—in the first 3 months after the diagnosis
   b. Persistent ITP—for 3–12 months
   c. Chronic ITP—more than 12 months
   d. Refractory ITP—when it persists even after splenectomy

8. Following seven drugs are responsible for this disease:
   i. Acetazolamide
   ii. Aspirin
   iii. Digoxin
   iv. Carbamazepine
   v. Phenytoin
   vi. Methyldopa
   vii. Quinidine

9. Immune thrombocytopenia can be classified into two forms:
   i. Acute form usually occurring in the children affecting both sexes following viral infection and will be resolved spontaneously within few months and may not require treatment.
   ii. Chronic form occurring in the age of 20–50 years with female ratio of 3:1 and not preceded by viral infection. Female preponderance may have relation with the prevalence of autoimmune disease in female.

10. Gestational ITP characteristics are the following:
    a. Count of platelets will be never below 70,000/cc.
    b. It usually does not cause bleeding.
    c. It is usually dilutional not consumptive.

11. Neonatal alloimmune thrombocytopenia occurs if the pregnant has been sensitized in the prior pregnancies by blood transfusion or if the previous child is platelet antigen positive though this time she is negative for platelet antigen.

12. Risks of pregnant patient with ITP are the following:
    a. Fetal loss
    b. Low fetal birth rate
    c. High incidence

13. Mechanism of drug-induced destruction by drugs:

Drugs absorbs to the platelet cell membrane

↓

Development of the antibody against the drug plus platelet complex

↓

This antibody antigen complex will be destroyed by the phagocytic system in the spleen as well as liver

14. In childhood, immune thrombocytopenia within few weeks of viral infection may be due to cross-immunization between the viral as well as platelet antigens leading to formation of immune complexes and destruction by the phagocytic system.

15. Following laboratory tests should be done in this disease:
    a. Platelet count is ≤40,000/cc
    b. Peripheral blood picture demonstrates tiny platelets fragment along with large platelets
    c. Bone marrow aspirates demonstrates large number of megakaryocytes
    d. Analysis of antibody to platelet glycoprotein IIb/IIIa, Ib/XI, and Ia/IIa is less sensitive event in presence of antiplatelet antibodies fixed to the platelet of the patient.
    e. Pool of normal donor platelet can be used to detect the free antiplatelet antibodies mainly antiglycoprotein IIb/IIIa antibodies in the serum.
    f. Other tests to detect the antiplatelet antibodies:
       - Lymphocytes activation by autologus platelets
       - Activation of lymphocyte by platelet antibody immune complexes.
       - Phagocytosis of the platelet-associated immunoglobulin G (IgG) by the competitive binding assays
       - Radiolabeled Coombs antiglobulin test
       - Fluorescein-labeled Coomb antiglobulin
       - Enzyme-linked immunosorbent assay (ELISA)
    g. Tests for systemic lupus erythematosus (SLE):
       - Antinuclear antibody test
       - Test for other autoantibodies:
         ○ Anti-dsDNA
         ○ Anti-Smith antibodies
       - Detection of C3 and C4
       - IgM, IgG, and IgA
       - Cryoglobulin
       - Serum protein electrophoresis
       - Lupus band test demonstrating IgG and C3/C4 deposits at the dermo-epidermal junction
    h. Test for HIV
    i. Test for anti-HCV antibody

16. Indications of active therapy are the following:
    a. Transfusion is not advisable if the platelet count is >30,000/cc and there is no active bleeding.
    b. Active therapy is advisable if there is cutaneous or mucosal bleeding indicating platelet count <20,000/cc.

   c. If the platelet count is <10,000/cc, there is chance of life-threatening hemorrhage like intracranial hemorrhage.

17. In case of severe condition, intravenous immunoglobulin at a rate of 400 mg/kg daily for 5 days and the response rate is 70% in 3–5 days. In case of active bleeding in children or adult, corticosteroid should be administered to reduce the destruction of platelet. In severe cases, there may be requirement of plasmapheresis.

18. In first trimester, steroid administration may produce cleft palate in very small number of cases. In late trimester, there is chance of:
   a. Abruptio placenta
   b. Rupture of fetal membrane

19. If the patient does not respond to corticosteroids for a month, in that case he or she should undergo splenectomy after administration of intravenous immunoglobulin to reduce the destruction of the platelets.

20. In case of neonatal thrombocytopenia, intravenous immunoglobulin is preferred over anti-D immunoglobulin as the latter may produce severe hemolytic transfusion.

21. In untreated cases in neonates, the transferred maternal antibodies will be destroyed in the neonates.

22. Following are the risks of rituximab administration:
   a. Hepatitis panel should be checked to prevent the reactivation of hepatitis B.
   b. Risk of progressive multifocal leukoencephalopathy
   c. COVID vaccination should not be gven within 6–12 months after administration of rituximab.
   d. Possible risk of hypergammaglobulinemia, if dexamethasone is administered with rituximab.
   e. This drug can cross the placenta leading to neonatal B cell depletion.

23. Anti-D immunoglobulin inhibits the destruction of antibody-coated platelets.
Its administration is limited in presence of spleen. Again anti-D globulin should not be given in pregnant woman as there is chance of neonatel jaundice and anemia.

24. The mechanisms of actions of the following drugs in this case are as follows:
   a. Fostamatinib is a splenic tyrosine kinase inhibitor which decreases the antibody-dependent phagocytosis in the spleen.
   b. Efgartigimod and rozanolixizumab are the antibody fragment which target the Fc receptor of neonates and thereby prevent recycling of IgG resulting in decreasing the half-life of IgG. The level of IgG becomes subpathogenic level.
   c. Sutimlimab, a humanized monoclonal antibody against C1s, thereby it will decrease the complement-mediated cytotoxicity leading to decrease in the destruction of the platelets.
   d. Rilzabrutinib, a Bruton tyrosine kinase inhibitor, will inhibit the Fc signal transduction leading to decreased phagocytosis as well as decreased production of autoantibody.

25. Thrombopoietin like eltrombopag, romiplostim, and avatrombopag stimulates the JAK-STAT pathway leading to:
   a. Proliferation of megakaryocyte
   b. Production of platelet
   Complication is development of thrombosis if:
   a. The patient is on oral contraceptives
   b. The patient has underlying antiphospholipid antibody issue
   c. The patient has other prothrombotic issue
In case of prolonged use, there is chance of fibrosis due to increased amount of reticulin deposition.

26. Following are the causes of consumptive thrombocytopenia:
   a. Thrombotic thrombocytopenic purpura
   b. Hemolytic-uremic syndrome
   c. Disseminated intravascular coagulation
   d. Sepsis by various mechanism:
      • Activation of complement
      • Release of histone
      • Activation of coagulation

27. Following are the causes of decreased production of platelet:
   a. Suppression of bone marrow by:
      • Drugs
      • Alcohol
      • Infections
      • Toxins
   b. Aplastic anemia
   c. Leukemia and other bone marrow malignancy
   d. Megaloblastic anemia
   e. Preleukemia
   f. Refractory anemia

CASE 8

A 32-year-old male having history of operation to correct anemia came to medical clinic with history of moderate exertional dyspnea, but he need not require blood transfusion as he can perform his usual activities normally. He is taking penicillin V 250 mg twice daily.

Hematological report demonstrated hemoglobin 8 g/dL with MCV of 110 fL, white blood cell count 8,000/cc, and platelet count 200,000/cc. Blood biochemistry demonstrated low haptoglobin level and increased level of 2,3-diphosphoglycerate. Osmotic fragility and direct Coomb test are negative. Peripheral blood picture demonstrated:

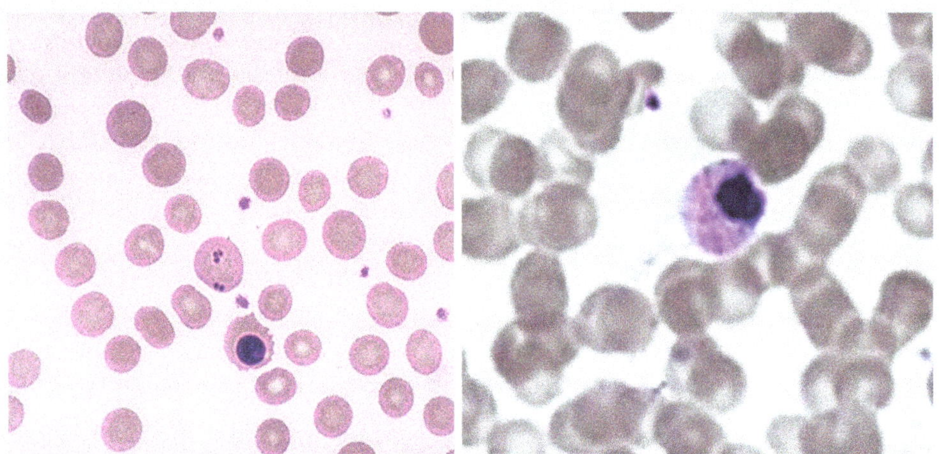

1. **Describe the above pictures.**
2. **Interpret the blood report.**
3. **What is your diagnosis?**
4. **Which red blood cells are mostly affected?**
5. **How this disease is inherited?**
6. **Which gene is responsible for this disease?**
7. **In which communities in the World, this disease is found?**
8. **What is the pathophysiology behind this disease?**
9. **What types of anemia will occur in this disease?**
10. **Why 2,3-diphosphoglycerate will be increased in the blood?**
11. **What will be the effect of this disease in newborn?**
12. **What type of anemia occurs in second trimester of pregnancy?**
13. **What is the significance of measuring the pyruvate kinase level in the blood?**
14. **Which is the major risk in this disease?**

Answers

1. The above pictures demonstrate:
   a. Right hand picture shows Howell–Jolly bodies
   b. Left hand picture demonstrates irregularly contracted cells known as contracted cells.
2. Blood picture demonstrates low hemoglobin and raised 2,3-diphosphoglycerate level in the blood. There is absence of target cells.
3. The diagnosis is hemolytic anemia due to pyruvate kinase deficiency.
4. Young RBC is mostly affected.
5. Pyruvate kinase deficiency is autosomal recessive.
6. This enzymatic activity is controlled by *PKLR* gene located in the chromosome 1q21. Mutation in this gene is responsible for this disease.
7. In Pennsylvania, Amish, and Romani communities, this disease is mostly found.
8. Integrity of RBC is maintained by membrane-bound ATPase which exchanges sodium and potassium to maintain the transcellular electrical neutrality, fluid

balance, and deformability. Absence of this enzyme will lead to:

a. Decrease in ATP production in the RBC leading to rigidity of the wall of the RBC

b. Loss of intracellular potassium leading to crenated cells

   As a result, there is extravascular hemolysis leading to development of hemolytic anemia.

9. Though there is extravascular hemolysis, but intra-vascular hemolysis will also occur.

10. Level of 2,3-diphosphoglycerate will be increased to compensate anemia.

11. Effect of this disease in the newborn:

a. As neonatal RBC consumes more ATP as compared to adult destruction of reticulocytes in the spleen, it will lead to hyperbilirubinemia leading to kernicterus which can be prevented by exchange transfusion.

b. Fetal hydrops can occur due to severe anemia in the uterus.

c. There may be occurrence of transfusion-dependent neonatal anemia.

12. There is dilutional anemia occur in second trimester of pregnancy because of increase in plasma volume as compared to red blood cell mass and it will improve the fetal outcome and minimize the postpartum blood loss.

13. Serum pyruvate kinase level may be low or normal. Hence, in this disease:

a. RBC age-corrected pyruvate kinase level should be measured which will be low.

b. Pyruvate kinase/hexokinase activity ratio should be measured which will be low.

14. Iron overload is the major risk in this disease. Hence, regular screening of the iron profile is indicated.

CASE 9

An 80-year-old nonsmoker male came to medical clinic with the complaint of progressively increasing numbness, pain, and coldness of the finger tips in the upper extremities. Physical examination is unremarkable. Hematological report demonstrated hemoglobin 8.5 mg/dL, total white blood cell count 15000/cc platelet count 1,200,000/cc. Peripheral blood picture demonstrated:

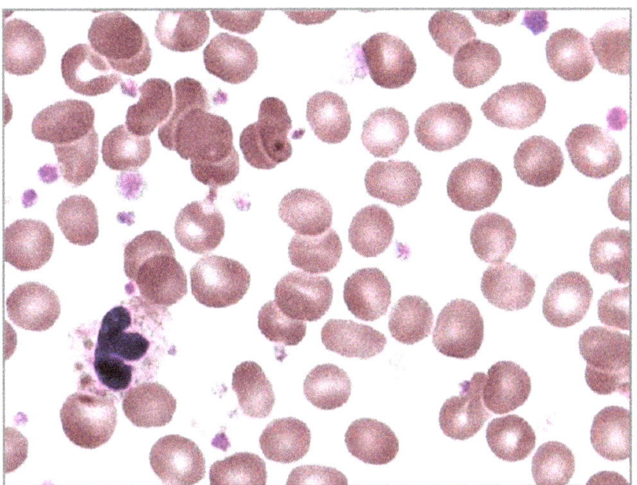

1. **Comment on the peripheral blood picture.**
2. **What is your diagnosis?**
3. **What are the causes of this abnormalities?**
4. **In what group, this diagnosis falls?**
5. **How can you define according to WHO?**
6. **What is the primary cause of this disease?**
7. **Which genetic mutation in this disease is associated with severe complications?**

8. **What are the other mutations associated with this disease?**
9. **What are the most common symptoms in this disease?**
10. **What are the diagnostic criteria in this disease according to WHO?**
11. **What are the investigations to be done to differentiate this disease from reactive cause?**
12. **Which receptors will be upregulated in reactive thrombocytosis?**
13. **Why genetic mutation types are required in this disease?**
14. **According to International Prognostic score, which are the risk factors for overall survival and how many treatment groups has been divided in this disease?**
15. **What is the caution during treatment with aspirin?**
16. **What are the mechanisms of action of different cytotoxic drugs used in this disease?**
17. **What are the complications in pregnant patient having this disease?**
18. **What are the treatments of choice in pregnant patient with this disease?**
19. **Why Busulfan is of limited choice in treating this disease?**
20. **What are the risks of use of imetelstat in this disease?**
21. **What is the pathophysiology of erythromelalgia and how it can be treated?**
22. **What is spurious thrombocytosis?**
23. **What is hereditary thrombocytosis?**
24. **What is the reported life expectancy in this disease?**
25. **What are the complications in this disease?**
26. **What are the therapeutic options involved in this case?**
27. **What are the toxicities of anagrelide?**

Answers

1. Peripheral blood picture demonstrates the increased number of platelets.
2. As the patient presented with pain, cold numb extremities, and peripheral blood showed thrombocytosis. The definite diagnosis is essential for thrombocytosis.
3. This abnormalities can be classified into two types:
   a. Primary thrombocytosis:
   b. Secondary thrombocytosis: This may be due to following causes:
      - Infection
      - Iron deficiency
      - Bleeding
      - Malignancy
      - Post splenectomy
4. It falls under myeloproliferative disorders which include:
   a. Polycythemia vera
   b. Primary myelofibrosis
   c. Essential thrombocythemia
5. According to WHO, essential thrombocytosis will occur when platelet count is >450,000/cc with presence of:
   a. JAK2 mutation, or
   b. Calreticulin mutation, or
   c. Myeloproliferative leukemia virus oncogene mutation
   d. Absence of clonal or reactive causes
6. Primary cause of this disease is uncontrolled proliferation of the hematopoietic cells as result of mutation of *JAK2, CALR* or *MPL* gene which are known as driver genes.
7. JAK2 mutation in this disease is associated with more severe complication as there is increased evidence of heparin-induced thrombocytopenia.
8. Following adverse mutations are associated with this disease:
   a. SH2B3
   b. SF361: It is associated with fibrosis.
   c. U2AF1: It is associated with fibrosis and platelet count is over million/cc.
   d. TP53: It predicts leukemic transformation
   e. IDH2
   f. EZH2: It is associated with platelet of >1,500,000/cc.
   g. 20q-
   h. –Y: It is due to loss of Y chromosome.
9. The most common symptoms in this disease are:
   a. Fatigue
   b. Insomnia

c. Migraine

d. Headache

e. Dizziness

10. According to WHO, the criteria in this disease are:

   a. Major criteria:

      i. Platelet count is ≥450,000/cc

      ii. Bone marrow specimen demonstrates proliferation of megakaryocyte lineage consisting increased number of enlarged mature megakaryocyte with hyperloculated nuclei. No significant increase or left shift in neutrophil granulopoiesis or erythropoiesis, very rarely a minor increase in the reticulin fibers.

      iii. The presentation does not meet WHO criteria for BCR-ABL1 + CML, PCV, myelofibrosis, myelodysplastic syndrome (MDS), or other neoplasms.

      iv. + JAK2, CALR, or MPL

   b. Minor criteria: There is presence of a clonal marker or absence of evidence of reactive thrombocytosis.

   Diagnosis is made if all four major criteria or first three major criteria and the minor criteria are met.

11. To differentiate this disease from reactive thrombocytosis, following investigations should be done:

   a. Acute phase reactant—CRP and ESR

   b. Serum iron profile

12. There is upregulation of TPO receptor and interleukin-6 in case of inflammatory or ischemic conditions.

13. In this disease, genetic mutation of *JAK2, CALR,* and *MPL* is required as these mutation determine:

   a. Survival of the patient

   b. Clinical feature of the disease

   c. Complication in this disease

14. According to International Prognostic score which are the risk factors for overall survival:

   a. Age ≥ 60 years

   b. Leukocyte count is ≥11,000/cc

   c. Cardiovascular risk factors:
      • Diabetes
      • Hypertension
      • Tobacco use

   d. Mutation of JAK2V617F

   e. History of prior thrombosis

   Essential thrombocytosis can be divided into three treatment groups:

   i. Low-risk group

   ii. Intermediate risk group

   iii. High-risk group

15. During treatment with aspirin caution should be taken regarding acquired von Willebrand syndrome when the platelet count is >1,000,000.

16. Mechanisms of action of the following drugs are:

   a. Hydroxyurea: It will reduce the number of both plates as well as leukocytes thereby reducing the incidence of myelofibrosis and thrombosis.

   b. Anagrelide: It will inhibit the differentiation and aggregation of platelets thereby reducing the incidence of thrombosis.

17. Complications in the pregnancy patient with essential thrombocytosis are:

   a. In the first trimester, fetal loss

   b. Placental complications:
      • Abruptio placentae
      • Eclampsia
      • Intrauterine growth retardation
      • Stillbirth

18. In pregnant patient with essential thrombocytosis, the treatment of choice are:

   a. Low molecular weight heparin during pregnancy and for 6 weeks after delivery

   b. Pegylated interferon for cytoreduction

   c. If the platelet count is >1,500,000 and the action of interferon is slow to reduce the platelet count, in that case plasmapheresis should be done.

19. Busulfan is of limited use in this disease because of its hematologic toxicity like high-grade transformation to myelodysplastic syndrome and acute leukemia.

20. Imetelstat, a telomerase inhibitor, has the following risks if it is used in this disease:

   a. Neutropenia

   b. Thrombosis

   c. Abnormal liver function test

21. Erythromelalgia is characterized by painful sensation of the both hands and feet due to abnormal interaction between the small blood vessels and platelets. The treatment of choice is aspirin.

22. Spurious thrombocytosis is characterized by miscount of platelet-like structure as platelet but not originally platelets. These are cryoglobulin crystals, cytoplasmic fragments, circulating leukemic cells, and bacteria.

23. Hereditary thrombocytosis, autosomal dominant variety with variable penetrance is characterized by hepatosplenomegaly and thrombocytosis. It will affect gene with TPO or its receptor MPL. In the bone marrow, there is megakaryocytosis and increased activation of platelets.

24. The reported life expectency in essential thrombocytosis is average 33 years and in below the age of 60 years.
25. Complications in this disease are the following:
    a. Thrombosis in:
        - Hepatic vein: Budd–Chiari syndrome
        - Coronary artery: Acute coronary syndrome
        - Cerebral artery: Transient ischemic attack or stroke
    b. Hemorrhage
26. Therapeutic option in essential thrombocytosis include:
    a. Plasmapheresis to reduce the platelet count mechanically
    b. Use of myelosuppressive agents:
        - Hydroxyurea
        - Radiophosphorus
    c. Maturation modulators:
        - Interferon-α
        - Anagrelide
    d. Antiplatelet agents
27. Toxicities of anagrelide:
    a. Headache
    b. Fluid retention
    c. Palpitation

All the side effects will occur within 2–4 weeks of therapy.

CASE 10

A 72-year-old male suffering from chronic lymphatic leukemia came to clinic with weakness, sudden increase in the size of the axillary lymph nodes, progressive abdominal distention, and lethargy.

On examination, there was pallor, pedal edema, axillary and inguinal lymphadenopathy, and ascites. Blood report demonstrated features of leukemia, blood urea 88 mg/dL, creatinine 2.8 mg/dL, and lactate dehydrogenase 640 mg/dL. Following are the hematological, bone marrow, and CT scan picture in this patient:

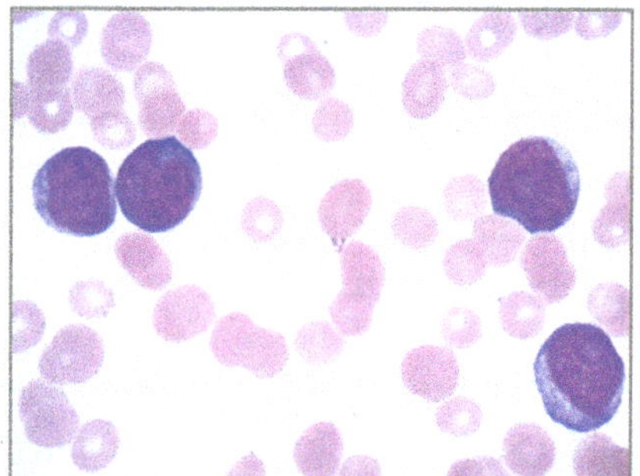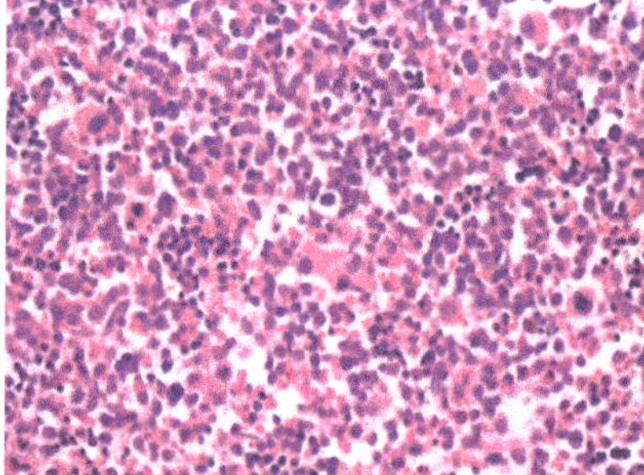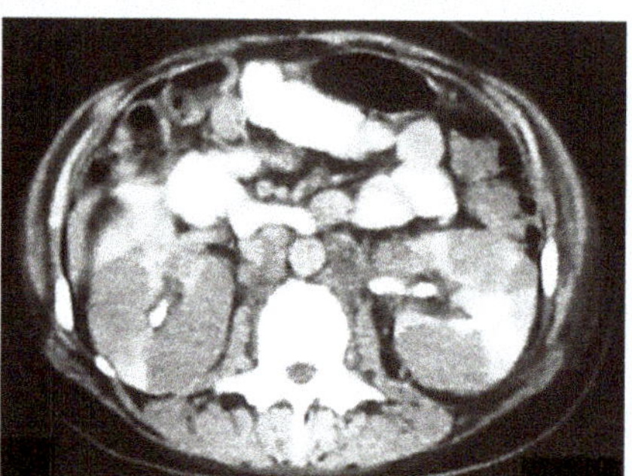

1. **Describe the peripheral blood picture.**
2. **Describe the picture in the bone marrow.**
3. **Describe CT scan of abdomen.**
4. **Describe the clinical, hematological, and biochemical correlation in this patient?**
5. **What is your diagnosis?**
6. **How can you define this disease?**
7. **What are the most common symptoms in this disease?**
8. **What are the sites of the extranodal involvement?**
9. **What are the risk factors for this disease?**
10. **What are the specific investigations to be done in this case for diagnosis?**
11. **Comment on the flow cytometric study in this disease?**
12. **What are the favorable prognostic factors in this disease?**
13. **What are the unfavorable prognostic factors in this disease?**
14. **How can you manage this case?**

Answers

1. Peripheral blood picture demonstrating large cells with large amount of basophilic cytoplasm—indicating immunoblastic transformation of chronic lymphocytic leukemia (CLL).

2. Bone marrow demonstrating hypercellularity with pleomorphic lymphocytes

3. CT scan of the abdomen demonstrates retroperitoneal lymphadenopathy.

4. In the back ground of CLL, there is sudden increase in the size of the gland, raised lactate dehydrogenase, and presence of lymphoblast in the peripheral blood picture suggestive of transformation of CLL to B cell lymphoma.

5. The patient has been suffering from Richter's syndrome.

6. This disease can be defined as transformation of CLL to B cell lymphoma or Hodgkin lymphoma characterized by rapid enlargement of lymph nodes, raised lactate dehydrogenase level, and, on positron emission tomography, presence of active nodal disease.

7. The most common symptoms in this disease are:
   a. Sudden clinical deterioration of the symptoms
   b. Development of systemic symptom
   c. Rapid enlargement of the lymph nodes
   d. Extranodal manifestations

8. Following extranodal sites are involved:
   a. Gastrointestinal system
   b. Central nervous system
   c. Skin
   d. Testes
   e. Eye
   f. Lung
   g. Kidney

9. Following are the risk factors for this disease:
   a. Clinical:
      - Advanced Rai stage at the time of diagnosis
      - Size of the lymph node is >3 cm in diameter.
      - Heavily pretreated CLL
   b. Associated poor prognostic factors:
      - Del(11q)
      - Del(17p)
      - Unmutilated immunoglobulin heavy-chain variable region gene
      - High expression of ZAP70 and CD49d
      - CD38
   c. Increased risk of transformation with mutation of *NOTCH1* gene

10. Following specific investigations should be done in this case:
    a. Laboratory assessment:
       - Lactate dehydrogenase
       - Complete blood count
       - Peripheral blood picture
    b. Radiological imaging:
       - CT scan of abdomen
       - PET-CT
    c. Biopsy of the involved nodes

11. In classic CLL, T-cell marker CD5 and mature B-cell marker CD19, CD20, and CD23 positive but FMC7 negative. But after transformation to B cell lymphoma, FMC7 becomes positive and CD5 becomes negative. There is also absent expression of CD52 and CD62L. Diffuse large B cell lymphoma variety will retain the expression of CD23 and CD5.

12. Following are the favorable prognostic factors in this disease:
    a. Clonal unrelated CLL
    b. Richter syndrome diffuse B cell lymphoma

13. Following are the unfavorable prognostic factors:
    a. Platelet count < 100,000/cc
    b. Trisomy 12
    c. TP53
    d. Lactate dehydrogenase >1.5 times the upper limit of normal
    e. Size of the tumor >5 cm
    f. More than one time prior treatment
    g. After induction failure to achieve complete remission

14. Treatments of this syndrome are:
    a. In Richter syndrome, diffuse B cell lymphoma:
       - R-CHOP or R-CHOP-like regimen
       - In case of young fit patient, stem cell transplantation
       - Emerging immunotherapy:
         ○ Bruton's tyrosine kinase inhibitors: Ibrutinib and acalabrutinib
         ○ BCL2 inhibitors: Venetoclax
         ○ PD-1 receptor inhibitors: Pembrolizumab
    b. Richter syndrome—Hodgkin lymphoma type: ABVD (adriamycin, bleomycin, vinblastine, dacarbazine) consisting of the following:
       - Adriamycin
       - Bleomycin
       - Vinblastine
       - Dacarbazine

CASE 11

A 65-year-old female came to medical outpatient department with exertional respiratory distress and tiredness for 10 days. On examination, there was pallor, and right colonic area tender. Clinical hematological report demonstrated hemoglobin 7.8 g/dL, white blood cell count 6,200/cc, platelet count 480,000/cc, and MCV 68 fL.

Peripheral blood picture and colonoscopic picture demonstrated as below:

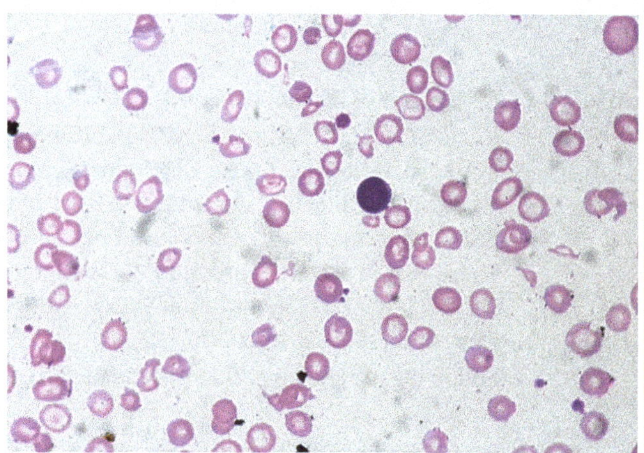 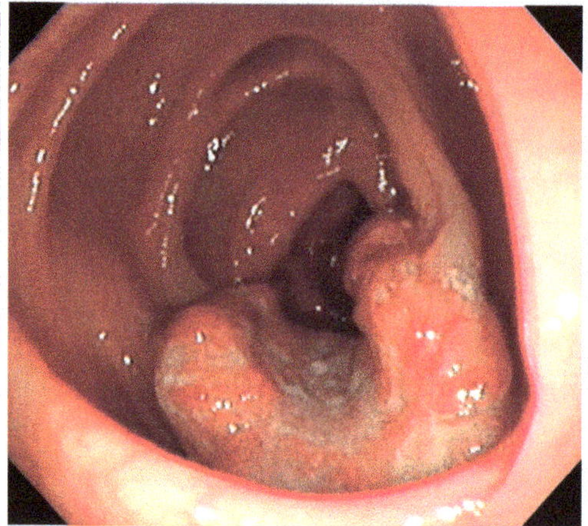

1. **What has been demonstrated in the peripheral blood picture?**
2. **Interpret the hematological report.**
3. **What is the colonoscopic picture?**
4. **What is your diagnosis?**
5. **What should be the bone marrow picture in this disease?**
6. **What are the physiological causes of this disease?**
7. **How can you differentiate between the absolute and functional deficiency of this disease?**
8. **What is the significance of reticulocyte hemoglobin in this disease?**
9. **What biochemical parameter reflects this diagnosis?**
10. **In case of microcytosis if MCV falls below normal, what should be the hemoglobin level?**
11. **What is the level of hepcidin in this disease?**
12. **What are the different stages in the development of this disease?**
13. **What is Mentzer index and what is its significance?**
14. **What are the drugs producing decreased absorption of iron?**
15. **What are the dietary factors responsible for reduced absorption of iron?**
16. **How can you calculate requirement of oral iron?**
17. **Mention the complications in this disease.**

Answers

1. Peripheral blood picture demonstrates:
   a. Hypochromia, i.e., more than one-third is central pallor.
   b. Microcytosis, i.e., size of the red blood cell is smaller than the nucleus of small mature lymphocytes.
   c. Anisocytosis
   d. Poikilocytosis
   e. Pencil-shaped red blood cells
   f. Pessary form of red blood cells, i.e., presence of thin rim of hemoglobin just beneath the membrane.
2. Hematological report demonstrates very low hemoglobin count, low mean corpuscular hemoglobin (MCH), and increased platelet count.

3. Colonoscopic picture demonstrates carcinoma involving ascending colon
4. The patient has been suffering from iron-deficiency anemia due to bleeding from carcinoma of the colon.
5. Bone marrow picture demonstrates:
   a. Erythroid hyperplasia—which is less as compared to bone marrow.

b. Presence of micronormoblast characterized by smaller size and ragged margin
c. <10% normoblast in sideroblast
6. Following are the physiologic causes of this disease:
   a. Pregnancy
   b. Lactation
   c. Infants

7. Following are the differences of absolute and functional iron deficiency:

Parameters	Iron-deficiency anemia	Functional anemia
Red blood cells	• Microcytic and hypochromic • Microcytosis more pronounced • Hypochromia follows microcytosis	• Hypochromia more pronounced • MCV <72 fL is rare • Hypochromia precedes microcytosis
Anisocytosis	Prominent	Less
Poikilocytosis	Prominent	Less
Red cell width	Increased	Normal
Total iron-binding capacity (TIBC)	Increased	Normal
% Saturation	Very low	Low
Ferritin	Low	Normal/increased
Soluble transferrin receptor	Increased	Normal
Serum hepcidin	Decreased	Increased

8. Reticulocyte hemoglobin is a part of automated profile of reticulocytes. As the half-life of the mature erythrocytes is long in the circulation, reduced hemoglobin content in the reticulocytes can assess acute iron deficiency as well as it can monitor the response to iron repletion therapy.
9. Following biochemical parameters indicate this iron-deficiency anemia:
   a. Serum iron will be reduced to 15 µg/mL.
   b. Total iron-binding capacity will be raised up to 500 µg/mL.
   c. Transferrin saturation is reduced to <16%.
   d. Serum ferritin will be reduced to <12 µg/dL indicating iron store is nil. If it is >100 µg/dL, it will exclude iron-deficiency anemia.

e. Soluble transferrin receptor level will be increased correlating with erythropoiesis.
f. Free erythropoietic protoporphyrin is raised to >200 µg/dL. As it binds with zinc, it is known as zinc protoporphyrin. It is very sensitive test in this disease.
g. Reticulocyte hemoglobin content: It is the earliest sensitive indicator of iron-deficiency anemia.
h. Percentage of hypochromic red blood cells will be reduced to <6%.
10. In case of microcytosis if MCV falls below normal, the hemoglobin level should be 10 g/dL.
11. Hepcidin level will be reduced in this disease.

12. Following are the different stages of development in iron-deficiency anemia:

Stages	Iron store	Serum ferritin	Serum iron	TIBC	FEP	Transferrin saturation	Hemoglobin	RBC
Stages of iron depletion	Low or absent	<20	Normal	Normal	Normal	Normal	Normal	Normochromic
Iron-deficient erythropoiesis	Absent	<12	Low	Normal/increased	Increased	Decreased	Normal	Normochromic
Iron-deficiency anemia (IDA)	Absent	<12	Low	Increased	Increased	Decreased	Decreased	Microcytic hypochromic

13. Mentzer index can be calculated as MCV/number of red blood cells million/μL.
    a. If the value is >13, it indicates iron-deficiency anemia.
    b. If the value is <13, it indicates β-thalassemia.
14. Following drugs are responsible for less absorption of iron:
    a. Antacids
    b. Proton pump inhibitors
    c. Tetracycline
    d. Quinolones
    e. Pancreatic enzyme supplements
    f. Cholestyramine
15. Following dietary factors are responsible for reduced absorption of iron:
    a. Coffee
    b. Milk
    c. Dietary fibers
    d. Phosphate-containing beverages
    e. Supplements containing calcium, manganese, or copper
16. Calculation of total iron requirement based on the total blood volume and hematocrit:
    Total iron deficit:
    Deficit of iron stores + hemoglobin iron deficit
    Deficit of iron store = 500 – 1,000 mg
    Hemoglobin iron deficit = Total body weight (lb) × (Target hemoglobin – Actual hemoglobin), where target hemoglobin is 14 g/dL
    Oral iron supplement in mg = 10 × total iron deficit
17. Complications in this disease are the following:
    a. Increased risk of infection
    b. Heart conditions
    c. Developmental delay in children
    d. Complications in pregnancy
    e. Depression

CASE 12

A 5-year-old male child came to medical clinic with tiredness, exertional dyspnea, and yellowish discoloration of urine and heaviness in the left upper abdomen for 3 weeks. On examination, patient is pale, jaundice, soft systolic murmur, and abdominal examination revealed palpable spleen 6 cm below the left costal margin. Hematological report demonstrated hemoglobin 7 g/dL, white blood cell 15,000/cc, platelet count 120,000/cc, and reticulocyte count 20%, hemoglobinuria and low haptoglobin. Liver function test demonstrated total bilirubin 6 mg/dL with unconjugated portion 4.5 mg/dL but normal serum glutamic-oxaloacetic transaminase (SGOT) and serum glutamic-pyruvic transaminase (SGPT).

Peripheral blood picture demonstrated:

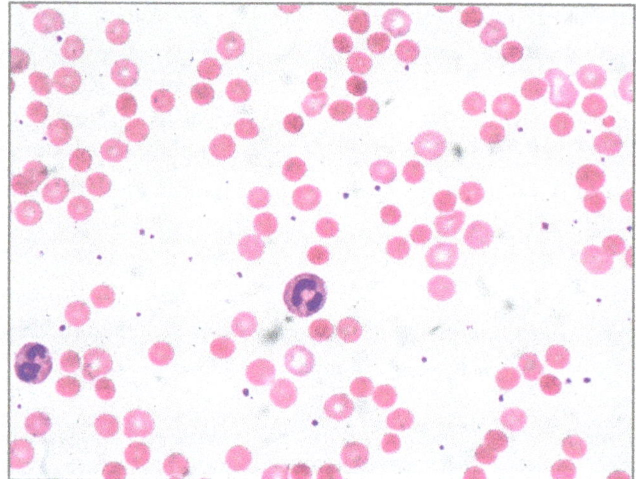

1. **What does the above picture demonstrate?**
2. **What is the interpretation of hematological and biochemical blood report?**
3. **What is your diagnosis?**
4. **Classify this disease.**

5. **Which drug is responsible for this disease?**
6. **What are the infectious causes of this disease in children?**
7. **How can you treat this disease?**

Answers

1. Peripheral blood picture demonstrates anisocytosis, poikilocytosis, presence of spherocytes, and nucleated red blood cells.
2. The hematological and biochemical report demonstrate low hemoglobin, high unconjugated bilirubin, low haptoglobin, hemoglobinuria, and increased amount of lactate dehydrogenase.
3. Above report and peripheral blood picture confirmed that this patient has been suffering from autoimmune hemolytic anemia.
4. There are two types of autoimmune hemolytic anemia:
   i. Warm antibody hemolytic anemia
   ii. Cold antibody hemolytic anemia
5. Purine nucleoside analog is responsible for this warm antibody hemolytic anemia.
6. Following infections are responsible for this disease in children:
   a. Epstein–Barr virus
   b. *Cytomegalovirus*
   c. Parvovirus
   d. *Mycoplasma pneumoniae*
7. Treatment:
   a. Prednisolone 1 mg/kg of body weight is the first line of treatment.
   b. Other drugs are azathioprine, cyclophosphamide, and cyclosporine.
   c. Anti-CD20 monoclonal antibody like rituximab
   d. Splenectomy:
      - It will reduce the red blood cell destruction.
      - It will remove the site of autoantibody production.

But, it should be avoided in children below the age of 5 years because of increased risk of infection. But, following preoperative vaccination should be administered:
   a. Meningococcal vaccine
   b. Pneumococcal vaccine
   c. *Haemophilus influenzae* vaccine
      Long-term penicillin prophylaxis is also required.

CASE 13

A 55-year-old man having history of long-standing anemia came to medical clinic with exertional respiratory distress, weakness, and red-colored urine. His peripheral blood film was demonstrated as below. His blood reports demonstrated hemoglobin 9 g/dL, MCV 70 fL, and white blood cell count 4,500/cc. Sucrose lysis test was positive.

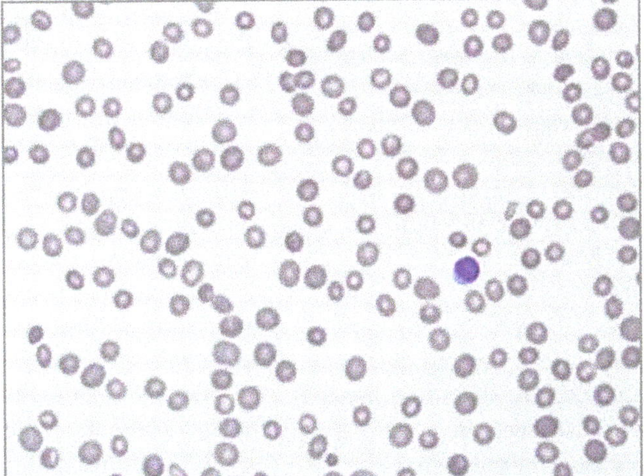

1. **Interpret the blood picture.**
2. **What is the most likely diagnosis?**

3. **What should be the confirmatory test and what is the method of doing that test?**
4. **Mutation of which gene is responsible for this disease?**
5. **What protein is responsible for this disease?**
6. **What is the clinical triad in this disease?**
7. **Why there is red-colored urine in this patient?**
8. **What is the mechanism of hemosiderinuria in this disease?**
9. **What are the precipitating factors for exacerbation of this disease?**
10. **Which factors are responsible for hemolysis in this disease?**
11. **Mention the significance of percentage of defective RBC in this disease?**
12. **Why there is pancytopenia in this disease?**
13. **What factors are responsible for thrombosis in this disease?**
14. **What are the different blood disorders associated with this disease?**
15. **What are the main organs involved in this disease?**
16. **What are the evidences of intravascular hemolysis in this disease?**
17. **What are the features in urine analysis in this disease?**
18. **Which monoclonal antibody is used to treat this disease and what are the precautions to be taken prior to its administration?**
19. **What is the role of nitric oxide in this disease?**
20. **What are the effects of this disease on the kidney?**
21. **What are the significance of fluorescein-labeled proaerolysin (FLAER) assay in this disease?**
22. **What are the types of flow cytometry used in this disease?**
23. **How can you classify this disease based on the clinical picture and laboratory test?**
24. **What is the significance of imaging in this disease?**
25. **What are the complications in this disease?**

Answers

1. Peripheral blood picture demonstrates evidence of anisocytosis, poikilocytosis, and polychromasia.
2. As this patient is sucrose lysis test positive, he is suffering from paroxysmal nocturnal hemoglobinuria (PNH).
3. Acidified serum test or Ham test is the specific for the diagnosis of this disease. In this process at 37°C, the red blood cells of patient is exposed to acidified normal serum at an optimum pH, i.e., 6.5–7 for lysis because in the acidified serum compliment will be activated in the alternate pathway and binds to abnormal red blood cells and lyse because these cells are unusually susceptible to complement.
4. Mutation of the X-linked gene phosphatidylinositol glycan class A leads to deficiency of protein glycosylphosphatidylinositol which usually binds to other protein moieties on the erythrocyte surface.
5. Following proteins are responsible for this disease:
   a. Decay accelerating factors CD55 which inhibits enzyme C3 convertase leading to prevention of spontaneous activation of the alternate pathway of complement
   b. Membrane inhibitor of reactive lysis CD59 which inhibits membrane attack complex, i.e., C5 to C9 of the complement pathway. It is more potent in protecting the red blood cells.
   c. Acetylcholinesterase
   d. Neutrophil alkaline phosphatase (ALP)
6. The clinical triad in this disease is:
   a. Recurrent episodes of intravascular hemolysis
   b. Venous thrombosis
   c. Cytopenias associated with bone marrow failure
7. During sleep, there is fall in plasma pH due to retention of carbon dioxide in the blood which is responsible for activation of the alternate pathway of the complement resulting in intravascular hemolysis and hemoglobinuria and hence morning sample of urine will be red color.
8. Most of the hemoglobin in urine will be reabsorbed by the proximal tubular epithelium and absorbed iron will be accumulated in the proximal tubular cells as hemosiderin. This hemosiderin-containing proximal tubular cells will be shaded in the tubular lumen and excreted as hemosiderinuria.

9. This disease will be exacerbated by:
    a. Infection
    b. Surgery
10. Degree of hemolysis depends upon the defective cells which are very sensitive to complement-mediated hemolysis. There are three types of defective red blood cells according to Rosse et al.:
    a. Very sensitive red cells, i.e., type III cells which are more sensitive to complement-mediated lysis when compared to normal cells.
    b. Medium sensitive red cells, i.e., type II cells which are 3–5 times more potent as compared to normal red blood cells.
    c. Nearly normal sensitive red cells to complement, i.e., type I cells
11. In case of active chronic hemolysis, the number of type III cells are >50%. Whereas, in case of mild hemolysis, the number of defective red blood cells are <20%.
12. As because the mutation of the gene occurs in the pluripotent hematopoietic stem cells, hence white blood cells and platelets are also affected.
13. Following factors are responsible for thrombosis in this disease:
    a. Activation of the platelets is the main culprit in the thrombosis.
    b. Toxicity of the free hemoglobin
    c. Depletion of the nitric oxide
    d. Absence of other glycosylphosphatidylinositol-linked proteins:
        • Urokinase type plasminogen activator receptor
        • Endothelial dysfunction
14. Following blood disorders are associated with PNH:
    a. Aplastic anemia
    b. Sideroblastic anemia
    c. Myelodysplastic syndrome
    d. Myelofibrosis
    e. Acute myeloid leukemia
15. Following main organs are involved in this disease:
    a. Hepatomegaly having central zonal necrosis
    b. Kidney becomes brownish due to deposition of hemosiderin.
    c. Dysphagia
    d. Male impotence
16. Following are the evidences of intravascular hemolysis:
    a. Serum level of lactate dehydrogenase will be increased.
    b. Serum level of indirect bilirubin will be increased.
    c. Serum level of haptoglobin will be increased.
    d. Hemoglobinuria
    e. Hemosiderinuria
17. Following are the features of urine analysis:
    a. Dark brown-colored urine which is benzidine positive due to active hemolysis.
    b. Hemosiderinuria can be diagnosed by Pearls' test.
    c. Hemoglobinuria can be detected by spectro-scopic examination.
    d. Urobilinogen in urine: It is positive in 1:20 dilution.
    e. Deposits in the urine which is yellow brown in color, known as tobacco yellow in color.
    f. Albuminuria
    g. Hyposthenuria
18. Eculizumab is a monoclonal antibody against active component of C5 which will reduce the incidence of clinical thrombosis. But, following precautions should be taken:
    a. Meningococcal vaccine should be administered at least 2 weeks prior to administration of this drugs.
    b. Prophylactic antibiotics should be administered prior and during this drug administration.
19. Role of nitric oxide in this disease:
    a. Nitric oxide is responsible for relaxation of the smooth muscle leading to vasodilatation.
    b. In case of depletion of nitric oxide, smooth muscle of the esophagus will be dystonic resulting in esophageal spasm, dysphagia, and abdominal pain.
    c. In case of nitric oxide depletion, smooth muscles in the corpora cavernosa unable to dilate leading to erectile dysfunction in male.
    d. Nitric oxide depletion leads constriction of pulmonary vascular smooth muscles resulting in pulmonary hypertension, symptom being shortness of breath.
20. Following types of kidney injury occur in this disease:
    a. This patient is prone to develop chronic kidney disease six times more as compared to normal patient.
    b. During the period of hemolysis, free heme is developed which is toxic to kidney leading to development of acute renal failure.
    c. In case of chronic hemolysis, iron will be deposited in the renal tissue leading to:
        • Renal scarring
        • Renal infarct
        • Dysfunction of the proximal tubule

21. Significance of FLAER in this disease: In the gold standard method of this disease, flow cytometry, monoclonal antibody, and special reagent known as fluorescent aerolysin reagent (FLAER) are used. The later will bind to directly glycosylphosphatidylinositol-anchored protein thereby can detect CD55 and CD59 with high sensitivity and specificity.

22. Two types of flow cytometry tests are available in this disease:
    i. Low sensitivity: It is adequate for the diagnosis of PNH.
    ii. High sensitivity: It can better detect this PNH in presence of another marrow disorder.

23. Based on the clinical picture and laboratory tests, this disease can be classified into following types:
    a. Classic PNH
    b. PNH with another bone marrow disorder like aplastic anemia, myelofibrosis or myelodysplastic syndrome
    c. Subclinical PNH: Here, there is no clinical or laboratory evidence of hemolysis.

24. Following are the significance of imaging in this disease:
    a. Echocardiography to detect the pulmonary hypertension
    b. Doppler abdominal ultrasound to evaluate to assess the hepatic blood flow or to detect thrombosis.
    c. Pulmonary angiography to detect pulmonary hypertension
    d. CT scan of abdomen to detect the Budd–Chiari syndrome
    e. MRI of head to detect the cerebral thrombosis

25. Following are the complications in this disease:
    a. Thrombosis in the:
       - Hepatic vein or artery
       - Cerebral vein or artery
       - Abdominal vein or artery
    b. Acute or chronic renal disease
    c. Pulmonary hypertension
    d. Erectile dysfunction
    e. Dysphagia

CASE 14

A 35-year-old chronic alcoholic male came to medical clinic with extreme tiredness, axillary swelling, fever with night sweat and progressive weight loss, and cough in spite of taking antibiotics. On examination, there was pallor, axillary lymphadenopathy which became tender on taking alcohol.

Blood investigation demonstrated hemoglobin 8.8 g/dL, MCV and MCH are all within normal limit, WBC 9,500/cc, ESR raised, bilirubin 4.8 mg/dL, SGPT 140 IU/L, ALP 260 U/L, and γ-glutamyl transferase (GGT) 250 U/L.

Bone marrow trephine biopsy and CT scan of abdomen demonstrate the following features:

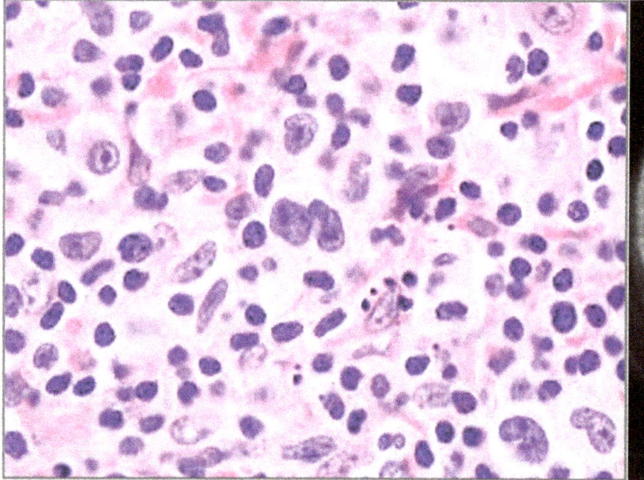 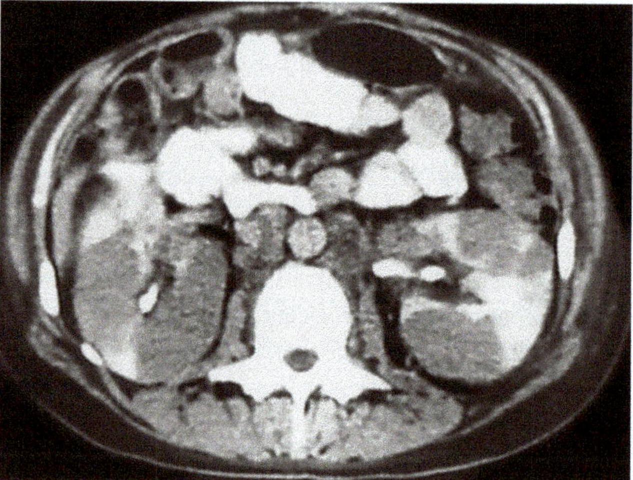

1. **Interpret bone marrow picture and CT scan of abdomen.**
2. **Interpret the hematological report.**
3. **What is the diagnosis?**
4. **What is the significance of sex in this disease?**
5. **What is the significance of Epstein–Barr virus in this disease?**
6. **What is the role of latent membrane protein-1 in this disease?**
7. **What is the activity of the specific cell in this disease?**
8. **What are the factors used in the classification of this disease?**
9. **How can you classify this disease?**
10. **Upon what base subtypes of this classical disease differ?**
11. **What are the morphological types of the specific cells found in different subtypes?**
12. **Mention the stage in this disease.**
13. **What are the immunophenotypes present in all the subtypes of classical disease?**
14. **Mention the prognostic features in this disease.**
15. **This patient can be subdivided into how many treatment groups?**
16. **What are the treatment schedules in different treatment groups?**
17. **How many patterns of relapses occurring in this disease?**
18. **Mention the prognostic factors in case of relapse of this classical disease?**
19. **What are the treatment-related complications in this disease?**
20. **What are the etiological factors in this disease?**
21. **What are the incidence of subtypes of this disease?**
22. **Which immunophenotypes are positive and negative for specific cells in this disease?**

Answers

1. Bone marrow trephine biopsy picture demonstrates presence of Reed–Sternberg giant cells. CT scan of abdomen demonstrates presence of retroperitoneal lymphadenopathy.
2. Hematological report demonstrates low hemoglobin, raised ESR, and derranged liver function test.
3. This patient has been suffering from Hodgkin disease.
4. In all subtypes of Hodgkin disease, male:female ratio is 1.4:1 except in the nodular sclerosis variety the ratio is 1:1.
5. Role of Epstein–Barr virus in this disease:
   a. This virus is found in most of the cases of mixed cellularity and lymphocytic depletion variety of lymphoma.
   b. In case of HIV infection, immunosurveillance loss will lead to development of Epstein–Barr virus associated classical lymphoma.
   c. In case of tropical country, there is 100% association of Epstein–Barr virus and this disease.
   d. B cell infected by Epstein–Barr virus which lead to expression of latent membrane protein-1 which is associated with this disease.
   e. There is presence of fractions of this virus found in the Reed–Sternberg giant cells.
6. Role of latent membrane protein-1 in this disease:
   a. Latent membrane protein-1 will interact with the receptor of tumor necrosis factor leading to activation of $\kappa\beta$ nuclear factor as well as terminal kinase pathways resulting in activation and proliferation of B cells.
   b. This protein prevents apoptosis of B cells through the induction of BCL-2 expression.
   c. This protein blocks phosphorylation of tyrosine thereby preventing reactivation of virus and promoting survival of B cells.
7. Reed–Sternberg giant cells will secrete interleukin-5, 6, and 13 and tumor necrosis factor and granulocyte-monocyte colony-stimulating factor leading to collection of various inflammatory cells which will support as well as survival of the tumor cells.
8. This disease can be classified based on:
   a. Clinical features
   b. Behavior
   c. Composition of the cellular back-ground
   d. Other morphological features
   e. Immunophenotyping
9. Hodgkin disease can be subclassified into two types:
   i. Classical Hodgkin lymphoma:
      - Nodular sclerosis
      - Mixed cellularity

- Lymphocyte rich
- Lymphocyte depletion
  ii. Nodular lymphocyte predominant Hodgkin lymphoma
10. The subtypes of classical Hodgkin lymphoma differ based on the following:
    a. Clinical features
    b. Growth patterns
    c. Morphological features of the Reed–Sternberg giant cells
    d. Cellular background
11. Following morphological Reed-Sternberg giant cells found in different subtypes of the classical Hodgkin lymphoma:
    a. Classical Reed-Sternberg giant cells are seen in mixed cellularity Hodgkin lymphoma.
    b. Lacunar cells are seen in nodular sclerosis variant of Hodgkin lymphoma.
    c. Hodgkin cell: It is not specific of Hodgkin lymphoma.
    d. Mummified cells—condensed eosinophilic cytoplasm along with pyknotic reddish nuclei
    e. Pleomorphic Reed-Sternberg cell—bizarre lobulated nuclei having variable shape and size, variable and prominent nucleoli, and eosinophilic cytoplasm. It is found in lymphocyte-depleted Hodgkin disease.
    f. Popcorn cells—large cells with large nucleus having folded and multilobulated nuclei resembling popcorn kernels. It is found in nodular sclerosis Hodgkin lymphoma.
12. Following are the stages of this disease:
    a. Stage I: Involvement of single lymph node region or a single extranodal organ or site (IE) like spleen, thymus, and Waldeyer ring.
    b. Stage II: Involvement of two or more lymph node regions on the same side of the diaphragm or localized involvement of a single extranodal organ or site along with one or more lymph node regions on the same side of the diaphragm.
    c. Stage III: Involvement of the lymph node regions on the both side of the diaphragm which may be associated with localized involvement of spleen (IIIS) or extranodal organ or site (IIIE) or both (IIISE).
    d. Diffuse or disseminated disease of one or more extranodal organs (involvement of liver and bone marrow) with or without involvement of lymph node.

These stages are further subdivided into:
    a. Without any symptom, i.e., asymptomatic
    b. Presence of constitutional symptoms like:
       - Night sweat
       - Unexplained fever of >38°C
       - Loss of >10% of body weight in the last 6 months
13. Following immunophenotypes present in all subtypes of Hodgkin cells:
    a. CD30+
    b. CD15+
14. Following are the bad prognostic factors in this disease:
    a. Age > 45 years
    b. Male sex is bad.
    c. Extent of the disease—it is worse in advanced stage.
    d. Constitutional symptoms—B types are bad.
    e. White blood cells > 15,000/cc
    f. Lymphocyte < 600/cc
    g. Albumin < 4 g/dL
    h. Hemoglobin < 10.5 g/dL
15. The patients have been subdivided into two treatment groups:
    i. Early stage classical Hodgkin lymphoma characterized by stage I to II (nonbulky) with favorable features
    ii. Advanced stage classical Hodgkin lymphoma characterized by stage III to IV (bulky tumor)
16. Treatment schedules are the following:
    a. For early stage group, it should be treated by chemotherapy with localized radiotherapy.
    b. For advanced stage, chemotherapy for 6–8 courses and later on involved field radiotherapy
17. Three patterns of relapsed and primary refractory classical Hodgkin lymphoma:
    a. Primary progressive classical Hodgkin lymphoma: It is characterized by failure to achieve complete remission or relapse within 3 months of the initial therapy.
    b. Early relapsed classical Hodgkin lymphoma is characterized by relapse within 12 months of complete remission.
    c. Relapse after 12 months following initial therapy, it is also known as late relapse.
18. Following are the prognostic factors in case of relapse:
    a. Time of relapse
    b. Poor performance status
    c. Age > 50 years
    d. Failure to obtain initial temporary remission

19. Treatment-related complications are the following:
    a. Gonadal toxicity
    b. Cardiac toxicity like cardiomyopathy
    c. Secondary neoplasm like acute myeloid leukemia and myelodysplastic syndrome
    Late complications of radiotherapy:
    a. Cardiovascular disease
    b. Secondary neoplasm:
       - Lung cancer
       - Breast cancer
       - Non-Hodgkin lymphoma
       - Soft tissue tumor
       - Bone tumor
       - Gastrointestinal tumor
       - Thyroid cancer
    c. Thyroid dysfunction

20. Etiological factors in this disease are the following:
    a. Epstein–Barr virus
    b. HIV infection
    c. Immunosuppression
    d. Autoimmune disorders
    e. Familial predisposition

21. Incidence of subtypes of Hodgkin lymphoma:
    a. Nodular sclerosis: 70%
    b. Mixed cellularity: 25%
    c. Lymphocyte rich: 5%
    d. Lymphocyte depletion: <1%

22. Immunohistochemistry stain of Reed–Sternberg cells demonstrates:
    a. CD15 and CD30 are positive.
    b. CD20 and CD45 are negative.

CASE 15

A 60-year-old female came to medical clinic with extreme tiredness, pain in small joint, and morning stiffness. On examination, there was pallor and swelling of the small joints of the hand with deformities. Hematological and biochemical reports demonstrated hemoglobin 7.5 g/dL, MCV, MCH, and mean corpuscular hemoglobin concentration (MCHC) were normal, ESR 52 mm/1st hour, WBC 8,000/cc, and platelet count 192,000/cc. Serum iron is low and serum ferritin is high. Following are the peripheral bood picture and picture of the joints:

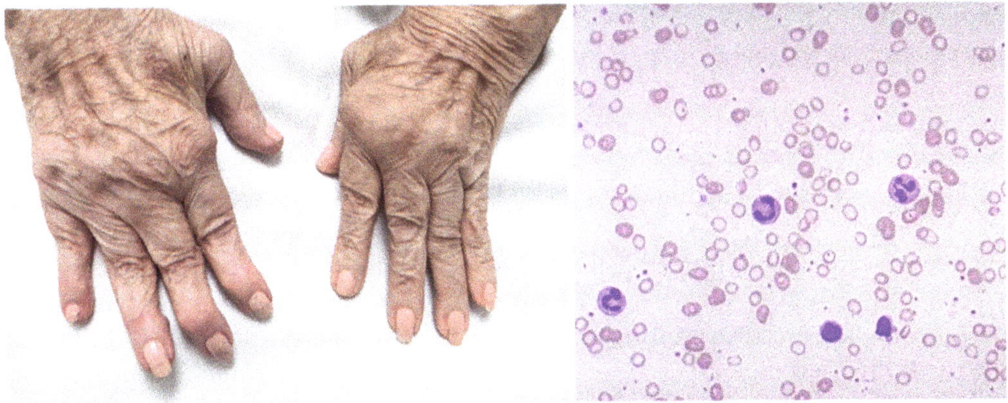

1. **Describe the above pictures.**
2. **What is the interpretation of the hematological and biochemical report?**
3. **What is your diagnosis?**
4. **Mention five infectious and five noninfectious inflammatory causes of this disease?**
5. **Why red blood cell survival is shortened in this disease?**
6. **Why there is impaired marrow response to anemia?**
7. **Why stored iron fails to release free iron into the circulation?**
8. **What is the most specific test to differentiate this disease from iron-deficiency anemia?**
9. **How can you define anemia?**
10. **How can you grade anemia?**
11. **Where the anemia is more prevalent?**
12. **How can you differentiate microcytic anemia based on iron studies?**

Answers

1. The left hand picture demonstrates evidence of rheumatoid arthritis involving metacarpophalangeal (MCP), proximal interphalangeal (PIP), and distal interphalangeal (DIP) joints. There is swan neck as well as boutonniere deformity. Right hand picture demonstrates evidences of anisocytosis, poikilocytosis, and polychromasia.

2. Hematological report demonstrates low hemoglobin, normal MCV, MCH, MCHC, low iron, and high ferritin.

3. This patient has been suffering from chronic anemia as a consequence of rheumatoid arthritis.

4. Five infectious causes of chronic anemia:
   i. Pulmonary tuberculosis
   ii. Lung abscess
   iii. Empyema
   iv. Pneumonia
   v. Osteomyelitis

   Five noninfectious inflammatory causes of chronic anemia are the following:
   i. Rheumatoid arthritis
   ii. SLE
   iii. Sarcoidosis
   iv. Crohn's disease
   v. Dermatomyositis

5. Red blood cell survival will be shortened due to following causes:
   a. Hyperplasia and activation of mononuclear phagocytic system
   b. Release of certain cytokines and tumor necrosis factor

6. Impaired marrow response to anemia due to following causes:
   a. Direct inhibitory effect of certain cytokines on the erythroid progenitor cells
   b. Low production of the erythropoietin, as a result marrow will fail to respond.
   c. Erythropoietin production will be suppressed by interleukin-2, interferon-α and tumor necrosis factor-α.

7. Stored iron fails to release iron to transferrin in the following mechanisms:
   a. Interleukin-1 increases the synthesis of apoferritin which combines with the available iron to form ferritin and will be stored in the macrophages.
   b. During phagocytosis or interleukin-6 it will release lactoferrin that combines with the iron more avidly as compared to lactoferrin, as result this lactoferrin fails to release iron to erythriood progenitor cells during erythropoiesis.
   c. Interleukin-6 increases the synthesis of hepcidin which in turn destroys ferroportin and thereby inhibits the transport of iron from the macrophages.
   d. Available low amount of iron will not be fully utilized by the erythroid precursor because either they have less number of receptors for transferrin or acute phase reactant inhibits binding of iron with the transferrin receptors.

8. Following specific tests should be performed to differentiate chronic anemia from iron-deficiency anemia:
   a. Soluble transferrin receptors—increased in iron-deficiency anemia but normal in anemia of chronic disease
   b. Serum hepcidin—decreased in iron-deficiency anemia but increased in anemia of chronic disease
   c. Bone marrow iron stores—depleted in iron-deficiency anemia but increased in anemia of chronic disease

9. Anemia can be defined as reduction of hemoglobin <13.5 g/dL in male and 12 g/dL in female or hematocrit level < 41% for male or 36% for female.

10. Anemia can be graded as following:
    a. Mild: Hemoglobin 10 g/dL to lower limit of normal
    b. Moderate: Hemoglobin 8–10 g/dL
    c. Severe: Hemoglobin 6.5–7.9 g/dL
    d. Very severe: Hemoglobin < 6.5 g/dL

11. Anemia is more prevalent in:
    a. Developing countries as a result of malnutrition and absence of proper medical care.
    b. In women due to menstrual bleeding and in pregnancy
    c. African and American people due to sickle cell disease or glucose-6-phosphate deficiency
    d. In case of old or late adulthood—with comorbidities like chronic kidney disease, medications, and malignancies

12. Differentiation of microcytic anemia based on iron studies:

Type of anemia	Serum iron	TIBC	Ferritin
Iron-deficiency anemia	Low	High	Low
Anemia of chronic disease	Low	Low	High
Sideroblastic anemia	High	Normal	High
Thalassemia	Normal	Normal	Normal

CASE 16

A 70-year-old man having recent past history of completed chemotherapy for indolent form of leukemia came to medical clinic with history of headache followed by drowsiness. On examination, there was pallor, jaundice, axillary lymphadenopathy, splenomegaly, increased neck stiffness, and bilateral generalized hyperreflexia.

Hematological report demonstrated pancytopenia. Peripheral blood picture and CT scan of brain are demonstrated as below:

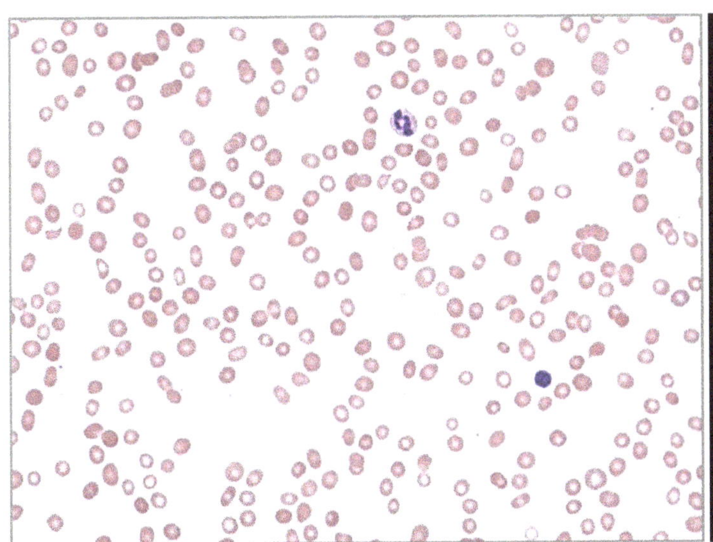
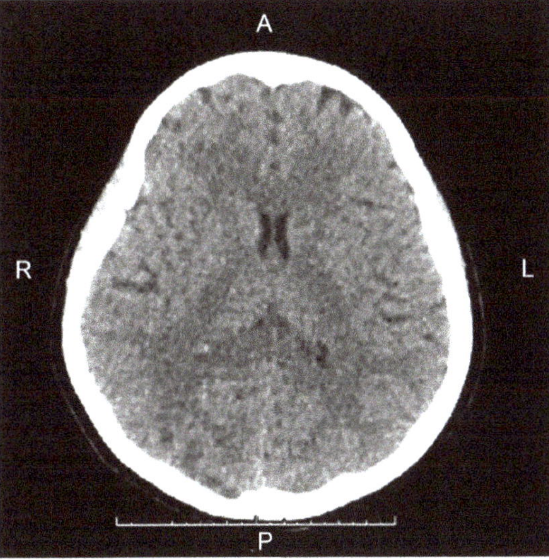

1. **What is shown in the peripheral blood picture?**
2. **Describe the CT scan of brain.**
3. **What is your diagnosis?**
4. **What are the tests to be done to diagnose this case?**
5. **How can you define this disease of this patient?**
6. **What are the risk factors for developing this disease?**
7. **What is the pathophysiology behind it?**
8. **What will be shown in the flow cytometric analysis?**
9. **What is the most typical skin involvement in chronic lymphocytic leukemia (CLL)?**
10. **What are the characteristic features in the immunophenotypic analysis in CLL?**
11. **What should be evaluated in this patient in the form of cytogenic evaluation of the peripheral blood picture prior to treatment?**
12. **Which cytogenic abnormalities in this patient require special attention?**
13. **What are the significance of 17p and 11q in this disease?**
14. **Mention the staging of chronic lymphocytic anemia.**
15. **What is Binet staging system in CLL?**
16. **What are the bad prognostic factors in CLL?**
17. **What are the indications of treatment with rituximab in this disease?**
18. **How this patient can be treated?**

Answers

1. Peripheral blood picture demonstrates decreased number of white blood cells, platelet, red blood cells, anisocytosis, poikilocytosis, polychromasia, and spherocytes.
2. CT scan of brain demonstrates low attenuation in the temporal and occipital region.
3. This patient has been suffering from autoimmune hemolytic anemia in the background of CLL.
4. Following tests should be done to diagnose this disease:
   a. Direct antiglobulin test
   b. Reticulocyte count
   c. Lymphoid cell flow cytometric analysis
   d. Bone marrow examination
5. Chronic lymphocytic leukemia can be defined as monoclonal lymphoproliferative disease which is characterized by proliferation followed by accumulation of the morphologically mature but immunologically dysfunctional B lymphocytes like smudge cells seen in the peripheral smear.
6. Following are the risk factors for this disease:
   a. Genetic factors
   b. Environmental factors:
      - Rubber factories
      - Exposure to benzene
      - Heavy solvent
      - Tobacco
   c. Occupational exposure like:
      - Chemicals
      - Radiations
      - Uranium miner
7. Pathophysiology behind this disease: CLL is a two-step processes leading to clonal replication of the malignant B lymphocytes (MBLs).
   a. In the first step, there is development of MBL due to several factors like:
      - Genetic mutation
      - Antigenic stimulation
      - Cytogenic abnormalities
   b. Second step is the progression of the MBL to CLL/SLL due to insult in the clone of B cells due to:
      - Further genetic abnormalities
      - Changes in the microenvironment in the bone marrow

Ultimately expression in the B cell antigen receptor induces antigen-independent cell-autonomous signaling.

8. Flow cytometric analysis demonstrates:
   a. B cells positive for B-cell markers such as CD19, CD20, CD21, and CD23
   b. Presence of low-density surface membrane immunoglobulin
   c. Predominant one light chain—either κ chain or λ chain
   d. B cells also demonstrates T-cell marker CD5.
9. Most important skin manifestation in this disease is leukemia cutis which is characterized by appearance of macules, papules, plaques, nodules, and blisters in the face which can be diagnosed by skin biopsy. Other skin lesions occur due to bleeding or vasculitis or infection.
10. Characteristic immunophenotypic features in this disease are the following:
    a. Low level of immunoglobulins—mostly IgM and sometimes IgM and IgD
    b. Expression of B cell-associated antigens such as CD19, CD20, CD21, CD23, and CD24, of which most common are CD5, CD19, and CD23.
    c. Expression of CD5 antigen which is T cell-associated antigen.
11. Following cytogenic abnormalities should be evaluated prior to treatment:
    a. Deletion of 13q
    b. Deletion of 11q
    c. Trisomy of 12q
    d. Deletion of 17p
    e. Deletion of 6q
12. 11 deletion is associated with rapid progression and poor survival.
    a. Trisomy 12q: Atypical disease and aggressive disease.
    b. 17p deletion: Drug resistant, very poor prognosis.
    c. 6q deletion—is associated with progression of the disease.
13. The significance of 17p and 11q in this disease:
    a. 17p deletion: Morphology is CLL and prolympho-cytic leukemia. Very poor prognosis.
    b. 11q deletion: Marked lymphadenopathy, rapid progression of the disease, and poor prognosis.
14. Staging of the disease according to Rai staging system: There are three stages:
    a. Stage 0:
       - No lymphadenopathy
       - Absence of splenomegaly or hepatomegaly
       - Presence of lymphocytosis
       - Normal red blood cell and platelet count

b. Stage I:
- Lymphadenopathy
- Absence of splenomegaly and hepatomegaly
- Lymphocytosis
- Normal red blood cell and platelet count

c. Stage II:
- Splenomegaly and may be hepatomegaly
- Presence or absence of lymphadenopathy
- Lymphocytosis
- Normal red blood cell and platelet count

d. Stage III:
- Presence or absence of lymphadenopathy
- Absence of hepatomegaly or splenomegaly
- Anemia
- Near normal platelet count

e. Stage IV:
- Lymphadenopathy
- Hepatomegaly and splenomegaly
- Anemia
- Lymphocytosis
- Thrombocytopenia

Stage 0: Low risk, median survival < 10 years.

Stage I and II: Intermediate risk, median survival 7–9 years.

Stage III and IV: High risk, median survival 1.5–5 years.

15. Binet staging system of CLL based on number of the affected group of lymphoid tissue in the lymph nodes of neck, inguinal region, axillary region, spleen, and liver:

a. Stage A:
- Involvement of fewer than three areas of lymphoid tissue
- Absence of anemia or thrombocytopenia
- Median survival is >10 years.

b. Stage B:
- Involvement of three or more areas of lymphoid tissue
- Absence of anemia or thrombocytopenia
- Median survival is 7 years.

c. Stage C:
- Any number of lymphoid tissue is involved.
- Anemia, hemoglobin < 10 g/dL
- Thrombocytopenia having platelet count <100,000/cc
- Median survival is 2–5 years.

16. Following are the bad prognostic factors for CLL:

a. Male sex

b. Age > 70 years

c. Clinical stage: Rai stage III and IV and Binet stage B or C

d. Lymphocyte count > 12,000/cc

e. Atypical lymphoid cells

f. Number or smudge cells < 30%

g. Pattern of marrow trephine infiltration is diffuse.

h. Lymphocyte doubling time < 12 months

i. Expression of CD38 is positive in ≥20% cells.

j. Expression of ZAP-70 is positive in ≥20%.

k. *IgVH* gene status is unmutated.

l. Raised serum markers like lactate dehydrogenase and β2 microglobulin

m. Genetic abnormalities are 11q deletion/17p deletion/trisomy 12q.

17. Indications of rituximab are the following:

a. Development of anemia and thrombocytopenia indicating progressive marrow failure

b. Massive enlargement of lymph nodes size being 10 cm in the longest diameter or progressive or lymphadenopathy

c. Massive splenomegaly— palpable 6 cm below the left costal margin or progressive or symptomatic splenomegaly

d. Progressive lymphocytosis of >50% over 2 months

e. Lymphocytic doubling time <6 months

f. Autoimmune anemia and/or thrombocytopenia which is poorly responsive to corticosteroids.

g. Any one or more constitutional symptoms:
- Unintentional loss of weight of ≥10% in the previous 6 months
- Significant fatigue
- Fever of >38°C for two or more weeks in absence of infection
- Night sweat for >1 month.

18. Drugs used commonly are chlorambucil, or rituximab or fludarabine.

a. Rai stage 0/1: No treatment is required.

b. Rai stage 2–3: No treatment is required unless symptoms are severe.

c. Rai stage 4–6: Treatment should be started unless totally asymptomatic.

d. Rai stage 7–10: Therapy with novel drugs like bcl-2 antagonist or kinase inhibitor should be started.

CASE 17

A 40-year-old male on antitubercular treatment with isoniazid, ethambutol, and rifampicin in association with pyridoxine came to medical clinic with purpuric spot throughout the body. Hematological report demonstrated platelet count 10,000/cc, hemoglobin 11 g/dL, and WBC 12,000/cc. Peripheral blood picture demonstrated as below. Bone marrow also demonstrated as below:

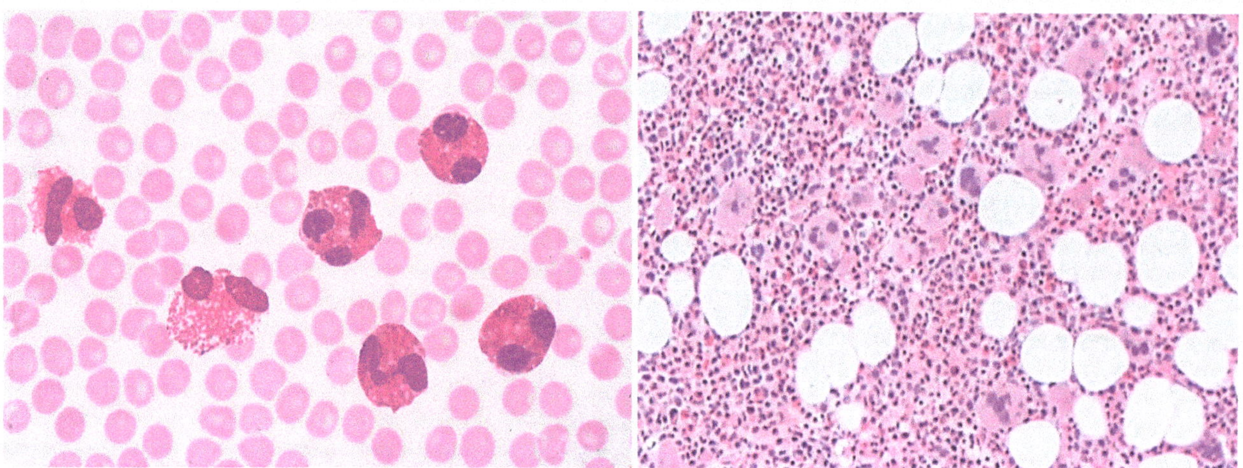

1. **Describe the peripheral blood picture and bone marrow picture?**
2. **What is your most likely diagnosis?**
3. **What is the most likely cause of this condition?**
4. **What are the drugs responsible for this condition?**
5. **Name two drugs responsible for decreased production of platelets?**
6. **How can this patient be treated?**

Answers

1. Peripheral blood picture demonstrates increased number of eosinophils and decreased platelet count. Bone marrow picture demonstrates increased number of megakaryocytes.
2. The most likely diagnosis is drug-induced thrombocytopenia with drug allergy.
3. Immune destruction of the platelets due to the drugs is responsible for this disease.
4. Other drugs responsible for this condition are:
   a. Heparin
   b. Sulfonamide
   c. Thiazide diuretics
5. Following two drugs are responsible for decreased production of platelets:
   i. Immunosuppressive drugs
   ii. Chemotherapeutic drugs
6. This patient should be treated by stoppage of the offending drugs and administration of steroids.

CASE 18

A 48-year-old male came to medical clinic with progressive tiredness and exertional respiratory difficulty and persisted productive cough inspite of taking amoxicillin. His chest X-ray is demonstrated as below. Peripheral blood picture is as demonstrated below:

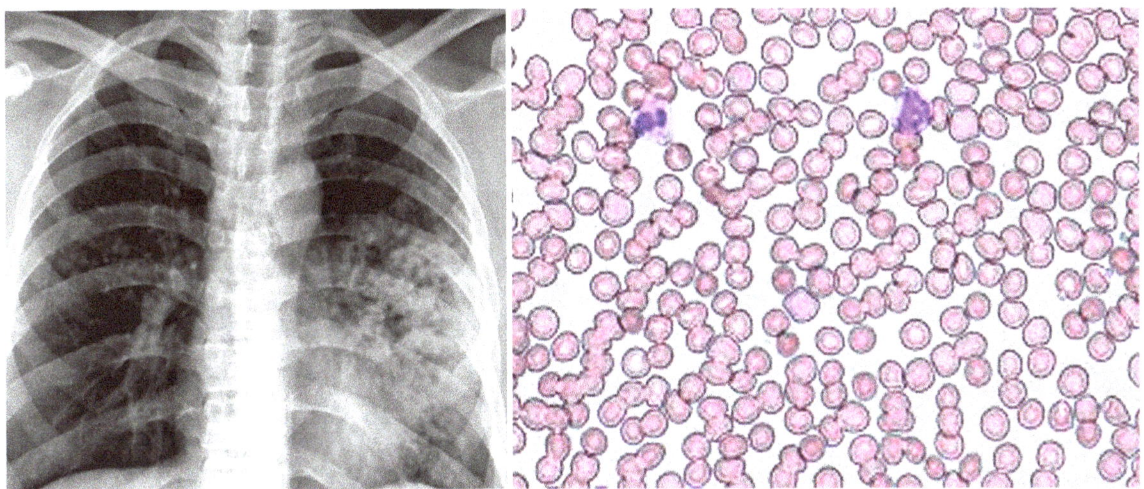

1. **Describe the chest X-ray.**
2. **Describe the peripheral blood picture.**
3. **What is the most likely diagnosis?**
4. **What will be the condition of the finger of the patient in this condition?**
5. **What are the diseases associated with this antibody?**
6. **Which antibody is responsible for this condition?**
7. **Why IgG is "incomplete antibody" and IgM is "complete antibody"?**
8. **How can you treat this patient?**
9. **What is the possible clue to the diagnosis?**

Answers

1. Chest X-ray demonstrates evidence of patchy consolidation in the left lower zone of the lung.
2. Peripheral blood picture demonstrates marked auto-agglutination indicating presence of cold agglutinin.
3. This patient has been suffering from autoimmune hemolytic anemia due to cold agglutinin as the patient has been suffering from mycoplasma pneumonia.
4. Patient's finger develops acrocyanosis as well as Raynaud's phenomenon as the acral part of the body is cold as compared to core temperature.
5. Acute cold antibody-associated agglutination occurs due to:
   a. *Mycoplasma* pneumonia
   b. Infectious mononucleosis

   Chronic clod agglutination occurs due to:
   a. Lymphoma
   b. Chronic lymphocytic leukemia
   c. Waldenström macroglobulinemia
6. Here, IgM antibodies react with the I antigen normally expressed on the red blood cells.
7. IgM because of its pentameric structure agglutinate spontaneously, hence these antibodies are called "complete antibody", whereas IgG will require antihuman globulin for agglutination of red blood cells.
8. This disease can be treated by simply avoidance of exposure to cold. But four weekly infusion of rituximab and anti-CD20 monoclonal antibody.
9. Clue to the diagnosis is the presence of acrocyanosis and livedo reticularis.

CASE 19

A 70-year-old male came to medical clinic with sudden loss of vision in one fine morning and ophthalmologist diagnosed this condition as branch of retinal artery thrombosis and presence of hemorrhage along with swelling in the left side of the neck. Blood test revealed hemoglobin level of 9.9 g/dL, ESR 100 mm/1st hour, and total protein 9.5 g/dL with globulin portion of 5.3 g/dL. Protein electrophoresis revealed IgM-κ. Bone marrow demonstrated as below:

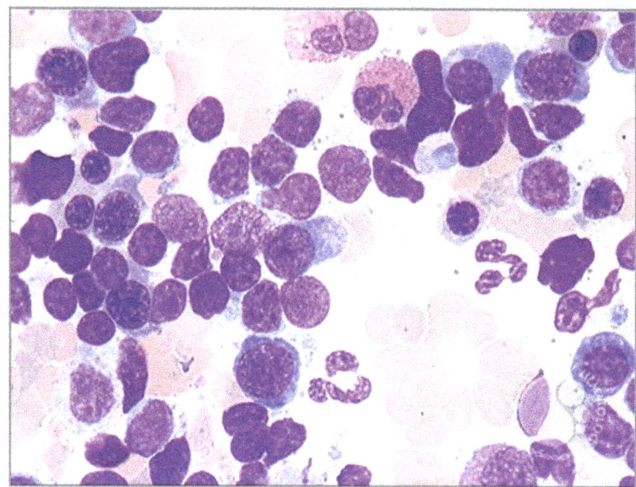

1. **What is shown in the bone marrow picture?**
2. **What is the most likely diagnosis?**
3. **Why there is visual disturbances?**
4. **What should be the normal viscosity of the blood? What occurs in this disease?**
5. **Why there is bleeding in this disease?**
6. **What may occur in the finger of this patient?**
7. **What is the most specific method of differentiating this disease from mantle cell lymphoma?**
8. **What should be clinical picture in the bone marrow examination?**
9. **How can you predict the prognostic score in this disease?**
10. **What are the complications occurring in this disease?**

Answers

1. Bone marrow picture demonstrates lymphoplasmacytic picture
2. The most likely diagnosis is Waldenström macroglobulinemia.
3. Visual disturbance is due to:
   a. Constricted and dilated retinal veins leading to appearance of "string of sausage".
   b. Retinal hemorrhage
   c. Blurring of vision
4. Normal viscosity of the blood is 1.4–1.8 cP. In this disease, the viscosity will be 6–8 cP.
5. Bleeding in this disease is due to:
   a. Adherence of macroglobulin to the platelet thereby preventing their aggregation
   b. Interference with the other coagulant factors
6. In the finger, there is evidence of Raynaud's phenomenon as the flow of the blood will be slow in this disease and during exposure to cold the patient may develop necrosis at the fingertip.
7. Flow cytometry can differentiate this disease from mantle cell lymphoma as this disease is positive for cyIgM, CD19, CD20, and CD22, whereas CD10 and CD23 are negative.
8. Bone marrow is typically highly cellular. Normal hematopoietic will be largely replaced by lymphoplasmacytic cells. Other cells found in the marrow are plasmacytoid lymphocytes, immunoblast, normal mast cells, plasma cells, and basophils.
9. Following are the predictors of poor outcome in this disease:
   a. Age > 65 years
   b. Hemoglobin of ≤11.5 g/dL

c. Platelet count of ≤100,000/cc

d. β2 microglobulin > 3 mg/L

e. Serum concentration of monoclonal protein >70 g/L

Risk categories are the following:

a. Low: ≤1 adverse variable except age

b. Intermediate: Two adverse characteristics or age > 65 years.

c. High: >2 adverse characteristics

10. Complications in this disease are the following:

a. Fever

b. Weight loss

c. Night sweat

d. Peripheral neuropathy

e. Amyloidosis

f. Renal failure

g. Cryoglobulinuria

CASE 20

A 28-year-old male came to medical clinic with following condition of the gum. On routine examination, following peripheral blood picture was found.

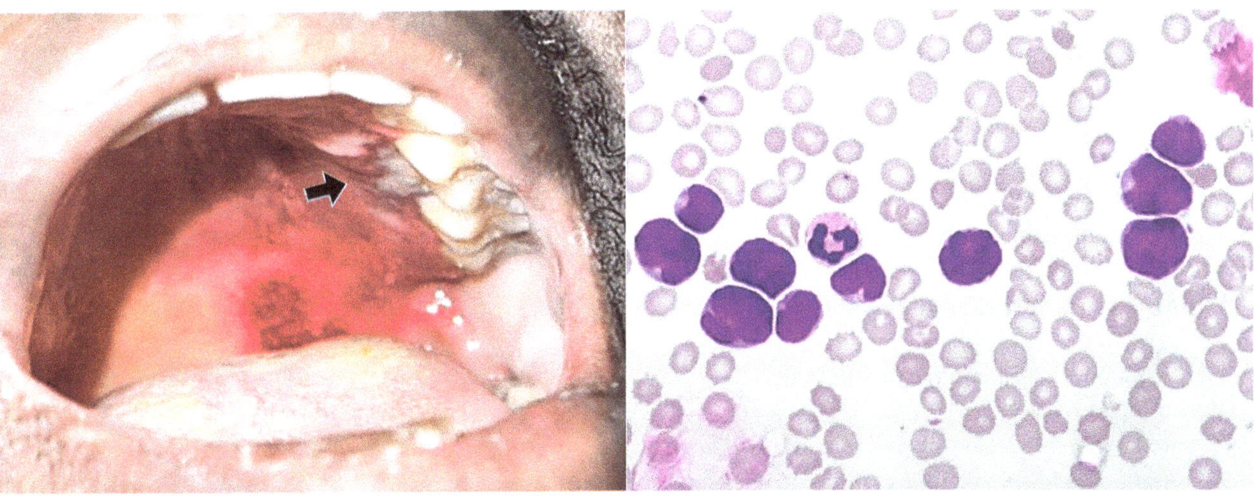

1. **What are shown in the above pictures?**

2. **What is your diagnosis?**

3. **Why there is gum bleeding?**

4. **Classify this disease. In which subvariety it is found?**

5. **What are the clinical features of this disease?**

6. **What are the laboratory investigations to be done in this disease?**

7. **What are the prognostic factors in this disease?**

8. **Name five favorable risk factors in this disease?**

9. **Mention five unfavorable risk factors in this disease?**

10. **What is induction chemotherapies in this disease?**

11. **Who will get better advantages with consolidation therapy? What is the drug of choice?**

12. **What are the causes of clinical relapse in this disease?**

13. **If the pregnant patient develops this disease, which drug should be avoided and why?**

14. **What are the CD markers in myeloid and monocytic variety of this disease?**

15. **How can you differentiate the prognosis by examining the morphology of the cells in the peripheral blood picture?**

Answers

1. The above pictures demonstrate bleeding in the gum and right-sided peripheral blood picture demonstrates multiple myeloid blast cells. These cells have:
   a. Plentiful gray cytoplasm
   b. Prominent nucleoli
   c. Cytoplasm contains vacuoles and sparse cytoplasm
2. This patient has been suffering from acute myeloid leukemia of monoblast subtype.
3. Gum bleeding is due to tissue infiltration with monoblast cells in the gum.
4. Acute myeloid leukemia can be classified into the following subvarieties:
   a. M0: Acute myeloid leukemia with minimal differentiation.
   b. M1: Acute myeloid leukemia with minimal differentiation
   c. M2: Acute myeloid leukemia with maturation
   d. M3: Acute promyelocytic leukemia
   e. M4: Acute myelomonocytic leukemia
   f. M5: Acute monoblastic leukemia
   g. M6: Acute erythroid leukemia—erythroid/myeloid
   h. M7: Acute megakaryoblastic leukemia—pure erythroid

   Acute myeloid leukemia can be again classified according to WHO:
   a. Acute myeloid leukemia and related neoplasms
   b. Acute myeloid leukemia with recurrent genetic abnormalities
   c. Acute myeloid leukemia with myelodysplasia-related changes
   d. Therapy-related myeloid neoplasms
   e. Acute myeloid leukemia not otherwise classified
   f. Myeloid sarcoma
   g. Myeloid proliferations related to Down syndrome
   h. Acute leukemias with ambiguous changes
   i. Myeloid neoplasms with germline predisposition
5. Clinical features related to marrow failure:
   a. Shortness of breath
   b. Fever
   c. Fatigue
   d. Focal bacterial infection
   e. Petechiae
   f. Severe bleeding indicates acute promyelocytic variety
   g. Bruising

   Features due to involvement of tissue:
   a. Bone pain—tenderness over the bone
   b. Gingival hyperplasia, there may be gum bleeding.
   c. Involvement leading to dysfunction of the central nervous system
   d. Visual abnormalities in the form of papilledema and retinal hemorrhage

   Rarely:
   a. Sweet syndrome
   b. Chloroma
6. Following laboratory abnormalities are found in acute myeloid leukemia:
   a. Hematologic features:
      - Increased number of white blood cells with increased number of blast cells
      - Granulocytopenia
      - Anemia
      - Thrombocytopenia
      - Disseminated intravascular coagulation
   b. Biochemical features:
      - Hyperuricemia
      - Increased level of lactate dehydrogenase
      - Increased serum level of blood urea, nitrogen, and creatinine
      - Hypokalemia
      - Leukostasis leading to lactic acidosis
      - Hypercalcemia
      - Spurious hypoxemia
      - Spurious hypoglycemia
   c. Imaging studies:
      - Intracranial hemorrhage due to hyper-viscosity
      - Thickened nerve sheath
      - Infiltrates in the lung
7. Following are the clinical prognostic factors in this disease:
   a. Age > 60 years
   b. Acute myeloid leukemia originating from myelo-dysplastic syndrome
   c. Treatment-related acute myeloid leukemia
   d. Molecular genetic abnormalities
   e. Performance status
   f. Extramedullary involvement
8. Following are the five favorable prognostic factors in this disease:
   a. Inv(6) or t(16,16)
   b. t(8,21)

c. t(15,17)

d. Normal karyotype with neoplasm 1

e. Normal karyotype with isolated biallelic CEBPA mutation

9. Following are the poor risk factors associated with this disease:

   a. Monosomal karyotype

   b. -5,5q-, -7,7q-

   c. Inv(3), t(3,3)

   d. t(6,9)

   e. t(9,22)

10. Most common therapy in this patient should be combination of 100–200 mg/m^2 cytarabine by continuous intravenous infusion over a period of 7 days and 3 days of 60–90 mg/m^2 daunorubicin or 12 mg/m^2 of idarubicin resulting in complete remission of >60%. Addition of 5 mg/m^2 cladribine, granulocyte colony-stimulating factors will improve the remission rate.

11. Consolidation therapy with high-dose cytarabine can be better in the following patients:

    a. Younger than 60 years of age

    b. Better-risk cytogenetics

    c. Core-binding factor mutations of t(8,21) and inv(16)

       The drug of choice is high-dose cytarabine using daily dose of 1–6 g/m^2 in divided doses in day 1, 3, and 5.

12. Causes of clinical relapse are the following:

    a. Chemosensitive disease which was partially treated, but later on return with additional genetic mutations.

    b. Subclone derived from same founder predominant clone presenting with low frequency and having same advantages during treatment, but later on it develops decreased sensitivity to chemotherapy.

    c. De novo generation of acute myeloid leukemia which is treatment related.

13. If pregnant patient develops acute myeloid leukemia. ATRA should not be administered in the first trimester because there may be chance of developing central nervous system or cardiovascular malformation. If this drug is administered in the second or third trimester, teratogenesis may not develop.

14. In case of myeloid variety of leukemia:

    a. CD33

    b. CD13

    c. CD15

In case of monocytic variety of leukemia:

    a. CD14

    b. CD64

    c. CD11b

15. One can differentiate the prognosis by examining the morphology of the cells in the peripheral blood picture:

Morphology	Favorable prognosis	Unfavorable prognosis
Auer rods	Present	Absent
Eosinophils	Present	Absent
Presence of megaloblastic erythroid cells	Absent	Present
Dysplastic megakaryocytes	Absent	Present

CASE 21

A 65-year-old male came to medical clinic with complaint of pain in the back of the neck associated with tingling and numbness of the hand. On examination, there was pallor and tenderness at the T7 vertebra level

Hematological and biochemical picture demonstrate hemoglobin 9 g/dL, platelet count 130,000/cc, white blood cell count 8,500/cc, ESR 90 mm/1st hour, plasma bilirubin level 1 mg/dL but SGOT and SGPT were normal, and plasma protein 9.2 g/dL with portion of globulin of 5.1 g/dL. CT scan picture of the dorsal spine demonstrated extradural tumor at the level of dorsal spine.

Following two pictures demonstrated:

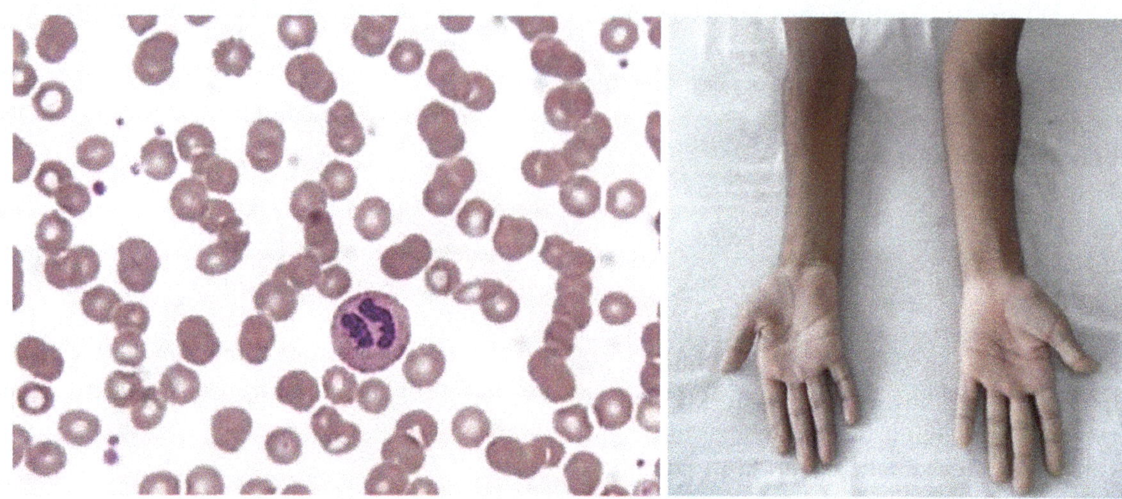

1. What have been demonstrated in the above pictures?
2. What is the interpretation of the blood report?
3. What is your diagnosis?
4. What is the significance of the demography of this disease?
5. What are the predisposing factors in this disease?
6. What are the cytokines involved in this disease?
7. Which cytokine is most important and what is its role in this disease?
8. Which cytokine is secreted by the abnormal cells in this disease?
9. What are the diagnostic criteria in the spectrum of this disease?
10. How the changes in the bone marrow will lead to development of this disease in future?
11. What are the bone involved in this condition?
12. What are the spectra of presentation in this lesion?
13. What are the causes of anemia in this disease?
14. What are the causes of recurrent infection and what are the organisms responsible?
15. What are the causes of bleeding tendency in this disease?
16. What is hyperviscosity syndrome occurring in this disease?
17. What are the mechanisms by which kidney will be involved?
18. What should be the classical blood picture in this disease?
19. What is the characteristic feature of classical abnormal cell found in this disease?
20. What are the other morphologically variant cells found in this disease?
21. In the bone marrow trephine biopsy, what are the pattern of these specific cells around the arteriole and what are the associated bony changes seen?
22. What should be the pattern of serum protein electrophoresis in this disease?
23. How can you detect the nature of this abnormal protein?
24. What are the percentages of the different immunoglobulin and light chain of this abnormal protein in the serum or urine?
25. Who are declared as "nonsecretors" and "nonproducers" in this disease?
26. What is plasma cell labeling index?
27. What is the significance of cytogenetics in this disease?
28. What are the bad prognostic factors in this disease?
29. What are the indicators of progression of this disease?

Answers

1. Peripheral blood picture reveals microcytic anemia along with rouleaux formation in the red blood cells. Second picture demonstrates the wasting of the hands involving both upper limbs.
2. Blood report demonstrates low hemoglobin, high ESR, and low platelet high protein along with increased production of globuln.

   In the peripheral blood, there is increased formation of rouleaux formation, presence of extradural tumor, and wasting of the small muscles of the hand—all are pointer to the diagnosis of multiple myeloma.
3. This patient has been suffering from multiple myeloma with complications like compression of the spinal cord by dorsal extradural tumor resulting in tingling numbness and wasting of the small muscles of the hand.
4. Demographic risk factors are the following:
   a. Age: Median age at diagnosis is 69 years. Highest incidence is between 65 and 74 years.
   b. Male sex: Male-to-female ratio is 1.4:1
   c. Race: It is more common in African American as compared to Caucasians.
   d. Familial: Its incidence is 3.7 times more common in the first-degreee relatives suffering from this disease.
5. Predisposing factors are the following:
   a. Its incidence is high among the survivors of Japanese atom bomb.
   b. Its risk is two times more common among the radiologist as compared to physicians.
   c. Its risk is increased in persons exposed to herbicides, pesticides, and workers in metal industries.
   d. Monoclonal gammopathy of undetermined significance:
      • Risk of progression of this disease toward multiple myeloma is increased if the plasma myeloma protein is >25 g/L as compared to the level of <5 g/L.
      • Risk of progression is increased if the immunoglobulin subtype is either IgA or IgM.
   e. Chronic antigenic stimulation by various infections, inflammatory condition, connective tissue disorders as well as autoimmune diseases will enhance the risk of multiple myeloma.
   f. Following virus infections such as HIV, herpesvirus-8, and hepatitis C will increase the risk of multiple myeloma.

6. Following cytokines are involved in this disease:
   a. Interleukin-6
   b. Vascular endothelial growth factor
   c. Tumor necrosis factor-α
   d. Interleukin-1
   e. Lymphokines
   f. Insulin-like growth factor-1
   g. Macrophage inflammatory protein-α
   h. Receptor activator of NF-$\kappa\beta$
   i. Interleukin-1β
   j. β-fibroblastic growth factor
7. Most important cytokine involved in this disease is interleukin-6, it is responsible for:
   a. Increased proliferation as well as survival of the myeloma cells in the bone marrow.
   b. It will reduce the apoptosis of the tumor cells leading to increased longivity of the cells.
   c. It will increase the osteoclastic activity associated with other factors like interleukin-1β, tumor necrosis factor-α, and macrophage inflammatory protein-1α.
8. Interleukin-1β is produced by all the patients of multiple myeloma responsible for:
   a. Increased osteoclast-activating factor activity leading to lytic bony lesion
   b. Increased expression of the adhesion molecules leading to homing of the myeloma cells in the bone marrow.
   c. Induction of production of interleukin-6
9. Diagnostic criteria in the plasma cell disorder are the following:
   a. Monoclonal gammopathy of unknown significance:
      • Myeloma protein < 3 g/dL
      • Bone marrow demonstrates monoclonal plasmacytosis of <10%
      • No evidence of other B cells of malignancy
      • Myeloma-related end organ disease is negative.
   b. Smoldering multiple myeloma:
      • Myeloma protein of ≥3 g/dL
      • Chronic plasmacytosis of >10% but <80%
      • No disease-related symptoms in the host:
         ○ No anemia
         ○ No hypercalcemia
         ○ No bone disease
         ○ No renal insufficiency

c. Multiple myeloma:
- Clonal bone marrow plasma cells of ≥10% or biopsy-proven bony or extramedullary plasmacytoma.
  Plus
- Any one or more of the myeloma defining events:
  - Myeloma defining events—evidence of damage of end organ that can be attributed to the underlying disorder of plasma cell proliferation.
  - Hypercalcemia—serum calcium > 1 mg/mL higher than the upper limit of normal or >11 mg/dL.
  - Renal insufficiency, i.e., creatinine clearance > 2 mg/dL
  - Anemia, i.e., hemoglobin level > 2 g/dL below the lower limit of normal or hemoglobin level is <10 g/dL.
  - Bone lesion—one or more osteolytic lesion on skeletal radiography, CT scan, or PET-CT
- Any one or more of the following biomarkers of malignancy:
  - Clonal bone marrow plasma cell percentage ≥ 60%
  - Involved: uninvolved serum free light chain ratio ≥ 100
  - One focal lesion on MRI studies (each focal lesion must be ≥5 mm in size).

10. Multiple destructive lesions as a result of deposition of myeloma cells present in the bone containing marrow followed by involvement of the cancellous bone and finally destroys the cortical bones.

11. Following bones are involved in this condition:
    a. Vertebrae
    b. Ribs
    c. Skull bones
    d. Pelvis
    e. Femur
    f. Clavicle
    g. Scapula

12. Following are the spectra of presentation in the bony lesion:
    a. Bone pain
    b. Pathological fractures
    c. Paraplegia due to compression in the spinal cord
    d. Polyneuropathy due to compression of cauda equina or on the cranial nerve by a big mass
    e. Suppression of the normal hematopoiesis due to infiltration of the bone marrow by the plasma cells

13. Anemia in this disease due to the following causes:
    a. Normal hematopoietic cells will be replaced by the malignant cells.
    b. Overactive cytokines interleukin-1 and tumor necrosis factor-α inhibit erythropoiesis.
    c. Reduced production of erythropoietin as a result of renal damage
    d. Bleeding
    e. FAS ligand reduces erythropoiesis

14. Following are the causes of recurrent infection:
    a. Suppression of the bone marrow
    b. Reduction of the normal humoral activity
    Following organisms are responsible for recurrent infection:
    a. *Staphylococcus aureus*
    b. *Streptococcus pneumoniae*
    c. *Haemophilus influenzae*
    d. Gram-negative bacilli like *E. coli*

15. Following are the causes of increased bleeding tendency:
    a. Presence of abnormal protein coats the platelet leading to decreased aggregation of platelet and interfering with clotting system
    b. Infiltration of the bone marrow by the myeloma cells leading to thrombocytopenia
    c. Uremia
    d. Hyperviscosity

16. High concentration of myeloma protein leads to increased viscosity of the blood.

17. Following factors will lead to renal damage:
    a. Deposition of Bence Jones protein in the glomerular mesangium
    b. Hypercalcemia leads to development of nephrocalcinosis
    c. Dehydration
    d. Hyperuricemia
    e. Nephrotoxic drugs
    f. Acute or chronic pyelonephritis
    g. Infiltration of the myeloma cells in streaks or nodules
    h. Filtration of the light chain particularly κ throughout the glomerulus
    i. AL type amyloid deposits usually λ chain

18. The peripheral blood picture demonstrates:
    a. Low hemoglobin—normocytic normochromic anemia
    b. White blood cells are normal or reduced.
    c. Platelet count is normal or reduced.
    d. Presence of rouleaux, i.e., red blood cells stick to one another in the form of linear array
    e. Presence of large number of plasma cells
19. Feature of classical anormal cell: It looks like normal plasma cell with eccentric nucleus having "spoke wheel" chromatin in the midst of basophilic cytoplasm and clear perinuclear.
20. Following are the morphologically variant plasma cells found in this disease:
    a. Flame cells with intense eosinophilic cytoplasm
    b. Mott cells or morula cells containing pale blue white grape-like accumulation of cytoplasm
    c. Russel bodies: These contain cherry-red refractile round bodies or hyaline globule.
    d. Dutcher bodies are intranuclear inclusions seen by PAS staining
    e. Crystalline rods in cytoplasm
21. In the bone marrow trephine biopsy, myeloma cells arrange in three more patterns around the arterioles:
    a. Interstitial with or without seams of plasma cells—it is least aggressive.
    b. Nodular or broadband type
    c. Diffuse fully packed cells replacing fully the hematopoietic cells
22. Following five different components seen in the serum protein electrophoresis:
    a. Albumin
    b. $\alpha2$-globulin
    c. $\alpha1$-globulin
    d. β-globulin
    e. γ-globulin
23. In multiple myeloma, electrophoretic pattern of the serum protein is characterized by tall, narrow, and sharply defined peak as a result of homogeneous protein in large amount. This protein can be detected by:
    a. Different methods of immunoelectrophoresis
    b. Serial radial immunodiffusion
    c. Immunofixation

24. Percentages of myeloma protein are the following:
    a. IgG: 52%
    b. IgA: 20%
    c. IgD: 2%
    d. IgM: <1%
    e. Free light chain: 16%
25. In some cases, there is no detectable myeloma protein. These cases are known as nonsecretory protein. In these cases, cytoplasmic myeloma protein can be detected by immunohistochemistry in 85% cases. Again in 15% of cases, there is no detectable cytoplasmic myeloma protein. These cases are known as nonproducers.
26. Plasma cell labeling index is used to detect the proliferating activity of the tumor cells and this can be measured by thymidine labeling. If this index is low, i.e., <1%, it indicates the low number of actively growing plasma cells but their survival is longer which is opposite to that and is seen if this index is >1%.
27. Significance of cytogenetics in this disease:
    a. Common chromosomal translocation is in the heavy chain locus on chromosome 14q32 in the 55% cases.
    b. Monosomy or partial deletion of the chromosome number 13 has adverse prognosis.
    c. In case of t(4,14) and t(14,16), worst prognosis
28. Following are the bad prognostic factors in this disease:
    a. High β_2 microglobulin level, i.e., >5.5 mg/L
    b. High CRP
    c. Raised level lactate dehydrogenase
    d. Plasmablastic morphology
    e. Serum albumin level of <3.5 g/dL
    f. High plasma cell labeling index
    g. Secretion of λ chain
    h. Large number of cytogenic abnormalities like t(4,14), t(14,16), t(14,20), del(13q), and hypoploidy
29. Progression of this disease can be characterized by:
    a. Pancytopenia
    b. Unexplained fever
    c. Hypercellular marrow
    d. Extramedullary plasmacytoma

CASE 22

A 5-year-old child came with severe weakness having longtime history of anemia for which blood was given. On physical examination, there was pallor and hepatosplenomegaly. His blood picture and facies were demonstrated as below:

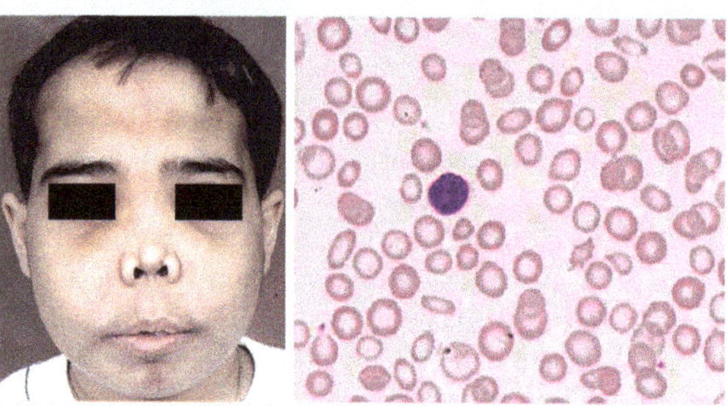

1. **What do the above pictures demonstrate?**
2. **What is your diagnosis?**
3. **How can you classify this disease?**
4. **What is the pathophysiology behind this disease?**
5. **What are the functional and structural abnormalities seen in this disease and why?**
6. **What are the effects of anemia in the patient?**
7. **What is the genetic mutation in this disease?**
8. **What are the causes of hypercoagulability in this disease?**
9. **Why there is osteoporosis in this disease?**
10. **How can you perform prenatal diagnosis?**
11. **How can you diagnose where blood has already been transfused?**
12. **How can you differentiate this disease from iron-deficiency anemia?**
13. **What are the abnormal cells seen in the peripheral blood picture?**
14. **What are the causes of raised hemoglobin A2 level other than this disease?**
15. **What are the nutritional sequelae that occur in this disease?**
16 **What are the complications of this disease?**

Answers

1. Facies demonstrate:
   a. Large and deformed skull
   b. Frontal and posterior bossing
   c. Depression of the nasal bridge
   d. Prominent zygomatic bones
   e. Overgrowth of maxilla leading to malocclusion of bones

   Peripheral blood picture demonstrates hypochromic macrocytic anemia, anisocytosis, target cells, and teardrop cells.

2. This patient has been suffering from β-thalassemia major.

3. β-thalassemia major can be classified into the following three types:
   a. β-thalassemia major—homozygous disease requiring regular blood transfusion
   b. β-thalassemia minor—heterozygous state requiring intermittent blood transfusion
   c. β-thalassemia intermedia—requiring no regular blood transfusion

4. Hemoglobin, tetramer, is composed of two α-globin chains combining with two β-globin chains. Fetal hemoglobin is composed of two α-globin chains combining with two γ-globin chains. Adult hemoglobin is mainly hemoglobin A consisting of two α- and two β-globin chains, and little A2 containing two α-chains and two δ-chains.

   So, pathophysiology of β-thalassemia is of two folds:
   a. Decreased concentration of hemoglobin A and increased concentration of hemoglobin A2 and F leading to decreased synthesis of normal hemoglobin resulting in anemia.
   b. In case of β-thalassemia major as well as intermedia, there is relative excess α-chain leading

to formation of insoluble inclusion of α-chain resulting in marked intramedullary hemolysis and ineffective erythropoiesis.

5. Following are the functional and structural abnormalities in the red blood cells due to precipitation of α-chains in the cells:

a. Membrane damage of the red blood cells leading to increased rigidity and decreased deformability resulting in destruction of the cells.

b. Alteration of the protein band-3 in the membrane of red blood cells leading to creation of neoantigen resulting in its removal by immune process.

c. Ineffective erythropoiesis

d. Increased surface exposure of anionic phospholipids, procoagulants leading to increased generation of thrombin resulting in hypercoagulability of the blood

6. Effects of anemia in this patient: It has two effects:

a. Repeated blood transfusion leading to increased iron overload resulting in accumulation of iron in the:

   - Liver resulting cirrhosis
   - Heart resulting cardiomyopathy
   - Pancreas resulting diabetes mellitus

b. Tissue hypoxia leading to increased production of erythropoietin resulting in massive erythroid hyperplasia in the bone marrow, it has two effects:

   i. Bony abnormalities—prominent maxilla and crew cut appearances in the skull

   ii. Extramedullary hematopoiesis resulting in splenomegaly, as result pooling of blood due to increased size and anemia results.

7. β-*globin* gene is present in the chromosome number 11. This mutation is usually point mutation, which is of two types:

a. Nondeletion defect:

   - Alteration in the β gene transcription
   - Affection of mRNA processing
   - Affection of translation of mRNA

b. Deletion defect: Removal of 3' end of the β-*chain* gene which is common in population of Punjab and Sindh.

8. Following are the causes of hypercoagulability:

a. Increased surface exposure of anionic phospholipids, procoagulants leading to increased generation of thrombin resulting in hypercoagulability of the blood

b. Activation of platelets

c. Endothelial cell injury

d. Peroxidative status

9. Following are the causes of osteoporosis in this disease where the bone density is ≥ 2.5:

a. Expansion of bone marrow

b. Iron overload

c. Endocrine dysfunction

10. Prenatal diagnosis can be done getting fetal DNA by chorionic villus sampling in the first trimester and analysis of DNA by PCR methods.

11. If the patient has already received blood transfusion, in that case, analysis of globin chain should be done in the peripheral blood leukocytes where the ratio of severe α/non-α balance is usually >2.

12. Red blood cell distribution width can differentiate this disease from iron-deficiency anemia as this will be increased in the later but decreased in the former.

13. Following cells are found in the peripheral blood picture:

a. Teardrop cells

b. Basophilic stippling

c. Target cells

d. Howell–Jolly bodies

14. Following are the causes of raised hemoglobin A2 level other than this disease:

a. Antiretroviral therapy

b. Vitamin B12 or folate deficiency

c. Hyperthyroidism

15. Following are the nutritional sequelae that occur in this disease:

a. Iron overload

b. Folate deficiency

c. Calcium depletion

d. Vitamin C deficiency

16. Complications in this disease are the following:

a. Due to iron overload in:

   - Heart leading to heart failure
   - Endocrine glands leading to:
     - Thyroid gland resulting in hyperthyroidism or hypothyroidism
     - Pancreas leading to diabetes mellitus
     - Gonads leading to hypogonadism

b. Thromboembolic events leading to pulmonary thromboembolism and recurrent occlusion of arteries

c. Effects of hypersplenism

d. HIV infection

e. HBV hepatitis—transfusion related

CASE 23

A 25-year-old female came to medical clinic with extreme tiredness, bruising, and menorrhagia. Her peripheral blood picture, bone marrow, and CT scan demonstrated as below:

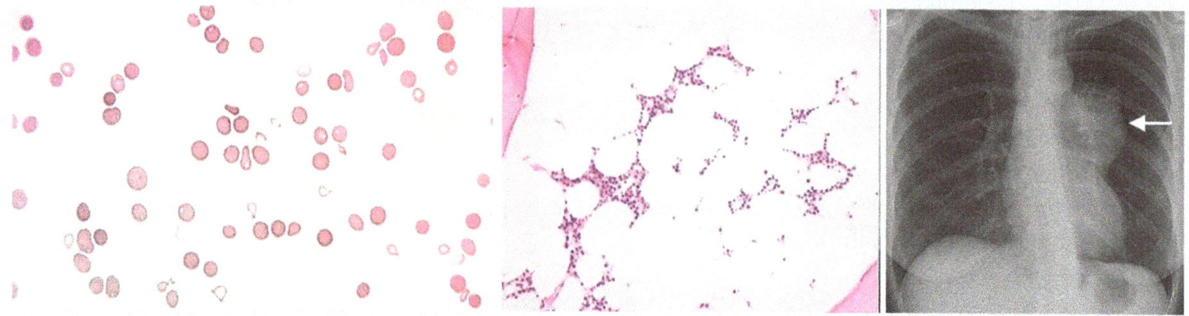

1. **What are shown in the above pictures?**
2. **What is your most likely diagnosis?**
3. **Mention eight drugs responsible for this blood picture.**
4. **How can you differentiate this disease from constitutional anemia?**
5. **How can you differentiate aleukemic leukemia from this disease?**
6. **How can you differentiate this disease from myelofibrosis?**
7. **Name four chemicals responsible for this disease.**
8. **What is the pathophysiology in this disease?**
9. **What are the probabilities regarding the fates of hematopoietic stem cells?**
10. **What are the criteria for defining the this disease?**
11. **What are the criteria for severe type of this blood picture?**
12 **Mention immunotherapies in this disease.**

Answers

1. The above pictures demonstrate:
   a. Extreme left hand picture demonstrates features of deficient red blood cells, hypochromia, scarcity of white blood cells, and platelet.
   b. Middle picture demonstrates hypocellularity mainly plasma cells, mast cells, and residual lymphocytes.
   c. Right hand chest X-ray demonstrates widening of anterior mediastinum, most likely thymoma.
2. The patient has been suffering from aplastic anemia probably due to thymoma.
3. Following eight drugs are responsible for aplastic anemia:
   a. Antibiotics
   b. Allopurinol
   c. Furosemide
   d. Corticosteroids
   e. Indomethacin
   f. Antithyroid drugs
   g. Nonsteroidal anti-inflammatory drugs (NSAIDs)
   h. Sulfonamides

4. The causes of constitutional anemia are the following:
   a. Fanconi anemia:
      - Distinguishing characteristics:
        - Younger patient
        - Family history
        - Physical abnormalities such as short stature, café-au-lait spots, anomalies in the thumb, and upper limbs
        - Diagnostic tests: Chromosomal analysis of the stressed blood lymphocytes culture
   b. Dyskeratosis congenita:
      - Distinguishing characteristics:
        - Younger patient
        - Family history
        - Physical abnormalities such as nail changes and leukoplakia
        - Diagnostic test: Mutation of short telomere in TERC, TERT, RTEL, TINF2, and DKCI
5. From aleukemic leukemia:
   a. Distinguishing features: Extremes of age
   b. Diagnostic tests: Presence of blast cells in the buffy coat smear.

6. From myelofibrosis:
   a. Distinguishing feature:
      - Hepatosplenomegaly
      - Leukoerythroblastic blood picture
   b. Diagnostic test: Fibrosis in the bone marrow biopsy
7. Following four chemicals are responsible for this disease:
   i. Benzene
   ii. Glues
   iii. Commercial solvents
   iv. Pentachlorophenol
8. Pathophysiology in this disease: There are two theories in this disease:
   i. Extrinsic immune-related suppression of hematopoietic stem cells: Damaged hematopoietic stem cells will mature into self-reactive T helper cells leading to release of interferon and tumor necrosis factor which suppress the hematopoietic stem cells. The exact antigen is not known but it appears to be glucose phosphate inositol which is linked to red blood cell membrane. There is upregulation of the genes for apoptosis.
   ii. Intrinsic abnormality of marrow progenitors: Inability to differentiation of stem cells into red blood cells leads to clonal evolution of the hematologic neoplasm like myelodysplastic syndrome. There is inability of the stem cells to proliferate leading to increased clone of premature hematopoietic stem cells.
9. Following are the probabilities of fates of the hematopoietic stem cells:
   a. The number of hematopoietic stem cells (CD34+)
   b. There is failure of proliferation and differentiation of the pluripotent or committed stem cells due to drugs, chemicals, or irradiations.
   c. Defective microenvironment in the bone marrow prevents the hematopoietic stem cells to populate for normal hematopoiesis
   d. One clone of stem cells interacts with other clone to inhibit the growth of the cells
   e. CD8+ cytotoxic cells or humoral antibody via autoantibody injure immunologically the hematopoietic stem cell
10. For defining the aplastic anemia at least two of the following criteria should be filled:
    i. Hemoglobin is < 10 g/dL
    ii. Absolute count of the neutrophil should be <1,500/cc.
    iii. Platelet count is <50,000/cc.
11. These are the criteria of severe aplastic anemia:
    a. Bone marrow cellularity:
       - <25%
         Or,
       - 25–50% with 30% residual hematopoietic cells
    b. In the peripheral blood (any two of the following):
       i. Absolute neutrophil count < 500/cc
       ii. Platelet count < 20,000/cc
       iii. Reticulocyte count is <20,000/cc on manual count or <60,000/cc on automated count or corrected reticulocyte count is <1%.
12. The immunosuppressive therapy in aplastic anema: Antithymocyte globulin along with cyclosporine A should be of choice if no suitable donor of bone marrow transfusion is available. There are two types of antithymocyte globulin:
    i. Horse antithymocyte globulin 40 mg/kg daily for 4 days
    ii. Rabbit antithymocyte globulin 3.5 mg/kg daily for 5 days
       Corticosteroid should be administered for first 2 weeks to treat the serum sickness if any.
       In case of relapse or refractory case, second dose of immunosuppression can be given. In refractory case, rabit antithymocyte globulin or alemtuzumab should be given to obtain hematologic response of 30–40%.

CASE 24

A 65-year-old male presented with progressively increasing tiredness, three episodes of infections treated with antibiotics within the span of 5 months. On examination, there was pallor and basal crepitations indicating persisting infection and just palpable spleen. His peripheral blood picture demonstrated hemoglobin 7.8 g/dL, white blood cell count 3,000/cc, platelet count 85,000/cc. Bone marrow tapping was tried but failed. Peripheral blood picture demonstrated:

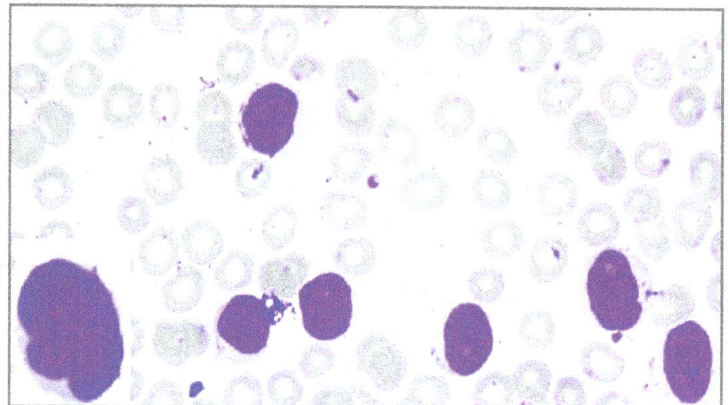

1. **What is shown in the above picture?**
2. **What is your diagnosis?**
3. **How can you define this disease?**
4. **What should be the characteristics of the neoplastic cells in the bone marrow?**
5. **Why there is dry tap in this case?**
6. **What is the importance of immunohistochemistry in this case?**
7. **What is the specific marker of this case?**
8. **What is the importance of immunophenotyping in this case?**
9. **What is the genetic relation with this disease?**
10. **How can you treat this disease?**

Answers

1. The peripheral blood picture demonstrates abnormal lymphoid cells, decreased clump of platelets, and hypochromic red blood cells.
2. This patient has pancytopenia, abnormal circulating lymphoid cells, splenomegaly, and failure of bone marrow aspiration suggests the diagnosis of hairy cell leukemia.
3. This disease can be defined as neoplasm of small mature B lymphocytes having abundant cytoplasm and hairy projections from the wall involving the peripheral blood, bone marrow, and the splenic pulp.
4. In the bone marrow, the infiltration is interstitial and patchy. The cell has honeycomb appearance with surrounding clear halo. The nuclei are oval or indented; abundant cytoplasm having prominent outline looking like "fried frog" in appearance.
5. The dry tap is due to increased amount of reticulin fibers along with diffuse infiltration of hairy cells.
6. In this case, the cells are positive for strong granular tartrate-resistant acid phosphatase in immunohisto-chemistry.
7. This cell is positive for antigen A1 because it is not expressed in other B lymphoid neoplasm.
8. This disease is CD19, CD20, CD22, CD25, CD103, and CD11c positive.
9. There is mutation of *V600E BRAF* gene of late activated memory B cells leading to development of this disease.

10. The drug of choice is cladribine as first line of chemotherapy as single dose can induce complete response in 90% of patients. But, as this patient is immunosuppressed, there is chance of infection.
    - Other drugs are chlorodeoxyadenosine, deoxycoformycin, or rituximab.
- In case of pregnant patient, interferon-α and in case of severe pancytopenia and other drug, treatment is contraindicated.
- In case patient with massive splenomegaly and severe pancytopenia, splenectomy is preferred.

CASE 25

A 50-year-old male having no history of prior liver disease came to medical clinic with heaviness in the left upper abdomen. On examination, patient was mildly anemic, huge splenomegaly, and sternal tenderness. His blood report revealed hemoglobin 12 g/dL, white blood cells 114,000/cc, and platelet count 420,000/cc. Peripheral blood picture, bone marrow picture, and cytogenic analysis demonstrated:

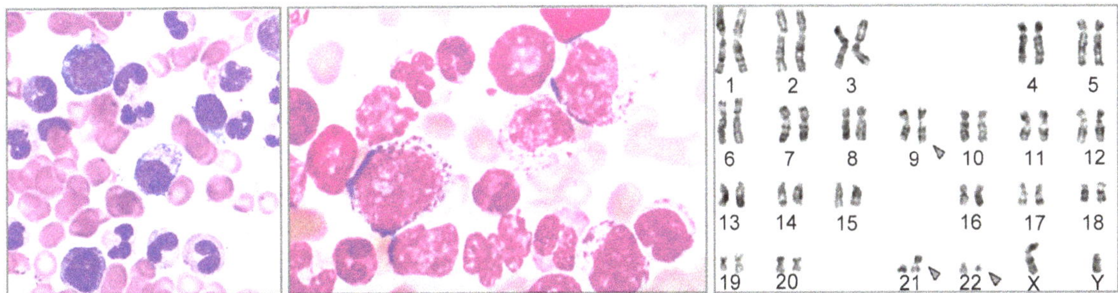

1. **What have been shown in the above pictures?**
2. **What is your diagnosis?**
3. **What are the stages of this disease?**
4. **What is the age incidence of this disease?**
5. **Why there is sternal tenderness?**
6. **Why patient may complaint of priapism?**
7. **What the patient may feel of pain in the left hypochondrium?**
8. **What should be the classical feature in the bone marrow in this disease?**
9. **What should be the level of neutrophil ALP in this disease?**
10. **Mention the criteria of the second phase in this disease.**
11. **What is the significance of lymphadenopathy in this disease?**
12. **When the patient will be diagnosed as he is in the third phase of this disease?**
13. **What are the different levels of responses to treatment in this disease?**
14. **How can you differentiate this disease from leukemoid reaction?**
15. **What are the aims of treating this patient in the first phase?**
16. **What are the drugs of choice for treating this patient?**
17. **How can you monitor this patient during treatment?**
18. **What are the criteria of treatment failure in this disease?**
19. **If there is sudden nonresponse during ongoing treatment what should be the cause?**
20. **What treatment should be given in female intending to have pregnancy?**
21. **What is the significance of leukostasis in this disease?**
22. **How can you grade the side effects of the tyrosine kinase inhibitors?**

Answers

1. The above pictures demonstrate:
   a. Peripheral blood picture demonstrates neutrophilic leukocytosis, immature granulocytes in the form of metamyelocytes, myelocytes, myeloblasts, but no immature erythroid cells. It suggests myeloproliferative disorder.
   b. Bone marrow picture demonstrates hypercellular, presence of <5% blast cells.
   c. Cytogenic analysis demonstrates translocation of the chromosome material between 9 and 22 chromosomes which are known as Philadelphia chromosome.

2. The patient has been suffering from chronic phase of chronic myeloid leukemia.

3. There are three stages of this disease:
   i. Chronic phase
   ii. Accelerated phase
   iii. Blast phase

4. The age incidence is in the fifth to sixth decade of this disease.

5. The sternal tenderness is due to:
   a. Increased cellularity
   b. Irritation of the periosteum

6. Patient developed priapism due to leukostasis.

7. Pain in the region of spleen due to splenic infarction as a result of leukostasis and leukemic cell infiltration in the vasculature.

8. Bone marrow in the chronic phase demonstrates:
   a. Hypercellularity with marked proliferation of the granulocytic series
   b. Blast cells are <5%.
   c. Decreased amount of erythroid precursors with increased myeloid to erythroid ratio
   d. The number of megakaryocytes is normal or increased. Size of megakaryocytes is dwarf or hypolobate morphologically.
   e. Evidence of immature granulocytes in a thickened band of 5–10 cells

9. Level of neutrophil ALP is low or near to zero but its level will be increased if it is associated with infection.

10. Accelerated phase of chronic myeloid leukemia if any one or more of the hematologic or cytogenetic criteria is/are present:
    a. Hematological:
       - Persistent or increasing white blood cells and/or
         Persistent or increasing splenomegaly not responding to therapy
       - Persistent thrombocytosis of >1,000,000/cc unresponsive to therapy
       - Persistent thrombocytopenia of <10,000/cc not related to therapy
       - ≥20% basophils in the peripheral blood
       - 10–19% blast cells in the peripheral blood
    b. Cytogenetic:
       - Additional clonal chromosomal abnormalities in the Philadelphia+ (Ph+) cells at the time of diagnosis that include "major route" abnormalities:
         o Second Ph
         o Trisomy 8
         o Isochromosome 17q
         o Trisomy 19
         o Complex karyotype or abnormalities of 3q26.2
       - Any new clonal chromosomal abnormality in Ph+ cells occurring during therapy

11. Cervical lymphadenopathy indicates:
    a. Poor prognosis
    b. The early entry into the blast crisis

12. Following are the criteria that can diagnose the patient as he is in the third phase:
    a. Blast cells ≥ 20% in the peripheral blood or of the nucleated cells in the bone marrow.
    b. Evidence of proliferation of the blast cells in the form of:
       - Myeloid sarcoma
       - Chloroma in the:
         o Skin
         o Central nervous system
         o Bone
         o Lymph nodes

13. Following are the levels of responses to treatment:
    - Hematologic response
    - Cytogenic response
    - Molecular response

14. In case of leukemia, neutrophil ALP level will be low but will increase in presence of infection. In case of leukemoid reaction, this level will be increased.

15. Aims of treatment in the first phase of the disease are:
    a. Debulking of the tumor
    b. Obtaining the hematological remission
    c. Subsequent therapy aims at cure of the residual disease

16. Drugs of choice are as follows:
    a. First-generation tyrosine kinase inhibitor: Imatinib—400 mg daily

b. Second-generation tyrosine kinase inhibitors:
- Bosutinib: 500 mg daily
- Dasatinib: 100 mg daily
- Nilotinib: 300 mg twice daily

c. Third-generation tyrosine kinase inhibitor: Ponatinib—45 mg daily

If the patient has >80,000/cc–100,000/cc white blood cell count, then 0.5–2.5 g hydroxyurea daily should be given to reduce the count along with 300 mg allopurinol daily to reduce the incidence of tumor lysis syndrome.

17. Following are the types of response to treatment:

a. Every 2 weeks full blood count should be monitored until complete hematological response and it should be confirmed on two occasions.

b. Aspiration of the bone marrow is every 6 months for assessing the cytogenic response. Complete cytogenic response should be Ph 0%. It indicates prolonged disease-free survival. Once it will be achieved, it should be confirmed on two occasions.

c. Every 3 months quantitative BCR-ABL transcripts should be done to assess:
- If the transcript will decline, it indicates disease responding to treatment.
- Stable level of transcripts
- If the transcripts are increasing, the patient loosing response to treatment.

18. Following are the criteria of failure to treatment with tyrosine kinase inhibitors:

a. Absence of hematological response in 3 months

b. Absence of cytogenic response, i.e., Ph > 95% in 3 months

c. In 6 months, less than partial cytogenic response, i.e., Ph > 35%

d. In 6 months, BCR-ABL > 10%

e. BCR-ABL > 1% in 6 months

f. Absence of complete cytogenic response in 12 months

g. Development of tyrosine kinase inhibitor-resistant mutations.

h. Loss of previously achieved response:
- Loss of complete hematological response
- Loss of complete cytogenic response

19. If the patient develops sudden nonresponse to the drug it may be due to:

a. Point mutation in the *BCR-ABL* gene resulting from the changes in the amino acid in the catalytic domain of this BCR-ABL1 protein

b. Progression of the chronic phase to accelerated phase or blast phase

20. If the patient intends to become pregnant and she has been suffering from chronic myeloid leukemia, in that case, this disease should be under optimum control with the tyrosine kinase inhibitor before conceiving.
- Drug should be stopped for at least 3 months prior to conception and also throughout the pregnancy as there is report of fetal malformations.
- Leukopheresis should be performed if there is significant leukocytosis.
- Hydroxyurea and interferon-α can be used during pregnancy without any complication.

21. Leukostasis occurs in this patient with high leukocyte count of >300,000/cc and patient may develop priapism or central nervous system complications. This can be treated by emergency leukopheresis or large volume apheresis for lowering the leukocyte count.

22. Side effects of tyrosine kinase inhibitors should be graded into the following types:

a. Grade 1: Here tyrosine kinase inhibitor therapy should be continued but may require specific treatment.

b. Grade 2: The therapy should be withhold until the disease is severe, or the treatment should be continued if the symptom decreases in severity. If this grade 2 side effect recurs, the treatment should be continued in reduced dose.

c. Grade 3: The therapy should be withhold until the disease is severe, then the therapy will restarted in reduced dose or withhold till the side effect will come to grade 1.

   If there is no resolution of the side effects or the side effects are recurrent, in that case, drug has to be changed.

d. Grade 4: In this case, drug has to be changed.

CASE 26

A 32-year-old female came to medical clinic with painless swelling on the left side of the neck. On examination, there is mild pallor, nontender mobile soft to firm discrete lymph node in the left side of the neck, and nonpalpable liver and spleen. Hematological report demonstrated hemoglobin 11.9 g/dL, white blood count 9,900/cc, and platelet count 170,000/cc. Peripheral blood picture and lymph node biopsy demonstrated as below:

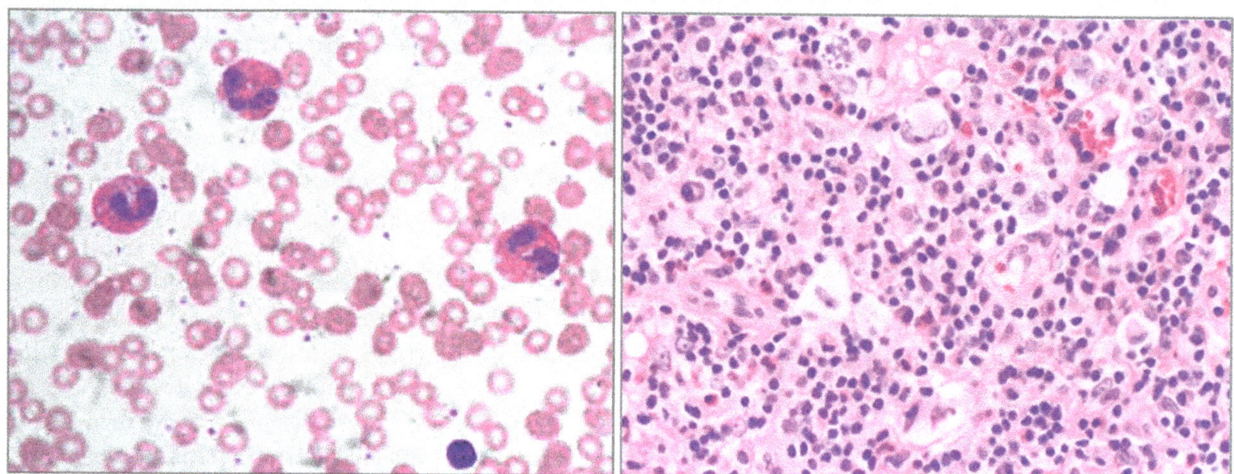

1. **What is seen in the above pictures?**
2. **What is your diagnosis?**
3. **What are the investigations to be done prior to commencement of treatment?**
4. **What is the age incidence in this disease?**
5. **What are the factors on which the prognosis depends?**
6. **What are the complications in this disease?**
7. **What are the relationships between the bone marrow transplantation in this disease?**

Answers

1. The above pictures demonstrate:
   a. Multiple eosinophils are demonstrated in the peripheral blood picture.
   b. Lymph node biopsy demonstrates Reed–Sternberg giant cells
2. This patient has been suffering from Hodgkin's lymphoma.
3. Following investigations have to be done in this case:
   a. Chest X-ray
   b. Thoracic CT scan
   c. Abdominal CT scan
   d. Bone marrow aspirate examination
   e. Full hematological examination
   f. Biochemical examination:
      - Liver function test
      - Lactate dehydrogenase
      - Calcium
      - Other electrolytes
      - Immunoglobulin
   g. PET scan
4. Age incidence in this disease: There is bimodal distribution between 20–40 years of age and >55 years of age.
5. Prognosis is bad if:
   a. >45 years of age
   b. Sex: Male
   c. Advanced disease, i.e., stage IV disease
   d. B types constitutional symptoms
   e. Hemoglobin level is >10.5 g/dL.
   f. Albumin level is <4 g/dL.
   g. Total leukocyte count is >15,000/cc.
   h. Lymphopenia or absolute lymphocyte count is ≤600/cc.

6. Complications in this disease are the following:
   a. Mantle radiotherapy:
      - Pericarditis
      - Valvular heart disease
      - Coronary artery disease
   b. Anthracyclines—cardiomyopathy
   c. Bleomycin and radiotherapy—pulmonary disease
   d. Alkylation therapy—myelodysplastic syndrome
   e. Other cancers may occur:
      - Breast cancer
      - Thyroid
      - Pancreas
      - Soft tissue
   f. Infertility
   g. Infectious complications
   h. Peripheral neuropathy
   i. Depression
   j. Disturbed sexual function
   k. Most common cancer following treatment of Hodgkin's lymphoma is lung cancer.

7. Two types of bone marrow transplantation can be done in this patient:
   i. Autologous transplantation is done in case of first relapse if the remain responsive to chemotherapy.
   ii. Allogenic bone marrow transplant can be done in case of second as well as subsequent relapse and the patient is at high risk.

CASE 27

A 27-year-old male came to medical clinic with his wife as she noticed the plethoric face of her husband for last 7 days. He complained of bruising in the thigh. On examination, face was puffy and plethoric with swollen eyelids.

On examination, his hemoglobin was 10 g/dL, white blood count 16,000/cc, and platelet count 310000/cc. His chest X-ray demonstrated as below. Peripheral blood picture demonstrated as below. These cells are acid phosphatase positive at their poles.

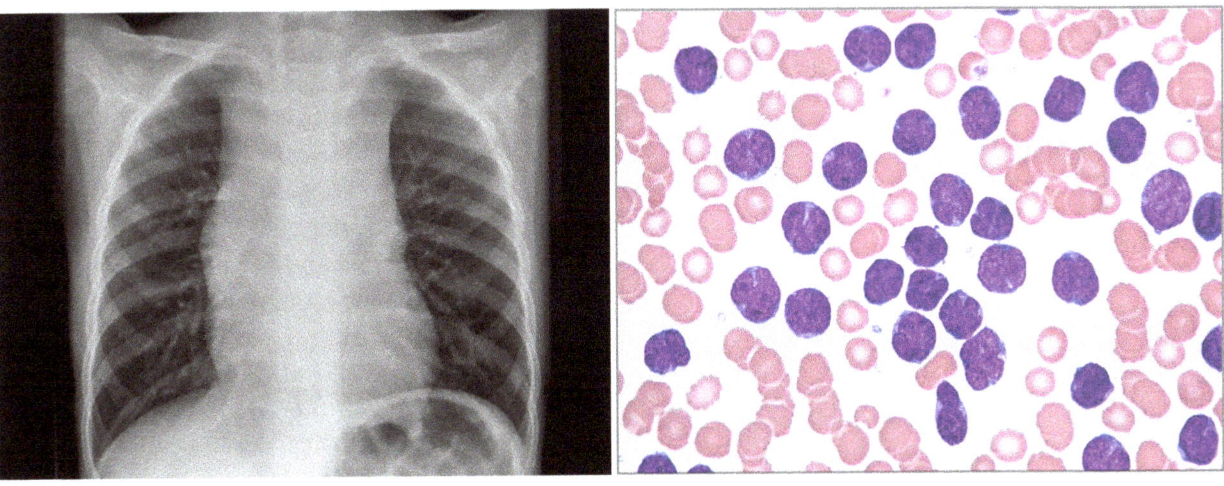

1. **What have been shown in the above pictures?**
2. **What is your diagnosis?**
3. **How can you differentiate between T and B cell variety in this disease?**
4. **In this variety of disease which cytogenic abnormality is favorable as well as unfavorable?**
5. **How can you classify central nervous system involvement in this disease?**
6. **How can you classify this disease according to French–American–British (FAB) classification?**
7. **What are the demographic, hematological, and morphologic determinants favorable for this disease?**
8. **Mention five emergency presentations of this disease and what are the interventions to be done in each case.**
9. **Mention the risk factors for this disease.**
10. **What are the induction regimens and how can you evaluate the response?**
11. **What are the pretreatment criteria in consolidation phase?**
12. **What is the drug in the consolidation phase in the 5th week?**

Answers

1. Above pictures demonstrate:
   a. Chest X-ray demonstrates anterior mediastinal mass
   b. Peripheral blood picture demonstrates:
      - Marked leukocytosis
      - Small to intermediate-sized atypical lymphoid cells
      - Irregular or convoluted nucleus
      - Scanty peripheral cytoplasm
2. Since the cells are positive for acid phosphatase at their poles, hence these are T cells. So, the patient has been suffering from T cells acute lymphoblastic lymphoma.
3. T cells are positive for CD3, CD2, CD5, CD7, CD1a, and terminal deoxynucleotidyl transferase (TdT) but negative for CD19. By these markers we can differentiate T and B cell diseases.
4. Following cytogenic abnormalities are unfavorable:
   a. t(9;22)(Ph+)
   b. t(v;11q23)
   c. B-ALL
   d. Hyperdiploid ALL
   e. t(1;19)
   Following cytogenic abnormality is favorable:
   a. B-ALL with hyperdiploidy
   b. t(12;21)
5. Classification central nervous system involvement in this disease:
   a. CNS1: No blast cell
   b. CNS2: WBC < 5/cc with blast cells
   c. CNS3: WBC ≥ 5 with blasts or symptomatic involvement of central nervous system like cranial nerve palsy.
6. FAB classification of acute lymphoblastic leukemia:
   a. L1: It is more common in children. It is small with high nucleocytoplasmic ratio and scanty cytoplasm
   b. L2: Variable size blast cells with moderate cytoplasm and irregular nuclear membrane containing 1–2 prominent nucleoli.
   c. L3: Large cell with basophilic vacuolated cytoplasm, low nuclear-cytoplasmic ratio with 1–2 prominent nucleoli.

7. Favorable demographic features are the following:
   a. Age: 1–10 years
   b. Ethnicity: White
   c. Gender: Female
   Favorable hematological features are the following:
   a. White blood cells 10,000/cc
   b. Hemoglobin < 7 g/dL
   c. Platelet count > 100,000/cc
   Favorable immunophenotyping features are:
   a. Early pre-B
   b. CD10+
8. Following five emergency presentations in this disease are as follows:
   a. Neutropenia with fever or infection—intravenous broad-spectrum antibiotics
   b. Thrombocytopenia—transfusion of platelets
   c. Airway obstruction:
      - Administration of oxygen
      - Administration of corticosteroids
      - Radiation
   d. Superior vena cava syndrome: Administration of corticosteroids with or without radiation.
   e. Ocular involvement: Radiation
9. Following are the risk factors:
   a. Trisomy 21
   b. Chromosomal breakage syndrome
   c. Immunodeficiency
   d. Environmental exposure
   e. Ionizing radiation
   f. Acquired chromosomal abnormalities
10. Induction regimens are as follows:
    a. Prednisolone 60 mg/day for 28 days
    b. Vincristine 1.5 mg intravenously weekly for 4 weeks
    c. Pegylated L-asparaginase 2,500 IU intravenously— single dose on day 4
    d. Intrathecal methotrexate:
       - CNS1: Every 1–2 weeks for three doses
       - CNS2 or CNS3: Weekly for at least four doses
    Evaluation of response:
    a. 14th day:
       - M1: Rapid early responder
       - M2 or M3: Slow early responder

b. 29th day: Bone marrow
- M1: Remission, continue as below
- M3: Failure of induction. Salvage reinduction is required.

11. Following are the pretreatment criteria of consolidation phase:
    a. Absolute neutrophil count ≥ 750/cc and platelet count ≥ 75,000/cc
    b. ALT less than two times of the upper limit of normal, direct bilirubin is normal for age.
    c. Serum creatinine is normal for age.
    d. Absence of active infection or life-threatening dysfunction of the organ.

12. In the fifth week, the drugs of consolidation phase of the treatment:
    a. Cyclophosphamide: Day 0 and 14
    b. Mercaptopurine: Daily for 28 days
    c. Vincristine: Intravenously at 14, 21, 42, and 49
    d. Cytarabine
    e. Intrathecal methotrexate weekly for doses.

CASE 28

A 16-year-old male came to medical clinic with colicky left upper abdominal pain, recurrent fever, and jaundice. His hematological and biochemical reports revealed hemoglobin 7.1 g/dL, white blood cell count 4,500/cc, platelet count 320,000/cc, and bilirubin 5.2 mg/dL. SGOT and SGPT were within normal limit. Peripheral blood picture and ultrasonography of upper abdomen demonstrated:

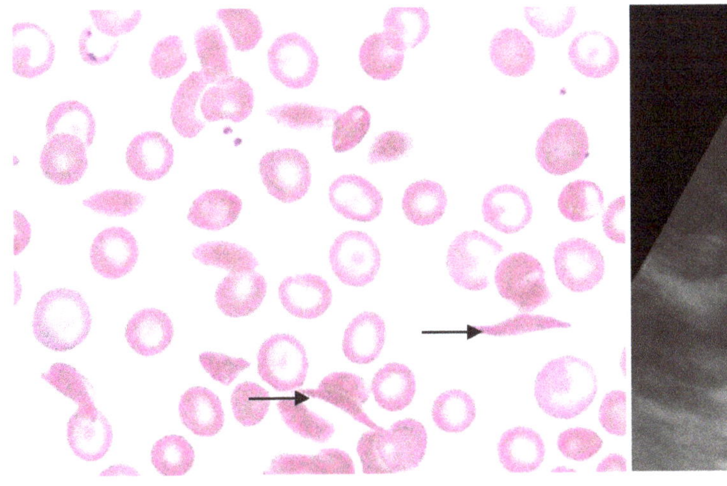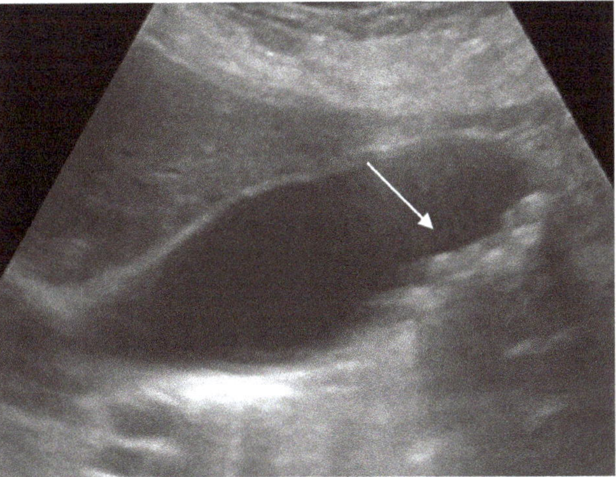

1. **What have demonstrated in the above pictures?**
2. **What is your diagnosis?**
3. **What is the disease distribution in the Indian subcontinent?**
4. **What is the genetic and molecular changes in this disease?**
5. **What is the result of genetic and molecular changes in the hemoglobin?**
6. **In heterozygous state of this disease, what is the effect of deoxygenation?**
7. **What is the effect of fetal hemoglobin in this disease?**
8. **In this specific disease deoxyhemoglobin can combine with which hemoglobins? Polymerizes from stronger to weaker manner?**
9. **Rate of polymerization depends upon hemoglobin concentration in red blood cells—justify.**
10. **What is the effect of transit time in microcirculation in this disease?**
11. **What is the effect of intracellular pH in this disease?**
12. **What are the clinical spectra of presentations in this disease?**
13. **What are the organs involved in vaso-occlusive crisis and what are the precipitating factors?**
14. **How leukocytes may contribute to the vaso-occlusive crisis?**
15. **What are the effects on the bones in this disease?**

16. **What are the organisms responsible for infection in this disease?**
17. **Which vessels are involved in the central nervous system and what are the factors that can prevent the cerebrovascular disease?**
18. **How autosplenectomy occurs in this disease?**
19. **What is megaloblastic crisis?**
20. **Which factor is mainly responsible for aplastic crisis in this disease?**
21. **What are the effects on cardiovascular system in this disease?**
22. **What are the effects on the kidney in this disease?**
23. **What are the effects on the hepatobiliary system in this disease?**
24. **What is the typical peripheral blood picture in this disease?**
25. **What are the tests for confirmation of this diagnosis?**
26. **What are the effective changes occurring in this disease after administration of hydroxyurea?**

Answers

1. Above pictures demonstrate:
   a. Peripheral blood picture demonstrates sickle cell, target cell, anisocytosis, and poikilocytosis
   b. Ultrasonography demonstrates presence of gallstones
2. This patient has been suffering from sickle cell anemia.
3. In Indian subcontinent, this disease is observed in Odisha, Andhra Pradesh, and Maharashtra.
4. Due to point mutation in the hemoglobin, there is substitution of thiamine for adenine in the sixth codon of the β gene.
5. GAG and GTG code for glutamic acid and valine respectively. Substitution of valine for the glutamic acid at the sixth position of β chain leading to altered solubility of the hemoglobin and in case of low oxygen concentration, this hemoglobin molecule will aggregate and polymerize resulting in formation of sickle hemoglobin.
6. In heterozygous state, the quantity of the hemoglobin S will be less in quantity and hemoglobin A interacts with hemoglobin S weakly during low oxygen concentration thereby hindering the aggregation and polymerization of hemoglobin S. So, this patient has no symptoms.
7. In infants in homozygous state, hemoglobin F will prevent aggregation as well as polymerization of hemoglobin S. Hence, in the first 6 months of life, the concentration of hemoglobin F is increased, but after 6 months, the concentration of fetal hemoglobin will be gradually fall to near normal adult level.
8. Deoxyhemoglobin S molecules will copolymerize with the other hemoglobin S, hemoglobin C, D, O, Arab, A, and F.
9. Role of polymerization of hemoglobin S depends upon the mean hemoglobin concentration per cells because:
   a. Increased MCHC can be seen in:
      - Intracellular dehydration or stasis
      - Slowing down of the blood flow as a result of aggregated sickle cells

      As a result, there is increased sickling.
   b. Decreased MCHC seen in:
      - Double heterozygous state of hemoglobin S
      - α-thalassemia

      As a result, there is reduced synthesis of globin leading to reduced concentration of hemoglobin; sickling will be reduced.
10. As sickling of the red blood cells will occur in the microvascular bed, reduced transit time in the capillaries will lead to decreased polymerization and the process of sickling.
11. Effect of intracellular pH in this disease: Low pH will decrease the affinity of the hemoglobin to oxygen leading to increase in the concentration of deoxygenated hemoglobin S resulting in further sickling. As a result, there is microvascular obstruction leading to tissue damage.
12. Following are the clinical spectra of presentations:
    a. Severe anemia
    b. Different forms of crises:
       - Vaso-occlusive crisis
       - Aplastic crisis
       - Megaloblastic crisis
       - Sequestration crisis
    c. Superadded secondary infections
    d. Hyperbilirubinemia

13. Following organs are mainly involved in the vaso-occlusive crisis:
    a. Bones
    b. Brain
    c. Kidneys
    d. Lungs
    e. Eyes
    f. Spleen
    g. Penis

    Following are the precipitating factors:
    a. Fever
    b. Acidosis
    c. Dehydration
    d. Exposure to cold

    There may not be any precipitating factor.

14. Leukocytes contributes to the vaso-occlusive crisis by the following mechanisms:
    a. Infections and other inflammation release various cytokines leading to adhesion of the red cells
    b. There is correlation of leukocytosis and disease severity.
    c. Leukocytes adhere to the vascular endothelium thereby interfering microvascular flow.

15. Effects on bones by this disease are the following:
    a. Painful swelling of the dorsal surface of the hands and feet due to destruction of the metacarpal, metatarsal bones, and proximal phalanges.
    b. Kyphosis
    c. Scoliosis
    d. Saber skin
    e. Towering skull
    f. Pathological fractures
    g. Bone infarcts
    h. Ischemic changes involving the central portion of the growth plate in the vertebrae
    i. Osteonecrosis of the hip

16. Following organisms are responsible for the infection in this disease:
    a. *Streptococcus pneumoniae*
    b. *Mycoplasma pneumoniae*
    c. Parvovirus
    d. *Chlamydia*
    e. H1N1

17. Following vessels are involved in the central nervous system:
    a. Anterior cerebral artery
    b. Middle cerebral artery

Following factors can prevent the cerebrovascular disease:
    a. Certain HLA allele
    b. Presence of α-thalassemia

18. Autosplenectomy means fibrotic as well as atrophic spleen leading to hypofunction of the spleen resulting in decreased activity of the macrophages and impaired immune response; as a result, the patients are very prone to infection with *Streptococcus pneumoniae*, septicemia, meningitis, and osteomyelitis due to *Salmonella typhi*. This autosplenectomy results from occlusion of the microcirculation leading to thrombus formation resulting in splenic infarction which ends in fibrosis.

19. Megaloblastic crisis occurs during pregnancy due to deficiency of folate that can be prevented by administration of folate.

20. Parvovirus B19 infection of the erythroblast leads to transient failure of erythropoiesis characterized by fall in the hemoglobin level and decreased reticulocyte count

21. Effects of cardiovascular system in this disease are the following:
    a. Enlarged heart in chest X-ray
    b. Presence of systolic murmur
    c. Multiple transfusions leading to hemosiderosis resulting in decreased cardiac function
    d. Different types of arrhythmias such as sinus tachycardia, extrasystole, and increased P-R intervals

22. Effects on kidney in this disease are the following:
    a. Hyposthenuria due to damage in the renal medulla
    b. Ischemic necrosis of the papillae leading to hematuria
    c. Nephrotic syndrome
    d. Renal failure

23. Effects on hepatobiliary system in this disease are the following:
    a. In early life, hepatomegaly
    b. Repeated blood transfusion leading to hemosiderosis
    c. Cholelithiasis
    d. Jaundice due to direct hyperbilirubinemia

24. Following features are found in the peripheral blood picture:
    a. During birth, the normal picture
    b. At the age of 6 months, few target cells and few sickle cells

c. In case of older children and adult:
- Normochromic and normocytic anemia
- Anisocytosis
- 5–50% sickle cells
- Few target cells
- Polychromatophils
- Basophilic stippling in few red blood cells
- Howell–Jolly bodies

d. In case of double heterozygous state, microcytosis only.

e. Reticulocyte count is increased to 5–20%.

25. Following tests are done for confirmation of diagnosis:
    a. Sickling test
    b. Solubility test
    c. Hemoglobin electrophoresis
    d. High performance liquid chromatography
    e. Estimation of fetal hemoglobin by alkali denaturation test
    f. Estimation of hemoglobin A2
    g. Estimation of globin chain to assess the genetic basis of the disease
    h. Prenatal diagnosis by analysis of fetal DNA by:
       - Amniocentesis at 16–20 weeks
       - Biopsy of chorionic villi at 10–12 weeks of gestation

26. Administration of hydroxyurea will reduce sickling by:
    a. Increases the hemoglobin F level in the red blood cells thereby interferes with the hemoglobin S polymerization. Again this hemoglobin S reduces tissue hypoxia as this hemoglobin carries more oxygen.
    b. It will increase the MCV and thereby reduces the concentration of hemoglobin S.
    c. It will reduce the blood viscosity thereby reduces the incidence of vaso-occlusive crisis.
    d. As it acts as anti-inflammatory agent, hence it will reduce the inflammation and thereby reduces the sickling episodes.
    e. It will produce nitric oxide by oxidizing the heme group and thereby reduces pain crisis.

CASE 29

A 78-year-old female having history of repeated blood transfusion came to medical clinic with extreme tiredness and easy bruising. Her face is grayish pigmented. Peripheral blood picture and bone marrow demonstrated the following:

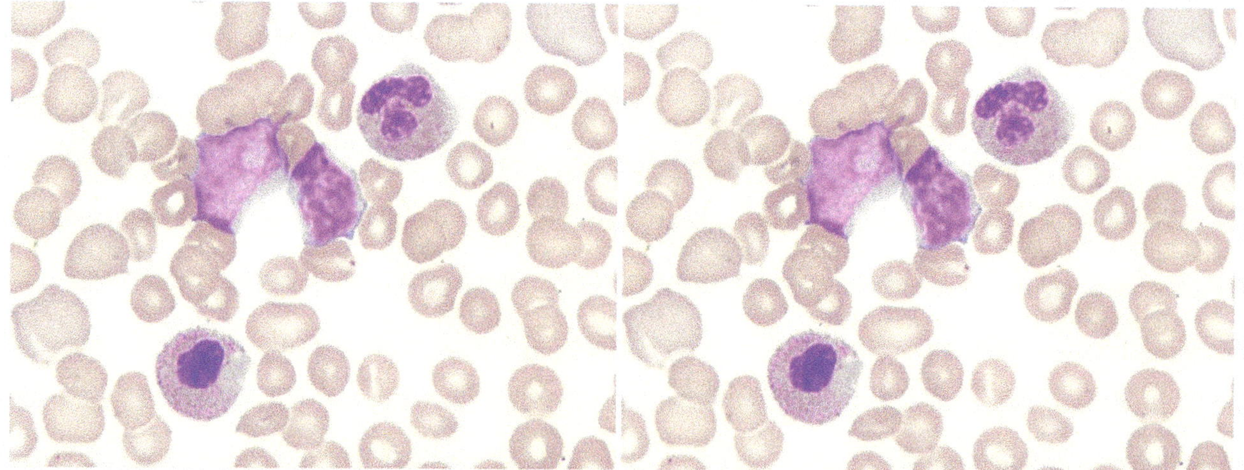

1. **What are demonstrated in the above pictures?**
2. **What is your diagnosis?**
3. **How can you define the disease?**
4. **Which genetic mutation responsible for this disease with ring sideroblast?**
5. **If this disease is associated with 5q deletion, what are the typical clinical and hematological pictures?**
6. **What are the characteristic features in dyserythropoiesis in this disease?**
7. **What are the characteristic features in dysgranulopoiesis in this disease?**

8. **What are the characteristic features of dysmegakaryopoiesis in this disease?**
9. **What are the relation between the prognosis and cytogenic abnormalities in this disease?**
10. **What are the clonal myeloid neoplasms having features of both dysplasia and proliferation of one or more myeloid lineages?**
11. **What are the features of atypical chronic myeloid leukemia?**
12. **How can you determine the prognosis in this disease?**

Answers

1. Above pictures demonstrate:
    a. Peripheral blood picture demonstrates:
        - Hyposegmented neutrophils
        - Hypogranularity in the neutrophils
        - Occasional blast cells
    b. Perl stain in the bone marrow demonstrates increased deposition of the hemosiderin
2. This patient has been suffering from myelodysplastic syndrome.
3. Myelodysplastic syndrome is a group of clonal hematopoietic disorder involving stem cells characterized by:
    a. Hemoglobin < 10 g/dL, absolute neutrophil count < 1,800/cc, and platelet count < 100,000/cc.
    b. Evidence of dysplasia involving one or more cell lines:
        - ≥10% of the erythropoietic and granulocytic series demonstrating dysplasia
        - ≥10% of megakaryocytes demonstrating dysplasia during evaluation of at least 30 megakaryocytes
    c. Ineffective erythropoiesis
    d. There is increased risk of developing into chronic myeloid leukemia
4. There is evidence of recurrent mutation of spliceosome gene *SF3B1* which is associated with myelodysplastic syndrome with ring sideroblast.
5. If the patient with this disease having genetic disorder having 5q deletion, the features are as follows:
    a. Women are frequently affected.
    b. Anemia
    c. Thrombocytosis
    d. In bone marrow, megakaryocytic hyperplasia with nonlobated or hypolobated forms of neutrophils
6. Characteristic features of dyserythropoiesis are the following:
    a. Nucleus:
        - Budding
        - Karyorrhexis
        - Multinuclearity
        - Internuclear bridging
        - Megaloblastoid features
    b. Cytoplasm:
        - Ring sideroblast having ≥5 granules of iron present in the perinuclear area encircling ≥1/3rd of the nucleus.
        - Vacuolated cytoplasm
        - PAS positivity
7. Characteristic features of dysgranulopoiesis in this disease are the following:
    a. Nucleus is either unusually small or unusually large
    b. Hypogranularity in the cytoplasm
    c. Irregular hypersegmentation of the nucleus
    d. Presence of Auer rods
    e. In case of refractory anemia with excess blast, the blast cells are seen in aggregates or in the form of clusters.
8. Characteristic features of dysmegakaryopoiesis in this disease are the following:
    a. Presence of micromegakaryocytes which are smaller to promyelocytes containing hypolobated nuclei.
    b. Multinucleation with widely separated nuclei
    c. Presence of monolobated or hypolobated nuclei
9. Following are the correlation between the cytogenic abnormalities and the prognosis of this disease:
    a. 5q deletion—good prognosis
    b. Complex or 7q deletion—bad prognosis
    c. Mutation of TP53—aggressive disease
    d. –Y, 11 deletion—very good prognosis
10. Following are the clonal myeloid neoplasms having features of both dysplasia and proliferation of one or more myeloid lineages:
    a. Atypical chronic myeloid leukemia
    b. Chronic myelomonocytic leukemia
    c. Juvenile myelomonocytic leukemia
    d. Myelodysplastic syndrome with ring sideroblast and thrombocytosis

11. Following are the features of atypical chronic myeloid leukemia:
    a. Occurs in seventh to eighth decade
    b. Negative for BCR-ABL1
    c. Low hemoglobin
    d. Low platelet count
    e. Leukocyte count of >20,000–90,000/cc due to increased number of neutrophils
    f. Blast cells are <5% and always <20% of total white blood cell count.
    g. Hypercellular bone marrow with myeloid hyperplasia and dysgranulopoiesis with/without dysmegakaryopoiesis.
    h. In 50% cases of dyserythropoiesis
    i. Prognosis is poor and aggressive disease

12. The prognosis of this disease can be determined by:
    a. Degree of cytopenia
    b. Proportion of the blasts cells in the blood and bone marrow
    c. Nature and extent of the cytogenetic changes

    In case of patient with early myelodysplasia, i.e., refractory anemia with or without ring sideroblast, no therapy is required. Median survival is 4–6 years.

    In case of patient with chronic myelomonocytic leukemia or refractory anemia with ring sideroblast, median survival is 1 year.

    In case of patient having 20% blast cells in the bone marrow and transformation to refractory anemia with ring sideroblast or 30% blast cells in the bone marrow having chronic myeloid leukemia should be treated with the drugs given in acute myeloid leukemia.

CASE 30

A 29-year-old male having history of working in the plumbing in corporate house came to medical clinic with acute colicky abdominal pain, recurrent nausea, and vomiting. His peripheral blood picture demonstrated as below:

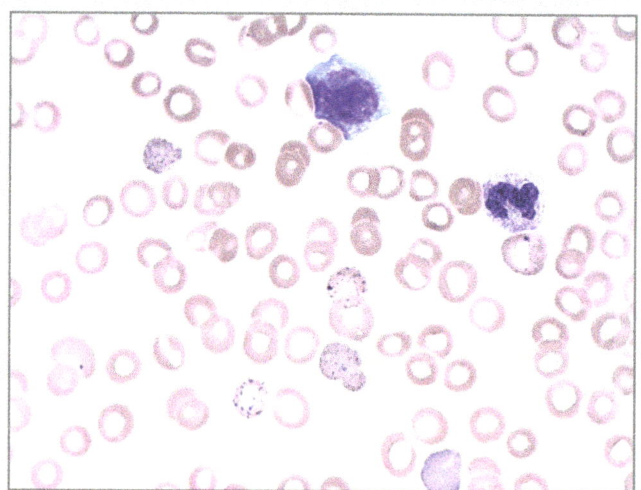

1. What has been shown in the above picture?
2. What is the most likely diagnosis?
3. What are the investigation you can do in this patient?
4. What are the causes of this type of peripheral blood picture?
5. What is the ppm limit for this causative agent?
6. What is the normal blood level of this causative agent?
7. What is the safe level of this causative agent?
8. Which vitamin can remove this agent from the body and how?
9. Which is the antidote for this causative agent?
10. What is the toxic limit of this causative agent?
11. What is the causes of the specific feature in peripheral blood picture?
12. What are the pathophysiology behind this disease?

Answers

1. Peripheral blood picture demonstrates evidence of basophilic stippling.
2. This patient has been suffering from lead poisoning.
3. Following investigations should be done:
   a. Serum lead level > 75 µg/dL
   b. Urinary δ-aminolevulinic acid and copro-porphyrin—active lead poisoning
   c. Very high level of protoporphyrin of >300 µg/dL indicates chronic lead poisoning.
   d. Urinary lead level of >0.1 mg/dL—it will confirm the diagnosis.
4. Following are the causes of basophilic stippling:
   a. Lead poisoning
   b. Thalassemia
   c. Myelodysplastic syndrome
   d. Immune hemolytic anemia
   e. Alcohol intoxication
   f. Congenital enzymopathies
   g. Megaloblastic anemia
   h. Sideroblastic anemia
5. The ppm limit of lead is 400 ppm in bare soils in the play areas and 1,200 ppm in nonplay areas.
6. Normal blood level of lead is 1 µg/dL.
7. There is no safe level of lead in this poisoning.
8. Vitamin C inhibits the uptake of lead at the cellular level thereby reducing the toxicity to the organs in the body.
9. 2,3-dimercaptosuccinic acid is more specific having wider therapeutic index and it is currently available for lead intoxication.
10. Blood level of >0.2 ppm indicates exposure to lead and >0.35 ppm indicates lead toxicity.
11. Basophilic stippling is due to fused ribosomes due to deficiency of pyrimidine 5′-nucleotidase leading to impaired degradation of RNA.
12. Here the defective synthesis of heme is due to:
    a. Deficiency of δ-aminolevulinic acid or ferrochelatase or coproporphyrin oxidase.
    b. Decreased activity of pyrimidine 5′-nucleotidase enzyme.

CHAPTER 8

Infectious Diseases

A 36-year-old female having history of hypothyroidism on 112.5 µg daily, hypertension, asthma on metered dose inhaler, allergic to penicillin came to the medical outdoor with rapid onset of fever with chill, myalgia, nasal congestion, occasional cough, backache, and nausea with several times vomiting prior to coming to hospital.

On examination, temperature is 102°F, pulse rate 88 beats/min, blood pressure 120/80 mm Hg, and respiratory rate 18 breaths/min.

Laboratory investigation demonstrated white blood cell count 8,000/cc and hemoglobin 15.2 g/dL. Liver, renal function test, and serum electrolytes were within normal limit.

1. **What is the most likely diagnosis?**
2. **What are the features suggestive of this disease?**
3. **What are the laboratory tests which should be done for the diagnosis in the emergency department?**
4. **Why viral culture should not be done here?**
5. **Why rapid cell culture should not be undertaken here?**
6. **Who are at risk of complications?**
7. **Which is the drug of choice in this patient?**
8. **Why baloxavir is not the drug of choice?**
9. **Why zanamivir is not used to treat this disease?**
10. **In this patient, what should be the duration of treatment?**
11. **In which conditions longer duration of treatment is required?**
12. **In which severe cases bacterial superinfection can be suspected?**
13. **Who should take postexposure chemoprophylaxis?**
14. **Who should receive preexposure chemoprophylaxis?**
15. **Which is the drug of choice of chemoprophylaxis and duration of administration of this drug?**
16. **What are the FDA-approved indications of influenza vaccine?**
17. **What are the indications of vaccination of influenza?**
18. **What are the possible adverse effects of this vaccination?**
19. **What is the time of administering the antiviral drug if the patient received this vaccine?**

Answers

1. The most likely diagnosis is influenza.
2. Points in favor of this diagnosis are the following:
   a. Rapid onset of fever, cough, and nasal congestion
   b. Body ache
   c. Myalgia
   d. Absence of tachycardia
   e. Severe lethargy
3. Two laboratory tests should be done in this patient for rapid diagnosis:
   a. Rapid molecular assay: It produces results within 15–20 minutes.

b. Rapid antigen detection test: It can detect the antigen within 10–15 minutes.

Both the tests are highly specific but rapid molecular assay test is highly sensitive because it can detect influenza A and B, whereas rapid antigen detection test has low or moderate sensitivity.

4. Though the viral culture is highly sensitive and highly specific, but it takes 3–10 days for giving the results.

5. Rapid influenza cell culture though highly sensitive and specific, it can produce the results within 1–3 days.

6. Following are the risk factors for developing complications:
   a. Immunosuppressed patients
   b. Presence of comorbidities
   c. Children of <2 years of age
   d. Adult of >65 years of age
   e. Pregnant woman
   f. Woman within 2 weeks of postpartum

7. Drug of choice is oseltamivir.

8. Baloxavir is not the drug of choice because:
   a. The administration of this drug has to be separated from polyvalent cations like calcium and magnesium.
   b. It is not recommended for hospitalized patients.

9. Zanamivir is not recommended because it is used as chemoprophylaxis. It is not given in:
   a. In case of severe influenza infection
   b. Pregnancy because as this drug is given through the inhalation, in this case due to low lung volume, there will be reduced distribution in the lung and there is increased chance of bronchospasm.

10. This patient requires 5 days course of treatment.

11. In following cases, longer duration of treatment is required:
    a. Immunocompromised patient
    b. Severe infection
    c. Critical illness

12. In following severe cases, bacterial superinfection can be suspected:
    a. Extensive pneumonia on imaging
    b. Respiratory failure
    c. Hypotension
    d. Fever
    e. Deterioration following initial improvement on antiviral agent

13. Following subjects should take postexposure prophylaxis:
    a. Children <5 years old
    b. Elder subject of > 65 years of age
    c. Pregnant woman
    d. Postpartum woman
    e. Morbid obese
    f. Nursing home residents
    g. Patients having chronic pulmonary disease
    h. Chronic cardiac disease
    i. Metabolic disease

14. Following persons should receive pre-exposure prophylaxis:
    a. Patient of 3 years old or more who are at risk of severe complications or in whom hematopoietic stem cell transplantation was done within last 6–12 months.

15. Chemoprophylactic drug of choice is oseltamivir at a dose of 30 mg twice daily. In case of pre-exposure prophylaxis, the duration of this disease activity in that community. In case of postexposure prophylaxis, the drug should be given for 7 days after exposure to influenza.

16. Following are the FDA-approved indications of influenza vaccine:
    a. Prevention of influenza A in subjects of ≥6 months
    b. Prevention of influenza B in subjects of ≥6 months

17. Following are the indications of vaccination:
    a. All the children between 6 and 59 months
    b. All the persons of ≥50 years of age
    c. Pregnancy
    d. Immunocompromised patients
    e. Patients with pulmonary disease and cardiac disease
    f. Children and adults between 6 months and 18 years who are on aspirin containing medications which are associated with increased risk of developing Reye syndrome.
    g. Nursing home residents
    h. Alaska native subjects or American Indian individuals
    i. Morbid obese

18. Following are the possible side effects of vaccination:
    a. Fever
    b. Irritations at the site of injection
    c. Irritability
    d. Drowsiness
    e. Myalgia

    By nasal spray:
    a. Upper respiratory tract infection
    b. Lower respiratory tract infection
    c. Fever
    d. Vomiting

    Rare:
    a. Allergic reaction
    b. Anaphylaxis

19. Time of administering the antiviral drug if the patient wants to take this vaccine:

a. Oseltamivir or zanamivir should be administered before to 2 weeks after getting live attenuated influenza vaccine-4.

b. Baloxavir should be administered 17 days before to 2 weeks after receiving the live vaccine.

c. Peramivir should be administered 5 days before to 2 weeks following administration of live attenuated vaccine.

CASE 2

An 85-year-old man admitted with fractured neck of the femur and operated. On the third postoperative date, patient developed cough with expectoration, for which he was treated with cephalosporin. But after 3 days, he developed severe loose motion along with cramping abdominal pain. He was undergone long colonoscopy which demonstrated:

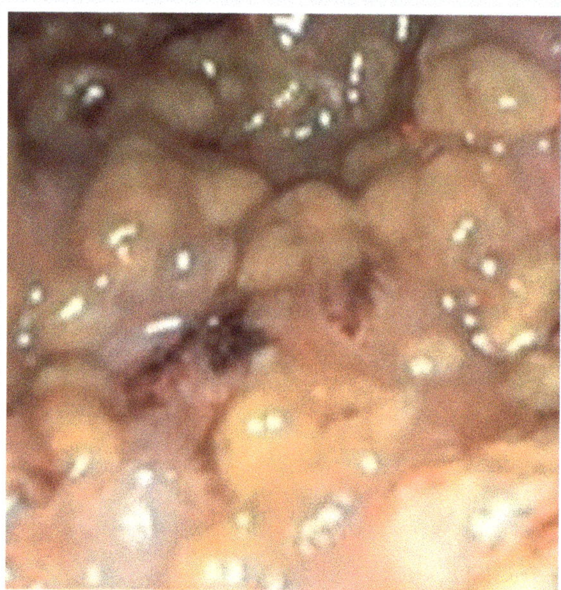

1. What specific investigation you will do to diagnose this case?
2. If the above test will be positive what will be your specific diagnosis?
3. What is the causative organism?
4. What are the toxins produced by that organism?
5. How the nonpathogenic organism can be converted into virulent strain?
6. Which factors regulate the toxin production?
7. What is hypervirulent mutant?
8. What are the methods of typing of *Clostridium difficile*?
9. What are the clades of *C. difficile*?
10. How it will enter into the body and spread?
11. How person to person spread will occur?
12. What are the immunoglobulins produced in this infection and what is its significance?
13. What are the inflammatory mediators which are produced by the toxins?
14. What are the ominous signs seen in this disease?
15. What is the antibiotic administration strategy in this disease?
16. What is the treatment of recurrence in this disease?

Answers

1. The stool should be sent for *C. difficile* toxin.
2. If the above test will be positive, the specific diagnosis is pseudomembranous colitis caused by *C. difficile.*
3. The organism is *C. difficile.*
4. This organism produced three toxins: These are TcdA, TcdB, and CDT.
5. Group V sigma factor, i.e., TcdR regulates toxin production, at the same time TcdC, antisigma factor, which acts directly on TcdR, will be inhibited. As a result, TcdR will increase its own production leading to increased production of toxin. Thus hypervirulent strain will be produced which increases the production of A and B toxins through the deletion of single nucleotide.
6. Following factors regulate toxin production:
   a. Sugar
   b. Amino acids
   c. Sporulation
   d. Low level of biotin
   e. Thioacetone quorum-signaling system regulating the expression of toxin independent of TcdC.
7. Hypervirulent mutant is TcdC which produces increased amount of A and B toxins.
8. Following are the methods of typing for this organism:
   a. Pulse field gel electrophoresis
   b. Ribotyping
   c. Multilocus enzyme electrophoresis
9. Five clades of *C. difficile* are the following:
   a. Defective trehalose metabolism clade
   b. TcdA-negative/TcdA-positive clade
   c. Two other human clades
   d. One animal clade
10. Spores of *Clostridium* from the infected feces or contaminated environment will enter in to the gastrointestinal tract and colonizes in the colon. Dysbiosis is the predisposing factor for this colonization and is enhanced by the antibiotics.
11. Methods of spreading of this infection from person to person are the following:
    a. Patients having diarrhea along with fecal incontinence is responsible for unidirectional spread in the hospital.
    b. Spores of the *Clostridium* in the environment floors and around the toilet
12. Following immunoglobulins are produced in this infection:
    a. High levels of immunoglobulin A (IgA) and IgM occur in the initial stage infection and indicate low risk of recurrence
    b. Low level of IgA relates to prolonged disease and high risk of recurrence
    c. High IgG level will protect the subject from this disease. But if this disease occurs, in that case, high level after 12 days indicates low level of recurrences.
13. Following inflammatory mediators are produced by the toxins:
    a. A and B toxins induce following mediators:
       - Interleukin-8
       - Interleukin-6
       - Tumor necrosis factor-alpha
       - Leptin
       - Substance P
    b. TcdA stimulates:
       - Vanilloid receptor
       - VR1 leading to release of substance P
14. The ominous sign in this disease is little or absence of diarrhea with predominant pain abdomen.
15. Treatment in this disease:
    a. In case of first disease with mild-to-moderate attack, metronidazole 400 mg thrice daily should be given for 10–14 days.
    b. Severe disease should be treated with vancomycin orally 125 mg four times daily or fidaxomicin 200 mg twice daily for 10–14 days. Fidaxomicin will reduce the incidence of recurrences.
    c. In case of nonresponse and suspected colitis, this patient should be treated with 500 mg vancomycin orally along with intravenous metronidazole 500 mg thrice daily.
    d. If the condition worsens, intracolonic vancomycin 500 mg four times daily along with intravenous immunoglobulin at a dose of 400 mg/kg.
16. Recurrence of the disease can be treated by:
    a. If the recurrence is not severe, this can be treated by orally fidaxomicin 200 mg twice daily.
    b. Oral vancomycin 125 mg four times daily for 7 days, then 125 mg thrice daily for next 1 week, then twice daily for next 7 days, once daily for fourth week, 125 mg at alternate day for fifth week and lastly every third day in the sixth week.
    c. Fecal transplant from close family member can be very effective.
    d. Human monoclonal antibody against toxin A, actoxumab, and against toxin B, i.e., bezlotoxumab reduces the recurrence through the binding with C-terminal repetitive binding domain.

CASE 3

A 20-year-old girl having history of termination of pregnancy 3 years ago and on birth control pills as she has one boyfriend who came to clinic with complaint of midcycle bleeding. On examination, cervical mucosa was friable and evidence of mucopurulent discharge. There was also evidence of keratoconjunctivitis. Cervical swab was taken and was seen under microscope.

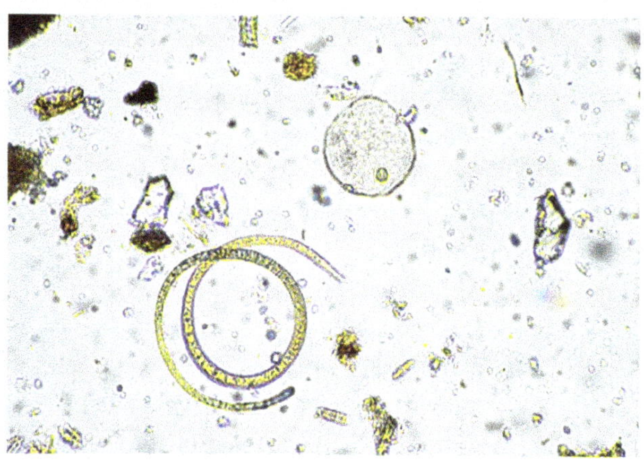 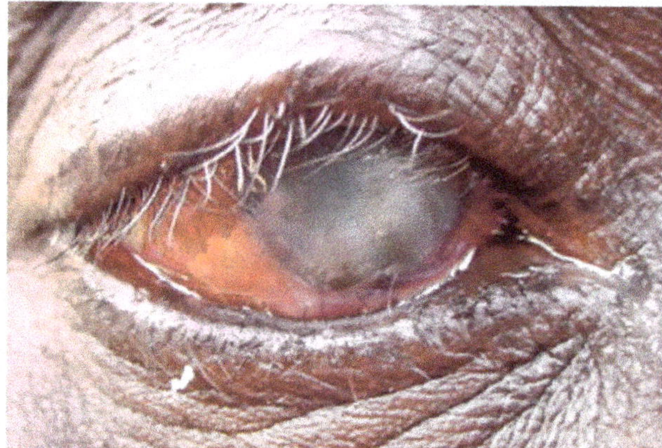

1. **Identify the pictures above.**
2. **What is your diagnosis?**
3. **What are the pathogenic varieties in this organism?**
4. **What are the biological variants in this organism?**
5. **What are the serological variants in this organism?**
6. **What are the developmental cycles in this organism?**
7. **What is the effect of vertical transmission of this organism in the child?**
8. **What are the methods of eye involvement in this disease?**
9. **What is the immunity in this disease?**
10. **How the organism evades the host immune response?**
11. **What are the methods of tissue damage by this organism?**
12. **What are the serovars responsible for what types of diseases in the human being?**
13. **What is trachoma?**
14. **What are the clinical indicators used in the diagnosis of the genital infection?**
15. **What are the stages of lymphogranuloma venereum?**
16. **How can you treat this disease?**
17. **What are the samples to be collected?**

Answers

1. The left hand picture demonstrates keratoconjunctivitis and right hand picture demonstrates *Chlamydia trachomatis*.
2. The diagnosis is that the patient has been suffering from keratoconjunctivitis along with cervicitis due to infection with *C. trachomatis*.
3. Following are the pathogenic varieties of the organism:
   a. *C. trachomatis*
   b. *Chlamydia pneumoniae*
   c. *Chlamydophila psittaci*
4. There are two human biological variants (biovar) of *C. trachomatis*:
   a. Trachoma and lymphogranuloma venereum
   b. *C. pneumoniae* infecting mice
5. Following are the serological variants (serovars):
   a. In the trachoma biovar: A–K, Ba, Da, Ia, and Ja
   b. In the LGG biovar: L1, L2, L2a, and L3
6. Following are the developmental cycles in this organism:
   a. Elementary body of the organism infects nonciliated columnar, cuboidal, or transitional epithelial cells and also macrophages

- Directly via cellular proteoglycans through electrostatic interactions
- Indirectly through the binding with the fibroblastic growth factor 2 leading to internalization into the cells.

So, *Chlamydia* enters into the cells through:

- Phagocytosis
- Receptor-mediated endocytosis
- Pinocytosis

b. Early intracellular phase: Within the cells, elementary body containing vacuole fused with each other through the membrane phospholipid but not with lysosomes to prevent intracellular destruction leading to formation of single fusion vacuole containing multiple elementary bodies. This homotypic fusion is the characteristic feature in *C. trachomatis* only. If the vacuole contains multiple serovars, there is chance of genetic exchange. They move toward the microtubular organization center to get nutrients from host cell Golgi apparatus.

c. Development of inclusion: Within the vacuole, elementary body is transformed into reticulate body which in turn multiplies by binary fission leading to formation of 500–1,000 progeny, occupying 90% of the cytoplasm. After several rounds of fission, the reticulate body will be reverted back into elementary body and released to infect adjacent cells.

7. Vertical transmission from the infected mother during birth occurs while the fetus passes through the infected birth canal leading to development of:
   a. Ophthalmia neonatorum
   b. Chlamydial pneumonia

8. Following are the methods of eye involvement:
   a. Eye to eye through the infected fingers
   b. Shared clothes
   c. Shared towels
   d. Eye-seeking flies
   e. Droplets through the coughing or sneezing

9. There are three types of immunity:
   a. Innate immune response: At the site of acute inflammation, there are accumulation of polymorphonuclear cells and macrophages along with release of cytokines and chemokines mainly interleukin-8 from the infected epithelial cells and it will attract neutrophils further. There are also accumulation of B cells, T cells, and dendritic cells in the submucosal areas resulting in T cell response and antibody response.

   b. Antibody response: There are increased production of mucosal secretory IgA and circulating IgG and IgM responses specific for major outer membrane protein (MOMP) and Hsp60. The antibodies bound to MOMP result antibody-dependent cellular cytotoxicity.

   c. Cellular response: At the site of infection, some antigen-presenting cells will engulf and process elementary body thereby presenting the peptides of the organism to major histocompatibility complex class II-mediated pathway, as a result CD4+ T cells are activated leading to production of interferon-γ, which is major inhibitory cytokine for Chlamydia.

10. *Chlamydia* evades the host immune response through the following mechanisms:
    a. Intracellular location protects the organism from the host antibodies and complements
    b. The organism downregulates the major histocompatibility complex class I molecules on the surface of the infected cells
    c. Fusion of phagosomes containing pathogens with the host cell lysozyme will be prevented
    d. Infected macrophages will induce T cell apoptosis through the paracrine effects as well as tumor necrosis factor-alpha.

11. Tissue damage occurs as a result of:
    a. Host inflammatory response to the infection
    b. Direct damage of the infected cells by the bacteria
    c. Production of cytotoxin which will deliver cytotoxicity to the infected host cells.

12. Following serovars are responsible for following types of diseases:
    a. A, B, Ba, and C: Ocular trachoma
    b. D, Da, E, F, G, H, I, Ia, J, Ja, and K: Oculogenital disease
    c. L1, L2, and L3: Lymphogranuloma venereum

13. Trachoma is characterized by:
    - Conjunctival lymphoid follicles containing germinal centers containing:
      ○ B lymphocytes
      ○ CD8+ T lymphocytes present in the para-follicular region
    - Inflammatory infiltrate containing:
      ○ Plasma cells
      ○ Dendritic cells
      ○ Macrophages
      ○ Polymorphonuclear leukocytes
      ○ In the scar tissue, there is expansion of CD4+ T lymphocytes

14. Following are the indicators for the diagnosis of genital infection as well as screening in women:
    a. Sexually active women having <25 years of age
    b. If there is more than one sexual partner
    c. Presence of mucopurulent vaginal discharge
    d. Burning sensation during passage of urine
    e. Friable cervical mucosa or presence of bleeding after sexual intercourse or in-between the normal menstrual periods
    f. Presence of lower abdominal pain or pain during the sexual intercourse

15. Following are the stages of lymphogranuloma venereum:
    a. Evidence of painless primary lesion present in the glans penis, labia, wall of the vagina or cervix, or in the oral cavity during incubation period.
    b. Secondary lesion, i.e., lymphadenitis in the inguinal or femoral region leading to bubo formation which ulcerates followed by discharge of pus.
    c. Tertiary stage, i.e., genitoanorectal syndrome.

16. Treatment of this infection:
    a. In adult:
       - Orally doxycycline 100 mg twice daily for 7 days
       - Orally azithromycin 1 g single dose
       - Levofloxacin 500 mg orally once daily for 7 days
    b. In case of pregnancy:
       - Orally azithromycin 1 g single dose
       - Orally amoxicillin 500 mg thrice daily for 7 days
    c. In neonates: Orally azithromycin 50 mg/kg daily orally in divided doses for 14 days

17. Following samples are collected from the infected subject:
    a. Mucopurulent vaginal discharge
    b. Urine in case burning sensation during micturition

CASE 4

A 40-year-old male having past history of recurrent history of endocarditis and operation to correct mycotic aneurysm came to clinic with tingling with pain during walking in the lower extremities. On examination, there are absent pulses in the popliteal, posterior tibial, and artery dorsalis pedis. Arteriography demonstrated occlusion in the distal aorta. During operative correction, the debris from the operative site demonstrated:

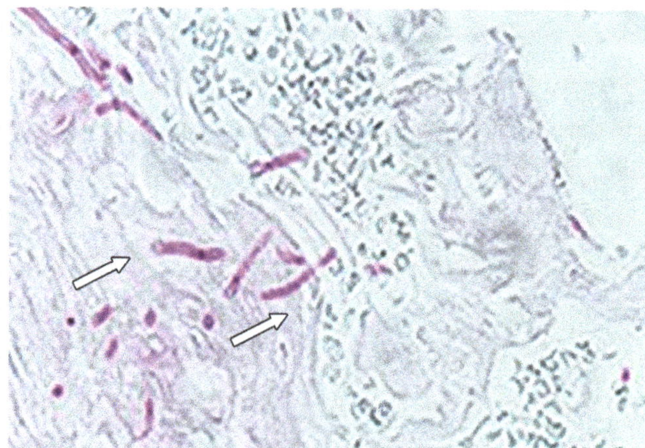

1. What is demonstrated in the slide?
2. What are the morphological forms in this organism?
3. What the factors regulating morphogenesis?
4. During birth which organs may be involved by this organism?
5. Which factors balance the opportunistic infection and commensal colonization?
6. How the organisms reach the internal organs?
7. In case of low iron condition, what will happen to this organism?
8. In the internal organs, the morphological transformation depends upon which factors?

9. **What is the role of innate immunity in this organism in human being?**
10. **What is the role of adaptive immunity in the human being against this organism?**
11. **During invasion, how the organism resists anoxia?**
12. **Mention the risk factors in case of mouth involvement.**
13. **Describe the typical features in case of mouth involvement.**
14. **Mention the risk factors in case of invasive disease.**
15. **In the cell culture, which subspecies of this organism grows and how can you differentiate them?**
16. **What is the antigen detected in this case and what are the drawbacks of this antigen?**
17. **What are the nanodiagnostic panels used for this organism?**
18. **What are the vaccines for *Candida* in the trial?**

Answers

1. There is evidence of unicellular budding along with pseudohyphae indicating *Candida albicans*.
2. There are two reversible morphological forms in this organism:
   a. Unicellular budding yeast
   b. Filamentous form—hyphae and pseudohyphae
3. Following factors regulate morphogenesis:
   a. Temperature
   b. pH
   Higher temperature and neutral pH favors hyphae
   Lower temperature and acidic pH favors yeast form
4. During passage through the birth canal, skin and gastrointestinal tract are colonized by this organism.
5. Following factors balance the opportunistic infection and commensal colonization:
   a. Innate immune response
   b. Resident microbiota
6. *Candida* will adhere to the endothelial lining of the blood vessel through the expression of adhesins like $\alpha M\beta 2$ and
   a. Interact with intracellular adhesion molecule such as ICAM-1 and ICAM-2
   b. Interact with platelet endothelial cell adhesion molecule-1
   c. Agglutinin like protein 3 interacts with N-cadherin
7. In case of low iron environment, *Candida* decreases its mitochondrial activity leading to changes in the cellular metabolism resulting in increased lactase production.
8. In the internal organs, the morphological transformation depends upon complex interaction of the internal signaling pathways like:
   a. Cyclic adenosine monophosphate-protein kinase A (cAMP-PKA)
   b. Mitogen-activated protein (MAP) kinase
   c. Protein kinase C (PKC)
   d. External environmental conditions such as temperature and pH
9. Innate immunity prevents invasion of *C. albicans* through phagocytosis by macrophages and polymorphs. Dectin-1, a C-type lectin pathogen recognition receptor of phagocytic cells, recognizes the fungal β-glucans leading to activation of phagocytosis and release of proinflammatory cytokines such as tumor necrosis factor, interferon-γ, and reactive oxygen species (ROS).
10. Adaptive immunity against this fungi will be generated through:
    a. T helper-11 cells: It will regulate the integrity of the epithelial barrier to maintain the equilibrium between the bacterial and fungal commensals.
    b. T helper-1 cells: Interleukin-18 drives protective Th1 response.
    c. T helper-2 cells: Interleukin-33 promotes Th2 response and suppresses the Th1 immunity.
11. During invasion, *Candida* adopts anoxia through the repression of the transcription factor of the filamentous growth Efg1.
12. Following are the risk factors in case of mouth involvement:
    a. Wearing dentures
    b. Smoking
    c. Antibiotic intake
    d. Corticosteroids intake for asthma
    e. Medications responsible for dry mouth
    f. Immunodeficiency
    g. Diabetes
    h. HIV infection
    i. Cancer patients undergoing treatment for cancer
13. Typical features in case of mouth involvement:
    a. Evidences of white patches or sores in the insides of the cheek, tongue, and roof of the mouth
    b. Cracked, eroded, and inflamed corner of the mouth

   c. Cotton like feeling in the mouth, taste loss, and odynophagia

14. Risk factors in case of invasive disease:
   a. Acquired immunodeficiency
   b. Neutropenia
   c. Stem cell transplantation
   d. Prolonged stay in intensive care unit
   e. Central nervous system catheters
   f. Parenteral nutrition
   g. Patients on hemodialysis in case of renal failure
   h. Patients on broad-spectrum antibiotics
   i. Preterm baby
   j. Low birth weight baby

15. In the cell culture, many subspecies of *Candida* will grow.
   a. But after incubation in plasma or serum at 37°C for 3 hours, *C. albicans* and *Candida dubliniensis* can grow but other cannot.
   b. Again, incubated in corneal agar, only *C. albicans* can grow but *C. dubliniensis* cannot grow.

16. *Candida* antigens like cell wall component "mannan" and anticandidal antibodies can be detected in the serum. But, the drawbacks of the detection of the antigen are:
   a. Decreased serum concentration of the antigen
   b. Rapid clearance of these antigens
   c. Low sensitivity in immunosuppressed host

17. Following are the nanodiagnostic panels:
   a. Fluorescence in situ hybridization by using peptide nucleic acid probes targeting species-specific RNA in the *Candida*.
   b. Latex agglutination test for detecting different antigen of *Candida* like Hsp90, Enol-1, Mp65, and Sap-1/2.
   c. Loop-mediated isothermal amplification based on the usage of specific primers for the DNA of *Candida*.

18. Two vaccines of *Candida* are in the trial:
   a. PEV7—containing an enzyme secreted by Candida recombinant aspartyl-proteinase 2 which is delivered via virosomes
   b. NDV-3—containing recombinant N-terminal of *C. albicans* agglutinin like sequence 3 protein

CASE 5

A 32-year-old corporate worker having history of bloody diarrhea 2 weeks ago following intake of heavy alcohol along with food in a renowned hotel and treated with antibiotics came to clinic with complaint of ascending weakness of both the lower limbs starting from his feet within a span of few days. Stool culture demonstrated:

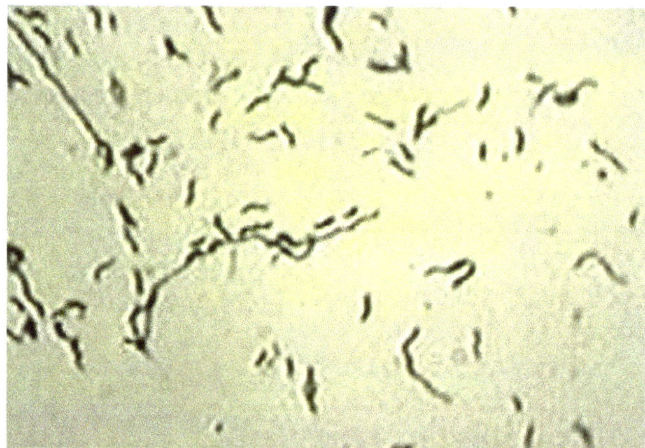

1. **What has been demonstrated in the picture above?**
2. **What is your diagnosis?**
3. **In which serogroup these organism lie?**
4. **In which method these organisms can be typed?**
5. **What are the other types of these organisms responsible for human disease?**
6. **What are the sources of infection by this organism?**
7. **What are the sites of adhesion in human being by this organism?**

8. **What are the antigens in this organism responsible for adaptive response by human being?**
9. **Which antibiotics are responsible for which neurological manifestations?**
10. **Which antibodies are responsible for protection against this infection?**
11. **What are the surface proteins essential for initial colonization in the gastrointestinal tract?**
12. **What are the complications in this disease?**
13. **What are the methods of diagnosis of this disease?**
14. **What are the leading contenders of vaccine against this disease?**

Answers

1. This picture demonstrates "seagull" morphology of the *Campylobacter* jejuni in the slide stained by silver stain.
2. The patient has been suffering from the neurological complications of *C. jejuni* infection.
3. *Campylobacter* jejuni has been subdivided into:
    a. "Penner" serogroup based on capsular polysaccharide antigen which is heat stable.
    b. "Lior" serogroup based on capsular as well as lipooligosaccharide antigen which is heat labile.
4. *Campylobacter* is typed different molecular methods:
    a. Restriction fragment length polymorphism
    b. Multilocus enzyme electrophoresis
    c. Whole genome sequencing
5. Following *Campylobacter* other than *C. jejuni* are responsible human diseases:
    a. *Campylobacter fetus*—intestinal and systemic infections in case of immunocompromised individual or subjects working with animals
    b. *Campylobacter concisus*—part of oral flora and associated with inflammatory bowel disease
    c. *Campylobacter showae*—part of oral flora and associated with inflammatory bowel disease
    d. *Campylobacter curvus*: It is associated with gastroenteritis, abscesses, and bacteremia
    e. *Campylobacter hyointestinalis*: It is found in the pork intestine and opportunistic diarrheal infection in human being.
    f. *Campylobacter sputorum*: It is associated with gastroenteritis, abscesses, and bacteremia.
6. Following are the sources of infection with this organism:
    a. Raw contaminated milk
    b. Contaminated water sources
    c. Close contact with the animals like:
        - Children's zoos
        - Infected dogs
        - Excreta of birds
    d. Sexual contact

7. Following are the sites of adhesion in the human being by this organism:
    a. Terminal ileum
    b. Colon
        The organism penetrate the mucus layer of the intestine to adhere with the enterocytes
8. The antigen of this organism responsible for the adaptive immunity:
    a. Flagella
    b. Outer membrane proteins
    c. Lipooligosaccharide
9. Following antibodies will cross-react with the myelin components in the nerve fibers leading to development of neurological manifestations:
    a. Antibodies to outer membrane proteins
    b. Lipooligosaccharides
    Following neurological manifestations will develop:
    a. Guillain–Barré syndrome
    b. Miller Fisher syndrome
10. Secretory antibody IgA in the maternal milk and intestinal secretions are responsible for protection against further infections as well as in case of children to develop severe disease.
11. Following are the surface proteins essential for adhesion and colonization in the gastrointestinal tract:
    a. CadF and FlpA are responsible for binding with the fibronectin and followed by invasion
    b. CapC involved in the adhesion and inflammation
    c. CiaB is internalized in the gastric cells.
    d. iamA, i.e., invasion-associated marker regulates the virulence of *Campylobacter*
    e. Cas9 regulates the virulence of *Campylobacter*
12. Complications in this disease are the following:
    a. Enterocolitis
    b. Toxic megacolon
    c. Cholecystitis
    d. Pancreatitis
    e. Hemolytic uremic syndrome

f. IgA nephropathy
g. Interstitial nephritis
h. Guillain–Barré syndrome
i. Miller Fisher syndrome

13. Following are the methods of the diagnosis in this disease:
    a. Isolation of this organism in the feces

b. Antigen detection by:
    - Polymerase chain reaction (PCR)
    - Immunochromatographic assay

14. Following are the leading contenders of the vaccine against this disease:
    a. Capsule-conjugate vaccine
    b. DNA-based vaccine

CASE 6

A 28-week-old female having history of intake of ham and cheese came to clinic with myalgia, headache, and fever for 2 days. Her total blood count was raised. Blood culture in blood agar demonstrated multiple brownish colony. Gram stain and electron microscopy demonstrated:

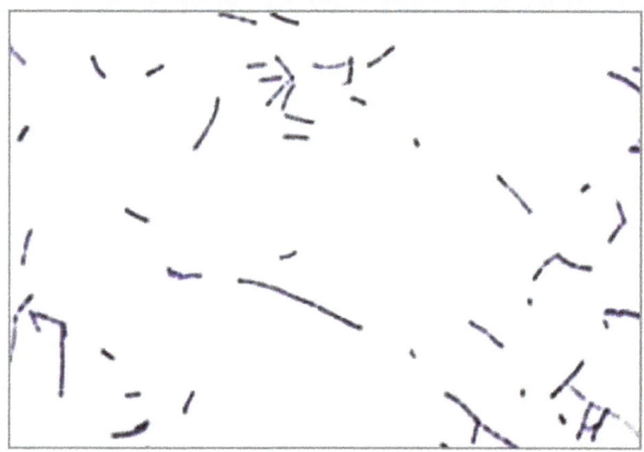
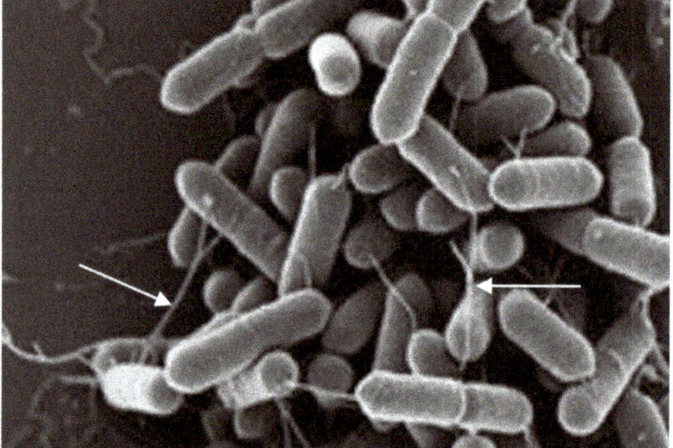

1. **Describe the above pictures.**
2. **In which clade the organism is included?**
3. **Into how many serotypes this organism has been subdivided?**
4. **Which serotypes are responsible for this disease?**
5. **What are the natural sources of this organism?**
6. **Which contaminated foods are responsible for this disease?**
7. **What are the most common presentations in this disease?**
8. **Which are the virulence factors in this organism?**
9. **What are the functions of the virulence factors of this organism in the human beings?**
10. **In the central nervous system, which cells are being penetrated by this organism?**
11. **What are the typical clinical presentations in this disease?**
12. **Which serotypes are β-hemolytic and how can you diffrentiate these serotypes?**

Answers

1. The above picture demonstrates gram-positive rods. Electron microscope demonstrates rods with flagella suggestive of *Listeria monocytogenes*.
2. In the clade Listeria sensu stricto, this organism has been included.
3. *Listeria monocytogenes* has been divided into 14 serotypes based on the flagellar antigen (H) and cell wall antigen (O).
4. The following serotypes are responsible for majority of the disease:
    a. 1/2a
    b. 1/2b
    c. 4b
5. Following are the natural sources of this organism:
    a. Soil
    b. Water
    c. Animal
    d. Vegetables

6. Following contaminated food are responsible for this disease:
   a. Fish
   b. Salad
   c. Pate
   d. Soft cheese
   e. Salami
   f. Ham
   g. Coleslaw
7. Most common presentations in this disease are follows:
   a. Meningitis
   b. Septicemia
8. Two virulence factors in this organism are as follows:
   a. Listeria adhesion protein (LAP)
   b. Internalin A (InlA)
9. Following are the functions of the virulence factors in this organism:
   a. LAP binds with Hsp60 receptors present on the enterocyte leading to activation of:
      - Nuclear factor kappa B (NF-κB) which activates inflammatory reaction
      - Myosin light-chain kinase which reconfigures of the intercellular tight junction as well as reconfigures of the adherens junction.
   b. InlA binds to the receptors E-cadherin present in the enterocytes, epithelial cells, and goblet cells
10. In the central nervous system, *L. monocytogenes* penetrates following cells through insect invasion of the endothelial cells and blood:
    a. Microglia
    b. Astrocytes
    c. Oligodendrocytes
11. Following are the clinical presentations in this disease:
    a. In pregnant patient:
       - Febrile flu-like illness
       - In 25% cases, fetal death
    b. Neonatal infection:
       - Early onset of bacteremia
       - Late onset meningitis
12. *Listeria monocytogenes*, *Listeria seeligeri*, and *Listeria ivanovii* are β-hemolytic. Former two zones show narrow zone hemolysis whereas last one demonstrates wide and double zone of hemolysis.

CASE 7

A 40-year-old female came to dermatology clinic with history of persistent rash throughout the body along with pain and needle in the upper limb. Physical examination demonstrated hypopigmented lesion present on the nasal bridge, cheeks, arms, abdomen, and legs. Biopsy from the lesion demonstrated:

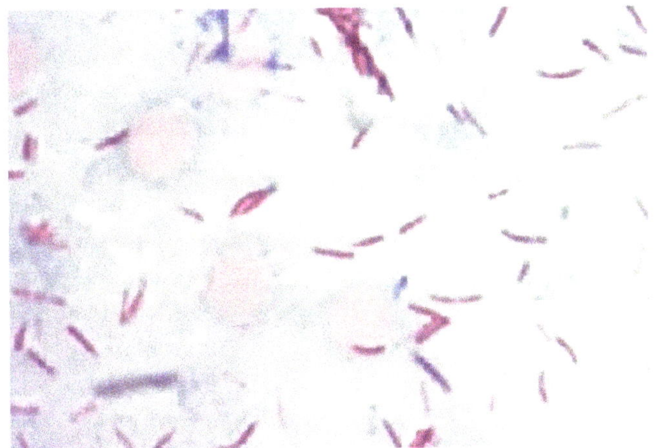

1. **What has been demonstrated in the slide?**
2. **What is your diagnosis?**
3. **Name the reservoir of this organism.**
4. **What are the genomes for this organism?**
5. **What are the proteins present on the cell wall of the organism?**
6. **What are the routes of entry of this organism?**

7. What are the processes through which the bacteria spread through the hematogenous route?
8. How the Schwann cells are infected by this organism?
9. How many days this organism takes for one division?
10. What are the areas in the body in which they use to grow and why?
11. How the bacteria invade keratinocytes?
12. How the bacteria invade Schwann cells?
13. In case of person to person spread, what are the risks in different forms of this disease?
14. What are the host responses to infection in the tuberculoid form?
15. What are the host response to infection in lepromatous form?
16. What cytokine imbalance is responsible for clinical form of this disease?
17. What is the role of dendritic cells in the immune response in this patient?
18. What is the role of IgA in this disease?
19. What is the role of genetic polymorphism in this disease?
20. How many types of hypersensitivity reactions found in this disease?
21. What are the bacterial antigens involved in the formation of immune complex?
22. What are the different clinical forms in this disease?
23. What is inderminate type in this disease and what is its progression?
24. What is paucibacillary type and why it is so called?
25. What is tuberculoid form and what is its progression?
26. What are the nerves affected in this disease?
27. What are types of sensory loos occurring in this disease?
28. What are the eye lesions in this disease?
29. What are the panels of clinical diagnostic criteria in this disease?
30. What is morphological index?
31. What are the two tests can be used to diagnose nerve injury?
32. What is the significance of serological tests in this disease?
33. What is the treatment of this disease according to World Health Organization (WHO)?
34. Why vaccine is not the priority in this disease?
35. Which drug administration is beneficial for this patient?

Answers

1. Stained slide demonstrates acid-fast rod-shaped bacilli.
2. The patient has been suffering from leprosy due to *Mycobacterium* infection.
3. The major reservoirs of this bacteria are:
   a. Human being
   b. Apes rarely
   c. Some species of monkeys
   d. Chimpanzee
   e. Nine-banded armadillo
   f. Mangabey monkeys
   g. Cynomolgus macaque
4. Sequencing of *Mycobacterium leprae* demonstrates 1605 that codes proteins and 50 genes for the stable RNA molecules.
5. Cell wall of the *Mycobacterium leprae* contains:
   a. Species-specific phenolic glycolipid used for the serodiagnosis of lepromatous leprosy
   b. Genus-specific lipoarabinomannan
6. Following are the routes of entry of this organism:
   a. Nasal epithelial cells
   b. Poorly differentiated keratinocytes
   c. Fibroblast
   d. Endothelial cells of the skin
7. The hematogenous spread occurs through macrophages and dendritic cells.
8. In the Schwann cells, *Mycobacterium leprae* bind to phenolic glycolipid-1 that attaches to the G-domain of the α2-chain of the laminin-2 isoform which is present in the basal lamina of this cells and this is restricted to the peripheral nerve. Subsequent uptake by this cell by the α-dystroglycan, a receptor present on the cell membrane

9. *Mycobacterium* takes 10–12 days for one division
10. Following are the areas in the body where this bacteria can grow due to lower body temperature:
    a. Skin
    b. Superficial nerves
11. In case of minor injuries in the epidermis, the bacteria attach to the keratinocytes via laminin-5 thereby prompting the keratinocytes to initiate innate immune response.
12. Schwann cells survive by the following factors:
    a. Insulin-like growth factor 1
    b. 2'-5'-oligoadenylate synthetase-like molecule which is responsible for autophagy.
13. Following are the risks in different forms of this disease:
    a. 8–10 times higher in case of lepromatous leprosy
    b. 2–4 times higher in case of tuberculoid form of leprosy
    Following factors will play a role:
    a. Frequent contact
    b. Genetic background
    c. Immunologic background
14. Following are the host cell responses in the tuberculoid form:
    a. Schwann cells expresses HLA class II molecules that stimulates CD4+ T cells and γ-interferon that produces CD4+ T cells in the lesion leading to formation of granuloma containing epithelioid cells and giant cells
    b. This bacteria interacts with toll-like receptors present on the Schwann cells thereby induce apoptosis leading to the damage of the nerve
    c. If the lesion will be chronic, there is swelling of the perineural areas leading to ischemia and fibrosis and axonal death.
    d. Infected keratinocytes present with the CD4+ T cells leading to production of γ-interferon which in turn activates keratinocytes further in the involved lesion
    e. T cell immunity will be enhanced by T helper cytokine pathway involving interleukin-2, 15, 12, and interferon-γ.
15. Following are the host immune responses in case of lepromatous leprosy:
    a. Phenolic glycolipid in the cell wall stimulates the IgM antibody production which down regulate the cell mediated immunity.
    b. These antibody forms immune complexes which will deposit in the tissue leading to attraction of neutrophils thereby activating complement. As a result, intense tissue or organ damage occurs.
    c. Th2 cytokine pathway involving interleukin-4, 5 and 10 will be activated in lepromatous form.
16. Following cytokine imbalance are responsible for clinical form of this disease:
    a. T cell immunity will be enhanced by T helper (Th1) cytokine pathway involving interleukin-2, 15, 12 and interferon-γ.
    b. Th2 cytokine pathway involving interleukin-4, 5, and 10 will be activated in lepromatous form.
17. Role of dendritic cells in the immune response in this patient: Dendritic cells fight against the bacilli in the nasal mucosa of the skin abrasion and thereby regulate the balance of Th1/Th2 cell-mediated immunity
18. IgA by clearing the bacteria efficiently in the respiratory tract mucosa will provide protection against this infection.
19. Following genetic polymorphisms are associated with these types of disease:
    a. HLA-DR2 and HLA-DR3 are associated with tuberculoid form of the disease.
    b. HLA-DQ1 is associated with lepromatous form of this disease.
20. There are two types of hypersensitivity reactions in this patient:
    a. Type 1 reaction or reversal reaction or delayed hypersensitivity reaction increases the cell-mediated immune response. It is the characteristic of tuberculoid leprosy.
    b. Type 2 reaction leads to deposition of the immune complexes in the involved tissue resulting in infiltration of neutrophils and development of high fever and edema.
    c. In case of untreated lepromatous leprosy, there may be development of Lucio phenomenon which also demonstrated type 2 hypersensitivity reaction.
21. Following bacterial antigens are involved in the formation of immune complexes:
    a. Phenolic glycolipid-1
    b. Lipoarabinomannan
    c. Major membrane protein II
22. Following are the clinical forms of this disease:
    a. Tuberculoid leprosy
    b. Borderline tuberculoid leprosy
    c. Mid-borderline leprosy
    d. Borderline lepromatous leprosy
    e. Lepromatous leprosy

23. In case of indeterminate type of leprosy:
    a. No sensory loss
    b. One or several hypopigmented areas in the skin
    c. Erythematous macules
       Some cases will heal spontaneously or in some cases, there may be immature response leading to progression to other forms of the disease.
24. In indeterminate or tuberculoid form of leprosy, the skin lesions are less than five and smear test demonstrates no bacilli. Hence, these forms of disease are known as paucibacillary leprosy.
25. Tuberculoid form of leprosy:
    a. One or more erythematous plaques are seen on the face and limbs but absent on the scalp and intertriginous areas.
    b. Loss of sensation
    c. Alopecia
    d. Tender and thickened peripheral nerves leading to loss of function
    Progression of the disease:
    a. It may resolve spontaneously.
    b. It will progress to borderline leprosy.
    c. In rare condition, it will progress to lepromatous form.
26. Following nerves are affected in this disease:
    a. Posterior tibial nerve
    b. Ulnar nerve
    c. Median nerve
    d. Lateral popliteal nerve
    e. Facial nerve
    f. Dermal nerves leading to hypoesthesia
27. Following are the types of sensory loss:
    a. Hypoesthesia
    b. Anhidrosis
    c. Loss of sensation in the glove and stocking distribution
28. Following eye lesions occur in this disease:
    a. Bacterial invasion leading to blindness
    b. Loss of corneal sensation
    c. Dryness of the conjunctiva and cornea
    d. Increased risk of microtrauma as well as corneal ulceration
29. Following are the three major criteria for the diagnosis:
    a. Hypopigmented or reddish patch on the skin along with loss of sensation
    b. Detection of the acid-fast bacilli in the biopsy or from the skin smears
    c. Thickening of the peripheral nerves

30. Morphological index is calculated as number of viable bacilli per 100 bacilli.
31. Following two tests are used to diagnose nerve injury:
    a. Histamine sweat test, where a drop of histamine diphosphate is placed on the both affected as well as nonaffected skin. In the normal skin, it will produce wheal, whereas in the affected skin, the wheal will be absent due to absence of peripheral nerves.
    b. Methacholine sweat test, where intracutaneous injection of methacholine demonstrates presence of sweating in the normal skin, whereas in the affected skin, there is no sweating.
32. Importance of serological tests in this disease:
    a. High titer of antibodies is found in case of untreated lepromatous leprosy.
    b. Antibodies to phenolic glycolipid are present in 90% of lepromatous leprosy patient but 50% of tuberculoid leprosy patients and 5% of healthy individual.
33. Following are the line of treatment according to WHO:
    a. In case of one lesion paucibacillary leprosy: 600 mg rifampicin single dose or 400 mg ofloxacin single dose or 100 mg minocycline single dose orally should be given.
    b. In case of more than one lesion and paucibacillary group, 6 months treatment is required in the form:
       • 100 mg self-administered dapsone orally daily
       • Monthly supervised 600 mg rifampicin orally
    c. In case of multibacillary leprosy, total treatment will be 24 months in the form:
       • 100 mg self-administered dapsone and 100 mg clofazimine orally daily
       • Monthly supervised 600 mg rifampicin and 300 mg clofazimine orally
34. Vaccine development is not the priority because:
    a. Dormant nature of *Mycobacterium leprae*
    b. Long incubation period
    c. Effective treatment with multidrugs
    d. Low prevalence of leprosy
    e. Insufficient funding
35. For *Mycobacterium leprae*, BCG as well as *Mycobacterium* indicus pranii is effective.

CASE 8

A 20-year-old adult having 1 day history of headache and fever was found on the next morning as drowsy and moaning. On physical examination, his temperature was 102°F, pulse rate 132 beats/min, blood pressure 110/60 mm Hg, presence of neck rigidity, and presence of purpuric rash on the legs, trunk, and wrist. Laboratory examination demonstrated white blood count 27,000/cc with predominant neutrophilic leukocytosis and thrombocytopenia. Blood culture demonstrated growth which on Gram stain showed:

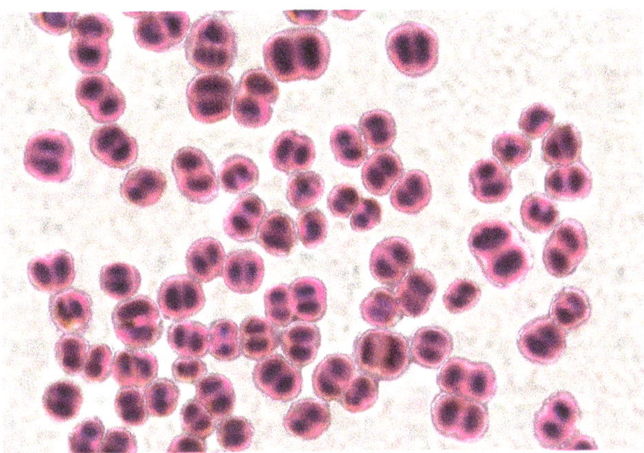

1. **What is demonstrated in the slide?**
2. **What is your diagnosis?**
3. **What are the three principal causes of this condition?**
4. **How these organism look like in the Gram Stain?**
5. **Which forms outer membrane protein in this organism?**
6. **What is the importance of phase variation of the outer membrane protein?**
7. **Which type of protein is present on the cell surface villi?**
8. **How many classes of outer membrane protein are there in this organism?**
9. **What are the functions of class V protein in this organism?**
10. **How many domains are present in this class V protein and what are their functions?**
11. **Class V subtype outer membrane protein can be subdivided into how many types and based on which?**
12. **How these variants of class V protein react with the human cells?**
13. **Which capsular strains are responsible for invasive disease?**
14. **What are the compositions of the above capsular serogroups?**
15. **How the organism spreads in the human body?**
16. **What is the role of innate immunity in the human being against this organism?**
17. **What is the function of acquired immunity against this organism?**
18. **In the blood stream, how this organism can be killed?**
19. **What is the role of immunity in case of neonates to child against this organism?**
20. **What are the featured outcomes of meningococcemia?**
21. **What is the role of lipopolysaccharide of this organism in the pathogenesis?**
22. **What is the nature and progression of rashes in this disease?**
23. **In the invasive disease produced by this organism, the patients can be separated into how many groups?**
24. **What are the complications in this disease?**
25. **What is the specific media for the recovery of this organism?**
26. **How can you differentiate Neisseria by utilization of sugars?**
27. **How different enzymes can detect this organism?**
28. **Which individual can spread this infection to normal individual?**
29. **What are the drugs for prophylaxis used for the prevention of this disease?**
30. **What are the processes of prevention from this disease?**

Answers

1. The above picture demonstrates gram-negative diplococci seen in pairs having adjacent sides flattened looking like coffee bean in appearance.

2. This patient has been suffering from meningo-coccemia leading to meningococcal meningitis complicated by decreased sensorium.

3. The three principal causes of meningitis are:
   a. *Neisseria meningitidis*
   b. *Streptococcus pneumoniae*
   c. *Haemophilus influenzae*

4. In the Gram stain, they look like gram-negative diplococci seen in pairs having adjacent sides flattened looking like coffee-bean appearance.

5. Outer leaflet of its outer membrane protein is formed by lipooligosaccharide where O antigen is absent.

6. Phase variation in this lipooligosaccharide will lead to interconversion between invasive antibody and complement-resistant phenotypes in this organism.

7. Pili present on the surface of the cells in this organism contain structural protein pilin which attaches with nasopharyngeal mucosal epithelium to make the organism resistant to phagocytosis

8. Based on descending molecular weight, this organism has been subdivided into five classes:
   a. Class I is PorA
   b. Class II is PorB
   c. Class III is PorB
   d. Class IV is reduction modifiable protein.
   e. Class V is opacity associated protein.

9. Functions of the class V protein are as follows:
   a. Ability of the organism to adhere tightly with the epithelium
   b. Ability to dictate the tissue tropism of this organism
   c. Ability to be up taken by the host epithelial cells.

10. There are two hypervariable domains present in the extracellular portion of this class V molecule giving rise to new class V variant because of:
    a. Point mutation
    b. Modular exchange domains between the different class V proteins

11. Based on the cellular receptors to which this class V proteins bind, they are subdivided into two major groups:
    a. O_{paHS} proteins: They will bind to heparan sulfate and fibronectin and vitronectin present in the extracellular matrix.
    b. O_{paCEA} protein: They will bind to carcino-embryonic antigen or related molecules.

12. O_{paHS} protein helps the human cells to internalize the meningococci:
    a. Directly through engaging the heparan sulfate proteoglycans present on the epithelial cells
    b. Indirectly through use of the fibronectin or vitronectin to make bridge between the O_{paHS} protein and cell surface integrins and cellular cytoskeleton

13. Virulence of this bacteria can be determined by six capsular strains:
    a. A
    b. B
    c. C
    d. Y and W-135
    e. X in West Africa

14. Virulent capsules are composed of:
    a. Serogroup A: It is composed by N-acetyl-mannosamine-1 phosphate
    b. Capsule B, C, Y, and W-135: These are composed of polysialic acid or sialic acid linked to glucose or galactose.
    c. Capsule X: It is composed of polymers containing $\alpha 1$ through 4 linked to N-acetylglucosamine-1 phosphate.

15. Nasopharyngeal mucosa takes up the bacteria and internalize by receptor-mediated endocytosis. From there, these bacteria enter into the subepithelial space and then into the blood stream. Here, capsule production is very important for their survival. Through the blood stream they reach meninges, joints, and the skin.

16. Innate immunity of the nasopharynx prevents the bacteria to attach with the nasal mucosal epithelium and thereby reaching the lower respiratory tree. Anatomy of the nasal cavity make the airflow turbulent by the nasal airy bones to make the contact of the bacteria with the nasal hairs and the mucus containing antimicrobial factors like lysozyme, lactoferrin, and overlying the mucosal epithelium for maximum time. Nasal mucosal epithelium is transitional and pseudostratified beneath which there is thick, vascular, and erectile glandular lamina propria. The humidified warm air will help to bind the bacteria through polysaccharide capsule. Trapped microorganism in the mucus are moved backward into the throat and swallowed on to the stomach.

17. Acquired immune response should be mediated by secretory IgA as its functions in these cases are:
    a. Prevention of the adherence of the organism with the mucosal surfaces
    b. Prevention of invasion of the mucosal epithelium

c. It will neutralize the exotoxins as well as microbial enzymes.

d. It can clear the pathogen mediated by mucociliary ladder.

e. It can help to agglutinate the microbial organisms in the nasopharyngeal secretions

18. These bacteria produce IgA1 protease which cleaves at IgA1 at the hinge region to produce Fc and Fab segments. But most of the secretory IgA is subclass 2 at the mucosal surface which is resistant to the protease enzyme.

    But after invasion of these bacteria, mannose-binding protein and alternate complement pathways help in the killing of the bacteria. So in case of the deficiency of this membrane-attack component, the subject will be susceptible to invasive disease.

19. As a result of transplacental transfer of the IgG antibodies, the neonates will be resistant to this disease up to 6 months after that they will be extremely susceptible to this infection. But, antibodies are induced in the body of the child years by the intermittent carriage of *N. meningitidis* but this carriage is rare under the age of 6 years.

20. Following are the outcomes of meningococcemia:

    a. Shock

    b. Meningitis

    c. Disseminated intravascular coagulation

    d. Myocardial dysfunction

21. Functions of lipooligosaccharides are as follows:

    a. Lipooligosaccharides are released from the meningococcus in blebs and activate complement cascade.

    b. One component of this lipooligosaccharide will bind to CD14/TLR4/MD2 receptor present on the macrophage or other cell surfaces to release a number of cytokines tumor necrosis factor-alpha and interleukin-1, 6, 8, 10, and 11, granulocyte monocytes colony-stimulating factors, and interferon-γ which will increase the severity of infection resulting in death.

    c. This lipooligosaccharide also binds to macrophages in the liver, spleen, and other sites leading to vasodilatation resulting in fall in blood pressure which will be responsible for fluid and electrolytes loss.

22. The rashes start as petechiae or maculopapule starting in the trunk and extremities and progresses to involve the whole body. The rashes progress to pustules and bullae and lastly hemorrhagic with central necrosis.

23. In case of invasive meningococcal disease, the patients will fall into four groups:

    a. Patients with bacteremia without shock

    b. Patients with bacteremia without feature of meningitis

    c. Patients with shock and meningitis

    d. Patient with meningitis alone

24. Complications in this disease are the following:

    a. Seizures

    b. Increased intracranial pressure

    c. Cerebral venous thrombosis

    d. Sagittal sinus thrombosis

    e. Hydrocephalus

    f. Cerebral herniation

    g. Communicating hydrocephalus leading to:
    - Difficulty in gait
    - Changes in the mental status
    - Incontinence
    - Hearing loss

    h. Fulminant meningococcemia leading to disseminated intravascular coagulation resulting in bleeding in the:
    - Lung
    - Urinary tract
    - Gastrointestinal tract

    i. Suppurative complications:
    - Septic arthritis
    - Pericarditis
    - Endophthalmitis
    - Pneumonia

25. Specific media for recovery of the organism:

    a. Chocolate agar

    b. Blood agar

    c. Thayer–Martin medium for specimen obtaining from the mucosal surface, the media contains antimicrobial agents to suppress the growth of the commensal gram-negative and gram-positive bacteria and fungal organisms.

26. By utilization of glucose, maltose, lactose, and sucrose, one can differentiate pathogenic *N. meningitidis* as it will utilize glucose and maltose only.

27. Meningococcus is oxidase positive and catalase positive.

28. Following individuals being in close contact during a week before the onset of the disease are:

    a. Household members

    b. Day care contact

c. Cellmates

d. Individuals exposed to infected nasopharyngeal secretions through:
- Kissing
- Mouth-to-mouth resuscitation

29. The chemoprophylaxis are as follows:
    a. Rifampin
    b. Ciprofloxacin
    c. Ceftriaxone

30. The disease can be prevented by following means:
    a. Tetravalent meningococcal capsular polysaccharide protein conjugate vaccine protects the disease caused by A, C, Y, and W-135 serogroups
    b. Conjugate vaccine MCV4: T cell-dependent immunogen protects and develops hard immunity in infants through reduction of nasopharyngeal carriage
    c. C conjugate vaccine is given three doses at 3, 4, and 12 months of age.

CASE 9

A 60-year-old male having history of chronic lymphocytic leukemia on chemotherapy as well as immunotherapy for 6 years came to medicine clinic with cough and expectoration with respiratory distress and diagnosed as pneumonia on contrast-enhanced computed tomography (CECT). Bronchoalveolar fluid examination demonstrated:

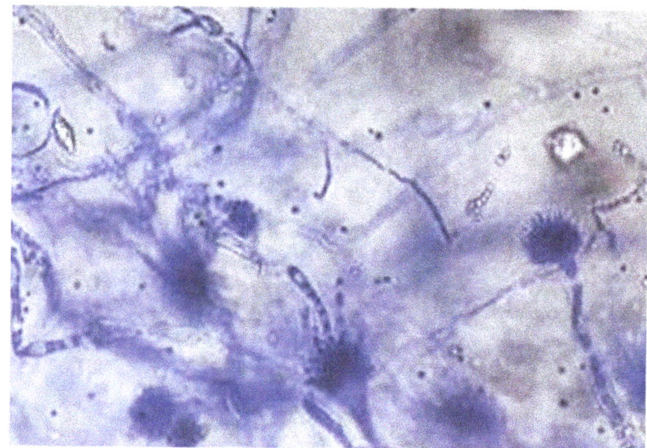

1. What is demonstrated in the above slide?
2. What is your diagnosis?
3. Where these organisms are found in nature?
4. Why the cell wall of this organism is rigid?
5. What are the species of this organism responsible for pulmonary allergic disorder?
6. Why only one species of this organism is responsible for pulmonary allergic disorder?
7. Which species of this organism is responsible for chronic granulomatous disease in children?
8. What are the different morphologies of conidia in the organism and which is most virulent?
9. What are the different routes through which the spore will infect and lodge in which organ?
10. Which enzyme of this organism is responsible for invasion into the respiratory tissue?
11. In immunocompetent individual, what is the role of innate immunity against this organism?
12. In cystic fibrosis, why this infection will occur?
13. What are the cells in the respiratory tract which defense against this organism?
14. Which subtypes of toll-like receptors act as adjuvant against bronchopulmonary aspergillosis?
15. What are the fungicidal methods going in the lungs provided by the neutrophils?
16. Why the defense mechanism of the neutrophil is rapid as compared to that of macrophage?
17. What are the causes that impair the functions of neutrophils against this organism?
18. What is the role of platelets in the defense mechanism against this organism?

19. **What are the levels increased by this organism during invasion?**
20. **What are the functions of resting conidia of this fungus?**
21. **In adaptive immunity, what factors provide resistance to this disease?**
22. **What are the functions of proinflammatory cytokines in this disease?**
23. **How the balance between Th1 and Th2 cell production is maintained in this disease?**
24. **What is the antibody response in this disease?**
25. **What are the functions of most potent toxin of this organism?**
26. **What are the different types of reactions demonstrated in this infection?**
27. **Clinical types of this infection can be classified based on which factors?**
28. **What are the factors associated with chronic necrotizing pulmonary aspergillosis?**
29. **What are the hematological diseases that are susceptible to this invasive disease?**
30. **What are the types of invasive diseases that occur in this infection?**
31. **What are the diseases of lung predispose to this infection?**
32. **What are the organisms responsible for mycetoma?**
33. **What are the compositions of fungal ball?**
34. **What are the other sites where you can get aspergilloma?**
35. **What are the diagnostic criteria of allergic bronchopulmonary aspergillosis (ABPA)?**
36. **What are the shadows found radiologically in ABPA?**
37. **What are the characteristic features in chest radiography in aspergilloma?**
38. **What is the novel treatment in ABPA?**
39. **What are the postoperative complications in aspergilloma?**

Answers

1. Gram-stained slide demonstrates smooth-walled conidiophores having swollen flask-shaped vesicles which are covered by single row of phialides on the upper half of the vesicles suggestive of *Aspergillus fumigatus*.

2. This patient has been suffering from broncho-pulmonary aspergillosis by *A. fumigatus*.

3. These organisms are found in the following areas in the nature:
   a. Soil
   b. Decaying vegetation
   c. Hay
   d. Stored grain
   e. Compost piles
   f. Mulches
   g. Sewage facilities
   h. Bird excreta
   i. Storage tank
   j. Fireproofing materials
   k. Bedding
   l. Pillows
   m. Air conditioning

4. Rigid wall of this organism is due to:
   a. Newly synthetized β(1-3)-glucans
   b. Other polysaccharides such as chitin, galactomannan, and β(1-3)-, β(1-4)-glucans

5. Following species of *Aspergillus* are responsible for pulmonary allergic disorder:
   a. *Aspergillus fumigatus*
   b. *Aspergillus niger*
   c. *Aspergillus terreus*
   d. *Aspergillus flavus*
   e. *Aspergillus clavatus*
   f. *Aspergillus nidulans*
   g. *Aspergillus oryzae*

6. *Aspergillus fumigatus* is thermotolerant within 15–55°C and can survive up to 75°C. Hence, this species can grow within the mammalian respiratory tract.

7. In children, *A. nidulans* can produce chronic granulomatous disease.

8. *Aspergillus fumigatus* having greenish-blue conidia and conidiophores originating from greenish phialides indicates accumulated metabolites and recognized as more virulent as compared to nonpigmented conidia and conidiophores.

9. Spores of the *Aspergillus* can enter through the respiratory tract to reach the lung and sinuses.

10. The enzyme proteases through the digestion of lung matrix invade the respiratory tract.

11. In case of immunocompetent host:
    a. Goblet cells in the epithelial layers in the respiratory tract lining secrete mucus where fungal spores are trapped and it moves by ciliated cells toward the upper respiratory tract from where the fungus is either coughed out or swallowed.
    b. In the smaller airways, surfactant protein A and D by the type II pneumocytes which act as opsonins and bind the spores and present to neutrophils and macrophages

12. In patient with cystic fibrosis, this infection will occurs because:
    a. Mucociliary function is impaired.
    b. Mucus is highly viscus which further affects the ciliary movement.

13. Macrophages and neutrophils in the respiratory tract defense against *A. fumigatus* by attacking conidiophores and developing hyphae respectively

14. Agonists of membrane-associated toll-like receptors 3 and 9 act as adjuvants against bronchopulmonary aspergillosis.

15. Neutrophils because of the large size of the hyphae of *Aspergillus* cannot engulf them rather accumulate around the hyphae in clusters and starts:
    a. Secretion of ROS
    b. Release of lysozymes
    c. Secretion of neutrophil cationic peptides
    All lead to degranulation of neutrophil.

16. Defense mechanism of neutrophil is rapid because:
    a. Polysaccharide hydrolases release glycoprotein from the cell wall of *aspergillus*
    b. Defensins also play a role in the hyphal damage

17. Following are the causes of neutrophilic dysfunction against this organism:
    a. Chemotherapy-induced neutropenia
    b. Corticosteroid-based treatment
    c. Purine analogs like fludarabine
    d. Some monoclonal antibody treatment like anti-CD52

18. Platelets can protect against aspergillosis by the following mechanism: They will be activated by attaching with the cell wall of the hyphae leading to direct damage of the cell wall.

19. Following levels are increased during invasion of the *A. fumigatus*:
    a. Serum fibrinogen
    b. C-reactive protein
    c. Other acute phase proteins

20. The functions of the resting conidia are as follows:
    a. Activation of alternate complement pathway
    b. Induce neutrophil chemotaxis
    c. Deposition of complement components on the surface of the fungus

21. Following factors provide resistance to this disease:
    a. Th1 cellular response with strong cellular immune component
    b. Increased level of interferon-γ
    c. Increased level of granulocyte and granulocyte-macrophage colony-stimulating factor
    d. Tumor necrosis factor-alpha
    e. Interleukin-1, 6, 12, and 18

22. Following are the functions of proinflammatory cytokines:
    a. Tumor necrosis factor-alpha increases the capacity of the neutrophils to damage hyphae
    b. Interferon-γ, neutrophil, and monocyte colony-stimulating factors increase the activity of neutrophils and monocytes against the hyphae
    c. Interleukin-5:
       • Increases the damage of hyphae
       • Increases release of interleukin-8 by neutrophils
    d. Interleukin-8:
       • Increases the recruitment of neutrophils at the site of inflammation
       • Mediates the antimicrobial peptide release

23. Nature of antigen will maintain the balance between the beneficial Th1 and damaging Th2 because conidia primes the dendritic cells which in turn activates Th1 CD4+ T cells, whereas priming dendritic cells with hyphae will enhance the Th2 cell response.

24. In case of bronchopulmonary aspergillosis, the serum contains high level of IgE isotypes and IgG, because B cells will secrete IgE, whereas interleukin-5 will recruit eosinophils. The infiltration of eosinophils, degranulation of basophils, and mast cells will lead to release of proinflammatory cytokines which in turn further increases the eosinophilic chemotaxis.

25. Functions of most potent toxin of *A. fumigatus*, i.e., gliotoxin are:
    a. It will affect the synthesis of the fungal DNA, RNA, and proteins.
    b. It will impair the host cellular function
    c. It will suppress the T-cell response
    d. It will inhibit the phagocytosis by the macrophages
    e. It will inhibit the phagocytosis by neutrophils by inhibiting production of NADPH and ROS.

26. There are following types of reactions occurring by this organism:
    a. Immediate type 1 hypersensitivity reaction in case of bronchopulmonary aspergillosis
    b. Late Arthur type of reaction occurs to *Aspergillus* antigen due to IgE-mediated mast cell activation
    c. Type III hypersensitivity reaction occurs by immune complexes and complement activation
27. Following are the clinical types of pulmonary aspergillosis:
    a. Allergic bronchopulmonary aspergillosis
    b. Chronic *Aspergillus* necrotizing pneumonia
    c. Invasive aspergillosis
    d. Pulmonary aspergilloma
28. Following lung diseases or factors are associated with chronic necrotizing pulmonary aspergillosis:
    a. Steroid-dependent chronic obstructive pulmonary disease
    b. Interstitial lung disease
    c. Previous thoracic surgery
    d. Alcoholism
    e. Chronic corticosteroid therapy
29. Following hematological diseases are susceptible to invasive aspergillosis:
    a. Leukemia
    b. Neutropenia
    c. Multiple myeloma
    d. Allogenic bone marrow transplantation
30. Following are the types of invasive disease occurring due to this infection:
    a. Acute or chronic pulmonary aspergillosis
    b. Tracheobronchitis and obstructive bronchial disease
    c. Acute invasive rhinosinusitis
    d. Disseminated diseases to brain, kidney, heart, skin, and eyes
31. Following lung diseases are those which are cavity forming diseases:
    a. Tuberculosis
    b. Cystic fibrosis
    c. Lung abscess
    d. Sarcoidosis
    e. Emphysematous bullae
    f. Chronic obstructive paranasal sinuses
32. Following organisms are responsible for forming mycetoma:
    a. *Aspergillus fumigatus*
    b. Fusarium
    c. Zygomycetes

33. Fungal ball consists of:
    a. Mass of hyphae
    b. Surrounded by proteinaceous matrix
    c. At the periphery dead tissue, mucus, and sporulating structures
34. Following sites also contain aspergilloma:
    a. Brain
    b. Various sinuses in the face
    c. Ear canals
    d. Kidneys
    e. Urinary tract
    f. Heart valves
35. Following are the diagnostic criteria of ABPA:
    a. Rosenberg–Patterson criteria:
       - Eight major criteria:
         i. Asthma
         ii. Presence of transient pulmonary infiltrate
         iii. Immediate cutaneous reactivity to *A. fumigatus*
         iv. Elevated total serum IgE
         v. Precipitating antibodies against *A. fumigatus*
         vi. Peripheral blood eosinophilia
         vii. Elevated serum IgE and IgG to *A. fumigatus*
         viii. Central/proximal bronchiectasis with normal tapering of distal bronchi
       - Three minor criteria:
         i. Expectoration of golden-brown sputum plugs
         ii. Positive sputum culture of *Aspergillus* species
         iii. Arthur types of delayed skin reaction to *A. fumigatus*
36. Following are the shadows found radiologically in ABPA:
    a. Finger in glove opacity indicating impaction of mucus in the dilated bronchi
    b. Tramline shadows suggestive of parallel linear shadows extending from the hilum in the bronchial distribution
    c. Toothpaste shadow indicating impaction of mucus in the bronchi
    d. Ring shadow indicating dilated bronchi inflamed bronchial wall
37. Radiological features in the aspergilloma are the following:
    a. Solid ball of water density within the spherical or ovoid cavity
    b. Solid ball may be mobile.
    c. The ball should be separated from the wall by an air space.
    d. Pleural thickening

38. Novel treatment in ABPA:
    a. Anti-IgE: Omalizumab, ligelizumab, and quilizumab
    b. Anti-interleukin-5: Mepolizumab, and reslizumab
    c. Anti-interleukin-5 receptor: Benralizumab
    d. Toll-like receptor (TLR) agonists can be used as adjuvants.

39. Postoperative complications in case of aspergilloma are as follows:
    a. Hemorrhage
    b. Bronchopleural fistula
    c. Residual pleural space
    d. Empyema

CASE 10

A 25-year-old male came to medical clinic with fever and common cold for 3 days. On examination, the throat was congested and cervical lymphadenopathy. The doctor prescribed ampicillin to prevent secondary infection. But after 3 days, he came again with worsening of fever along with maculopapular rashes throughout the body.

1. **What is your diagnosis?**
2. **What is the composition of the envelope of this organism?**
3. **Where is the site of latency of this organism?**
4. **In the body, this organism presents in how many states?**
5. **In which group this organism belongs to and what are the other organisms present in this group?**
6. **What are the cancers associated with this organism?**
7. **What are the gene products of this organism and what are their functions?**
8. **How this organism will be endocytosed in human being?**
9. **What is the proof of significant tropism of this organism in human being?**
10. **What is the difference between virions derived from B cells and epithelial cells?**
11. **What are the sites of replications of the organism in human being?**
12. **How this organism replicates in the B cells in the human being and what is its significance?**
13. **How the organism spreads through the infected B cells into the whole body?**
14. **What is the incubation period of this infection?**
15. **What is the other name of this disease and why?**
16. **What is the basic difference of age of infection in the developing and developed world?**
17. **What are the protective factors in the oral mucosa against this infection?**
18. **After entering mucosal epithelium, what is the difference between the childhood and adulthood in behaving with the organism?**
19. **What is the function of the natural killer cells against this infection in human being?**
20. **What are the antigens in the organism and when antibodies appear against them?**
21. **In primary infection, what is the role of CD4+ T cells against this organism in human being?**
22. **In primary infection, what is the role of CD8+ T cells against this organism in human being?**
23. **What are the strategies of this organism to evade immunity of the host and also to avoid CD8+ T cells?**
24. **What are the types of rashes in this infection?**
25. **What are the hematological complications in this infection?**
26. **What is X-linked lymphoproliferative disease (XLPD) in this infection?**
27. **What do you mean by chronic active infection with this organism?**
28. **Why it is not a case of cytomegalovirus or streptococcal infection or primary HIV infection?**
29. **What is the most specific antibody should be done and by which method?**
30. **Which test can detect remote infection with this organism?**
31. **Which test can differentiate the primary infection from reactivation by this organism?**
32. **What are the aims of vaccination against this organism?**

Answers

1. The patient has been suffering from infectious mononucleosis caused by Epstein–Barr virus.

2. Envelope of this virus is composed of viral glycoprotein which presents on its surface and that includes gp350, gB, gH, gp42, and gL.

3. The site of latency of this virus is lymphocyte.

4. Epstein–Barr virus exists in two states:
   a. In case of lytic replication, the resultant virion has linear DNA.
   b. In case of latency, the viral genome will be circular episome which replicates in the dividing cells with the help of cellular enzymes.
   a. This virus belongs to γ-herpesvirus. Other organisms present in this group: Human herpesvirus B which is also known as Kaposi sarcoma associated virus.

5. Following cancers are associated with the Epstein–Barr virus:
   a. Gastric carcinoma
   b. Burkitt lymphoma
   c. Nasopharyngeal cancer
   d. Hodgkin's lymphoma
   e. T-cell lymphoma
   f. Primary central nervous system lymphoma

6. Following are the gene product in this virus and their functions:
   a. *EBNA1*: Maintenance of Epstein–Barr virus gene
   b. *EBNA2*: It will activate Epstein–Barr virus expression and host B cell gene.
   c. *EBNA3*: It will repress the expression of tumor suppression gene which will promote transformation of B lymphocyte into lymphoblastoid cell line.
   d. *LMP1*: It will activate and proliferate B cells and it also inhibits cell apoptosis.
   e. *LMP2*: It mimics signaling of B cell receptor.

7. gp350 on the surface of the virus binds to cellular receptor for the complement component C3d. gp42 glycoprotein on viral surface binds to major histocompatibility complex of class II molecule. Then the viral cell membrane will be fused with the host cell membrane mediated by gH/gL and gB.

8. By the above mechanisms virus will be endocytosed.

9. There is evidence of significant tropism of this virus in case of nasopharyngeal carcinoma and oral hairy leukoplakia seen in HIV patient due to unchecked lytic replication of squamous epithelium.

10. Epstein–Barr virus produced by B cells binds to major histocompatibility complex class II molecule during budding from the infected cells whereas virus produced by epithelial cells has no major histocompatibility complex class II molecule but has high level of gp42. So, this virus is better at infecting B cell.

11. Epstein–Barr virus will replicate in oral epithelial cells which will lead to infection of mucosal B cell.

12. Epstein–Barr virus undergoes lytic replication in the oropharyngeal cells leading to production of latently infected virions. These infected B lymphoblasts undergo continuous proliferation in the cell cycle. This process is known as transformation or immortalization. As a result, there is increase in the pool of infected B lymphocytes.

13. Epstein–Barr virus-infected cells are transported through the afferent lymphatic channels to cervical lymph nodes to infect more and more B cells. From there these infected B cells enter the blood stream through the thoracic duct to reach the other lymph nodes and spleen leading to development of splenomegaly and generalized lymphadenopathy.

14. Incubation period in this disease is 4–8 weeks.

15. This disease is also known as "kissing disease" because this disease can spread from infected to noninfected person through kissing.

16. In the developing world, all the children will be infected at the age of 2–4 years. This disease will be asymptomatic or very mild. So, it may be undiagnosed. In contrast, in the developed world due to high standard of living and proper hygiene, the age of onset of infection will be delayed and it is seen among the affluent individual.

17. Following are the protective factors in the oral mucosa:
    a. Saliva: It will protect, hydrate, and thereby lubricate the oral mucosal epithelium.
    b. Mucin: It will aggregate and remove the organism as well as antimicrobial peptide like defensins.

18. After entering the mucosal epithelium, this Epstein–Barr virus will be exposed to intraepithelial lymphocytes mainly natural killer cells which will kill the infected cells having decreased expression of class II major histocompatibility complex on the surface. These natural killer cell populations are high in case of childhood and early adulthood. Hence, primary infection is asymptomatic in infant and in adult. High CD8+ T cells are required to control this infection.

19. Invariant natural killer cells have invariant T cell receptors that can recognize glycolipids which are presented by nonclassical major histocompatibility complex class I molecule CD1d. Some of these cells having CD8 marker either directly kill the virus-

infected cells along with produce interferon-γ to increase Th1 response.

20. The lytic and latent antigens are present in this disease, these are:
    a. Early antigens (EAs): It will express during lytic replication.
    b. Late antigens: These are:
       - Virus capsid antigens (VCAs)
       - Envelope antigens
       - Gp350
    c. Latency antigens:
       - Epstein–Barr antigens
       - Latent membrane proteins

21. In early infection, T cells respond to virus in the form of proliferation of CD4+ T cells and CD8+ T cells which will outnumber the B cells at a ratio of 50:1.

22. Roles of CD8+ T cells in the primary infection:
    a. CD8+ T cells will recognize the Epstein–Barr virus encoded peptides which are presented by the B cells leading to release of proinflammatory cytokines and thereby intensify inflammatory response.
    b. In early infection, CD8+ T cell specific lytic antigens predominate but during convalescence period, there is shift toward T cells which recognize latent antigens mainly EBNA3, it is expressed by B cells.
    c. Cytotoxic CD8+ T cells kill the virus-infected cells, but continuous shedding of virus in the throat occurs which may be due to poor recruitment of CD8+ T cells to the tonsils.
    d. Few virus-infected cells will be in the resting state thereby preparing a pool of memory cells.
    e. After recovery from the primary infection, cytotoxic memory CD8+ T memory cells pool will remain and it will increase in number with age.

23. The strategies of Epstein–Barr virus that help to evade the immune system to avoid the attack by CD8+ T cells:
    a. Few Epstein–Barr virus containing latent virus will downregulate the antigens of the viruses will evade immune response.
    b. In any dividing memory cell, this virus should express EBNA1 to ensure that the genome must be replicated. To prevent this targeting protein, EBNA1 should contain the sequence of glycine-alanine repeat which is not necessary for the maintenance of genome.
    c. Envelope protein gp42:
       - Is shed actively as soluble truncated molecule at the time of lytic infection.

- It binds to the major histocompatibility complex class II molecule/peptide complexes
- It will inhibit activation of CD4+ T cells which is required for CD8+ T cells generation.

    d. The immune modulator BCRF1 secreted by the Epstein–Barr virus during lytic cycle is viral homolog of cytokine interleukin-10. As a result of inhibition of function of Th1 cells, there is shift toward Th2 cells. These cells promote B cells but do not promote CD8+ T cells for killing the cells containing Epstein–Barr virus.

24. Rashes are as follows:
    a. Macular, petechial, and scarlatiniform rashes
    b. Urticarial
    c. Erythema multiforme
    d. If the patients receives ampicillin, 90% may develop maculopapular rashes within 10 days of administration

25. Hematological complications are as follows:
    a. Mild thrombocytopenia
    b. Aplastic anemia
    c. Severe idiopathic thrombocytic purpura

26. Patients suffering from XLPD are extremely susceptible to Epstein–Barr virus infection. In case of primary infection, this disease is severe at onset with huge expansion of B cells infected with this virus along with infiltration of T cells in the liver and other organs in the body. This patient has following abnormalities in the immune system:
    a. Defective natural killer cells activity
    b. Absence of invariant natural killer cells
    c. Overactivity of Th1 cells
    d. Poor Th2 cells response
    All the above leads to:
    a. CD8+ T cells overexpansion as well as
    b. Overproduction of Th1 inflammatory cytokines
    c. Macrophage activation
    d. Hemophagocytosis
    The defect is in the small cytoplasmic protein SAP which is involved in the signaling of T lymphocytes and natural killer cells.

27. Chronic active Epstein–Barr virus infection is rare condition common in Asia and South America presents with:
    a. Interstitial pneumonia
    b. Hemophagocytosis
    c. Lymphadenitis
    d. Uveitis
    e. Persistent hepatitis

Pathogenesis results from immune defect resulting in proliferation of Epstein–Barr virus-infected T cells or natural killer cells.

It can be diagnosed by elevated antibodies VCA-IgG and EA IgG against Epstein–Barr virus antigen. These patients die within few years from:

a. Severe pancytopenia
b. Hypogammaglobulinemia
c. NK/T cell nasal lymphoma

28. It is not a case of cytomegalovirus infection because:
    a. Sore throat is less severe
    b. Absent or minimal lymphadenopathy
    c. Specific antibody against cytomegalovirus
    It is not a case of streptococcal infection because:
    a. Splenomegaly and hepatomegaly are not present.
    b. Fatigue is less prominent.

29. Anti-VCA-IgM antibody will be present early in the illness due to Epstein–Barr virus infection but declines rapidly over 3 months and it should be estimated by enzyme-linked immunosorbent assay (ELISA) and also by immunofluorescence assay by using Epstein–Barr virus-infected lymphoblastoid cell line as antigenic substrate.

30. In case of remote infection with this virus, anti-VCA-IgG antibody will present throughout the life.

31. Antibody to Epstein–Barr nuclear antigen (EBNA) is not present in early infection but will persist thereafter for indefinite period. Hence, it can differentiate the primary infection from reactivation from the primary infection.

32. Aim of the vaccination against this infection:
    a. To protect adolescents and young adult, the debilitating consequences of infectious mononucleosis
    b. It will reduce the incidence of Epstein–Barr virus positive Hodgkin's lymphoma.
    c. To prevent nasopharyngeal carcinoma and Burkitt lymphoma in the high-risk population
    d. To prevent lymphoproliferative disease (LPD) in case of seronegative patient with XLPD
    e. To prevent LPD in patient who received transplants from seropositive donor subject

CASE 11

A 65-year-old man from Bihar came to clinic with high fever, malaise, weight loss, and anorexia. On examination, there is hepatosplenomegaly. Peripheral blood demonstrated polymorphonuclear leukocytosis and bone marrow demonstrated:

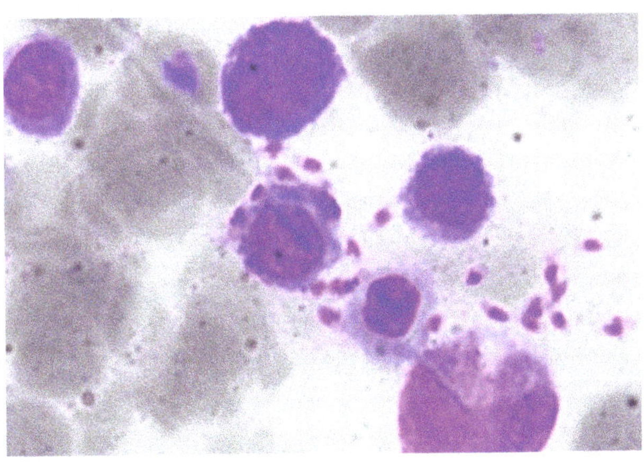
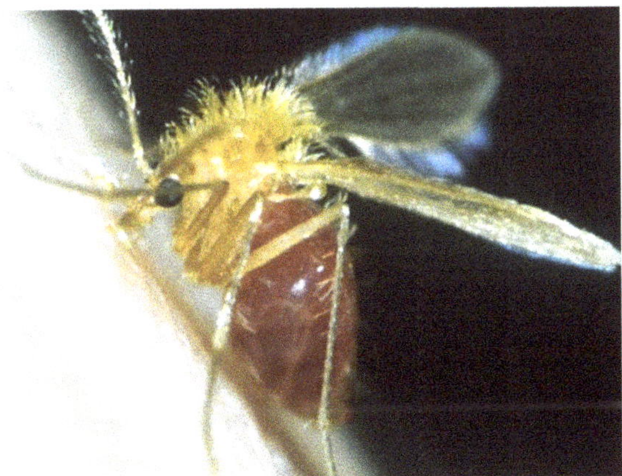

1. **What do the above pictures describe?**
2. **What is your diagnosis?**
3. **What are the forms of this organism?**
4. **What are the different types of spread of this organism in different diseases?**
5. **Name species of organisms producing cutaneous disease.**
6. **Name two species of this organism producing mucocutaneous disease.**
7. **Which form of this disease is produced through the relapse of infection?**
8. **Name five reservoirs of this disease.**

9. **Name the vectors for this disease and mention four natures of this vector.**
10. **How the organism propagates within the vector?**
11. **Provide schematic of the life cycle of this species in human being and the vector.**
12. **After entry into the skin how the organism will be lysed within the phagocytes?**
13. **After being activated what phagocytes will do?**
14. **What will be the activity of the organism to survive within the cells?**
15. **Which proinflammatory cytokines will increase the susceptibility to this infection and by which mechanism?**
16. **Write five characteristic features of the cutaneous form of this disease.**
17. **In case of strong immune response of the host, what types of skin lesions we can get?**
18. **Name four characteristic features of mucocutaneous form of this disease.**
19. **Why this disease is so named?**
20. **In case of cutaneous lesion, how the samples may be collected?**
21. **What is the rapid dipstick used to diagnose this disease?**
22. **Which antibody level will be increased in case of *Leishmania tropica*?**
23. **What is the treatment in this disease?**

Answers

1. The pictures demonstrate:
    a. *Leishmania donovani* body in the bone marrow
    b. Right hand picture demonstrates sand fly
2. The patient has been suffering from kala-azar or visceral leishmaniasis.
3. This organism has two forms:
    a. Intracellular form known as amastigote form
    b. Extracellular flagellated form known as promastigote form
4. Following are the different forms of spread:
    a. *Leishmania braziliensis* and *Leishmania panamensis*: There is cutaneous spread followed by involvement of mucous membrane of mouth and nose.
    b. *Leishmania donovani* and *Leishmania infantum* spread deeply to mononuclear phagocytic system present in the bone marrow, liver, and spleen.
5. Species of the organisms producing cutaneous disease are:
    a. Old World cutaneous leishmaniasis is caused by:
        - *Leishmania major*
        - *Leishmania aethiopica*
        - Dermotropic *L. infantum*
    b. New World cutaneous leishmaniasis is caused by:
        - *Leishmania mexicana* complex comprising of:
            - *L. mexicana*
            - *Leishmania amazonensis*
            - *Leishmania venezuelensis*
        - *L. braziliensis* complex comprising of:
            - *Leishmania guyanensis*
            - *L. panamensis*
            - *L. braziliensis*
            - *Leishmania peruviana*
6. Two species of organisms producing mucocutaneous disease are:
    a. *L. panamensis*
    b. *L. braziliensis*
7. Relapse of infection can be manifested as cutaneous disease known as post-kala-azar dermal leishmaniasis.
8. Following are the reservoirs of this disease:
    a. Rodents
    b. Gerbils
    c. Hyraxes
    d. Sloths
    e. Domestic dog
9. The vectors are:
    - Sand fly—the *Phlebotomus* species in the old World
    - Sand fly—the *Lutzomyia* species in the new World
    Four natures of the vectors are:
    a. They bite at dusk or at night
    b. The sandflies do not fly to greater height above the ground
    c. They bite the person lying close to the ground
    d. They carry the infection from the local population of drug

10. The organism propagates within the vector in the following ways:

> Sand fly bites the targeted host and takes the blood meal
>
> ↓
>
> Amastigotes that are ingested from the skin of the host will be changed into promastigote form
>
> ↓
>
> The promastigote form will pass into the midgut, proliferate
>
> ↓
>
> Leading to damage of the gastrointestinal tract
>
> ↓
>
> Then they will be regurgitated into the mouth parts i.e. Proboscis
>
> ↓
>
> Then it will be transported into the host skin during bite

11. In the human body:

> During taking the blood meal the sandfly will inject the promastigote into the human skin
>
> ↓
>
> Promastigotes are phagocytosed by the macrophages
>
> ↓
>
> There is transformation of promastigote to amastigote form in the macrophages
>
> ↓
>
> Amastigotes will proliferate in the various tissues including macrophages

In the vector:

> Sand fly bites the targeted host and takes the blood meal
>
> ↓
>
> Amastigotes that are ingested from the skin of the host will be changed into promastigote form
>
> ↓
>
> The promastigote form will pass into the midgut, proliferate
>
> ↓
>
> Leading to damage of the gastrointestinal tract
>
> ↓
>
> Then they will be regurgitated into the mouth parts i.e. proboscis
>
> ↓
>
> Then it will be transported into the host skin during bite

12. When the promastigote form will be ingested by the phagocytes known as phagosomes, this phagosomes will be fused with the lysozymes followed by the discharge of the contents of lysosome mainly lysozymes which ultimately lyse the susceptible pathogens.

13. After engulfment of the amastigotes, the phagocytes will be activated:
    a. To produce ROS as well as reactive nitrogen metabolites. The activated phagocytes also release tumor necrosis factor-alpha.
    b. By the Th1 helper cells through interferon-γ
    c. By the antigen presenting cells mainly by dendritic cells
    d. Secrete interleukin-12.

14. To survive this organism, the following conditions may occur:
    a. Surface membrane metalloproteinase lipophos-phoglycan, the molecule of Leishmania and activated C kinase receptor of leishmanial homolog will suppress the macrophage activation and ROS and nitrogen intermediates.
    b. Leishmanial lipophosphoglycan will inhibit the complement-induced opsonization and it also promotes to attract the neutrophils at the site of entry leading to release of proinflammatory cytokines.
    c. *Leishmania* resists:
        • Attack by lysozyme
        • Compromise the function of dendritic cells
    d. Activated C kinase receptor of leishmanial homolog induces Th2 response

15. Interleukin-10, 13, and tumor growth factor-β increase the susceptibility to infection with this organism.

16. Five characteristic features of the cutaneous form of this disease:
    a. This disease occurs in the exposed part of the disease as the sand fly bites in these areas.
    b. The lesion is found in the:
        • Legs
        • Face
        • Arms
    c. Lesion appears within 2–6 weeks
    d. The lesion starts as red papule which evolves into painless papulonodular lesion, which may be secondarily infected by the bacteria.
    e. In case of weakened response, there may be diffuse cutaneous leishmaniasis with high burden of parasites. Lesion may be multiple and popular lesions.

17. In case of strong immune response along with low parasite burden, the condition that produces *Leishmania recidivans*, as this response clears effectively the initial infection site.

18. Four characteristic features of mucocutaneous leishmaniasis are:
    a. Cutaneous lesion first appears which will self-heal but parasite will be present within the body.
    b. After several years of interval, there is reemergence of the parasites in the mucous membrane of the nose and mouth.
    c. The infection will progress backward toward larynx and pharynx.
    d. There may be secondary infection in the upper or lower respiratory tract.

19. In India dark skin the combination of anemia and hormonal effect of chronic infection makes the condition of the individual as graying complexion. Hence, the disease is so named as kala-azar.

20. In case of cutaneous lesion, the lesion should be squeezed. The nick should be given over the lesion to collect the tissue-fluid and impress over the glass K39 antigen as this stick will be impregnated with this antigen.

21. rK39 is the rapid dip stick used to diagnose this disease.

22. Serum level of anti-α-gal IgG will be increased in case *L. tropica* and *L. major* infection.

23. Treatment of the visceral leishmaniasis:
    a. Sodium stibogluconate 20 mg/kg of body weight intramuscularly or as intravenous infusion for 28–30 days.
    b. Amphotericin B deoxycholate—15 intravenous infusion at a dose of 0.75–1 mg/kg of body weight daily or alternate day in the region of antimony refractory.
    c. If there is amphotericin B-related adverse reaction, liposomal amphotericin B can be used at a dose of 10–15 mg/kg of body weight single administration to prevent organ toxicity with cure rate of 95%.
    d. Miltefosine 50 mg twice daily orally in adult having weight of ≥25 kg and 25 mg for <25 kg for 28 days. It cannot be used in case of pregnancy because of its teratogenic effect.
    e. Paromomycin, an aminoglycoside, a highly effective drug should be used at a dose of 15 mg/kg of body weight for 21 days.
    f. Multidrug regimen consisting of liposomal amphotericin B 5 mg/kg single dose followed by orally miltefosine for 7 days or paromomycin for 10 days with a cure rate of 97%.

CASE 12

A 45-year-old male came to gastroenterology clinic with history of upper abdominal pain, nausea, and lethargy which was relieved by taking food and antacids. He has family history of stomach cancer. Endoscopy was performed along with biopsy of the stomach tissue in hematoxylin demonstrated:

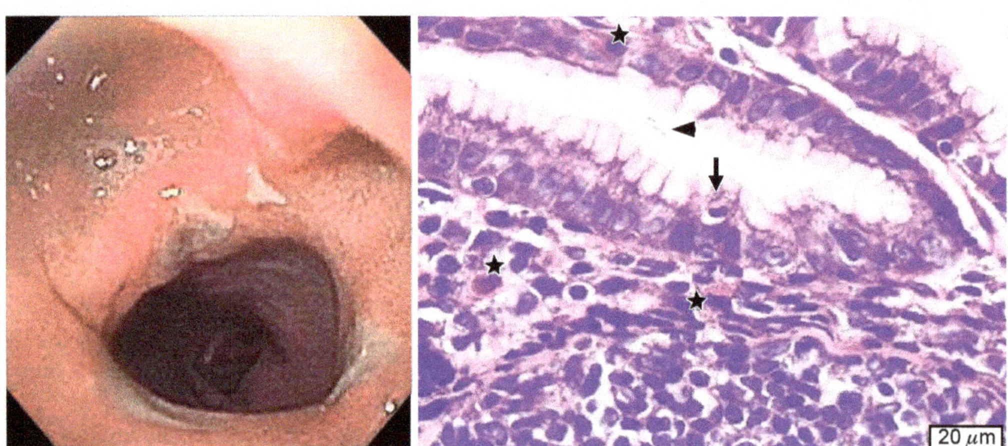

1. **What has been shown in the above pictures?**
2. **What is your diagnosis?**
3. **What is "pathogenic island"?**
4. **What is the importance of "pathogenic islands" in this organism?**
5. **Why this organism is called microaerobic?**

6. **Which specific enzyme is present in this organism and what is its importance?**
7. **Which specific species of this organism is responsible for producing gastroenteritis in human being?**
8. **What are the routes of entry of this organism into human body?**
9. **What factors are responsible for the penetration of this organism into the mucus layer of stomach?**
10. **What are the adhesins present on the surface of the organism?**
11. **Which factor in the host is triggered against this organism and what is its effect?**
12. **What are the differences in the infection rate between industrialized and nonindustrialized countries and why?**
13. **What are the functions of gastric epithelial cells against this organism?**
14. **How dendritic cells become activated in the gastric mucosa and what is its function?**
15. **What are the mechanisms of evasion of the immune system of the organism in the human body?**
16. **What are the effects of colonization of this organism in the stomach mucosa?**
17. **What is the function of vacuolating cytotoxin in the gastric mucosa?**
18. **What are the functions CagA of this organism in the gastric epithelial cells?**
19. **On what factor duodenal or gatric mucosal invasion depends?**
20. **What are the risk factors for gastric carcinogenesis in this case?**
21. **What is the cause of ITP in case of infection with this organism?**
22. **What is "hit-and-run" model in this infection?**
23. **What are the extragastrointestinal manifestations due to this organism?**
24. **What are the conditions that will be protected by this organism?**
25. **What are the serious consequences of this organism?**
26. **What is the recent development in the molecular diagnostics for identifying this organism?**
27. **Which biomarker is very common with gastric cancer in this organism?**
28. **In the primary care setting, what are the important noninvasive tests for detection of this organism?**
29. **What are the sequential therapies for killing of this organism?**
30. **What are the approaches being assessed in this treatment?**
31. **What are the barriers in the development of vaccine against this organism?**

Answers

1. The pictures above demonstrate:
   a. There are evidence of ulcers in the pyloric channel at 4 and 11 o'clock position.
   b. Right hand picture demonstretes evidence of *Helicobacter pylori* in the biopsy taken from gastric mucosa.

2. This has been suffering from *Helicobacter*-induced pyloric channel ulcer.

3. *Helicobacter pylori* is highly polymorphic. The genome of this organism has five regions that may be acquired from the other organism by lateral transfer of DNA. These are known as "pathogenic islands" carrying virulent genes.

4. *Helicobacter pylori* contains Cag pathogenicity island (Cag-PAI) containing 30 genes responsible for production of type IV secretion system and it is used for transferring Cag protein as well as other bacterial factors into the host cells.

5. As this organism grows in the atmosphere of 5–15% oxygen, 5–12% carbon dioxide, and 70–90% nitrogen, hence this organism is called microaerobic organism and it will take 5 days to grow in the horse blood agar.

6. This organism contains urease both on the surface as well as in the cytoplasm and regulates pH and can survive in the acid environment transiently though it is not acidophilic.

7. *Helicobacter cinaedi* is responsible for gastroenteritis in human being.

8. Following are the routes of entry of this organism into the human body:
   a. Fecal-oral route through the sweage contamination of the water supplies.
   b. Oral-oral route

9. After the entry of the organism into the stomach, it survives the acid environment for short period because it will be killed by the acid. But, the urease enzyme present on the surface of the bacteria will resist by hydrolyzing urea and producing ammonium,

thereby provide sufficient time to penetrate mucous layer of the stomach mucosa.

10. Following adhesins present on the surface of the organism:
    a. Sialic acid-binding adhesin
    b. Oip adhesin
    c. Blood group-binding adhesin:
        - It is the principal adhesin which binds to the Lewis blood group antigen present on the gastric epithelial cells.
        - It will anchor the bacterial secretion system with the host cell surface to inject efficiently the bacterial factors in the the cytoplasm of the gastric epithelial cells.

11. When blood group-binding adhesin is attached with the gastric epithelial cells, it will trigger TSS system host cell to induce transcription of the gees thereby enhancing the inflammation which ultimately develops intestinal metaplasia may be associated with precancerous transformation.

12. In the industrialized countries such as Western Europe and North America, the incidence of this disease is 5–10% in the first decade which will be increased to 60% in the sixth decade. It may be due to:
    a. Improved social standards of housing
    b. Portable water supply
    c. Sweage disposal
    d. Cohort effect

    In the nonindustrialized countries such as Africa, South America, and Middle East, the incidence in the first decade will be 60–70% with little increase with age.

13. When these bacteria penetrate the gastric epithelial cells:
    a. Epithelial cells express toll-like receptor 2 (TLR2) and TLR4 which interact with the microbial-associated molecular pattern present on the bacteria to produce defensins and other antimicrobial peptides.
    b. Many interleukins including interleukin-8 as well as chemokines produced by the gastric epithelial cells recruit monocytes, neutrophils as well as macrophages into the submucosa to induce the inflammatory response.
    c. Various pattern recognition receptors including toll-like receptors present in the epithelial cells induced by various microbial products produce proinflammatory cytokines leading to further amplification of the acute inflammatory response.

14. Dendritic cells after being activated through the pattern recognition receptors of the *H. pylori*:
    a. Upregulate their CD86

    b. Increase the expression major histocompatibility complex class II molecule
    c. Release proinflammatory cytokine-like interleukin-12
    d. Carry processed antigen from the *H. pylori* to local draining lymph nodes to produce IgA and IgG antibodies

15. Following are the mechanisms of evasion of the immune system by *H. pylori*:
    a. Evasion of the recognition by toll-like receptors, RIG-like receptors, and C lectin-like receptor
    b. Lipopolysaccharides of low immunogenicity
    c. CagA and other protein material transferred by type IV recognition system which:
        - Suppresses phagocytosis
        - Decreases production of antimicrobial peptides through gastric epithelial cells
        - Induces teratogenic dendritic cells thereby suppressing the T cells and blocking the effector T cells
    d. Vacuolating toxin A:
        - It will suppress phagocytosis.
        - Induces teratogenic dendritic cells and blocking T cell effector response
    e. γ-glutamyl transpeptidase: It induces teratogenic dendritic cells and blocking T cell effector response.
    f. Cholesterol-α-glucosyltransferase: It will suppress the phagocytosis.
    g. Catalase superoxide dismutase: It will suppress the production of nitric oxide and ROS.
    h. Arginase:
        - It will suppress the production of nitric oxide and ROS.
        - It will block the effector T-cell response.

16. Colonization of *H. pylori* in the gastric mucosa will lead to:
    a. Increased production of acid in the stomach mucosa
    b. Hypergastrinemia
    c. Hyperpepsinogenemia

    All the above will lead to gastric atrophy. Acid secreting mucosa will be destroyed will lead to hypoacidity and ultimately gastric cancer.

17. Vacuolating toxin, a multimeric pore-forming protein has several effects:
    a. Disrupts mitochondria thereby promoting phagocytosis
    b. It affects autophagy
    c. It will disrupt the tight junction between the cells.

d.   It blocks the T cell proliferation

e.   It will disrupt the acid production by oxyntic cells.

18.   CagA, a phospholipid at tyrosine residue will be activated thereby activates SHP-2 as well as Csk.

  a.   Activation of SHP will change the shape of the cells to hummingbird phenotype.

  b.   Activated Csk will activate Src tyrosine kinase forming Csk-CagA protein complexes which in turn produce negative feedback on the further activation of CagA.

  c.   CagA-SHP complex leads to apoptosis of the infected cells

  Nonphosphorylated CagA will interact with PAR1, which regulates polarity of the cells and tight junction followed by induction of the scarring cells.

  The net effect is complex array of cellular alteration that leads to stem cells of the epithelial cells into gastric carcinogenesis.

19.   Gastric and duodenal ulcer depends upon interaction between the host and polymorphism of the organism.

  a.   In case of route of duodenal ulcer, high acid and low cancer risk

  b.   In case of gastric ulcer route, low acid, pangastritis, and high cancer risk

20.   Risk factors for gastric carcinogenesis are the following:

  a.   Atrophic mucosa of the stomach

  b.   Decreased consumption of dietary antioxidant

  c.   Increased consumption of salt

21.   Idiopathic thrombocytopenic purpura: It is an extragastric effect due to presence of autoantibodies.

22.   In the "hit-and-run" model even after removal of *H. pylori* infection, the process of carcinogenesis will be continued and is unstoppable.

23.   Following are the extragastrointestinal manifestations due to *H. pylori*:

  a.   Coronary artery disease

  b.   Migraine

  c.   Stroke

  d.   Rosaceae

  e.   Behçet's disease

  f.   Gallbladder disease

  g.   Idiopathic thrombocytopenic purpura

  h.   Iron-deficiency anemia

  i.   Vitamin B12 deficiency

24.   *Helicobacter pylori* is protective for:

  a.   Reflux esophagitis

  b.   Barrett's esophagus

  c.   Esophageal cancer

  d.   Gastroesophageal reflux-induced asthma

25.   Most serious consequences of this infection are development of:

  a.   Gastric adenocarcinoma but not cancer originating from cardia or gastroesophageal junction

  b.   Mucosal-associated lymphoid tissue lymphoma

26.   Recent development of molecular diagnostics is the detection of miRNA found in the body tissue or fluid which involved in the regulatory systems, whose deregulation will lead to development of a panel of biomarkers like mir-223 which can identify either gastric cancer of *H. pylori.*

27.   The biomarker mir-223 is very common with gastric cancer.

28.   In the primary care setting, following noninvasive tests are done to detect this organism:

  a.   Stool antigen test by using either monoclonal or polyclonal antibodies

  b.   Urea breath test

29.   Sequential therapies are proton pump inhibitor and amoxicillin for 10 days followed by addition of clarithromycin or metronidazole for additional 7 days.

30.   Additional approaches being assessed in this treatment are as follows:

  a.   Addition of the prebiotics with the antibiotic regimen

  b.   Administration of antibiotic cocktail directly to the stomach mucosa during endoscopy

  c.   Plant-derived phytochemicals:

  •   Antibiofilm medication derived from the *Acorus calamus*

  •   Inflammatory 7,8-dihydroxycoumarin from the Changbai daphne

31.   Following are the barriers to the development of the vaccine:

  a.   Ability of the organism to avoid the response of the host with no obvious protein, inhibition of this may erradicate the organism.

  b.   Extensive polymorphism of *H. pylori*

  c.   Variation of the genomic sequence of *H. pylori*

CASE 13

A 55-year-old woman having history of rheumatoid arthritis on weekly methotrexate, steroid, and monthly infliximab came to respiratory clinic with respiratory distress, cough with scanty expectoration, high resolution CT scan demonstrated reticulonodular infiltrate. Bronchoalveolar lavage dmonstrated as below. Her urine is also positive for that organism.

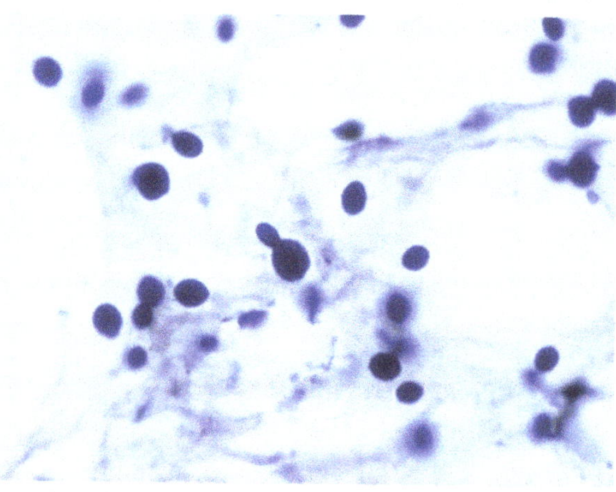

1. What has been described in the above pictures?
2. What is your diagnosis?
3. What is the other name of this disease and why it is so named?
4. What are the types of variant of this organism? Name them along with the disease they are responsible for.
5. In what forms they survive the temperature in the environment and for this survival what are they called?
6. Why birds are resistant to the organism and in that case how they carry organism?
7. Where the organism can grow?
8. At what temperature they grow in what form in media?
9. What is the growing pattern in the media at different temperatures?
10. How they can enter the body and which cell they will encounter?
11. How the organism spreads throughout the body?
12. What is the factor in this organism leads to how many clades of this?
13. In which places of this world the clades of this organism are distributed?
14. In which cell the organism replicates?
15. How the organism can resist their destruction in the cells?
16. How the organism enhances its growth intracellularly?
17. How the macrophage responds to ingested organism?
18. After lysis of the macrophage, what is the activity of the intracellular organism?
19. In the macrophage, how the intracellular growth of the organism will be inhibited?
20. What is the role of fraction of IgG on the organism?
21. Which type of immunodeficiency is associated with dissemination of this disease?
22. How T cells provide protective immunity against this organism?
23. In the acute phase of response, what will occur against this organism?
24. If there is deficiency of tumor necrosis factor-α, what will be the result of immunity against this infection?
25. What is the function of granuloma in this disease?
26. What happens in case of X-linked hyperimmunoglobulin M immunodeficiency?
27. What are the rheumatologic manifestations in this disease?
28. Why pericarditis occurs due to this infection?
29. What are the effects of compression by enlarged lymph nodes in the body?

30. **What is the effect of enlarged mediastinal lymph nodes in the thoracic cavity in acute pulmonary infection in this infection?**
31. **In chronic case, what are the other diseases involved with this infection?**
32. **What is the solitary pulmonary nodule in this case?**
33. **In case of progressive disseminated infection, what other organs are involved in acute condition?**
34. **In subacute form of progressive dissemination, what are the extrapulmonary organs involved?**
35. **What are the sites of ulcer in chronic disseminated form of this disease?**
36. **What are the susceptible persons develop progressive disseminated form of disease?**
37. **What is the typical eye involvement in this disease?**
38. **What are the specimens which should be obtained for analysis in this infection?**
39. **What is the importance of M and H bands in the serological tests for this organism?**
40. **Which is the most powerful tool for the diagnosis of disseminated form of this disease?**
41. **What types of PCR can be done in this infection using what primary sets?**
42. **How can you manage chronic progressive form of this disease?**
43. **What are the surgeries required in this disease?**
44. **How can you prevent this disease?**

Answers

1. The above picture demonstrates evidence of budding in the macrophage in the slide stained by Gomori–Grocott stain.
2. This patient has been suffering from pulmonary histoplasmosis in a patient of rheumatoid arthritis on immunosuppressive therapy.
3. The other name of this disease is Darling's disease under the name of Samuel Darling, a pathologist.
4. There are three varieties of histoplasmosis:
    a. *Histoplasma capsulatum* var. capsulatum—common histoplasmosis
    b. *Histoplasma capsulatum* var. duboisii—African histoplasmosis
    c. *Histoplasma capsulatum* var. farciminosum—produces lymphangitis
5. Histoplasma is thermally dimorphic ascomycete because they survive in different temperature:
    a. At temperature below 30°C, it will be present in mycelial saprophytic mold form.
    b. In the mammalian body at 37°C, it is present as parasitic yeast form.
6. Birds are not infected by this organism because of their high body temperature of 40°C, in that case they carry the organism in their feathers.
7. This organism is found in:
    a. Bird droppings
    b. Excreta of bats
    c. Chicken droppings
    d. Starling droppings
    e. Poultry house litter
    f. Caves
    g. The areas harboring bats
    h. Bird roosts
8. At 25°C, this organism can grow in Sabouraud dextrose agar or in brain-heart infusion agar which will be supplemented by 5–10% sheep blood.
9. At 25°C, this organism demonstrates as suede-like cotton granular colonies—color being white initially followed by brown to pale yellow-brown or yellow-orange reverse.

    At 37°C, it will demonstrate round to oval budding yeast which is in the form of creamy smooth moist, white colonies.
10. This organism will enter through inhalation of the aerosol into the bronchioles and alveolar spaces and encounter with the phagocytes.
11. In the lung, the microconidia bind to $\beta(1,3)$-glucans, integrins CD11/CD18 through the complement receptor 3 and pattern recognition receptor Dectin-1. They spread to the draining lymphatics and blood stream through the pulmonary macrophages and reaches many organs such as liver, spleen, and regional lymph nodes containing mononuclear phagocytes.
12. Based on the 5–7 chromosomes in this organism, 8 clades have been founded which are distributed throughout the World.
13. Distribution of the clades in different parts of the World:
    a. Two are North American clades
    b. Two are South American clades
    c. One Australian clade

d. One Indonesian clade
e. One African clade
f. One Eurasian clade

14. After ingestion, the organism resides and replicates in the phagocytes every 15–18 hours.

15. The organism can reduce their intracellular killing by inhibiting the fusion of the phagosomes and thereby preventing exposure to hydrolytic enzymes in the lysosome.

16. At pH 6.5, the fungus will enhance its growth due to availability of the iron as it is required for its growth.

17. Macrophage of the human being responds to intracellular organism by oxidative burst which is mediated by:
    a. NADPH oxidase
    b. Release of nitric oxide
    c. Nitrogen intermediates

18. After lysis of the macrophages, the organisms are released and again ingested by the other newly recruited macrophages and neutrophils at the site of infection. In the immunocompromised subject, these cycles are repeated several times.

19. Intracellular growth of the organism will be inhibited by:
    a. Interleukin-3
    b. Granulocyte-macrophage colony-stimulating factor inhibits via production of zinc-sequestering metallothioneins.
    c. Macrophage colony-stimulating factor

20. Fraction of the IgG in infected patient containing complement fixing antibodies and precipitating antibodies are associated with progressive disease paradoxically.

21. There is susceptibility of this disease in associated with T cell immunodeficiency.

22. By following methods T cells provide protective immunity against this organism:
    a. Specific T cells through the production of cytokines which will activate the phagocytes along with tumor necrosis factor-α and interferon-γ
    b. Invariant natural killer cells also produce interferon-γ and interleukin-12.

23. In acute phase of infection following events will occur:
    a. Interleukin-12, tumor necrosis factor-α and interferon-γ will be released which will help in the influx of the white blood cells along with T and B cells into the lungs.
    b. Granulocyte-macrophage-colony stimulating factor produces interferon-γ, tumor necrosis factor-α, and nitric oxide which will downregulate Th2 cytokines, interleukin-4, and 12.

24. Deficiency of tumor necrosis factor-α will lead to dramatic elevation of interleukin-10 and 4 in the lungs thereby increased dissemination of the infection.

25. Long-lasting infection resulting for weeks or months from the inflammatory response leads to formation of fibrinous granulomatous lesion containing caseous necrosis at the center which will later on become calcified. It may recur from impaired cell-mediated immunity. The function of this granuloma is to restrict fungal growth.

26. The formation of the granuloma requires the generation of tumor necrosis factor-α, interleukin-17, and 4, in absence of any one of the above will lead to depressed cell-mediated immunity resulting in dissemination of this disease. In case of X-linked hyperimmunoglobulin M immunodeficiency, there is deficiency of interleukin-17 resulting in development of disseminated histoplasmosis.

27. Rheumatologic manifestations in this disease are as follows:
    a. Arthritis
    b. Erythema multiforme
    c. Erythema nodosum

28. Pericarditis may occur in this disease due to following factors:
    a. Granulomatous inflammatory response in the mediastinal lymph nodes which is adjacent to pericardium
    b. Granulomatous infection within the pericardium due to Histoplasma capsulatum infection

29. Compression of the hilar and mediastinal lymph nodes produces following features:
    a. Superior vena cava syndrome due to compression of the superior vena cava
    b. Obstruction of the venous drainage in the brain leading to:
       • Tinnitus
       • Headache
       • Visual disturbances
       • Alteration of the consciousness
    c. Compression of the pulmonary circulation and airway leads to:
       • Cough
       • Hemoptysis
       • Chest pain
    d. Compression of the esophagus will lead to dysphagia

30. In case of acute pulmonary histoplasmosis, enlarged mediastinal lymph nodes will lead to:
    a. Retraction of the airways
    b. Postobstructive pneumonia as well as bronchiectasis

31. Chronic pulmonary histoplasmosis coexists with the following diseases:
    a. Sarcoidosis
    b. Pulmonary tuberculosis
    c. Actinomycosis
    d. Other mycosis
32. In case of chronic fungal infection, there is development of a solitary pulmonary nodule with a rim of calcification that can be visualized in the chest X-ray. Fungus in this nodule is calcified. If the nodule is old, it will contain central caseation looking like tuberculosis which will be occupied by the fungi.
33. In case of acute progressive disseminated histoplasmosis, following organs are involved:
    a. Central nervous system:
       - Meningitis
       - Cerebritis
    b. Hematopoietic system:
       - Anemia
       - Leukopenia
       - Thrombocytopenia
    c. Liver
    d. Spleen
    e. Eye: Uveitis
    f. Bone marrow
    g. Adrenal glands
    h. Skin:
       - Papular rash
       - Nodular rash
    i. Genitourinary tract
    j. Adrenal gland
34. In the subacute form of progressive dissemination, following organs are involved:
    a. Gastrointestinal tract—diarrhea and abdominal pain
    b. Cardiac involvement—valvular disease, cardiac insufficiency, pericarditis, and pleural effusion
    c. Central nervous system involvement—headache, visual disturbance, gait disturbances, confusion, and seizures
    d. Mouth and gum pain
35. Following are the sites of ulcers in chronic disseminated form of the disease:
    a. Oropharyngeal mucosa
    b. Buccal mucosa
    c. Gingiva
    d. Tongue
    e. Larynx
36. Following are the susceptible persons for progressive disseminated histoplasmosis:
    a. Children of <3 years
    b. Elderly
    c. People exposed to large inoculum
37. Following are the types of eye involvement in this disease:
    a. Retinal damage leading to development of scar resulting in leakage from the retina and loss of vision
    b. Histo spot characterized by atrophic scar along with infiltration of the lymphocytic cells present in the posterior to the equator of the eye, it is bilateral.
    c. Retinal hemorrhage
    d. Macular scarring
38. Following specimens are obtained from this patient for analysis:
    a. Blood
    b. Sputum
    c. Bronchial lavage
    d. Cerebrospinal fluid in case of suspected central nervous system involvement
    e. Tissue biopsy from lung tissue, lymph nodes through bronchoscopy or thoracoscopy
39. Complement fixing antibodies with antigen extract of mycelial form of Histoplasma capsulatum, known as histoplasmin to detect the presence of M and H precipitin bands.
    a. If the titer of complement fixing antibodies to both yeast as well as mycelial form is >1:8, then it is considered as positive.
    b. If the titer is >1:32, it suggests acute histoplasmosis.
    c. If the antibody is against Y antigen, it suggests primary infection.
    d. If the antibody is against M antigen, it suggests late infection. If this band appears in acute infection, it will persist for months to years and also in chronic form.
    e. H band usually appears after M band and disappears early
    f. Presence of both M and H band suggests active histoplasmosis
40. Detection of capsular antigen of Histoplasma capsulatum in the urine is a very powerful tool for the diagnosis of disseminated histoplasmosis.
41. Nested PCR should be done with multiple primer sets:
    a. Histoplasma capsulatum rDNA and 100 kDa like protein which is unique to Histoplasma.
    b. N-acetylated α-linked acidic dipeptidase and internal transcribed spacer antigen

42. Management of chronic progressive histoplasmosis:
    a. For asymptomatic patient, no treatment is required.
    b. In case of mild interstitial pneumonitis with or without thin-walled cavities, serial chest X-ray monitoring at an interval of 2–4 months
    c. In case of persistent symptoms or presence of thick-walled cavities, medical treatment should be started.
43. Following surgeries may be required in this disease:
    a. Resection of the thick-walled cavities in the lung
    b. Repair of the infected heart valves
    c. Repair of the aneurysm
44. a. Avoid exposure to endemic areas and bird dropping of bat, pigeon, calves and contaminated soil.
    b. Use of N95 mask to reduce the above exposure.
    c. Before starting immunosuppressive therapies screening of potential exposure to this organism by taking proper travel history to endemic areas, baseline serological and antigen testing for this organism.
    d. Use of minimum effective dose of the steroids or other immunosuppressive therapies.
    e. Antifungal prophylaxis prior to TNF inhibitors or high dose of corticosteroids.

CASE 14

A 35-year-old man came to medical clinic with alternate day spiky rise in the temperature for 6 days that was relieved with sweating each time. Physical examination demonstrated tachycardia, tachypnea, and high temperature, and there was just hepatosplenomegaly.

Blood slide in thin film stained by hematoxylin and eosin demonstrated:

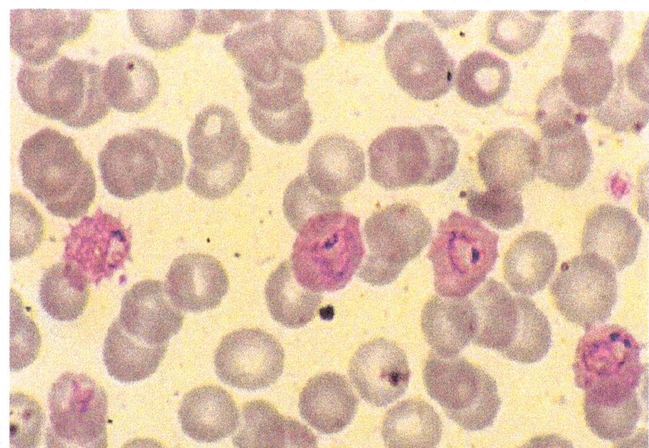

1. **Describe the above picture.**
2. **What is your diagnosis?**
3. **What are the species of this organism that will infect the human being?**
4. **Which species is most virulent and which species is most dominant?**
5. **How this organism enters the human body in which form and by whom?**
6. **What are the types of spread of this organism from the site of entry?**
7. **In the liver, how this form of organism cross the sinusoidal cells to enter the hepatocytes?**
8. **In the liver stage of infection when the cell ruptures?**
9. **What is a special stage occurring in the liver and by whom?**
10. **What factors help in successful migration of this organism into the hepatocytes?**
11. **In the erythrocyte, what are the steps of invasion by this organism and in which stage?**
12. **If all the steps of invasion will be passed, what will be the process of entry into the cell and what will be formed in the erythrocyte?**
13. **How the most common species of this parasite invades erythrocyte?**
14. **After rupture of each erythrocyte, how many number of daughter parasites are released at the end of asexual reproduction?**
15. **During taking the blood meal, mosquito will take what types of erythrocyte for spreading the disease?**
16. **What are the stages of development of this parasite in the mosquito?**

17. **What are the mode of spread of this disease other than mosquito?**
18. **What are the six countries in the World accounted for half of the all malarial death?**
19. **What are the proposed mechanisms to explain the resistance to the disease?**
20. **Why in COVID-19 pandemic there was increased incidence of the disease?**
21. **If any child is attacked with this disease, what will be the future fate of that child?**
22. **What are the mechanisms responsible for immunity in the liver stage?**
23. **What are the mechanisms of immunity in the erythrocytic stage?**
24. **What are the escape mechanisms of the parasite in the liver stage?**
25. **What are the escape mechanisms of the parasite in the erythrocytic phase?**
26. **Mention the pathogenic mechanisms responsible for the clinical features of this disease.**
27. **What is the cause of cyclical temperature elevation in this disease?**
28. **What are the complications in this disease?**
29. **What are the different morphologies of these parasites under the microscope?**
30. **Mention the treatment of this disease both uncomplicated and complicated form.**
31. **What is the mechanism of infection of recently approved artemisinin-based combination therapy?**
32. **Name the companion drugs for artemisinin derivatives.**
33. **What are the drugs for radical cure of this disease?**
34. **What are the approved insecticides for next treatment?**
35. **How can you control the larval stage of the mosquito?**
36. **What are the proposed vaccine strategies against this parasite?**

Answers

1. The above picture demonstrates presence of multiple ring stage of the parasites within one red blood cells and the cells are larger than the other cells—it indicates the *Plasmodium vivax* infection.

2. The patient has been suffering from benign tertian malaria.

3. Five species of *plasmodium* are infect the human being:
   a. *Plasmodium falciparum*
   b. *Plasmodium vivax*
   c. *Plasmodium ovale*
   d. *Plasmodium malariae*
   e. *Plasmodium knowlesi*

4. *Plasmodium falciparum* is the most common parasite and *P. vivax* is the most common parasite.

5. *Plasmodium* parasite in the sporozoite form will enter the blood stream of the human being by Anopheles mosquito while taking the blood meal.

6. After entry of the organism into the human being, some will be present in the dermis for some time, some will enter into the blood stream following crossing the vascular endothelial cell into the blood stream and some will enter into the draining lymph nodes.

7. In the liver, surface circumsporozoite protein on the surface of the sporozoite reacts with the highly sulfated heparan sulfate proteoglycans present on the sinusoids to enter the hepatic sinusoids.

8. The parasite after entering the hepatocyte crosses the several hepatocytes to switch into replicative form. To avoid the lysosomal enzymes, they will be present in the parasitophorous vacuole and increase in their number to form asexual stage called schizonts with 2 weeks and ultimately release into the blood stream in the form of merozoites through the rupture of the liver cells.

9. In the liver cell, the *P. vivax* and *P. ovale* produce a resting stage called hypnozoites because some sporozoites do not develop into the schizonts immediately but remain in the uninucleate stage hypnozoites.

10. Small vacuole in the sporozoites releases special substance in a coordinated way to help in the migration and invasion into the hepatocytes and formation of merozoites.

11. In the erythrocyte stage, the merozoites will invade the erythrocytes in multiple steps:
    a. Binding of merozoites
    b. Reorientation
    c. Discharge of secretory organelles known as rhoptries and micronemes
    d. Formation of an electron-dense tight junction between apical end of merozoites and membrane of erythrocytes.

12. If all the steps are passed successfully, then there is actinomycin-powered entry of the parasite into the erythrocytes followed by formation of membrane

bound parasitophorous vacuole and revealing of the membrane of the erythrocytes. The parasite will enter the erythrocyte through the attachment of membrane surface protein anchored by glycophosphatidylinositol (GPI) along with few erythrocyte binding ligands. In the erythrocyte ring form of parasite will be formed.

13. Most common form *P. vivax* attaches with reticulocytes through the reticular-binding protein but cannot attach with the matured erythrocytes. This parasite is able to attach with the Duffy blood group antigen on the erythrocytes through the Duffy-binding protein present on the surface of the erythrocytes.

14. In the erythrocyte at the end of asexual reproduction schizonts are formed and lastly the erythrocytes rupture releasing 16 to 23 merozoites in the blood.

15. During taking blood meal, the mosquito will take male and female gametocytes containing erythrocytes that will be in sexual development phase in this vector.

16. Within the gut of the mosquito:
    a. Exflagellated microgametocyte will fuge with the macrogametocyte to form zygote.
    b. The zygote becomes ookinete which after invading the intestinal wall form oocyte.
    c. These oocyte develop into thousands of sporozoites
    d. These sporozoites will reach the salivary gland of the mosquito.

17. There are the two types of spread:
    a. Person to person spread: Through the bite of female mosquito sporozoites are injected into the the blood.
    b. Nonmosquito spread:
       • Blood transfusion
       • Sharing of the hypodermic needles
       • Accidental pricking of the needles
       • From mother to fetus

18. Six countries are accounted for the half of the malarial death in the World:
    a. Nigeria
    b. Democratic Republic of Congo
    c. United Republic of Tanzania
    d. Burkina Faso
    e. Mozambique
    f. Niger

19. Following are the proposed mechanisms for explaining the resistance to malaria:
    a. Sickling of the infected cells
    b. Increased splenic phagocytes
    c. Premature hemolysis and death of the parasites

    d. Impaired digestion of the hemoglobin
    e. Weakened cytoadherence
    f. Acquired immunity of the host
    g. Translocation of the hemoglobin S-specific growth of the parasite inhibiting microRNAs
    h. Induction of heme oxygenase 1
    i. Glucose-6-phosphate dehydrogenase deficiency
    j. Polymorphisms in the Fc receptor γ gene

20. During COVID-19 pandemic, there was >20% rise in the morbidity and >50% increase in mortality in malaria due to:
    a. Reduction of routine malaria control measure
    b. Increased malnutrition
    c. Poverty
    d. Social instability

21. If the child faces early attack, he becomes resistant to the severe disease about the age of 5 years and after that age the level of parasitemia decreases progressively until the adulthood when its level becomes negligible.

    Maternal IgG antibodies against the blood stage of parasite are transferred into the fetus through the placenta thereby limiting the evel of parasitemia thus limiting the severity of the disease.

    Again, in absence of antigenic stimulation in a year, the immunity will be lost gradually because this stimulation is required for maintaining the level of immunity.

22. Following mechanisms are responsible for the immunity in the liver stage of the parasite:
    a. During entry into the blood stream and lymph nodes, sporozoites should be blocked by the species-specific antibodies.
    b. Antibodies to surface circumsporozoite protein and sporozoite prevent blocking of the binding of the parasites to the hepatocytes.
    c. Activates complement factor by the antibodies
       • Activates complement
       • Activates phagocytosis
       • Activates natural killer cells induced lysis through the Fc receptors
       • Recognizes neoantigens on the parasites that is present on the surface of the hepatocytes and kills the parasites by Kupffer cells and natural killer cells through the cell-mediated mechanism.
    d. In the clinically silent liver stage, since the parasites grow within the hepatocytes unnoticely, the DNA of the parasites stimulates the pattern recognition receptors seen on the surface of

the hepatocytes will be activated leading to interferon-γ production resulting the recruitment of:
- Macrophages
- Neutrophils
- Lymphocytes

    e.   Intrahepatic parasites kill cytotoxic CD8+ T cells through the interferon-γ production

    f.   Natural killer cells, natural killer T cells, and γδ T cells are also kill the parasites through the interfern-γ and types 1 interferon.

23. Following mechanisms are responsible for the immunity in the liver stage of the parasite:
    a. In the blood stream, the antibodies target merozoites at the site of attachment on the erythrocytes thereby preventing the entry of parasites.
    b. GPI, a major microbe-associated molecular pattern, toll-like receptor-2 present on the macrophage induces proinflammatory cytokines like interleukin-1 and tumor necrosis factor-α.
    c. In the erythrocyte, antiparasite antibodies mediate destruction of infected erythrocyte by:
       - Cellular killing
       - Block adhesion
       - Neutralize the toxin of parasite

    It will reduce the induction of excessive inflammation.
    d. Complement also will lyse the infected red blood cells.
    e. CD4+ T cells kill the infected erythrocyte by activated macrophages
    f. Natural killer cells can kill the plasmodium-infected erythrocytes by inducing proinflammatory cytokines like interferon-γ, perforins, and granzymes.
    g. Antibodies also kill the male and female gametocytes in the blood stream
    h. FcRY present on the many immune cells can kill the infected erythrocytes by antibody-mediated destruction.

24. Following are the escape mechanisms of the parasites to avoid immune response against the parasite in the liver stage:
    a. During inasion of the hepatocytes, surface circumsporozoite protein of erythrocytes binds to Kupffer cells of sinusoids leads to formation of high level of cAMP at the intracellular level therby ROS formation will be prevented.
    b. Downregulation of inflammatory Th1 cytokines and upregulation of anti-inflammatory Th2 cytokines when the sporozoites will come in contact with Kupffer cells.
    c. There is induction of Kupffer cell apoptosis along with reduction of expression of major histocompatibility complex-1.
    d. In the hepatocytes, parasitophorous vacuole prevents degradation of the parasite
    e. Heme oxygenase 1 of the host through the modulation of the host inflammatory response will enhance the development of intrahepatic parasites.

25. Following are the escape mechanisms of the parasites to avoid immune response against the parasite in the erythrocytic phase:
    a. Intracellular parasites will prevent direct interaction with the immune cells.
    b. Absence of major histocompatibility complex-1 molecule on the erythrocyte will avoid recognition by CD8+ T cells.
    c. Evasion of the host immune response can be helped by the expression of variable antigenic surface protein present on the infected erythrocytes
    d. Pigment, hemozoin of the *P. falciparum*, hinders phagocytic function of the activated macrophages
    e. Hemozoin pigment also reduces the production of the radical oxygen intermediates

26. Following are the pathogenic mechanisms for the clinical features of this disease:
    a. Mononuclear phagocytic system induces the release of proinflammatory cytokines from the host cells such as tumor necrosis factor-α, interleukin-1 as well as endogenous pyrogens.
    b. Release of toxins like hemozoin pigment following rupture of infected erythrocytes is responsible for the cyclical fever.
    c. Anemia develops as a result of:
       - Release of toxins like hemozoin pigment and defective production of erythrocytes
       - Antibody-mediated destruction of the infected erythrocytes due presence of antigen on the surface of the erythrocytes
    d. Less deformable red blood cells due to modification of the red blood cell membrane are trapped and destroyed by the spleen leading to development of splenomegaly.
    e. In case of *P. falciparum*, capillaries will be obstructed by parasitized erythrocytes because membrane of the erythrocytes will be modified as adhesin molecules on the capillary endothelium

27. Causes of cyclical temperature in this disease are rupture of infected erythrocytes followed by release of merozoites in the blood stream leading to release of toxin and hemozoin pigments as well as GPI fragments

into the circulation. So, there is release of pyrogenic cytokines like interleukin-1β and interleukin-6 by the macrophages.

28. Complications of this disease are as follows:
    a. Cerebral complications mainly occur in case of *P. falciparum* infection
    b. Nephrotic syndrome
    c. Bilious remittent fever
    d. Algid malaria due to parasitic congestion of the adrenal gland followed by necrosis and destruction of this gland
    e. Acute respiratory distress syndrome
    f. Disseminated intravascular coagulation
    g. Black water fever due to intravascular hemolysis resulting in hemoglobinuria leading to renal failure
    h. Burkitt's lymphoma in case of combined infection with *Plasmodium* and Epstein–Barr virus infection

29. Different morphologies in different stages of the parasites in the erythrocytes under microscope:
    a. In the ring stage:
       - In *P. falciparum*: Purple spot with a thin ring
       - In *P. vivax*: Purple spot with deformed body
       - In *P. ovale*: Ring with large purple spot
       - In *P. malariae*: Purple spot with thick body
       - In *P. knowlesi*: Purple spot with an amorphous thick ring
    b. In the trophozoite stage:
       - *Plasmodium falciparum*: Growing bigger spot around a smaller spot
       - *Plasmodium vivax*: A misshapen circle containing extended spot
       - *Plasmodium ovale*: Oval circle sometimes having smaller corners containing a purple spot having undefined shape
       - *Plasmodium malariae*: Basket or band shaped
       - *Plasmodium knowlesi*: Purple-branched spot
    c. Schizont stage:
       - *Plasmodium falciparum*: Not yet established
       - *Plasmodium vivax*: Ill-defined purple spots inside a circle
       - *Plasmodium ovale*: More than one spot inside an oval circle
       - *Plasmodium malariae*: Duffuse purple spots around a darker spot
       - *Plasmodium knowlesi*: Countable defined purple spots

    d. Gametocyte stage:
       - *Plasmodium falciparum*: Banana or sausage shaped
       - *Plasmodium vivax*: Extended big spot
       - *Plasmodium ovale*: Row of accumulated spots
       - *Plasmodium malariae*: Almost filled up big-stained spot
       - *Plasmodium knowlesi*: Big spot containing small spots

30. Treatment of malaria:
    a. Uncomplicated *P. falciparum* and *P. malariae* which is chloroquine sensitive:
       - Chloroquine phosphate 600 mg as a loading dose followed by 300 mg at 6, 24, and 48 hours
         Or
       - Hydroxychloroquine 620 mg as loading dose followed by 310 mg at 6, 24, and 48 hours
    b. Uncomplicated *P. falciparum* and *P. malariae* but chloroquine resistant:
       - Atovaquone + proguanil—250 +100 mg—four tablets daily for 4 days
         Or
       - Artemether + lumefantrine—20 + 120 mg—four tablets as initial dose, then after 8 hours followed by twice daily for 2 days
         Or
       - Quinine sulfate 542 mg thrice daily for 3 days, *plus* doxycycline 100 mg daily for 7 days, *or* tetracycline 250 mg 250 daily for 7 days, *or* clindamycin 20 mg/kg/day in three divided doses for 7 days
       - Mefloquine 684 mg as loading dose followed by 456 mg every 6–12 hours for total dose of 1,250 mg
    c. Uncomplicated *P. vivax* and *P. ovale* chloroquine-sensitive patient:
       - Treatment as above *plus* primaquine phosphate 30 mg daily for 14 days or tafenoquine 300 mg once only.
    d. Uncomplicated *P. vivax* and *P. ovale* chloroquine-resistant patient:
       - Quinine sulfate *plus* either doxycycline or primaquine or tafenoquine as per above dose
         Or
       - Atovaquone + proguanil as above dose *plus* either primaquine, or tafenoquine
         Or
       - Mefloquine as above *plus* primaquine or tafenoquine as above dose

e. Uncomplicated any species of chloroquine-sensitive malaria in pregnant woman: Chloroquine or hydroxychloroquine as per above doses

f. Uncomplicated any species of chloroquine-resistant malaria in pregnant woman:
    - In first, second, and third trimester, quinine sulfate as per above dose *plus* either clindamycin or mefloquine as above dose
    - In second and third trimester, artemether *plus* lumefantrine as per above dose

g. Complicated malaria in case of unstable nonpregnant women: Intravenous artesunate 2.4 mg/kg of body weight at 0, 12, 24, and 48th hours plus either artemether + lumefantrine, atovaquone + proguanil, doxycycline, or mefloquine as per above dose

31. Artemisinin-based combination therapy acts:
    a. Asexual blood stage to alleviate symptoms
    b. Gametes to reduce the spread of the disease

32. The companion drugs for artemisinin derivatives are the following:
    a. Lumefantrine
    b. Mefloquine
    c. Amodiaquine
    d. Sulfadoxine + pyrimethamine
    e. Chlorproguanil + dapsone

33. Primaquine is used for radical cure as this drug acts on the hypnozoite stage of the parasite.

34. Following are the approved insecticides for next treatment:
    a. Pyrroles
    b. Pyrethroids

35. Following are the methods of controlling the larval stage of the mosquito:
    a. Application of oil at the surface to make the larvae suffocated
    b. Toxins from the bacterium *Bacillus thuringiensis* var. israelensis
    c. Insect growth regulators like methoprene—it is specific to mosquito.

36. Proposed vaccine strategies of *P. falciparum* include:
    a. Whole sporozoite antigens using whole attenuated sporozoites
    b. Liver stage vaccine: Here thrombospondin-related adhesin protein which is linked to multiepitope string which is inserted to adenovirus of chimpanzee.
    c. Blood stage vaccine: Here antigen from immuno-modulant nonpolymorphic merozoite is used.
    d. Transmission blocking vaccine

CASE 15

A 45-year-old female working at cafeteria in the school came to doctor's clinic with burning sensation during micturition, pain in the loin, and spiking fever. On examination, there is tenderness in the renal angle as well as suprapubic tenderness. During investigation, there is neutrophilic leukocytosis. Urine examination demonstrated pus cells and protein in the urine. Urine dipstick was positive for nitrite and pus cells. Urine culture demonstrated:

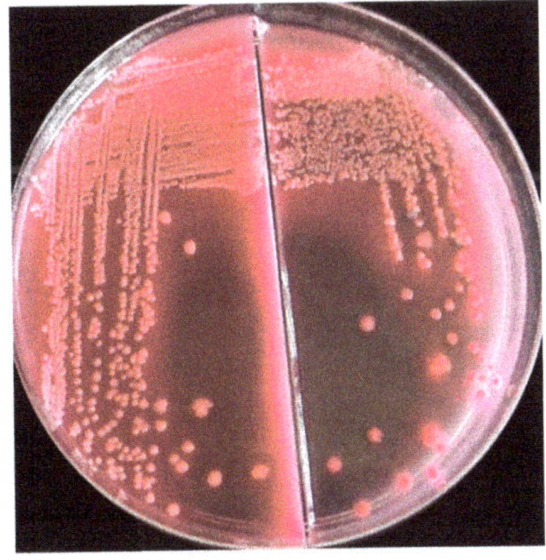
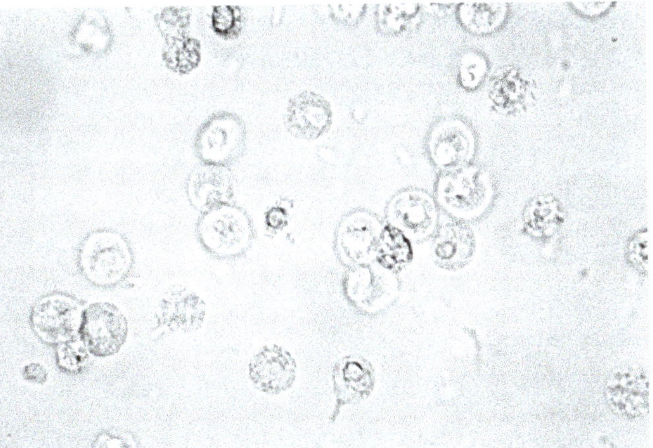

1. **What has been shown in the above pictures?**
2. **What is your diagnosis?**
3. **What is its outer membrane is composed of?**

4. **Name the fatty acids present on the inner lipid A.**
5. **What are the functions of endotoxin of this organism?**
6. **Urinary tract infection is caused by which strain of the organism?**
7. **What are the other species of *Enterobacteriaceae* responsible for urinary tract infection?**
8. **When this organism starts colonizing in the human being and through which route?**
9. **How this organism spreads in the female genitourinary tract?**
10. **Is there any chance of getting person to person spread?**
11. **In neonate, which sex is common to get infected with this organism?**
12. **What are the risk factors for getting this infection?**
13. **What are the characteristic features of uropathogenic type of this organism in case of this urinary tract infection?**
14. **What are the characteristic features of P fimbriae responsible for which type of UTI?**
15. **What are the functions of the fimbriae other than P fimbriae?**
16. **What is the effect of this organism in the urinary bladder?**
17. **In the renal medulla, what are the factors enhancing infection with this organism?**
18. **What are the host protective responses against this organism from local and systemic point of view?**
19. **What is the importance of cell-mediated immunity in urinary tract infection?**
20. **How this organism damages the renal tissue?**
21. **What is the adaptive immune response of the host in case of pyelonephritis?**
22. **What is the clinical presentation in this disease in different age group?**
23. **What are the complications in this infection?**
24. **What is reinfection and relapse in UTI?**
25. **What are the automated methods for assessing bacteriuria?**
26. **What is the treatment protocol in asymptomatic bacteriuria?**
27. **What is the treatment protocol in men in urinary tract infection?**
28. **What is the treatment in case of pregnant woman in UTI?**

Answers

1. The above pictures demonstrate:
   - MacConkey agar demonstrates growth of *Escherichia coli*
   - The other picture demonstrates red blood cell cast in the urine under microscope
2. This patient has been suffering from acute pyelonephritis.
3. The outer hydrophobic membrane of *E. coil* is composed of lipopolysaccharide.
4. Lipid A of the lipopolysaccharide has the following fatty acids:
   a. Hexanoic acid
   b. Dodecanoic acid
   c. Tetradecanoic acid
   d. Hexadecanoic acid
   e. Octadecenoic acid
   These fatty acids are linked by ester amide bonds to ketodeoxyoctanoate via N-acetylglucosamine.
5. Lipopolysaccharides, the endotoxin has following functions:
   a. Dramatic effects on clotting as well as kallikrein cascades
   b. Complement activation
   c. Production of cytokine
6. Urinary tract infection is caused by K12 strain of *E. coli.*
7. Other members of Enterobacteriaceae responsible for UTI are:
   a. *Enterobacter*
   b. *Klebsiella*
8. Within few hours to few days after birth gastrointestinal tract will be colonized by *E. coli*. This organism comes through the contaminated food or water from other individual directly.
9. In female, the *E. coli* with appropriate virulence factors will attach with the vaginal epithelium and colonize in the introitus, from there the bacteria enter the urinary tract through the urethra and infect the urinary bladder producing cystitis. In presence of vesicoureteric reflux, the bacteria enter the renal tissue leading to development of pyelonephritis.

10. Enteropathogenic *E. coli* can produce gastroenteritis spreading through the fecal-oral route.

11. In case of neonates, most commonly males are affected.

12. Risk factors responsible for urinary tract infection are as follows:
    a. Age
    b. Pregnancy
    c. Sexual intercourse
    d. Condom and spermicidal jelly
    e. Use of diaphragm
    f. Delayed postcoital micturition
    g. Menopause
    h. History of recent urinary tract infection
    i. In-hospital catheterization

13. Following are the virulence characteristics of uropathogenic *E. coli* to cause urinary tract infection:
    a. P fimbriae capable of binding with P blood group antigen which is present on the uroepithelial cells.
    b. Specific capsular antigens like K1 associated with serum resistance
    c. Hemolysin production
    d. Cytotoxic necrotizing factor
    e. Secreted autotransported toxin
    f. Siderophore receptors
    g. TonB iron uptake mechanism

14. P fimbriae are composed of:
    a. Main fimbrial protein
    b. Adhesin—PapG: It has several allele variants:
       - Allele II variant binds to globoside and is responsible for pyelonephritis
       - Allele III variant binds to Forssman antigen and is responsible for asymptomatic bacteriuria and cystitis in children and woman.

15. The other types of fimbriae except P fimbriae in uropathogenic *E. coli* are:
    a. Type 1 fimbriae: They bind to mannose receptors on the uroepithelial cells.
    b. S fimbriae: They bind to sialyllactose residue which is present on the renal tubules and glomeruli.
    c. Dr fimbriae: They bind to decay accelerating factor and type IV collagen and are responsible for cystitis in children, pyelonephritis in case of pregnant woman, and gastroenteritis.
    d. Curli fimbriae: They are a type of amyloid which provides firm adhesion by binding with phosphoethanolamine cellulose secreted by strains of *E. coli*.

16. *E. coli* binds with the uroepithelial cells in the urinary bladder leading to widening of the junctions between the squamous epithelium and thereby exposing the basal cells with which the *E. coli* binds. This adhesion of the *E. coli* leads to increased stimulation of Th1 cytokine synthesis in the uroepithelium, increased production of interleukin-1, 6, and 8 which in turn recruits granulocytes and macrophages, patient develops temperature.

17. In the renal medulla, following factors favoring the infections with *E. coli*:
    a. High concentration of ammonia
    b. Osmolarity
    c. Low pH

    All the factors lead to immune paresis

18. Following are the protective responses of host against this organism:
    a. Host secretes defensins from the uroepithelium as well as Tamm–Horsfall protein. It will bind to *E. coli* and thus removes the bacteria.
    b. There is exfoliation of the epithelium along with *E. coli* which is found in the urine.
    c. Host also develops acquired immune response against this organism in the upper urinary tract leading to production of all isotypes of organism.

19. Cell-mediated immunity against this infection is less important in this infection except secretion of the cytokines.

20. Increased number of granulocytes accumulated in the urinary tract leading to release of oxygen free radicals as well as proteolytic enzymes which ultimately damage the renal tissue in the form of necrosis and induces further renal inflammation.

21. Though adaptive immune response is of less importance, but secretory IgA inhibits the binding of the uroepithelial cells with the *E. coli*.

22. Different types of presentation in different age groups:
    a. In neonates: Fever, vomiting, and floppy infants
    b. In older children and adult:
       - Suprapubic pain, fever, frequency, dysuria, and urine may contain blood indicating cystitis.
       - Presence of fever with rigor, loin pain, frequency, and dysuria indicating acute pyelonephritis.
    c. Elderly patients: Fever, incontinence, dementia, and features chest infection

23. Complications in this infection are as follows:
    a. Renal scarring
    b. Septicemia
    c. Papillary necrosis
    d. Renal abscess
    e. Perinephric abscess
    f. Renal failure
24. Reinfection is infection due to different organisms which are drug susceptible. Relapse is infection with the same organism which is drug resistant.
25. Following are the automated methods for assessing bacteriuria:
    a. Turbidimetry
    b. Bioluminescence
    c. Electrical impedance
    d. Flow cytometry
    e. Radiometric test
26. Treatment protocol in case of asymptomatic bacteriuria:
    a. In case of nonpregnant woman and elderly, no treatment
    b. In case of pregnant woman and children with evidence of vesicoureteral reflux, treatment is required as there is chance of renal scarring and renal failure.
27. Treatment of urinary tract infection in men: Goals are:
    a. Eradication of infection of prostate
    b. Treatment of infection in the bladder
    In case of acute bacterial prostatitis:
    a. Antibiotics has to be given according to the culture/sensitivity reports and should be continued for 2–4 weeks.

    In case of documented chronic bacterial prostatitis, 4–6 weeks antibiotic treatment should be recommended.

    In case of chronic prostatitis with recurrent infection of the urinary tract, 12 weeks antibiotic treatment should be recommended.
28. In case of pregnant women:
    a. Ampicillin and cephalosporin are the drug of choice.
    b. In overt pyelonephritis, parenteral β-lactam antibiotic therapy with or without aminoglycoside should be recommended.

CASE 16

A 25-year-old male having history of frequent intake of hotel food came to medical clinic with complaint of fever with loose stool having offensive smell and stick to the pan. Stool examination demonstrated:

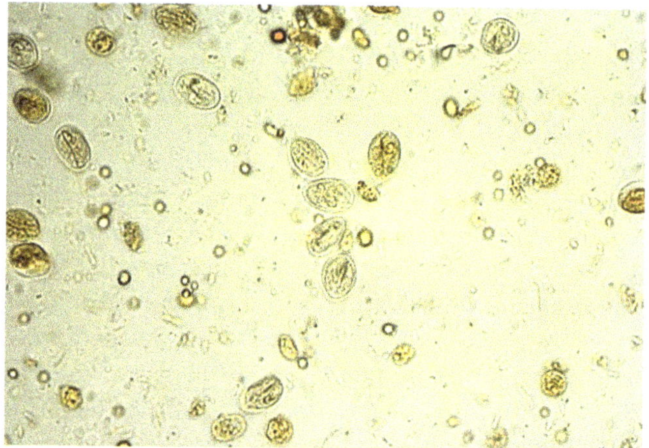

1. **What has been described in the above picture?**
2. **What is your diagnosis?**
3. **What are the stages in the life cycle of this parasite and describe them?**
4. **What are the genomic ploidies occurring during the life cycle?**
5. **What are the characteristic features of the prokaryote present in the eukaryote of this parasite?**
6. **What are the genotypes of this parasite responsible for infection in human being?**
7. **How this cycle of this parasite is going on in the human body?**

8. **How many cycles are necessary for infection in the human being?**
9. **What are the routes of spread in case of person to person infection?**
10. **What is "Backpacker's" diarrhea?**
11. **What is the nonimmunologic defense against this parasite in the human being?**
12. **What are the factors responsible for innate immunity in the human being against this parasite?**
13. **Which proinflammatory cytokine is of major importance in the clearance of this parasite?**
14. **Which proinflammatory cytokine is T cell responsive and which T cell is responsible?**
15. **What is the importance of Th17 cells in this infection?**
16. **What is the effect of depletion of CD4+ T cells in this infection?**
17. **How the antibody to this parasite will be developed in the human being?**
18. **What are the types of antibodies developed against this parasite?**
19. **What are the fluids containing secretory antibody?**
20. **What are the immunologic proteins of this parasite that is responsible for production of IgG?**
21. **How the antigenic variation occurs in this organism?**
22. **What are the causes of diarrhea and malabsorption occurring in this infection?**
23. **What are the main pathophysiologies behind this parasitic infection?**
24. **How this parasite produces dysbiosis after colonization?**
25. **What are the factors responsible for variable clinical presentation in the human being?**
26. **Describe the typical stool in this infection.**
27. **What are the clinical features in children in this infection?**
28. **What are the factors responsible for serious complications in this infection?**
29. **How can you increase the percentage of visualization of this parasite?**
30. **What are the stains used for detection of this organism?**
31. **What is the special test can be done to increase the incidence of detection of this parasite?**
32. **What are the drugs can be given to treat this infection?**
33. **Which drug can be given during pregnancy?**

Answers

1. The above picture demonstrates the cysts of *Giardia lamblia* in the stool
2. This patient has been suffering from giardiasis.
3. There are two phases in the life cycle:
    a. Trophozoite form:
        - Flagellated
        - Pear-shaped
        - Two nuclei
        - There is a sucking disk on the ventral surface in the body and median bodies.
        - Rigid cytoskeleton containing microtubules as well as microribbons
    b. Cystic form:
        - Smooth-walled
        - Oval-shaped
4. There are five chromosomes having different sizes and variations in the number of genome. This variation is very important in the regulation and differentiation of the genes.
5. Giardia is the oldest eukaryote having the characteristics and metabolism of prokaryote but no mitochondria.
6. Though there are eight genotypes from A to H, but major human pathogens are A and B.
7. Cyst after ingestion from the contaminated food or water becomes opened up releasing trophozoites in the intestinal lumen. These trophozoites are multiply by binary fission and colonize in the epithelial surfaces leading to diarrhea. The trophozoites are attached with the intestinal wall through the sucking disk to take nutrition from the host. Again, following detachment from the intestinal wall they will move toward the colon. During passage, some trophozoites will become encysted forming cysts and come out through the feces along with the trophozoites.
8. At least 10–25 cycles are necessary to produce infection.
9. Person to person spread occurs through:
    a. Ingestion of the contaminated food and water through the fecal-oral route, hands, and fomite.

    b.   Sexual transmission occurs occasionally in case of homosexuals

10. Backpacker's diarrhea or traveler's diarrhea as this infection occurs in a person traveling from the developing country and transmitted from beavers to man.

11. Following are the nonimmunologic defense of the host:
   a. During replacement of the epithelial cells, every 3–5 days. Trophozoites are also detached and excreted through the feces.
   b. Mucus secreted from the intestinal goblet cells will impede the attachment of the trophozoites with the intestinal epithelial cells.

12. Following factors are responsible for the innate immunity against this parasite:
   a. Antimicrobial peptides secreted from the intestinal epithelial cells like defensins as well as cathelicidins have antigiardia activity.
   b. Intestinal epithelial cells secrete nitric oxide which will inhibit excystation and encystation of this parasite.
   c. Monocytes and macrophages will kill the parasites in vitro but within the intestine they have negligible role.
   d. Mast cells can destroy this parasite through the release of mast cell protease.
   e. Dendritic cells are activated and matured by Giardia lysates, excretory and secretory products, and other proteins leading to increased release of proinflammatory cytokines, interleukin-12 and 6, and tumor necrosis factor-α.
   f. Activated dendritic cells also release immunomodulatory cytokines

13. Interleukin-6 produced by dendritic cells is mostly responsible for clearance of Giardia.

14. In *Giardia* infection, the strong protective adaptive immune response will be developed and the main cells are CD4+ T lymphocytes including Th1, Th2, and Th17. Increased ratio of T17 cells and Treg lymphocytes will give increased resistance to this infection.

15. Th17 T cells produce interleukin-17 in the blood providing increased resistance to this infection.

16. Depletion of CD4+ T cells will lead to development of chronic giardiasis; on the other hand, increased CD8+ T cells will protection against giardiasis.

17. Antigenic products of *Giardia lamblia* penetrate the mucosal barrier and pass through the M cells present in the Peyer's patches or dendritic cells having intraepithelial processes within the lumen of the intestine into the blood to produce antibodies against this parasite.

18. There are two types of antibodies produced in this infection: secretory IgA antibody in the mucosal epithelium and IgG antibody present in the serum.

19. Secretory IgA antibodies are found in human fluid like breast milk and saliva.

20. Following immunologic proteins are responsible for production of IgG antibodies:
   a. Variant-specific surface proteins
   b. Cytoskeletal proteins unique to *Giardia* like α-tubulin, β-tubulin, α-giardin, and β-giardin
   c. Enzymes like arginine deaminase, ornithine carbamoyltransferase as well as enolase

21. Each trophozoite expresses only one type of variant-specific surface protein but they can switch this protein through the interference RNA and messenger RNA.

22. In giardiasis, the mechanisms of diarrhea are:
   a. Damage to the endothelial brush border
   b. Enterotoxins
   c. Immunologic reactions
   d. Changes in the motility of the gut
   e. Hypersecretion of fluid through the increased activity of adenylate cyclase

23. Main pathophysiologies behind this infection are:
   a. Loss of brush border surface area in the intestinal wall
   b. Flattening of the intestinal villi
   c. Inhibition of disaccharide activities
   d. Overgrowth of enteric bacterial flora

24. Increased population of Proteobacteria and decreased population of Firmicutes leading to dysbiosis in this infestation.

25. Following factors will lead to variable presentation in this infection:
   a. Virulence of the particular strain of Giardia
   b. Genotypes like A and B in this parasite
   c. Number of cysts ingested
   d. Age of the host
   e. State of immunity

26. Typical stool in this infection is loose, yellowish, and foul smelling which floats on the surface of water due to its high fat content.

27. In case of children, there will be malabsorption along with protein loosing enteropathy leading to failure to thrive and stunted growth.

28. Following factors will lead to serious complications:
   a. Patients with HIV
   b. Cancer

c. Transplants

d. Elderly

e. Hypochlorhydria due to *H. pylori* infection

29. Following methods can increase the chance of detection of the parasite in the stool:

a. Concentration method for prior visualization under microscope

b. Formalin-ether concentration method

c. Sucrose gradient concentration method

30. Following stains are used for staining the parasites:

a. Iodine

b. Methylene blue

c. Trichrome

31. Following special tests are used to increase the detection of the organism in the patients:

a. ELISA

b. Direct fluorescence assay

32. Following drugs can be given to treat this infection:

a. Nitroimidazole derivatives:
   - Metronidazole
   - Tinidazole
   - Secnidazole
   - Ornidazole

b. Benzimidazole derivatives:
   - Albendazole
   - Mebendazole

c. Nitrofurantoin derivatives: Furazolidone

d. Acridine compound:
   - Mepacrine
   - Quinacrine

e. Aminoglycosides: Paromomycin

f. Nitazoxanide

33. In case of pregnancy, following are the treatment protocols:

a. Drugs should be avoided in the first trimester of pregnancy

b. Mild symptomatic patient should be treated after delivery but adequate hydration as well as proper nutrition should be maintained.

c. But, in case of early pregnancy, paromomycin is considered as safe during first trimester of pregnancy.

CASE 17

A 40-year-old male homosexual having multiple male partners and no history of not taking protection during sex came to medical clinic with shortness of breath during exertion and low-grade fever. Physical examination demonstrated in the mouth (picture below), occasional basal crepitations in the chest bilaterally. Chest X-ray demonstrated following picture bronchoalveolar lavage demonstrated as below:

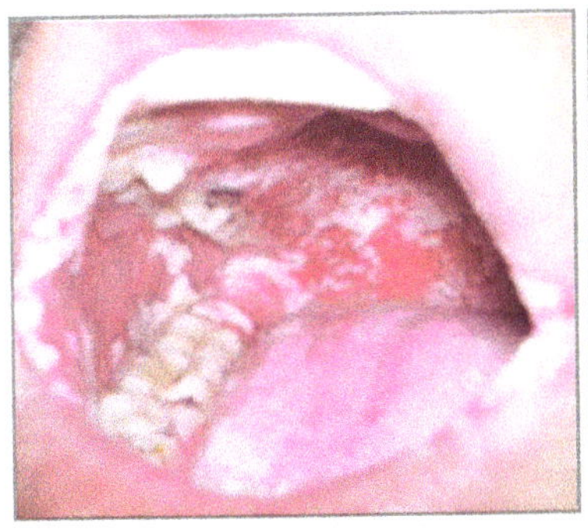
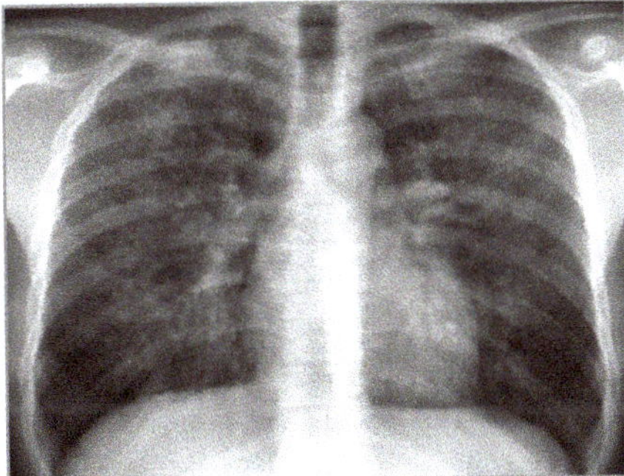
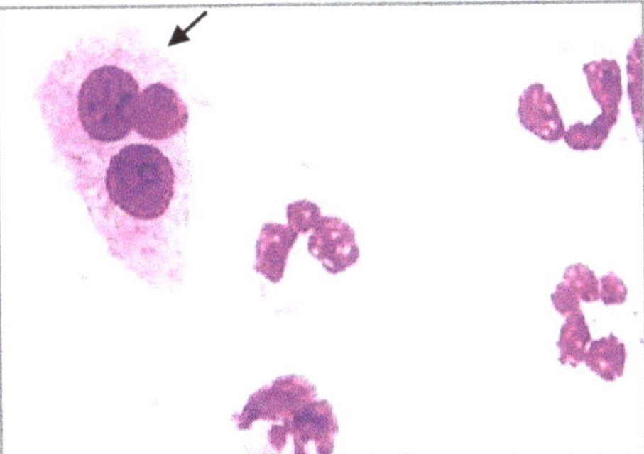

1. **What has been shown in the above pictures?**

2. **What is your diagnosis?**

3. **What are the species of the organism based on what factors?**

4. **What are the similarities between these species of this organism?**

5. **What are the genes included in the most common type of organism?**

6. **Single-stranded RNA in this organism is covered by how many structures?**

7. **By which methods viral structures will be released into cytoplasm?**

8. **After entry into the cells, what is the role of viral RNA?**

9. **In the nucleus, how the provirus is formed?**
10. **When the provirus will be reverted back to cellular cytoplasm and what is its destiny?**
11. **What is the function of proteases of both host cells and virus?**
12. **After formation of the mature infectious virus, what is its destiny?**
13. **What are the routes of transmission of the virus from person to person?**
14. **Who are resistant to sexual transmission and why?**
15. **Which strain of the organism is not readily transmitted from person to person?**
16. **Which cells are the specific terget of this organism and why?**
17. **After entry into the human body, how it can spread into the blood stream?**
18. **Which type of sexual intercourse is not protected from this infection and why?**
19. **Why sexually transmitted disease is a risk factor for infection with this organism?**
20. **What are the routes of vertical transmission?**
21. **What are the actions of the mucosa in the vagina and rectum against this infection?**
22. **What are the functions of the dendritic cells in the lamina propria of mucosa?**
23. **What is transinfection?**
24. **Why male person is susceptible to this infection?**
25. **Why infected cells are not destroyed by complement mediated lysis?**
26. **What is the nature of innate immune response on the virus-infected cells?**
27. **Within how many days after the entry of the virus lymph node will be attacked?**
28. **During viremia, how the viral load can be decreased?**
29. **What is seroconversion in this infection?**
30. **What do you mean by "set point" at the end of acute phase in this infection?**
31. **In case of variants of this virus, where is the variation commonly seen?**
32. **What is the importance of clinical latency phase in this infection?**
33. **When the full-blown syndrome of this disease will start?**
34. **What is the key point in immunodeficiency in this disease and what is the mechanism?**
35. **Which cell types control the function of immunologic cell types?**
36. **Which types of T helper cells mediated immunity at the mucosal surface and what are the effects of loss of these cells from the gut?**
37. **What are the functions of the dendritic cells in this disease?**
38. **What changes will occur in primary lymphoid organ in case of immunodeficiency?**
39. **What are the changes in the lymph nodes in this disease and why?**
40. **What are the typical clinical spectra of presentation in this disease?**
41. **Mention five examples in each category of this infection defining illness.**
42. **Describe five characteristic features of the most common neoplasm occurring in this infection.**
43. **Describe the opportunistic infection according to CD4 cell count.**
44. **During detection of viral RNA, what are the extra features to be assessed?**
45. **From which sites, sample should be taken for detection of antibody to this organism in rapid testing?**
46. **Which antigen is detected during screening of this organism?**
47. **In case of infants, which special test to be done to detect the positivity?**
48. **For staging of this disease, what should be tested?**
49. **Name the drugs according to site of action.**

Answers

1. The pictures demonstrate:
   a. Extensive oropharyngeal candidiasis.
   b. Straight X-ray demonstrates bilateral shadowing extending from hilum to periphery of the lung.
   c. Bronchoalveolar lavage demonstration multiple polymorphonuclear cells, trophozoites of *Pneumocystis carinii*, and a lymphocyte.
2. The patient having an HIV disease has been suffering from *P. carinii* infection along with extensive oropharyngeal candidiasis.

3. There are two species of HIV—HIV-1 and HIV-2 being differ in origin and nucleotide sequence.

4. The similarities between the two species of HIV are:
   a. Replication cycle
   b. Transmission

5. The following genes are included in this virus:
   a. For capsid and matrix, *Gag* gene
   b. Three enzymes required for replication of the virus, *Pol* gene
   c. For envelope glycoprotein, *Env* gene
   d. For regulation of synthesis and processing of the viral RNA, *Rev* and *Tat* gene
   e. For combating cellular intrinsic defense, *Nef, Vif, Vpr*, and *Vpu* genes

6. Viral RNA is covered by two layers:
   a. RNA is enclosed within a conical core which is made of a capsid protein p24.
   b. The conical core is surrounded by matrix protein
   c. It is surrounded by lipid envelope containing:
      - Envelope glycoprotein
      - Transmembrane protein gp41
      - Surface protein gp120
      - Glycosylated viral protein

7. Surface envelope glycoprotein gp120 will bind to CD4 cells leading to conformational changes within the virus which allows the virus to engage with cellular cytokine receptor CCR5 and CXCR4. This interaction will lead to changes in the transmembrane protein gp41 of virus so that hydrophobic peptide will be inserted into the target cellular membrane and this fusion will allow viral capsid to be released into the cytoplsm of the host cell.

8. After entry into the cell, viral RNA will be protected by the viral capsid from being recognized by toll-like receptor and thereby initiating the innate immunity. Now, the viral transcriptase will convert viral RNA to double-stranded DNA, then viral capsid transmitted into the nucleus through the nuclear pore.

9. In the nucleus, capsid will be disassembled and the enzyme integrase inserts the HIV DNA into the chromosome of the host to form provirus.

10. As the viral DNA produces, multiple RNA transcripts and these are transported into the cytoplasm, and few will be encapsidated as the viral genome progeny and some will form:
    a. Envelope glycoprotein gp160
    b. Polyprotein Pol
    c. Polyprotein Gag

11. Host cell protease furin breaks the envelope glycoprotein gp160 into transmembrane protein gp120 and surface protein gp40. As a result, assembly of the viral protein and viral genome will start at the plasma membrane containing envelope glycoprotein and immature virus will come out as budding.

    HIV protease breaks Gag and Pol polyproteins into the remaining components like p17, p24, and viral enzymes thereby facilitating the assembly of viral nucleocapsid, as a result mature virus will be formed.

12. After completion of the replication of the virus, some of them will be in the resting state within the cells and rest will come out to spread the infections.

13. HIV virus will enter the body of the human being through the mucosal surface present in the vagina and rectum and rarely by mouth. The viruses will cross the epithelium and enter the cells interacting with the receptors CCR5 and CD4. Routes of transmission of this vrus are as follows:
    a. Direct contact with the body fluids like semen, vaginal, and cervical secretion
    b. Amniotic fluid
    c. Breast milk
    d. Blood and blood products
    e. Use of contaminated needles in case of intravenous drug users

14. The subjects who are lack in CCR5 are resistant to infection with this virus by sexual transmission.

15. HIV strain that uses CXCR4 is found in late during infection and is not readily transmitted from person to person.

16. Memory CD4+ T cells are the primary target of this HIV virus as these cells have high expression of CCR5. But, dendritic cells and monocytes/macrophages lineage express both CD4.

17. After entry into the body, the virus-infected T cells and dendritic cells will reach the lymph nodes where the virus multiply leading increase in the viral population. Now, the virus-infected CD4+ T cells will reach the throracic duct from there they will reach the blood stream.

18. Vaginal epithelium is covered by stratified columnar epithelium and hence these epithelium can deal with the frictional forces. But, rectal mucosa is covered by single layer columnar epithelium which cannot resist the friction during sexual intercourse through the rectum.

19. Sexually transmitted disease is a great risk factor for transmission of HIV infection as the genital herpes will disrupt the epithelial lining leading to the entry of the HIV virus into the subepithelial mucosa.

20. Vertical transmission occurs during:
    a. Late pregnancy
    b. During delivery
    c. During breastfeeding
21. Vaginal epithelium is covered by stratified columnar epithelium and hence these epithelium can deal with the frictional forces. But, rectal mucosa is covered by single layer columnar epithelium which cannot resist the friction during sexual intercourse through the rectum.
22. Dendritic cells in the lamina propria have several functions:
    a. In the stratified squamous epithelium, dendritic cells display pathogen recognition receptors like C-type lectins which will bind to high mannose glycans. Here dendritic cells are known as Langerhans cells.
    b. Dendrite from the intraepithelial immature dendritic cells to capture HIV from the lumen through the binding of C-type lectins or langerin thereby transferring the virus on the surface to CD4+ T cells on the surface of memory CD4+ T cells present in the lamina propria.
    c. Mature dendritic cells containing HIV viruses will migrate to the regional lymph nodes where they will present these peptides to CD8+ T and CD4+ T cells via major histocompatibility complex class I and II, respectively.
23. Transinfection means transmission of infection through the release of the virus from the dendritic cells to infect neighboring CD4+ T cells
24. Penile shaft and outer surface of the prepuce known as foreskin will be covered by keratinized stratified squamous epithelium; as a result, it will act as protective barrier against the HIV infection. But, inner mucosa of the foreskin is enriched with dendritic cells and not keratinized; as a result, this mucosa is very susceptible to HIV virus.
25. HIV virus has regulator of complement activation during the budding process which prevents spontaneous host cell destruction and at the same time protects the virus from lysis.
26. Innate immune response paradoxically will recruit activated CD4+ T cells leading to progression of infection, and at the same time, it will increase the cellular immunity as well as type-1 interferon response.
27. At least 7–14 days is required for the HIV virus to travel to draining lymh nodes from the entry sites.
28. During the stage of viremia, there is increased level of CD8+ cytotoxic T cells which will kill this virus-infected cells by attacking p24 peptides thereby reducing the viral load 10–100-fold over few months.
29. Seroconversion to HIV virus ensues as cytotoxic cell response will start and it is marked appearance of p24 antibodies targeting viral proteins like envelope protein and this will persist for long time.
30. "Set point" at the end of acute infection means a balance between the new virus production and control by the immune system. But, it is not possible to clear the virus completely because replication of the virus will continue thereby development of reservoir of latently infected T cells and macrophages.
31. In case of variants of HIV virus, variation is mostly marked in:
    a. Variable region of the envelope protein
    b. Protein gp120
    c. Target virus neutralizing antibodies—it will generate escape mutants in the hypervariable region of gp120 protein.
32. The length of the clinical latency phase depends upon "set point" which varies person to person. If the level is high, the duration of latent phase is shorter prior to ensue of AIDS. During this phase, viremia gradually increases and level of CD4+ T cells will gradually decrease.
33. Full-blown syndrome of AIDS occurs within few months to >10 years when CD4+ T cell counts will reach below 200/cc.
34. The key points resulting in immunodeficiency are death of CD4+ T cells due to following causes:
    a. Directly via HIV infection
    b. Apoptosis of CD4+ T cells mediated by the CD8+ T cytotoxic cells that recognize infected CD4+ T cells
35. CD4+ T cells conducts the immunologic orchestra together with the dendritic cells and controls the development and function of the immunologic cells.
36. T helper 17 cells mediate immunity at the mucosal surface against bacterial and fungal pathogens. The loss of these cells at the mucosal surface leads to:
    a. Increase in the intestinal permeability
    b. Translocation of the microbial products from the lumen of the intestine
    c. Increase immune activation leading to irreversible damage of the mucosal barrier
37. Functions of the dendritic cells are as follows:
    a. CD4+ T cells along with dendritic cells control and the development of the immunologic cell types.
    b. This cell is involved in the transinfection of the CD4+ T cells along with HIV virus.

c. Infected dendritic cells affect the differentiation of T0 cells to Th1, Th2, and Th17 cells thereby disrupts all the immune responses.

38. In the primary lymphoid organs like in thymus:
    a. The thymocytes will be infected with HIV leading to decreased output of CD4+ T cells.
    b. Stromal cell function will be changed.
    c. The architecture of the cells will be changed.

39. Following are the changes in the lymph nodes:
    a. Polyclonal activation of CD8+ T cells and B cells
    b. Reduction in the number of CD4+ T cells

40. Clinical spectra of the diseases are:
    a. Completely asymptomatic
    b. Acute seroconversion syndrome characterized by maculopapular skin rash, night sweat, fever, malaise, lymphadenopathy, diarrhea, mouth ulcers, genital ulcer, and different neurogic diseases.
    c. Persistent generalised lymphadenopathy characterized by enlarged lymph nodes in two or more areas of the body for at least 3 months
    d. Full blown syndrome—AIDS defining diseases

41. Five examples of each category of AIDS defining disease are as follows:
    a. Neoplasm:
        - Cervical cancer
        - Primary lymphoma of central nervous system
        - Lymphoma: Burkitt's lymphoma or immunoblastic lymphoma
        - Kaposi sarcoma
    b. Viral infections:
        - Cytomegalovirus retinitis
        - Herpes simplex ulcers of >1 month
        - Progressive multifocal leukoencephalopathy—opportunistic JC virus infection
        - HIV-associated dementia
    c. Bacterial infections:
        - Pulmonary and extrapulmonary tuberculosis
        - *Mycobacterium avium* complex (MAC)
        - Two or more episodes of pneumonia in 12 months
        - *Salmonella septicemia*
    d. Parasitic infections:
        - Cerebral toxoplasmosis
        - Diarrhea due to *Cryptosporidium*
        - Atypical disseminated leishmaniasis
        - Reactivation of American trypanosomiasis
    e. Fungal infections:
        - *Pneumocystis carinii* pneumonia

- Esophageal candidiasis
- Extrapulmonary cryptococcosis
- Disseminated extrapulmonary histoplasmosis

42. The most common neoplasm of the skin is known as Kaposi sarcoma having following five characteristic features:
    a. It commonly occurs in me.
    b. It is found in the skin and oral cavity.
    c. Lesion of the skin is violaceous due to formation of new blood vessels.
    d. It is invasive and it will slowly progress to visceral form.
    e. Human herpes virus 8 or Kaposi sarcoma-associated herpes virus—it is found in TMR tissue.

43. Opportunistic infections according to CD4 T cell count:

CD4+ T cell count in 10^6/L	Infections
250–500	• Tuberculosis • Oral candidiasis
150–200	• Kaposi sarcoma • Lymphoma • Cryptosporidiosis
75–125	• *Pneumocystis jirovecii* pneumonia • Cryptococcal meningitis • Toxoplasmosis • Esophageal candidiasis • Disseminated MAC infection • Recurrent herpes simplex virus infection
<50	• Cytomegalovirus retinitis • Progressive multifocal leukoencephalopathy • Cryptosporidiosis • Cryptococcal meningitis

44. During detection of viral RNA, following extra features should be assessed:
    a. Viral antibodies
    b. Viral antigens
    c. Viral neucleic acid
    d. Proviral DNA
    e. Viral resistance testing

45. From the following areas, samples should be collected for detection of antibodies against this organism:
    a. Plasma
    b. Saliva
    c. Serum

46. Following antigens or antibody combination immunoassay should be detected during screening:
    a. HIV-antibodies
    b. p24, antigen during window phase when antibodies cannot be detectable.
47. In case of infants, direct detection of virus is necessary from the whole blood for proviral DNA in the cells as the antibodies against this virus will be available for up to 15 months in case of HIV-positive mothers.
48. For staging of the disease:
    a. Viral load: It will determine the destruction rate of the immune sysatem.
    b. CD4+ T cells: It will indicate the degree of immunodeficiency which will indicate the chance of opportunistic infections.
49. The name of the drugs according to the site of actions:
    a. Attachment inhibitors: Active metabolite of fostemsavir—temsavir which binds to gp120 to stabilize the protein thereby preventing binding to CD4+ T cells to attach and replicate.
    b. CCR4 inhibitor or chemokine coreceptor inhibitor: Maraviroc will block the binding of this virus with the coreceptor thereby preventing the virus to enter the cells.
    c. Fusion inhibitors: Enfuvirtide will bind to gp41 subunit of the viral envelope thereby preventing conformational changes which is required for the fusion of the viral envelope with the membrane of the host cell.
    d. Reverse transcriptase inhibitors: These are of two types:
       - Nucleosides: These drugs bind competitively to this reverse transcriptase to prevent the conversion of ssRNA to dsDNA.
         - Abacavir
         - Emtricitabine
         - Zidovudine
         - Lamivudine
       - Nucleotide: This drug will bind to reverse transcriptase away from the active site.
         - Tenofovir

       Integrase inhibitor: Non-nucleoside reverse transcriptase inhibitors—
       - Efavirenz
       - Rilpivirine
    e. Integrase inhibitors: It will block the viral integrase thereby preventing the provirus from forming the chromosome of the host cells.
       - Cabotegravir
       - Elvitegravir
       - Dolutegravir
    f. Protease inhibitors: These drugs will bind to active sites of the viral protease thereby inhibiting their function as well as preventig posttranslational clevage of polyproteins.
       - Atazanavir
       - Darunavir
       - Ritonavir

CHAPTER **9**

Neurology

A 72-year-old man came to medical outdoor with complaints of tremor at rest and difficulty in walking for last 3 months and during walking he tends to fall in front.

On examination, his vitals were normal, face is mask like, and tremor is of pill-rolling type, posture stooped, and gait was short shuffling type.

1. **What is the most likely diagnosis?**
2. **Is Myerson's sign is reliable in this case?**
3. **What is blepharoclonus and how can this be demonstrated?**
4. **Name five motor abnormalities in this patient.**
5. **Describe the classical tremor occurring in this disease.**
6. **Where cogwheel rigidity can be demonstrated?**
7. **If the gait is not narrow-based, what are the other differential diagnoses?**
8. **Which sign may be the earliest in this disease?**
9. **What are drugs responsible for this disease?**
10. **What is found in this disease in the brain and is it specific for this disease?**
11. **What is Parkinson-plus syndrome?**
12. **How can you differentiate this disease from this type of syndrome?**
13. **Why COMT is used with levodopa?**
14. **Why are the surgical procedures used to treat this disease?**

Answers

1. The most likely diagnosis is Parkinson's disease.
2. Myerson's sign is also known as glabellar tap reflex that involves tapping the forehead of the patient leads to few blinking followed by stop blinking. But in this disease, patient will continue blinking.
3. Blepharoclonus is also known as tremor of the eyelids and this can be easily demonstrated when the eyes are gently closed, but not if the eyes are closed tightly.
4. Five motor abnormalities are:
   a. Short shuffling narrow-based gait
   b. Continuous pill-rolling tremor that occurs at rest with reduced swinging of the arms
   c. Postural instability with propulsion as well as retropropulsion
   d. Lead pipe rigidity in absence of tremor and cogwheel rigidity in presence of tremor
   e. Synkinesia, i.e., increased rigidity of one arm will be increased when the other arm moves voluntarily.
5. Classical description of the tremor:
   a. Speed: 4–6 Hz
   b. In 20% cases, there may not be any tremor.
   c. It can be easily demonstrated by asking the patient to keep his arm in rest in his lap in semiprone position.
   d. This tremor is associated with jaw tremor or foot tremor.
   e. It will be aggravated by emotional stress or by walking and disappears during sleep.

  f. This tremor is not associated with head tremor as the latter is associated with essential tremor.

6. Tremor with rigidity or cogwheel tremor can be demonstrated in the wrist by asking the patient to manipulate the hand in a circular motion in the wrist.

7. If the gait is not narrow-based, the alternative diagnoses are:

  a. Multiple system atrophy

  b. Cerebellar degeneration

8. The earliest sign in this disease is reduced swing of the arm.

9. Following drugs are responsible for parkinsonism:

  a. Chlorpromazine

  b. Prochlorperazine

  c. Metoclopramide

  d. Methyldopa

  e. Sodium valproate

10. The inclusion bodies found in this disease are Lewy bodies which are characterized by spherical and eosinophilic inclusion bodies found in the cellular cytoplasm in the brain stem. It consists of dense core surrounded by the halo, made of radiating fibrils. In the other, Lewy body found in cortex contains no halo. It is not specific for this disease as it is also found in:

  a. Lewy body dementia

  b. Alzheimer's disease

  c. Hallervorden-Spatz disease

11. Parkinson-plus syndrome is characterized by involvement of different neuronal systems through different pathological processes and it includes:

  a. Poor response to levodopa

  b. Early onset of:

   • Dementia

   • Early falls

   • Hallucination

   • Symptoms of autonomic dysfunction

  c. Pyramidal signs that cannot be explained by previous strokes or any pathology in the spinal cord

  d. Cerebellar signs

  e. Gaze palsies or nystagmus

12. Differentiation between Parkinson's disease and Parkinson's syndrome:

Clinical features	Parkinson's syndrome	Parkinson's disease
Signs of distribution	It is symmetrical	It is asymmetrical
Progression of the disease	Rapidly progressive	Slowly progressive
Response to levodopa	Poor	Good
Plus sign	May occur	Absent

13. Catechol-O-methyl transferase (COMT) inhibitors are such as tolcapone and entacapone used in this disease as it will prevent breakdown of levodopa in the gastrointestinal tract thereby help to reduce the dose of levodopa. As a result, "off" time will be increased and "on" time will be decreased, thus reducing the wearing-off effect.

14. Following procedures are involved in this disease:

  a. Thalamotomy involves destruction of ventral intermediate nuclei of thalamus for relief from contralateral tremor.

  b. Pallidotomy which involves destruction of globus pallidus interna to improve the features of Parkinson's disease

  c. Subthalamotomy involves destruction of a portion of overactive subthalamic nucleus to give relief from contralateral cardinal features of Parkinson's disease

  d. Deep brain stimulation which replaces the surgeries

  e. Transplantation of dopamine producing cells has been evaluated.

CASE 2

A 45-year-old man came to medical outdoor with limping gait. On examination, the patient has pes cavus and claw toes. The motor system examination demonstrated distal symmetrical wasting of muscles with diminished tendon reflexes with reduced sensation in gloves-and-stocking distribution, palpable lateral popliteal nerves, and gait is high steppage, and positive Romberg test. However, proximal thigh muscles are normal.

1. **What is the most likely diagnosis?**

2. **What are the features to look for prior to examine this patient?**

3. **What should be the lower limbs look like?**

4. **What is the differential diagnosis of foot drop and for that what should be searched for?**

5. **Is there any importance of lateral popliteal nerve in this disease?**
6. **What is the importance of pes cavus in this disease?**
7. **What are the other causes of pes cavus?**
8. **What are the other foot deformities that may occur?**
9. **Which type of sensory loss usually occurs?**
10. **What are types of this disease according to nerve conduction velocity?**
11. **What may be the presentation in that family members?**
12. **Why peripheral nerve is thickened in this disease?**

Answers

1. The diagnosis is Charcot–Marie–Tooth disease.
2. Following should be watched toward the patient prior to examine the patient:
   a. Walking aids of the patient
   b. Look at the shoes of the patient
   c. Limping style of the patient
   d. Scuffing of the front of the shoe resulting from foot drop
3. Wasting of the distal part of the lower limb muscles on the anterolateral compartment with abrupt stoppage of the wasting at the lower one-third of the thigh and above two-thirds of thigh muscles being normal leading to appearance of "stork legs" or "spindle legs" or "inverted champagne bottle" appearance.
4. Peroneal nerve palsy is the important differential diagnosis and in that case trauma on the neck of the fibula should be searched for.
5. Lateral popliteal nerve should be thickened in 50% cases in type 1 disease.
6. Pes cavus is present in 70% cases in this disease and it will not flatten in spite of weight-bearing. It indicates that this disease is congenital and long-standing.
7. Other causes of pes cavus are as follows:
   a. Unilateral pes cavus:
      - Poliomyelitis
      - Spinal trauma
      - Burns
      - Tumors in the spinal cord
      - Malunion of fracture of calcaneus or talus
      - Sequelae of compartment syndrome
   b. Bilateral pes cavus:
      - Friedreich's ataxia
      - Cerebral palsy
      - Spinal muscular atrophy
      - Syringomyelia
      - Muscular dystrophies
      - Spinal cord tumors
8. Other foot deformities are as follows:
   a. High foot arches
   b. Hammer toes
   c. Achilles tendon contracture
9. Vibration sense and proprioceptive sense are mostly affected, but in some cases, pain sensation is reduced in gloves and stocking distribution. Pain fibers are not affected because these are unmyelinated nerve fibers.
10. There are three types of this disease:
    a. Type 1 disease: Primary demyelinating neuropathy along with nerve conduction velocity of less than 35 m/s.
    b. Type 2 disease: It is primary axonal neuropathy with nerve conduction velocity of more than 45 m/s.
    c. Type 3 disease: It is dominant intermediate form having nerve conduction velocity of 35 to 45 m/s and some members of that family may be affected.
11. Family members of this disease presents with pes cavus and absence of ankle jerk.
12. In case of demyelination, proliferation of Schwann cells to form concentric layer of demyelination and remyelination resulting in thick abnormal myelin around the axons leading to onion bulb appearance of the nerve. Hence peripheral nerve is thickened in this disease.

CASE 3

A 42-year-old man came to neurology outdoor with slurring of speech, difficulty in deglutition and nasal regurgitation, and progressive weakness of upper and lower limb muscles.

On examination, in the cranial nerve, there is absent of gag reflex and lower motor type of paralysis of the tongue.

Upper and lower limbs demonstrated wasting along with fasciculation of both lower and upper limb muscles along with wasting of the small muscles of the hand in presence of hypertonia and hyperreflexia and extensor plantar response, all modalities of sensation were normal.

1. **What is the most likely diagnosis?**
2. **Define the disease.**
3. **What are the forms of this disease?**
4. **What is the genetic basis of this disease?**
5. **What are the causes of fasciculation?**
6. **How can you differentiate this disease from syringomyelia?**
7. **How can you differentiate this disease from cervical myelopathy?**
8. **What are features of poor prognosis in this disease?**
9. **What do you mean by bulbar and pseudobulbar palsy?**
10. **Which nerve will never be involved in this disease?**
11. **What will be progression of the weakness in this disease?**
12. **What is the deformity in the hands in this disease?**

Answers

1. The most likely diagnosis is motor neuron disease.
2. Motor neuron disease can be defined as loss of neurons at all the motor systems distributed from cortex to brainstem along with anterior horn cells in the spinal cord.
3. Following are the forms of motor neuron disease:
   a. Amyotrophic lateral sclerosis demonstrates signs of upper and lower motor neuron
   b. Primary lateral sclerosis demonstrates predominantly upper motor neuron signs
   c. Progressive muscular atrophy demonstrates predominantly lower motor neuron signs
   d. Progressive bulbar palsy demonstrates predominant involvement of bulbar muscles leading to development of bulbar or pseudobulbar palsy
4. Genetic basis of this disease:
   a. Mutation of *SOD1* gene encoding copper-zinc superoxide dismutase in chromosome number 21—autosomal dominant pattern of inheritance
   b. Mutation of *ALS2* gene in chromosome 2—autosomal recessive pattern of inheritance
   c. Mutation of *SETX* gene in chromosome 2—autosomal dominant pattern of inheritance
   d. Mutation of *VAPB* gene in chromosome 20—autosomal dominant pattern of inheritance
   e. Mutation of *DCTN1* gene in chromosome 2—autosomal dominant pattern of inheritance

Following mutation of the gene leads to risk of developing motor neuron disease:

   a. Angiogenin in chromosome number 14
   b. Vascular endothelial growth factor in chromosome number 6
   c. Charged multivesicular body protein 2B in chromosome 2
   d. Survival motor neuron in chromosome number 5
   e. Neurofilament protein in chromosome number 22

5. Following are the causes of fasciculation:
   a. Thyrotoxic myopathy
   b. Syringomyelia
   c. Cervical spondylosis
   d. In case of healthy adult after exercise
   e. Hypokalemia
   f. Hypomagnesemia
   g. Hereditary motor and sensory neuropathy
   h. Neuralgic amyotrophy
   i. Syphilitic amyotrophy
   j. Spinal muscular atrophy
   k. Acute poliomyelitis
6. In case of syringomyelia, there is upper motor neuron lesion in the lower limbs and lower motor neuron

lesion in the upper limb along with dissociated sensory loss with or without evidence of Horner's syndrome.

7. In case of cervical spondylosis, sensory signs are present which are absent in motor neuron disease, whereas bulbar signs are absent in cervical myelopathy.

8. Following features indicate poor prognosis in motor neuron disease:
   a. Female sex
   b. Bulbar muscle involvement at onset
   c. Presentation at older age

9. Bulbar palsy can be demonstrated as upper and lower motor weakness of:
   a. Facial muscles
   b. Palatal muscles
   c. Muscles of the tongue with presence of fasciculation

Pseudobulbar palsy is characterized by:
   a. Emotional lability
   b. Stiff tongue
   c. Absence of fasciculation
   d. Brisk jaw jerk

10. Oculomotor nerve will never be involved in motor neuron disease.

11. Weakness to start with is unilateral in the early course beginning in the arms, legs, and oropharyngeal muscles and it will spread bilaterally. In some cases, the disease starts distally and progresses proximally; in that case, foot drop is the early sign.

12. There is:
   a. Dorsal guttering
   b. Hyperextension at the metacarpophalangeal joints
   c. Flexion in the interphalangeal joints
   So, hands look like claw hands.

CASE 4

A 45-year-old man came to medicine outdoor with reeling to the right and vertigo. On examination, there was intention tremor, impaired heel-knee test, and finger-nose testing on the right side and nystagmus having fast component toward right.

1. **What is the most likely diagnosis?**
2. **What is the fallacy of heel-knee test?**
3. **How tone is maintained by cerebellum?**
4. **What is cerebellar tremor?**
5. **What may be the pursuit abnormalities in this patient?**
6. **How can you check saccades?**
7. **What are the causes of cerebellar syndrome and how can you detect the causes?**
8. **What is scanning speech?**
9. **What are the signs that can localize the lesion in cerebellum?**
10. **What type of jerk can be elicited in the knee?**
11. **What are the causes and diagnostic points in paraneoplastic cerebellar degeneration?**

Answers

1. The most likely diagnosis is right cerebellar syndrome.
2. The fallacy of heel-knee test is that if the patient will rest the ankle over the shin, it will use the contour of the shin to guide its movement. As a result, the ataxia is masked. This can be overcome by placing the heel of one foot on the ankle of the other and drag it up to the shin of the knee.
3. In normal circumstances, deep cerebellar nuclei will send the reinforcing signals to motor cortex as well as cerebellar tract thereby the tone will be increased.
4. Cerebellar tremor is also known as intention tremor, where the tremor is not present at rest but increases during voluntary movement. It will be increased during approaching toward target.
5. Pursuit can be demonstrated when the patient is asked to follow the finger path of "H" fashion in front of the patient and the movement will be smooth. In case of cerebellar lesion, this smooth movement will be replaced by Jerky movement which is known as "broken pursuit". In case of internuclear ophthalmoplegia, there is impaired adduction of the

adducting eye associated with the nystagmus of the abducting eye.

6. Saccades can be demonstrated by asking the patient to keep his head in steady state and at the same time to look alternatively to the hands and the fingers placed in front of him wide apart. In this position, undershoots or hypometric saccades or overshoots or hypermetric saccades can be observed.

7. Causes of cerebellar syndrome are as follows:
   a. Demyelination in multiple sclerosis:
      • Internuclear ophthalmoplegia
      • Optic atrophy
   b. Alcoholic cerebellar degeneration:
      • Peripheral neuropathy
      • Features of liver disease
   c. Space occupying lesions in the posterior fossa:
      • Papilledema
      • Sixth nerve palsy: It is false localizing sign due to increased intracranial pressure due to compression of the fourth ventricle.
   d. Friedreich's ataxia:
      • Pes cavus
      • Signs of posterior column lesion in the legs
      • Absent ankle jerk
      • Extensor plantar response
   e. Paraneoplastic cerebellar degeneration:
      • Features of malignancy like:
         ○ Clubbing
         ○ Horner's syndrome
         ○ Lump in the breast in females
         ○ In male prostate cancer
      • Bilateral cerebellar signs
   f. Hypothyroidism:
      • Myxedematous facies
      • Delayed relaxation of the ankle jerk
      • Dry skin
      • Menorrhagia in females

8. Scanning speech means breaking the syllables. There is hesitancy to start the word.

9. Following are the signs that can localize the lesion in the cerebellum:
   a. In case of the lesion in the vermis, there is involvement of the muscles in the trunk and axis leading to truncal ataxia.
   b. In case of lesions in the cerebellar hemisphere, there is ipsilateral ataxia according to the site of involvement.

10. Pendular knee jerk can be elicited in this case, when there is swinging of the leg after hammer hitting the patellar tendon while the involved knee is allowed to hang over the other knee.

11. Causes of paraneoplastic cerebellar degeneration are malignancy of:
    a. Uterus
    b. Breast
    c. Ovary
    d. Small cell carcinoma of lung
    e. Hodgkin's lymphoma

This disease is immune mediated. This disease can be diagnosed by demonstrating the high titer of autoantibodies in the serum as well as cerebrospinal fluid (CSF). These autoantibodies develop as a result immune response to the tumor that will cross-react against the cells of the nervous system.

This cerebellar degeneration is always bilateral while cerebellar dysfunction due to other causes is always unilateral and according to the lesion.

CASE 5

A 52-year-old man came to medical outdoor with weakness of the hands and fine movements of the fingers. Also patient complained of inability to open the mouth after closure and there was difficulty in vision.

On examination, there is frontotemporal balding and wasting of the facial and neck muscles. There is wasting and weakness of the distal muscles with depressed deep. There was myotonia and high stepping gait.

1. **What is the most likely diagnosis?**
2. **What is the cause of visual abnormality?**
3. **What type of deformities will occur in the hand?**
4. **Why gripping will be absent in this patient in advanced cases?**
5. **What is myotonia?**
6. **How can you demonstrate myotonia?**
7. **What are the associated features?**
8. **Mention the genetic basis of this disease.**

9. **What are the other disorders involved in this genetic expansion?**
10. **What are the endocrinological complications?**
11. **What are the cardiovascular complications in this disease?**
12. **What are the types of this disease?**
13. **What are the channelopathies responsible for this disease?**

Answers

1. The most likely diagnosis is myotonic dystrophy.
2. The cause of visual abnormality is subcapsular cataract.
3. There is hyperextension of the metacarpophalangeal joints and hyperflexion of the interphalangeal joints producing claw hand.
4. In advanced cases of this disease gripping of the hand will be absent due to wasting of the small muscles of the hand.
5. Myotonia can be defined as continued contraction of the small muscles after cessation of voluntary contraction which is followed by impaired relaxation.
6. Myotonia can be demonstrated by gentle percussion at the hypothenar eminence when there is visible dent due to contraction of the muscles which will be filled slowly due to delayed relaxation.
7. Following are the associated features:
   a. Diabetes mellitus
   b. Hypogonadism as evidenced by gynecomastia and testicular atrophy
   c. Cardiomyopathy as evidenced by heart failure
   d. Mitral valve prolapse
   e. Conduction defects
   f. Atrial fibrillation
   g. Goiter as evidenced by nodular thyroid enlargement
8. Normal repeat of trinucleotide in the myosin protein kinase in chromosome 19 is 5 to 6 times, but in this disease the number of repeat is 2000 times. It will demonstrate expansion, i.e., increased severity of this disease with successive generation.
9. Following disorders involved in the repeat of expansion of trinucleotide are:
   a. Fragile X syndrome
   b. Friedreich's ataxia
   c. Huntington's chorea
   d. Spinocerebellar ataxia
   e. Dentataorubropallidolysian atrophy
10. Endocrinal complications in this disease:
    a. Diabetes mellitus
    b. Hypogonadism
    c. Nodular thyroid enlargement

11. Cardiovascular complications in this disease are as follows:
    a. Resting changes in ECG:
       • Prolonged PR interval
       • Prolonged QTC interval
       • ST-T wave changes
       • Low voltage P wave
       • Dominant R wave in V1
       • Widening of QRS complex
    b. Arrhythmias:
       • Supraventricular tachycardia
       • Ventricular tachycardia
       • Atrial flutter
       • Atrial fibrillation
    c. Conduction defect:
       • First-, second-, or third-degree atrioventricular (AV) block
    d. Mitral valve prolapse
    e. Cardiomyopathy:
       • Left ventricular hypertrophy
       • Myocardial myotonia
       • Cardiac fibro-fatty changes
12. There are two types of this disease:
    a. Type 1 myotonic dystrophy: Classical form
    b. Type 2 myotonic dystrophy: This is autosomal dominant. The clinical features are same as that in type 1, but there is proximal muscle wasting as well as weakness. Here, the genetic abnormality is repeat expansion of CCTG in the *ZNF9* gene on the chromosome number 3.
13. The causes of myotonia due to channelopathies are as follows:
    a. Myotonia congenita due to chloride ion channelopathy (CLC-1)
    b. Myotonia congenita, i.e., Becker's disease due to chloride ion channelopathy, autosomal recessive, late onset, and severe disease
    c. Paramyotonia congenita due to sodium ion channelopathy and autosomal dominant (SCN4A).
    d. Hyperkalemic periodic paralysis due sodium ion channelopathy and autosomal dominant
    e. Drugs like clofibrate

CASE 6

A 38-year-old smoker male came to medical outdoor with difficulty in walking and abnormal gait and callosities under the sole in both the feet. During walking, he also noticed abnormal movement of the knees.

On examination, there was lower motor type weakness of the involving both the lower limbs with depressed reflexes, sensory loss was in stocking distribution and also sensation carried by the posterior column, high stepping gait, and Romberg's sign was positive.

1. **What is the most likely diagnosis?**
2. **Prior to physical examination in the patient, what you have to look for in this patient?**
3. **What are the skin changes occur in this disease?**
4. **What are the sites for examining thickened peripheral nerve?**
5. **What are the common causes of thickened peripheral nerve?**
6. **What is the neuropathic joint?**
7. **Why wasting occurs distal toward proximal distribution?**
8. **In case of first involvement of the lower limb, when upper limb will start to be involved?**
9. **In small fiber neuropathy, why tendon reflexes will be intact?**
10. **Which sensory loss predicts which fiber neuropathy?**
11. **Why this patient has high stepping gait?**
12. **Is there any relation of high stepping gait with Romberg's gait?**
13. **What are the five causes of thickening of the peripheral nerves?**

Answers

1. The most likely diagnosis is peripheral sensorimotor neuropathy.
2. Prior to physical examination in this patient, following has to watch:
   a. Look for the walking aids
   b. Look for the walking shoes with ankle supports—it suggests foot drop
   c. Presence of scuffing in front of the shoes—it results from foot drop
   d. Presence of reduced manual dexterity like slip-on shoes and button on the clothes—it suggests distal motor neuropathy.
   e. Presence of any deformities like pes cavus—it indicates congenital neuropathy.
3. Following are the skin changes in this disease:
   a. Skin is dry and atrophic
   b. Hypopigmentation in the skin
   c. Ulcer formation
   d. Callosities under the sole
   e. Chronic infection due to repeated injuries and trauma leading to osteomyelitis
   f. Autonomic features such as warm, red and swollen, and pale and cold extremities due to loss of autoregulation of the blood vessels

4. Sites for examining the thickened nerves are as follows:
   a. At elbow for ulnar nerve
   b. At knee for common peroneal nerve
   c. On the dorsum of the foot for superficial peroneal nerve
5. Common causes of nerve thickening are as follows:
   a. Hereditary motor and sensory neuropathy
   b. Leprosy
   c. Amyloidosis
   d. Acromegaly
6. Neuropathic joint is characterized by swollen but painless joints with abnormal ranges of movements due to loss of pain sensation, there may be marked crepitus, and joints involved are ankle and elbow.
7. Wasting of the muscles occurs from distal to proximal distribution which is consistent with degeneration of length-dependent axon. Weakness starts in the toes and feet first, as the disease progresses, the disease will ascend upward.
8. When the wasting and loss of sensation reaches knee joints, the hands will start to be involved.
9. In case of small fiber neuropathy, sensory afferents from the muscle spindle will be spared; hence, the tendon reflexes will be intact.

10. In case of small fiber neuropathy, pain, temperature, and autonomic fibers will be affected.

    In case of large fiber neuropathies, vibration and proprioceptive senses will be affected.

11. This patient has loss of sensation in the ankle along with the foot drop due to motor neuropathy. This patient watches the ground carefully during walking to compensate the loss of position sense; hence, this patient demonstrates high stepping gait.

12. This patient has loss of sensation in the ankle along with the foot drop due to motor neuropathy. This patient watches the ground carefully during walking to compensate the loss of position sense. So, if the patient stands with his feet together with eye closed, the visual sensation will be off. The patient becomes unsteady and tends to fall.

13. Five causes of thickened peripheral nerves are:
    a. Amyloidosis
    b. Sarcoidosis
    c. Hypertrophic neuropathy
    d. Neurofibromatosis
    e. Acromegaly

CASE 7

A 38-year-old smoker male came to medical outdoor with ulcers and callosities under the feet and loss of hair up to the knee. On examination, bilateral symmetrical sensory loss was in stocking distribution and also sensation carried by the posterior column, high stepping gait, and Romberg's sign was positive.

1. **What is the most likely diagnosis?**
2. **What are the common causes of sensory neuropathy?**
3. **What are the causes of autonomic neuropathy?**
4. **What is small fiber neuropathy?**
5. **What are the causes of small fiber neuropathy?**
6. **Name seven causes of mononeuropathy multiplex.**

Answers

1. The most likely diagnosis is peripheral sensory neuropathy.
2. Common causes of sensory neuropathy are the following:
   a. Diabetes mellitus
   b. Hypothyroidism
   c. Uremia
   d. Vasculitis
   e. Vitamin B12 deficiency
   f. Infections:
      - Leprosy
      - Lyme disease
   g. Alcohol
3. Causes of autonomic neuropathy are the following:
   a. Guillain–Barré syndrome
   b. Human immunodeficiency virus (HIV) infection
   c. Amyloidosis
   d. Diabetes mellitus
   e. Botulism
4. Small fiber neuropathy is characterized by impaired small fibers carrying sensation. These fibers include:
   a. Thin myelinated A-delta fibers carrying cold, pain, and autonomic sensations
   b. Unmyelinated C fibers carrying temperature sensation
5. Following are the causes of small fiber neuropathy:
   a. Alcohol
   b. Diabetes
   c. Leprosy
   d. Hypothyroidism
   e. Amyloidosis
   f. Heavy metals:
      - Gold
      - Arsenic
6. Seven causes of mononeuritis multiplex are the following:
   a. Diabetes
   b. Rheumatoid arthritis
   c. Polyarteritis nodosa
   d. Sarcoidosis
   e. Lymphoma
   f. Wegener granulomatosis

CASE 8

A 42-year-old male came to neurology outdoor with difficulty in walking along with occasional tripping during walking on his right side. On examination, there is weakness of dorsiflexion and eversion at the ankle along with dorsiflexion of great toe on right side but preservation of inversion of the foot. Sensory examination demonstrated sensory loss on the dorsum of foot and lateral calf of right side. There is scar around the neck of the fibula.

1. **What is the most likely diagnosis?**
2. **What should you look for prior to physical examination of the patient?**
3. **What are the common causes of this disease?**
4. **What are the branches of the involved nerve?**
5. **What are the common causes of palsy of this nerve?**
6. **What are the predisposing factors for common peroneal nerve palsy?**
7. **What are the causes of mononeuropathy multiplex?**

Answers

1. The most likely diagnosis is common peroneal nerve palsy.
2. Following should be checked prior to physical examination of this patient:
   a. Walking aids
   b. Patient's shoes—to watch for the ankle supports or orthoses
   c. Scuffing at the front of the shoes resulting from the foot drop
3. Common causes of peroneal nerve palsy are the following:
   a. Extrinsic compression from short cast and braces
   b. Knee surgery
   c. Fracture of the fibula
4. There are two branches of the common peroneal nerve:
   a. Superficial peroneal nerve—responsible eversion of foot and carrying sensation on the lateral calf and dorsal surface of the foot.
   b. Deep peroneal nerve—responsible for dorsiflexion of foot and carrying sensation in the web space in between the first and second toe.
5. Causes of peroneal nerve palsy are the following:
   a. Extrinsic compression:
      - Short braces
      - Tourniquets
      - Cast of the plaster
      - Leg crossing

   - Sudden weight loss
   - Prolonged pressure on this nerve during surgery
   b. Trauma:
      - Fracture fibula
      - Direct trauma
      - Total arthroplasty of the knee
      - Proximal tibial osteotomy
6. Predisposing factors for common peroneal nerve lesion as follows:
   a. The peroneal nerve lies on the surface of hard bone where the nerve is covered by skin.
   b. Loss of pad of fat which is present over the fibular head as a result of sudden weight loss.
   c. The nerve can be tethered where it enters into the peroneus longus muscle. In this, this nerve is vulnerable to stretch-related injury.
7. Causes of mononeuritis multiplex are the following:
   - Leprosy
   - Diabetes mellitus
   - Polyarteritis nodosa
   - Churg–Strauss syndrome
   - Wegener granulomatosis
   - Rheumatoid arthritis
   - Systemic lupus erythematosus (SLE)
   - Sarcoidosis
   - Lymphoma
   - Sjögren's syndrome
   - Carcinoma
   - Lyme disease
   - Amyloidosis

CASE 9

A 55-year-old man came to medical outdoor with complaint in walking following sudden low back pain. On examination during walking, there was evidence of left-sided foot drop, weakness of inversion, eversion and dorsiflexion of foot, and dorsiflexion of the great toe and abduction of hip. Straight leg rising sign positive, sensation lost over the dorsum of the foot, and lateral side of the calf and lateral side of the thigh.

1. **What is the most likely diagnosis?**
2. **How can you differentiate this lesion from common peroneal nerve palsy?**
3. **What are the investigations that differentiate this lesion from common peroneal nerve palsy?**
4. **Mention the examples of the flaccid foot drop according to the site of the lesion.**
5. **Mention four causes of spastic foot drop.**

Answers

1. The most likely diagnosis is lesion in the L5 nerve root.
2. Following are the differentiating point between this lesion and common peroneal nerve palsy:

Clinical features	Common peroneal nerve palsy	L5 nerve root lesion
Ankle inversion	It is spared	It is affected
Abduction of hip	It is spared	It is affected
Sensory loss	Absent	Present
Presence of pain	Painless	Present
Inner hamstring jerk	Spared	Absent
Straight leg rising sign	Absent	Present

3. Following investigations differentiate this lesion from common peroneal nerve palsy:
   a. Neurophysiology: It can detect the common peroneal neuropathy and the site of lesion.
   b. Electromyography of tibialis posterior muscle to detect the L4/L5 lesion which is not innervated by common peroneal nerve.
   c. MRI of the spine that can detect the L5 lesion.
4. Examples of the flaccid foot drop according to site of lesion:

Sites of the lesion	Examples
Sciatic nerve	• Trauma • Surgery in the hip

Continued

Continued

Sites of the lesion	Examples
	• Neurofibroma • During intramuscular injection, damage of this nerve
Common peroneal nerve	• Short braces • Tourniquets • Plaster cast • Sudden loss of weight • Prolonged squatting
Involvement of L5 root	• Disk prolapse • Tumor in cauda equina • Neurofibroma
Cauda equina	Tumor
Lumbosacral plexus	Pelvic pathology
Lower motor neuron lesion	• Motor neuropathies • Motor neuron disease
Neuromuscular junction	Myasthenia gravis
Muscles	• Different myopathies • Spinal muscular atrophy

5. Following are the causes of spastic foot drop:
   a. Spinal cord: Spastic paraparesis
   b. Cauda equina: Tumor
   c. Parasagittal cortex: Tumor
   d. Internal capsule: Stroke

CASE 10

A 12-year-old male came to medical outdoor with slurring of speech, inability to walk, and swaying movement of the body on both sides during walking. On examination, patient has pes cavus, high-arched palate and kyphoscoliosis, wide-based gait, scanning speech, broken pursuit and hypermetric saccades in both directions, bilateral cerebellar signs, and pyramidal signs of both lower limbs with loss of knee and ankle jerks. There was bilateral posterior column sign along with positive Romberg's sign.

1. **What is the most likely diagnosis?**
2. **What are the points in favor of your diagnosis?**
3. **What may be the clinical clue to the cardiorespiratory cause of scoliosis?**
4. **What are the causes of high-arched palate?**
5. **Comment on the nystagmus in this patient.**
6. **How can you differentiate this disease from tabes dorsalis?**
7. **What are the other associated diseases may be present in this patient?**
8. **What is the genetic background in this disease?**
9. **Which nerves are involved and which nerves are not involved in this disease?**
10. **What are the clinicopathological correlations in this disease?**
11. **Mention the conditions where both knee and ankle jerks are absent but plantar extensor?**
12. **Mention the cardiac abnormalities associated with this disease.**
13. **What are the conditions where there is early onset recessive ataxia?**

Answers

1. The most likely diagnosis is Friedreich's ataxia.
2. Following points are in favor of this diagnosis:
   a. Young patient
   b. Features of cerebellar disease
   c. Congenital abnormalities:
      - Pes cavus
      - High-arched palate
   d. Pyramidal tract signs in the lower limb
   e. Depressed reflexes of ankle and knee jerks
   f. Extensor plantar response
   g. Peripheral neuropathy
3. Peripheral cyanosis may be the clinical clue to the severe scoliosis leading to cardiorespiratory morbidity.
4. Causes of high-arched palate are the following:
   a. Friedreich's ataxia
   b. Marfan syndrome
   c. Tuberous scoliosis
   d. Turner's syndrome
5. Cerebellar nystagmus is a horizontal coarse nystagmus having fast component toward the side of lesion.

   In case of bilateral cerebellar involvement, nystagmus will occur in both the directions on lateral gaze.

   In 20% patients, nystagmus is present in primary position that will be increased on lateral gaze.
6. In tabes dorsalis, there is:
   a. Absence of cerebellar signs
   b. Presence of Argyll Robertson pupil (ARP)
   These are absent in this disease.

7. The other associated diseases are present in Friedreich's ataxia:
   a. Diabetes mellitus
   b. Optic atrophy
   c. Hypertrophic cardiomyopathy
   d. Sensorineural deafness
8. This disease is autosomal recessive condition having genetic locus on chromosome 9q13, where mutation of trinucleotide repeats expansion of >200 times (normal 50 times) in this gene encoding a protein frataxin leads to abnormal regulation of iron as well as oxidative phosphorylation, as a result iron will be accumulated within the mitochondria of the affected cells. This accumulated iron leads to oxidative phosphorylation and formation of free radicals resulting in cellular death present in the spinal cord and peripheral nerves.
9. The following nerves are involved with there is demyelination of the nerve fibers:
   a. Pyramidal tract
   b. Spinal roots
   c. Posterior columns
   d. Corticospinal tract
   e. Spinocerebellar tract
   Following nerves are not involved:
   a. Unmyelinated fibers
   b. Sensory roots
   c. Peripheral nerves
10. Clinicopathological correlations in this disease are as follows:
    a. Degeneration of the posterior columns—loss of joint sense, position sense, and vibration sense
    b. Loss of the large nerve fibers in the dorsal root ganglia—absent or diminished reflexes

c.   Degeneration of the ventral spinocerebellar tract, dentate nucleus, dentate-rubral pathways, superior vermis, and Clarke column—cerebellar ataxia

d.   Involvement of corticospinal tract—upper motor neuronal lesion and extensor plantar response

11. In following conditions, there is depressed ankle and knee jerks but extensor plantar response:
   a.   Subacute combined degeneration
   b.   Tabes dorsalis
   c.   Friedreich's ataxia
   d.   Motor neuron disease
   e.   Conus medullaris lesion
   f.   Combination of conditions:
      - Peripheral neuropathy and stroke
      - Cervical myelopathy and peripheral neuropathy
      - Lumbar as well as cervical spondylosis

12. Following cardiac abnormalities are associated in this disease:
   a.   Left ventricular hypertrophy
   b.   Arrhythmias
   c.   Conduction defects
   d.   Chronic interstitial myocarditis
   e.   Inferolateral inversion of T wave in ECG
   f.   Myocardial fibrosis
   g.   Hypertrophic cardiomyopathy

13. Following are the early onset recessive ataxia:
   a.   Friedreich's ataxia
   b.   Ataxia telangiectasia
   c.   Refsum's disease
   d.   Abetalipoproteinemia

CASE 11

A 41-year-old man came to medical outdoor with slurred speech and tremor on the hand during work. On examination, speech was scanning, impaired adduction both eyes but abduction normal, and direct light reflex absent but consensual reflex is present. Cerebellar signs are present bilaterally. When abducting eye is closed, adduction of the opposite eye is normal. Hypermetric saccades along with nystagmus are seen in both the eyes. Position and joint sense were absent bilaterally. Fundoscopy demonstrated pale optic disk with distinct margin in the left eye.

1.   **What is the most likely diagnosis?**
2.   **What are the points in favor of this diagnosis?**
3.   **What are the sites where the demyelinating plaques have predilection for deposition?**
4.   **What are the organs that should be examined in this patient?**
5.   **Explain the eye lesions in this case.**
6.   **What is pseudoathetosis?**
7.   **If the cerebellar signs are associated with internuclear ophthalmoplegia, how can you differentiate these conditions?**
8.   **What do you mean by internuclear ophthalmoplegia?**
9.   **What are the causes of internuclear ophthalmoplegia?**
10. **What are the results of fundoscopy in this patient?**
11. **What are the different categories in this disease?**
12. **What is the most important shock-like sensory sign that may be present in this patient? What are the other conditions of this sign which may be present?**
13. **What are the drugs that prevent relapse?**

Answers

1.   The most likely diagnosis is multiple sclerosis.
2.   The points in favor of this diagnosis are:
   a.   Cerebellar signs
   b.   Pyramidal tract signs
   c.   Eye signs in fundoscopy
   d.   Dorsal column signs
3.   Following are the areas where there is predilection for deposition of the plaques:
   a.   Optic nerve leading to:
      - Optic atrophy
      - Afferent pupillary defect
   b.   Cerebellum leading to development of cerebellar signs

c. Brain stem leading to development of:
- Internuclear ophthalmoplegia
- Sensory loss in the face
- Upper motor neuron types of facial weakness
- Diplopia

d. Spinal cord leading to development of:
- Pyramidal tract signs
- Posterior column signs such as loss of vibration sense and position sense.

4. Following organs should be examined:
a. Eye for fundoscopy
b. Cerebellar signs in upper and lower limbs
c. Upper limb for pyramidal tract signs
d. Lower limb for pyramidal tract and posterior column signs

5. Eye lesions are:
a. Optic atrophy from optic neuritis
b. Afferent pupillary defect such as loss of direct light reflex and presence of consensual light reflex
c. In the affected eye, there is visual field defect like presence of central scotoma.

6. Pseudoathetosis is characterized by appearance of writhing movement of the finger when both the eyes are closed.

7. If there is presence of both cerebellar signs along with internuclear ophthalmoplegia, in that case:
a. Impairment of adduction is the key sign to diagnose internuclear ophthalmoplegia.
b. Nystagmus with fast phase toward the side of lesion in case of unilateral cerebellar lesion and both sides in case of bilateral cerebellar lesion
c. When the abducting eyes are closed, the adducting eyes will be normal.

8. Medial longitudinal fasciculus starts from below the posterior commissure and ends into the upper cervical cord connecting ipsilateral third nucleus (medial rectus for adduction) with the contralateral sixth nerve nucleus involving lateral rectus muscles for abduction. This tract maintains the conjugate eye movements.

Lesion of this fasciculus—there is loss of ipsilateral adduction. Normal abduction of the contralateral eye—there is divergence. As a result, the abducting eye will flick back toward the nose for correction followed by abduction resulting in few beats of nystagmus in the contralateral eye. So, the key feature of internuclear ophthalmoplegia is weakness in the ipsilateral adduction and nystagmus of the abducting eye.

9. Causes of internuclear ophthalmoplegia are as follows:
a. Multiple sclerosis
b. Systemic lupus erythematosus
c. Lesions in the brainstem:
- Infarction
- Tumors
- Aneurysm
d. Wernicke's encephalopathy
e. Miller Fisher syndrome
f. Overdose of the drugs:
- Tricyclic antidepressant (TCA)
- Phenytoin
- Barbiturates

10. Fundoscopy results in this patient: Disk is pale with clear and distinct margin.

11. Following are the categories in this disease:
a. Relapsing remitting: It is characterized by short-lasting acute attack followed by steady state in the baseline indicating remission for a period.
b. Secondary progressive: This is characterized by gradual progression in the course of the disease in the relapsing remitting form of this disease.
c. Primary progressive variety: It is characterized by gradual progression in the feature of this disease from its onset without any remission.
d. Progressive relapsing: It is characterized by progressive deterioration if this disease with superimposition of relapses.

12. Lhermitte's sign is characterized by electric shock such as sensation passing down the spine into the hands and legs indicating the involvement of the dorsal column in the spinal cord. The causes are:
a. Multiple sclerosis
b. Tumor in the cervical cord
c. Cervical myelopathy
d. Subacute combined degeneration of the spinal cord

13. Following drugs can prevent relapse:
a. Interferon-β:
- It will reduce the relapse rate.
- It will reduce the inflammatory activity by 50–80%.
- It will improve the cognitive function as well as quality of the life.
- It will results in the formation of neutralizing antibodies.

- The adverse effects:
  - Flu-like syndrome
  - Fatigue
  - Myalgia
- b. Glatiramer:
  - It will reduce the relapse rate by 35%.
  - It is a synthetic polypeptide.
  - It will compete with the autoantigen myelin basic protein.
  - There is 30–40% reduction in the inflammatory activity.
  - It can be easily tolerated.
- c. Mitoxantrone:
  - It is anthracenedione chemotherapeutic agent

- 67% relapse activity will be reduced.
- It can be used for 2–3 years because of its cumulative cardiotoxicity
- Adverse effects are:
  - Alopecia
  - Nausea
- d. Natalizumab:
  - It is monoclonal antibody acting against $\alpha 4$ integrin present on the leukocytes.
  - 67% relapse rate will be reduced.
  - 80–90% inflammatory activity will be reduced in MRI.

CASE 12

A 45-year-old man came to medical outdoor with left upper limb demonstrating upper motor neuron type of weakness. Cerebellar sign demonstrated intention tremor, dysdiadochokinesia, impaired finger-nose test, rebound phenomenon, and scanning speech. Posterior column demonstrated loss of vibration and proprioception.

1. **What will be the next examination?**
2. **What is the most likely diagnosis?**
3. **What type of atrophy occurs in this case?**
4. **Why pain and temperature sensation will not be affected in this patient?**
5. **If the lower limb is affected, what are the gait abnormalities may be found?**
6. **What are the features in the CSF in this case?**

Answers

1. Next examination is fundoscopic examination of the eye which will demonstrate optic atrophy. Visual field examination demonstrates central scotoma.
2. The most likely diagnosis is multiple sclerosis.
3. Disuse atrophy occurs in this disease
4. As pain and temperature are carried out by the unmyelinated sensory nerve fibers, hence these sensations are not affected in this patient.
5. If the lower limb is affected, the following gait abnormalities can be found:
   a. Cerebellar gait—wide-based ataxic gait
   b. Hemiplegic gait
   c. In case of bilateral pyramidal weakness, Scissor gait
   d. Sensory gait: It is wide-based ataxic gait where the patient will look at the ground carefully during walking because visual input compensates for the loss of joint and position sense. But in this case, ataxic gait is mainly cerebellar.
6. a. Total protein/albumin quotient is normal or slightly elevated.
   b. CSF: Serum glucose ration is normal.
   c. CSF leukocyte count in 98% cases is less than 50/cc.
   d. 90% are lymphocytes rarely monocytes
   e. Immunoglobulin are IgG by linear or non-linear formulae are elevated in 60% patients, in some cases IgM and IgA synthesis may be found.
   f. In 95% cases oligoclonal band may be found.

CASE 13

A patient presented with bilateral lower limb upper motor neuron type weakness with loss of sensations having a sensory level at thoracic spine 8.

1. **What is your most likely diagnosis?**
2. **What are the group of muscles that are affected in the lower limbs?**
3. **Prior to examination of the patient, what are the clues you may get in the surrounding of the patient?**
4. **What are the maneuvers that can demonstrate the plantar extension?**
5. **How can you diagnose associated cerebellar lesion in this patient?**
6. **What are the gaits you may see in this patient?**
7. **What are the features you may see in the anterior spinal artery occlusion?**
8. **What are the features of tropical spastic paraparesis?**
9. **What is transverse myelitis?**

Answers

1. The most likely the diagnosis is spastic paraparesis due to the lesion at the level of thoracic spine 8.
2. In the lower limb, following group of muscles are involved:
   a. Hip flexors
   b. Knee flexors
   c. Ankle dorsiflexors
   d. Muscles of ankle eversion
3. Prior to examining the patient, following can be seen in the surroundings of the patient:
   a. Walking aids
   b. Patient's shoes for ankle supports suggesting associated foot drop
   c. Scuffing in front of the shoes resulting from the foot drop
   d. Wheelchair indicating disability of the patient
   e. Indwelling catheter suggesting bladder involvement
4. Following maneuvers are involved to demonstrate the planter extension:
   a. Chaddock's maneuver: Here, the plantar extension can be elicited on the dorsolateral aspect of the foot.
   b. As the severity of the disease is increased, the plantar extension can be elicited from the whole sole of the foot.
   c. Oppenheim sign: Here, the extensor plantar response will be elicited by pressing the inner border of the tibia heavily.
   d. Gordon sign: Here extensor plantar response can be elicited by pinching the Achilles tendon.

5. Associated cerebellar involvement can be diagnosed by examining the worsening of the tremor when the heel will approaches the heel or knee.
6. There are two gaits can be seen in this patient:
   a. Scissor's gait—in case of bilateral spastic weakness of the both lower limbs
   b. High steppage gait—it suggests foot drop
7. In case of anterior spinal artery occlusion:
   a. There is loss of sensations related to spinothalamic tract.
   b. Preservation of sensations related to posterior column
8. Features of tropical spastic paraparesis are the following:
   a. HTLV-1-associated neuropathy in common endemic area such as Japan, Africa, South America, and Caribbean.
   b. Incubation period ranges from months to years
   c. Progressive spastic paraparesis
   d. Disturbances in the sphincter
   e. Mild sensory involvement
   f. Transmission through the:
      • Sexual contact
      • Needle sharing
      • Blood product
      • Vertical transmission
9. Features of transverse myelitis are the following:
   a. It is caused by inflammation of the spinal cord diffusely or one or multiple levels. The causes are as follows:
      • Bacteria

- Viral
- Demyelinating
- Radiation
- Anterior spinal occlusion
- Vasculitis

b. Bilateral involvement of:
- Motor deficit
- Sensory deficit
- Sphincter deficit

CASE 14

A patient came to medical outdoor with complaints in the upper limb—segmental wasting of biceps, depressed reflexes of biceps, and supinator jerk with inversion of exaggerated triceps jerks. Loss of all modalities of sensation in cervical 5–7 involved dermatomes.

1. **What is the most likely diagnosis?**
2. **What is myelopathy hand sign?**
3. **What are the muscles affected by in this lesion?**
4. **What do you mean by inversion?**
5. **What do you mean by "midcervical reflex pattern"?**
6. **What are the other signs can be seen in this patient?**
7. **What is the dorsal column sign in this patient?**
8. **What are the causes of this disease?**
9. **What are the structures present in the cervical canal?**
10. **Why plain cervical X-ray is required in this patient?**

Answers

1. The most likely diagnosis is cervical myelopathy.
2. Myelopathy hand sign can be described as in eye closed with outstretched and supinated hand there is abduction of the little finger and deficient adduction and/or extension of ulnar two or three fingers. This is also known as "finger escape sign".
3. Following muscles are involved:
   a. Biceps—elbow fraction
   b. Brachioradialis—forearm supination
   c. Deltoid—abduction of shoulder
4. Inversion means—absence of response in the biceps and brachioradialis along with the reflex contraction of the myotome that is innervated by the lower segments, i.e., finger flexors or triceps.
5. "Midcervical reflex pattern" can be described as combination of inverted supinator and biceps jerk (C5 and C6) and exaggerated triceps jerk (C7 to C8).
6. There are two other signs present in this patient:
   a. Grip and release test: Normal subject can open and close the fist up to 20 times within 10 seconds, but this patient with cervical myelopathy has difficulty in performing this maneuvers which may be slow and incomplete.
   b. Dynamic Hoffman's sign: This can be elicited by nipping the nail of the middle finger. During this time, there will be contraction of the thumb and index fingers. If this test is negative during rest, this should be elicited during active flexion as well as extension of the cervical spine and this will become positive during this maneuvers.
7. With closed eyes, there is writhing movements of the fingers in absence of sensory feedback in this cervical cord lesion which is known as pseudoathetosis. It is sign of dorsal column involvement.
8. Causes of cervical myelopathy are the following:
   a. Degenerative disease of the cervical disk in the cervical region:
   - Primary osteoarthritis
   - Rheumatoid arthritis
   - Ankylosing spondylitis
   - Acromegaly
   - Achondroplasia
   b. Trauma
   c. Tumor in the cervical cord
   d. Ossified posterior longitudinal ligament
9. Following structures present in the cervical canal:
   a. Nerves
   b. Meninges
   c. Ligaments
   d. Epidural fat

10. Straight X-ray of cervical spine in AP, lateral, and oblique view: It can evaluate—
    a. Intervertebral disk space
    b. Facet joints
    c. Formation of osteophytes
    d. Absolute sagittal diameter in the spinal canal

CASE 15

This patient came to medical outdoor with horizontal nystagmus having fast component to the right, broken pursuit, and hypermetric saccades.

1. **What is your diagnosis?**
2. **If the lesion is in the left side, what is your inference?**
3. **Why this nystagmus is not of vestibular origin?**

Answers

1. The most likely diagnosis is right cerebellar lesion.
2. If the lesion is left-sided, the fast component is away from the lesion.
3. In case of vestibular origin, nystagmus is of two types:
    a. In case peripheral variety:
        • The nystagmus is either horizontal rotatory type or horizontal.
        • It is always unidirectional with fast component being away from the side of lesion.
        • Nystagmus will be increased toward the direction of the fast component.
    b. In case of central type:
        • The nystagmus may be horizontal, rotatory, vertical, or mixed.
        • This nystagmus is bidirectional.
        • Component changes with the direction of gaze. So, the nystagmus is left-beating on the left gaze, whereas right-beating on the right gaze.

CASE 16

This patient has impaired adduction with nystagmus but abduction is normal in both eyes. But if abducting is covered, the adduction in the opposite eyes becomes normal. On lateral gaze, there is diplopia.

1. **What is the most likely diagnosis?**
2. **Where is the site of lesion?**
3. **What are the common causes of this lesion?**
4. **What are the types of impaired adduction?**
5. **What are the drugs responsible for this lesion?**

Answers

1. The most likely diagnosis is bilateral internuclear ophthalmoplegia.
2. The site of lesion is medial longitudinal fasciculus.
3. The common causes of lesion are the following:
    a. Multiple sclerosis
    b. Infarction
    c. Tumor
    d. Vasculitis
    e. Trauma
    f. Syphilis
    g. Aneurysm
    h. Wernicke's encephalopathy
    i. Arnold–Chiari malformation
4. There are two types of adduction:
    On attempted horizontal gaze impaired adduction may be:
    a. Complete, where the eyes will not cross the midpoint.
    b. Partial, where the adduction is slower than normal speed.
5. Following drugs are responsible for this internuclear ophthalmoplegia:
    a. Phenytoin
    b. TCA
    c. Barbiturate

CASE 17

A 39-year-old male presented with progressive weakness of the hands. On examination, all the intrinsic muscles including thenar and hypothenar eminences and claw hand. There was also weakness of wrist extensor are atrophied. Deep tendon reflexes were depressed. Sensory system as well as coordination was normal.

1. **What are the neural structures involved in this case?**
2. **What are the differential diagnoses?**
3. **How can you come to the final diagnosis?**
4. **What are the causes of claw hand?**
5. **What are the muscles involved in the flexion and extension of the small joints of the hand?**
6. **If there was sensory involvement in the specific dermatome related to C8 and T1 and presence of clubbing and Horner's syndrome, what is the diagnosis?**
7. **What are the actions of the muscles of the hand?**
8. **What is "split hand syndrome"?**
9. **What are the specific signs can dictate specific diagnosis?**

Answers

1. Following neural structures are involved in this case:
   a. Anterior horn cells
   b. Nerve roots
   c. Lower motor neurons originating from C8 to T1
2. The differential diagnoses are the following:
   a. Peripheral motor neuropathy
   b. Motor neuron disease, i.e., progressive muscular atrophy
3. Final diagnosis:
   a. If the wasting preferentially affects the ulnar or median nerve innervated muscles, the diagnosis is peripheral mononeuropathy.
   b. If the wasting involves all the nerves proportionately then the generalized wasting suggests involvement of anterior horn cells, nerve roots, or lower motor neurons which is known as motor neuron disease. Again, weakness of the wrist extensor suggests motor neuron disease.
4. The causes of the claw hand are:
   a. Hyperextension of metacarpophalangeal joints
   b. Flexion of the proximal and distal interphalangeal joints
5. Following muscles are involved in the flexion and extension of the small joints of the hand:
   a. Flexion:
      - Metacarpophalangeal joints:
        - Lumbricals
        - Interossei
      - Proximal interphalangeal joint: Flexor digitorum sublimis
      - Distal interphalangeal joint: Flexor digitorum profundus
   b. Extension:
      - Metacarpophalangeal joints: Extensor digitorum
      - Proximal interphalangeal joint:
        - Lumbricals
        - Interossei
      - Distal interphalangeal joint:
        - Lumbricals
        - Interossei
6. If there was sensory involvement in the specific dermatome related to C8 and T1 and presence of clubbing and Horner's syndrome, the diagnosis is Pancoast tumor.
   Features of Horner's syndrome are the following:
   a. Unilateral involvement
   b. Miosis
   c. Partial ptosis
   d. Facial anhidrosis
7. Following are the actions of the muscles of the hand:
   a. Abductor pollicis brevis—abduction of the thumb
   b. Opponens pollicis—opposition of thumb
   c. Palmar interossei—adduction of the fingers (PAD)
   d. Dorsal interossei—abduction of the fingers (DAB)
   e. Abductor digiti minimi—abduction of the little finger
8. In case of motor neuron disease, thenar muscles are more denervated as compared to hypothenar muscles. Again, first dorsal interossei are more denervated as compared to thenar muscles. As a result, muscles of the lateral aspect of the hand are more affected as

compared to medial aspect muscles. This is known as "split hand". This syndrome can also occur in case of spinal muscular atrophy and poliomyelitis.

9. Following specific signs can dictate the diagnosis if this patient presented with the above features:
    a. General features:
        - Rheumatoid arthritis—disuse atrophy
        - Presence of cervical collar—cervical myelopathy
    b. Face:
        - Specific facies—myotonic dystrophy
        - Fasciculation in the tongue muscles—motor neuron disease
    c. Eyes:
        - Presence of Horner's syndrome—Pancoast tumor and syringomyelia
        - Presence of ptosis—myotonic dystrophy
        - Internuclear ophthalmoplegia—syringomyelia
    d. Hands:
        - Clubbing—Pancoast syndrome
        - Myotonia—myotonic dystrophy
    e. Feet: Pes cavus—Friedreich's ataxia, old poliomyelitis, and hereditary motor neuropathy
    f. Legs: Inverted champagne bottle—hereditary motor as well as sensory neuropathy
    g. Gait—spastic paraparesis:
        - Syringomyelia
        - Cervical myelopathy
        - Motor neuron disease
        - Tumor

CASE 18

A 43-year-old male presented with wasting of the upper limb and swollen elbow joints moving abnormally. On examination, there is kyphoscoliosis, distal muscle wasting along with wasting of the small muscles of the hands, absent deep tendon reflexes, and dissociated sensory loss in the hands. There is scar in the midline in cervical region.

1. **What is the most likely diagnosis?**
2. **Why there is this type of deformity?**
3. **Why there is scar in the cervical region?**
4. **What do you mean by dissociated sensory loss?**
5. **What do you mean by Charcot joints?**
6. **What do you mean by "La main succulente"?**
7. **What is the result of extension of the syrinx?**
8. **What are the diagnostic points in favor of syringomyelia?**
9. **What are the other neurological structures that may be involved in this disease?**
10. **What are the causes of this disease?**
11. **How can you explain the clinical signs in this disease?**
12. **What are the other causes of dissociated sensory loss?**
13. **What are the treatment procedures in this disease?**

Answers

1. The most likely diagnosis is syringomyelia.
2. Kyphoscoliosis is due to involvement of the median motor nuclei innervating paraspinal muscles.
3. Cervical scar is due to either:
    a. Cervical laminectomy or
    b. Decompression of the syrinx
4. Dissociated sensory loss means the absence of pain and temperature with preservation of vibration and position senses.
5. Charcot joint means a neuropathic joint which is swollen deformed joint with abnormal range of movement which is due to loss of joint and position sense.
6. "La main succulente" means cold, edematous, and cyanosed hands due to trophic and vasomotor disturbances.
7. Extension of syrinx:
    a. Anterior extension into the anterior horn cells in the spinal cord will damage the lower motor

neurons leading to diffuse muscle atrophy beginning in the hands and progressing proximally to include forearm and shoulder girdles. There are dorsal guttering and claw hand.

b. Anterior extension will involve the decussating fibers of spinothalamic tract in the corresponding segments leading to loss of pain and temperature sensation in the hand with intact position and joint sense.

c. Posterior extension of the syrinx will involve posterior column leading to loss of position and joint sense.

8. Following points diagnose syringomyelia:

a. Lower motor neuron signs in the upper limb

b. Upper motor neuron sign in the lower limb

c. Dissociated sensory loss in the upper limb.

9. Following structures may be involved in this disease:

a. To determine the lowest point of the syrinx, sensation of the trunk beyond should be tested.

b. If Horner's syndrome is found, it suggests involvement of the sympathetic neurons in the intermediolateral cell column in the spinal cord indicating extension of the syrinx superiorly to C8 to T1

c. Involvement of cranial nerves 9th to 12th indicates the extension of the syrinx to bulb

d. Internuclear ophthalmoplegia, i.e., impaired adduction associated with nystagmus in the abducting eyes indicates involvement of medial longitudinal fasciculus.

e. Examination of facial sensation: Long nucleus of 5th cranial nerve—upper portion of the nucleus receives sensation from the inner part of the face and lower part receives sensation from the outer part of the face. So, the lower part of the nucleus will be involved by the syrinx before reaching medulla.

10. The causes of syringomyelia:

a. Idiopathic

b. Blockage of CSF: This is most common cause
   - Arnold–Chiari malformation
   - Basal arachnoiditis
   - Basilar invagination
   - Meningeal carcinomatosis
   - Arachnoid cyst
   - Meningioma at the foramen magnum

c. Injury to spinal cord

d. Intramedullary tumor

11. The clinical signs in this disease can be explained by the following methods:

As the syrinx extends throughout the cervical and thoracic segment of spinal cord, the signs can be subdivided into the following:

a. At the level of syrinx:
   - Anterior horn cells of the cord will be affected leading to damage of the lower motor neuron throughout the length of the tumor resulting in lower motor neuron signs in that levels.
   - Decussating fibers of the anterior spinothalamic tract throughout the level of the syrinx leading to loss of sensation of pain and temperatures in the affected segments but not involving the vibration and position sense.

b. Below the level of syrinx: Corticospinal tract will be involved at the level of syrinx leading to development of upper motor neuron signs in the lower half.

12. Causes of dissociated sensory loss are as follows:

a. Occlusion of anterior spinal artery

b. Small fiber neuropathies involving thin myelinated nerve fibers A-delta fibers responsible for cold, pain, and temperature and unmyelinated nerve fibers C fibers responsible for warmth

13. Following are the treatment in this disease:

a. Cervical decompression through the suboccipital craniectomy, C1 to C3 laminectomy, and duraplasty

b. Dorsolateral myelotomy

c. Shunt formation: Following are the shunt procedures:
   - Syringoperitoneal shunt
   - Syringosubarachnoid shunt
   - Ventriculoperitoneal shunt

CASE 19

In the swinging torch test, there is dilatation of the pupil but there is sustained constriction of the left pupil.

1. **What is your diagnosis?**
2. **What are the causes of this disease?**
3. **What is the result if the eyes are tested separately?**
4. **What is the aim of swinging torch test?**
5. **When this type of defect will occur?**

Answers

1. The patient has been suffering from relative afferent pupillary defect, i.e., Marcus Gunn pupil.
2. The causes of this disease are as follows:
   a. Disease of the optic nerve
   b. Disease of the retina
3. If the eyes are tested separately, both the direct and consensual reflexes are intact.
4. The aim of swinging torch test:
   a. In the normal condition putting the light on the pupil, both the pupils will constrict and it will persist throughout the examination period.
   b. In the case of afferent pupillary defect in the one eye, the function of the optic nerve will provide adequate direct reflex to the affected side and consensual reflex on the opposite side.
   c. During this swinging torch light test as the light will be switched back to the affected side, direct reflex on the affected side is weaker as compared to consensual reflex in the unaffected side. When the light is removed from the opposite eye, the consensual reflex pupil will dilate.
   d. When the torch light is shown to the affected side, there is abnormal pupillary dilatation.
5. Pupillary defect will occur in:
   a. Optic nerve disease
   b. Retinal disease
   c. Difference in the extent of this disease in-between the eyes. Because both the eyes are affected equally, there will be no apparent pupillary defect.

CASE 20

A 45-year-old man demonstrated:

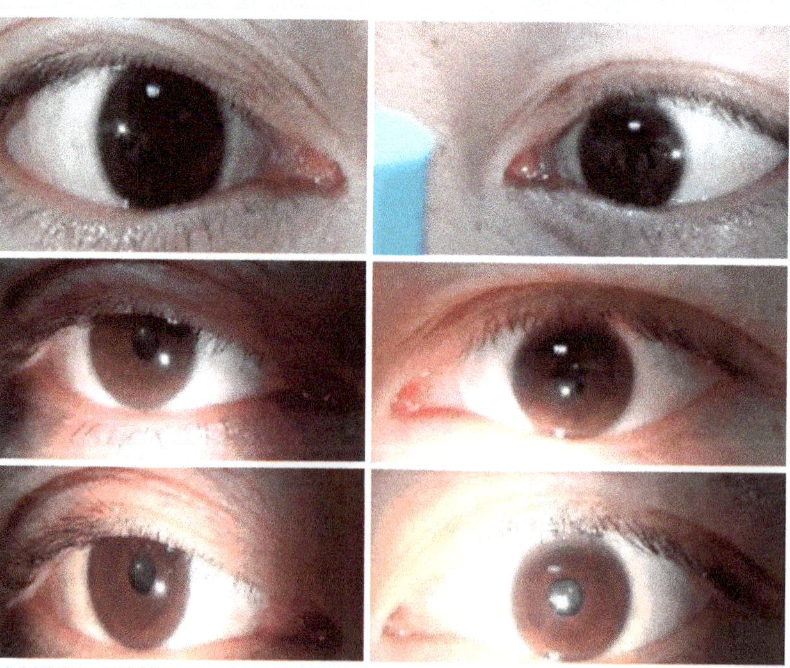

1. **What is shown in above pictures?**
2. **What is the most likely diagnosis?**
3. **What is the most common cause and what are the other features to look for to reach that diagnosis?**
4. **What are the other causes of this condition?**
5. **What is the site of lesion?**
6. **What is reversed of this pupil?**
7. **What is pseudotype of this pupil?**

Answers

1. The above pictures demonstrate:
   a. Both the pupils are small and unequal.
   b. Both the pupil normally accommodate to an object
   c. The pupils will not react to light.
2. The diagnosis is Argyll Robertson pupil.
3. The most common cause of ARP is syphilis. Following features should be checked to reach this specific diagnosis:
   a. Optic atrophy—syphilitic meningitis
   b. Charcot joints along with trophic ulcers—involvement of posterior column in this disease
   c. Sensory ataxia—indicates positive Romberg test
   d. 6th, 7th, and 8th cranial nerves are affected—suggest syphilitic meningitis
   e. Loss of joint sense as well as position sense—indicates posterior column lesion
   f. Loss of ankle jerk and plantar extensor—indicates tabes dorsalis
   g. Presence of dementia—indicates neurosyphilis
   h. Cardiac examination demonstrates murmur of aortic regurgitation—indicates syphilitic aortitis

4. Other causes of ARP are the following:
   a. Diabetes mellitus
   b. Lesions in the midbrain:
      - Infarction
      - Tumor
      - Hemorrhage
      - Syringobulbia
      - Sarcoidosis
      - Demyelination
   c. Wernicke's encephalopathy
   d. Brainstem encephalitis
   e. Lyme disease
5. The site of lesion is most probably in the pretectal region of the midbrain which is proximal to oculomotor nuclei. But, this cannot explain the contour of the pupil which may be due to local cause.
6. Reversed ARP means normal reaction to light but absence of accommodation to an object, which is seen encephalitis lethargica.
7. Pseudo-ARP means aberrant regeneration which follows complete 3rd nerve palsy leading to incomplete and abnormal recovery. This pupil looks like ARP but unresponsive to light and accommodation reaction will be preserved.

CASE 21

In eye examination, right eye constricts slowly to light and accommodation, but in response to the continuous stimulus the constriction was excessive, but after removal of the stimulus that pupil gradually dilated to normal.

1. **What is the most likely diagnosis?**
2. **How can you differentiate this pupil from ARP?**
3. **Mention the light pathways.**
4. **Mention the site of lesion.**
5. **What are the extra features you expect in Holmes–Adie syndrome?**
6. **What is the effect of 0.1% pilocarpine in this pupil?**
7. **What is the size of the pupil in older age and why?**

Answers

1. The most likely diagnosis is myotonic pupil.
2. The difference between ARP and myotonic pupil:

Features	ARP	Myotonic pupil
Size of the pupil	Small	Usually large
Accommodation reflex	Present	Delayed response
Light reflex	Absent	Delayed response
Affection of eye	Bilateral	Unilateral
Reaction to mydriatics	Poor response	Normal response
Reaction to weak cholinergic	Response absent	Hyperactive
Associated features	Other features of syphilis	Tendon reflexes absent

3. Light pathways: Optic nerve—optic chiasma—optic tract—bypassing lateral geniculate body to pretectal area of the midbrain—to Edinger-Westphal nucleus in the midbrain. From this nucleus, the efferent pathway starts through oculomotor nerve, which through the ciliary ganglion will reach ciliary muscles of the eye.

4. The site of lesion is at the postganglionic parasympathetic fibers in the ciliary ganglion.
5. In case extra features in Holmes–Adie syndrome:
   a. Absent deep tendon reflexes due to synaptic disorders in the spinal reflex pathways
   b. Diffuse or localized autonomic disturbances:
      - Postural hypotension
      - Hypohidrosis
      - Chronic diarrhea
6. 0.1% pilocarpine is a weak cholinergic agent having normal effect in the normal pupil. In myotonic pupil since there is parasympathetic denervation, acetylcholine hypersensitivity results in pupilloconstrictor response.
7. Size of the pupil depends upon the interaction between the sympathetic and parasympathetic stimulation. Activation of parasympathetic nerve mediates through the 3rd nerve and it is affected by light reflex pathways. Activation of the sympathetic nerve is the inherent property not activated by the external stimuli. In the extremes of age, sympathetic tone is less leading to physiologically smaller pupil.

CASE 22

Eye examination revealed:

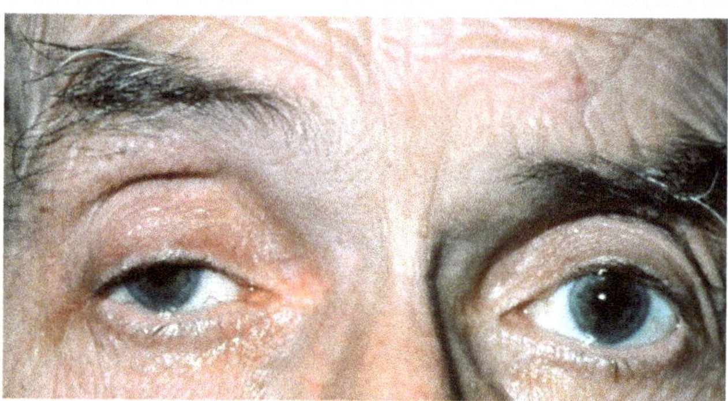

In this patient, light reflex and accommodation reflex are present along with ipsilateral anhidrosis on the face only. There was evidence of a scar on the right side of the neck.

1. **What is revealed in the above picture?**
2. **What is the most likely diagnosis?**
3. **What is the importance of scar?**
4. **How can you demonstrate anhidrosis?**
5. **What are the causes of miosis?**
6. **What is the response of the pupil to dim vision or far vision?**
7. **Why there is partial ptosis in this disease? What is the difference between partial and complete ptosis?**
8. **Is it true enophthalmos, if not, why?**
9. **Which movement can overcome this partial ptosis?**

10. **Describe sympathetic neuron in this case according to order?**
11. **How can you classify this lesion?**
12. **What is the pattern of anhidrosis according to the site of lesion?**
13. **What is the effect of 1:1,000 adrenaline on this different pattern of lesion?**
14. **What is the effect of 1% hydroxyamphetamine in this different pattern of lesion?**
15. **How can you diagnose the etiology of this syndrome clinically?**
16. **What are the causes of unilateral ptosis?**
17. **What are the causes of this disease?**

Answers

1. The features in the above picture are:
   a. Miosis
   b. Enophthalmos
   c. Ipsilateral anhidrosis over the face
2. The most likely diagnosis is Horner's syndrome.
3. The scar is due to previous neck surgery.
4. Anhidrosis can be demonstrated by stroking the skin over the face by the side of the pen and comparing with the other side. In case of anhidrotic skin, the pen will glide easily over the skin surface more freely. Prior to this testing, sweat test should be done. The areas in the body to be tested are face, neck, and upper trunk.
5. Miosis is due to involvement of the pupillodilator fibers.
6. As the sympathetic pupillodilator fibers are impaired, in response to dim light or far vision, pupil either does not dilate or slowly dilate.
7. Ptosis can be defined as when all parts of the pupil will be covered by the eyelid. It may be unilateral or bilateral. Upper eyelid is covered by levetor palpebrae superioris innervated by 3rd nerve but both the eyelids are controlled by Müller's muscles innervated by sympathetic fibers. In Horner's syndrome, the later muscle is affected in this disease due to involvement of sympathetic pupillodilator fibers, as a result upper eyelid will come down and lower eye will come up to some extent leading to production of the narrow palpebral fissure.
8. It is not true enophthalmos because the palpebral fissure is not involved in this case. Hence, it is partial enophthalmos.
9. Voluntary upward gaze can overcome the partial ptosis.
10. There are three order of neuron:
    a. First order of neuron: The nerve starts from hypothalamus to brain stem through the spinal cord to T1 root in the spinal cord.
    b. Second order of neuron: From T1 root in the spinal cord, second order of neuron will originate and runs along the cervical sympathetic chain to relay into superior cervical ganglion.
    c. Third order of neuron originates from superior cervical ganglion and reaches Müller's muscles, pupils, and sweat gland.
11. There are two types of lesion:
    a. Central lesion: It will affect the first order of neuron.
    b. Peripheral lesion: It will affect second and third order of neuron.
12. Pattern of anhidrosis according to site of lesion:
    a. Central lesion: There is anhidrosis in ipsilateral face, neck, and upper trunk.
    b. Peripheral preganglionic lesion: There is anhidrosis in ipsilateral face only.
    c. Peripheral postganglionic lesion: No anhidrosis
13. When 1:1,000 adrenaline eye drop is given:
    In case of postganglionic lesion, there is postganglionic denervation leading to depletion of amine oxidase; as a result, pupil is sensitized to adrenaline.
    In case of preganglionic and central lesion, amine oxidase will be present which breaks down the adrenaline rapidly before its accumulation in the cleft.
    So, in central, preganglionic lesion and normal condition, adrenaline has no effect whereas in postganglionic lesion, the pupil will be dilated.
14. Hydroxyamphetamine will stimulate the presynaptic region in the superior cervical ganglion. So in case of central and preganglionic lesion, the pupil will be dilated as that of normal pupil. If the lesion is in the postganglionic region, pupil will not dilate as that of normal pupil.
15. Etiology of this syndrome can be diagnosed in this method:
    a. In the neck:
       • Presence of scars:
         ○ Trauma
         ○ History of previous neck surgery
         ○ Central venous catheterization

- Masses:
  - Lymphadenopathy
  - Goiter
  - Tumor
- Aneurysm

b. In the hands:
- Stain of nicotine, clubbing, wasting of the muscles of the hand, and sensory loss at the level of C8 to T1—pancoast tumor
- Wasting in the small muscle of the hand, dissociated sensory loss, fasciculation in the small muscles in the hand—syringomyelia

c. Chest:
- Hemoptysis, bronchial breath sound, crepitation in the apical region—pancoast tumor
- Cervical rib
- Thoracotomy scar and sternotomy scar—past history of cardiothoracic surgery

16. Causes of unilateral ptosis are as follows:
   a. Horner's syndrome
   b. 3rd nerve palsy
   c. Myasthenia gravis
   d. Congenital lesion

17. Causes of Horner's syndrome are as follows:
   a. Central causes:
   - Brainstem tumor
   - Spinal cord tumor
   - Demyelination
   - Syringomyelia
   - Basal skull tumor
   - Basal meningitis
   - Arnold–Chiari malformation
   b. Peripheral preganglionic lesion:
   - Pancoast tumor
   - Cervical rib
   - Lymphadenopathy
   - Central venous catheterization
   - Cardiothoracic surgery
   - Aortic aneurysm
   - Surgery in the neck
   - Birth trauma
   c. Peripheral postganglionic lesion:
   - Dissection in the internal carotid artery
   - Caroticocavernous fistula
   - Herpes zoster

CASE 23

Speech is scanned, slurred, indistinct, jerky, variable length and tones, and there is respiratory whoops in-between the phrases.

1. **What is the most likely diagnosis?**
2. **Why the speech is slurred?**
3. **Why the speech is of variable length?**
4. **Demonstrate five signs of this parent disease.**

Answers

1. The diagnosis is ataxic dysarthria.
2. Speech is slurred because there is lack of coordination in-between phonation and articulation at the end of words, phrases as well as sentences.
3. Speech is of variable length because of lack of coordination between the phonation, articulation, and respiration; and hence, the speech is explosive also.
4. Five signs of the disease are:
   a. Pendular knee jerk
   b. Intension tremor
   c. Dysdiadochokinesia
   d. Abnormal heel-knee test and finger-nose test
   e. Nystagmus with first phase toward the site of lesion

CASE 24

In the neurological outdoor during examination, the speech of the patient is indistinct, nonmodulated, high-pitched, explosive, and not properly articulated and harsh.

1.   **What is the most likely diagnosis?**
2.   **What this specific dysarthria reflects?**
3.   **Why unilateral pyramidal tract lesion safe from the view of speech-related muscles?**
4.   **What are the cranial nerves that are not receiving bilateral pyramidal tract innervation?**

Answers

1.   The diagnosis is spastic dysarthria.
2.   Specific spastic dysarthria is due to upper motor neuron type of weakness involving the muscles of articulation and phonation.
3.   Most of the cranial nerves are bilaterally innervated from upper motor neuron in the form of corticobulbar tract. This is the safety mechanism in case of unilateral pyramidal tract lesion and hence articulating muscles will continue to function adequately in case of unilateral pyramidal tract damage.
4.   7th and 12th nerves will receive only contralateral innervation from the pyramidal tract. Hence, on unilateral pyramidal tract lesion, there is contralateral weakness of lower face and tongue protrusion.

CASE 25

Speech is slow, monotonous, low volume, low-pitched, and sometimes unnecessary pause followed by short outburst of rapid speech.

1.   **What is the most likely diagnosis?**
2.   **What is the etiological diagnosis and what are cardinal signs of this disease?**
3.   **What are the cardinal features in this disease?**

Answers

1.   The most likely diagnosis is spastic dysarthria.
2.   The etiological diagnosis is Parkinson's disease due to loss of dopaminergic output from the substantia nigra.
3.   The cardinal features in this disease are:
     a.   Bradykinesia
     b.   Rigidity
     c.   Tremor at rest

CASE 26

The patient was asked "what he took yesterday in dinner"? The patient did not understand the question but told some nonunderstandable words. His articulation was intact.

1.   **What is the diagnosis?**
2.   **What is the common site of lesion in this case?**
3.   **What type of answer he has given to you?**
4.   **What are the basic components of language function which should be tested to come to a diagnosis?**

Answers

1.   The diagnosis is sensory aphasia or Wernicke's aphasia.
2.   The lesion is in the fiber that connects Wernicke's area in the dominant hemisphere including posterior perisylvian area and posterior part of the dominant superior temporal gyrus.

3. He has given answers containing different words. This is known as phonemic paraphasia.
4. There are four basic components of language function:
   a. Fluency: In this type, the patient should complete the sentence containing 5–10 words.
   b. Comprehension: Patient should perform works without performing gesture. There are three stages in comprehension:
      - One stage: Close your eyes
      - Two stage: Close the eyes and touch your tongue
      - Three stage: Take the pencil from the table then keep it in the drawer and then shut the drawer
   c. Repetition: Tell a sentence containing both words and number and tell the patient to repeat it.
   d. Naming: The patient is shown an object and asks him to name it.

CASE 27

During examination of the speech abnormality, the comprehension of speech was normal, but speech was nonfluent, difficulty in finding words, repetition was impaired, and there was grammatical error.

1. **What is the diagnosis?**
2. **Where is the site of lesion?**
3. **What types of sentence the patient will utter?**
4. **Is the comprehension is really normal?**
5. **How can you differentiate dysarthria from dysphasia?**
6. **What do you mean by "semantic" and "syntax"?**
7. **Which cerebral hemisphere is involved in these lesions?**
8. **Which areas in the brain are Broca's and Wernicke's area?**
9. **Which are arcuate fasciculus and angular gyrus?**
10. **What is transcortical involvement?**

Answers

1. The patient has been suffering from Broca's aphasia or expressive aphasia.
2. The lesion affects the fibers connecting the Broca's area with the dominant precentral area and posterior part of inferior frontal gyrus.
3. The patient will tell the phrases which are:
   a. Short
   b. Telegraphic like sending the telegrams
   c. Agrammatic
   d. Omits articles, verbs, adverbs, conjunctions, and prepositions
   e. Morphologically inflected like pleural and past tense
   f. Retention of noun, verbs, and adjectives
4. During routine assessment the comprehension may be normal, but during minute examination, comprehension of the passive construction may be detected as abnormal like "the lady was attacked by robber" which will be interpreted as "the robber was attacked by the lady".
5. Dysphasia means "disorder of language", whereas dysarthria means "disorder of speech".
6. Semantic means "selection of words" and syntax means "phrase or sentence formulation".
7. In 97% right-handed individuals, dominant hemisphere is involved where in 60% left-handed individuals, dominant hemisphere is involved.
8. Broca's area is anterior to precentral gyrus and posterior part of inferior frontal gyrus.
   Wernicke's area is posterior pre-Sylvian area as well as posterior part of superior temporal gyrus.
9. Angular gyrus is present in the temporoccipital cortex which is present in the occipital lobe in the halfway between the Wernicke's area and visual cortex.
   Arcuate fasciculus connects Broca's and Wernicke's area through the occipital lobe.
10. Transcortical aphasia can be divided into three types:
    a. Transcortical motor aphasia affecting the communication between the Broca's area and premotor area, so, it is motor aphasia without the involvement of repetition.
    b. Transcortical sensory aphasia affecting the area behind the Wernicke's area at temporoccipital junction, so, it is like sensory aphasia without repetition area involvement.
    c. Mixed transcortical aphasia looking like global aphasia but sparing repetition.

CASE 28

From history:
There was double vision on extreme right lateral gaze, hearing loss in the right side, difficulty in mastication, and weakness of muscles.

From the examination:
- Impaired abduction of the right eye
- Diplopia in the extreme lateral gaze
- Lower motor type of weakness as well as sensation over the right side of the face
- Masticatory muscles are affected.
- Rinne's test is positive as there is laterization toward normal ear.
- Presence of nystagmus with fast component toward right
- There is broken pursuit with saccadic eye movement.
- Features of cerebellar signs

1. **What is the most likely diagnosis?**
2. **What are the points in favor of the diagnosis?**
3. **What is the earliest sign in this disease?**
4. **What are the features of facial nerve involvement?**
5. **What are the inspectory findings during opening of the mouth in this disease?**
6. **In case of large lesion, what are the cranial nerves can be involved in this patient?**
7. **What is the boundary of this area where the lesions will occur?**
8. **Mention five causes of this lesion?**
9. **What are the modalities of treatment in this patient?**

Answers

1. The most likely diagnosis is tumor in the cerebello-pontine angle.
2. Following points are in favor of this diagnosis:
   a. Presence of cerebellar signs
   b. Presence of 5th, 6th, 7th, and 8th nerve palsy
3. The earliest sign in this case is involvement of 5th nerve in the form of loss of cranial reflex.
4. Following are the signs of facial nerve involvement:
   a. Frontal belly of occipitofrontalis
   b. Loss of ipsilateral frowning due to weakness of corrugator supercilii
   c. Inability to close the eyes due to involvement of orbicularis oculi
   d. Loss of elevation of the angle of the mouth due to weakness of orbicularis oris
   e. Loss of taste in the anterior two-thirds of the tongue
   f. Reduced ipsilateral tearing
   g. Hemifacial spasm
   h. Hyperesthesia in the posterior wall of the external auditory meatus (Hitselberger sign)

5. During opening of the mouth or protruding the jaw, there is ipsilateral deviation of the jaw indicating the weakness of the muscles innervated by motor branches of 5th nerve.
6. If the lesion is very large, it involves lower cranial nerves as evidenced by:
   a. 9th nerve: Ipsilateral weakness of palate and deviation of the uvula toward normal side.
   b. 10th cranial nerve: Paresis of vocal cord leading to hypophonia
   c. 11th cranial nerve: Inability to elevate ipsilateral shoulder due to weakness of trapezius and inability to rotate the neck toward the same side due to ipsilateral weakness of sternocleidomastoid muscles.
   d. 12th cranial nerve: Deviation of the tongue toward the same side due to weakness of the ipsilateral muscles.
7. Boundary of the cerebellopontine angle:
   a. Medial boundary: Brainstem
   b. Lateral boundary: Petrous part of temporal bone
   c. Roof: Cerebellum
   d. Base: Lower cranial nerves

This space is lined by meninges and the space is filled up by CSF.

8. Five causes of this lesion are as follows:
    a. Acoustic neuroma
    b. Meningioma
    c. Cholesteatoma
    d. Hemangioblastoma
    e. Medulloblastoma

9. Treatment modalities in this disease:
    a. Complete surgical excision of the tumor for eradication
    b. Stereotactic radiotherapy, where multiple beams of radiation is directed toward the tumor leading to arrest of growth of tumor.
    c. Observation, where the tumor is small and the patient is asymptomatic and hearing is good.

CASE 29

Posture of the patient is flexed at left elbow, adduction and internal rotation at the left shoulder, semipronated forearm, and dystonic posture of the left hand. Left lower limb is extended at the knee joint and abduction at the hip.

1. **What is the specific diagnosis?**
2. **Prior to examining the patient, what are things you can get in that room which may favor the diagnosis?**
3. **By seeing the posture of the patient, what is your inference regarding the conditions of the muscles?**
4. **What is the classical posture of the upper arm and what should be the site of lesion?**
5. **What is pronator drift?**
6. **What is the Babinski's equivalent sign in the upper limb?**
7. **What is the classical hemiplegic gait?**
8. **What are the other examinations you want to perform in this patient?**
9. **How can you differentiate between brainstem stroke and cerebral stroke?**
10. **What are the features of posterior circulation stroke?**
11. **What is the significance of unilateral arm weakness over unilateral leg weakness?**

Answers

1. The diagnosis is left-sided hemiparesis.
2. Look for the following in that room:
    a. Walking aids
    b. Patient's shoes—scuffing in front of the shoes which results from foot drop
3. Upper limb is weak indicating the weakness of the extensor muscles. Lower limb is extended indicating weakness of the flexor muscles.
4. There is dystonic posturing of the hemiplegic side. Shoulder is adducted and internally rotated, elbow is flexed, wrist is flexed, and finger extended which can be demonstrated by asking the patient to perform mental arithmetic task. It indicates the lesion in the contralateral striatum and internal capsule.
5. Pronator drift is the most sensitive sign of unilateral upper motor neuron disease and this can be demonstrated where finger should be kept adducted and forearm fully supinated.
6. Babinski's equivalent sign in the upper limb is Hoffman's reflex which can be demonstrated by flicking the middle finger at the distal interphalangeal joint where looking for the remaining fingers including thumb for flexion.

7. Classical hemiplegic gait is affected limb which will be stiff and extended. During each step, the patient tries to tilt the pelvis to the other side; so, that affected leg will circumduct looking like semicircle. There may be foot drop along with scraping of the toes on the floor.
8. Other examinations to be performed in this patient are as follows:
    a. Complete neurological examination including upper and lower limb, cranial nerves, and higher function.
    b. Assessment of visual field to detect homonymous hemianopia
    c. Assessment of speech in case of right-sided hemiparesis involving right dominant hemisphere
    d. Fundoscopic examination to detect papilledema in case of any suspected space occupying lesion
    e. Measurement of blood pressure
    f. Examination of pulse in case of atrial fibrillation
    g. Auscultation of the carotid artery to detect any carotid bruit

9. In case of cerebral stroke, speech abnormalities, apraxia, neglect, homonymous hemianopia, and seizures should be present. In case of brainstem stroke, cerebellar dysfunction, abnormalities in the eye movement, Horner's syndrome, and presence of crossed signs in the form of right 3rd or 7th nerve palsies associated with left-sided hemiplegia should be present.

10. In case of posterior circulation stroke, there are cerebellar signs, brainstem sign along with homony- mous hemianopia, and problems in memory because posterior circulation involves occipital cortex, thalamus, and hippocampus.

11. Unilateral weakness suggests a lesion in the contra- lateral cerebral cortex involving precentral gyrus supplied by the middle cerebral artery.
   Unilateral limb weakness suggests a lesion contra- lateral cerebral cortex supplied by anterior cerebral artery covering the motor area responsible for movement of the legs.

CASE 30

A 42-year-old patient presented with nonrepetitive and nonstereotyped involuntary movements looking like dancing quality spreading from one side to other which was aggravated by the movements along with lip protrusion and indrawing.

1. **What is your diagnosis?**
2. **What is the special hand movement which may be seen in this patient?**
3. **What are the types of involuntary movements?**
4. **Which part of the body is affected in which types of the diseases?**
5. **What is the literal meaning of this disease?**
6. **What may be the presenting sign of the tongue in this disease?**
7. **What are the genetics in the congenital variety of this disease?**
8. **What are the features of congenital form of the disease?**
9. **How can you diagnose Wilson's disease?**
10. **What type of tremor occurs in Wilson's disease?**
11. **What are the nonneurological features in Wilson's disease?**

Answers

1. This is a case of chorea.
2. The special hand movement in this disease is "milkmaid's grip." It can be assessed by hand shake. There is alternate squeezing and gripping of the hands.
3. There are many types of involuntary movements:
   a. Chorea
   b. Choreoathetosis
   c. Athetosis
   d. Tardive dyskinesia
   e. Senile chorea
   f. Neuroacanthocytosis
   g. Sydenham's chorea
   h. Dystonia
   i. Myoclonus
   j. Hemiballism
   k. Akathisia
4. The upper part of the body is affected in:
   a. Huntington's disease
   b. Tardive dyskinesia
   c. Senile chorea
   Lower limb is involved in:
   a. Sydenham's chorea
   b. Neuroacanthocytosis
5. Literal meaning of chorea is "Greek word 'khoreia' "— means "choral dance."
6. Sign in the tongue is "harlequin's tongue" or "jack- in-the-box tongue"—means the tongue will appear to dart in and out of the mouth.
7. Huntington's chorea is autosomal dominant disease characterized by expansion of trinucleotide in the gene encoding the Huntington protein present on the chromosome 4. In case of normal subject, expansion repeats 9–34 times, if it is beyond this it is Huntington's disease.
8. Clinical features in Huntington's disease are the following:
   a. Rigidity of Westphal variant
   b. Chorea
   c. Bradykinesia

d. Dystonia
e. Ataxia
f. Myoclonus
g. Slow saccadic movements in the eye
h. Cognitive impairment
i. Psychiatric disturbances

9. Wilson's disease can be diagnosed by:
   a. Serum ceruloplasmin of <300 µg/L
   b. 24 hours excretion of urinary copper of >100 µg/day
   c. Liver copper will be high

10. Wing-beating tremor occurs in Wilson's disease which is characterized by coarse, irregular, and to-and-fro movement occurring at rest where the arm will held forward and flexed at the elbow, during action, or may be postural.

11. Nonneurological features in the Wilson's disease:
    a. Hepatic disease:
       • Hepatitis
       • Cirrhosis
       • Massive hepatic necrosis
    b. Metabolic:
       • Hypothyroidism
       • Renal tubular acidosis
    c. Others:
       • Hemolysis
       • Arthropathy

CASE 31

A 21-year-old male came with stereotyped repetitive movements of the tongue, jaw, and lips with protrusion of the tongue and facial grimacing along with opening and closing of the jaw.

1. **What is your diagnosis?**
2. **What do you mean by "dyskinesia"?**
3. **What is the pathophysiology of this disease?**
4. **What are the drugs responsible for this disease?**
5. **What is the treatment of this disease?**

Answers

1. The diagnosis is tardive dyskinesia.
2. Dyskinesia means involuntary movement and disorders
3. If the patient on long-term therapy with dopamine antagonist, it will lead to D2 hypersensitivity of the receptors situated in the basal ganglia. So, if the drug is stopped or the dose of the drug is reduced, in that case, there is rebound response of the postsynaptic D2 receptors to the dopamine even in low concentration leading to development of tardive dyskinesia.
4. Following drugs are responsible for this disease:
   a. Phenothiazines
   b. Metoclopramide
   c. Butyrophenones
5. Treatment of this disease:
   a. Cessation of the offending medications
   b. General pharmacotherapy will be ineffective.

CASE 32

A 39-year-old male presented with nasal quality and low volume of speech, nasal regurgitation of fluid, and slurring of the speech at the level of tongue and lips. On examination, jaw jerk is absent. There is mixed upper and lower motor neuron lesions with presence of fasciculation in the small muscles of the limbs.

1. **What is the most likely diagnosis?**
2. **How can you differentiate this disease from pseudobulbar palsy by demonstrating the soft palate function?**
3. **How can you differentiate this disease from pseudobulbar palsy by examining the tongue?**
4. **What are the causes of this disease?**

Answers

1. The most likely diagnosis is bulbar palsy following motor neuron disease.
2. During examination of soft palate, in both types of palsies, there is weakness of soft palate. But in case of bulbar palsy, there is absent or reduced gag reflex due to lower motor neuron type of palatal weakness, whereas in case of pseudobulbar palsy, there is upper motor neuron type of palatal weakness leading to exaggerated gag reflex.
3. If the patient is asked to protrude the tongue, in case of bulbar palsy, there is lower motor neuron type of weakness of the tongue muscles with presence of fasciculation and the tongue will be deviated toward the side of lesion. Whereas in case of pseudobulbar palsy, tongue muscles will be shrunken, immobile, and stiff and the patient will be unable to protrude the tongue outside the mouth.
4. Causes of bulbar palsy are as follows:
   a. Lower motor neuron type palsies (true bulbar palsy):
      - Motor neuron disease
      - Poliomyelitis
      - Syringobulbia
      - Basilar ischemia
      - Brainstem tumor
      - Neurosyphilis
      - Subacute meningitis
   b. Myasthenic bulbar palsy, i.e., disorder at the neuromuscular junction:
      - Myasthenia gravis
      - Botulism
   c. Myopathic bulbar palsy, i.e., disorder of muscles:
      - Muscular dystrophies
      - Polymyositis

CASE 33

The patient came with right-sided lower motor neuron type weakness with absent of plantar reflex and pes cavus.

1. **What is the diagnosis?**
2. **What is the pathophysiology behind it?**
3. **Mention the clinical syndrome of this disease.**
4. **What are the vaccines available for this disease?**

Answers

1. The most likely diagnosis is poliomyelitis.
2. The pathophysiology behind this disease is:

Transmission of the virus through the feco-oral route through the ingestion of the contaminated water

↓

Replication of the polioviruses in the oropharyngeal and gastrointestinal mucosa

↓

The viruses drain into cervical and mesenteric lymph nodes

↓

From these nodes the viruses will enter the blood stream

↓

Through the blood the viruses cross the blood–brain barrier

↓

Through the axonal transport to the peripheral nerves

3. The clinical syndromes in this disease are:
   a. Abortive poliomyelitis
   b. Nonparalytic poliomyelitis
   c. Paralytic poliomyelitis
   d. Paralytic poliomyelitis with bulbar involvement
   e. Encephalitis
4. Following vaccines are available for this disease:
   a. Inactivated poliovirus vaccine: Sabin vaccine containing all the three strains of inactivated or destroyed viruses.
   b. Oral live attenuated poliovirus vaccine: Salk vaccine containing all the three strains of live attenuated viruses. Dosages are orally 2, 4, and 6–18 months followed by booster dose at 4–6 years of age.

CASE 34

During neurological examination of a patient having history of exposure, demonstrates following features: swollen nontender deformed joints, painless ulcers in the plantar aspect of the feet, loss of vibration, position and joint sense, lower motor neuron type of weakness in the lower limbs but plantar extensor, and Romberg's sign is positive. Pupil demonstrates

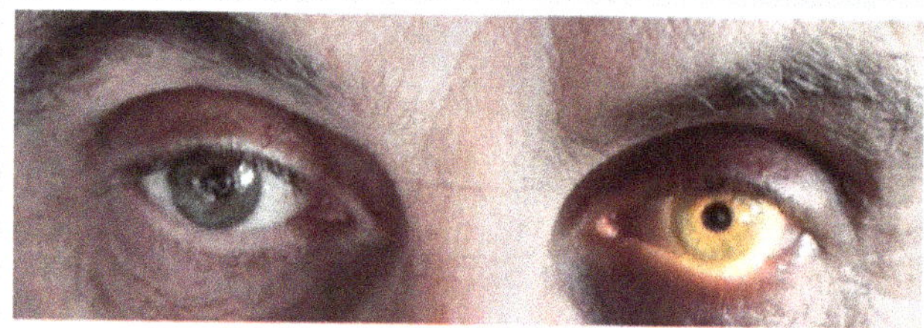

1. **What is the most likely diagnosis?**
2. **Why it is not tabes or GPI?**
3. **Mention five common conditions where the knee jerk is absent but plantar extensor?**
4. **Describe the pupil.**
5. **What are the phases in this disease?**
6. **Define neurosyphilis.**
7. **Mention five causes of false-positive venereal disease research laboratory (VDRL) test.**

Answers

1. The most likely diagnosis is taboparesis.
2. In case of tabes dorsalis, there is lower motor neuron type weakness, involvement of posterior column. In case of general paresis of insane, there is upper motor neuron type of weakness as a result of progressive frontotemporal meningoencephalitis along with cortical atrophy. But in taboparesis, there are features of both tabes dorsalis and GPI like loss of deep tendon reflexes along with plantar extensor.
3. There are five common conditions where knee jerk is absent but plantar is extensor:
   a. Subacute combined degeneration of the spinal cord
   b. Taboparesis
   c. Friedreich's ataxia
   d. Motor neuron disease
   e. Conus medullaris syndrome
4. The pupil is ARP which is characterized by:
   a. Bilateral small unequal pupil
   b. Accommodation reaction is present.
   c. Light reflex is absent.
   d. Wrinkling of the forehead resulting from compensatory overactive frontalis muscle.
5. There are three phases in this disease:
   a. Primary phase: It is characterized by painless ulcer in the penis and regional lymphadeno-pathy.

   b. Secondary phase: It is characterized by:
      - General features—acute febrile illness and general/lymphadenopathy
      - Skin as well as mucous membranes:
        ○ Scaly maculopapular rash in the palms and soles
        ○ Condylomata lata
        ○ Mouth ulcers
        ○ Alopecia
      - Eyes:
        ○ Iritis
        ○ Uveitis
        ○ Choroid retinitis
        ○ Optic atrophy
      - Nervous system:
        ○ Cranial neuropathy
        ○ Sensorineural deafness
      - Other features:
        ○ Arthritis
        ○ Hepatosplenomegaly
   c. Tertiary phase:
      - Cardiovascular manifestations
        ○ Aortic regurgitation
        ○ Aortic aneurysm
      - Neurovascular manifestations:
        ○ Meningovascular syphilis
        ○ Tabes dorsalis of insane
        ○ General paresis of insane

6. Neurosyphilis is characterized by invasion of the central nervous system in case of untreated syphilis and neurosyphilis where cerebrospinal spinal fluid white blood cells of >20/cc or a positive VDRL test.

7. Five causes of false-positive VDRL test are as follows:
   a. Rheumatoid arthritis
   b. SLE
   c. Pregnancy
   d. Malaria
   e. Autoimmune hepatitis

CASE 35

A 26-year-old male having history of common cold 2 days ago suddenly complained of weakness of closing the eye, secretions coming from the mouth, cannot elevate his head.

1. **What is your diagnosis?**
2. **What type of the lesion he has?**
3. **What are the causes of lesion?**
4. **What are the investigations to be done in this case?**
5. **What are the complications in this disease?**

Answers

1. The diagnosis is lower motor neuron palsy.
2. Patient has lower motor neuron palsy involving facial nerve.
3. The causes are as follows:
   a. Idiopathic in >95% cases
   b. Structural lesions in the brain:
      - Brainstem:
        ○ Stroke
        ○ Tumor
        ○ Demyelination in the brain
      - Cerebellopontine angle lesion: Acoustic neuroma
      - Infections in the middle ear
      - Parotid gland:
        ○ Infection
        ○ Tumor
        ○ Surgery
   c. Mononeuritis multiplex
4. In case of acute case developing within 1–2 days, no test is required. But in other cases, following tests are required:
   a. Blood tests:
      - C-reactive protein (CRP)
      - Erythrocyte sedimentation rate (ESR)
      - Serum angiotensin converting enzyme
      - Serology for:
        ○ Lyme disease
        ○ HIV
      - Antiganglioside antibodies
      - Autoantibodies
   b. Nerve conduction studies
   c. Lumbar puncture to detect:
      - Mononeuritis multiplex
      - Polyradiculopathy
      - Meningeal infiltration
5. Complications in this case are as follows:
   a. Corneal abrasion
   b. Persistent facial weakness
   c. Hemifacial spasm
   d. Sensory disturbances in the distribution of the facial nerve
   e. Crocodile tears due to aberrant reinnervation like abnormal tearing during eating

CASE 36

On examination, there is wasting of the facial muscles, absence of ptosis, eye movements are normal, no frontotemporal baldness, and there is wasting of the upper limb girdle muscles along with winging of the scapula. There is positive Beevor's sign and weakness in the dorsiflexion of the foot.

1. **What is your diagnosis?**
2. **What is Beevor's sign?**
3. **What type of facies is present in this case?**
4. **How the wasting of the muscles spread in the face?**
5. **What are the important negative findings when compared with myotonic dystrophy?**
6. **What is the important negative finding as compared to myasthenia gravis?**
7. **What do you mean by winging of the scapula?**
8. **What is the genetics in this case?**

Answers

1. The diagnosis is facioscapulohumeral dystrophy.
2. Beevor's sign: This sign detects the weakness of the lower abdominal muscles. When the patient asked to flex his neck and raise his head while the patient is in supine position, there is contraction of the upper and lower abdominal muscles normally thereby the position of the umbilicus will be in the central position. But in this case as the upper abdominal muscles are stronger as compared to lower abdominal muscles, the umbilicus will shifted upward. This is known as Beevor's sign.
3. In this patient, the facies will be expressionless which is known as myopathic facies.
4. Wasting of the facial muscles spread initially from the orbicularis oculi, orbicularis oris, and zygomaticus asymmetrically.
5. In case of myotonic dystrophy frontotemporal balding, eyelid muscles are involved which are absent in this case.
6. In case myasthenia gravis, extraocular muscles are involved which are absent in this case.
7. When the patient is asked to spread his arm in front of him, there is upward movement of the scapula due to weakness of the lower trapezius muscles. It is known as winging of the scapula.
8. This is autosomal dominant case. The chromosome involved is number 4 (4q35).

CASE 37

A 10-year-old child becomes wheelchair bound involving the proximal muscles of the upper and lower limb and flexors of the neck, whereas wrist extensors and tibialis anterior is mostly affected, pseudohypertrophy of the calf muscles. Deep tendon reflexes are reduced.

1. **What is your diagnosis?**
2. **What is the life expectancy in this patient?**
3. **Which can differentiate this patient from Becker's muscular dystrophy?**
4. **What is waddling gait?**
5. **What is the Gower sign?**
6. **What is the genetic basis of this disease?**
7. **What is the molecular basis in this disease?**

Answers

1. The diagnosis is Duchenne's muscular dystrophy.
2. The life expectancy in this patient is 20–25 years.
3. Ambulatory status can differentiate this patient from Becker's muscular dystrophy. This patient will manifest at the age of 3–6 years with waddling gait and becoming wheelchair bound by the age of 12 years. If the patient remains ambulant after the age of 13 years, the diagnosis may be doubtful. Whereas the patient diagnosed as Becker's muscular dystrophy will become nonambulant at the age of 30 years.
4. Waddling gait is wide-based gait where the trunk will move side to side. The pelvis will drop on the side when the foot is off the ground. There is forward tilt of the pelvis due to weakness of the hip extensors leading to hyperlordosis of the spine to maintain the posture.

5. Gower sign indicates proximal muscle weakness involving the hip extensor. As a result, the patient has to push his knees in order to stand erect.
6. This disease is X-linked recessive disorder due to mutation of the dystrophin gene (*Xp21*). Here, female is the carrier but males are affected as they are carriers of the affected gene.
7. Dystrophin, the largest gene, is present in 2% of X chromosome, expressed in the cardiac, skeletal, smooth muscle cells as well as in the brain and is responsible for maintaining the structural integrity of the muscle fibers. In this disease, loss of dystrophin leading to:
   a. Sarcolemmal breakdown
   b. Calcium influx into the muscles
   c. Oxidative stress and injury

   All the above will lead to death of the muscle cells.

CHAPTER 10

Pulmonary Function Tests

There are four possibilities in respect to FEV1, FVC, and FEV1/FVC ratio:

1. *Normal*: When all the values are within normal limit.
2. *Obstructive disease*: It can be defined as—
    a. FEV1—reduced
    b. FVC—relatively spared
    c. FEV1/FVC ratio—reduced
3. *Restrictive disease*:
    a. FEV1—low normal
    b. FVC—reduced
    c. FEV1/FVC—normal or increased
    d. In this case restrictive lung disease can be diagnosed by low total lung capacity which should be low.
4. Combined restrictive and obstructive lung disease can be diagnosed if the FVC is reduced out of proportion of FEV1/FVC ratio, i.e., FEV1/FVC ratio is 65% predicted and FVC is 40% predicted. Restrictive disease can be ruled by normal FVC.

Value of TLC, RV, and RV/TLC in lung disease: All will in the direction of restriction or obstruction. The interpretations are:

1. When all the values are normal—normal.
2. High volumes—indicate obstruction
    a. TLC increased—indicates hyperinflation. It can be more accurately determined if FRC is low.
    b. RV increased—indicates air trapping
    c. Ratio of RV/TLC—increased the degree of air trapping
3. Low volumes—in case of restrictive lung disease
    a. TLC decreased—indicates restrictive lung disease. It can help in the grading of restriction

Size and shape of the flow-volume curve (**Figs. 1A to H**):

1. Normal size and shape also known as "knee variant" (**Fig. 1A**)
2. Small and concave or scooped—suggestive of obstructive lung disease (**Fig. 1B**).
3. Small and steep slope with witch's hat shape: It indicates restriction at the parenchymal level (**Fig. 1G**).
4. Small but parallel slope as compared to predicted curve: It indicates restriction at the chest wall level (**Fig. 1H**).
5. Small and convex slope: It indicates poor effort of respiration suggestive of neuromuscular disease (**Fig. 1H**).
6. Small and flat of both expiratory and inspiratory component: Fixed inspiratory and inspiratory obstruction (**Fig. 1D**)
7. Small and flat at expiratory component: It indicates variable intrathoracic obstruction (**Fig. 1F**).
8. Small but flat inspiratory component: It indicates variable extrathoracic obstruction (**Fig. 1E**).

Interpretation of lung function test (**Flowchart 1; Tables 1 and 2**):

Step 1:
- FEV1/FVC is <70%—indicates obstructive pattern (chronic obstructive lung disease and asthma)
- ≥70%—indicates restrictive pattern

Step 2: Severity of obstruction:
- *FEV1*: 80–100% predicted (stage 1)
- *FEV1*: 50–80% predicted (stage 2)
- *FEV1*: 30–<50% predicted (stage 3)
- *FEV1*: <30% predicted (stage 4)
- *FEV1*: <50% with right-sided heart failure (stage 4)

Step 3:
- ≥12% increase and an absolute improvement of at least 200 mL after inhalation of β-agonist
- FEV1 or FVC is considered a significant response.

Step 4: Total lung capacity—normal range is 80–100% predicted.
- *TLC > 120%*: Hyperinflation
- *TLC < 80%*: Restrictive lung disease
- *70–80% predicted*: Mild restrictive lung disease
- *60–70% predicted*: Moderately restrictive lung disease

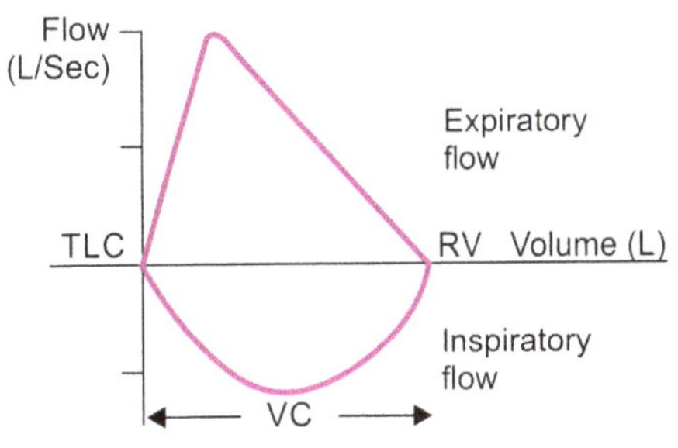

A. Normal

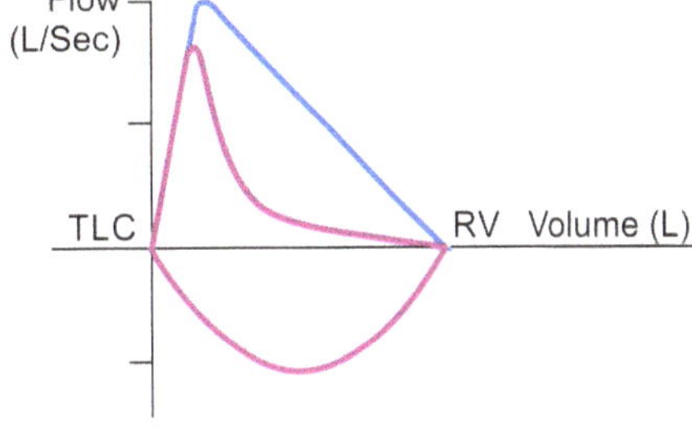

B. Emphysema

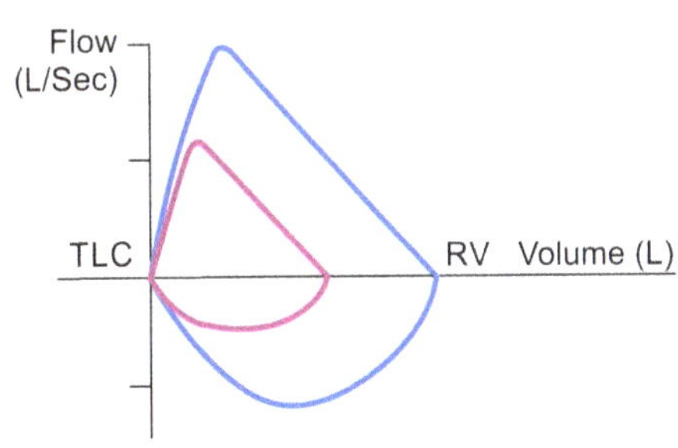

C. Unilateral main-stem bronchial obstruction

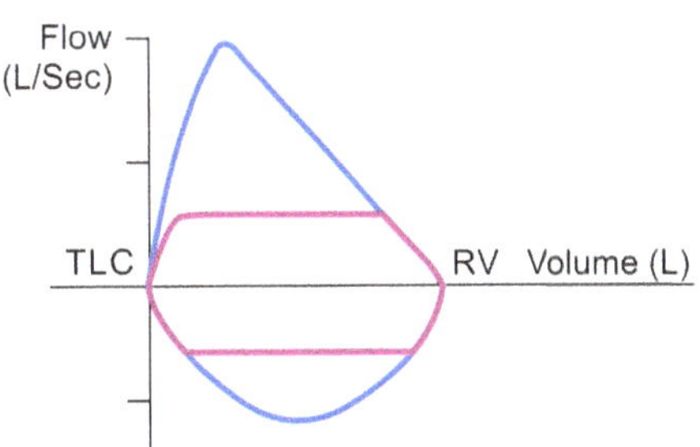

D. Fixed UAO

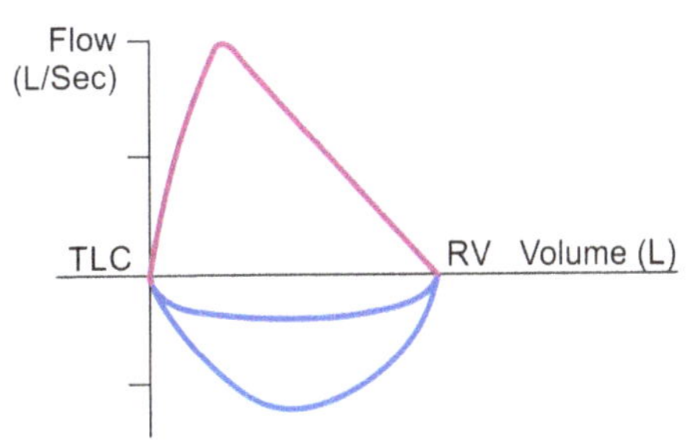

E. Variable extrathoracic UAO

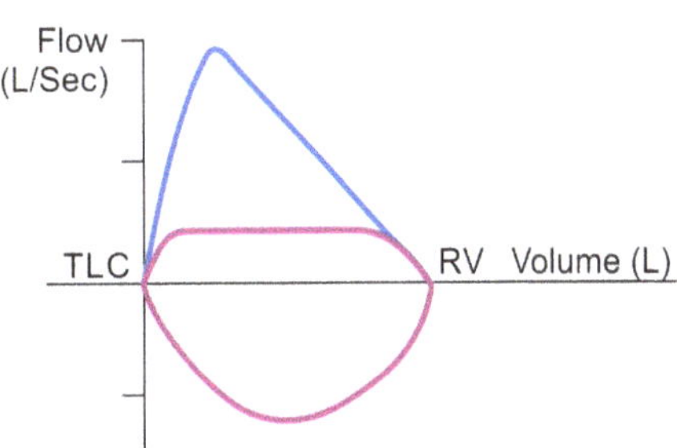

F. Variable intrathoracic UAO

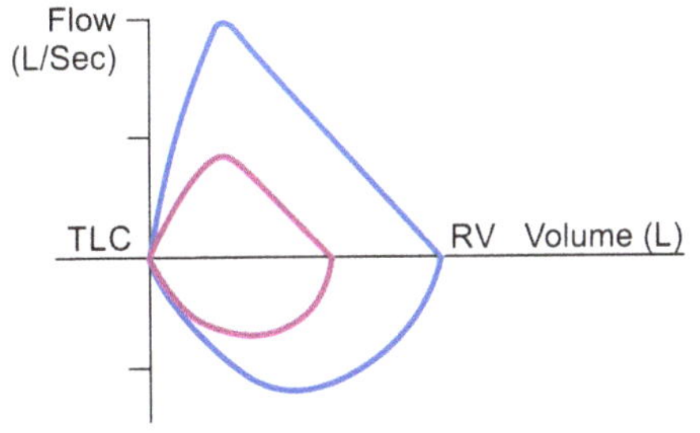

G. Restrictive parenchymal lung disease

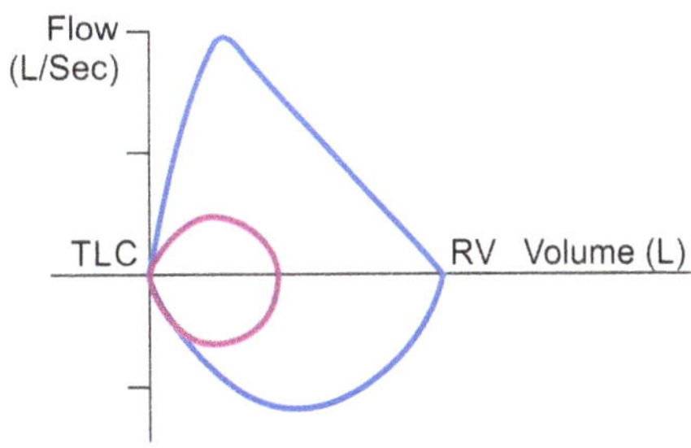

H. Neuromuscular weakness

FIGS. 1A TO H: Different size and shape of the flow-volume curves.

- *50–60% predicted*: Moderately severe restrictive lung disease
- *<50% predicted*: Severely restrictive lung disease

Step 5: RV/TLC ratio (normal is 80–120% predicted): RV/TLC ratio > 35% or more than predicted—indicates air trapping

Step 6: DLCO (normal range is 80–100% predicted):
- In obstructive lung disease:
  - Decreased in emphysema
  - Normal in chronic bronchitis
  - Normal in increased in case of asthma
- Restrictive lung disease:
  - Decreased in parenchymal lung disease
  - Normal in nonparenchymal disease

Stepwise approach:
1. Determination of FEV1/FVC ratio
2. Determination of FEV1—whether it is low or normal.
3. Severity of the abnormality should be graded.

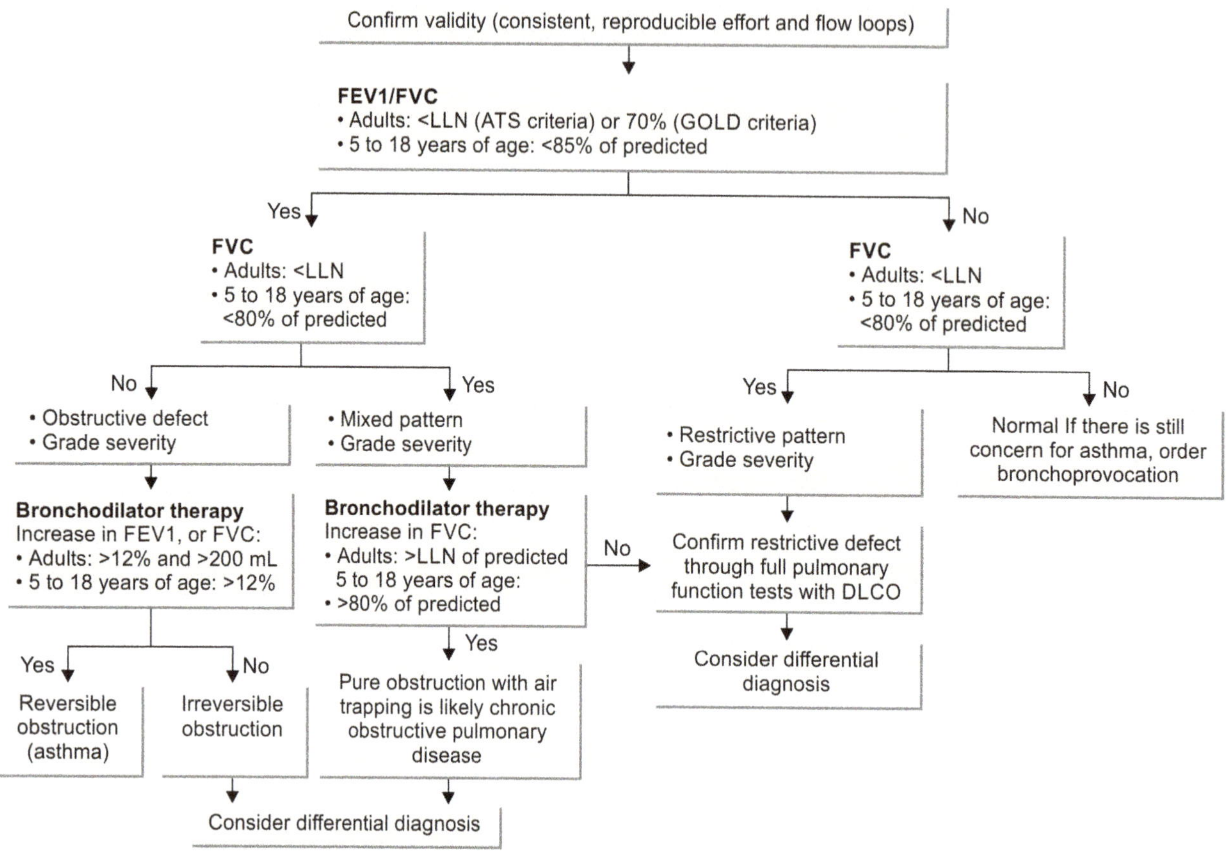

FLOWCHART 1: Interpretation of pulmonary function test.
(ATS: American Thoracic Society; GOLD: Global Initiative for Chronic Obstructive Lung Disease; LLN: lower limit of normal)

TABLE 1: Interpretation of pulmonary function test.

Test results based on age		Suggested diagnosis
FVC	**FEV1/FVC ratio**	
5–18 years: ≥ 80%	5–18 years: ≥ 85%	Normal
Adults: ≥ LLN	Adults: ≥ LLN or ≥ 70%	
5–18 years: ≥ 80%	5–18 years: < 85%	Obstructive defect
Adults: ≥ LLN	Adults: < LLN or < 70%	
5–18 years: < 80%	5–18 years: ≥ 85%	Restrictive pattern
Adults: < LLN	Adults: ≥ LLN or ≥ 70%	
5–18 years: < 80%	5–18 years: < 85%	Mixed pattern
Adults: < LLN	Adults: < LLN or < 70%	

(LLN: lower limit of normal)

TABLE 2: American Thoracic Society grades for severity of pulmonary function test.

Severity	FEV1, percentage of predicted
Mild	>70
Moderate	60–69
Moderately severe	50–59
Severe	35–49
Very severe	<35

4. Reversibility of the obstructive defect
5. Bronchoprovocation

In the tracings of spirometry usually three values are shown:

1. Predicted values which are expected normal values of any person with reference to age, sex, weight as well as height.
2. Measured values which are characterized by the actual values. These are shown by inspiration and expiration maneuvers.
3. Percentage of the predicted value can be calculated and expressed as the percentage of the predicted value, i.e., *(measured value/predicted value) × 100*.

Presence of airway abnormality can be diagnosed by the following measurement:

- *FEV1*: <80% of the predicted value
- *FVC*: <80% of the predicted value
- *FEV1/FVC ratio*: <75%

In case of obstructive disorder:
- *FEV1*: < 80% of the predicted value
- *FVC*: Reduced to <80% of the predicted value
- *FEV1/FVC ratio*: <75% of the predicted value
- Total lung capacity will be increased.
- Residual volume will be increased.
- RV/TLC will be increased.

In case of restrictive diseases:
- *FEV1*: <80% of the predicted value with proportion to FVC
- *FVC*: Reduced to <80% of the predicted value
- *FEV1/FVC ratio*: Normal or increased to >75% of the predicted value
- Total lung capacity will be reduced.
- Residual volume may or may not be reduced.
- RV/TLC will be normal.

Slow vital capacity: It is similar to FVC. In slow vital capacity, the patient can exhale slowly and completely, but in case of FVC, the patient will exhale forcefully, as a result of high flow through the airways that lead to excessive narrowing of the or closure of the diseased airways resulting in air trapping and the air cannot be exhaled completely **(Fig. 2)**.

Maximum volume ventilation: In this procedure the patient is asked in breathe as fast and as hard as possible for 6–12 seconds. The result will be extrapolated to 60 seconds in liter/minute.

Normal MVV = FEV1 × 30. If MVV is >FEV1 × 40, it suggests test is poorly performed.

Mixed obstructive-restrictive pattern: If the patient demonstrates reduced TLC—suggests restrictive lung disease, if FEV1/FVC ratio is increased—suggests obstructive lung disease. In this case to detect the degree of obstruction, percent reduction of FEV1 is required. Again, FEV1 is reduced due to reduction of TLC in the restricted lung disease. So to correct this, following is required: *Percent of predicted FEV1/Percent predicted TLC*. It may be moderate or moderately severe degree.

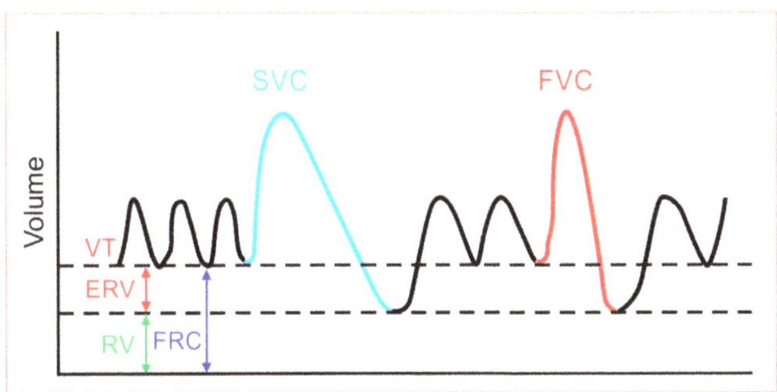

Fig. 2: Slow vital capacity and forced vital capacity.
slow vital capacity (SVC); Forced vital capacity (FVC)

CASE 1

A 50-year-old white smoker female came to respiratory clinic with chronic respiratory distress. Her spirometry done that demonstrated:

Parameters	Predicted	Pre	% predicted	Post
FVC	3.30	1.51	45.75	2.34
FEV1	2.69	0.4	14.86	0.55
FEV1/FVC		26.49		0.23
FEF25-75	2.84	0.12	4.22	

Lung volume:

Parameter	Predicted	Pre	% predicted
Total lung capacity	5.2	7.2	138.46
Residual volume	1.87	5.3	283.42
RV/TLC	35.96	73.61	

Diffusing capacity:

Parameter	Predicted	Pre	% predicted
DLCO	23	4	17.39
VA	5.25	2.25	42.85
DLCO/VA	4.38	1.77	40.41

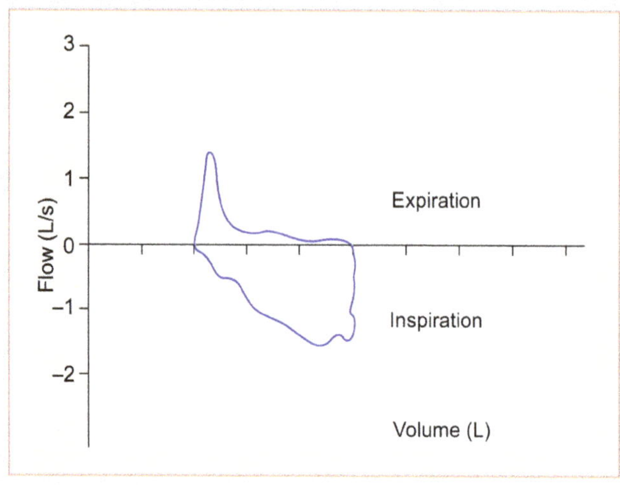

1. **What is shown in the result of spirometry?**
2. **What is the result shown in lung volume changes?**
3. **What are the changes in the flow-volume curve?**
4. **What is the interpretation of diffusion capacity?**
5. **What is your interpretation of the result?**
6. **How can you estimate air trapping?**

Answers

1. *Spirometry demonstrates*:
    a. FEV1 is reduced to very severe degree.
    b. *FVC*: Reduced
    c. *FEV1/FVC*: Reduced
    d. *FEF25-75*: It signifies obstruction
2. Lung volume demonstrates:
    a. Total lung capacity—severely increased
    b. Residual volume—severely increased
    c. RV/TLC—indicates air trapping along with evidence of hyperinflammation

3. Flow-volume curve demonstrates small and scooped out looking like "dog-leg appearance"
4. Diffusion capacity demonstrates that DLCO/VA is very low suggestive of defect in the diffusion.
5. Based on the results of spirometry, lung-volume and flow-volume curves are the diagnosis of obstructive lung disease with hyperinflammation and impaired gas exchanges suggestive of emphysema.
6. Air trapping can be estimated by following two ways:
    a. TLC – VA = 7.2 – 2.25 = 4.95 L
    b. RV (predicted) – RV (measured) = 5.3 – 1.87 = 3.43 L

CASE 2

A 70-year-old female came to respiratory clinic and pulmonary function test was advised:

Spirometry demonstrated:

Parameters	Predicted	Observed	% predicted
FVC	3.3	3.25	101.5
FEV1	2.4	2.6	108.3
FEV1/FVC		80	
FEF25–75	1.9	2.7	142

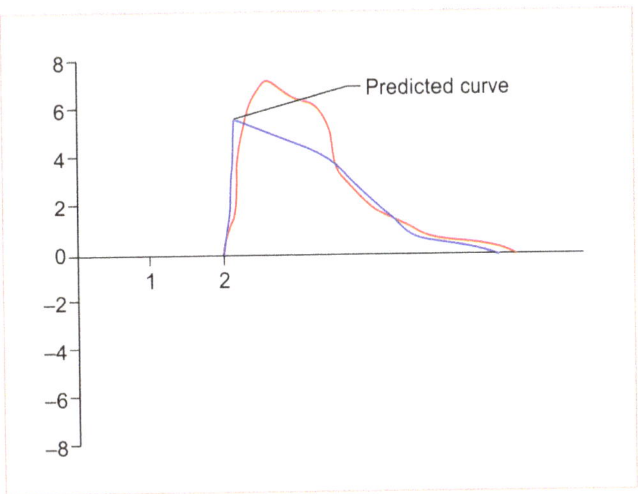

1. **How can you interpret the spirometry?**

2. **What is your diagnosis?**

Answers

1. FEV1, FVC, FEV1/FVC, and FEF25–75 are all within normal limit. Flow-volume curve demonstrates as normal with knee. This is normal variant and can be reproducible.

2. The spirometry of patient is normal.

CASE 3

A 60-year-old female came with history of progressively increasing respiratory distress. Her spirometry was performed:

Parameters	Predicted	Observed	% predicted
FVC	4.58	2.4	52.4
FEV1	3.6	1.92	53.3
FEV1/FVC		0.79	
FEF25–75	3.3	1.5	45.45

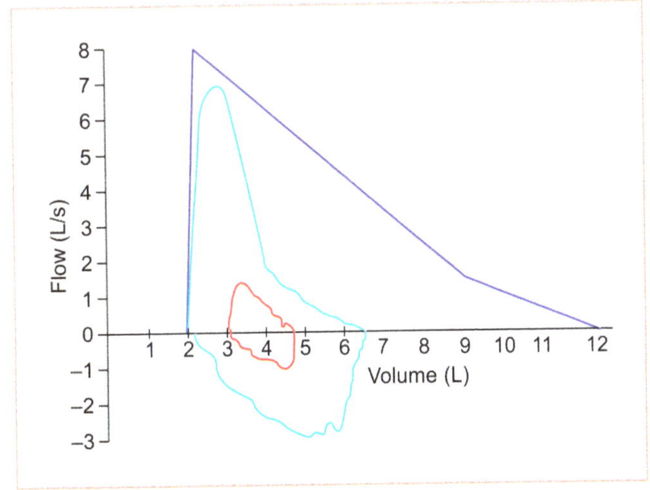

1. **Interpret the spirometry.**

2. **What is the diagnosis?**

3. **What are the causes of this disease extrinsic to lung?**

Answers

1. Interpretation of spirometry:
   a. FEV1 is reduced.
   b. FVC is reduced.
   c. FEV1/FVC ratio is in the lower limit of normal.
2. The patient has been suffering from the restrictive lung disease.
3. Following are the causes of restrictive disease extrinsic to lung:
   a. Kyphoscoliosis
   b. Obesity
   c. Pleural causes:
      - Pleural fibrosis
      - Pleural scarring
      - Pleural effusion
      - Asbestosis
   d. Ascites
   e. Neuromuscular disorders:
      - Amyotrophic lateral sclerosis
      - Muscular dystrophy
      - Poliomyelitis
      - Phrenic neuropathies

CASE 4

A 75-year-old Asian male came to respiratory clinic with history of respiratory distress.

Parameters	Predicted	Observed	% predicted
FVC	3.08	1.35	43.83
FEV1	2.4	0.6	25
FEV1/FVC		0.44	
FEF25–75	1.5	0.25	16.66

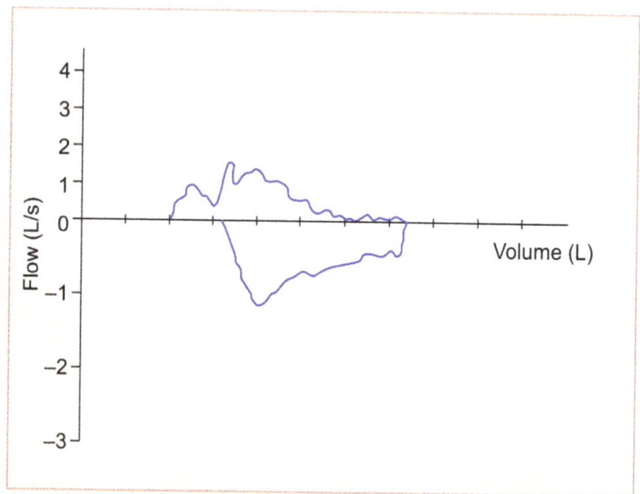

1. **Interpret the spirometry.**
2. **Describe flow-volume curve.**
3. **Why the shape of the inspiratory part of the flow-volume curve is like this?**
4. **Why the shape of the expiratory part of the flow-volume curve is like this?**
5. **Why both part of the curve are flattened?**
6. **What are the causes of this type of graph?**

Answers

1. Spirometry demonstrates:
   - Both FEV_1 and FVC are low.
   - FEV_1/FVC is low.

2. Flow-volume curve demonstrates the curve is flat in respect both the inspiratory and expiratory components indicating the presence of fixed airway obstruction.

3. It is flat due to extrathoracic obstruction above the level of sternal notch. Pressure within the larynx, pharynx, and extrathoracic portion of trachea will be negative as compared to pressure outside the airways (atmospheric pressure) during inspiration thereby curve of the inspiratory part of the curve becomes flat.

4. Obstruction intrathoracic part of trachea and main bronchi is compressed during expiratory phase of respiration by increased intrathoracic pressure thereby producing flattening in the expiratory phase flow-volume curve.

5. In case of fixed airway obstruction above or below the level of sternal notch. It will not be related to expiratory or inspiratory phase; hence, this curve does not depend upon the intrathoracic or extrathoracic part of the airways. Hence, both phase of flow-volume curve are flattened.

6. Causes of this type of graph are as follows:
   a. Fibrotic stricture in the upper airways
   b. Nonmovable tumor in the upper or lower airways

CASE 5

A 52-year-old white male with body mass index (BMI) of 30/m² came for routine test required for the service. Spirometry was advised.

Spirometry:

Parameters	Predicted	Observed	% predicted
FVC	5.12	4.72	92
FEV1	4.1	3.6	87.8
FEV1/FVC		0.76	
FEF25–75	1.95	0.98	50

Lung volumes:

Parameters	Predicted	Observed	% predicted
TLC	7.4	7.68	103.7
RV	2.09	2.48	
RV/TLC			

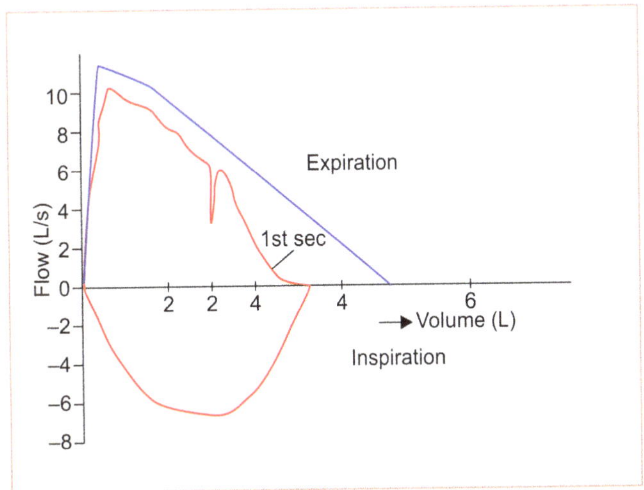

1. **Interpret the results of spirometry.**
2. **Interpret flow-volume loop.**
3. **What is your interpretation?**

Answers

1. Interpretation of spirometry results: All the values are within normal limit except FEF25–75 is low. It indicates obesity.
2. In the flow-volume curve—in the observed value the curve is little smaller as compared to predicted graph.

But, the expiratory curve is interrupted by sudden cough in the 1st second.

3. Patient has normal spirometry except mild isolated reduction in FEF25–75 indicating presence of obesity.

CASE 6

A 52-year-old male came to respiratory clinic with respiratory distress. His flow-volume curve demonstrated:
Straight X-ray of chest demonstrated:

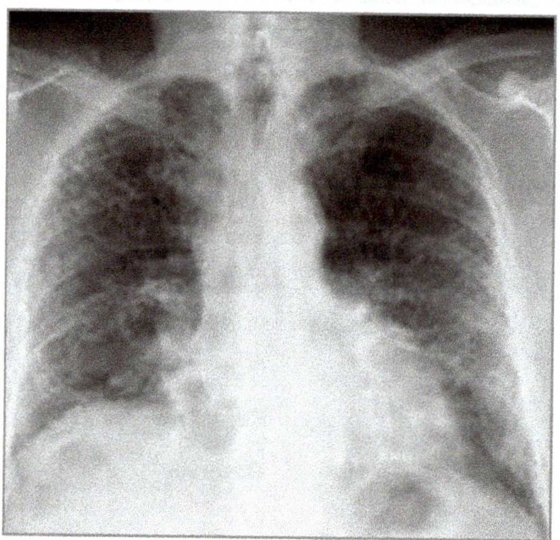

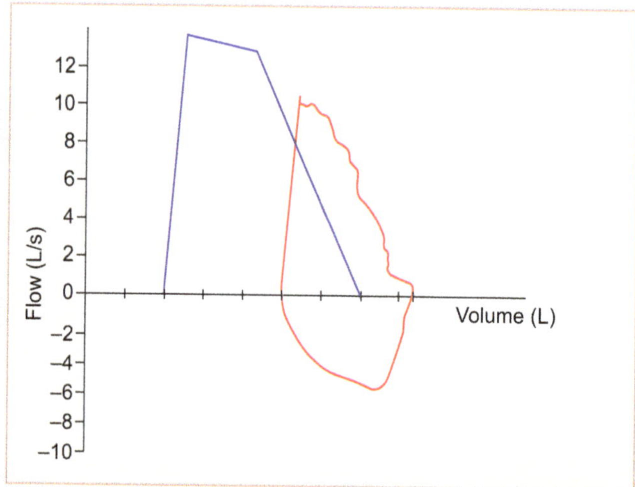

1. **Demonstrate flow-volume curve.**
2. **Describe the chest X-ray.**
3. **What is the diagnosis?**

Answers

1. Flow-volume curve demonstrates:
   a. Observed flow-volume curve is small but steep like Witch's hat.
   b. The width of the curve is low having normal ratio indicating restrictive lung disease.
   c. Observed curve is shifted to the right as compared to predicted curve indicating decreased total lung capacity and residual volume. This proves restrictive pattern of parenchymal disease like interstitial lung disease.

2. X-ray of chest demonstrates:
   a. Reticular pattern of the interstitial marking in the periphery of the lung bilaterally worst in the lung bases.
   b. There is bisection of the diaphragm by right fifth anterior rib indicating some loss of lung volume loss.

3. This patient has been suffering from interstitial lung disease.

CASE 7

An 80-year-old man admitted in emergency with severe respiratory distress. He was undergone pulmonary function test prior to and after administration of bronchodilator drugs.

Spirometry demonstrated:

Parameters	Predicted	Prebronchodilator	% predicted	Postbronchodilator	% predicted	Change
FVC	2.96	1.88	63	2.08	70.2	9.5%
FEV1	2.1	0.78	37.1	0.9	42.8	15.3
FEV1/FVC		41		44		
FEF25–75	1.46	0.23	15.7			

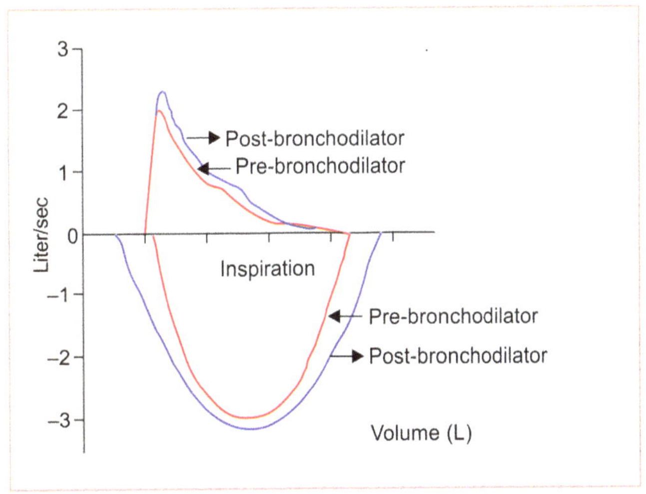

Flow-volume curve demonstrated:

1. **How can you interpret flow-volume curve?**
2. **How can you interpret spirometry?**
3. **What is your diagnosis?**

Answers

1. Flow-volume curve demonstrates:
   a. Pre- and postbronchodilator curves are small and scalloped.
   b. There is some improvement after administration of bronchodilator.
   c. Curve itself demonstrates either air-leak or poor initial breath in the postbronchodilator study.

2. Spirometry demonstrates:
   a. There is severe reduction in FEV1 and FEV1/FVC ratio—indicates obstructive lung disease.
   b. FEF25–75 is very low—indicating obstruction and air trapping.

c. There is only 15.3% change after administration of the bronchodilator which is <200 mL—it indicates insignificant bronchodilator response to bronchodilator.

3. Patient has been suffering from severe obstructive pulmonary disease and inadequate response to bronchodilator.

CASE 8

A 55-year-old female has been admitted with respiratory distress. Respiratory and cardiovascular system examinations were normal. So pulmonary function test was performed:

Parameters	Predicted	Observed	% predicted
FVC	2.9	2.5	86.2
FEV1	2.3	2.2	95.6
FEV1/FVC		0.88	
FEF25–75	2.34	2.24	96.5

Lung volume demonstrated:

Parameters	Predicted	Observed	% predicted
TLC	4.8	4.3	89.6
RV	1.95	1.75	89.7
RV/TLC	0.40	40.7	

Diffusion capacity:

Parameters	Predicted	Observed	% predicted
DLCO	20	11	55
DLCO/VA	4.22	2.4	56.8
VA	4.75	4.5	88.4

Picture of the hand in this patient demonstrated:

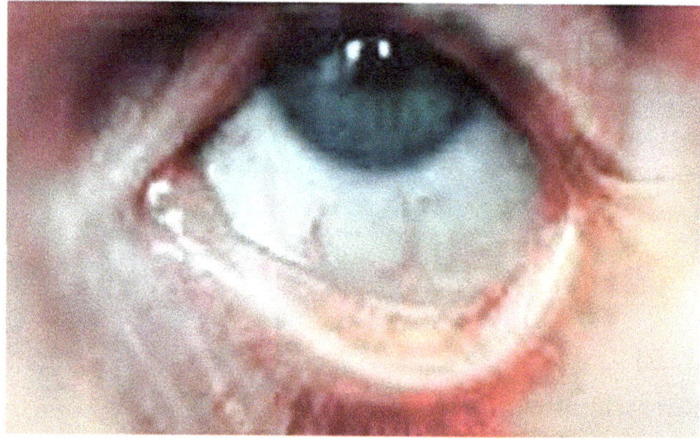

1. **Interpret the above pulmonary function test.**
2. **What are the causes of the respiratory distress?**
3. **What is the conclusion correlation with the above picture?**

Answers

1. Interpretation of pulmonary function tests:
   a. FEV1, FVC, and FEV1/FVC are within normal limit.
   b. TLC, RV, and RV/TLC are within normal limit.
   c. DLCO/VA is very low. It suggests abnormality in the gas exchange.

2. Causes of this abnormality are as follows:
    a. Early parenchymal lung disease
    b. Anemia
    c. Pulmonary vascular disease

3. As the respiratory and cardiovascular examination was normal, and the conjunctiva demonstrated anemia, the patient has been suffering from severe anemia leading to respiratory distress.

CASE 9

A 65-year-old female was admitted with severe respiratory distress with cough and expectoration. She was advised spirometry.

Parameters	Predicted	Prebronchodilator	% predicted	Postbronchodilator	Change
FVC	4.5	3.06	68%	3.15	2.9
FEV1	3.75	2.56	68.26	2.9	13.2
FEV1/FVC		0.83			
FEF25–75	4.5	2.5	55.5	3.1	24

Lung volume:

Parameters	Predicted	Observed	% predicted
TLC	5.5	4.2	76
RV	1.1	1.48	134.5
RV/TLC	20%	35.2	

Diffusion capacity:

Parameters	Predicted	Observed	% predicted
DLCO	28	22.1	78.92
DLCO/VA	5.09	5.39	105.9
VA	5.5	4.1	74.5

The chest X-ray of the patient:

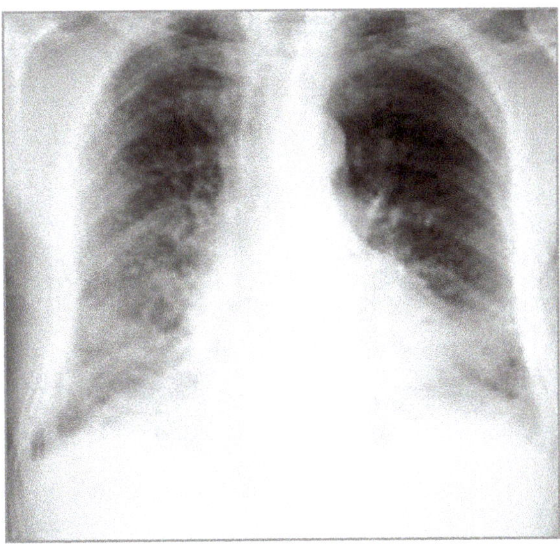

1. **Interpret the lung function test.**
2. **What is the most likely conclusion?**
3. **What is the above chest X-ray demonstrates?**
4. **What is the most likely diagnosis in this case?**

Answers

1. Interpretation of the lung function test:
   a. Spirometry demonstrates:
      - Restriction of FEV1, FVC with normal ratio of FEV1/FVC suggestive of restrictive pathology
      - Postbronchodilator response is negligible in all the parameters.
   b. Lung volume measurement demonstrates:
      - TLC is low. So, it is less likely restrictive only.
      - RV is increased suggestive of air trapping.
      - Lung volume study shows the feature of obstruction
   c. Diffusion capacity is nearly normal.
2. The conclusion is:
   a. Spirometry study demonstrates restrictive pathology
   b. Lung volume study demonstrates obstructive pathology

   So, combined defect is the most likely diagnosis.
3. The chest X-ray demonstrates:
   a. Interstitial reticular shadow bilaterally in the lung mainly right sided
   b. Reticulonodular shadow presents in the lung bases and subpleural region
   c. Trachea is shifted to right.
   d. Hyperinflation on the left lung field with reduction in the density of the left upper lung field.
4. The most likely diagnosis is interstitial fibrosis with emphysema.

CASE 10

A 50-year-old man came to respiratory clinic with history of respiratory distress and stridor.

His lung function test demonstrated:

Parameters	Predicted	Observed	% predicted
FVC	4.8	5.15	107.3
FEV1	3.8	3.4	89.4
FEV1/FVC		89	
FIF 50		0.56	
FEF 50		2.4	
FIF50/FEF50		0.23	

Lung volumes:

Parameters	Predicted	Observed	% predicted
TLC	6.95	6.8	97.84
RV	2.2	1.5	68.2
RV/TLC	0.31	0.22	70.96

Diffusion capacity:

Parameters	Predicted	Observed	% predicted
DLCO	25.6	27.1	105.8
DLCO/VA	3.75	3.79	101.06
VA	6.82	7.8	114.4

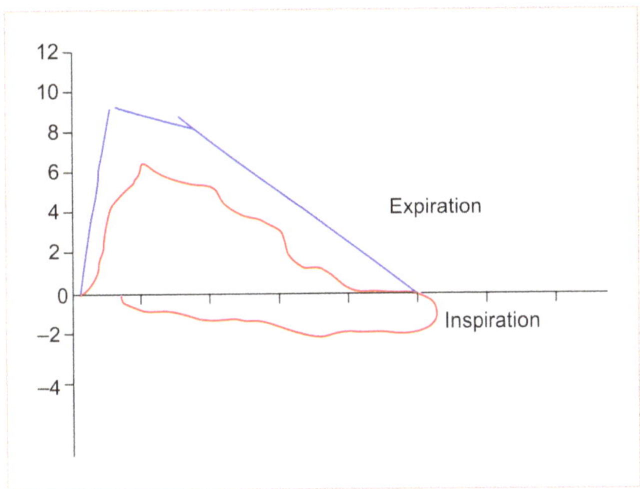

Flow-volume curve demonstrated the following:

1. **Interpret the lung function test.**
2. **What is your conclusion?**
3. **What are the causes of this type of graph?**

Answers

1. Interpretation of lung function test:
   a. Spirometry demonstrates:
      - Normal FVC, FEV1, and FEV1/FVC ratio are normal.
      - FIF50/FEF50 <1—indicates variable extrathoracic upper airway obstruction
   b. Lung volume demonstrates normal TLC, RV, and RV/TLC ratio
   c. Values of diffusion capacity are normal.
   d. Flow-volume curve demonstrates:
      - Curve is small.
      - Expiratory component is normal but small.
      - Inspiratory component is flat.
2. The conclusion is that the patient has been suffering from variable extrathoracic upper airway obstruction because:
   a. Flat inspiratory component of the flow-volume curve.
   b. Ratio of FIF50/FEF50 is <1.
   c. There is history of stridor.
3. Causes of extrathoracic upper airway obstruction are as follows:
   a. Blockage at the level of oral or nasal cavities or nasopharynx (stertor):
      - Hypertrophy of the nasal turbinate:
        ○ Allergic rhinitis
        ○ Nasal polyposis
        ○ Septal deviation
        ○ Foreign bodies in the nasal cavity
        ○ Adenoid hypertrophy
      - Upper airway obstruction:
        ○ Angioedema
        ○ Ludwig angina
        ○ Oropharyngeal cancer
        ○ Tonsillar hypertrophy
        ○ Parapharyngeal abscess
        ○ Retropharyngeal abscess
        ○ Peritonsillar abscess
   b. Blockage at the level of larynx:
      - Epiglottitis—bacteria, fungi, and mycobacteria
      - Laryngeal stenosis
      - Granulomatous polyangiitis
      - Amyloidosis
      - Sarcoidosis
      - Behçet's disease
      - Subglottic stenosis following prolonged intubation or trauma

CASE 11

A 60-year-old woman having BMI of 40 kg/m^2 went to respiratory clinic with history of occasional shortness of breath. She was advised lung function test.

Parameters	Predicted	Observed	% predicted
FVC	4.5	2.8	62.2
FEV1	3.4	2.1	61.7
FEV1/FVC	0.75	0.75	
FEF25–75	4.1	1.8	43.9

Lung volume:

Parameters	Predicted	Observed	% predicted
TLC	6.8	4.9	72
RV	2.51	1.59	63.3
RV/TLC	0.37	0.33	89.2

Diffusing capacity:

Parameters	Predicted	Observed	% predicted
DLCO	25.1	15.2	25.1
DLCO/VA	3.4	2.6	76.4
VA	7.3	5.9	80.8

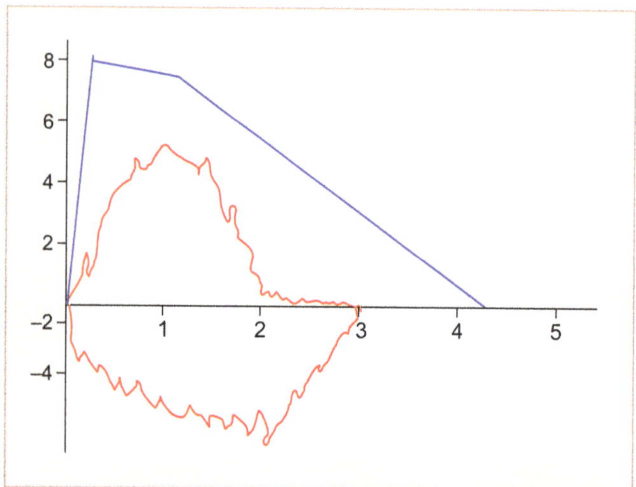

Flow-volume curve demonstrated the following:
1. **Interpret the lung function test.**
2. **What is your conclusion?**
3. **What is the cause of this disease?**

Answers

1. Interpretation of pulmonary function test:
   a. Spirometry demonstrates:
      - FVC and FEV1 are reduced.
      - But FEV1/FVC is normal.
   b. Lung volume study demonstrates:
      - TLC is reduced.
      - RV is reduced.
   c. DLCO is low.
2. The conclusion is that this patient has been suffering from restrictive lung disease.
3. As the BMI is 40 kg/m^2, hence, the cause of the restrictive lung disease is obesity. Decreased lung volume is due to central obesity.

CASE 12

A 70-year-old nonhypertensive old male having BMI of 40 kg/m^2 came to emergency department with shortness of breath. She was advised pulmonary function test, which demonstrated the following:

Parameters	Predicted	Observed	% predicted
FVC	4.4	1.5	34
FEV1	3.43	1.12	32.6
FEV1/FVC		0.74	
FEF25–75	3.98	0.9	22.6

Lung volume:

Parameters	Predicted	Observed	% predicted
TLC	6.8	3.2	47
RV	2.5	1.6	64
RV/TLC	0.37	0.5	136.2

Diffusing capacity:

Parameters	Predicted	Observed	% predicted
DLCO	27.23	15.54	57.06
DLCO/VA	4.2	4.73	112.61

Mean expiratory pressure (MEF) = 220 cm of water
Mean inspiratory pressure (MIF) = 26 cm of water
In the supine position, the FVC = 900 mL

1. **Interpret pulmonary function test.**
2. **What is your conclusion from this data?**
3. **What the most likely diagnosis?**

Answers

1. Interpretation of the date of the pulmonary function test:
   a. Spirometry demonstrates:
      - FVC is low.
      - FEV1 is low.
      - FEV1/FVC is normal.

      It suggests restrictive disease.
   b. Lung volume study demonstrates:
      - TLC is reduced.
      - RV is reduced.

      It suggests restrictive disorder.
   c. Diffusing capacity demonstrates:
      - DLCO is low.
      - DLCO/VA is normal.

      It suggests no diffusion abnormality.
2. The conclusion from the above interpretation is there is presence of restrictive lung disease with normal diffusion capacity.
3. As maximum inspiratory pressure is low but maximum expiratory pressure is normal, it indicates that there is weakness of the inspiratory respiratory muscles. Again in the supine position, the FVC is 900 mL. It indicates severe restriction of the diaphragmatic movement.

CASE 13

A 30-year-old male came to the emergency department with respiratory distress. He was advised pulmonary function test and chest X-ray.

Spirometry demonstrated:

Parameters	Predicted	Observed	% predicted
FVC	5.5	2.0	36.36
FEV1	4.6	1.6	34.78
FEV1/FVC		0.8	
FEF25–75	5	1.2	24

Lung volume:

Parameters	Predicted	Observed	% predicted
TLC	5.9	1.98	33.5
RV	1.6	0.32	20
RV/TLC	0.27	0.16	59.2

Diffusion capacity:

Parameters	Predicted	Observed	% predicted
DLCO	38.9	21.6	53.9
DLCO/VA	5.5	7.32	133.1

Flow-volume curve demonstrated:
Chest X-ray demonstrated:

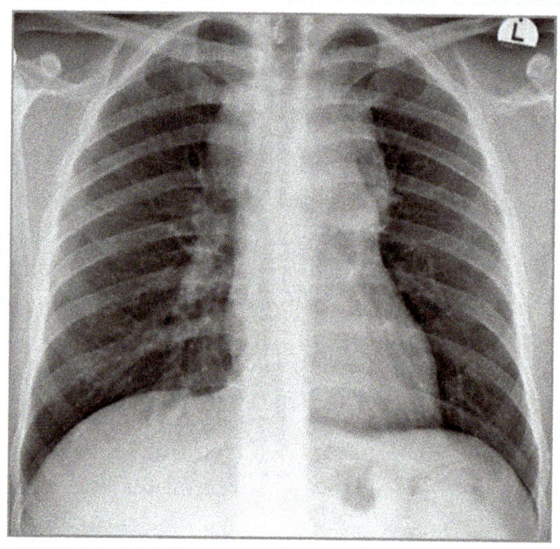

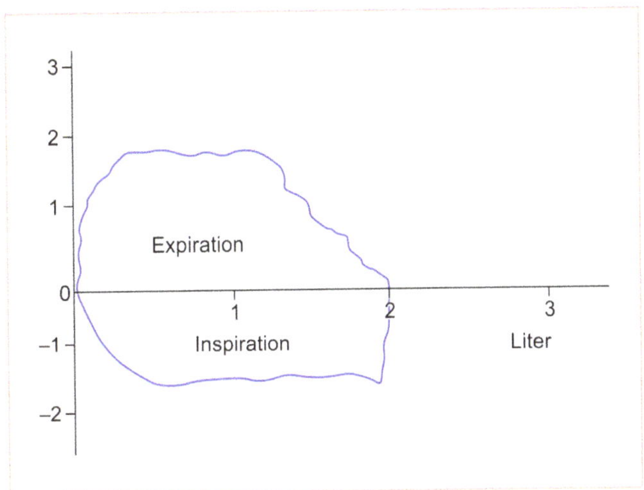

1. **Interpret lung function test.**
2. **Describe the chest X-ray.**
3. **What is your conclusion?**

Answers

1. Interpretation of the lung function test:
   a. Interpretation of spirometry:
      - FEV1 is low.
      - FVC is low.
      - FEV1/FVC is normal.

      It suggests there is restricted pattern of the disease.
   b. Flow-volume loop demonstrates:
      - Inspiratory flow is flat.
      - Expiratory flow is flat.

      It suggests fixed upper airway obstruction.
   c. Diffusing capacity:
      - DLCO is low but if VA is considered, then it overcorrects the diffusing capacity suggesting absence of parenchymal disease.
2. Chest X-ray demonstrates widening of the mediastinum
3. The diagnosis is fixed upper airway obstruction due to compression over the trachea due to paratracheal lymphadenopathy.

CASE 14

A 50-year-old man came to emergency department with respiratory distress. He was advised lung function test and chest X-ray.

Spirometry:

Parameters	Predicted	Observed	% predicted
FVC	4.5	2.56	56.8
FEV1	3.5	1.89	54
FEV1/FVC		73%	
FEF25–75	3.6	1.41	39.1
PEF	8.12	11.78	145.02

Lung volume:

Parameters	Predicted	Observed	% predicted
TLC	6.12	4.1	66.99
RV	2.1	1.3	61.9
RV/TLC	34.3	31.7	

Diffusing capacity:

Parameters	Predicted	Observed	% predicted
DLCO	29.2	18.2	62.32
DLCO/VA	6.25	4.01	64.16

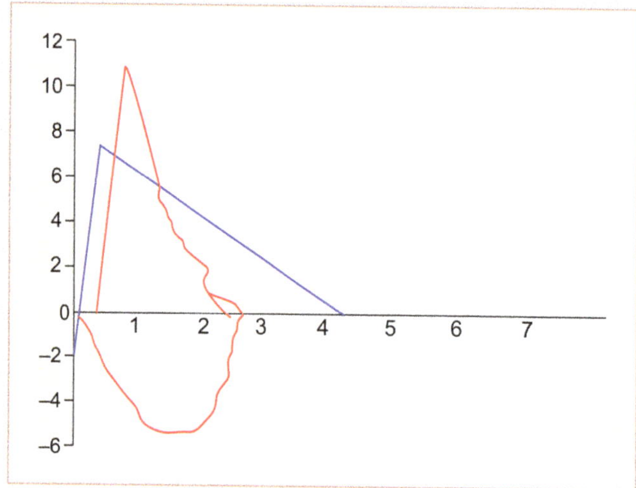

Flow-volume loop demonstrated:

Chest X-ray demonstrated:

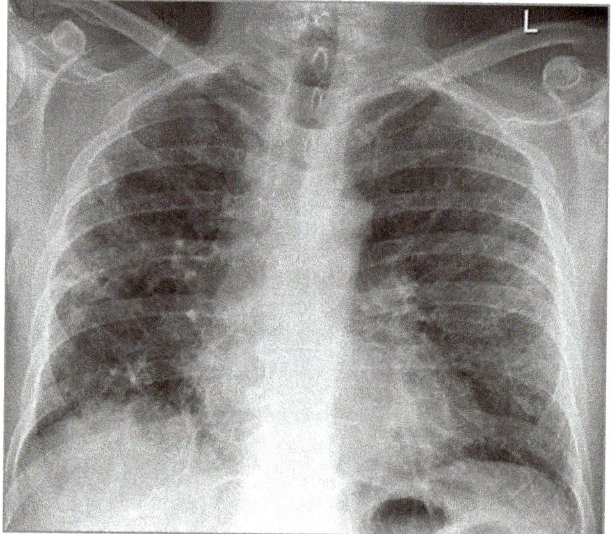

1. **Interpret lung function test.**
2. **Describe the chest X-ray.**
3. **What is your conclusion?**

Answers

1. Interpretation of the lung function test:
   a. Spirometry demonstrates:
      - Low FVC
      - Low FEV1
      - Ratio of FEV1/FVC will be normal.

   It indicates that the patient has restrictive disease.

   b. Lung volume demonstrates:
      - Low TLC
      - Low RV
      - Ratio of RV/TLC is normal.

c. Gas exchange demonstrates that ratio of DLCO/VA is low indicating there is defect at the parenchymal level.

d. Flow-volume curve demonstrates that the inspiratory and expiratory components are small, but expiratory component has steep slope like witch's hat appearance indicating low FVC.

2. Chest X-ray demonstrates:

a. Appearance of reticular shadowing at the periphery of the lung, it is more prominent at the lung bases.

b. The contour of the heart is shaggy in appearance. The diagnosis is interstitial pulmonary fibrosis.

3. This patient has been suffering from restrictive type pulmonary disease like interstitial lung disease leading to pulmonary fibrosis.

CASE 15

A 75-year-old man came to respiratory unit with severe respiratory distress. He was advised pulmonary function test.

Pulmonary function test demonstrated:

Parameters	Predicted	Observed	% predicted
FVC	4.26	2.56	60
FEV1	3.17	1.3	41
FEV1/FVC		50.8	
FEF25–75	7.6	4.9	64.5

Lung volume demonstrated:

Parameters	Predicted	Observed	% predicted
TLC	6.7	4.8	71.64
RV	2.55	2.46	96
RV/TLC	38	51.25	134.8

Diffusing capacity demonstrated:

Parameters	Predicted	Observed	% predicted
DLCO	24.1	9.97	41.36
DLCO/VA	3.7	2.58	69.7

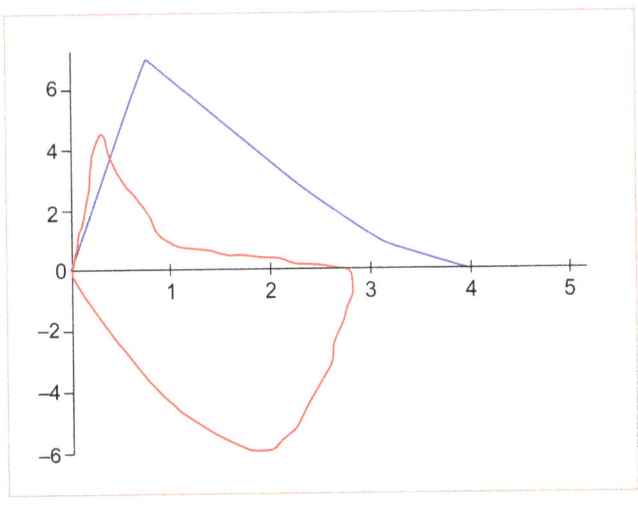

Flow-volume curve demonstrated:

1. **Interpret lung function test.**
2. **What is your diagnosis?**

Answers

1. Interpretation of lung function test:
   a. Spirometry demonstrates:
      - Reduced FVC
      - Reduced FEV1
      - Reduced FEV1/FVC ratio
      - FEF25–75 is also reduced.

      It suggests obstructive disorder.
   b. Lung volume demonstrates:
      - Mildly reduced TLC
      - RV is normal.
      - RV/TLC is increased.

   It suggests mild restrict disorder but there is evidence of air-trapping.
   c. DLCO is reduced. It suggests either obstructive or restrictive disorder.
   d. Flow-volume curve demonstrates:
      - Graph is small.
      - Expiratory curve is scooped out.

      It suggests obstructive disorder.
2. The conclusion is that this patient has been suffering from severe obstructive pulmonary disease with mild restrictive pattern.

CASE 16

A 50-year-old male came to respiratory clinic with respiratory distress and cough. He was advised pulmonary function test. He was advised pulmonary function test.

Parameters	Predicted	Prebronchodilator	% predicted	Postbronchodilator	Change
FVC	4.1	2.67	65.1	3.1	116.1%
FEV1	2.91	1.79	61.52	2.4	134.07%
FEV1/FVC		67.04		77.4	115.45%

1. **Interpret the pulmonary function test.**
2. **Classify the severity of the lung disease.**
3. **What is the conclusion?**

Answers

1. Interpretation of the lung function test: In prebronchodilator phase:
   a. FVC is 65% of predicted. So, it is low.
   b. At prebronchodilator state.
   c. FEV_1/FVC is low at postbronchodilator state.

   In postbronchodilator phase:
   a. There is change in FVC—116.1% change.
   b. There is improvement in FEV1—134.07%.
   c. FEV1/FVC improvement is 115.45%.

2. Classification of the severity of the disease:
   a. FEV1 in prebronchodilator phase is 61.52% predicted. So, degree of obstruction is moderate degree.
   b. There is good response to bronchodilator because changes in FEV1 and FVC are 34% and 16% respectively or >200 mL—indicates good response to bronchodilator.
3. This patient has been suffering from moderately severe bronchial asthma.

CASE 17

A 60-year-old hypertensive woman having past history of systemic lupus erythematosus on steroids and methotrexate came to emergency department with severe respiratory distress but no cough or expectoration. Her pulmonary function test was performed which demonstrated:

Parameters	Predicted	Observed	% predicted
FVC	4.1	1.95	47.5
FEV1	2.95	1.6	54.2
FEV1/FVC		82.05	

TLC	5.73	2.86	49.9
RV	1.5	0.73	48.66
RV/TLC		25.52	

1. **Interpret pulmonary function test.**
2. **What is the conclusion?**

Answers

1. Interpretation of the pulmonary function test:
   a. FVC is low.
   b. FEV1 is low.
   c. FEV1/FVC is normal.
   d. TLC is low.
   e. RV is low.

2. The conclusion is that this patient has been suffering from restrictive lung disease. Since this patient has history of collagen vascular disease. Hence, she most probably has been suffering from interstitial pulmonary fibrosis.

CASE 18

A 20-year-old male came to respiratory clinic with respiratory distress. His pulmonary function test was performed which demonstrated:

Parameters	Predicted	Observed	% predicted
FVC	4.79	3.2	66.8
FEV1	3.37	1.40	41.5
FEV1/FVC	70.35	43.75%	62.18%
FEF25–75%	4.7	1.1	23%

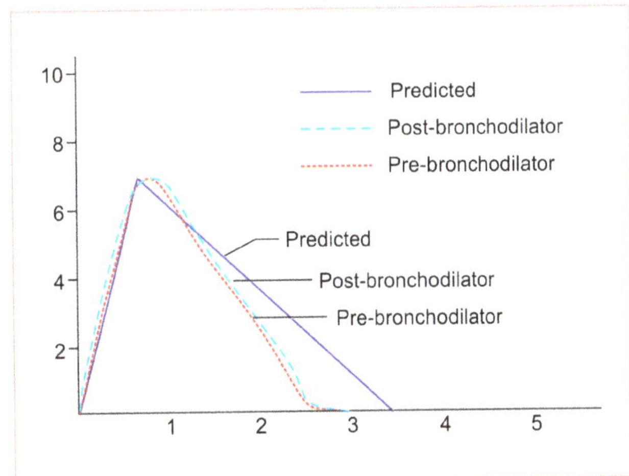

1. **Interpret the pulmonary function test.**
2. **What is your conclusion?**

Answers

1. Interpretation of spirometry:
   a. FVC is 66.8% predicted. So, it has moderate obstructive lung disease.
   b. FEV1 is 41.5%. So, it is <50%. So, it indicates moderately severe obstruction.
   c. FEV1/FVC is 62.18% predicted. So, it is obstructive lung disease.

2. This patient has been suffering from moderately severe obstructive lung disease.

CASE 19

A 45-year-old female, chronic smoker for >15 years, suffers from recurrent upper respiratory tract infection. Chest X-ray being normal and was referred for routine pulmonary function test.

Parameters	Predicted	Prebronchodilator	Predicted	Postbronchodilator
FVC	3.92	3.72	94.8	3.86
FEV1	3.2	2.91	90.9	3.0
FEV1/FVC	81.63	78.22	95.8	76.7
FEF25–75%	3.3	1.85	56	2

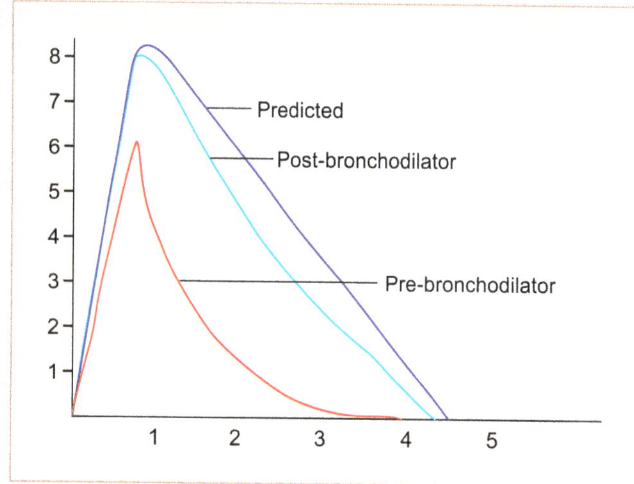

Flow-volume curve demonstrated:

1. **What is the interpretation of the pulmonary function test?**
2. **What is your conclusion?**

Answers

1. Pulmonary function test demonstrates:
   a. Flow-volume curve demonstrates:
      - Abnormally low flow at abnormally low lung volumes
      - There is no difference in the graph in pre- and postbronchodilation.
   b. Spirometry demonstrates that FVC, FEV1, and FEV1/FVC ratio are nearly normal and there is not much difference between pre- and postbronchodilator.
   c. FEF25–75 is abnormally low.

2. This is a case of small airway disease because:
   a. In the flow-volume curve there is abnormally low flow at the low lung volume.
   b. Normal FEV1
   c. FEF25–75% is abnormally low.
   d. There is no significant improvement in the function of the smaller airway after administration of the bronchodilator.
   e. History of smoking

CASE 20

A 20-year-old nonsmoker male came to respiratory clinics with chest tightness and cough in the early morning and during exercise and episodic wheeze. On examination, there was presence of scattered rhonchi throughout the chest. Pulmonary function test was advised, it demonstrated:

Parameters	Predicted	Prebronchodilator	% predicted	Postbronchodilator	% predicted
FEV1	4.4	2.54	57.7	3.51	72.36%
FVC	5.7	4.67	81.9	4.95	105.99%
FEV1/FVC	77.2	54.4		70.9	
FEF25–75%	4.6	2.3	50	4	173.91%

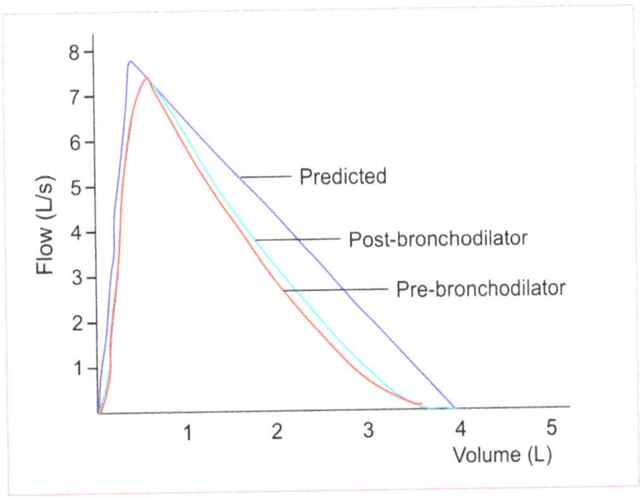

Flow-volume curve demonstrated:

1. **Interpret pulmonary function test.**
2. **What is the most likely diagnosis?**
3. **What is the pathophysiology behind it?**

Answers

1. Interpretation of the pulmonary function test:
   a. FEV1/FVC indicates obstructive lung pathology
   b. FEV1 is 57.7% predicted in prebronchodilator phase—indicated moderately severe obstructive lung disease.
   c. After administration of bronchodilator, there is substantial improvement in FEV1 from 57.7–72.36% predicted and also improvement in the ratio FEV1/FVC from 54.5–70.9%.
   d. Flow-volume curve demonstrates concavity inward in the expiratory flow looking like scooped, associated with low FEV1/FVC ratio indicates obstructive ventilatory defect
2. The most likely diagnosis is moderately severe bronchial asthma.
3. Three main pathophysiology in bronchial asthma:
   a. Constriction of the bronchial smooth muscles which is reversible.
   b. Inflammatory edema of the bronchial mucosa which is reversible with steroid.
   c. Thick mucus in the lumen of the bronchus.

CASE 21

A 40-year-old male having history of smoking for >16 years complained of recurrent upper respiratory tract infection and productive coughing for 3 months. On examination, there was presence of scattered crepitations in both the bases. He was advised pulmonary function test.

Parameters	Predicted	Prebronchodilator	% predicted	Postbronchodilator	% predicted
FEV1	3.7	2.61	70.5	2.85	77.02
FVC	4.7	4.2	89.3	4.34	92.34
FEV1/FVC	78.7	62.14		65.6	
FEF25–75%	3.6	2	55.5	2.2	61.4

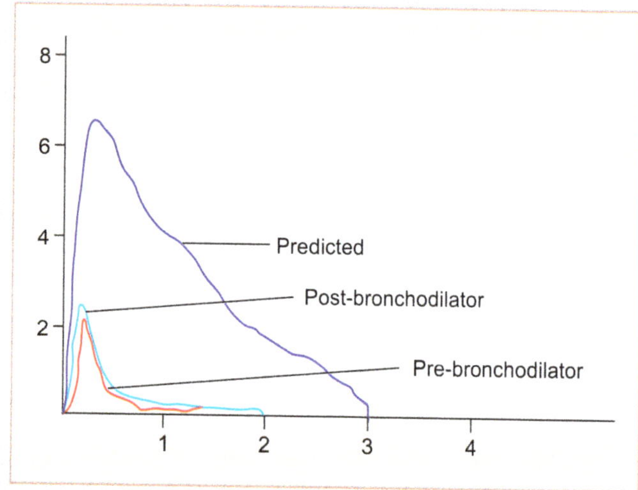

Flow-volume curve demonstrated:

1. **Interpret pulmonary function test.**
2. **What is your diagnosis?**

Answers

1. Interpretation of pulmonary function test:
   a. FEV1/FVC ratio is 62.14% which indicates obstructive pathology.
   b. FEV1 is 70.5% and FEF25-75%, and 55.5% indicates airflow obstruction.
   c. After administration of bronchodilator, there is mild improvement in FEV1 (from 70.5–77.02% predicted), FEV1/FVC ratio (from 62.14–65.6%) indicates little improvement in the pulmonary function.
   d. Flow-volume curve demonstrates expiratory component and has little scalloping inward.
2. Since patient has history of chronic smoking. Hence, the patient has been suffering from mild chronic obstructive pulmonary disease.

CASE 22

A 70-year-old male with history of smoking for >50 years and past history of hospital admission twice for respiratory tract infection and treated. This time patient admitted with type II respiratory failure.

On auscultation, there was evidence of consolidation on right base with evidence of hyperinflation bilaterally. Patient was advised pulmonary function test.

Parameters	Predicted	Prebronchodilator	% predicted	Postbronchodilator	% predicted
FEV1	2.5	0.8	32	0.96	38.4
FVC	3.4	2.0	58.8	2.2	64.7
FEV1/FVC	73.5	40		43.63	
FEF25–75%	1.7	0.88	51.76	0.9	52.9

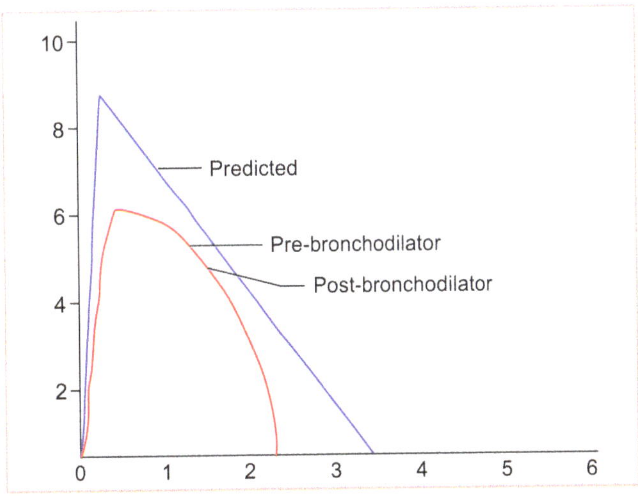

Flow-volume curve demonstrated:

1. **Interpret the pulmonary function test.**
2. **What is the most likely diagnosis?**
3. **What is the cause of limitation of airflow in this case?**

Answers

1. Interpret the pulmonary function test:
   a. Prebronchodilator FEV1 is very much low (32% predicted), FEV1/FVC ratio 40% predicted indicates severe obstructive ventilatory defect.
   b. Postbronchodilator FEV1 was not improved (38.4% predicted).
   c. FVC is reduced indicating closure of the airways.
   d. Flow-volume curve is small with expiratory component is deeply concave.

2. This patient has been suffering from severe chronic obstructive airway disease leading to secondary infection.

3. Airflow limitation in this case is due to:
   a. Inflammatory thickening as well as distortion of the walls of the airways—indication of small airway disease.
   b. Expiratory collapse of the small and large airways due to loss of elastic support

CASE 23

A 42-year-old nonsmoker female having history of rheumatoid arthritis came to respiratory clinic with exertional respiratory distress. On respiratory system examination, there was coarse crackles in the bases of the lungs bilaterally. Her chest X-ray demonstrated:

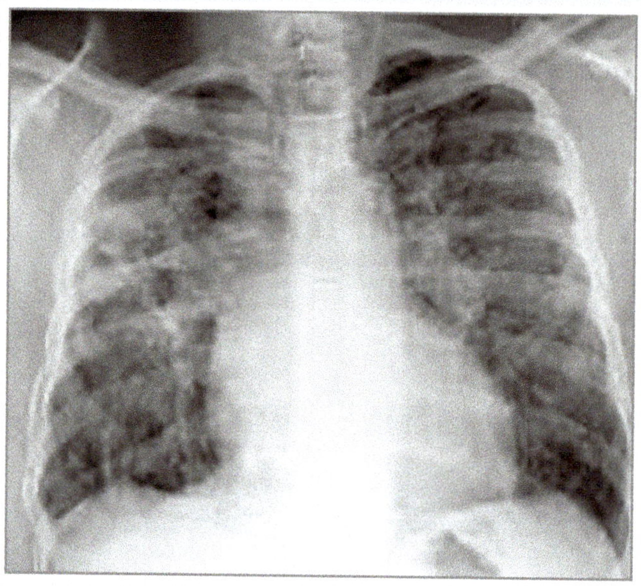

She was advised pulmonary function test:

Parameters	Predicted	Prebronchodilator	% predicted	Postbronchodilator	% predicted
FEV1	3.2	2.1	65.6	2.15	67.2
FVC	4.1	2.38	58	2.41	58.78
FEV1/FVC	78	88.2		89.2	
FEF25–75%	3.28	4.1	125	4.32	131.7

Flow-volume curve demonstrated:

1. **Interpret the pulmonary function test.**
2. **Describe the chest X-ray.**
3. **What is the likely diagnosis?**
4. **Why there is increased flow through the airways?**

Answers

1. Interpretation of pulmonary function test:
    a. FEV1 and FVC are reduced but FEV1/FVC ratio is normal indicating restrictive lung disease.
    b. FEF25–75% is supernormal indicating absence of airway obstruction.
    c. There is no change after administration of the bronchodilator.
    d. Flow-volume curve demonstrates small in size

2. Chest X-ray demonstrates reticular and reticulonodular shadow bilaterally throughout the lung indicating diffuse pulmonary infiltrate

3. Patient has been suffering from fibrosing alveolitis in a case of rheumatoid arthritis.

4. Supernormal flow rates are due to increased traction of the wall of the airways from the surrounding lung parenchyma leading to distention of the airways.

CASE 24

A 42-year-old female came to respiratory outpatient department with complaint of chest pain. On examination, her height was 154 cm and weight was 61 kg. Her pulmonary function test demonstrated:

Parameters	Predicted	Measured	Percentage
FEV1	2.36	1.95	82.62
FVC	2.75	2.65	96.36
FEV1/FVC ratio	85.8	73.58	85.75
PEF		2.78	
FEF25–75	3.48	1.36	39%

1. **Interpret this pulmonary function test.**
2. **What are FEV1 and FVC?**
3. **FEV1/FVC ratio—what is its importance?**
4. **Why FVC is important in the pulmonary function test?**
5. **Why FVC increases in case of pulmonary fibrosis?**

Answers

1. FEV1—82.62%, FVC—96.36%, and FEV1/FVC—85.75%. These values indicate normal spirometry. But, the FEF is 39% predicted. Hence in the face of all the normal values, FEF value suggests the presence of bronchial hyperresponsiveness to any allergen. So, the patient has been suffering from allergic rhinitis.
2. *FEV1*: It can be defined as forced expiratory volume in 1 second. FVC—it can be defined as forced vital capacity.
3. *FEV1/FVC ratio*: This ratio indicates the nature of the lung diseases. In case of obstructive and restrictive type of lung disease, this ratio will be reduced, but these two types can be differentiated by examining the total lung capacity which will be reduced in case of restrictive type and increased or normal in case of obstructive type of lung diseases.
4. FVC is important in pulmonary function test as any subject has unique limit to maximal air flow at any given lung volume and this limit can be reached with moderate expiratory efforts. Addition of force cannot increase the airway flow during expiration. Once the peak flow will be reached, the patient cannot exceed the air flow of 5.2 L/s regardless his or her effort.
5. In case of pulmonary fibrosis, airways will be distended due to increased lung tissue elasticity leading to increase in the maximal flow in spite of decreased lung volume. Hence, FVC will be increased.

CASE 25

A 42-year-old female has come to chest department with mild respiratory distress. On examination, her weight was 61 kg, height 152 cm, basal metabolic index 26.4 kg/m^2, chest examination demonstrated mild wheezing, and diminished breath sound with prolonged expiration. Pulmonary function test demonstrated:

Parameters	Predicted	Measured	Percentage
FEV1	2.38	1.88	78.99%
FVC	2.8	2.45	87.5%
FEV1/FVC ratio	85	78.78	92.68
PEF		3.12	

1. **How can you interpret this pulmonary function test?**
2. **What should be the condition of total lung capacity?**
3. **What the causes of lung diseases responsible for this abnormality in the lung function test?**
4. **What are the mechanisms of alveolar hypoventilation in obstructive lung diseases?**
5. **What are the causes of altered physiology in case of obstructive lung diseases?**

Answers

1. FEV1, FVC, and FEV1/FVC are 78.99% (<80%), 87.5%, and 92.68%, respectively. It indicates that this patient has been suffering from mild obstructive airway disease.

2. In this case, total lung capacity should be normal but as the disease will advance, this value will be gradually increased.

3. Following are the obstructive lung diseases:
   a. Bronchial asthma
   b. Chronic obstructive pulmonary diseases
   c. Emphysema

4. Mechanism of hypoventilation in the obstructive lung diseases:
   a. Increased work of breathing
   b. Ventilation/perfusion mismatch
   c. Abnormalities in the ventilatory drive
   d. Decreased effectiveness of the diaphragm

5. Following are the causes of the altered physiology in case of obstructive lung diseases:
   a. Increased residual volume:
      - Intrinsic increase:
        - In acute asthma, bronchial obstruction
        - In chronic obstructive due to lung disease or emphysema
        - In case of due to bronchiectasis or cystic fibrosis, bronchial obstruction
      - Extrinsic increase due to:
        - Tracheomalacia
        - Obese neck

CASE 26

A 35-year-old male came to emergency with severe respiratory distress, cough, and wheeze. On examination of the chest, there was diminished vesicular breath sound with prolonged expiration. His pulmonary function tests demonstrated as below:

Parameters	Predicted	Measured	Percentage
FEV1	3.35	1.10	33.33%
FVC	3.90	1.90	48.71%
FEV1/FVC ratio	85	57.89%	68.10%
PEF	8.4	2.8	33.33%
FEF25–75	4.3	0.9	20.93%

1. **Interpret the pulmonary function test.**
2. **What is your diagnosis?**
3. **How can you grade obstructive lung disease?**
4. **Why FVC will be decreased in case of bronchial asthma?**

Answers

1. FEV1 33.33% of predicted, FVC 48.71% of predicted, and FEV1/FVC 68.10%—suggest airway obstruction. FEF25–75 suggests obstruction as the level of smaller airways.

2. According to the definition of severity of obstructive lung disease, this patient has been suffering from moderately obstructive lung disease.

3. Gradation of the obstructive lung disease:
   a. *Grade 1*: Mild—
      - FEV1/FVC < 70% predicted
      - FEV1 > 70% predicted
   b. *Grade 2*: Moderate—
      - FEV1/FVC > 60% but <70% predicted
      - FEV1: 60–69% predicted
   c. *Grade 3*: Moderately severe—
      - FEV1/FVC: 50–59% predicted
      - FEV1: 50–59% predicted
   d. *Grade 4*: Severe—
      - FEV1/FVC: 35–49% predicted
      - FEV1: 35–49% predicted
   e. *Grade 5*: Very severe—
      - FEV1/FVC < 35% predicted
      - FEV1 < 35% predicted

4. In case of bronchial asthma, resistance to the maximal airflow will be decreased because of the following:
   a. Bronchial smooth muscle spasm
   b. Inflammation of the bronchial mucosa
   c. Mucosal edema
   d. Mucus plug on the bronchial wall

CASE 27

There are three values of spirometry from the three subjects:

Subject	FEF25–75 L/s	PEF L/s	FEF50 L/s	FEF75 L/s
Normal (1)	3.14	9	5.9	3.1
2	0.65	2.5	0.8	0.5
3	1.34	7.4	5	2.6

1. **How can you interpret the above value?**
2. **What are the three subjects suffering from?**
3. **Describe the meaning of the above parameters.**

Answers

1. FEF25–75 in second subject is 21% predicted, PEF is 27.77% predicted, FEF50 is 13.55% predicted, and FEF75 is 16.12% predicted.

   FEF 25 - 75 in third subject is 42.67% predicted, PEF is 82.22% predicted, FEF 50 is 84.74% predicted and FEF 75 is 83.87% predicted.

   So, in the first subject, all the values are within normal limit. In the second subject, all the observed values are far below the predicted value. In case of third subject, all the observed value are >80% of the predicted value.

2. The differential diagnoses are:
   a. First subject is normal.
   b. Second subject has been suffering from the obstructive lung diseases.
   c. Third subject has been suffering from restrictive lung diseases.

3. a. FEF25–75 is the middle 50% of the forced vital capacity and this can be measured from the spirogram. It will indicate the conditions of the smaller airways.
   b. *PEF*: It can be described as the highest airflow that can be achieved during full expiration. It can be used as short-term monitoring tool.
   c. *FEF5*: It is the flow of air after 50% of the forced vital capacity which has been exhaled.
   d. *FEF75*: It is the flow of air after 75% of the forced vital capacity which will be exhaled.

CHAPTER 11

Renal Medicine

An 80-year-old African hypertensive female on antihypertensive medications for 20 years came to medicine department with anorexia, nausea with occasional vomiting, weight loss for >10 kg body weight, lethargy, muscle cramps, pruritus, and tiredness. She has past history of cerebrovascular accidents.

On examination, the patient is anemic, pulse rate 90 beats/min, blood pressure 190/110 mm Hg, and pedal edema. Her cardiovascular and respiratory examinations were normal. Neurological examination demonstrated mild right-sided limb weakness with hyperreflexia.

Fundoscopy demonstrated:

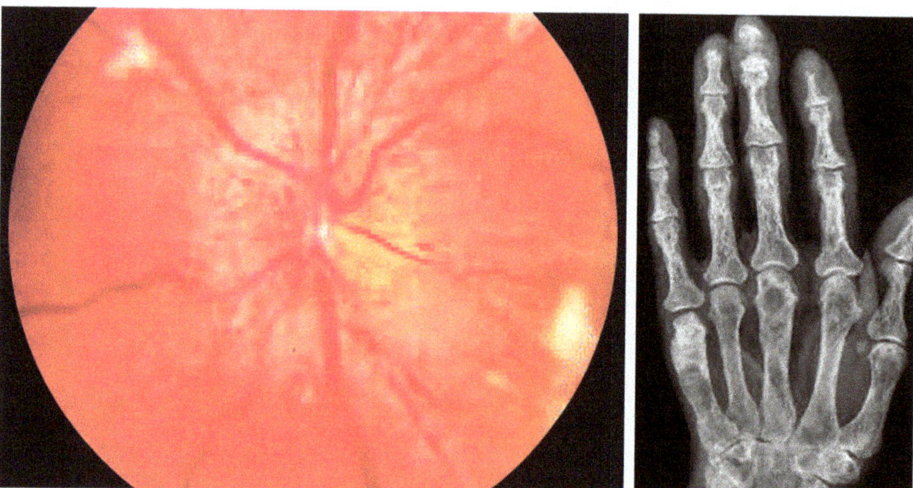

Her blood level demonstrated hemoglobin 7.8 g/dL, mean corpuscular volume (MCV) 85 fL, total white blood cell count 6,800/cc, liver function test demonstrated alkaline phosphatase 420 IU/L, calcium and phosphate level of 8 mg/dL, and phosphate 3.5 mmol/L.

1. **What is the above fundoscopic finding?**
2. **What do the above X-ray pictures demonstrate?**
3. **What is your diagnosis?**
4. **What are the features suggestive of the chronicity of the disease?**
5. **What are the features which may be found that are suggestive of chronic renal failure?**
6. **What are the familial diseases lead to chronic renal failure?**

Answers

1. Fundoscopic features are:
   a. Blurring of the optic disk
   b. Cotton-wool spot
   c. Presence of macular star
   d. Increased tortuosity of the arteries
2. Above X-ray pictures demonstrate:
   a. Erosion of the terminal phalanx
   b. Subperiosteal erosions of the middle phalanx of middle finger on its radial aspect.
3. The diagnosis is end-stage renal failure in a case of hypertensive chronic kidney disease associated with hypertensive retinopathy.
4. Following features are suggestive of chronicity of this disease:
   a. Positive history:
      - Normocytic normochromic anemia suggestive of erythropoietin deficiency
      - Raised alkaline phosphatase suggestive of hyperthyroidism due to decreased renal clearance of the phosphate and reduction of $1\alpha,25$-dihydroxycholecalciferol as a result of decreased synthesis of 1α-hydroxylase
      - Suggestive of X-ray feature
   b. Negative features:
      - Absence of sepsis
      - Absence of administration of the nephrotoxic drugs
      - Absence of prolonged period of hypotension
5. Following features may be found in the renal ultrasound: In chronic kidney disease:
   a. Polycystic kidney disease
   b. Bilateral ureteral obstruction leading to bilateral hydronephrosis
   c. Renovascular disease
   d. Reflux nephropathy
   e. Small size kidney of <8 cm bilaterally
   f. Increased echogenicity indicating increased tissue density
6. Following familial diseases lead to chronic renal failure:
   a. Autosomal adult polycystic kidney disease
   b. Autosomal recessive polycystic kidney disease
   c. Hypertension
   d. Chromosome 9, 10, 11, and 19 related renal segmental glomerulosclerosis
   e. Autosomal dominant tubulointestinal diseases
   f. Diabetes mellitus
   g. Alport syndrome
   h. Fabry disease
   i. Sickle cell nephropathy
   j. Familial hypercalcemic hypocalciuria
   k. Cystinuria
   l. Barakat syndrome or HDM syndrome syndrome related to mutation of GATA3 gene located chromosome 10p14 consisting of hypoparathyroidism, sensorineural hearing loss, and kidney disease
   m. Liddle syndrome
   n. Bartter syndrome
   o. Gitelman syndrome

CASE 2

A 30-year-old female came to medical outpatient department with high swinging temperature, progressively increasing pain in the loin, and nausea with occasional vomiting for 5 days. On examination, patient looked toxic, pulse rate 110 beats/min, temperature 104°C, blood pressure 110/75 mm Hg, on abdominal examination both the loin are tender, and other systems were normal.

Laboratory examination demonstrated white blood cell count 20,000/cc and C-reactive protein (CRP) 120 mg/L. Urine analysis showed >50 red and white blood cells/high power field (HPF).

Urine microscopy demonstrated:

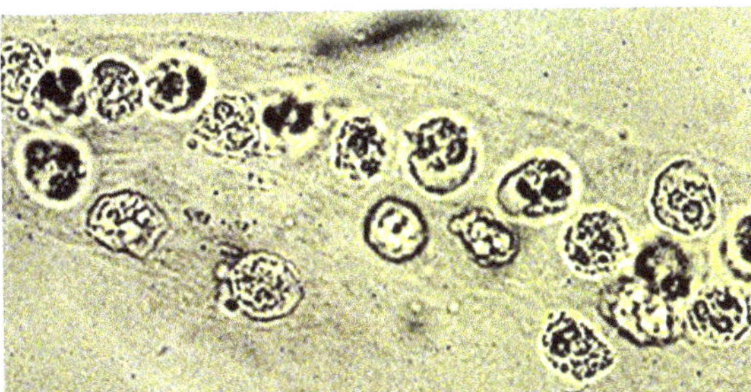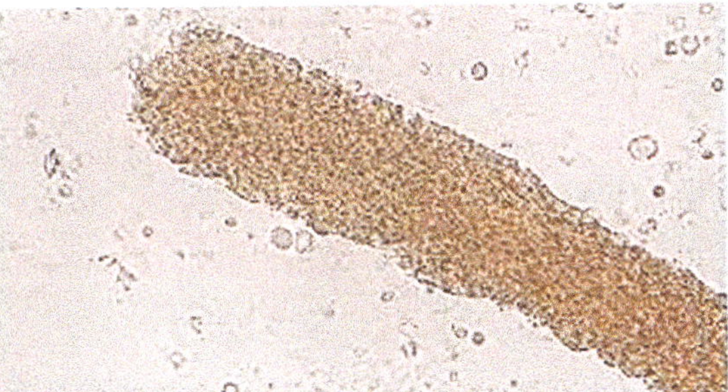

1. **Describe the above pictures found in the urine.**
2. **What is your diagnosis?**
3. **What are the cells found in the urine?**
4. **What is the normal cast found in the urine?**
5. **What are the types of cast found in the urine?**
6. **How can you prevent acute uncomplicated urinary tract infection?**
7. **How can you treat this case?**

Answers

1. Above pictures demonstrate:
   a. White blood cell casts
   b. Red blood cell casts
2. The patient has been suffering from acute pyelonephritis.
3. Following cells are found in urine:
   a. Squamous epithelial cells—15–20 per low power field indicates that the urine is contaminated.
   b. Transitional epithelial cells: It is found in:
      • Bladder catheterization
      • Bladder irrigation
      • Malignancy
   c. Renal tubular epithelial cells: It occurs in case of tubular injury.
   d. Red blood cells: >2 red blood cells/HPF suggest either infection or glomerulonephritis. If it is dysmorphic, it suggests upper urinary tract infection. If its shape is normal, it indicates lower urinary tract infection.
   e. White blood cells: 2–5 cells/HPF is considered normal but more than this indicates urinary tract infection or interstitial nephritis or in allergic nephritis.
4. Cast is formed by coagulated protein secreted by the tubular cells in the long, thin, and hollow distal convoluted renal tubules or collecting ducts.
5. Following types of cast are found in the urine:
   a. Hyaline cast: It is found in the normal individuals in case of:
      • Severe volume depletion
      • Morning urine sample
      • Acidic and concentrated urine
   b. Granular casts: It is found in acute tubular necrosis originating from break down of cellular casts.
   c. Waxy and broad cast: It occurs in advanced kidney disease.
   d. Red blood cell cast: It is found in—
      • Glomerulonephritis
      • Acute pyelonephritis
   e. White blood cell casts: It is found in—
      • Pyelonephritis
      • Tubulointerstitial nephritis
      • Renal tuberculosis
   f. Fatty casts: It looks like "Maltese cross" under polarized lamp. It is found in nephrotic syndrome.
6. This urinary tract infection can be prevented by following methods: This is required when woman experiences two infections within 6 months or three infections within a year.
   a. Postintercourse single dose:
      • Nitrofurantoin 100 mg
      • Trimethoprim 100 mg
      • Ciprofloxacin 125 mg
      • Norfloxacin 200 mg
      • Cephalexin 250 mg
   b. Long-term low dose (at bed time daily):
      • Nitrofurantoin 100 mg
      • Trimethoprim 100 mg
      • Ciprofloxacin 125 mg
      • Norfloxacin 200 mg
      • Cephalexin 500 mg
      • Trimethoprim/sulfamethoxazole 40/200 mg
7. This patient can be treated by the following regimen:
   a. First-line treatment:
      • Nitrofurantoin 100 mg twice daily for 5 days
      • Fosfomycin 3 g single dose
      • Pivmecillinam 400 mg twice daily for 5 days
   b. Second-line therapy:
      • Trimethoprim/sulfamethoxazole 160/800 mg twice daily for 3–5 days
      • Trimethoprim 100 mg twice daily for 3–5 days
      • Ciprofloxacin 500 mg twice daily for 3–5 days
      • Levofloxacin 500 mg daily for 3–5 days
      • Norfloxacin 400 mg twice daily for 3–5 days.
      • Amoxicillin plus clavulanic acid 625 mg twice to thrice daily for 7 days

CASE 3

A 75-year-old hypertensive male taking 50 mg metoprolol daily, consumer of 30 cigarettes daily, and 30 units of alcohol weekly came to outpatient department with progressively increasing swelling of both legs starting from feet up to sacrum and involving penis and scrotum along with swelling of the face in the morning and frothy urine for 2 months. For last 7 days, patient has exertional respiratory distress and spontaneous bruising. On examination, there was bilateral limb edema, bruising on forearm and periorbital purpura, other vitals were normal, and engorged pulsatile neck vein. Both lung bases are dull on percussion and inspiratory crackles. Other systems were within normal limit.

Laboratory investigation demonstrated that there is normochromic normocytic anemia, cholesterol 388 mg/dL, triglyceride 244 mg/dL, albumin 2.2 g/dL, and renal function test was within normal limit. Urinalysis demonstrated +++ protein but no blood.

1. **What are the causes of the edema in this patient?**
2. **What is the cause of periorbital bruises?**
3. **What is the most probable diagnosis?**
4. **What are the essential features in this disease?**
5. **What are the types of the etiological material?**
6. **How can you diagnose the etiology?**
7. **What are the other non-nephrogenic presentations of this etiology?**

Answers

1. Since the patient has bilateral limb edema along with periorbital edema, it indicates that the patient has been suffering from nephrotic syndrome.

2. Patient has periorbital purpura, bruising in the forearm along with normocytic, and has normochromic anemia which is suggestive of amyloidosis.

3. Patient has been suffering from nephrotic syndrome resulting from amyloid nephropathy.

4. The essential features are as follows:
   a. Deposition of acellular eosinophilic material arising from abnormal protein bound to amyloid P protein within:
      - Tubulointerstitium
      - Vessel wall
      - Glomeruli
   b. This is negative for Jones silver, lightly positive on periodic acid-Schiff (PAS), and blue-gray on trichrome staining.

5. There are following types of deposited materials:
   a. AL type caused by monoclonal gammopathy of light chain which is frequently associated with lambda light chain
   b. AA type characterized by serum amyloid A protein associated with:
      - Inflammatory conditions
      - Intravenous drug use
      - Connective tissue disorders
      - Infections
      - Inflammatory bowel disease
      - Paraneoplastic syndrome
   c. ALECT2 type is leukocyte cell-derived chemotaxin-2 amyloid protein most commonly involves kidney followed by the liver.
   d. Hereditary type is autosomal dominant with variable penetrance, most common being transthyretin type. Here, renal involvement is due to mutation of Val30Met.

6. Diagnosis can be done by:
   a. Visualization of the characteristic of deposits seen by special stains
   b. Confirmation by:
      - Orange-red color by Congo red stain
      - Apple-green birefringence when seen by polarized microscopy
   c. Potassium permanganate bleaches AA amyloid
   d. Specific immunohistochemistry can identify immunoglobulin light chains or amyloid A protein
   e. Electron microscopy can detect nonbranching randomly arranged amyloid fibrils, but it cannot distinguish AA, AL, or AH amyloids.
   f. Amyloid type can be confirmed by spectrometry and serum flow cytometry.

7. Other presentations according to organ involvement are:
   a. Restrictive cardiomyopathy
   b. Infiltrative liver disease
   c. Peripheral neuropathy due to carpal tunnel syndrome
   d. Macroglossia
   e. Primary hypoadrenalism

CASE 4

A 47-year-old hypertensive, nonalcoholic, and nondiabetic female came to emergency department with dull aching continuous pain in the loin for years and macroscopic hematuria for 2 days. She has past history of similar pain bilaterally for >22 years. She was hypertensive since her first pregnancy. Her father died due to subarachnoid hemorrhage. Her paternal uncle had history of renal transplantation.

On examination, her blood pressure was 190/110 mm Hg, rest of the vital was in normal limit. On abdominal examination, there were masses bilaterally in the loin, ballottable, right one being tender, and percussion note over the masses was tympanic. In laboratory examination, hematological and biochemical tests were normal.

Urine analysis demonstrated blood is strongly positive. Urine microscopy demonstrated >250 red cells and 15 white blood cells/HPF.

1. **What is the most probable diagnosis?**
2. **What are the points in favor of this diagnosis?**
3. **What are the genetic mutations occurred in this disease?**
4. **What are differences between the genes responsible for this disease?**
5. **What are the revised ultrasound criteria for diagnosis of this disease?**
6. **What are the revised ultrasound criteria to exclude this disease?**
7. **What are the common extra-renal manifestations in this disease?**
8. **Mention the frequent complications in this disease.**
9. **What are the mechanisms for hypertension in this disease?**
10. **What are the effects of uncontrolled blood pressure in this disease?**
11. **What are the prognostic tools for predicting the progression of the disease?**
12. **What are the indications of nephrectomy in this disease?**

Answers

1. The most probable diagnosis is autosomal dominant polycystic kidney disease (ADPKD).
2. Following are the points in favor of this diagnosis:
   a. Presence of ballottable masses in the loin bilaterally
   b. Presence of pain in the loin
   c. Macroscopic hematuria
   d. Hypertension
   e. Family history of death due to subarachnoid hemorrhage
   f. Family history of renal transplant
3. Mutations of the two following genes lead to development of ADPKDs:
   a. *PKD1* located on short arm of the chromosome 6 encoding polycystin-1
   b. *PKD2* located on chromosome 4 encoding polycystin-2

   Both the membrane-bound glycoproteins are present on the plasma membrane of primary cilia regulating calcium homeostasis.
   c. Mutation of *GANAB* gene encoding glucosidase II subunit responsible for 3% of these unresolved cases.
4. Mutation of *PKD1* gene leads to increased number of cyst formation but not the faster growth of these cysts as compared to the mutation of *PKD2* gene
5. Revised criteria for diagnosis of ADPKD are as follows:
   a. In 15–39 years of patients, ≥3 cysts—unilateral or bilateral
   b. In 30–39 years of patients, ≥3 cysts—unilateral or bilateral
   c. In 40–49 years of patients, ≥2 cysts in each kidney
   d. In >60 years of age, ≥4 cysts in each kidney

6. Revised ultrasound criteria to exclude this disease are as follows:
   a. 15–29 years of age: ≥1 cyst in kidney
   b. 30–39 years of age: ≥1 cyst in kidney
   c. 40–49 years of age: ≥2 cyst in kidney
7. Common extra-renal manifestations in this patient are as follows:
   a. Polycystic liver disease
   b. Pancreatic cysts
   c. Seminal vesicle cysts
   d. Vascular manifestations:
      - Intracranial aneurysms
      - Dolichoectasias
      - Dissection of cervicocephalic artery
      - Dissection of the thoracic aorta
      - Aneurysm of coronary artery
   e. Cardiac valvular abnormalities:
      - Mitral valve prolapse
      - Aortic regurgitation
      - Tricuspid valve prolapse
   f. Colonic diverticulosis
   g. Abdominal hernias:
      - Inguinal hernia
      - Paraumbilical hernia
      - Incisional hernia
8. Most common complications in this disease are as follows:
   a. Hypertension
   b. Pain in the loin
   c. Nephrolithiasis
   d. Urinary infection
   e. End-stage renal disease
9. Following are the mechanisms of hypertension in this disease:
   a. Activation of renin-angiotensin-aldosterone system
   b. Expansion of cysts
   c. Intrarenal ischemia
   d. Decreased expression levels of polycystin-1 and polycystin-2
   e. Decreased availability of nitric oxide
10. Uncontrolled blood pressure will lead to following effects:
    a. Increased mortality rates from:
       - Valvular heart diseases
       - Aneurysms
    b. Increases the risk of:
       - Proteinuria
       - Hematuria
    c. Increases the risk of speedy decline of renal function
11. Following are the tools for predicting the prognosis of this disease:
    a. CT or MR imaging:
       - Class I: Typically bilateral and diffuse presentation
       - Class II: Atypical and asymmetric distribution of cysts
    b. Mutant PKD1 is more worse than PKD2 mutation
    c. Male sex
    d. Truncating mutation is worse than nontruncating mutation in PKD1
    e. Diagnosis prior to age of 30 years.
    f. Hyperlipidemia
    g. Low high-density lipoprotein
    h. First episode of hematuria prior to age of 30 years
    i. Onset of hypertension prior to 35 years of age
    j. Sickle cell trait
12. Following are the indications of nephrectomy in this patient:
    a. Recurrent infection
    b. Severe infection
    c. Severe renal hemorrhage
    d. Intractable pain
    e. Renal carcinoma
    f. Pretransplant nephrectomy should be done in case of hugely enlarged kidney interfering with the site of implantation of the transplanted kidney.

CASE 5

A 37-year-old smoker taking 22 cigarettes daily, alcoholic taking 12 units weekly, hypertensive for 3 years resistant to four drugs came to hypertensive clinic. She had past history of pregnancy which was uneventful.

On examination, her vitals were normal except blood pressure was 95/105 mm Hg, absence of café-au-lait spot or neurofibroma, and no evidence of radiofemoral delay. All the systems were in normal function.

Laboratory investigations demonstrated urea 88 mg/dL and creatinine 1.54 mg/dL. Ultrasound of kidney was normal. Renal angiogram demonstrated:

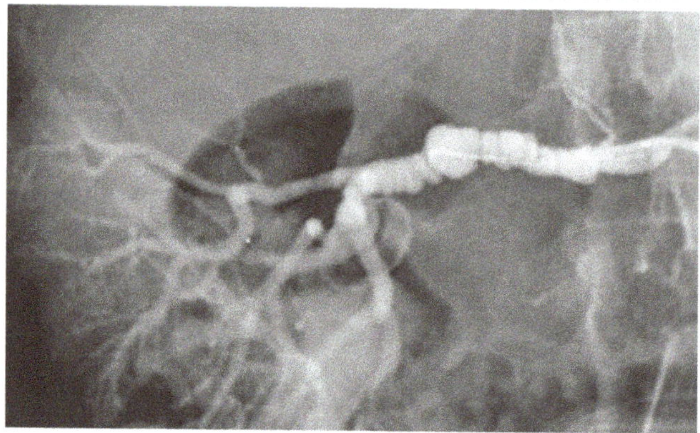

1. **What is the finding in the above picture?**
2. **What is your diagnosis?**
3. **What are the types of this etiology?**
4. **Which clinical syndromes are associated with this etiology?**
5. **What are the features to be screened in this disease?**
6. **What are the risk factors for this disease?**
7. **What is resistance index and how can you use it to manage this case?**
8. **Which group of patients cannot be benefited from revascularization?**
9. **What are the imaging investigations to be done in this case?**
10. **How renal angiography helps in detecting functionally significant lesion?**
11. **What are the characteristics of the patients get benefit from revascularization?**

Answers

1. Above picture demonstrates "string of beds" appearance in the mid portion of the right renal artery

2. The patient has been suffering from refractory hypertension due to renovascular disease resulting from fibromuscular dysplasia.

3. There are following causes of renal artery stenosis:
   a. Atherosclerotic renal artery stenosis—most common type
   b. Fibromuscular dysplasia—second most common type
   c. Others are:
      - Thromboembolic disease
      - Aortic dissection
      - Infrarenal aortic aneurysm
      - Takayasu arteritis
      - Berger's disease
      - Polyarteritis nodosa
      - Type 1 neurofibromatosis
      - Retroperitoneal fibrosis

4. Typical syndrome associated with renal artery stenosis consist of:
   a. Renovascular hypertension
   b. Progressive loss of renal function due to ischemic nephropathy
   c. Recurrent flushing pulmonary edema occurring in case of bilateral renal artery stenosis or unilateral renal artery stenosis involving solitary kidney

5. Following are the features suggestive of renal artery stenosis:
   a. Sudden onset of hypertension at 30 years of age or older than 50 years of age
   b. Recurring episodes of flushing pulmonary edema
   c. Renal failure of unknown cause
   d. Unilateral atrophic kidney
   e. Sudden worsening of the previously well-tolerated hypertension
   f. Renal failure precipitated by angiotensin-converting enzyme inhibitor (ACEI) or angiotensin receptor blockers (ARBs)

g. Present of abdominal bruit on auscultation

h. Unexplained hypokalemia

i. Presence of associated atherosclerosis involving the other renal artery

6. Following are the risk factors in this disease due to atherosclerosis:
   a. Hypertension
   b. Diabetes mellitus
   c. Smokers
   d. Older age
   e. Dyslipidemia

7. Resistance index is characterized by measurement of velocity of relative blood flow both during systole and diastole in renal artery by Doppler ultrasonography which can be calculated by the following:

$$\text{Resistance index} = (1 - \text{enddiastolic velocity}/\text{maximal systolic velocity}) \times 100$$

   This index will correlate with changes in the blood pressure following revascularization.

   If the index is >89, it suggests extensive atherosclerotic disease involving smaller vessels and this cannot be recovered after revascularization.

8. Following groups of patients cannot be benefited from revascularization:
   a. Preexisting long-standing hypertension for >3 years well controlled with medical therapies
   b. Kidney size is <8 cm.
   c. Preexisting chronic kidney disease which is stable but progresses over time.
   d. Insignificant stenosis physiologically on noninvasive imaging, i.e., stenosis <70%

9. Following imaging investigations should be done in this disease:
   a. Renal ultrasound with Doppler study:
      - Peak systolic velocities

- Renal to aortic ratio: It is the ratio of peak systolic velocities in the renal artery to the aorta. This ratio of >3.5 correlates with significant renal artery stenosis.
- Resistive index: It can be defined as (peak systolic velocity, end-diastolic velocity)/peak systolic velocity. It indicates resistance to blood flow in the microcirculation.

   b. Spiral computed tomography and CT angiography: It is highly sensitive and specific method for detecting the renal artery stenosis.
   c. Magnetic resonance angiography: It will use gadolinium contrast which may lead to nephrogenic systemic fibrosis in case of advanced kidney injury if GFR is <30 mL/min/m^2.
   d. Renal angiography
   e. Captopril radionuclide angiogram

10. Following translational pressure gradient can help to detect the functionally significant lesion:
   a. Ratio between the pressure in the distal and proximal to the stenosis of <0.9
   b. Resting mean pressure gradient of >10 mm Hg
   c. Hyperemic systolic gradient of >20 mm Hg

11. Following types of patients may get benefit from revascularization:
   a. Recent onset of resistant or accelerated or malignant hypertension who have stable control of previous blood pressure.
   b. Recent onset of acute or subacute deterioration of the renal function who are suffering from stable chronic kidney disease.
   c. After administration of ARBs or ACEI, there is significant rise in creatinine.
   d. Sudden and recent increase in the dose as well as number of antihypertensive medications who have stable blood pressure previously.

CASE 6

A 65-year-old nonsmoker, nonhypertensive, and nondiabetic female was developed prolonged ileus and abdominal pain after right hemicolectomy on two broad-spectrum antibiotics followed by spiky temperature, for which gentamicin was added. In spite of that temperature was continued, blood culture was negative. After 1 day, patient gradually became hypotensive with systolic blood pressure 90 mm Hg and oliguria.

On examination, her pulse rate was 120 beats/min and respiratory rate 32 breaths/min. There is localized guarding in the right iliac fossa and absent bowel sound.

Investigation demonstrated white blood count 24,000/cc, hemoglobin 8 g/dL, sodium 128 IU/L, potassium 6 mEq/L, creatinine 5.9 mg/dL, urea 102 mg/dL, bilirubin 5.5 mg/dL, alanine aminotransferase (ALT) 63 IU/L, serum gentamicin level 4.9 mg/dL (normal <2 mg/dL), and serum glucose 54 mg/dL.

1. **What is your diagnosis?**
2. **What are the manifestations of septicemia?**
3. **Why liver function test has been altered?**
4. **What are the risk factors associated with aminoglycoside nephrotoxicity?**
5. **How the dose of this drug can be modified?**

Answers

1. This patient has been suffering from acute kidney injury due to intra-abdominal sepsis with amino-glycoside toxicity progressing toward multiorgan dysfunction syndrome.

2. Following are the manifestations of septicemia in this case:
   a. Localized guarding due to anastomotic leak leading to localized peritonitis
   b. Fever
   c. Tachycardia
   d. Hypotension
   e. Metabolic acidosis
   f. Oliguria
   g. Hypoglycemia
   h. Raised white blood cell count

3. Liver function test has been altered due to ischemia leading to jaundice.

4. Following are the risk factors associated with aminoglycoside nephropathy:
   a. Dose of the drug
   b. Duration of therapy
   c. Advanced age
   d. Use of other nephrotoxic agents
   e. Sepsis
   f. Hypotension
   g. Dehydration
   h. Use of intravenous contrast agents
   i. Preexisting renal insufficiency
   j. Liver failure

5. Usually, 5% of the administered dose is accumulated with the epithelial cells after filtration through the glomerulus. This accumulation is saturable phenomenon. So, uptake will be limited after the single administration. So, single dose is preferred as compared to the multiple doses. So, if the dose can be extended to >24 hours, the nephrotoxicity will be reversed.

CASE 7

A 29-year-old patient chronic alcoholic being heroin addict for last 5 years and sharing needles with other addicts was found unconscious on the floor in left lateral position by her maidservant coming after 3 days in her house as she had no touch with her family for years. She had neither any medical illness nor any psychiatric problem.

On examination, she has bradycardia, bradypnea, and evidence of left lower zone consolidation. She was unconscious rousable with painful stimuli and other neurological finding was normal. Her left hand was swollen and painful.

Laboratory investigation demonstrated hemoglobin 9 g/dL, serum sodium 139 mmol/L, potassium 7 mmol/L, urea 119 mg/dL, creatinine 7.01 mg/dL, bicarbonate 13 mmol/L, creatinine 46,000 IU/L, and calcium 7.5 mg/dL. Arterial blood gases demonstrated pH 7.2, PCO_2 84 mm Hg, and PO_2 60 mm Hg. Urine color on catheterization was:

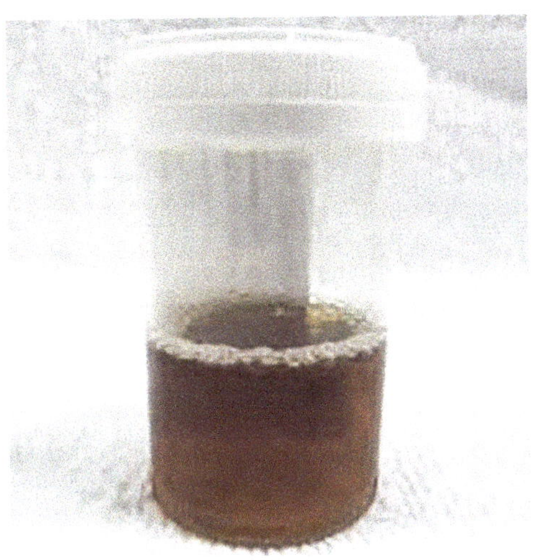

ECG demonstrated:

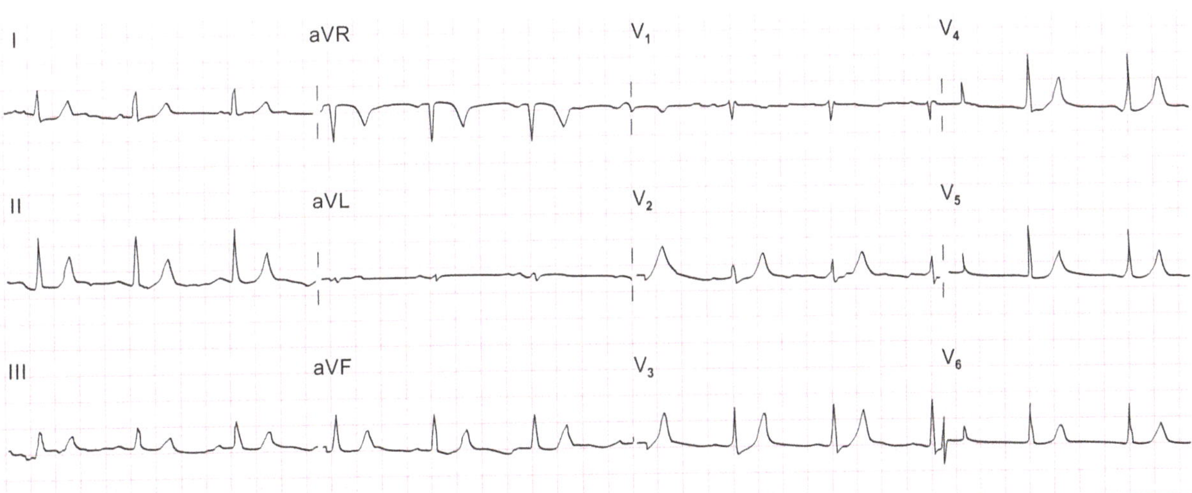

1. **Describe the above pictures.**
2. **What is your interpretation regarding arterial blood gases?**
3. **Why the color of urine is black colored?**
4. **How can you differentiate it from hemoglobinuria?**
5. **What are the causes of this disease producing this urine?**
6. **What is your diagnosis?**
7. **What are the effects of muscle damage in this patient?**
8. **Why there was hypocalcemia?**
9. **What are the complications of the muscle damage?**
10. **What is the cause of this ECG changes?**

Answers

1. Demonstration of the above pictures:
   a. First picture demonstrates black-colored urine
   b. Second picture of ECG demonstrates absent P wave, peaked T wave, and prolongation of PR interval

2. Arterial blood gases demonstrate:
   a. Low pH suggestive of acidosis
   b. Bicarbonate is low indicating metabolic acidosis.
   c. High PCO_2 indicating associated respiratory acidosis

   So, patient has been suffering from mixed metabolic and respiratory acidosis.

3. Black-colored urine is due to release of myoglobin from the severe pressure-related ischemic damage of the muscles of the left limb for 3 days.
4. Myoglobinuria can be differentiated from hemoglobinuria by ammonium sulfate test:
    a. Colored precipitate in case of hemoglobinuria
    b. Colored supernatant in case of myoglobinuria
5. Causes of rhabdomyolysis are as follows:
    a. Trauma
    b. Illicit drug use
    c. Infection
    d. Heat stroke
    e. Metabolic disorders
    f. Inflammatory myopathy
    g. Excessive exercise
    h. Severe hypokalemia
    i. Crush injuries
6. The diagnosis is acute renal injury secondary to rhabdomyolysis resulting in hyperkalemia.
7. Following are the effects of muscle damage:
    a. Massive elevation of creatine kinase
    b. Rise in potassium
    c. Rise in phosphate level in the blood
8. Hypocalcemia occurred due to sequestration of calcium into the muscle in the oliguric phase which will be reverted in the recovery phase leading to rebound hypercalcemia.
9. Complications of the severe muscle damage are as follows:
    a. Electrolyte abnormalities
    b. Hypoalbuminemia
    c. Hyperuricemia
    d. Compartment syndrome
    e. Acute kidney injury
    f. Disseminated intravascular coagulation
10. ECG changes in hyperkalemia:
    a. Peaked T wave
    b. Flattening of P wave
    c. Prolongation of PR interval
    d. Sinus bradycardia
    e. Conduction block
    f. Widening of QRS complexes
    g. Development of sine wave
    h. Ventricular fibrillation
    i. Complete asystole

CASE 8

A 50-year-old chronic smoker and chronic alcoholic male has been referred to nephrologist to investigate the cause of microscopic hematuria following 3 days of sore throat and fever, but no past history of macroscopic hematuria or any urinary symptom. He has no visual problem and no significant family history of renal disease.

On examination, his pulse rate is 76 beats/min, blood pressure 160/105 mm Hg, and otherwise all the findings related to different systems were normal.

Laboratory investigation demonstrated blood urea 78 mg/dL, creatinine 1.9 mg/dL, and γ-glutamyltransferase (GGT) 222 IU/L. Urine analysis demonstrated ++ protein, ++ blood, microscopic analysis demonstrated >100 red blood cells/cc, and 24 hours urinary protein 1.4 g.

Histopathology of kidney demonstrated:

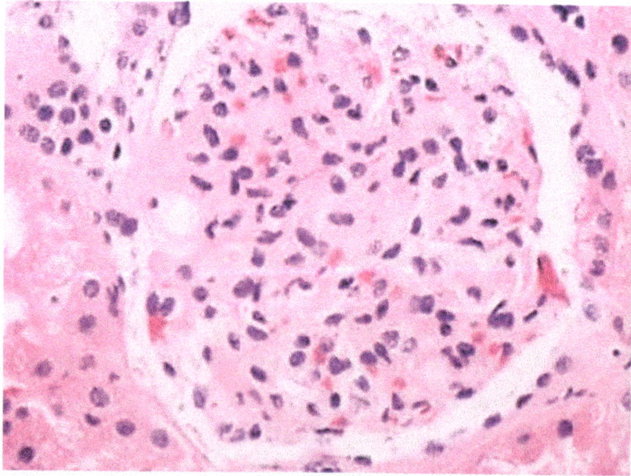 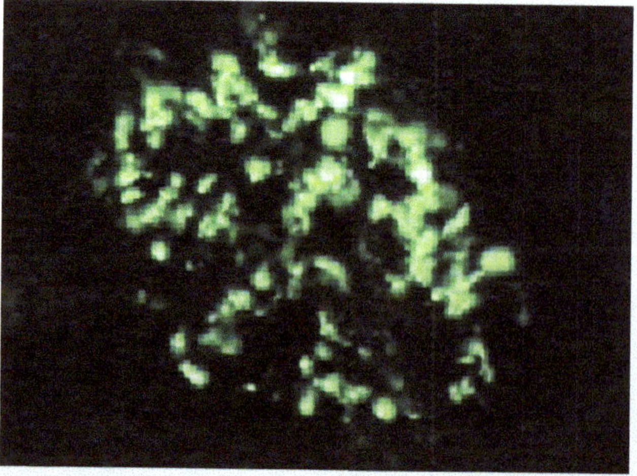

1. **What is the description of the above histopathological pictures?**
2. **What are the most probable differential diagnoses?**
3. **What is the definite diagnosis?**
4. **Why it is not thin basement membrane disease?**
5. **Why it is not the case of Alport syndrome?**
6. **What are the pathophysiological consequences in this disease?**
7. **What are the other conditions associated with this disease?**
8. **How can you classify this disease?**
9. **What is the prognosis in this disease?**
10. **What are the risk factors in this disease?**
11. **What are the indications of giving immunosuppressive therapy to these patients?**
12. **How you treat the patient in high-risk group?**
13. **What are the types of etiological factors?**
14. **What are the factors to be considered in the equation at the time of biopsy?**
15. **What are the conditions responsible for acute worsening of the renal function?**

Answers

1. Above left hand picture demonstrates:
    a. Increased mesangial matrix
    b. Increased mesangial hypercellularity
    Above right hand picture demonstrates increased amount of immunoglobulin A (IgA) deposited in the mesangium
2. Most probable differential diagnoses are:
    a. IgA nephropathy
    b. Thin basement membrane disease
    c. Alport syndrome
3. Definite diagnosis is IgA nephropathy because of the following points:
    a. Prior episodes of upper respiratory tract infection
    b. There is history of chronic alcohol intake with raised GGT.
    c. Presence of microscopic hematuria
    d. Presence of IgA deposits in the mesangium
4. It is not thin basement membrane disease because:
    a. It is familial disorder.
    b. Isolated microscopic hematuria
    c. No history of antecedent throat infection
    d. Diffuse thinning of the glomerular basement membrane in electron microscopy

5. This is not the case of Alport syndrome because:
    a. It is progressive glomerular disease.
    b. Presence of deafness
    c. Ocular blindness
6. Deposited of underglycosylated IgA subclass 1 in the mesangium will bind to the Fc receptor of these cells leading to formation of the immune complexes. These complexes activate mesangial cells to liberate proinflammatory cytokines as well as fibroblastic growth factors leading to cellular injury.
    This deposited IgA activates complement system leading to deposition of C3 complement.
7. Other conditions associated with this disease are as follows:
    a. Alcoholic and virus-mediated cirrhosis
    b. Celiac disease
    c. Human immunodeficiency virus (HIV) infection
    d. Henoch–Schönlein purpura
    e. Inflammatory bowel disease
    f. Some rheumatic diseases:
        • Spondyloarthropathies
        • Dermatitis herpetiformis
        • Psoriasis
    g. Minimal chain disease
    h. Membranous nephropathy
    i. Antineutrophil cytoplasmic antibody (ANCA)-positive vasculitis

8. This disease can be classified according to Oxford classification MEST criteria:

Pathologic features	Scores		
	1	**2**	**3**
Mesangial hypercellularity	<50% glomeruli demonstrate hypercellularity	>50% glomeruli demonstrate hypercellularity	Not applicable
Endocapillary hypercellularity	Nil	Any glomeruli demonstrating endocapillary hypercellularity	Not applicable
Segmental sclerosis	Nil	Any glomeruli showing segmental sclerosis	Not applicable
Tubular atrophy/ interstitial fibrosis	≤25% tubular atrophy/interstitial fibrosis	>25–50% tubular atrophy/ interstitial fibrosis	>50% tubular atrophy/interstitial fibrosis
Crescents	Nil	10–25% glomeruli demonstrate cellular/fibrocellular crescents	>25% of glomeruli have cellular/fibrocellular crescents

9. Prognostic features in this disease are as follows:
    a. Patient with isolated hematuria—there is very low risk of progression.
    b. In patients with persistent proteinuria of 500–1,000 mg daily, 25–30% require renal replacement therapy within 20–25 years.
    c. In patients with persistent proteinuria of 2,000–3,000 mg/day in presence or absence of hypertension should require renal replacement therapy.
    d. Poor prognostic factors:
        • Impaired renal function
        • Heavy proteinuria of >3 g/day
        • Difficult to treat hypertension
        • Tubulointerstitial and glomerular fibrosis
        • Rapidly progressive crescentic IgA nephropathy

10. Risk factors in this disease are as follows:
    a. Low risk factors:
        • Normal renal function
        • Episodic macroscopic hematuria
        • Proteinuria < 1 g/day
        • No hypertension
    b. Medium risk factors:
        • Older age
        • Proteinuria > 1 g/day
        • Hypertension
    c. High risk factors:
        • Impaired renal function
        • Heavy proteinuria of >3 g/day
        • Difficult to treat hypertension
        • Tubulointerstitial and glomerular fibrosis
        • Rapidly progressive crescentic IgA nephropathy

11. Following are the indications of administering the immunosuppressive therapies:
    a. Persistent proteinuria
    b. Nephrotic syndrome
    c. Accelerated decline in glomerular filtration rate
    d. Resistant disease
    e. Relapse of this disease
    f. Advanced disease

12. In case of advanced disease, the treatment will be the following:
    a. If the proteinuria is within the nephrotic range: Prednisolone 0.5–1 mg/kg/day for 8 weeks.
    b. In case crescentic IgA nephropathy:
        • Prednisolone 0.5–1 mg/kg/day for 8 weeks
        • Cyclophosphamide 2 mg/kg/day for 8 weeks

13. IgA is second most abundant immunoglobulin having a role on mucosal immunity. There are two subclasses:
    a. IgA1: Spleen and lymph node being nonsecretory lymphoid organs produce IgA1.
    b. IgA2: It is found in the gut associated lymphoid tissue.

14. Following factors are considered in the equation at the time of biopsy:
    a. Age
    b. Race
    c. Use of ACEI/ARBs
    d. Systolic blood pressure
    e. Diastolic blood pressure
    f. Proteinuria
    g. Use of immunosuppression
    h. Effective glomerular filtration rate
    i. MEST score

15. Following factors are responsible for acute worsening of the kidney function in IgA nephropathy:
    a. Accelerated hypertension
    b. Tubular obstruction due to heavy glomerular hematuria
    c. Crescentic IgA nephropathy
    d. Acute tubular toxicity resulting from heavy glomerular hematuria—free radical damage
    e. Other causes of acute kidney injury

CASE 9

A 26-year-old man came to outpatient department with anorexia, fatigue, polyuria, backache, and recurrent burning sensation during micturition for 2 months.

Laboratory investigation demonstrated hemoglobin 10 g/dL, erythrocyte sedimentation rate (ESR) 55 mm/1st hour, urea 24 mg/dL, creatinine 1.1 mg/dL, sodium 140 mEq/L, chloride 115 mEq/L, potassium 2.6 mEq/L, calcium 8.5 mg/dL, phosphate 1.1 mmol/L, bicarbonate 14 mmol/L, and sugar 117 mg/dL. Urine pH was 5.5.

1. **What are the metabolic abnormalities demonstrated here?**
2. **What is the most probable diagnosis?**
3. **Why this patient has been suffering from this disease?**
4. **Classify the variants of this disease.**
5. **Which is the most common variant of this disease?**
6. **What are the causes of this common variant?**
7. **What is the pathophysiology in this disease suffering from?**
8. **What are the metabolic effects in this disease demonstrated here?**
9. **What are the biochemical abnormalities that can differentiate this disease from other types?**
10. **Which specific test can differentiate this disease from other types?**

Answers

1. Here, biochemical abnormalities demonstrated hypokalemia, hyperchloremia, low bicarbonate, low calcium, and phosphate level. So, this is consistent with high anion gap of (140 + 2.5 – 115 = 27.5) hyperchloremic hypokalemic metabolic acidosis.

2. As there is hyperchloremic, hypokalemic high anion gap metabolic acidosis, and urine pH is 5.5, so there is failure to acidify the urine. The diagnosis is distal renal tubular acidosis.

3. Patient failed to acidify the urine because:
    a. Defect in the excretion of the hydrogen ion by the distal tubule
    b. Defect in the absorption of the bicarbonate ion by the proximal tubule

4. Renal tubular acidosis has been classified into four types:
    a. Distal renal tubular acidosis
    b. Proximal renal tubular acidosis
    c. Mixed renal tubular acidosis
    d. Hyporeninemic hypoaldosteronism

5. Most common variant is the distal renal tubular acidosis.

6. The causes of this common variant are as follows:
    a. Connective tissue diseases:
        - Systemic lupus erythematosus (SLE)
        - Sjögren's syndrome
        - Systemic sclerosis
        - Rheumatoid arthritis
    b. Primary biliary cirrhosis
    c. Genetic: Both autosomal dominant and autosomal recessive disease due to mutation of the genes encoding the chloride-bicarbonate exchanger or hydrogen-ATP pump subunit.
    d. Tubointerstitial disease
    e. Nephrocalcinosis
    f. Drugs: Lithium, amphotericin B, and nonsteroidal anti-inflammatory drugs (NSAIDs)
    g. Hypergammaglobulinemia: Multiple myeloma and monoclonal gammopathy

7. Pathophysiology of distal renal tubular acidosis:
    a. Damage of the α-intercalated cells of distal tubule fails to generate new bicarbonate ion and also new hydrogen ion. So, kidney will be unable to excrete acidic urine in the distal tubule thereby raising the pH of the urine even in case of metabolic acidosis.

b. Decreased functioning of hydrogen-ATPase

c. Increased leakage of the proton from the tubules back into the lumen in case of toxicity of amphotericin B

d. Damage of the α-intercalated cells in the distal tubules decreases the reabsorption of sodium decreases the secretion of the potassium.

8. Following metabolic abnormalities are demonstrated here:

a. Hypercalciuria leading to hypocalcemia resulting in osteomalacia as evidenced by bone pain

b. Alkaline urine leading to nephrocalcinosis

c. Hypocitraturia

d. Metabolic acidosis

e. Recurrent urinary tract infection

9. Following biochemical abnormalities can differentiate this disease from the other types:

Features	Type 1	Type 2	Type 4
Bicarbonate	<10–20 mEq/L	12–18 mEq/L	>17 mEq/L
Serum potassium	Low	Low	High
Urine pH	Alkaline > 5.5 in presence of metabolic acidosis	Alkaline if the bicarbonate is above the threshold for reabsorption (12–18 mEq/L) Otherwise, it is <5.5	<5.5

10. Acid load test:

a. In case healthy subject, urine pH will be decreased as acid will excrete through the urine.

b. In case of distal renal tubular acidosis, urine will be alkaline, i.e., >5.5 in spite of acidic serum and plasma bicarbonate should be below 21 mEq/L.

CASE 10

A 60-year-old female suffering from long-standing rheumatoid arthritis for 20 years on methotrexate and sulfasalazine presented to medical outdoor with weakness, anorexia, and swelling of her face, legs, and abdomen.

On examination, her face is puffy, pallor moderate, pitting pedal edema, blood pressure 170/105 mm Hg, hepatosplenomegaly, and mild ascites.

Laboratory investigation demonstrated hemoglobin 8 g/dL, white blood cell count 2,600/cc, creatinine 1.36 mg/dL, urea 39.6 mg/dL, ALT 230 IU/L, alkaline phosphatase (ALP) 185 IU/L, albumin 2.9 mg/dL, and urine protein +++.

Rectal biopsy and renal biopsy demonstrated:

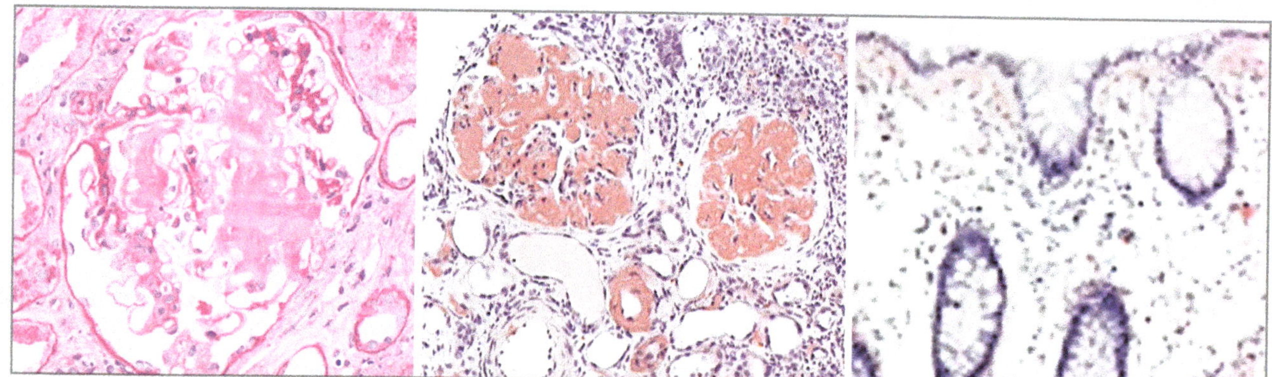

1. **Describe the above histopathological pictures?**
2. **What is your diagnosis?**
3. **Which protein is involved in this disease?**
4. **What are the other diseases where this protein is deposited?**
5. **What are the other types of proteins that may be deposited in kidney?**

Answers

1. Description of the above histopathological pictures:
   a. Pale eosinophilic PAS-positive amorphous extracellular material involving the basement membrane.
   b. Second one is stained by Congo red stain in the kidney tissue.
   c. Congo red staining of the rectal mucosa demonstrated presence of greenish birefringence in the muscularis propria in the subepithelial area.
2. The probable diagnosis is nephrotic syndrome as a remote complication of rheumatoid arthritis.
3. The amyloid protein AA is involved in this disease.
4. In case of following diseases, this protein will be deposited in the kidney:
   a. Rheumatoid arthritis
   b. Inflammatory bowel disease
   c. Other connective tissue disorders
   d. Drugs
   e. Intravenous drugs
   f. Paraneoplastic syndrome
5. Other types of protein deposited in kidney:
   a. AL type of amyloid leading to primary amyloidosis
   b. Leukocyte cell-derived chemotaxin-2 amyloid or LECT-2 amyloid involving the liver and kidney
   c. Hereditary amyloidosis
   d. Dialysis related amyloidosis: In this case, β2 microglobulin that cannot be removed and will be deposited in the bone, heart, and kidney.

CASE 11

A 5-year-old smoker, alcoholic male presented in the medical outdoor with low-grade fever, backache, anorexia, weight loss for 3 months, and painless hematuria for 2 days.

On examination, patient's face was plethoric, enlarged hard nontender discrete supraclavicular lymph node, left enlarged ballottable mass in the right loin, and enlarged firm liver.

Laboratory investigation demonstrated hemoglobin 18 g/dL and platelet count 450,000/cc.

Routine urine analysis showed 25–30/HPF WBC and plenty of red blood cells along with red blood cell cast.

1. **What are the probable diagnoses?**
2. **What is your most likely diagnosis?**
3. **What are the points in favor of your diagnosis?**
4. **Why there is fever in this case?**
5. **What are the risk factors in this disease?**
6. **What are the hereditary diseases that may lead to this disease?**
7. **What are the workplace exposures that are related to this disease?**
8. **What are the histological subtypes in this disease?**
9. **What are the paraneoplastic syndromes associated with this disease?**
10. **What are the stagings in this disease?**
11. **What are the common sites of metastasis in this disease?**
12. **What are the agents used to treat this metastasis?**

Answers

1. The probable diagnoses are:
   a. Renal cell carcinoma
   b. Renal tuberculosis
2. The most likely diagnosis is renal cell carcinoma.
3. Following points are favor of this diagnosis:
   a. Painless hematuria
   b. Loin pain
   c. Palpable ballottable mass in the loin
4. Fever in this case due to release of pyrogen from the tumor.
5. Following are the risk factors in this disease:
   a. African-American race
   b. Older age
   c. Obesity
   d. Hypertension
   e. Chronic renal failure
   f. Dialysis treatment

g. Polycystic kidney disease
h. Sickle cell disease
i. Renal stones

6. Following hereditary diseases are associated with this disease:
    a. Von Hippel–Lindau syndrome
    b. Birt-Hogg-Dube syndrome
    c. Hereditary papillary renal carcinoma
    d. Hereditary leiomyomatosis

7. Following workplace exposures are associated with this disease:
    a. Cadmium
    b. Herbicides
    c. Asbestos
    d. Trichloroethylene

8. Following are the histological subtypes in this disease:
    a. Clear cell: Here, the cell contains glycogen and lipid-rich cytoplasm. It is most common.
    b. Chromophilic masses: It is bilateral and associated with trisomy 7 or 17.
    c. Chromophobic lesions contain large polygonal cells
    d. Oncocytoma lesions consist of predominant eosinophilic cells. This lesion is most likely to spread.
    e. Collecting duct cell cancer: This is very aggressive.

9. Following are the paraneoplastic syndromes associated with renal cell carcinoma:
    a. This disease secretes following hormones:
        - Erythropoietin
        - Insulin
        - Gonadotropin
        - Renin
        - Placental lactogen

        As a result, following clinical and biochemical features are produced:
        - Polycythemia
        - Hypercalcemia
        - Hypertension
        - Hypokalemia
        - Stauffer's syndrome

10. Following are the stagings of this disease:
    a. Robson staging:
        - Stage I: Limited to kidney
        - Stage II: Involvement of perinephric fat but remains limited to Gerota's fascia.
        - Stage III:
            - IIIa: Renal vein involvement
            - IIIb: Nodal involvement
            - IIIc: Both IIIa and IIIb
        - Stage IVa: Direct invasion of adjacent organ structure
        - Stage IVb: Distant metastasis
    b. TNM classification:
        - T1:
            - T1a: Limited to kidney, >4 cm
            - T1b: Limited to kidney, >4 cm but <7 cm
        - T2:
            - T2a: Limited to kidney, >7 cm but <10 cm
            - T2b: Limited to kidney, >10 cm
        - T3: Tumor or tumor thrombus extension into major veins or perinephric tissues but not into ipsilateral adrenal gland or beyond the Gerota fascia
            - T3a: It spreads to renal vein
            - T3b: It spreads to infradiaphragmatic inferior vena cava.
            - T3c: It spreads to supradiaphragmatic inferior vena cava or invades the wall of the vena cava.
        - T4: It involves ipsilateral adrenal gland or invades beyond the Gerota fascia.
        - N0: No nodal involvement
        - N1: Metastatic involvement of the regional lymph node
        - M0: No distant metastasis
        - M1: Distant metastasis

        Stage I: T1 N0 M0
        Stage II: T2 N0 M0
        Stage III: TIII or N1 with M
        Stage IV: T4 or M1

11. Following are the common sites of metastasis:
    a. Lung
    b. Brain
    c. Bone
    d. Liver
    e. Adrenal gland

12. Following agents are used to treat metastasis:
    a. Immunotherapy: It is divided into the following:
        - Cytokine-based treatment:
            - Interferon-α
            - High-dose interleukin-2
        - Check point inhibitors: Nivolumab

b. Targeted therapy:
- Inhibitors of vascular endothelial growth factor—monoclonal antibody like bevacizumab

- Tyrosine kinase inhibitors:
  - Sunitinib
  - Pazopanib
  - Sorafenib
  - Axitinib

CASE 12

A 19-year-old male presented in the outpatient department with fever, frequency of micturition, and headache for 12 days. He was prescribed cephalexin. After 15 days, he suddenly developed pain in the eye along with blurred vision, puffiness in the face, swelling in the legs, and rashes in the skin.

On examination, his blood pressure was 180/100 mm Hg, pulse rate 110 beats/min, pitting pedal edema, temperature 100°F, and skin rashes in different areas in the body. Slit-lamp examination demonstrated "diffuse ciliary flush and white blood cells flares in the anterior chamber of the eye".

Laboratory examination demonstrated hemoglobin 10 g/dL, white blood cell count 12,000/cc, ESR 100 mm/1st hour, creatinine 9.4 mg/dL, urea 53.21 mg/dL, bicarbonate 17 mmol/L, potassium 6.2 mEq/L, sodium 132 mmol/L, and chloride 91 mmol/L.

1. **What is the most probable diagnosis?**
2. **What are the metabolic disturbances present in this patient?**
3. **What are the points in favor of your diagnosis?**
4. **Define this disease.**
5. **What are the criteria to diagnose this disease?**
6. **What are the causes of this disease?**
7. **What is the gold standard of diagnosis in this disease?**

Answers

1. This patient has been suffering from acute kidney injury due to acute interstitial nephritis as a result of administration of antibiotics along with uveitis. This is also known as tubulointerstitial nephritis and uveitis syndrome or TINU.
2. Patient has been suffering from increased anion gap metabolic acidosis with hyperkalemia.
3. Following are the points in favor of this diagnosis:
   a. Presence of skin rashes within few days after administration of the antibiotics
   b. Puffiness in the face
   c. Pedal edema
   d. Eye involvement
   e. Features of uremia
4. This disease can be defined as a type of hypersensitivity reaction which is characterized by inflammation of the interstitium without involvement of glomeruli.
5. Following are the criteria to diagnose TINU:
   a. Presence of typical uveitis and interstitial nephritis on renal biopsy

   Or,

   b. Typical features of uveitis along with meeting all the three criteria:
      - Abnormal creatinine or reduced creatinine clearance
      - Abnormal urine analysis:
        - Low-grade proteinuria
        - Microscopic hematuria
        - Sterile pyuria
        - White blood cell casts
        - Eosinophiluria
        - Raise $\beta2$ microglobulin
      - Systemic illness for >2 weeks:
        - Fever
        - Weight loss
        - Fatigue
        - Elevated ESR
        - Anemia
        - Abnormal liver enzyme
6. Following are the pathophysiology of this disease:
   a. Drugs act as haptens binding to the cytoplasmic or extracellular components of the tubular epithelial cells leading to generation of immunological response resulting in increased serum level of IgE. This is type 1 hypersensitivity reaction.

b. In some cases, there is increased latent period between the exposure to the drug and appearance of rashes and positive skin test. This is type 4 hypersensitivity reaction.

7. The gold standard of diagnosis in this disease is kidney biopsy which demonstrates:

a. Edematous interstitium infiltrated with T cells and macrophages present surrounding the blood vessels

b. There may be granulomatous infiltration.

c. There may be the presence of eosinophils and neutrophils.

d. Glomeruli are normal.

e. Effacement of podocytes in case of NSAID-induced interstitial nephritis

CASE 13

A 20-year-old male having well controlled insulin-dependent diabetes mellitus on insulin therapy has presented with severe weakness, polyuria, along with anorexia for 5 days.

On examination, his blood pressure was 95/60 mm Hg, pulse rate 120 beats/min, moderate pallor, and no jaundice.

Neurological examination demonstrated diminished power, tone, and reflexes but sensory systems were normal.

Laboratory examination demonstrated hemoglobin 10 g/dL, white blood cell count 12,000/cc, ESR 80 mm/1st hour, serum potassium 3 mEq/L, sodium 136 mEq/L, chloride 114 mEq/L, bicarbonate 13 mmol/L, pH 7.26, urea 42 mg/dL, creatinine 2 mg/dL, serum lactate 3.1 mmol/L. Urine pH was 5.4.

1. **Describe the metabolic abnormality in this case.**
2. **What are the three conditions associated with this biochemical event?**
3. **What is the disease the patient is suffering from?**
4. **Why is there neurological abnormality?**
5. **What should be the ECG feature in this disease?**

Answers

1. The patient has been suffering from normal anion gap (136 – 114 – 13 = 9) metabolic acidosis.
2. Following are the three conditions associated with this biochemical abnormality:
   a. Distal renal tubular acidosis
   b. Ureterosigmoidostomy
   c. Therapy with acetazolamide
3. This patient is suffering from distal renal tubular acidosis.
4. This neurological abnormality is due to hypokalemia.
5. ECG features of hypokalemia:
   a. Increased amplitude of P wave
   b. Prolongation of PR interval
   c. Widespread depression of ST segment
   d. Flattening or inversion of T waves
   e. Prominent U wave
   f. Apparent long QT interval due to fusion of T and U waves

CASE 14

A 30-year-old chronic smoker came to chest department with productive cough with recurrent hemoptysis and respiratory distress for 10 days.

On examination, patient's face was puffy, moderate pallor, pitting edema, blood pressure 160/110 mm Hg, and pulse rate 100 beats/min.

Laboratory investigation demonstrated hemoglobin 9 g/dL, white blood cell count 14,000/cc, ESR 85 mm/1st hour, serum bilirubin 1.65 mg/dL, urea 45 mg/dL, creatinine 4.8 mg/dL, serum bicarbonate 16 mmol/L, potassium 5.8 mmol/L, and albumin 21 g/dL.

Urine analysis demonstrated plenty of red blood cell, red blood cell casts, and heavy proteinuria. Chest X-ray demonstrated the following:

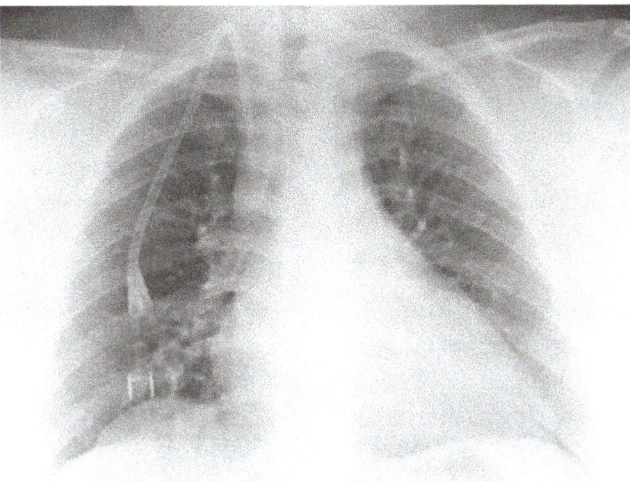

1. **What is described in the above picture?**
2. **What are the differential diagnoses?**
3. **What is the most likely diagnosis?**
4. **Which human leukocyte antigens (HLAs) are strongly associated with this disease?**
5. **Which HLAs are associated with reduced frequency of this disease?**
6. **Which HLAs are strongly associated with this disease?**
7. **What are the environmental factors that may lead to this disease?**
8. **What is the possible pathophysiology in this case?**
9. **What are the spectra of pathological changes seen in the kidney biopsy in this patient?**
10. **In the serological testing, which specific target should be used to prevent false-positive result?**
11. **What should be the treatment in this case?**

Answers

1. Above picture demonstrates bilateral coalescent opacities in the airspaces.
2. The differential diagnoses are as follows:
    a. Goodpasture syndrome
    b. Granulomatosis with polyangiitis
    c. Systemic lupus erythematosus
    d. Microscopic polyangiitis
3. The most likely diagnosis is Goodpasture syndrome.
4. Following HLAs are increasingly prevalent in this disease:
    a. HLA-DR15
    b. DRB1*03
    c. DRB1*04
5. Following HLAs have reduced frequency in this disease:
    a. DRB1*01
    b. DRB1*07
6. Following HLAs are strongly associated with this disease:
    a. DRB1*1501
    b. DRB1*1502
7. Following environmental factors are associated with this disease:
    a. Drug—alemtuzumab by causing lymphocyte depletion
    b. Cocaine inhalation
    c. Infection—influenza
    d. Smoking
    e. Exposure to metal dust
    f. Extracorporeal shock wave lithotripsy
8. Possible pathophysiology in this disease:
    a. In case of healthy individual, alveolar epithelium acts as barrier to the environmental factors or antibasement membrane antibodies. Main component of the basement membrane is type 4 collagen having six different chains from $\alpha1$ to $\alpha6$.

But in case of any insult, as the alveolar capillary permeability increases, it leads to trespassing of the autoantibodies resulting in binding with the basement membrane. Following factors are responsible for increasing the capillary permeability:

- Tobacco smoking
- Bacteremia
- Endotoxemia
- Exposure to volatile hydrocarbons
- Upper respiratory tract infection
- Higher inspired oxygen
- Increased capillary hydrostatic pressure

9. Following are the spectra of pathophysiological changes in kidney biopsy in this patient:
   a. Expansion of segmental mesangial matrix and hypercellularity—earliest change
   b. Focal and segmental necrosis along with aggressive destruction of the capillaries with increased number of neutrophils
   c. In advanced cases, diffuse nephritis with segmental and total necrosis with extensive crescent formation
   d. Presence of myeloperoxidase-positive ANCA antibodies in 10–15% of patients
   e. Immunofluorescent study demonstrates linear capillary wall anti-glomerular basement membrane (anti-GBM) antibodies

10. In serological testing, specific target should be used to prevent false-positive result in detection of antibodies to α-3 NC1 domain of collagen type 4.

11. Treatments in this case are following:
    a. Pulse methylprednisolone 0.5–1 g in 100 mL of normal saline to be given over 30 minutes for 3 days followed by oral prednisolone 60 mg/day. Cyclophosphamide 1–2 mg/kg daily
       This combination should be continued for 3–6 months.
    b. Plasma exchange: 8–10 treatments in <2 weeks
       Serum anti-GBM antibodies should be measured to screen the efficacy of the treatment.

CASE 15

A 16-year-old boy having recent past history of bloody diarrhea with fever along with abdominal pain has come to outpatient department with respiratory distress, severe headache, and decreased level of consciousness.

On examination, patient looked toxic, blood pressure 180/105 mm Hg, moderate pallor, and temperature 100.8°F, pulse rate 110 beats/min, respiratory rate 32 breaths/min, and purpuric spot on the body.

On investigation, his hemoglobin is 8 g/dL, white blood cell count 14,000/cc, mean corpuscular volume 104 fL, increased reticulocyte count, creatinine 6 mg/dL, and urea 85 mg/dL.

Urine analysis demonstrated moderate proteinuria and red blood cell casts.

1. **What is your most likely diagnosis?**
2. **How can you come to the diagnosis of this disease?**
3. **Define this disease.**
4. **What are the types of this disease?**
5. **What is the pathophysiology in this disease in this patient?**
6. **What are the drugs responsible for this disease?**
7. **Mention the genetic predisposing in this disease.**
8. **Is all the mutation in the genes regulating the complement pathway lead to this disease?**
9. **What are the triggering factors in the atypical variety of this disease?**
10. **How can you treat the atypical variety of this disease?**
11. **In this case, why antibiotic should be used?**
12. **What is the result of renal transplantation in the atypical variety of this disease?**
13. **Which genetic factors are associated with good outcome in the renal transplantation in the atypical variety of this disease?**
14. **Which genetic factors are associated with worse outcome in the renal transplantation in the atypical variety of this disease?**

Answers

1. The most likely diagnosis s hemolytic uremic syndrome.
2. By following methods, the diagnosis should be confirmed:
   a. To confirm the diagnosis:
      - Renal function test
      - Complete blood count
      - Peripheral blood culture:
        - Schistocytes
        - Reticulocyte count
        - Haptoglobin
        - Lactate dehydrogenase
   b. To rule out the differential diagnosis:
      - Direct comb test
      - Antiphospholipid antibodies
      - Antinuclear antibodies (ANAs)
      - Antineutrophil cytoplasmic antibodies
      - Antibodies to *Leptospira*, HIV virus
      - Polymerase chain reaction (PCR) for detecting:
        - *Cytomegalovirus*
        - Epstein–Barr virus
   c. For detecting the underlying etiology:
      - *Shigella* shiga toxin by:
        - Stool culture
        - Rectal swab culture
        - Polymerase chain reaction
      - For detecting the genetic disorders:
        - Serum level of complement C3
        - Enzyme-linked immunosorbent assay (ELISA) test for complement factor H and I
        - Flow cytometry for membrane cofactor protein CD46
        - ELISA for antifactor H antibodies
      - Sequencing of genes that encode factor H, I, B, C3, and CD46
      - For *Streptococcus pneumoniae* associated thrombotic microangiopathy:
        - Blood culture
        - Positive T cell antigen
      - In case of suspected defective metabolism in cobalamin by high performance liquid chromatography:
        - Serum homocysteine
        - Serum methionine
      Tandem mass spectrometry to detect urine methylmalonic acid

   - In case of suspected thrombocytopenic purpura:
     - ADAMTS13 activity
     - ADAMTS13 antigen
     - ADAMTS12 antibodies

3. This disease is characterized by lesion in the microvasculature characterized by:
   a. Detachment as well as swelling of the endothelium
   b. Deposition of amorphous material in the subendothelial space
   c. Platelet aggregation in the vascular lumen leading to microthrombosis resulting in partial of complete obstruction of the vessel lumen
4. There are two types of this disease:
   a. Diarrhea associated with hemolytic uremic syndrome due to shiga exotoxin or *Escherichia coli* (strain O157:H7)
   b. Diarrhea not associated with hemolytic uremic syndrome
5. Pathophysiology in case of diarrhea associated with hemolytic uremic syndrome:

The shiga exotoxin or *E. coli* (0157:H7) adhere to the gut mucosa through binding with 97-kD outer membrane protein

↓

Translocate across the inflamed colonic mucosa

↓

Binds to intrarenal vasculature as well platelets

↓

Damage to the vascular endothelial cells

↓

Leading to release of von-Willebrand factor multimers and prothrombotic factors

↓

Renal failure

Pathophysiology of hemolytic uremic syndrome without diarrhea:

It occurs as a result of uncontrolled activation of alternate pathway of complement

↓

Leads to formation of membrane attack complex

↓

Injury to the normal cells resulting renal failure

6. Following drugs are responsible for atypical variety of this disease:
   a. Quinine
   b. Tacrolimus

    c. Cyclosporine
    d. Rapamycin
    e. Ciprofloxacin
    f. Oral contraceptive pills

7. Hereditary hemolytic uremic syndrome occurs due to:
   a. Loss of functional mutation of the following regulatory gene:
      - Complement factor H: It is most common.
      - Complement factor I
      - Thrombomodulin
      - Membrane cofactor protein
   b. Gain of functional mutation of the following effector genes:
      - Complement factor B
      - C3

8. Not all the genetic mutations are associated with this disease because many family members are heterozygous and remain asymptomatic.

9. Following are the triggering factors in this atypical variety of this disease:
   a. HIV virus infection
   b. Bacterial infections like:
      - *Streptococcus pneumoniae*
      - *Mycoplasma pneumoniae*
   c. Pregnancy
   d. Malignancy

10. Following are the treatment options:
    a. Anticoagulant therapy is the standard therapeutic option in this patient.
    b. Monoclonal antibody, eculizumab, acts against the C5 of complement cascade thereby preventing its activation and formation of C5a-C5b-9 membrane attack complex. But, its use may be limited in case of patients with C5 mutations.
    c. In case of autoantibodies to complement factor H, eculizumab can be used conjointly with corticosteroids.
    d. Plasmapheresis should be the treatment of choice in case delay in the diagnosis or nonavailability of the eculizumab.

11. Antibiotics should be used in case of hemorrhagic colitis because:
    a. It will shorten the duration of diarrhea.
    b. It will decrease the duration of the complications.
    c. It will reduce the risk of transmission.
    d. It will shorten the duration of bacterial shedding.

12. Following are the results of renal transplantation in atypical variety of hemolytic uremic syndrome:
    a. Results of transplantation outcome are worse.
    b. The incidence of recurrence of this disease in the transplanted kidney is 50%.
    c. Graft failure occurs in 80–90% of patients
    d. Even if the genetic screening is negative, living-related renal transplantation will be contraindicated because of unidentified genetically susceptibility factors.

13. In case mutation of membrane cofactor, protein is associated with best outcome because:
    a. Low rate of recurrence
    b. Long-term graft survival

14. Mutations of complement factor H and complement factor I are associated with worse outcome because of 70–90% recurrence.

CASE 16

A 9-year-old healthy boy came to casualty department vomiting for 3 days followed by decreased urination and purplish rash in the lower extremities for 1 day. On examination, there was pallor, and petechial rashes in the lower limbs and also in the trunk.

1. **What is your diagnosis?**
2. **What is the most common genetic mutation associated with this disease?**
3. **Why this mutation is associated with this disease?**
4. **Which gene is associated with atypical hemolytic uremic syndrome (HUS)?**
5. **By which method, the genes are analyzed?**
6. **What are the findings in the renal biopsy?**
7. **How can you treat this case?**
8. **In which cases, eculizumab may be recommended in patient already received plasma exchange?**
9. **What do you mean by hematological remission and relapse in this disease?**

Answers

1. This patient has been suffering from atypical variety of hemolytic uremic syndrome.
2. Most common genetic mutation associated with this disease is mutation of complement factor H which is the prime fluid phase regulator in the alternate complement pathway.
3. In 95% patients with anticomplement factor H, antibodies have complete deficiency of two proteins like complement factor-related protein 1 and 3 as a result of deletion of CFHR1-R3.
4. Mutation of chromosome number 6 is associated with increasing susceptibility to suffer from this disease.
5. By following methods, the genes are analyzed:
   a. Direct sequencing
   b. Multiplex ligation-dependent probe amplification for detecting the hybrid complement factors H genes as well as copying the number of variations in the genes that encode complement factor H and complement factor-related proteins.
   c. Screening of diacylglycerol kinase ε genetic mutation.
6. Following are the features in the renal biopsy:
   a. Thrombi composed of fibrin, platelet, and von Willebrand factor are present in the renal and interlobular arteriole.
   b. Thickening of the glomerular capillary wall
   c. Thickening and narrowing of the capillary lumens
   d. Expansion of the mesangium
   e. Mesangiolysis
   f. Cortical necrosis in severe cases

7. The drug of choice is eculizumab which should be started within 24–48 hours of the onset of disease. But as eculizumab is not available in India, the next therapeutic option is plasma exchange.

Daily exchange of double volume of plasma (75 mL/kg of body weight) until the hematological remission

↓

60 mL/kg of body weight alternate day for four sessions

↓

Then 60 mL/kg of body weight plasma exchange twice weekly for next six sessions

↓

Then this plasma exchange should be stopped in case of factor H antibody disease, but this may be required in children for maintaining the hematological remission

8. In following cases, eculizumab may be recommended who already received plasma exchange:
   a. In spite of 5–7 plasma exchange there is no remission.
   b. Appearance of life-threatening complications such as seizures and myocardial dysfunction
   c. Complications associated with access to the vessels or plasma exchange
   d. Disease due to genetic mutations
9. Hematological remission can be defined as:
   a. Platelet count is >150,000/cc
   b. Absence of schistocytes
   c. Normal lactate dehydrogenase (LDH) level

   Hematological relapse after being normal for at least 2 weeks can be defined as:
   a. Presence of microangiopathic hemolytic anemia
   b. Thrombocytopenia

CASE 17

The patient in case number 16 again has been admitted after 2 years with oliguria and rashes all over the body. On examination, there was pallor, petechial rashes all over the body but mainly in the lower limbs. He already received 12 plasma exchanges and was on antihypertensives.

In addition to the questions described above, following are the new questions:

1. **What is your diagnosis?**
2. **Which factors are mostly responsible for this recurrence?**
3. **Mention five factors to be estimated in this patient in case of relapse.**

Answers

1. The most probable diagnosis is recurrence of hemolytic uremic syndrome.
2. Following factors are responsible for complement factor 3 and complement factor H.
3. Following five most commonly genes are responsible for relapse:
   a. Complement factor H
   b. Complement factor I
   c. Membrane cofactor protein
   d. Complement factor 3
   e. Complement factor B

CASE 18

A 10-month-old patient has been admitted with vomiting of 2 days duration along with excessive irritability and decreased micturition. On examination, patient is irritable, blood pressure 16/95 mm Hg, presence of bluish purple rashes all over the body, urea 88 mg/dL, and creatinine 4.7 mg/dL.

1. **What is your diagnosis?**
2. **What are responsible metabolic defect may be responsible for this disease?**
3. **What are the screening required in this patient?**
4. **After treatment, what are the residual defects may have in this patient?**

Answers

1. This patient has been suffering from atypical variety of hemolytic uremic syndrome.
2. Following metabolic defects may be present:
   a. Mutation of diacylglycerol kinase
   b. Defective metabolism of cobalamin
   c. Inherited deficiency of ADAMTS13 deficiency
3. Following screening are required in this patient:
   a. Genetic sequencing for complement factor H, I, B, C3, and CD46
   b. Activity of ADAMTS13
   c. Activity of diacylglycerol kinase
   d. Measurement of serum homocysteine and methionine by:
      - High performance liquid chromatography
      - Tandem mass spectrometry
4. After treatment, following residual defects may have in this patient:
   a. Deranged renal function test
   b. Proteinuria
   c. Hypertension

CASE 19

A 50-year-old man presented in the emergency department with progressively increased swelling of both lower limbs for 3 months along with shortness of breath and decreased urination for 3 days. There was history of passing frothy urine. In last 1 day, he developed hematuria and left loin pain.

On examination, there was pedal edema, blood pressure 160/95 mm Hg, and bilateral basal crackles in both bases.

Laboratory examination demonstrated hemoglobin 11 g/dL, serum protein 4.3 g/dL with albumin 1.3 g/dL, urea 68 mg/dL, creatinine 1.2 mg/dL, and +++ protein in urine.

1. **What is the most likely diagnosis in this patient?**
2. **Define this disease.**
3. **What are the causes in adult?**
4. **What are the different types of proteinuria?**
5. **How can you differentiate it from overflow proteinuria?**
6. **What are the findings in renal biopsy in this patient?**
7. **How can you stage the patient based on electron microscopy findings?**
8. **What are the antibodies found in this patient's serum?**
9. **What are the typical biopsy features suggestive of secondary causes?**
10. **What are the factors associated with poor outcome in this disease?**
11. **What are features to be evaluated in case of rapid loss of kidney function?**
12. **What are the complications in this disease?**
13. **Can anticoagulant be given in this disease?**
14. **What are the causes of renal vein thrombosis?**

Answers

1. The most likely diagnosis is membranous nephropathy leading to left renal vein thrombosis.
2. The disease can be defined as constellation of features like >3.5 g/day or urine protein/creatinine ratio of 3 g/g, hypoalbuminemia, peripheral edema, hyperlipidemia, and lipiduria with or without hypertension.
3. Causes of nephrotic syndrome are as follows:
   a. Primary glomerulonephritis:
      - Membranous glomerulonephritis
      - Focal segmental glomerulosclerosis
      - Minimal change disease
      - Membranous glomerulonephritis
      - C3 glomerulopathy
      - IgA nephropathy
   b. Secondary glomerular diseases:
      - Diabetic nephropathy
      - Amyloidosis
      - Collagen vascular disease
      - Poststreptococcal glomerulonephritis
      - Preeclampsia
      - Infection:
         - Hepatitis B
         - Hepatitis C
         - Malaria
         - Syphilis
      - Lymphoma
      - Multiple myeloma
   c. Drugs:
      - NSAIDs
      - Gold
      - Penicillamine
   d. Congenital:
      - Alport syndrome
      - Fabry's disease
      - Nail-patella syndrome
4. Different types of proteinuria are as follows:
   a. Glomerular proteinuria: It results from the disruption of the glomerular filtration barrier leading to increased amount of filtration that will exceed the tubular capacity to absorb. This protein is mainly albumin.
   b. Tubular proteinuria: It results from inadequate absorption of low molecular weight protein $\beta2$ microglobulin or lysozyme due to defect in the proximal tubular function.
   c. Overflow proteinuria: It results from excessive production of abnormal small molecular weight protein like light chain or multiple myeloma or lysosome in case of myelomonocytic leukemia that will exceed the absorption of the proximal tubule.
5. Overflow of proteinuria can be differentiated from nephrotic syndrome by discordance by:
   a. Urine sulfosalicylic acid test: This is strongly positive in overflow proteinuria.
   b. 24 hours urine protein
   c. Dipstick—weakly positive or negative in case of overflow proteinuria
6. Findings in the renal biopsy are as follows:
   a. Thickening of the glomerular basement membrane demonstrating presence of spikes by silver or PAS stain
   b. Immunofluorescence microscopy demonstrated granular immunoglobulin G (IgG) and C3 deposits along the capillary walls
   c. On electron microscopy, there is subepithelial deposit.
7. Membranous nephropathy can be staged according to electron microscopic features:
   a. Stage I: Sparse small deposits in absence of thickening of the glomerular basement membrane.
   b. Stage II: More extensive subepithelial deposits along with formation of basement membrane spikes in-between the thickened glomerular basement membrane and deposits.
   c. Stage III: Combination of stage II along with deposits completely surrounded by basement membrane (intramembranous deposits).
   d. Stage IV: Incorporation of deposits in the glomerular basement membrane along with irregular thickening of the glomerular basement membrane.
8. Following antibodies are found in primary membranous nephropathy:
   a. In 70% cases, M type phospholipase A2 receptor (PLA2R) presents on the human podocytes will lead to production of antibodies against this antigen.
   b. In 10% cases of membranous nephropathy, antibodies are produced against another podocyte antigen. Thrombospondin type 1 domain-containing 7A—these patients are negative for PLA2R.
   c. In rare cases, both the above antibodies are found.

9. Following biopsy features can lead to the diagnosis of autoimmune etiology:
   a. Proliferative features suggest mesangial or endocapillary cause
   b. Full-house pattern of immunoglobulin staining or presence of C1q in immunofluorescence microscopy
   c. In immunofluorescence microscopy, presence of glomerular deposits containing immunoglobulin (Ig) other than IgG4.
   d. In the subendothelial region of the capillary wall and mesangium or along the wall of the tubular basement membrane, presence of electron-dense deposits.
   e. On electron microscope endothelial tubulo-reticular inclusions.

10. Following factors are associated with the poor outcome in this disease:
    a. Age > 50 years
    b. Male sex
    c. High blood pressure
    d. Chronic kidney disease
    e. Severity of initial proteinuria
    f. Persistent proteinuria of >4 g/day—strongest predictor of the progressive kidney disease
    g. Histological changes:
       • Tubular atrophy
       • Interstitial fibrosis
       • Glomerulosclerosis
    h. Elevated β2 microglobulin

11. In case of rapid loss of kidney function, following factors should be evaluated:
    a. Acute tubular necrosis
    b. Acute interstitial nephritis
    c. Renal vein thrombosis
    d. Obstruction of the urinary tract
    e. Antiglomerular basement membrane disease
    f. ANCA-associated vasculitis

12. Following are the complications in this disease:
    a. Hypogammaglobulinemia
    b. Increased risk of infection such as pneumococcal pneumonia and sepsis
    c. Hypovitaminosis D as a result of loss of vitamin D-binding protein
    d. Increased risk of thromboembolic event
    e. Increased risk of cardiovascular event in presence of severe nephrosis
    f. Loss of thyroid-binding globulin leading to low T3 and T4
    g. Loss of transferrin
    h. Loss of iron

13. Anticoagulant can be given in this patient having severe nephrotic range of proteinuria having >10 g/day and serum albumin < 2.5 g/dL in absence of any contraindication.

14. Renal vein thrombosis occurs due to:
    a. Loss of fibrinolytic factors in the urine
       • Antithrombin III
       • Protein C
       • Protein S
    b. Increased synthesis of clotting factors:
       • Factor V
       • Factor VIII
       • Fibrinogen
    c. Thrombocytosis
    d. Over diuresis leading to:
       • Dehydration
       • Reduction of renal blood flow
       • Increased viscosity

CASE 20

A 68-year-old man admitted in the emergency department with severe and continuous vomiting, loose motion following intake of outside foods for 2 days leading to oliguria, and confusion for last 6 hours.

On examination, his blood pressure was 90/60 mm Hg, pulse rate 120 beats/min, and cold, calmmy extremity.

Laboratory investigations demonstrated sodium 115 mmol/L, potassium 3 mmol/L, chloride 85 mmol/L, bicarbonate 16 mmol/L, creatinine 5.1 mg/dL, and urea 19 mg/dL.

1. **What is the most likely diagnosis?**
2. **Define this disease.**
3. **What is the relation between urea and creatinine?**
4. **What are the causes of high urea/creatinine ratio?**
5. **What are the causes of low urea/creatinine ratio?**
6. **Why blood level of urea decreased?**
7. **What are the complications in this disease?**

Answers

1. This patient has been suffering from acute renal injury due to prerenal cause.
2. According to Kidney Disease: Improving Global Outcomes (KDIGO), acute kidney injury can be defined as:
   a. Increase in serum creatinine by 0.3 mg/dL or more within 48 hours
   b. Increase in serum creatinine to 1.5 times or more baseline within the prior 7 days
   c. Urine volume < 0.5 mL/kg/h for at least 6 hours
3. Urea/creatinine ratio:
   a. In some cases, urea is high but creatinine is normal. It is not indicative of renal failure.
   b. Where urea is low but creatinine is high—indicate renal failure.
4. Causes of high urea/creatinine ratio are as follows:
   a. High-protein diet
   b. Dehydration
   c. Gastrointestinal hemorrhage
   d. Treatment with steroid
5. Causes of low urea/creatinine ratio are as follows:
   a. Vomiting leading to increased loss of urea
   b. In case of liver disease due to nonfunction of urea cycle, urea is not produced.
   c. Peritoneal and hemodialysis leading to leaking of urea into dialysate
   d. Rhabdomyolysis
   e. Protein-restricted diet leading to decreased formation of urea
   f. Trimethoprim intake
6. a. In acute gastroenteritis due to anorexia and vomiting protein intake will be decreased.
   b. In acute gastroenteritis there increased loss of protein with stool.
   c. Due to hypotension reduced hepatic perfusion and hepatic dysfunction leads to decreased synthesis of urea in the liver.
7. Following are the complications in this disease:
   a. Hyperkalemia
   b. Metabolic acidosis
   c. Hyperphosphatemia
   d. Pulmonary edema
   e. Heart failure
   f. Gastrointestinal bleeding

CASE 21

A 60-year-old nondiabetic, nonhypertensive male having no significant past medical history came to outdoor with complaint of inability to rise from sitting position, increased volume of micturition as well as pain all over the body for 5 months.

On examination, his blood pressure was 130/85 mm Hg, pulse rate 90 beats/min, and weakness in the proximal muscles.

Laboratory investigation demonstrated raised ESR, blood glucose 127 mg/dL, serum sodium 138 mEq/L, potassium 2.9 mEq/L, bicarbonate 12 mmol/L, chloride 112 mEq/L, urea 13 mg/dL, calcium 8.2 mg/dL, and creatinine 1 mg/dL. Urine analysis demonstrated ++++ protein and +++ glucose.

1. **What are the important features here?**
2. **What is your most likely diagnosis?**
3. **Why there is increased excretion of bicarbonate?**
4. **What are the causes in this disease?**
5. **What should be the urine pH?**
6. **What is the usefulness of acid loading test in this disease?**
7. **How can you administer bicarbonate in this patient?**

Answers

1. In above case, there is proteinuria, glycosuria, hypokalemia, hyperchloremia, low bicarbonate level in presence of polyuria, and proximal muscle weakness.
2. The most likely diagnosis is proximal renal tubular acidosis.
3. Increased excretion of bicarbonate results from decreased reabsorption of the bicarbonate from the proximal tubule leading to metabolic acidosis
4. The causes of proximal renal tubular acidosis are:
   a. Fanconi syndrome
   b. Wilson's disease
   c. Cystinosis

    d.   Hyperparathyroidism

    e.   Multiple myeloma

    f.   Amyloidosis

    g.   Degraded tetracycline

    h.   Heavy metal poisoning:
   - Lead
   - Mercury
   - Cadmium

    i.   Drugs:
   - Ifosfamide
   - Carbonic anhydrase inhibitors

5.   Urine pH is variable. It may be below 5.3 if reabsorptive threshold of bicarbonate is high or it may be above 5.3 if reabsorptive threshold is low.

6.   Acid loading test can be defined as the ability of a kidney to excrete acids in the urine in case of high acid load. In case of distal type, urine pH is always >5.3; whereas, in type II, urine pH will be variable depending upon its absorption of bicarbonate from the tubular space.

7.   The amount of bicarbonate to correct acidosis can be calculated from this equation:

$$HCO_3^- \text{ deficit} = HCO_3^- \text{ space (L)} \times$$
$$(\text{Desired } HCO_3^- - \text{actual } HCO_3^-)$$

where, HCO_3^- space = 0.5 – 0.8 × body weight in kg. In case normal person, this space is 50% of the body weight; but it can be increased to 80% in case of severe acidosis, where bicarbonate level is <10 mEq/L.

CASE 22

A 15-year-old boy presented in medicine outdoor with history of polyuria along with nocturia, weakness, muscle cramp, weight loss, increased weakness after strenuous exercise, and extreme fatigue for nearly 8 years. He has also history of occasional spasm of the hand and foot muscles.

On examination, his blood pressure was 110/70 mm Hg, pulse rate 88 beats/min, lower limb muscle demonstrated diminished tone and power and hyporeflexia.

Laboratory investigation demonstrated serum potassium 2.4 mEq/L, bicarbonate 40 mmol/L, calcium 8.8 mEq/L, glucose 92 mg/dL, urine protein +, and urine potassium 40 mmol/L.

1. **What is the most likely diagnosis?**
2. **Define this disease.**
3. **What are the genetic mutations responsible for this disease?**
4. **What are the definite investigations required for this disease?**
5. **What are the other two most common differential diagnoses?**

Answers

1.   The most likely diagnosis is Gitelman syndrome.

2.   Gitelman syndrome is an autosomal recessive tubular disorder due to mutation of the genes that encode sodium, magnesium, and chloride carriers present in the distal convoluted tubules characterized by presence of:

    a.   Normal blood pressure

    b.   Hypokalemia

    c.   Metabolic alkalosis

    d.   Hypocalciuria

    e.   Hypomagnesemia

    f.   High renin in the blood

    g.   High aldosterone in the blood

Magnesium channel is also downregulated in the duodenal cells.

3.   Following genetic mutations are responsible for this disease:

    a.   *SLC12A3* gene encoding thiazide-sensitive sodium chloride cotransporter

    b.   *TRPM6*: It is responsible for distal tubular magnesium transport.

4.   Definite investigations required are:

    a.   Serum potassium: It should be <3 mmol/L.

    b.   24 hours urine potassium: It should be >20 mmol/L.

    c.   Hypocalciuria

    d.   Hypomagnesemia

    e.   High serum level of renin

    f.   High serum aldosterone level

5.   Other common differential diagnoses are:

    a.   Bartter syndrome: In this disease, hypocalciuria and hypomagnesemia are absent.

    b.   Diuretic abuse

CASE 23

A 48-year-old nondiabetic, nonhypertensive female has come to outdoor with complaint of dull aching pain in the right loin radiating to right groin and inner thigh that cannot be relieved with analgesics and low-grade fever and nausea and vomiting for 5 days. Patient used to lie on right lateral position with flexed right limb.

On examination, her pulse rate is 112 beats/min, blood pressure 135/90 mm Hg, severely tender right loin, and groin.

Laboratory investigation demonstrated hemoglobin 12 g/dL and white blood count 24,000/cc with polymorphonuclear leukocytosis.

1. **What is the probable diagnosis?**
2. **What are the risk factors in this disease?**
3. **What are the mucosal defense mechanisms in this patient?**
4. **What is the pathophysiology of this disease?**
5. **Why this disease is most common in females?**
6. **What are the complications may occur in this case?**
7. **Which genes increase the tendency of this disease in this patient?**
8. **What are reinfection recurrences in this disease?**

Answers

1. The most probable diagnosis is acute pyelonephritis.
2. The risk factors in this disease are as follows:
   a. Age
   b. Sex
   c. Pregnancy
   d. Sexual intercourse
   e. Use of diaphragm
   f. Condom
   g. Spermicide gel
   h. Delayed postcoital micturition
   i. Menopause
   j. Past history of urinary tract infection
3. Following are the defense mechanisms in this patient that have been hampered:
   a. Urine:
      - Acidic pH
      - High osmolarity of urine
      - Urinary inhibitors of bacterial adherence
      - Competitive inhibitors of attachment to the uroepithelium cells
      - Mechanical flushing by urine flow
   b. Mucosal immunity:
      - Secretion of chemokines and cytokines by uroepithelial cells
      - Mucosal IgA
      - Mucopolysaccharide lining: It will increase the difficulty of bacterial penetration.

4. Pathophysiology in this case:

   a.

These organisms colonize in the periurethral area, then ascend through the urethra to urinary bladder
↓
P-fimbriae of most common organism *E. coli* attach with the receptors present on the uroepithelial cells followed by penetration
↓
After penetration, bacteria multiply and thereby form biofilm
↓
After sufficient colonization of sufficient bacteria, they will ascend along the ureter toward kidney with the help of fimbria and also bacterial toxins preventing the flow of urine
↓
When they will reach renal parenchymal tissue start inflammatory response leading to development of pyelonephritis

   b. Bacteria also infect the renal parenchyma through the hematogenous spread

   As inflammation starts, inflammatory cascade will be switched on leading to acute pyelonephritis.

5. This disease is most common in females because:
   a. Shorter urethra
   b. Close proximity to anus
   c. Hormonal changes in females
6. Following complications may occur in this case:
   a. Perinephric abscess
   b. Renal vein thrombosis
   c. Sepsis
   d. Papillary necrosis
   e. Acute renal failure
   f. Emphysematous pyelonephritis: It is the most serious complication.

7. Following genes increase the familial to infection in the urinary tract:
   a. *CXCR1*
   b. *TLR4*
   c. TNF-α
   d. Uromodulin (THP)

8. Reinfection: It can be defined as recurring infection but due to separate organisms, which are usually susceptible to drugs.
   Relapse can be defined as recurring infection due to drug-resistant organisms.

CASE 24

A 32-year-old nonhypertensive and nondiabetic female presented in the clinic with low-grade fever, pain in the loin, frequency of micturition, and anorexia and generalized weakness for 3 months. She had a course of broad-spectrum antibiotics but without any help.

On examination, patient was pale, blood pressure 100/60 mm Hg, pulse rate 112 beats/min, toxic-looking, and temperature 100°F.

Laboratory investigation demonstrated hemoglobin 10 g/dL, white blood cell count 13,000/cc, and raised ESR. In the urine, there were plenty of pus cells and mild proteinuria but urine culture showed no growth.

1. **What are the two possible diagnoses?**
2. **What are the tests to the diagnosis?**

Answers

1. As the patient has been suffering from sterile pyuria, the possible two diagnoses are:
   a. Partially treated urinary tract infection
   b. Renal tuberculosis
2. Following tests are to be done for excluding renal tuberculosis:
   a. Purified protein derivative (PPD) skin test
   b. Urine studies:
      - Solid media: Löwenstein–Jensen media provides results within 4 weeks.
      - Radiometric media: Here, BACTEC 460 media provides results within 2–3 days.
   c. Nucleic acid amplification test: This test can be classified into three different tests:
      i. Polymerase chain reaction: This result will be available within 6 hours. Following tests are available—
         - Genus-specific 16S rRNA PCR test
         - Species-specific IS6110 PCR test
         - Roche Amplicor *Mycobacterium tuberculosis* (MTB) PCR test
         - Amplified *M. tuberculosis* direct detection test
      ii. Ligase chain reaction
      iii. Xpert MTB/RIF: It will give results within 2 hours.
   d. Imaging studies:
      - Chest X-ray
      - Spine X-ray
      - Kidney, ureter, and bladder (KUB)
      - CT scan
      - MRI

CASE 25

A 60-year-old woman having history of long-standing rheumatoid arthritis taking medicines and recurring urinary tract infection came to emergency department with polyuria, thirst, weight loss for 1 month, and severe pain bilaterally in the loin for 12 hours.

On examination, her pulse rate was 110 beats/min, sweating, blood pressure 160/95 mm Hg, bilaterally tender loin, deformed metacarpophalangeal joints of both upper and lower limb with swan neck deformity.

Laboratory investigation demonstrated hemoglobin 9.5 g/dL, blood sugar 121 mg/dL, creatinine 3.52 mg/dL, urea 28 mg/dL, sodium 120 mEq/L, chloride 75 mEq/L, and bicarbonate normal. Urine analysis demonstrated mild proteinuria and plenty of pus cells with white blood cell cast, but no growth on culture.

1. **What is the most likely diagnosis?**
2. **What is the pathophysiology behind this disease?**
3. **What are the histopathological changes seen in this case?**
4. **What are the features of nonenhanced CT scan in this case?**
5. **What are the complications in this disease?**

Answers

1. The most likely diagnosis is analgesic-induced tubulointerstitial nephritis.
2. Prostaglandin due to its vasodilatory effect improves renal blood flow. But the analgesics inhibit this pathway leading to hypoperfusion of the kidney resulting in medullary ischemia. As a result, there is papillary necrosis. There are also interstitial tubular necrosis and interstitial nephritis.
3. Histopathological changes are as follows:
   a. Mononuclear to eosinophilic infiltration in the interstitium
   b. Interstitial fibrosis
   c. Papillary calcification
   d. Deposits of metabolite in the medullary interstitium

4. Following are the CT scan features in this case:
   a. Decreased renal mass
   b. Renal scarring
   c. Reduction of the volume of the kidney with irregular surface on the kidney.
   d. Papillary calcifications
   e. Parenchymal thinning
5. Following are the complications in this disease:
   a. Urinary tract obstruction due to soughing of renal papilla
   b. Recurrent urinary tract infection
   c. Salt loosing nephropathy
   d. Sterile pyuria
   e. Tumor of uroepithelium

CASE 26

A 20-year-old boy has come to emergency department with severe headache, fever, and intractable vomiting for 8 hours and not passed any urine for last 8 hours. At once, he was admitted and catheterization done. Only 70 cc urine was drained.

On examination, his pulse rate is 112 beats/min, blood pressure 140/90 mm Hg, temperature 100°F, and mildly pitting edema.

Laboratory investigation demonstrated hemoglobin 8 g/dL, white blood cell count 14,000/cc, serum sodium 133 mmol/L, potassium 5.1 mEq/L, creatinine 4.6 mg/dL, and urea 85 mg/dL. Urinary sodium 92 mmol/L, urinary urea 392 mg/dL, serum and urine osmolarity 300, and serum osmolarity 320 mOsmol respectively.

1. **What is the most likely diagnosis?**
2. **What are the points in favor of this diagnosis?**
3. **What are the conditions responsible for failure of autoregulation in this disease?**
4. **What is the prognosis in this disease?**

Answers

1. Patient has been suffering from acute tubular necrosis due to prerenal cause.
2. Following points are in favor this diagnosis:
   a. Increased excretion of sodium >60 mmol/L
   b. Ratio of urine osmolarity: Plasma osmolarity 1:1.1
   c. Urinary excretion of urea <448 mg/dL

3. Normally, afferent arteriole dilates and efferent arteriole constricts to maintain the intraglomerular filtration pressure. But following mechanisms are responsible for impairing the autoregulation:
   a. Advanced age
   b. Atherosclerosis
   c. Chronic kidney disease

d. Hypertension
e. NSAIDs
f. Constriction of the afferent arteriole by:
- Sepsis
- Hypercalcemia
- Hepatorenal syndrome
- Cyclosporine
- Tacrolimus
g. Dilatation of the efferent arteriole:
- ACEI
- ARBs

4. Prognosis in this disease: Survival rate in this disease is 50%. Following factors are associated with increased mortality:
   a. Male sex
   b. Poor nutritional status
   c. Oliguria
   d. Seizures
   e. Strokes
   f. Acute myocardial infarction
   g. Need for the mechanical ventilation

CASE 27

A 5-year-old male child has come to medicine clinic with puffiness of the face for 14 days and diminished micturition and swelling of the feet for 3 days.

On examination, his pulse rate is 90 beats/min, regular, blood pressure 120/80 mm Hg, and bilateral pedal and parietal edema.

Laboratory investigations are all within normal limit except serum albumin 2.1 g/dL and cholesterol 195 mg/dL. Protein in urine was +++ and no red or white blood cell and cast in urine.

1. **What is your diagnosis?**
2. **Define this disease.**
3. **What are the causes of this disease?**
4. **What is heavy proteinuria?**
5. **In case of presence of red blood cell in urine, what do you suspect?**
6. **What are the indications of kidney biopsy in this patient?**
7. **What are the histologic findings found in this patient?**
8. **What are the extrarenal manifestations in this patient?**
9. **What are the primary metabolic profiles should be done in this patient?**
10. **What are the unique findings to be searched in this patient?**
11. **Mention the genetic distribution in this disease.**
12. **What are the proteins involved in the pathogenesis of this disease?**
13. **How can you treat this disease?**
14. **How can you define steroid-resistant syndrome?**
15. **What is called remission?**

Answers

1. This patient has been suffering from nephrotic syndrome.
2. Nephrotic syndrome can be defined as massive proteinuria, hypoalbuminemia having serum protein <2.5 g/dL, hyperlipidemia having serum cholesterol of >200 mg/dL, and edema with or without hypertension.
3. The causes of this disease are as follows:
   a. Primary causes of nephrotic syndrome:
      - Minimal change disease
      - Focal segmental glomerulosclerosis
      - Membranous nephropathy
      - Membranoproliferative glomerulonephritis
   b. Secondary causes of nephrotic syndrome:
      - Poststreptococcal glomerulonephritis (PSGN)
      - Systemic lupus erythematosus
      - Medications
      - Diabetes mellitus
      - Amyloidosis
      - Infections—hepatitis B, C, and HIV virus
      - Henoch–Schönlein purpura

4. Heavy proteinuria can be defined as:
   a. Presence of +++ or ++++ protein in urine by dipstick method in the early morning sample of urine for 3 consecutive days.
   b. Spot urine protein/creatinine ratio of >2 mg/g
   c. Excretion of protein in urine >40 mg/m^2/hour on timed sample.
5. Presence of microscopic hematuria with or without presence of red blood cell cast indicates:
   a. PSGN
   b. Proliferative glomerulonephritis
6. Following are the indications of renal biopsy in this patient:
   a. Age of onset is <9 months or >16 years.
   b. Gross hematuria
   c. Persistent microscopic hematuria
   d. Low serum C3
   e. Suspicion of secondary cause
   f. Renal failure not due to hypovolemia
   g. Sustained severe hypertension
   h. In case of resistance to steroid
   i. Planning for calcineurin therapy
7. Histopathological features in this patient are as follows:
   a. On light microscopy, absence of any glomerular abnormalities
   b. On immunofluorescence microscopy, there is absence of any glomerular deposit.
   c. On electron microscopy, there is effacement of podocytes and disruption of disorganized actin filaments.
8. Following are the extrarenal manifestations in this patient:
   a. Peritonitis
   b. Thromboembolic events
   c. Acute kidney injury due to:
      - Intrarenal edema
      - Tubular obstruction
      - Severe contraction of extracellular intravascular compartment
   d. Atherosclerotic as well as cardiovascular diseases due to:
      - Persistent hypercholesterolemia
      - Unremitting nephrotic syndrome
9. Following are the primary metabolic profiles done in this patient:
   a. Quantification of urine protein to detect the nephrotic range
   b. Hypoalbuminemia
   c. Hypercholesterolemia
   d. Hypocalcemia secondary to low albumin level
   e. Hyponatremia in case of excess absorption of water as compared to sodium
   f. C3 level should be measured in case of suspicion of membranoproliferative glomerulonephritis
   g. Complete blood count in case of any systemic illness or malignancy
10. Following are the different unique laboratory tests to be done in case of this disease:
    a. Antistreptolysin O titer
    b. ANA
    c. Double-stranded DNA (dsDNA)
    d. HIV test
    e. Hepatitis B and C serology
    f. In case of idiopathic minimal change:
       - M-type phospholipase A2 receptor (PLA2R)
       - Thrombospondin type 1 domain-containing 7A
       - Venography in case of new-onset membranous nephropathy
11. Following are the genetic distribution in this disease:
    a. In 5% cases of minimal chain disease, familial pattern is seen.
    b. In 30–40% cases of primary focal sclerosing glomerulonephritis, following mutation of the following proteins are seen:
       - Podocin and podocyte protein
       - α-actinin-4
       - CD2AP
       - Wilms tumor 1
       - Phospholipase C epsilon 1
       - TRPC6
       - Inverse forming gene interferon-2
       - Mitochondrial transport protein
       - Nuclear transport protein
    c. In case of congenital nephrotic syndrome, mutation of:
       - Nephrin gene
       - Laminin β2
    d. In case of type II membranoproliferative glomerulonephritis, there is genetic mutation of alternate pathway complement.
12. Following proteins are involved in the pathogenesis of this disease:
    a. Interleukin-13
    b. Soluble urokinase plasminogen activator receptor
    c. Urinary CD80
    d. Vascular endothelial growth factor

13. Treatment schedule: 2 mg/kg or 60 mg/m^2 (maximum 60 mg) prednisolone should be given orally daily in divided doses for 6 weeks.

    Then 40 mg/m^2 or 1.5 mg/kg prednisolone should be given orally daily in divided doses for next 6 weeks, then it should be stopped.

14. If the patient fails to achieve proteinuria in spite of getting treatment by steroid with adequate dose for 4–8 weeks, then this patient can be diagnosed as steroid-resistant nephrotic syndrome.

15. Remission can be defined if any one will occur after testing for 3 consecutive days.
    a. Nil urine albumin or trace
    b. Proteinuria of <3 mg/m^2/hour
    c. Spot urine protein/creatinine ratio <0.2 mg/g

CASE 28

A 1-year-old female child with steroid-dependent nephrotic syndrome on 0.5 mg/kg/alternate day prednisolone for 1 year came to the clinic with two relapses. On examination, patient was hypertensive and iatrogenic Cushingoid facies.

1. **What do you define relapses?**
2. **What do you define steroid dependence?**
3. **What are the types of relapses?**
4. **How can you treat relapses?**
5. **What are the recommendations of adding alternative agents?**
6. **What are the drugs used as alternative agents?**
7. **Who are steroid sparing agents and why?**

Answers

1. Relapse can be defined as relapse if the patient can follow any of the following criteria:
   a. Urine albumin +++ or ++++
   b. Proteinuria of >40 mg/m^2/hour
   c. Spot protein to creatinine ratio of >2 mg/g

2. Steroid dependence can be defined as two consecutive relapses in the patient on alternate day steroids or within 2 weeks of the discontinuation of steroids.

3. There are two types of relapses:
   a. Frequent relapse: It can be defined as two or more relapses in the first 6 months or >3 relapses in 1 years.
   b. Infrequent relapse: It can be defined as ≤3 relapses within 1 year.

4. Patient should be treated in the following manner:
   a. In case of infrequent relapse: Patient should be treated with 2 mg/kg/day prednisolone in divided doses for each relapse till remission. Then 1.5 mg/kg orally at alternate day for another 4 weeks followed by discontinuation of treatment.
   b. In case of frequent relapse: This patient requires long-term treatment with steroid at a dose of 0.5–0.7 mg/kg at alternate day to maintain remission for 9–12 months. This relapse can be triggered by upper respiratory tract infection. This relapse can be tackled by adding steroid as daily dose for 5–7 days along with the antibiotics.

5. Following are the recommendations of adding alternative agents:
   a. If the dose of prednisolone is higher than 0.5–0.7 mg/kg on alternate day, it fails to maintain remission.
   b. If there are features of corticosteroid toxicity such as growth failure, hypertension, or cataract.

6. Following drugs are used as alternative agents:
   a. Levamisole at a dose of 2–2.5 mg/kg at alternate day
   b. Cyclophosphamide at a dose of 2–2.5 mg/kg daily
   c. Mycophenolate mofetil at a dose of 600–1,200 mg/m^2
   d. Cyclosporine at a dose of 4–5 mg/kg daily
   e. Tacrolimus at a dose of 0.1–0.2 mg/kg/day
   f. Rituximab at a dose 375 mg/m^2 twice weekly

7. Following are the steroid sparing agents:
   a. Cyclophosphamide
   b. Mycophenolate mofetil
   c. Rituximab

CASE 29

An 11.5-year-old male child has come to pediatric clinic with history of periorbital puffiness. From history, it has been found that patient was on steroid at 2 mg/kg for 6 weeks then 1.5 mg/kg for 2 weeks. On examination, patient developed iatrogenic Cushingoid facies and mild pedal edema. Urine analysis demonstrated +++ protein and serum albumin 2 g/dL.

1. **What is the most likely diagnosis?**
2. **How can you define this disease?**
3. **What is the role of renal biopsy in this disease?**
4. **What are the genetic mutations associated with this disease?**
5. **Genetic testing should be done in which syndrome occurring in the childhood?**
6. **In which types of patient genetic testing should be done?**
7. **What is the recommendation of vaccination in this patient?**

Answers

1. This patient has been suffering from steroid-resistant nephrotic syndrome.

2. If the patient fails to achieve proteinuria in spite of getting treatment by steroid with adequate dose for 4–8 weeks, then this patient can be diagnosed as steroid-resistant nephrotic syndrome.

3. Following are the indications of renal biopsy in this patient:
   a. Minimal change disease patient will respond satisfactorily to this therapy.
   b. Focal segmental glomerulosclerosis along with changes in the tubulointerstitium responds less satisfactorily.
   c. Membranoproliferative glomerulonephritis, membranous nephropathy, IgA nephropathy, amyloidosis, and Alport syndrome require different management.

4. Following are the genetic mutations for which testing should be done in this patient:
   a. Podocyte protein constituting the slit diaphragm
   b. Proteins of podocyte cytoskeleton
      These are NPHS1, NPHS2, CD2AP, TRPC6, and ACTN4
   c. Protein present on glomerular basement membrane—LAMB2
   d. Protein present on the mitochondria—COQ2
   e. Transcription factor for normal development—WT1 and LMX1B

5. Genetic testing should be done in the following syndrome occurring in the childhood:
   a. Denys–Drash syndrome: Here, diffuse mesangial sclerosis and Wilms tumor may occur.
   b. Frasier syndrome
   c. Pierson syndrome

6. Genetic testing should be done in following types of patients:
   a. Congenital nephrotic syndrome where the symptom onset is below 3 months of age.
   b. Family history of steroid-resistant nephrotic syndrome
   c. Girls having initial steroid resistance
   d. Sporadic initial steroid-resistant patient not responding to cyclophosphamide or calcineurin inhibitors
   e. Syndromic forms like:
      - Denys–Drash syndrome
      - Frasier syndrome
      - Pierson syndrome

7. Following recommendation regarding vaccinations for this patient:
   a. Oral polio, varicella vaccines, and other live vaccine should be given to this patient while the patient is off from immunosuppressive therapy for at least 4 weeks.
   b. If required, live vaccine can be given while the patient is on alternate day steroid therapy. Dose being 0.5 mg/kg.
   c. Patient should receive pneumococcal vaccine as per recommendation of pediatric association. It should be given 2 months after administration of conjugate vaccine in the child of >2 years of age.
   d. In case of relapse of nephrotic syndrome, another course of pneumococcal vaccine should be given 5 years after the primary vaccination.

CASE 30

A 9-year-old male child having recent past history of recovery from fever and upper respiratory tract infection 3 weeks back by antibiotics came to medicine outdoor with complaints of hematuria, headache, and facial puffiness for 3 days. No history of arthralgia or skin rash.

On examination, there was periorbital edema, blood pressure 140/95 mm Hg, pulse rate 112 beats/min, normal jugular venous pressure, and absence of crackles on auscultation.

Laboratory investigation demonstrated hemoglobin 12.5 g/dL, white blood cell count 1,000/cc, sodium 136 mEq/L, and potassium 6.1 mEq/L. Urine analysis demonstrated protein ++ and plenty of red blood cells.

1. **What is the most likely diagnosis?**
2. **What are the points in favor of diagnosis?**
3. **How can you differentiate this disease from the nephrotic syndrome?**
4. **What are the strains of streptococci responsible for this disease?**
5. **What is the pathogenesis in this disease?**
6. **What are the indications of renal biopsy in this disease?**
7. **What are the histopathologies in this disease?**

Answers

1. The most likely diagnosis is poststreptococcal nephritic syndrome due to previous upper respiratory infection in recent past.
2. Following points are in favor of diagnosis:
   a. Features of renal involvement such as hematuria, edema, hypertension, and oliguria
   b. Presence of hyperkalemia
   c. Presence of preceding upper respiratory infection 3 weeks back
3. Following points differentiate nephritic syndrome from nephrotic syndrome:

Nephrotic syndrome	Nephritic syndrome
Age 1–12 years	
Absence of hematuria	Presence of cola-colored urine indicating gross hematuria
Gross edema leading to ascites, pedal edema, and parietal and periorbital edema	Periorbital edema and pedal edema
Hypertension may not be present	Hypertension present
There must be hypoalbuminemia	May not be hypoalbuminemia
>3 g/day	<3 g/day
Hypercholesterolemia and hypertriglyceridemia	Normal level of cholesterol and triglyceride
Potassium level will be normal	There is hyperkalemia
Absence of cast	Presence of red blood cell casts

Continued

Continued

Nephrotic syndrome	Nephritic syndrome
Presence of free lipid droplet	Lipid droplet is absent
Absence of red blood cells	Red blood cell is dysmorphic

4. Following streptococcal strains are responsible for acute nephritic syndrome:
   a. In case of respiratory tract infection: 1, 3, 4, 12, 25, and 49
   b. In case of dermatological infection: 2, 49, 55, 57, and 60
5. Pathogenesis in this disease: Streptococcal antigen binds to IgG antibody and to form immune complexes and deposits on the glomerular basement membrane with following two receptors:
   a.

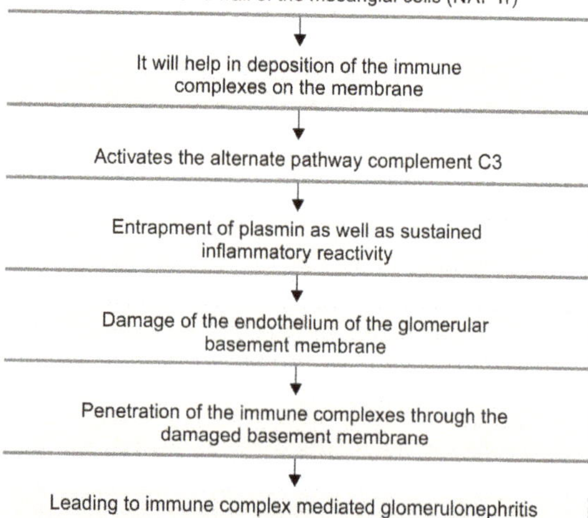

b.

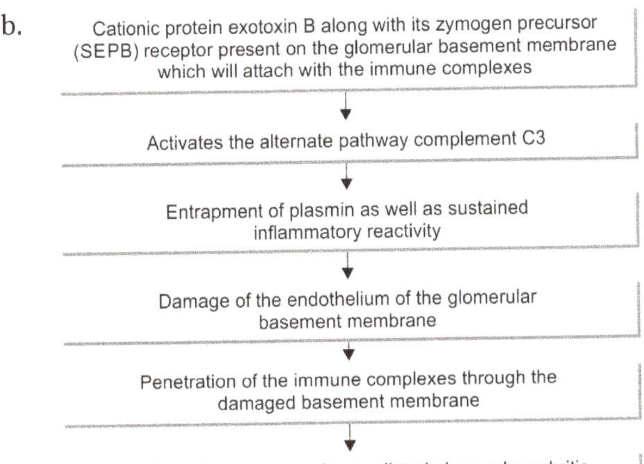

6. Indications of renal biopsy are as follows:
   a. If function of the kidney fails to recover in more than 7–10 days
   b. If the kidney function will decline rapidly.
   c. Persistent low level of C3 for >12 weeks
   d. Persistent proteinuria beyond 6 months
   e. If the systemic features suggest autoimmune disease
   f. If the C3 level is normal, predicting IgA nephropathy
   g. Absence of serological evidence of streptococcal infection
   h. Persistence of gross hematuria >4 weeks
   i. Persistence of microscopic hematuria >1 year

7. Following are the histological features in this case:
   a. Light microscopy demonstrates:
      - Diffuse exudative proliferative glomerulonephritis
      - Prominent proliferation of endocapillaries with accentuation of the lobar pattern
      - Infiltration with numerous neutrophils
      - Hypercellularity as a consequence of proliferation of both the mesangial and endothelial cells
   b. Immunofluorescence microscopy demonstrates deposition of the complement factor C3 and IgG along the glomerular basement membrane. There are three types of patterns described:
      i. Starry pattern: Irregular distribution of the fluorescent activity along the basement membrane.
      ii. Garland pattern: It refers to distribution of elongated and thicker deposits along the wall of the capillary.
      iii. Mesangial pattern: It refers to the distribution of the fluorescent activity along the mesangial walls.
   c. Electron microscopy: It will demonstrate subepithelial deposits or humps in scattered pattern on the glomerular basement membrane in absence of surrounding reaction on the basement membrane.

CASE 31

A 12-year-old male child having recent past history of low-grade fever, weight loss, myalgia, and night sweat 3 weeks back came to emergency department with fever, hematuria, headache, and facial puffiness for 4 days.

On examination, his pulse rate was 100 beats/min, blood pressure 140/95 mm Hg, febrile, and pedal edema.

Laboratory investigation demonstrated white blood count 14,000/cc with neutrophilic leukocytosis, hemoglobin 10 g/dL, and potassium 6 mEq/L. Transthoracic echocardiogram demonstrated the following:

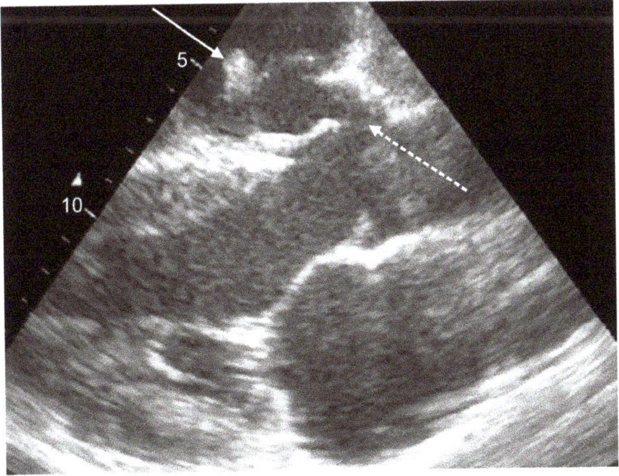

1. **What is shown in the above picture?**
2. **Why there was fever?**
3. **What is the most likely diagnosis?**
4. **What are the organisms responsible?**
5. **Mention the pathophysiology.**
6. **How can you manage this case?**

Answers

1. Above picture demonstrates the ventricular septal defect.
2. Low-grade fever in the background of ventricular septal defect indicates that this patient is suffered from subacute bacterial endocarditis.
3. The most likely diagnosis is acute nephritic syndrome due to subacute bacterial endocarditis in a patient with persistent ventricular septal defect.
4. Following organisms are responsible:
   a. *Streptococcus viridans*
   b. *Staphylococcus epidermidis*
   c. *Staphylococcus aureus*
   d. *Streptococcus pyogenes*
   e. *Streptococcus pneumoniae*
   f. *Salmonella* typhi
   g. *Brucella* species
5. This is an immunologically mediated disease where microbial antigen deposits on the glomerular basement membrane and mesangium along with the antibody and complement factor C3 leading to release of inflammatory cytokine resulting in acute nephritic syndrome.
6. Treatment of subacute bacterial endocarditis as per bacterial culture and sensitivity for 4–6 weeks will improve the renal outcome.

CASE 32

A 10-year-old girl having recent past history of skin infection and taken one course of antibiotic 6 weeks back admitted with puffiness of the face and cola-colored urine for 1 week.

On examination, there was periorbital edema, pulse rate 100 beats/min and blood pressure 155/105 mm Hg. Laboratory investigation demonstrated urea 90 mg/dL, creatinine 7.2 mg/dL, and total count of white blood cell 10,000/cc. Urine analysis demonstrated plenty of red blood cells along with red blood cell cast and protein ++.

1. **What is the possible diagnosis?**
2. **Define this disease?**
3. **What are the microscopic features in this disease?**
4. **What are the indications of renal biopsy in this disease?**

Answers

1. This is a case of postinfectious glomerulonephritis with progressing worsening of renal function leading to rapidly progressive renal failure.
2. Rapidly progressive glomerulonephritis can be defined as severe form of injury to the glomeruli leading to glomerular capillary loop rupture with accumulation of the leukocytes as well as blood constituents in the Bowman capsular space inducing proliferation of visceral epithelial cells which together forming cellular crescents.
3. Microscopic features in this disease are as follows:
   a. Light microscopy demonstrated hypercellularity in the glomeruli consisting of inflammatory cells and endothelial and mesangial cells.
   b. Electron microscopy demonstrated presence of subepithelial humps which is characterized by deposits of electron-dense material in the subepithelial space near the glomerular basement membrane.
   c. Immunofluorescence microscopy demonstrated evidence of deposits of IgM and C3 within first 2 weeks of the disease.
4. Usually, the patients with poststreptococcal glomerulonephritis do not require renal biopsy, but in the following conditions, the renal biopsy may be required:
   a. Anuric renal failure
   b. If the level of complement is normal.
   c. If there is progressive decline in the renal function.
   d. If there is no rise in the antistreptococcal antibodies

CASE 33

A 55-year-old diabetic male having recent past history of recovery from fever and urinary tract infection 1 week back by antibiotics came to medicine outdoor with complaints of hematuria, headache, and facial puffiness for 3 days. No history of arthralgia or skin rash.

On examination, there was periorbital edema, blood pressure 170/105 mm Hg, pulse rate 112 beats/min, normal jugular venous pressure, and absence of crackles on auscultation.

Laboratory investigation demonstrated hemoglobin 12.5 g/dL, white blood cell count 1,000/cc, sodium 136 mEq/L, and potassium 6.1 mEq/L. Urine analysis demonstrated protein ++ and plenty of red blood cells.

1. **What is the most likely diagnosis in this case?**
2. **What are the differences in the presentation in this case as compared to PSGN?**
3. **What are the typical features in the histology in this case?**
4. **In this case, what are the serological tests that should be done in this case?**
5. **Mention the treatment in this case.**
6. **What is the progression in this case.**

Answers

1. The most likely diagnosis is *Staphylococcus*-associated acute glomerulonephritis.
2. Following are the differences in the presentation in this present as compared to PSGN:
   a. No specific strain of *Staphylococcus* is responsible.
   b. Location of the infection is urinary tract.
   c. There is no latent period.
   d. It usually occurs in older adult
   e. There is preexisting morbidity like diabetes mellitus.
3. Following are the typical features in the renal histology:
   a. On immunofluorescence, there is deposit of IgA at the site of the deposits. If IgG is present, it will be overshadowed by IgA.
4. Following are the serological tests in this case:
   a. Culture of urine, sputum, and blood for positivity of *Staphylococcus aureus*.
   b. Low C3 and C4
5. The main aim is to stop the antigenemia through the increased production of the immune complexes. Hence, immunosuppressive therapy will be absolutely contraindicated as the staphylococcal infection may lead to sepsis in this case.
6. Following are the progression of the disease:
   a. In 50% case, residual kidney disease will be present and it depends upon the bacterial elimination and this consists of hematuria, proteinuria, and persistent reduction of glomerular filtration rate.
   b. Some patients progressing toward the end-stage renal failure requiring dialysis
   c. Presence of comorbidity like diabetes mellitus also determines the disease course

CASE 34

A 30-year-old man with no comorbidities having recent past history of fever subsided after taking over-the-counter antibiotics came to emergency department with erythematous rashes all over the body along with progressively increasing creatinine level to 7 mg/dL in presence of normal output. In the emergency, intravenous fluid was started.

On laboratory investigation, complete blood count, liver function test, serum electrolytes, and serum protein electrophoresis were within normal limit.

Urine analysis demonstrated protein++, 9–10 red blood cells/HPF and 4–5 white blood cells/HPF. Kidney size in ultrasound was normal. Renal biopsy was performed which demonstrated:

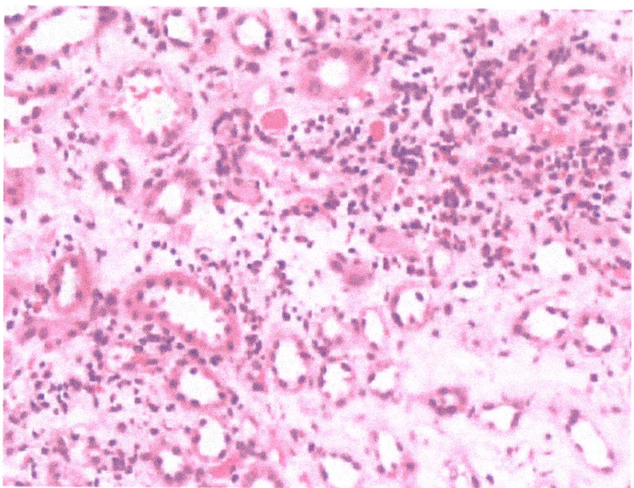

1. **What are the features demonstrated in the histology picture?**
2. **What is the most likely diagnosis?**
3. **What are the clues to the diagnosis?**
4. **What are the cases where urinary sediment may be absent?**
5. **What are the cases where eosinophils may be present in urine?**
6. **What are the causes of this diagnosis?**
7. **What type of hypersensitivity occurs in this disease?**
8. **What are the causative factors for this type of hypersensitivity reaction?**
9. **What are the categories of antigen that can induce this disease?**
10. **What is the pathophysiology in case of NSAIDs-induced disease?**
11. **What are the urine biomarkers?**
12. **What are the characteristic histopathological findings in this disease?**
13. **By imaging, how can you differentiate between this disease and acute tubular necrosis?**
14. **What are the features in the immunofluorescence microscopy?**
15. **What are the supportive measures to be taken in this disease?**
16. **What are the risk factors leading to progression to chronic kidney disease?**

Answers

1. The histological picture in case of renal biopsy demonstrated the following:
   a. Infiltration of the inflammatory cells in the tubular interstitium
   b. Edema in the wall of the tubule
   c. Glomeruli are not involved.
2. This patient has been suffering from rapidly progressive renal failure due to acute tubulointerstitial nephritis.
3. Following are the clues to this diagnosis:
   a. Presence of active urinary sediments
   b. Normal size of the kidney
   c. Presence of rashes all over the body
   d. Intake of over-the-counter drugs for subsidence of fever
4. In the following cases, urinary sediment may be absent:
   a. Acute tubulointerstitial nephritis
   b. Atheroembolic renal failure
   c. Pelvic mass
   d. Retroperitoneal fibrosis
5. In the following cases, eosinophil may be present in urinary sediment:
   a. Acute tubulointerstitial nephritis
   b. Atheroembolic renal failure

6. Following are the causes of this diagnosis:
   a. Drugs
   b. Infection
   c. Autoimmune systemic disease
   d. Idiopathic disease
7. It is a type of cell-mediated delayed hypersensitivity reaction occurring in this disease.
8. Following are the causative factors for this type of hypersensitivity reaction in this disease:
   a. It occurs in small percentage of individuals
   b. It may be associated with extrarenal manifestations of hypersensitivity.
   c. Presence of granuloma in the renal biopsy
   d. This disease may recur after accidental reexposure to the same offending drug or to a closely related drug.
9. Three major categories of antigens capable inducing this acute tubulointerstitial nephritis:
   a. Components of tubular basement membrane protein such as glycoprotein 3M-1 and TIN-Ag/TIN1
   b. Tubular protein secreted such as Tamm–Horsfall protein
   c. Extrarenal protein such as immune complexes
10. Pathogenesis in this disease:
    a. It occurs as a result of cell-mediated delayed hypersensitivity reaction which is characterized by infiltration of CD4+ T cells.
    b. There may be also antibody-mediated response against basement membrane protein as evidenced by high IgE levels in the blood.
11. Following are the biomarkers in the urine in acute tubulointerstitial nephritis:
    a. Tumor necrosis factor-alpha
    b. Interleukin-9
    c. Monocyte chemotactic peptide-1

12. Following are the characteristic findings in this disease:
    a. Interstitium is infiltrated with inflammatory cells.
    b. Interstitial edema
    c. Evidence of tubulitis
    d. Presence of granulomas in the interstitium
    e. Presence of antitubular basement membrane antibodies
    f. Diffuse foot process effacement in case of NSAID-induced minimal change disease
    g. Glomeruli are normal.
    h. Intrarenal blood vessels are normal.
13. Gallium scan can differentiate between acute tubular necrosis and acute tubulointerstitial nephritis because in the later case gallium-67 will bind to lactoferrin that is expressed on the inflammatory cell surfaces.
14. Immunofluorescence microscopy demonstrates linear deposits of IgG and complement on the tubular basement membrane
15. Following are the supportive measures to be taken in this disease:
    a. Adequate hydration should be maintained.
    b. Volume depletion or volume overload should be avoided.
    c. Proper identification and correction of the electrolyte abnormalities
    d. Rash should be treated symptomatically.
    e. Drugs that impair the renal blood flow should be avoided.
    f. Drug dose should be adjusted according to the status of the renal function.
16. Following are the risk factors that aid in the progression to the chronic renal disease:
    a. Elderly age
    b. Baseline chronic kidney disease
    c. Dependent on initial dialysis
    d. Recovery within the first month
    e. Degree of fibrosis in the renal biopsy

CASE 35

A 28-year-old female came to outpatient department with rash, fever, and joint pain. Her blood test demonstrated ESR 100 mm/1st hour, ANA 3+ and speckled pattern, and dsDNA > 405 IU/mL. Her urine only demonstrated microscopic hematuria and protein 400 mg/day. The patient was on 60 mg/day prednisolone, but is very irregular. Again, all the above symptoms recur after 1 year and the patient came to outpatient department.

This time, on examination, all her vitals were normal and rashes on the faces. All the systemic examinations were normal.

Laboratory examination demonstrated hemoglobin 8.5 g/dL, white blood cell count 4,000/cc, and platelet count 110,000/cc, serum albumin 2 g/dL, and cholesterol 320 mg/dL. Urine analysis demonstrated +++ protein, 24 hours estimated >3.5 g/day.

Above serologies remained are strongly positive and low C3 and C4. Hemolysis workup was within normal limit.

1.   **What is your most likely diagnosis?**
2.   **What are the points in favor of your diagnosis?**
3.   **What are the immunologic serologies that should be done to determine that the lupus is active?**
4.   **How do you classify this disease?**
5.   **What are the histopathological features in this disease?**
6.   **What are the typical histologic features present in this disease?**
7.   **What are the full-house patterns in this disease?**
8.   **What are the types of vascular lesions seen in this disease?**
9.   **How can you suspect the transformation of stages clinically?**
10. **What percentage of patients will enter into rapidly progressive renal failure?**
11. **Is there any involvement of tubules in this disease?**
12. **What are the treatment options in this case?**
13. **How can you monitor this patient during treatment?**
14. **What are the possible outcomes in treating lupus nephritis?**
15. **What are the poor prognostic factors in this disease?**
16. **How can you treat a case of unsatisfactory response to treatment?**

Answers

1. Patient has been suffering from stage III to IV lupus nephritis.

2. Following are the points in favor of diagnosis:
    a.   Young female within the reproductive group
    b.   Presence of butterfly rashes on the face
    c.   Polyarthritis
    d.   Presence of edema and hypertension
    e.   Macroscopic proteinuria
    f.   Microscopic hematuria

3. Following immunological serology should be determined if the lupus is active:
    a.   ANA
    b.   Anti-Smith antibody
    c.   Anti–Sjögren's-syndrome-related antigen A (anti-SSA) antibody
    d.   Anti–Sjögren's-syndrome-related antigen B (anti-SSB) antibody
    e.   Antiribonucleoprotein
    f.   Anti-dsDNA
    g.   Complement components
    h.   Rheumatoid factor
    i.   Antiphospholipid antibodies

4. Classification of the disease:
    a.   Class I: Minimal mesangial lupus nephritis
    b.   Class II: Mesangial proliferative lupus nephritis
    c.   Class III: Focal lupus nephritis involving <50% of glomeruli
    d.   Class IV: Diffuse lupus nephritis involving ≥50% of glomeruli—
        •   IV-S: Diffuse segmental lupus nephritis involving <50% glomerular surface area
        •   IV-G: Diffuse global lupus nephritis involving ≥50% glomerular surface area
    e.   Class V: Membranous lupus nephritis
    f.   Class VI: Advanced sclerosing lupus nephritis

5. Following are the histopathological features in this disease:
    a.   Class I:
        •   Normal glomeruli in light microscopy
        •   Immunofluorescence microscopy— mesangial immune deposits
    b.   Class II: Class I plus—
        •   On light microscopy: Mesangial hyper-cellularity along with or without mesangial expansion
    c.   Class III:
        •   Active focal or segmental endo- or extracapillary glomerulonephritis
        •   Focal subendothelial deposits with or without mesangial alterations
        •   Wire-loop deposits with little or no glomerular proliferation.

Focal lesions:
- III A: Active lesions
- III A/C: Active and chronic lesions
- III C: Chronic lesions

d. Class IV:
- Active diffuse endo- or extracapillary glomerulonephritis
- Diffuse subendothelial deposits with or without mesangial alterations
- Wire-loop deposits with little or no glomerular proliferation.
  Diffuse:
  - IV S: Segmental (<50% of one glomerular tuft is involved)
  - IV G: Global (>50% of one glomerular tuft is involved)
  - IV A: Active lesions
  - IV A/C: Active and chronic lesions
  - IV C: Chronic lesions

e. Class V: Subepithelial immune deposits in light microscopy involving 50% of the glomerular capillary loops along with or without mesangial alterations.

f. Class VI: ≥90% glomeruli will be globally sclerosed without any residual activity.

6. Following typical histologic features are present in this disease:

a. Hallmark is deposition of immune complexes in the mesangium, subepithelial, or subendothelial areas.

b. Wire-loop lesion which is characterized by deposition of the immune complexes involving peripheral circumference of the glomeruli.

c. Hyaline thrombi characterized by large intracapillary deposition of immune complexes

d. Segmental fibrinoid necrosis characterized by rupture of glomerular basement membrane leading to typical segmental deposition of fibrin

e. Nuclear dust characterized by apoptosis of the infiltrating neutrophils leading to formation of Karyorrhectic nuclear debris

f. Hematoxylins bodies: It is tissue equivalent of lupus erythematosus (LE) bodies present only 2% of cases, but truly it is the only pathognomonic sign.

7. Following are the full-house patterns in case of lupus nephritis:

a. Immunofluorescence patterns—presence of all the following immunoreactants like:
- IgG
- IgM
- IgA
- C1q: It is fairly specific for lupus nephritis.
- C3

b. Subclasses of IgG: It usually demonstrates—
- Dominant IgG1 and IgG3
- Mild IgG2
- Minimal IgG4

8. Following types of vascular lesions seen in this disease:

a. Uncomplicated vascular immune complex deposits

b. Thrombotic microangiopathy

c. Noninflammatory necrotizing vasculitis

d. Inflammatory vasculitis

9. By following methods, class transformation can be judged clinically:

a. Transformation from class III to IV can be diagnosed by:
- Worsening of proteinuria
- Active urinary sediments
- Decreased glomerular filtration rate

b. In case of class V, if there are presence of active sediments and worsening of glomerular filtration rate, it will indicate proliferative lupus.

10. 10–20% patients will enter into rapidly progressive renal failure. Prognosis is very poor in case of crescentic glomerulonephritis.

11. Regarding tubular abnormalities:

a. In dysfunction of proximal tubule, there is increased excretion of:
- β2 microglobulin
- Light chain protein

b. In case distal tubular dysfunction:
- Distal renal tubular acidosis
- Hyporeninemic hypoaldosteronism
- Normotensive hyperreninemia
- Decreased excretion of potassium

12. Treatment options in this patient are as follows:

a. In induction phase:
- Methylprednisolone 0.25–0.5 g/day for 1–3 days followed by oral prednisolone 0.6–1 mg/kg/day but not exceeding 80 mg/day for 4–8 weeks plus any one of the following:
  - Cyclophosphamide 2 mg/kg orally daily for 6–12 weeks—dose has to be adjusted monitoring blood count.

- ○ High-dose intravenous cyclophosphamide 0.5–1.0 mg/m^2 monthly for 6 months—dose has to be adjusted monitoring blood count.
- ○ Low-dose intravenous cyclophosphamide 500 mg every 2 weeks for total 6 doses—dose has to be adjusted monitoring blood count.
- ○ Mycophenolate mofetil 2–3 g daily orally in divided doses for 6 months
  b. Maintenance phase:
     - Mycophenolate mofetil 0.5–2 g daily in two divided doses with tapering dose of prednisolone
     - Azathioprine 1–3 mg/kg daily along prednisolone in tapering dose
     - Oral cyclosporine 2–4 mg/kg daily with prednisolone in tapering dose
     - Low-dose prednisolone should be continued with slow tapering to attain the minimal dose for controlling symptoms.

13. Monitoring of the patient during treatment:
    a. During induction therapy:
       - Monthly serum creatinine
       - Routine urine analysis
       - Urine protein creatinine ratio (UPCR)
       - Monitoring of blood pressure
    b. At 3 months along with above parameters, following should be done:
       - C3
       - C4
       - dsDNA
       - Albumin level
    c. If above parameters are improving, therapy should be continued. It the parameters deteriorate, change of therapy should be considered.
    d. At 6 months, in addition to above parameters, 24 hours urine protein should be measured. Based on this result, further therapy should be considered.
    e. In case of no response, either renal biopsy should be done to detect its chronicity or treatment should be changed.
    f. During the maintenance therapy, every 3 months following should be considered:
       - Serum creatinine
       - Routine urine analysis
       - UPCR

    g. In case of any abnormality in the above tests, following should be done:
       - C3
       - C4
       - dsDNA

14. According to KDIGO, there are three types of outcomes that are noted:
    a. Complete response: It is characterized by following within 6–12 months of starting of the therapy but not >12 months:
       - Reduction of proteinuria by <0.5 g/g
       - Stabilization of the function of the kidney (10–15% of baseline)
    b. Partial response within 6–12 months of starting of the therapy but not >12 months: Reduction of proteinuria by 50% at least to <3 g/g
    c. No response: It is characterized by failure to achieve complete or partial response within 6–12 months after stating of the therapy.

15. Following are the poor prognostic factors in this disease:
    a. Demographic factors:
       - Young age
       - Male sex
       - Black race
    b. Clinical factors:
       - Raised serum creatinine
       - Class IV—diffuse proliferative nephritis
       - Anemia
       - Response to therapy
       - Thrombocytopenia

16. Following are the methods of treatment in case of unsatisfactory response to treatment:
    a. Adherence to treatment should be verified.
    b. Drug should be administered in adequate dose with measuring the plasma level of that drug.
       - Measurement of mycophenolic acid in case of analogs of mycophenolate
       - Infusion records of administration of cyclophosphamide
    c. If chronic nephritis or other diagnosis thrombotic thrombocytopenic purpura, renal biopsy is indicated.
    d. There may be switching to alternate second-drug regimen.
    e. Combination of mycophenolic acid and calcineurin inhibitors
    f. Addition of biological therapies such as rituximab
    g. Extended course of intravenous cyclophosphamide can be administered.

CASE 36

A 28-year-old female suffering from stage III lupus nephritis on regular cyclophosphamide along with steroid for 4 months in induction phase. Now, she wants to take pregnancy.

1. **What types of contraception are required during the period of treatment?**
2. **What are the mechanisms by which the fertility will be affected?**
3. **What are the measures to be taken to prevent infertility due to cyclophosphamide?**
4. **What are the risks associated with pregnancy?**
5. **What monitoring should be done in pregnant lupus patient?**
6. **What are the drugs which should be altered during pregnancy?**
7. **What are the drugs which should be started or continued?**
8. **What are the factors indicating bad pregnancy outcome?**

Answers

1. Following are the effective contraceptive methods which can translate into uncomplicated pregnancy in the inactive phase of lupus nephritis and the patient is on nonteratogenic medication:
   a. Progesterone intrauterine device
   b. Progesterone subdermal implant
   c. Estrogen-containing oral contraceptives: It should not be given in case of active disease or patient has been suffering from antiphospholipid antibodies.
   d. Barrier method: Though it is less effective, but during active phase of illness, patient has to rely upon this method.
2. Following are the methods of affecting the fertility in this disease:
   a. There is autoimmune SLE-related menstrual dysfunction which produces amenorrhea in lupus associated with anticorpus luteum antibodies in patient with high disease activity.
   b. Cyclophosphamide-related ovarian failure in female is dose and age dependent. Dose of ≥15 pulses is associated with nearly 100% ovarian failure. In case of 20–30 years female, chance of gonadal failure is >40%, whereas in >30 years of age, this failure becomes nearly 100%. Gonadotoxicity is irreversible as the number of oocytes is fixed throughout the life.
   c. There are incidences of sexual dysfunction in this patient because of psychological factors.
   d. Alteration of the hypothalamic–pituitary–gonadal axis in case of progressive lupus nephritis leading to renal failure results infertility.

3. Following measures should be taken in female to prevent infertility:
   a. If possible altered immunosuppressive agents like mycophenolate mofetil should be taken.
   b. Cyclophosphamide should be taken for shorter duration in lower doses.
   c. Intravenous administration of cyclophosphamide should be avoided.
   d. Concomitant administration of monthly protective agents like growth hormone-releasing hormone such as leuprolide should be administered to prevent ovulation but with accepted risk of osteoporosis and menopausal symptoms.
   e. Cryopreservation of oocyte should be done as hormone stimulation during collection of oocyte may flare the lupus.
4. Following are the risks associated with pregnancy in SLE patient:
   a. Disease activity during pregnancy:
      - There are renal as well as hematological flares.
      - Active disease during first 6 months
      - Discontinuation of hydroxychloroquine may lead to disease flare.
   b. Pregnancy-related complications:
      - 3–5 times higher rate of preeclampsia as compared to normal population
      - History of lupus
      - Presence of antiplatelet antibodies
      - Hypocomplementemia
      - Thrombocytopenia

c. Outcome in fetus:
- Fetal loss
- 50% preterm birth
- Intrauterine growth retardation
- Hypertension
- Antiphospholipid antibodies
- Thrombocytopenia
- Lupus nephritis

5. Following monitoring should be done in pregnant lupus patients:
   a. Complete remission of lupus nephritis for at least 6 months
   b. Following drugs should be used during pregnancy:
      - Low-dose steroid
      - Azathioprine up to 2 mg/kg/day
      - Mycophenolate mofetil
      - Cyclosporine
      - Tacrolimus
   c. Preconception period counseling
   d. Assessment and evaluation of maternal and fetal risk factors
   e. Estimation of sets of autoantibodies

6. Following drugs should be altered or stopped during pregnancy:
   a. Cyclophosphamide should be stopped 3 months prior to pregnancy for minimum period of 6 weeks.
   b. Methotrexate
   c. Mycophenolate mofetil should be stopped 3 months prior to pregnancy.
   d. ACEI or ARBs should be stopped better before early pregnancy and must be stopped during second and third trimester of pregnancy.

7. Following drugs should be started or continued during pregnancy:
   a. Aspirin should be started before 16 weeks of pregnancy.
   b. Azathioprine
   c. Cyclosporine or tacrolimus: There is increased risk of gestational diabetes mellitus mostly associated with steroids.
   d. Prednisolone: It is mostly inactivated by placental enzyme. But, betamethasone and dexamethasone can cross the placenta.
   e. Hydroxychloroquine:
      - If continued, it:
         - Prevents flare
         - Reduces the risk of clots
         - Improves the long-term survival
      - If stopped, it:
         - Increases risk of flare
         - Reduces risk of congenital heart block in Ro-positive women
         - Reduces intrauterine growth retardation

8. Following factors indicate bad outcome in pregnancy during pregnancy:
   a. During first trimester:
      - High blood pressure needs medications
      - Lupus becomes most active
      - Positive results of lupus anticoagulant
   b. During second trimester:
      - More active lupus disease
      - Lupus flare

In absence of any risk factor in first trimester, pregnancy outcome will be 8%.

CASE 37

A 58-year-old lady having no comorbidities admitted in medicine emergency with joint pain, low-grade fever, generalized weakness and progressively decreasing urination, and bilateral lower limb swelling for 4 weeks. She had history of erythematous rashes in the lower limb and low-grade fever 5 years ago which was treated by antiallergic drugs.

On examination, there was anemia, blood pressure 145/95 mm Hg, bilateral pedal edema, serum glutamate pyruvate transaminase (SGPT) 222 IU/L, serum glutamic oxaloacetic transaminase (SGOT) 302 IU/L, hemoglobin 10 g/dL, urea 110 mg/dL, and creatinine 4.5 mg/dL. Serology demonstrated hepatitis C virus (HCV) positive, hepatitis

B surface antigen (HBsAg) negative, HIV negative, ANA, and ANCA negative but rheumatoid factor positive. Serum cryoglobulins were positive.

Urine analysis demonstrated +++ protein and red blood cells and white blood cells 25–30 and 10–12/HPF, respectively. Kidney biopsy done which demonstrated:

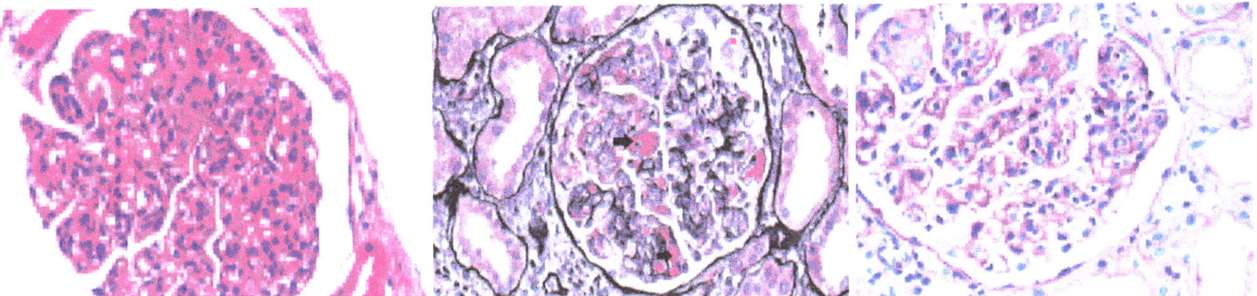

1.   **What are shown in the above pictures?**
2.   **What is the most probable diagnosis?**
3.   **What do you mean by cryoglobulinemia?**
4.   **What are the types of cryoglobulin and this patient has been suffering from what type?**
5.   **What are the types of cryoprecipitate found in the blood??**
6.   **What is the association of complement with cryoglobulinemia?**
7.   **What are the types of typical histopathological changes occur in this disease?**
8.   **What are the classical types based on the ultrastructural mechanism?**
9.   **What are the predictors of mortality in this disease?**

Answers

1. Description of the microscopic picture:
   a. Light microscopy demonstrated glomerular hypercellularity and lobular accentuation of the glomerular tuft
   b. Silver staining of the biopsy material demonstrated immune deposits in the capillary wall and presence of cryoglobulin in the lumen
   c. Third picture is the PAS-stained renal tissue demonstrating:
      - Mesangial expansion
      - Endocapillary proliferation
      - Thickening of glomerular basement membrane.

2. The most likely diagnosis is membranoproliferative glomerulonephritis due to cryoglobulinemia resulting from hepatitis C virus infection.

3. Cryoglobulin is the type of immunoglobulin as well as complement components that precipitate at temperature of <37°C and will be redissolved in the warm condition in vitro and this is known as cryoprecipitation. Presence of this cryoglobulin in the blood is known as cryoglobulinemia.

4. There are three types of cryoglobulins present based on the types of immunoglobulin:
   a. Simple or type 1 cryoglobulin: It is either monoclonal immunoglobulins such as IgG and IgA or monoclonal free light chain.
   b. Mixed or type 2 cryoglobulin: It is either monoclonal immunoglobulin such as IgG, IgM, and IgA or polyclonal free light chain.
   c. Mixed or type 3 cryoglobulin: It is polyclonal immunoglobulins of all isotypes.

   This patient has been suffering from type 2 cryoglobulinemia.

5. Two types of cryoprecipitate found in the blood:
   a. Cryoglobulins: These are the antibodies that will precipitate at <37°C and will be dissolved in the warm conditions. They are responsible for inflammation and the organ damage.
   b. Cryofibrinogen: It will get precipitated from the refrigerated plasma. It consists of mixture of fibrinogen, fibroactin, fibrin, and fibrin degradation products.

6. Cryoglobulinemia is associated with cryoglobulin containing immune complexes.
   a. Type I cryoglobulin is responsible for very few complement abnormalities.
   b. Type II and III are associated with reduction of serum level of total hemolytic complement (CH50) and early complement C1q, C2, and C4. C3 is not affected because it is the late complement.
7. Following are the typical histological changes in this mesangioproliferative glomerulonephritis:
   a. Mesangial and endothelial cell proliferation with expansion of the mesangial matrix
   b. Peripheral capillary wall thickening by subendothelial immune deposits with or without intramembranous dense deposits
   c. Evidence of interposition of mesangial cells into the capillary wall giving rise of tram-track double-contour appearance in the light microscopy
8. Following types are found according to the ultrastructural appearance:
   a. Type I: Subendothelial deposits
   b. Type II: Presence of dense deposits in the glomerular basement membrane
   c. Type III: Presence of subepithelial or subendothelial deposits
9. Following are the predictors of mortality in this disease:
   a. Age
   b. Male gender
   c. Circulating cryoglobulin
   d. Immunosuppressive treatment
   e. Cutaneous ulceration
   f. Chronic hepatitis
   g. Widespread vasculitis
   h. Advanced renal failure

CASE 38

A 42-year-old lady having no previous comorbidities but having history of two consequent abortion followed by preterm delivery admitted previously with severe abdominal pain and constipation and subsequently diagnosed as subacute intestinal obstruction. Her upper and lower gastrointestinal endoscopy and CT scan of abdomen were normal. She was treated conservatively and released. But again, she readmitted within 4 days with similar complaints along with fever and bilateral bluish discoloration of both the lower limbs. Laboratory investigations demonstrated leukocytosis, high lactate level, serum creatinine 4 mg/dL, activated partial thromboplastin time (APTT) prolonged, positive lupus anticoagulant and anti-β2 glycoprotein 1 IgG but negative for anticardiolipin antibody, ANA, and dsDNA.

Urine analysis demonstrated presence of plenty of red blood cell and red blood cell cast. Straight X-ray of the abdomen demonstrated the following features.

She was subsequently undergone laparotomy.

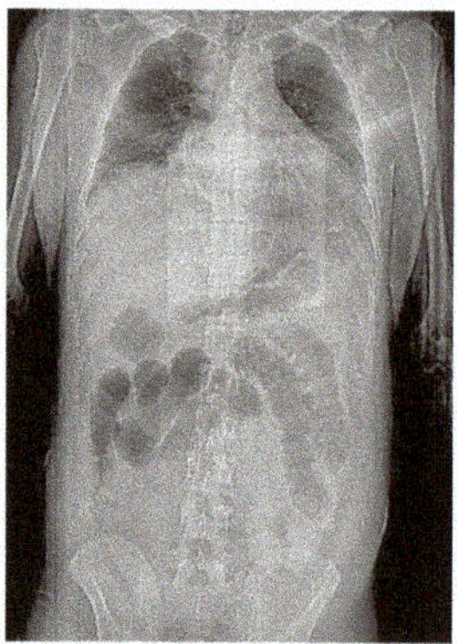 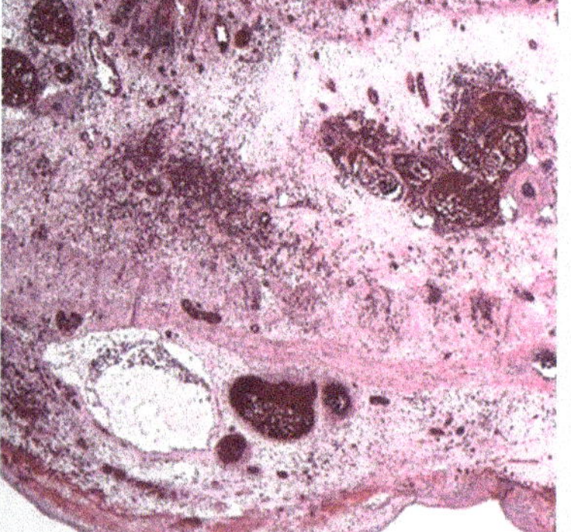

1. **What is your diagnosis?**
2. **What is the most likely diagnosis?**
3. **What are the criteria in this etiology?**
4. **What are the criteria of the catastrophic type of this disease?**
5. **What is the skin lesion described here?**

6. **What is the final diagnosis in this patient on which points?**
7. **What are types of renal involvement due to this etiology?**
8. **What are the guidelines regarding the screening of the lupus anticoagulant?**
9. **What are the treatments of choice in this case?**

Answers

1. Straight X-ray of abdomen demonstrates the features suggestive of superior mesenteric venous thrombosis:
   a. There is significant dilatation of proximal bowel loops
   b. Edema in the wall of the intestine
   c. Concertina sign
   d. Absence of air-fluid levels
   e. Presence of nasogastric tube in situ
   Histopathological features in this case are thrombosis of the superior mesenteric vessels.

2. The most likely diagnosis is membranoproliferative glomerulonephritis due to antiphospholipid syndrome.

3. Diagnostic criteria of antiphospholipid antibody syndrome are as follows:
   Any one of clinical criteria plus one laboratory criteria:
   a. Clinical criteria:
      - Vascular thrombosis involving any vein, artery, or small vessel in any organ proven by imaging or histology, but presence of superficial venous thrombosis does not fit the criteria.
      - Pregnancy morbidity:
         ○ ≥1 unexplained death of morphologically normal fetus at ≥10 weeks of gestation
         Or,
         ○ ≥1 premature births of neonate of <34 weeks due to eclampsia or placental insufficiency
         Or,
         ○ Three consecutive pregnancy loss of <10 weeks that are unexplained by chromosomal, anatomical, or hormonal cause.
   b. Laboratory criteria:
      - Presence of ≥1 antiphospholipid antibodies on ≥2 occasions at 12 weeks apart:
         ○ IgG and/or IgM anticardiolipin antibodies in moderate-to-high titers of >40 units by ELISA test.
         ○ IgG and/IgM anti β-2 glycoprotein in moderate to high titers of more than 40 units by ELISA test.
         ○ Lupus anticoagulant

4. Following are the criteria of the catastrophic type of the disease:
   a. Involvement of ≥3 organs/tissues
   b. Histological evidences of intravascular thrombosis
   c. Development of the manifestation in <1 week
   d. Presence of antiphospholipid antibodies

5. Skin lesion demonstrated here is livedo reticularis.

6. Following are the points on which the final diagnosis was made as primary catastrophic antiphospholipid syndrome of primary variety:
   a. Recurrent abortion
   b. Presence of preterm birth
   c. Presence of mesenteric venous thrombosis
   d. Progressively worsening renal failure may be due to thrombotic microangiopathy.

7. Following types of renal involvement occur in primary antiphospholipid syndrome:
   a. Thrombotic microangiopathy
   b. Membranous nephropathy
   c. Minimal change nephropathy
   d. Pauci-immune glomerulonephritis

8. Guidelines recommended for the screening of lupus anticoagulant with ≥2 phospholipid-dependent coagulation assays are:
   a. Activated partial thromboplastin time
   b. Dilute Russell's viper venom time
   c. Kaolin/silica clotting time

9. Treatments of choice are:
   a. Low molecular weight heparin is preferred over conventional heparin.
   b. In case of pregnancy, heparin should be given as it will cross the placenta.
   c. Pulse dose of steroid
   d. Plasmapheresis to remove the antibodies
   e. Intravenous immunoglobulin
   f. Rituximab or eculizumab

CASE 39

A 34-year-old lady having past history of eclampsia delivering male baby at 36 weeks of gestation admitted this time at 28th weeks of gestation with severe diarrhea, vomiting, and abdominal pain for 2 days. There was family history of pregnancy-induced hypertension.

On examination, the blood pressure was 185/105 mm Hg. Ultrasound demonstrated abruption of placenta, and the patient delivered stillbirth baby following spontaneous membrane rupture. Prior to expulsion of the baby patient also developed generalized seizures and diminished urination which progressed toward anuria. Laboratory investigation demonstrated dropping of hemoglobin from 13 to 8 g/dL with fragmented red blood cells in the peripheral blood, dropping of platelet count from 160,000 to 55,000/cc, and rise in creatinine from 1.5 to 6.5 mg/dL. Serum haptoglobin low and lactate dehydrogenase 5,400 IU/L and rise in SGPT from 49 to 641 IU/L.

1. **What is the most likely diagnosis?**
2. **What are the changes in kidney occurring during pregnancy?**
3. **What is preeclampsia?**
4. **Mention the causes of acute kidney injury in case of pregnancy.**
5. **What are the risk factors in preeclampsia?**
6. **What type of anemia occurred in this case?**
7. **What are the pathophysiologic mechanisms in this case?**

Answers

1. Patient has been suffering from acute kidney injury complicated by hyperkalemia due to pregnancy-induced eclampsia along with thrombotic microangiopathy.

2. Following changes occur in the pregnancy:
   a. Size of the kidney:
      - Length of the kidney will be increased by 1–1.5 cm.
      - Volume of the kidney will be increased by 30%.
   b. Hydronephrotic changes in the kidney: It is characterized by dilatation of the kidney in >85% of the pregnant woman.
   c. Blood flow in the kidney will be increased by 80% from the baseline.
   d. Glomerular filtration rate will be increased to 150–200 mL/min
   e. Due to increased flow of urine, serum creatinine will be decreased to 0.4–0.5 mg/dL.
   f. Due to increased excretion of uric acids, level of uric acid falls to 2 mg/dL.
   g. Due to dilution of the urine, its osmolarity will be reduced to 260 mOsmol/kg.
   h. Due to increased excretion of sodium through the urine, there may be mild hyponatremia.
   i. Due to hyperventilation, there is respiratory alkalosis leading to decreased level of bicarbonate.

3. According to the American College of Obstetricians and Gynecologist 2013 guidelines, preeclampsia can be defined as newly diagnosed systolic blood pressure of ≥140 mm Hg or diastolic blood pressure of ≥90 mm Hg for at least two occasions at 4 hours apart after 20 weeks of gestation in previously normotensive individual or systolic and diastolic blood pressure of ≥160 and ≥110 mm Hg, respectively confirmed within short interval for facilitating timely antihypertensive medication.

Plus

Proteinuria in the form of spot urine protein/creatinine >0.3 mg/mg or >300 mg/day or, ++ on testing with dipstick

Or,

In absence of proteinuria, new-onset hypertension, following other features of like organ dysfunction:
   a. Platelet count <100,000/cc
   b. Renal dysfunction in the form of serum creatinine >1.1 mg/dL or doubling of the concentration of serum creatinine in absence of other kidney disease
   c. Appearance of pulmonary edema
   d. Persistent cerebral symptoms
   e. Persistent visual symptoms
   f. Impairment of liver function test in the form of increased serum SGPT at least twice the normal level.

4. Causes of acute renal injury in pregnancy are as follows:
   a. Obstetrical complications:
      - Septic abortion
      - Placenta previa

- Uterine hemorrhage
- Abruptio placentae
- Puerperal sepsis
- Intrauterine fetal death

b. Disorders related to pregnancy:
  - Acute fatty liver of pregnancy
  - Preeclampsia
  - Eclampsia
  - HELLP syndrome
  - Thrombotic microangiopathy
  - Hyperemesis gravidarum
  - Thrombotic thrombocytopenic purpura
  - Atypical hemolytic uremic syndrome

c. Causes not related to pregnancy:
  - Lupus nephritis
  - Dehydration
  - Acute postinfectious glomerulonephritis
  - Lupus nephritis

5. Risk factors of preeclampsia are as follows:
  a. Paternal obstetric factors:
     - Father born from preeclampsia
     - Family history of preeclampsia (fetal HLA variant)
  b. Maternal risk factors:
     - Molar pregnancy
     - Nulliparity
     - History of preeclampsia
     - Prior placental abruption
     - Artificial reproductive technology
     - Prior history of intrauterine growth retardation
     - Hydrops fetalis
     - Gestational diabetes
  c. Maternal comorbidities:
     - Chronic hypertension
     - Pregnancy-induced diabetes
     - Preexisting chronic kidney disease
     - Obesity
     - Antiphospholipid antibody syndrome
     - Polycystic ovarian syndrome

- SLE
- Age > 40 years

d. Maternal genetic factors:
  - Thrombophilia
  - Preeclampsia in case of first-degree relative

6. In this case, microangiopathic hemolytic anemia occurs.

7. Pathophysiology of kidney disease in this case:
  a. Incomplete remodeling of the uterine spiral arteries results in the ischemia in the placenta leading to production and release into circulation of:
     - Antiangiogenic factors in high amount
     - Soluble fms-like tyrosine kinase
     - Soluble endoglin
  b. At the same time, level of vascular endothelial growth factor and placental growth factors (PGFs) will be low.
  c. Soluble fms-like tyrosine kinase antagonizes the vascular endothelial growth factor and PGF

     As a result, there is diffuse renal vasoconstriction leading to glomerular endothelial damage.

     Preeclampsia is characterized by diffuse renal vasoconstriction, platelet activation, disseminated intravascular coagulation along with contraction of the maternal plasma volume.
  d. Abnormal placentation due to various genetic, immunologic, and various environmental factors is the fundamental cause leading to the development of preeclampsia. In case of normal healthy pregnancy, uterine spiral arteries lose their muscular layer leading to formation of the large capacitance of low-resistant vessels that invades the myometrium resulting in increased blood flow to the placenta. But in case of preeclampsia, total mechanism fails leading to decreased blood flow into the placenta resulting in placental hypoperfusion. As a result, widespread maternal vascular endothelial injury leading to increased capillary permeability occurs due to oxidative stress. This systemic vascular injury leads to maternal syndrome.

CASE 40

A 28-year-old female having history of lupus-induced stage 3 chronic kidney disease came to clinic with 12 weeks of pregnancy. She has complaint related to kidney disease.

On examination, her blood pressure was 140/80 mm Hg, pulse rate 90 beats/min, regular, and mild pallor only.

Laboratory examination demonstrated hemoglobin 10.5 g/dL, creatinine 2 mg/dL, electrolytes normal, and spot urine/creatinine ratio 0.6. Ultrasonography demonstrated increased echogenicity bilaterally in the kidney and antinuclear factor was negative. She has past history of intake steroid and rituximab for treating lupus nephritis and on antihypertensive drugs such as metoprolol and amlodipine.

1. **What is the most likely diagnosis?**
2. **What are the adverse effects of pregnancy in this patient?**
3. **What are the effects of pregnancy on chronic kidney disease?**
4. **What are the effects of kidney disease on pregnancy?**
5. **Why prepregnancy contraception is required in this patient?**
6. **What are the effects on neonates in pregnant patient with kidney disease?**
7. **What are the causes of adverse neonatal outcome in this patient?**
8. **What are the antenatal cares to be taken in this patient?**
9. **What are the infections may occur in this patient?**
10. **What are the factors that determine the timing of delivery in case of patient with chronic kidney disease?**
11. **What are the drugs that can be used safely in pregnancy?**

Answers

1. Most likely diagnosis is lupus-induced nephritis leading to stage 3 chronic kidney disease in a patient with first trimester of pregnancy.

2. Following are the adverse effects of pregnancy in patient with chronic kidney disease:
   a. Preeclampsia
   b. Intrauterine fetal growth retardation
   c. Preterm delivery
   d. Deterioration of maternal renal function

3. Pregnancy will hasten the condition of chronic kidney disease depending upon the following risk factors:
   a. Baseline glomerular filtration rate
   b. Proteinuria
   c. Hypertension

   Following are the effects on kidney disease:
   a. Proteinuria is increased.
   b. Worsening of hypertension
   c. Worsening of anemia
   d. Risk of preeclampsia will be increased.
   e. Worsening of renal function

4. Following are the effects of kidney disease on the pregnancy:
   a. Degree of function of the kidney determines the outcome in this patient.
   b. Inability to use ACEI and ARBs in this case
   c. Absence of hypertension decreases the incidence of poor outcome in this patient
   d. Proteinuria of >1 g/day and glomerular filtration rate of <40 mL/min are associated with poor outcome of mother and fetus.

5. Following contraception should be done in this patient:
   a. If patient is taking teratogenic medication.
   b. If patient is taking cytotoxic medication.
   c. Patients with active lupus nephritis
   d. In case of first year of renal transplantation

6. Following are the effects on neonatal outcome in pregnant patients with chronic kidney disease:
   a. Premature birth
   b. Small for gestational edge
   c. Neonatal mortality
   d. Stillbirth

7. Following are the causes of adverse neonatal outcome in pregnant patient with chronic kidney disease:
   a. Blood pressure of >140/90 mm Hg
   b. Effective glomerular filtration rate of <40 mL/m^2
   c. Nephrotic range of proteinuria
   d. Women with active kidney disease
   e. Women with lupus nephritis
   f. Female having renal transplant
   g. Past bad obstetric history

8. Following antenatal care should be taken in patient with chronic kidney disease:
   a. Patient should undergone trisomy screening.
   b. If patient is on teratogenic drug, she should be referred to fetal medicine department for detection of any fetal abnormalities.
   c. Patient should undergo scan for assessing the growth and wellbeing of the fetus in the third trimester.
   d. Disease activity of the parent SLE should be assessed.

e. Fasting glucose and glycosylated hemoglobin should be monitored in this patient if the patient is on steroid or calcineurin inhibitors.

f. If the patient has already received renal transplantation, she should be screened for dysfunction of the graft; in that case, dose of the Immunosuppressive drugs should be adjusted.

g. All the patients should receive standard vaccination.

9. Following types of infections occur in this patient:
   a. Urinary tract infection
   b. Viral infection such as *Cytomegalovirus* and herpes simplex

10. Following are the factors that determine the timing of delivery in patient with chronic kidney disease:
    a. Deterioration of renal function
    b. Symptomatic hypoalbuminemia
    c. Pulmonary edema
    d. Preeclampsia
    e. Refractory hypertension

11. Following medications are safely used in pregnancy:
    a. Low-dose aspirin
    b. Low molecular weight heparin
    c. Labetalol
    d. Nifedipine
    e. Methyldopa
    f. Hydralazine
    g. Prednisolone
    h. Cyclosporine
    i. Tacrolimus
    j. Azathioprine
    k. Hydroxychloroquine

CASE 41

A 60-year-old man having history of chronic kidney disease complained of low back pain and pain in the hip for >5 months. His creatinine was 5.8 mg/dL, blood urea 88 mg/dL, hemoglobin 8.5 g/dL, intact parathyroid hormone (PTH) 865 ng/mL, alkaline phosphatase 350 IU/L, vitamin D3 level 12 ng/mL, low-density lipoprotein (LDL) level 138 mg/dL, triglyceride 242 mg/dL, phosphate 6.5 mg/mL, calcium 8.5 mg/mL, and bicarbonate level 18 mEq/L. Ultrasonography demonstrated small kidney bilaterally. Patient's abdominal X-ray demonstrated aortic calcification. His X-ray of the shoulder and vertebra demonstrated:

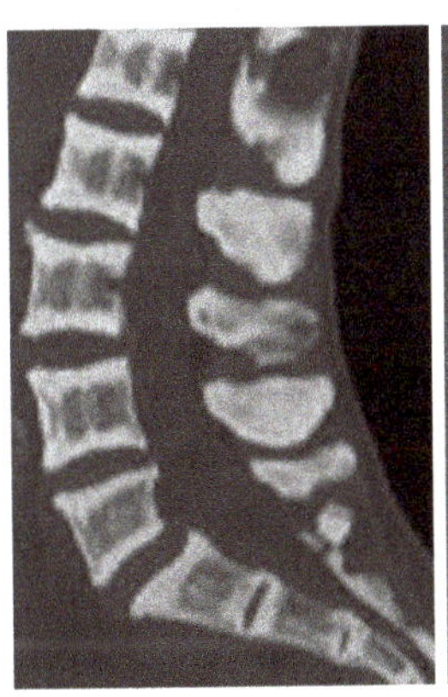
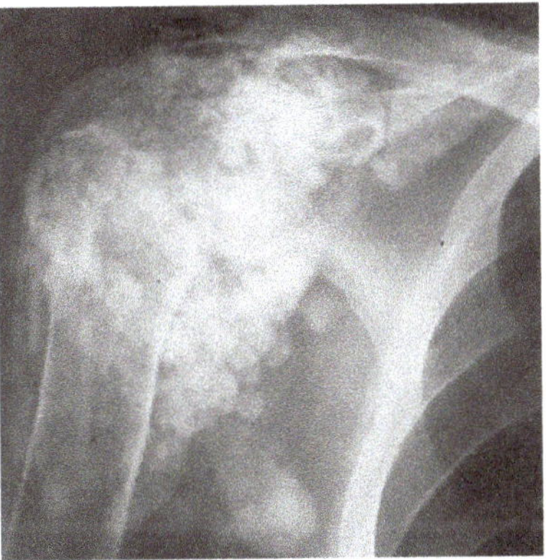

1. **What do the above pictures demonstrate?**
2. **What is your diagnosis?**
3. **Justify your diagnosis.**
4. **What is the cause of mineral bone disease in chronic kidney disease?**
5. **What are the risk factors of vascular calcification?**
6. **What is the pathology of vascular calcification?**
7. **What are the causes of hyperparathyroidism?**
8. **What are the causes of retention of phosphate?**
9. **In early stage of chronic kidney disease serum phosphate level will not be increased?**

10. **What are the pathogenic mechanisms for hyperphosphatemia-induced hyperparathyroidism?**
11. **What are the causes of low calcitriol in chronic kidney disease?**
12. **What are the causes of hypocalcemia in chronic kidney disease?**
13. **What is the gold standard method of diagnosis of the above bone disease in chronic kidney disease?**
14. **What are the types of bone disorders occuring in chronic kidney disease?**
15. **How the different types of mineral bone disease can be differentiated?**

Answers

1. Above pictures demonstrate:
   a. Presence of sclerotic band on the superior and inferior end plates of the vertebral bodies — it represents excess accumulation of osteoid tissue. It appears opaque because of its increased volume as compared to normal bone.
   b. Ectopic calcification in the muscles and subcutaneous tissue in the right shoulder girdle

2. The most likely diagnosis is stage 5 chronic kidney disease with mineral bone disease in the form of Rugger–Jersey spine and ectopic calcification in the right shoulder girdle.

3. Points in favor of this diagnosis are as follows:
   a. Effective glomerular filtration rate is:
      - According to CLD-EPI, 11 mL/min/m^2
      - According to Modification of Diet in Renal Disease (MDRD) equation, 12 mL/min/m^2
   b. Ultrasonography demonstrated bilateral small kidney
   c. Serum phosphate level is high.
   d. Serum calcium level is low.
   e. Serum intact parathormone level is high.
   f. Vitamin D deficiency level is low.
   g. Features of mineral bone disease

4. The most important cause is hyperparathyroidism leading to:
   a. Hyperphosphatemia
   b. Hypocalcemia
   c. Low 1,25-dihydroxyvitamin D
   d. High level of fibroblastic growth factor 23 (FGF23)
   e. Acidosis

5. Following are the risk factors of vascular calcification:
   a. Uremia
   b. Increased product of calcium and phosphate
   c. Increased parathormone level
   d. Caucasian race
   e. Use of warfarin in the dialysis
   f. Deficiency of protein C and S
   g. Diabetes mellitus
   h. Malnutrition

6. Uremic calcific arteriopathy is a small vessel vasculopathy due to mural calcification, intimal proliferation, fibrosis and thrombosis involving vessels of the skin, soft tissue, and visceral organ.

7. Following are the causes of hyperparathyroidism:
   a. Retention of phosphate
   b. Serum free ionized calcium concentration is decreased.
   c. Decreased 1, 25-vitamin D3 (calcitriol)
   d. Increased level of FGF23
   e. Following changes occur in the parathyroid gland:
      - Decreased vitamin D receptors
      - Decreased calcium sensing receptors
      - Decreased fibroblast growth factor receptors
      - Decreased klotho in the gland

8. Following are the causes of retention of phosphate:
   a. Hypocalcemia
   b. Increased expression of parathormone gene
   c. Decreased formation or decreased activity of calcitriol

9. In early chronic kidney disease, there is reduced reabsorption of phosphate from the renal tubule mediated by increased level of serum PTH and FG23 resulting increased excretion of phosphate through the urine.

10. Following are the pathogenic mechanisms of hyperphosphatemia-induced hyperparathyroidism:
    a. Decreased level of serum calcium
    b. Decreased formation or decreased activity of calcitriol
    c. Directly through the reduction of PTH: Messenger RNA concentration via increasing the stability of posttranscriptional PTH messenger RNA.
    d. Stimulation of FGF23 secretion that will suppress the parathormone.

11. Following are the causes of low calcitriol in chronic kidney disease:
    a. Reduced renal mass
    b. Increased serum level of phosphate
    c. Increased concentration of FGF23
    d. Retention of phosphate leading to suppression of 1α-hydroxylase

12. Following are the causes of hypocalcemia in chronic kidney disease:
    a. Retention of phosphate
    b. Decreased concentration of calcitriol
    c. Resistance to calcemic action of parathormone on the bone as concentration of the serum parathormone is inversely proportional to serum level of calcium.
13. Gold standard method of the diagnosis as well as classification of the mineral bone disease in chronic kidney disease is bone biopsy which can be taken from the iliac crest after administering two tetracycline markers separated by 21 days.
14. There are three types of mineral bone disease:
    a. Increased bone turnover due to secondary hyperparathyroidism
    b. Adynamic bone disease due to disorders affecting bone volume which includes osteoporosis and osteopenia
    c. Mineralization due to defective bone mineralization leading to development of osteomalacia
15. Goldner–Masson trichrome staining can differentiate mineralized lamellar bone and osteoid which is nonmineralized. Osteoid nonmineralized tissue stains red brown with this stain and mineralized lamellar bone stains blue and can be seen under light microscopy.

CASE 42

A 60-year-old diabetic and hypertensive male having no past history of kidney disease admitted with chest pain, respiratory distress, and diagnosed as acute myocardial infarction. Primary angioplasty was performed. Laboratory investigation prior to angioplasty demonstrated creatinine 1.4 mg/dL and urea 65 mg/dL. Within 1 day after this angioplasty patient though nonoliguric but rising creatinine to 4.8 mg/dL. Patient was treated conservatively with proper hydration and creatinine decreased to 1.6 mg/dL.

1. **What is the most probable diagnosis?**
2. **Define this disease.**
3. **What are the mechanisms of this disease?**
4. **What are the risk factors associated with this disease?**
5. **What is the risk scoring system in this disease?**

Answers

1. The most probable diagnosis is contrast-induced nephropathy.
2. Contrast-induced nephropathy can be defined as impaired renal function that is measured as either 25% increase in serum creatinine from the base line or 0.5 mg/dL increase in the absolute value of creatinine within 2–3 days after the administration of intravenous contrast.
3. There are two mechanisms in this contrast-induced nephropathy:
    a. Direct mechanism: It is defined as direct injury to the tubular epithelium leading to loss of function of the tubular cells, apoptosis, and ultimately necrosis.
       - Early in this case, Na^+/K^+-ATPase will be redistributed from the basolateral membrane to the luminal surface leading to abnormal transport of ion across the cells and increased delivery of the sodium to the distal tubule. This will lead to renal vasoconstriction through tubuloglomerular feedback.
       - With the progression of the disease, tubular cells will be damaged and detached from the basement membranes leading to luminal obstruction resulting in increased intratubular pressure which ultimately decreases the glomerular filtration rate.
    b. Indirect mechanism:
       - Local release of endothelin, nitric oxide, and prostaglandin produce vasoconstriction leading to decrease in the flow of blood through the glomerulus resulting in ischemic injury to the tubular cells.
       - Increased blood viscosity further reduces the microcirculatory flow and alters the

plasma osmolarity which leads to impairment of the deformability of the red blood cells—it results microvascular stasis leading to thrombosis.

4. Following are the risk factors associated with this disease:
   a. Type of contrast material: High osmolarity contrast material is associated with this disease whereas low osmolarity agent reduces the risk of this nephropathy.
   b. Amount of contrast material: High volume of >350 mL or >4 mg/kg or repeated administration of the contrast material within 3 days is associated with increased risk of this nephropathy.
   c. Preexisting chronic renal disease
   d. Indications for the use of contrast: Risk increases with types of clinical presentation. Following clinical presentations are associated with increased risk of contrast-induced nephropathy:
      - Acute myocardial infarction
      - Shock with hemodynamic instability
      - Coronary artery bypass grafting
      - Valve replacement
      - Age > 75 years
      - Anemia
      - Diabetes mellitus
      - Creatinine level is >1.5 mg/dL.
      - Congestive heart failure

5. Roxana Mehran scoring system for prediction of contrast-induced nephropathy:

Risk factors	Score
Hypotension	5
Advanced congestive heart failure	5
Impaired renal function	
Serum creatinine > 1.5 mg/dL	4
Or	
Effective glomerular filtration rate	
40–60 mL/min/m^2	2
20–40 mL/min/m^2	4
<20 mL/min/m^2	6
Age > 75 years	4
Anemia	3
Diabetes	3
Volume of contrast media per 100 mL	1
Elective use of intra-aortic balloon pump	5
Risk stratification: Scores 0–5: 7.5% Scores 6–10: 14% Scores 11–16: 26.1% Scores >16: 57.3%	

CASE 43

A 45-year-old male having history of stage 5 chronic kidney disease with history of hypertension and diabetes for 12 years on continuous ambulatory peritoneal dialysis (CAPD) came to nephrology clinic with abdominal pain, fever, and coming out turbid fluid for 4 days. Peritoneal fluid demonstrated turbid fluid and white blood cell count of 600/cc with neutrophils 75%. He was treated with intraperitoneal vancomycin and intravenous ceftazidime.

1. **What is the diagnosis?**
2. **How can you prevent this type of infection?**
3. **Mention the risk factors for this type of peritonitis.**
4. **What are the criteria of diagnosing this infection?**
5. **What are the common antibiotics to be given in this peritoneal infection?**
6. **What are the different types of this peritoneal infection?**
7. **What are the indications of removal of catheter?**
8. **What type of tube is recommended for preventing this infection?**

Answers

1. The most likely diagnosis is CAPD-induced peritonitis.
2. Following are the procedure to prevent CAPD-induced peritonitis:
   a. Proper hand hygiene
   b. Exit site should be clean by antibiotic ointment.
   c. Prompt treatment of the exit site infection
3. Following are the risk factors for peritoneal dialysis-induced peritonitis:
   a. Social smoking
   b. Presence of pets
   c. Obesity
   d. Hypokalemia
   e. Depression
   f. Hypoalbuminemia
   g. Gynecological intervention
   h. Colonoscopy
   i. Prior hemodialysis
   j. Peritoneal dialysis against choice of the patient
   k. Infusion of contaminated peritoneal fluid
   l. Carrier state of staphylococcal infection
   m. Exit site of infection
4. Following are the criteria of peritoneal dialysis-induced peritonitis:
   a. Clinical features consisting with the features of peritonitis, like:
      - Fever
      - Abdominal pain
      - Peritoneal fluid becomes cloud.
   b. White blood cell count in the peritoneal fluid of >100/cc
   c. >50% is polymorphonuclear neutrophils.
   d. Positive culture in the effluent fluid
5. Common antibiotics to be given in this CAPD-induced peritonitis:
   a. Empiric antibiotic should cover both gram-positive and gram-negative antibiotics.
   b. Choice of antibiotics:
      - Vancomycin or first-generation cephalosporin
      - Third-generation cephalosporin or aminoglycoside for gram-negative antibiotics
   c. Choice of route should be intraperitoneal method unless there is sepsis. Vancomycin should be instilled intraperitoneally once daily 3–5 days to maintain the serum level of this drug at above 15 µg/cc.
   d. Dose should be intermittent.
   e. Antibiotic-containing fluid should be dwelled for at least 6 hours for proper action.
6. Following are the different types of intraperitoneal infection:
   a. Recurrent peritonitis: This is described as an episode occurring within 4 weeks of the completion of therapy of a prior episode but with the different organism.
   b. Relapsing peritonitis: This is described as an episode occurring within 4 weeks of the completion of therapy of a prior episode but with the same organism.
   c. Repeat peritonitis: This is described as an episode occurring >4 weeks after the completion of therapy of a prior episode but with the same organism.
   d. Refractory peritonitis: This can be defined as failure of the effluent to clear after 5 days administration of the antibiotics.
   e. Catheter-related peritonitis: This can be defined as incidence of peritonitis in conjunction with the exit site of infection.
   f. Tunnel infection: This is characterized by the presence of the inflammation and/or ultrasonographic evidence of collection along the catheter tunnel.
7. Following are the indications of catheter removal:
   a. Refractory peritonitis
   b. Fungal peritonitis
   c. Relapsing peritonitis
   d. Repeat peritonitis
   e. Infection at the tunnel site
   f. Refractory exit site infection
   g. Mycobacterial peritonitis
   h. Polymicrobial infection
8. Y connection system is recommended because of the flush before fill design in case of CAPD.

CASE 44

A 70-year-old man having history of type 2 diabetes mellitus for 15 years came to medical department with progressive weakness, easy fatigability, and bilateral lower limb swelling for 1 month. 3 years back his creatinine level was 0.9 mg/dL and albumin-creatinine ratio (ACR) 190 mg/g. During recent examination, his blood pressure was 160/105 mm Hg, serum creatinine 4.2 mg/dL, urine volume 600 mL/day, urine ACR 550 mg/g, serum potassium 5 mEq/L, HbA1c 8%, and absence of urinary sediment. His fundoscopy demonstrated:

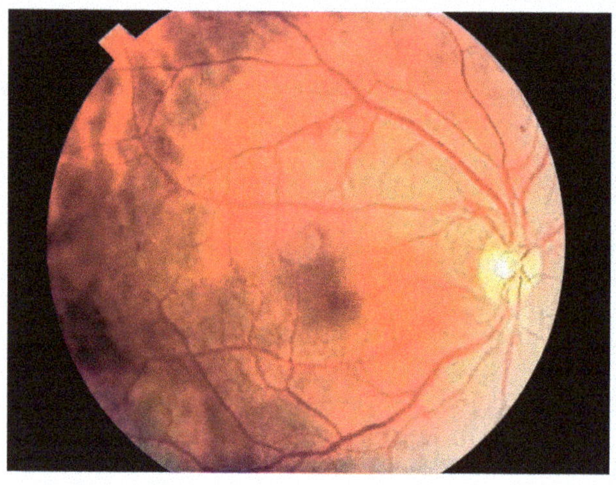 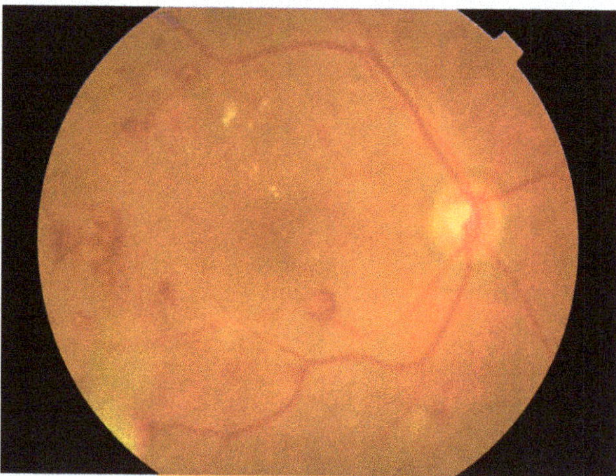

1. **What is the description of the above pictures?**
2. **What are the different types of retinal involvement in this disease?**
3. **What is the diagnosis in this case?**
4. **What are the stages of this disease?**
5. **What are the risk factors in this disease?**
6. **What are the histopathological stages in this disease?**
7. **What are the relations between the eye and kidney involvement in this disease?**
8. **What are the screening to be done in this patient?**
9. **What are the clues for diagnosis of nondiabetic kidney disease?**
10. **What are the indications of renal biopsy in diabetic nephropathy?**
11. **What are the oral antidiabetic drugs which are contraindicated in this disease?**
12. **What is the goal of low-density lipoprotein in this patient?**
13. **What are the dietary restrictions to be done in this case?**
14. **What are the strategies to be taken to retard the disease progression?**
15. **What are the special problems can be faced relating to vascular access in this patient?**

Answers

1. Above pictures demonstrate:
   a. Left picture demonstrates multiple microaneurysms
   b. Right one demonstrates neovascularization, macular edema, and hemorrhage.
2. There are two types of retinal involvement in diabetes:
   a. Nonproliferative retinopathy:
      - Mild: Presence of at least of one microaneurysm
      - Moderate: Presence of—
        - Microaneurysm
        - Hemorrhage
        - Hard exudates
      - Severe: Presence of—
        - Hemorrhage and microaneurysm in the four quadrants
        - Venous beading at least two quadrants
        - Intrarenal microvascular abnormalities in one quadrant.

b. Proliferative retinopathy:
- Hallmark of proliferative retinopathy is neovascularization.
- Preretinal hemorrhage: It is characterized by pockets of blood in-between retina and posterior hyaloid space. Here hemorrhage looks like boat shaped.
- Vitreous hemorrhage: It is characterized by clumps of blood within the gel.
- Proliferation of the fibrovascular tissue: This area appears avascular when the vessels are regressed.
- Tractional detachment of retina: Retina looks like tented up, immobile, and concave
- Presence of macular edema

3. Patient has been suffering from diabetic nephropathy along with diabetic retinopathy.

4. There are five stages of diabetic nephropathy:
   a. Stage 1: It is characterized by hyperfunction of the kidney as evidenced by:
      - Hyperfiltration
      - Increased size of the kidney by 20%
      - Renal plasma flow will be increased by 10–15%.
      - Absence of albuminuria
      - Normal blood pressure
   b. Stage 2: Early histological changes, but clinically silent.
   c. Stage 3: Incipient diabetic retinopathy—in this stage, presence of microalbuminuria and blood pressure starts rising.
   d. Stage 4: Overt diabetic nephropathy—it is characterized by persistent proteinuria of >0.5 g/day, declining in the renal function, and rise in blood pressure.
   e. Stage 5: It is end-stage renal failure.

5. Following are the risk factors in this case:
   a. Genetic susceptibility: Its incidence is increased in the patients with diabetic sibling.
   b. High blood pressure
   c. Glycemic control: This nephropathy occurs in patients with poor diabetic control.
   d. Race: Its incidence associated with type 2 diabetes mellitu will be three- to five-fold increase in:
      - Black as compared to Caucasians
      - Pima Indians
      - Mexican Americans

e. Obesity: High body mass index is vulnerable to develop diabetic nephropathy.
f. Smoking: It is associated with following adverse effects in diabetic patients:
   - Increase in the albuminuria
   - Risk of end-stage renal failure
   - After starting the dialysis, survival will be decreased.
g. Dyslipidemia
h. Insulin resistance
i. High dietary intake of protein
j. Preeclampsia
k. Periodontal disease

6. Following are the histopathological stages in this disease:
   a. Thickening of the basement membrane: It is the earliest change.
   b. Loss of negatively charged filtration material heparan sulfate from the glomerular basement membrane resulting in increased filtration of negatively charged albumin
   c. Expansion of mesangium due to accumulation of extracellular matrix correlating with the clinical manifestations
   d. Development of eosinophilic PAS-positive nodules known as nodular glomerular sclerosis. The name of the nodule is Kimmelstiel–Wilson nodules.
   e. Deposition of IgG or complement: It is seen by immunofluorescence microscopy.
   f. Prominent vascular changes characterized by hyaline and hypersensitive arteriosclerosis

7. Relations between diabetic nephropathy and diabetic retinopathy are as follows:
   a. In case of type 1 diabetes mellitus, patient with nephropathy almost always developed microvascular disease like retinopathy.
   b. In case of type 2 diabetes mellitus, 50–65% patients with diabetic nephropathy developed retinopathy.

8. Following screening should be done for the diagnosis:
   a. Fasting and postprandial glucose
   b. Glycosylated hemoglobin
   c. Urine albumin excretion:
      - In case of type 1 diabetes mellitus, if the diabetes is >5 years.
      - In case of type 2 diabetes mellitus, at the onset of diagnosis of diabetes mellitus

   d. Annual estimation of glomerular rate

   e. Annual estimation of serum creatinine

   f. Macroscopic and microscopic analysis of urine

   g. Annual fundoscopic examination

   h. Ultrasonographic examination of the kidney size along with the examination of the patency of the renal arteries

   i. Bimonthly measurement of the blood pressure

9. Following are the clues to the diagnosis of nondiabetic kidney disease:

   a. Absence of diabetic retinopathy

   b. In case of type 1 diabetes mellitus, duration of diabetes is <5 years.

   c. Sudden and rapid onset proteinuria

   d. Sudden development of nephrotic syndrome without antecedent microalbuminuria

   e. Presence of active sediments of red blood cell cast, WBC casts, and dysmorphic red blood cell

   f. Presence of other systemic disease

   g. Rapid decline in renal function whereas in case of diabetic nephropathy, decline in the renal function by 0.5–1.5 mL/min/m^2

10. Following are the indications of renal biopsy in case of diabetic nephropathy:

   a. Presence of retinopathy

   b. Presence of urinary sediments in urine microscopy like dysmorphic red blood cell, red blood cell cast, and WBC cast

   c. Rapidly increasing proteinuria

   d. Symptoms suggestive of multisystem disorders

11. Following oral antidiabetic drugs are contraindicated in this disease:

   a. Metformin: It is contraindicated if the effective glomerular filtration rate is <30 mL/min/m^2.

   b. Sodium-glucose cotransporter-2 (SGLT-2) inhibitor is contraindicated if the effective glomerular filtration rate is <45 mL/min/m^2.

   c. Thiazolidinediones: As it causes retention fluid leading to heart failure, hence in patients with chronic kidney disease, it should not be given. Again, there is risk of fracture in chronic kidney disease; hence, it should not be given.

   d. Glucagon-like peptide-1 (GLP-1) receptor antagonist should not be given if effective glomerular filtration rate is <30 mL/min/m^2.

   e. α-glucosidase inhibitors are contraindicated if serum creatinine level is >2 mg/dL.

12. Goal of low-density lipoprotein cholesterol in diabetic patient:

   a. <100 mg/dL, in case of diabetic patients in general

   b. <70 mg/dL, in case of diabetic patients with cardiovascular disease

13. Following are the dietary restrictions in diabetic nephropathy:

   a. In the early stage of diabetic nephropathy, protein restriction is 0.8–1 g/kg/day of body weight

   b. In the late stage of diabetic nephropathy, protein restriction is 0.8 g/kg/day.

   c. Low sodium diet—2.3 g/day or 100 mEq/day

14. The strategies to be taken to retard the disease progression of this disease:

   a. Maintain the HbA1c to <7%

   b. Blood pressure control:

     • It should be maintained below 140/90 mm Hg if there is <1 g/day proteinuria.

     • It should be maintained at below 130/80 mm Hg if proteinuria is >1 g/day.

     • Smoking should be avoided.

     • Serum cholesterol should be maintained below 170 mg/dL.

     • Body weight should be reduced according to race, sex, and age.

     • Daily aerobic exercise for 30 minutes for at least 4 days per week

     • In case of albuminuria, ARBs should be administered

     • Animal protein intake should be restricted.

15. Following special problems can be faced relating to vascular access in this patient:

   a. In diabetic patient, there is higher incidence of failure of arteriovenous fistula

   b. Longevity of the fistula will be less.

   c. Infection is very high.

   d. Maturation time of the fistula will be very high.

   e. There is chance of secondary failure of the fistula.

   f. Digital ischemia is due to steal phenomenon.

CASE 45

A 72-year-old nonhypertensive man having history of diabetes for 10 years came to routine checkup where he was diagnosed as hypertensive. His blood pressure was 185/105 mm Hg and peripheral pulses. Cardiovascular and respiratory systemic examinations were normal. Laboratory examination demonstrated urea 60 mg/dL and creatinine 1.8 mg/dL. Ultrasound demonstrated bilateral echogenicity in both the kidneys and slow flow pattern in the renal arteries. In spite of administration of three antihypertensive drugs, blood pressure was not controlled and again came to emergency department with respiratory distress. On auscultation, there was presence of fine crepitation in both lung bases.

1. **What is the most likely diagnosis?**
2. **What is the definition of renovascular hypertension?**
3. **What amount of stenosis is required to develop renovascular hypertension?**
4. **What are the points of suspicion for renovascular hypertension?**
5. **What are the roles of vasoactive factors in this disease?**
6. **What are the features of significant renal artery stenosis?**
7. **How can it be diagnosed captopril renogram?**

Answers

1. The most likely diagnosis is the patient suffering from resistant hypertension due to renovascular cause with type 2 diabetes mellitus.
2. Definition of renovascular hypertension: It is secondary hypertension due to decreased renal perfusion in presence of high blood pressure when the occlusion of luminal diameter will be 70–80%.
3. As 50–60% occlusion of the renal arteries can maintain the parenchymal blood flow, so at least 70–80% of luminal narrowing to produce ischemia in the renal tissue.
4. Following are the points of suspicion of renovascular hypertension:
   a. Presence of atherosclerosis in the vessels
   b. Diastolic bruit in the abdomen
   c. Onset of hypertension in patient of <30 years old or >55 years old
   d. Sudden deterioration of the previously controlled hypertension
   e. Unilateral small-sized kidney and the difference in the size of both the kidneys are >1.5 cm.
   f. Sudden increase in the blood pressure in spite of taking three antihypertensive drugs
   g. Presence of recurrent pulmonary edema
   h. Presence of severe hypertensive retinopathy
   i. Inhibition of reticuloendothelial system leads to deterioration of the renal function
5. Following are the vasoactive factors involved in this disease:
   a. Increased concentration of nitric oxide in the poststenotic segment of the renal artery due to decreased renal perfusion—it has vasodilatory action.
   b. Increased production of endothelin peptides produced by the vascular endothelial cells and renal epithelial cells as a result of upgradation of transforming growth factor-beta (TGF-β), interleukin-1, and tumor growth factor.
   c. Increased production of prostacycline and prostaglandin-E2 due to tissue hypoperfusion—these are renoprotective.
   d. Thromboxane-A2 decreases glomerular filtration rate by decreasing the renal blood flow, it also modulates the vascular permeability.
   e. Antithrombin-II: It has hemodynamic properties.
6. Following features are suggestive of significant renal artery stenosis:
   a. Elevated peak systolic velocities: Velocities in the stenotic segment >1.8–2 m/s—correlate with >60% reduction of the vessel diameter.
   b. Renal artery/aorta ratio: If it is >3.5, it indicates >60% stenosis of the renal artery.
   c. Acceleration time: If it is >0.07 seconds, it correlates with >60% stenosis in the renal artery.
   d. Loss of early systolic peak: In case of proximal stenosis, changes in the intrarenal waveform along with loss of early systolic peak—demonstrating "tardus parvus" appearance.
7. Captopril renogram can differentiate the function of both kidneys one having normal and other having stenotic renal artery.

   Captopril is an ACEI. After hour of oral intake of 25–50 mg of captopril, radioisotope was injected.
   a. If there is decline of glomerular filtration rate, it indicates that kidney has stenotic renal artery.
   b. If there is increase in the glomerular filtration rate, it indicates normal renal artery.

CASE 46

A 62-year-old man having history of type 2 diabetes mellitus for 10 years and hypertension for 8 years on five antihypertensive drugs having family history of both hypertension and diabetes came to outdoor with progressively increasing fatigue, swelling of the both legs, and occasional chest pain.

On examination, blood pressure was 170/105 mm Hg in right hand and 165/100 mm Hg in left hand, no orthostatic hypotension, and body mass index 30 kg/m^2.

Laboratory investigation demonstrated liver function test and serum electrolytes were within normal limit, only serum creatinine was 2.5 mg/dL, and urea was 55 mg/dL. Ultrasonography of abdomen was normal.

1. **What is the most likely diagnosis?**
2. **What is the definition of this disease?**
3. **What the fundoscopic finding in this case?**
4. **What are the drugs responsible for this disease?**
5. **What are the investigations should be done to exclude the secondary causes?**
6. **What is the lifestyle modification should be done for controlling blood pressure?**
7. **What should be instructed in this patient to prevent renal dysfunction?**

Answers

1. This patient has been suffering from resistant hypertension with renal dysfunction in the background of long-standing type 2 diabetes mellitus and long-standing hypertension on four antihypertensive drugs.

2. Definition of the resistant hypertension:
   a. Resistant hypertension: If the patient is on three antihypertensive drugs at optimum doses with complementary mechanism of action but cannot achieve control of blood pressure or
   b. Blood pressure control can be achieved by ≥4 antihypertensive medications.
   c. Controlled resistant hypertension: Blood pressure controlled to the patient's individualized target while receiving the treatment with ≥4 antihypertensive drugs including one diuretic with maximum optimal dose without any intolerable side effects.
   d. Uncontrolled resistant hypertension: It can be defined as failure to achieve control blood pressure in spite of taking four antihypertensive drugs including a diuretic.
   e. Refractory hypertension: It can be defined as blood pressure of >140/90 mm Hg despite the use of ≥5 antihypertensive drugs including a diuretic and one mineralocorticoid antagonist at optimal dose.

3. Fundoscopic findings in this case are as follows:
   a. Arteriovenous crossing changes:
      - Salus's sign: Deflection of the retinal vein as it will cross the arteriole.
      - Gunn's sign: Tapering of retinal vein on either side of the arteriovenous crossings
      - Bonnet's sign: It is characterized by banking of retinal vein distal to arteriovenous crossing.
   b. Arterial changes:
      - Decrease in the arteriovenous ratio to 1:3 whereas normal ratio is 2:3.
      - Changes in the arteriolar light reflex: Here, light reflex appears as copper and/or silver wiring
   c. Retinal changes:
      - Retinal hemorrhages:
         ○ Dot-blot hemorrhages: It is characterized by bleeding in the inner retinal layer.
         ○ Flame-shaped hemorrhage: It is characterized by bleeding in the superficial retinal layer.
      - Retinal exudate:
         ○ Hard exudates: It is characterized by deposits of lipid in the retina.
         ○ Soft exudate: It is characterized by cotton-wool spots appearing due to ischemia of the nerve fibers.
   d. Macular changes: It is characterized by macular star formation due to deposition of hard exudates around the macula.
   e. Optic nerve swelling: There is swelling of the optic disk.

4. Following drugs are responsible for this disease:
   a. Anabolic steroids
   b. Glucocorticoids
   c. NSAIDs

d. Sympathomimetic

e. Erythropoietin

f. Antidepressants

g. Calcineurin inhibitors

h. Inhibitors of vascular endothelial growth factor

i. Tyrosine kinase inhibitors

j. Amphetamines

k. Cocaine

l. Anabolic steroids

m. Caffeine

5. Following investigations should be done to exclude secondary hypertension:

Causes of secondary hypertension	Investigations
• Renal artery stenosis • Atherosclerotic stenosis	• Ultrasound of abdomen • Duplex Doppler ultrasound • MRI • CT scan • Conventional angiography
Cushing syndrome	• Dexamethasone suppression test • Estimation of excretion of 4 hours urine cortisol • Measurement of salivary cortisol
Obstructive sleep apnea	• Berlin questionnaire • Overnight oximetry • Polysomnography
• Primary aldosteronism • Secondary hyperaldosteronism	• Estimation of serum sodium and potassium • Serum aldosterone concentration to plasma renin activity ratio • Response of blood pressure to mineralocorticoid receptor antagonist • Genetic testing • Contrast-enhanced CT scan of the adrenal gland • Adrenal gland venous sampling
Congenital adrenal hyperplasia	• Clinical studies • Hormonal studies
• Gordon syndrome • Liddle syndrome • Apparent excess of mineralocorticoids	• Clinical diagnosis • Low level of serum aldosterone and renin • Serum electrolytes
Pheochromocytoma	• Measurement of plasma free metanephrines • Estimation of 24 hours urine metanephrines and catecholamines
Hyperthyroidism	Thyroid-stimulating hormone

Continued

Continued

Causes of secondary hypertension	Investigations
Coarctation of aorta	• Echocardiogram • Clinical diagnosis • Thoracic MR angiography
Acromegaly	• Clinical diagnosis • MRI scan of the pituitary gland

6. Lifestyle modification for controlling the blood pressure:

Modification of dietary factors	Description	Systolic blood pressure reduction
Reduction of weight	BMI is ≤25	5–20 mm Hg/ 10 kg reduction of weight
DASH diet (dietary approaches to stop hypertension)	Enriched with: • Fruits • Vegetables • Reduction of saturated and total fat • Low fat dairy • Low intake of sodium	8–15 mm Hg
Low intake of dietary sodium	3.8–6 g daily	2–8 mm Hg
Increased physical activity	Daily 30 minutes aerobic exercise	4–10 mm Hg
Increased intake of potassium	4.7 g daily	Variable
Moderate intake of alcohol	• Less than two drinks daily for men • Less than one drink daily in women	2–4 mm Hg
Others	Yoga, meditation, acupuncture	2–10 mm Hg

7. Following instructions should be given to the patient:

a. Lifestyle modification:

- Low-salt diet
- Exercise
- Reduction of weight
- Water restriction

b. Medications:

- Oral furosemide 40 mg twice daily to reduce the body weight by 4–5 kg
- Clonidine 0.1 g thrice daily to maintain the blood pressure 130/75 mm Hg
- Other drugs can be added:
  ○ Alpha-blocker: Prazosin
  ○ Vasodilator: Hydralazine
  ○ Mineralocorticoid antagonist: Spirono-lactone

CASE 47

A 40-year-old nondiabetic and nonhypertensive man came to emergency with the complaints of high-grade fever, nausea, vomiting, arthralgia, headache, oliguria, and yellowish discoloration of urine for 2 days. On examination, there was jaundice, orientation normal, blood pressure 110/65 mm Hg, tachypnea, and temperature 102°F. Chest auscultation demonstrated crackles. In abdomen, there was no organomegaly. Laboratory examination revealed hemoglobin 10 g/dL, white blood cell count 17,000/cc, blood urea 120 mg/dL, creatinine 4 mg/dL, sodium 125 mEq/L, bicarbonate 20 mEq/L, bilirubin 9 mg/dL, SGPT 120 IU/L, and SGOT 100 IU/L.

Axilla demonstrated the following feature:

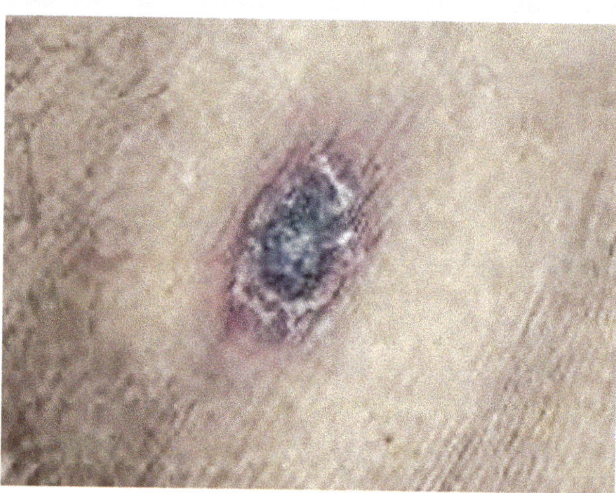

1. **Describe the above skin lesion.**
2. **What is the most likely diagnosis?**
3. **What are the clues to the diagnosis?**
4. **What is the etiology of this diagnosis?**
5. **What is the incubation period?**
6. **Describe the typical rash in this case.**
7. **Are there any biomarkers that help in the prognosis of this kidney involvement?**
8. **How the diagnosis will be confirmed?**
9. **Provide the calculation of fluid overload-adjusted creatinine.**
10. **Does the patient require dialysis?**
11. **What are the diseases producing jaundice with acute kidney injury?**

Answers

1. The above picture demonstrates large ulcerated lesion in the right axilla covered with the exudates.
2. The most likely diagnosis is this patient has been suffering from acute kidney injury with volume overload, with hepatitis due to infection with scrub typhus.
3. Following are the clues to the diagnosis:
   a. Presence of ulcerated eschar in the axilla
   b. Presence of jaundice
   c. Oliguria
   d. Fever
4. The etiology is scrub typhus caused by *Orientia tsutsugamushi*, a coccobacillus. It is distinct from *Rickettsia* antigenically.
5. The incubation period is 7–10 days.
6. Bite mark "eschar" occurs at the site of chigger feeding appearing as ulcer that enlarges, ulcerates and ultimately undergoes necrosis leading to formation of black crust. Common sites are:
   a. Neck
   b. Axillary region
   c. Infra-axillary region
   d. Other areas are below the umbilicus in front of the body.
   e. In women, mammary and inframammary region

7. Following are the biomarkers that help in the diagnosis and prognosis:
   a. The molecules upregulated in the tubular injury:
      - Neutrophil gelatinase-associated lipocalin
      - Kidney injury molecule-1
   b. Low molecular weight protein that is reabsorbed by the tubules:
      - $\beta 2$ microglobulin
      - Cystatin C
   c. Inducers of cell cycle arrest:
      - Tissue inhibitor of metalloproteinase-2
      - Insulin-like growth factor-binding protein-7
   d. Macrophage release products—interleukin-18
   e. Fatty acid metabolism markers—liver-type fatty acid-binding protein

8. Diagnosis is confirmed by:
   a. IgG antibody to scrub typhus: It will take 7–10 days to become positive. Titer of 1:64 is 90–100% sensitive and specific.
   b. IgM antibody will rise earlier in recent infection but false-positive test may occur.

9. Calculation of fluid overload-adjusted creatinine:

Adjusted creatinine = (initial creatinine × admission weight in kg × 0.6 + cumulative 3 days fluid balance)/ admission weight × 0.6.

10. This patient requires dialysis if:
    a. Serum creatinine is increased by >2 mg/dL.
    b. Serum urea is >100 mg/dL.
    c. Serum potassium is >6 mEq/L.
    d. Serum bicarbonate is <15 mEq/L.

11. Following diseases produce jaundice along with acute kidney injury:
    a. Infections:
       - Malaria
       - Leptospirosis
       - Dengue
       - Scrub typhus
    b. Drugs:
       - Rifampicin
       - INH
       - Pyrazinamide
       - Chloroquine
    c. Toxins:
       - Alcohol intake
       - Viper bite
       - Yellow phosphorus
       - Poisoning with hair dye

CASE 48

A 5-year-old child having history of 2 days vomiting came to medicine clinic with generalized weakness and inability to sit for 3 days. She had no significant past history including visual and hearing loss except the child uses of taking nearly 4.5 L of water daily and constipation. She had no history of craving for salt.

On examination, patient looked dehydrated, generalized hypotonia, obtunded sensorium, acidotic breathing, short for age, and features of rickets which were progressive.

Laboratory investigation demonstrated serum sodium 132 mEq/L, potassium 1.4 mEq/L, bicarbonate 7 mEq/L, chloride 114 mEq/L, calcium 8 mEq/L, urea 104 mg/dL, creatinine 0.9 mg/dL, and pH 7.21 mEq/L. Urine pH 7.3 and hypercalciuria.

1. **What is the clinical diagnosis?**
2. **What are the differential diagnoses?**
3. **What is the reason that children are prone to develop deformities in the bone?**
4. **What is urinary anion gap?**
5. **What are the points in favor of your specific diagnosis?**
6. **How can you differentiate renal and nutritional rickets?**
7. **What is Dent's disease?**

Answers

1. Clinical diagnosis is rickets and may be of familial, renal, or non-nutritional cause.
2. Differential diagnoses are as follows:
   a. Renal tubular acidosis
   b. Chronic kidney disease
   c. Hypophosphatemic rickets
3. In the growing bone, additional 1–3 mmol/kg acid will be generated from the hydroxyapatite leading to increased acid load to buffer.
4. Urinary anion gap = Urine sodium + urine potassium – urine chloride
5. The following points are in favor of diagnosis of distal renal tubular acidosis:
   a. Polyuria
   b. Polydipsia
   c. Features of rickets
   d. Growth retardation
   e. Anion gap = 11
   f. Metabolic acidosis
   g. pH 7.21 mEq/L

   h. Hyperchloremia
   i. Hypokalemia
6. Differences between the nutritional and renal rickets:

Features	Nutritional	Renal cause
Age of onset	6 months to 2 years	>2 years
Polyuria and polydipsia	Absent	Present
Short stature	Absent	Present
Deformities in the lower limb	Less likely	Hypophosphatemic variety
Fracture of bone	Uncommon	Common
Dental abscess	Absent	Present
Weakness in the muscles	Present	Present
Tetany	Uncommon	Common
Family history	Absent	Present

7. Dent's disease is X-linked recessive syndrome due to mutations of *CLCN5* gene resulting in phenotypic proximal tubular wasting of solute, nephrocalcinosis, renal stones, and hypercalciuria leading to renal failure resulting in rickets in some cases

CASE 49

A 22-year-old female came to medical clinic with nocturia for 1 year and headache, fatigue, vomiting, and loss of appetite but no oliguria for 3 weeks. She has no complaint related to joint pain, rashes, fever, oral ulcers, hematuria or frothy urine, respiratory distress, or swelling of the legs. She had no problem related to micturition and no bowel incontinence.

During infant age, he developed recurrent fever and some operation at the ureter was done that her family cannot recollect.

On examination, there was pallor, pulse rate 80 beats/min, blood pressure 165/90 mm Hg, respiration rate 28 breaths/min, mild pedal edema, and other systemic examination was unremarkable.

Laboratory examination demonstrated serum urea 68 mg/dL, creatinine 5.8 mg/dL, and hemoglobin 6.8 g/dL.

1. **What is the possible diagnosis?**
2. **What are the points in favor of this diagnosis?**
3. **Why the anemia is disproportionate in this case?**
4. **At what stage of red blood cell formation, erythropoietin and iron are required?**
5. **How can you classify the etiological diagnosis?**
6. **What are the causes responsible for this chronic involvement of the kidney?**
7. **How can you grade this etiology?**
8. **What are the indications of surgery in this etiology?**
9. **What are the procedures can be done to correct the etiology in childhood?**
10. **What are the causes of chronic renal disease in this etiology?**

Answers

1. This young patient has been suffering from chronic kidney disease due to chronic interstitial nephritis which may be secondary to primary vesicoureteral reflux.

2. Following are the points in favor of this diagnosis:
   a. Chronic kidney disease because serum creatinine is 5.8 mg/dL, urea is 68 mg/dL, and blood pressure is 165/90 mm Hg.
   b. Chronic interstitial nephritis because there are:
      - Anemia
      - Nocturia
      - Absence of oliguria
      - Absence of fluid overload
   c. Vesicoureteral reflux is the main etiology because:
      - There was history of recurrent fever in infant age
      - There was an operation in the kidney after which the reflux was corrected.

3. The anemia is disproportionate because:
   a. Loss of erythropoietin because of interstitial fibrosis and atrophy of the tubule leading to peritubular fibroblast as this is the site of erythropoietin production.
   b. There may be associated with iron deficiency and vitamin B12 deficiency.

4. Hematopoietic stem cell leads to development of erythroid series

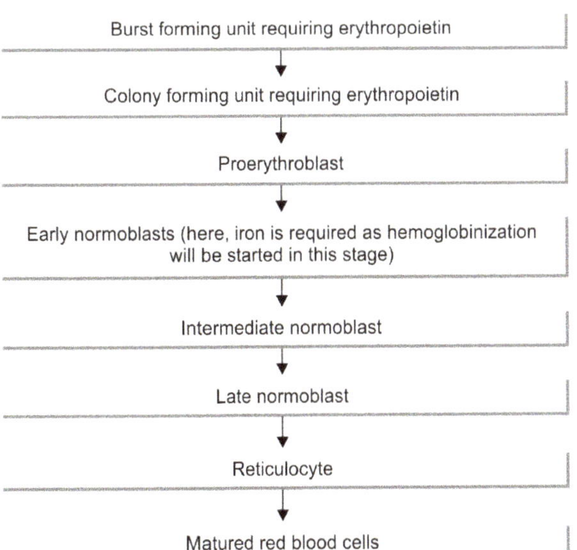

5. Classification of the vesicoureteral reflux:
   a. Primary cause
   b. Secondary cause:
      - Neurogenic bladder
      - Bladder dysfunction
      - Bowel dysfunction
      - Bladder outlet obstruction

6. Following are the causes of chronic involvement of the kidney:
   a. Chronic glomerulonephritis
   b. Chronic interstitial nephritis
   c. Vesicoureteral reflux
   d. Alport syndrome
   e. Fabry's disease
   f. Autosomal recessive polycystic kidney disease
   g. Nephrolithiasis

7. Gradation of the vesicoureteral reflux:
   a. Grade I: Reflux into the ureter
   b. Grade II: Reflux up to the renal pelvis without dilatation
   c. Grade III: Moderate dilatation of pelvis and ureter but with no or slight blunting of the fornices
   d. Grade IV: Moderate dilatation of the calyces, pelvis, and ureter along with obliteration of the fornices but maintenance of papillary impression in majority of calyces
   e. Grade V: Ureter, pelvis, and calyces are grossly dilated with blunting of the fornices and loss of papillary impressions.

8. Indications of surgery in case of vesicoureteral reflux are as follows:
   a. Patient with breakthrough infection
   b. Noncompliant patients
   c. Serial dimercaptosuccinic acid (DMSA) demonstrating new scars
   d. Severe grades persisting even after 2 years
   e. Patients requiring surgery

9. Techniques of surgery are as follows:
   a. Endoscopic techniques:
      - Periorificial injection of Teflon or Deflux (dextranomer/hyaluronic acid)
   b. Open surgical techniques:
      - Lich-Gregoir (extravesical ureteroneocystostomy)
      - Cohen (extravesical and cross-trigonal reimplantation)
      - Politano-Leadbetter technique (intravesical ureteroneocystostomy and extravesical mobilization as well as transection of ureter which is followed by reimplantation)

10. Bilateral scarring in the kidney along with progressive loss of renal function in case of vesicoureteral reflux are due to following mechanism:
    a. Reflux-related recurrent pyelonephritis
    b. Abnormal development of the kidney—congenital renal dysplasia or hypoplasia

CASE 50

A 6-year-old type 2 diabetic female child having history of long-standing history of nonalcoholic steatohepatitis-related cirrhosis came to emergency department with black stool, diminished micturition, swelling of legs, and progressive increasing abdominal distension for 2 weeks and altered sensorium for 3 days. There was no history of abdominal pain, hemoptysis, diarrhea, dysuria, frothy urine, recurrent urinary tract infection, arthralgia, limb weakness, and abuse of drugs.

On examination, patient is disorientated, pallor, pitting edema, afebrile, pulse rate 92 beats/mins, blood pressure 100/70 mm Hg, and respiratory rate 36 breaths/min. Abdominal examination demonstrated tense ascites and asterixis.

Laboratory investigation demonstrated hemoglobin 8.5 g/dL, platelet count 70,000/cc, polymorphonuclear leukocytosis, urea 210 mg/dL, and creatinine 8 mg/dL. Liver function test demonstrated 12 mg/dL, SGPT 235 IU/L, SGOT 210 IU/L, albumin 2.2 g/dL, ammonia 220 µg/dL, INR 2.2, and serology was negative. Ultrasonography demonstrated small shrunken liver, normal-sized kidney, and huge ascites.

1. **What is the most likely diagnosis?**
2. **What are the points in favor of diagnosis?**
3. **What are the diagnostic criteria in this disease?**
4. **What are the types of this disease?**
5. **What is the pathophysiology in this disease?**
6. **What are the roles of albumin in this disease?**
7. **What are the roles of the drugs in this disease?**
8. **What are guidelines of combined transplantation of both liver and kidney in this disease?**
9. **How can this disease be prevented in case of cirrhosis?**

Answers

1. Patient has been suffering from hepatorenal syndrome leading to acute kidney injury in a case of chronic hepatic disease with evidence of hepatocellular failure.

2. Following are the points in favor of this diagnosis:
   a. Rapid progression of oliguria
   b. Presence of ascites
   c. Acute worsening of the kidney function in the background of chronic kidney disease
   d. Evidence of gastrointestinal bleeding
   e. Diminished micturition

3. Following are the diagnostic criteria according to the American Association for the Study of Liver Disease:
   a. Chronic or acute hepatic disease with advanced hepatic failure and portal hypertension
   b. Acute kidney injury defined as an increase in the serum creatinine of ≥0.3 mg/dL within 48 hours or increase from the baseline of ≥50% within 7 days
   c. The absence of any other apparent cause for the acute kidney injury including shock, current or recent intake of nephrotoxic drugs, and the absence of ultrasonographic evidence of obstruction or parenchymal renal disease
   d. Spontaneous bacterial peritonitis is complicated by acute kidney injury that may be reversible in 30–40% of patients. It can be associated with acute tubular necrosis but it is also a major precipitant of the hepatorenal syndrome.

4. There are two types of hepatorenal syndromes:
   a. Type I hepatorenal syndrome: It can be defined as at least twofold increase in the serum creatinine of >2.5 mg/dL in <2 weeks.
   b. Type 2 hepatorenal syndrome: It is characterized by presence of ascites that are resistant to diuretics. It is also termed as HRS-nonacute kidney injury that can be defined as effective glomerular filtration rate of <60 mL/min/m^2 for >3 months with initial fulfilment of International Club of Ascites criteria for the diagnosis of acute kidney injury.

5. Pathophysiology of hepatorenal syndrome: The main characteristic features which are playing the central role in this disease are:
   a. Portal hypertension
   b. Splanchnic vasodilatation: In early stage of the disease, i.e., in the compensated state, reduction in the systemic blood pressure will be compensated by the increased cardiac output to preserve the renal function. But as the liver

function deteriorates, circulatory changes in the systemic blood vessels lead to decreased vascular resistance resulting in increased cardiac output. There is splanchnic arterial vasodilatation due to:

- Increased synthesis of the nitric oxide
- Increased synthesis of systemic vasodilatory mediators

So, there is decrease in the central hypovolemia which leads to activation of the systemic vasoconstrictors, like:

- Release of arginine vasopressin
- Renin-angiotensin-aldosterone system (RAAS)
- Activation of sympathetic system

As a result, arterial pressure and the renal perfusion will be maintained. But, there is retention of water and sodium leading to ascites, pitting edema, and impaired excretion of free water. This tense ascites results decreased renal perfusion leading to decrease in the glomerular filtration rate, as a result hepatorenal syndrome-related acute kidney injury developed.

6. Infusion of albumin, a volume expander, is beneficial in this disease because of the following proposed mechanisms:
   a. Binding of albumin with the vasodilators such as nitric oxide, interleukin-6, and tumor necrosis factor-α leading to increased cardiac preload and peripheral vascular resistance
   b. There is reduced level of inflammatory markers in the plasma as well as ascitic fluid.
   c. It will increase the survival.

7. Roles of drugs in this disease are as follows:
   a. 100 g 20% salt-poor albumin should be given initially followed by 20–40 g/day.
   b. 0.5–1 mg terlipressin every 4–6 hourly intravenously for 3 days along with albumin having response rate of 45–75%.
   c. Noradrenaline, α-adrenergic agonist, is effective in the treatment of hepatorenal syndrome.
   d. Midodrine, α-adrenergic agonist, plus somatostatin analog, octreotide, along with infusion of albumin should be given in case of type I hepatorenal syndrome.

8. Following are the guidelines of combined transplantation of both liver and kidney in this disease:
   a. Chronic kidney disease defined as effective glomerular filtration rate of ≤60 mL/min/m^2 along with at least one of the following:
      - Most recent glomerular filtration rate of ≤30 mL/min/m^2
      - Has initiated chronic dialysis for the end-stage renal disease
   b. Acute kidney injury having combination of any one of the following for 6 consecutive weeks (it must be documented every 7 days):
      - Glomerular filtration rate of ≤25 mL/min/m^2
      - Requiring acute treatment with dialysis
   c. Metabolic disease, like:
      - Methylmalonic aciduria
      - Hyperoxaluria
      - Familial nonneuropathic systemic amyloidosis
      - Atypical hemolytic uremic syndrome as a result of mutation of either factor H or I

9. Following are the methods of prevention of this disease:
   a. Identification and removal of the potential precipitating factors in the development of this disease
   b. Volume expansion by:
      - Blood in case of severe bleeding
      - Albumin in case of large volume paracentesis or SBP
   c. Early administration of broad-spectrum antibiotics for treating the infection
   d. Discontinuation of nephrotoxic drugs and diuretics
   e. Discontinuation of the contrast agents

CASE 51

A 60-year-old type 2 diabetic male for 3 years on oral antidiabetic drugs came to emergency department with swelling of legs, distention of the abdomen, and frothy urine for 2 and half months. There was no history of joint pain, skin rashes, hemoptysis, cough, and no abuse of nephrotoxic drugs.

Physical examination demonstrated pulse rate 72 beats/min, blood pressure 122/75 mm Hg, respiratory rate 18 breaths/min, pedal pitting edema, ascites, absence of diabetic retinopathy, and other systemic examination was normal.

Laboratory examination demonstrated 24 hours urine protein 9 g, fasting blood sugar 180 mg/dL, HbA1c 9.5%, and creatinine 2 mg/dL. Serum electrolytes are normal except serum bicarbonate 20 mEq/L, cholesterol 480 mg/dL, serum albumin 1.6 mg/dL, uric acid 7.4 mg/dL, and blood urea nitrogen (BUN) 45 mg/dL.

Ultrasonography demonstrated enlarged kidney with distinct differentiation of corticomedullary region.

1. **What is the most likely diagnosis?**
2. **What are the points in favor of your diagnosis?**
3. **What are the differential diagnoses?**
4. **In this disease, what are the features of nondiabetic kidney disease?**
5. **What are the serological tests to be done in this case?**
6. **What are the indications of renal biopsy in diabetes with kidney disease?**
7. **What are the types of involvement of kidney in diabetes mellitus?**
8. **Mention the points that will lead to suspect the glomerular disease in patient with diabetes mellitus.**
9. **What are the genes in case of diabetic nephropathy?**
10. **Mention the lesions that may be present in patient coexisting with diabetes nephropathy.**

Answers

1. The most likely diagnosis is adult-onset nephrotic syndrome in a patient with diabetic nephropathy without any microvascular complications.

2. Following are the points in favor of this diagnosis:
   a. Presence of nephrotic range of proteinuria
   b. Presence of hypoalbuminemia
   c. Abdominal distention
   d. Pedal edema
   e. Hypercholesterolemia
   f. Serum creatinine is 2 mg/dL
   g. Urea/creatinine is >20 mg/dL along with high level of uric acid suggestive of depletion of intravascular volume.

3. Following are the differential diagnoses:
   a. Membranous nephropathy leading to adult-onset nephrotic syndrome
   b. Diabetic nephropathy

4. Following features are in favor of the nondiabetic kidney disease in this case:
   a. Absence of retinopathy
   b. Diabetes mellitus is of short duration.
   c. Atypical clinical course—abrupt onset
   d. Massive pedal edema and ascites leading to hypoalbuminemia

5. Following serological tests to be performed in this case:
   a. Detection of anti-PLA2R antibody along with staining of PLA2R in the kidney tissue in the biopsy

   b. Complement C3
   c. Antinuclear antibody—immunofluorescence
   d. Viral serology
   e. Serum protein electrophoresis
   f. Assay for serum light chain
   g. Serum immunoelectrophoresis

6. Following are the indications of renal biopsy in diabetes along with kidney disease:
   a. Diagnostic definition in all suspected patients of nondiabetic renal disease for the presence of at least one or more of the following features:
      - Duration of the type 1 diabetes is <5 years.
      - Active urinary sediment
      - Particularly in type 1 diabetes mellitus absence of retinopathy
      - Rapid onset and progressive albuminuria or sudden onset of nephrotic syndrome
      - Clinical suspicion of other nephropathies such as amyloidosis or vasculitis
      - Following are the positive markers of the other systemic diseases:
        ○ ANCA
        ○ Cryoglobulinemia
        ○ Double-stranded DNA
        ○ Low complement
        ○ Antinuclear antibody
      - Rapid declining in renal function and/or albuminuria
        ○ Expected declining rate of glomerular filtration rate in untreated type 1 diabetic

- patient and Pima Indians with type 2 diabetes mellitus is 7–12 mL/min/m^2.
  - ○ Expected decline in glomerular filtration rate in patient on inhibitors of renin-angiotensin system is 3–6 mL/min/m^2.
  - b. In suspected case of diabetic nephropathy
7. Following are the spectrum of renal involvement in diabetes mellitus:
   a. Nondiabetic kidney disease:
      - IgA nephropathy
      - Immune complex glomerulonephritis
      - Antiglomerular basement membrane disease
      - Amyloidosis
      - Drug-induced acute kidney injury
      - Interstitial nephritis
   b. Albuminuric diabetic kidney disease characterized by increased secretion of albumin with or without fall in glomerular filtration rate
   c. Diabetic cystopathy
   d. Renal stone disease
   e. Ischemic renal disease
      - Bilateral renal artery stenosis
      - Diffuse atherosclerosis
   f. Normoalbuminuria diabetic kidney disease— characterized by normal excretion of albumin with fall in the glomerular filtration rate
   g. Complicated urinary tract infection:
      - Emphysematous pyelonephritis
      - Renal papillary necrosis
   h. Pregnancy-related kidney disease:
      - Preeclampsia
      - High birth weight babies

8. Following points can give clues for diagnosis of nondiabetic glomerular disease in diabetic patient:
   a. Sudden onset of nephrotic range of proteinuria
   b. If the fall in the glomerular filtration rate is >10 mL/min/m^2
   c. Duration of type 1 diabetes is <5 years
   d. Active urinary sediment
   e. Presence of renal dysfunction which is associated with other systemic diseases.
   f. Indigenous or unknown nephrotoxic drugs
   g. In case of type 1 diabetic retinopathy, absence of retinopathy
   h. Without any phase of microalbuminuria, there is development of gross and overt proteinuria.
9. Following genes may be present in diabetic nephropathy:
   a. Angiotensin-converting enzyme
   b. Apolipoprotein E
   c. Myosin heavy chain 9
   d. Peroxisome proliferator-activated receptor-γ
   e. Acetyl-CoA carboxylase-β
   f. Aldo-keto reductase family 1, number B1
10. Following lesions may be present in coexisting diabetic nephropathy:
    a. Hypertensive nephrosclerosis
    b. Focal segmental glomerulosclerosis
    c. IgA nephropathy
    d. Membranous glomerulonephritis
    e. Pauci-immune glomerulonephritis
    f. Acute tubular necrosis

CASE 52

A 55-year-old nondiabetic and nonhypertensive male has come to emergency department with sudden decrease in the volume of urine along with nausea, vomiting, and puffiness of the face. No history of drug ingestion, joint pain, skin rash, loose motion, fever, or upper urinary tract infection.

On examination, his blood pressure is 145/95 mm Hg, pulse rate 80 beats/min, pedal pitting edema, no pallor, jaundice, and systemic examination disclosed no abnormality.

Hematological investigations were normal. Serum biochemistry only demonstrated liver function tests, electrolytes, and lipid profile were normal, and uric acid was 9.2 mg/dL.

Urine analysis demonstrated red blood cells 2–3/HPF, white blood count 10–12/HPF, no cast, and oxalate crystals 12–14/HPF.

Ultrasonography demonstrated normal corticomedullary differentiation with normal echogenicity.

1. **What is the most probable diagnosis?**
2. **What are the causes of hyperoxaluria?**
3. **What is the composition of oxalate in urine?**

4. **What are common plant toxins responsible in this renal failure?**
5. **What are the general measures to be taken in this case?**
6. **What are the specific measures to be taken in hyperoxaluria due to the genetic defect?**
7. **What is the significance of oxalate in the urine in this patient?**
8. **How djenkol beans produce nephropathy?**
9. **What is the mechanism of mushroom-related renal failure?**

Answers

1. The most probable diagnosis is acute kidney injury due to hyperoxaluria.
2. Causes of hyperoxaluria:
   a. Primary hyperoxaluria (PH):
      - Inborn error of metabolism:
        o PH1: Deficiency of alanine-glyoxylate aminotransferase
        o PH2: Glyoxylate/hydroxypyruvate reductase deficiency
        o PH3: 4-hydroxy 2-oxoglutarate aldolase deficiency
   b. Secondary hyperoxaluria:
      - Gastrointestinal disorders:
      - Toxins:
        o Ethylene glycol
        o Plant toxins
3. Composition of oxalate in urine:
   a. In case of PH, 95% calcium oxalate monohydrate
   b. In case of secondary hyperoxaluria, mixed stone—whewellite and weddellite
4. Following plant toxins are responsible for acute kidney injury:
   a. Mushroom poisoning
   b. Djenkol beans
   c. Chinese herb nephropathy
   d. Sap of the marking-nut tree
   e. *Averrhoa bilimbi*
   f. Plant containing colchicine
5. Following general measures should be taken in this case:
   a. In case of PH:
      - Daily fluid intake >3 L/day
      - Pyridoxine in case of type PH1 defect
      - Urinary alkalinization
      - Thiazide diuretics in PH3 defect
      - In case of end-stage renal failure, renal replacement therapy
   b. In case of secondary hyperoxaluria:
      - Hydration with alkalinization
      - In case of end-stage renal failure, renal replacement therapy
6. Specific measures should be taken in this case:
   a. Primary hyperoxaluria:
      - No role of dietary restriction as the intestinal absorption is <5%.
      - Transplantation:
        o PH1: Combined or sequential liver and kidney transplantation
        o PH2: Isolated renal transplant
        o PH3: Isolated renal transplant
        o Isolated renal transplant in case of pyridoxine-sensitive adults
   b. In case of secondary hyperoxaluria:
      - Dietary restriction because here >40% absorption occurs through the gastro-intestinal tract.
      - Limited data regarding the transplantation in this case
7. Urine should be freshly examined to detect the oxalate crystals in the urine because if the urine is kept for long lime, urate conglomerate to form crystals and it is found under microscopy.
8. Consumption of 10 or more beans leads to nephrotoxicity within few hours as toxins of djenkolic acid form crystals in the urinary system. Symptom is suprapubic pain. Sometimes it may lead to obstructive uropathy.
9. Amatoxin, i.e., α-amanitin of *Amanita phalloides* mushroom present in the mushroom leads to severe gastrointestinal complications resulting in oliguric prerenal failure. Occasionally, other types of mushroom poisoning lead to rhabdomyolysis resulting in acute tubular necrosis.

CASE 53

A 60-year-old smoker for 35 years came to medical clinic with facial puffiness, progressive increasing swelling of abdomen, and lower limbs for 4 months. He has no history of fever, hemoptysis, jaundice, hematuria, chest pain and lower urinary tract infection, loss of appetite, joint pain or skin rash, or intake of over-the-counter medications. Physical examination demonstrated bilateral pedal edema, blood pressure 170/95 mm Hg, pulse rate 78 beats/min, and puffy face. Systemic examination demonstrated ascites and other systems were normal. Laboratory examination demonstrated platelet count 370,000/cc, total count 6,700/cc, serum electrolytes normal, LDL 190 mg/dL, triglyceride 210 mg/dL, albumin 2.3 g/dL, and liver function test was within normal limit. Urine analysis demonstrated 24 hours protein 8.5 g/day, serum C3, C4, and ANA were normal. Serum antiphospholipase A2 receptor antibody was 300 RU/mL.

Chest X-ray and ultrasonography of whole abdomen were normal. Renal biopsy demonstrated:

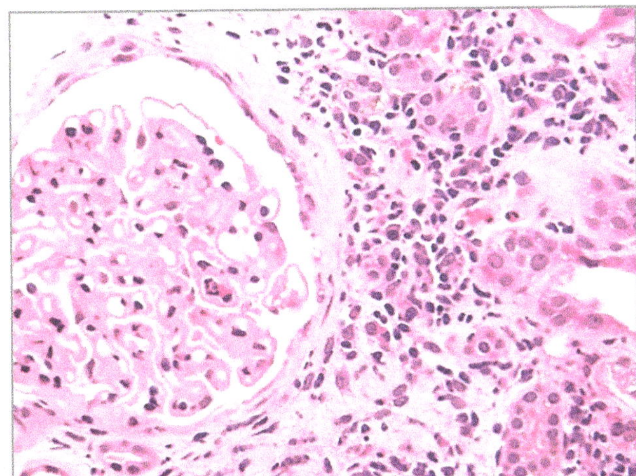 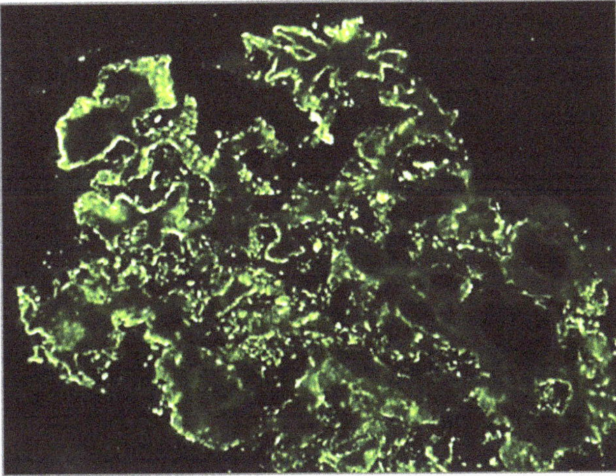

1.   **What are the histological pictures seen above?**
2.   **What is your most probable diagnosis?**
3.   **What should be the typical immunofluorescence findings in this case?**
4.   **How can you classify electron microscopic finding of dense deposit digits in this disease?**
5.   **What are the diagnoses to be confirmed by kidney biopsy?**
6.   **What are the risk factors for the rapid progression of membranous nephropathy?**
7.   **What are the major steps in the pathogenesis in membranous nephropathy?**
8.   **What are podocyte antigens seen on the podocyte membrane?**
9.   **What are the radiological investigations to be done in this disease?**
10. **What are the immunosuppressive therapies to be administered in this disease?**

Answers

1.   Above histological pictures demonstrate:
     a.   Light microscopy demonstrated the following features:
          - Thickening of the basement membrane with spike formation along with mesangial hypercellularity
          - No focal or segmental glomerulosclerosis
          - Absence of collapsed glomerular tuft
          - Mild interstitial inflammation
          - Blood vessels are normal.
     b.   Immunofluorescence microscopy demonstrates:
          - Diffuse effacement of foot process
          - Absence of subendothelial or mesangial deposits
          - Fine granular deposits of IgG

2.   The patient has been adult-onset nephrotic syndrome due to membranous nephropathy associated with PLA2R.

3.   Typical immunofluorescence microscopic findings are the following:
     a.   Fine granular diffuse deposits of IgG, kappa, and lamda

b. 1+ positivity for C3 along the wall of the capillary loop

c. Negative for C1q, IgA, and IgM

d. Antiphospholipase A2 receptor antigen along the loop of the glomerular capillary

e. Subclasses of IgG present are mostly IgG4 as compared to IgG1, IgG2, and IgG3.

4. Classification of the electron microscopic features of electron-dense deposits in membranous nephropathy:

a. Stage 1: Small sparse and electron-dense deposits on the epithelial side of glomerular basement membrane.

b. Stage 2: Large electron-dense deposits leading to thickening of the glomerular basement membrane along with effacement of the foot process giving the pattern of spike and dome pattern.

c. Stage 3: Stage 2 plus intramembranous coarse granular deposits with formation of "neomembrane".

d. Stage 4: Presence of irregular thickening and dissolution of the deposits leading to formation of holes and sclerosis of the glomerular basement membrane.

5. Following etiologies can be excluded by renal biopsy:

a. Focal sclerosing glomerulonephritis

b. Amyloidosis

c. Idiopathic glomerulosclerosis

d. Minimal change disease

6. Following are the risk factors for the rapid progression of membranous nephropathy:

a. Clinical factors:
   - Age of onset >60 years
   - Male sex
   - Hypertension
   - Hyperlipidemia

b. Laboratory investigations:
   - Proteinuria > 8–10 g/day
   - Persistent nephrotic proteinuria of >3.5 g/day
   - $\beta2$ microglobulinuria > 250 mg/day
   - IgG/albumin clearance > 0.2
   - Urinary IgG excretion >1 µg/min
   - Urinary excretion of $\alpha1$ microglobulin >40 µg/min
   - Serum albumin < 2.5 g/dL
   - Anti-PLA2R antibody titers > 50 RU/mL

c. Histopathologic picture:
   - Advanced glomerulosclerosis—typically >50% glomeruli demonstrate sclerosis
   - Collapse of glomerular tuft—any
   - Vascular hyalinosis—any

7. Following are steps in the pathogenesis of membranous nephropathy:

a. Expression of antigenic protein on the cell membrane of podocytes

b. Activation of complement and injury to podocytes

c. HLA class II molecules are responsible for the presentation to the immune system.

d. In situ deposition of immune complex at the base of the membrane of podocytes

8. Following antigens are present on the podocyte membrane:

a. Antiphospholipase A2 receptor acting as receptor for secreted phospholipase A enzymes

b. Thrombospondin type 1 domain-containing 7A

c. Neutral endopeptidase

d. Nerve epidermal growth factor like 1

e. Semaphorin 3B

f. Exotoxin 1 and 2

g. Neural cell adhesion molecule 1

9. Following are the radiological investigations to be done in this disease:

a. Ultrasonography to detect:
   - Any alteration in the kidney size
   - Evidence of obstruction
   - Renal vein thromboembolism

b. Renal vein Doppler study and CT scan and magnetic resonance angiography to demonstrate renal vein thrombosis

c. CT angiogram of pulmonary artery to detect pulmonary embolism

d. Lower extremity Doppler study to demonstrate leg vein thrombosis

10. Following regimen should be administered in this disease:

a. Ponticelli regimen (6 months):
   - Month 1, 3, and 5 month: 1 g intravenously × 3 days followed by 0.4 mg/kg/day oral prednisolone × 27 days
   - Month 2, 4, and 6: 2 mg/kg/day cyclophosphamide orally × 30 days

b. Modified Ponticelli regimen (6 months):
   - Month 1, 3, and 5 months: 1 g intravenously × 3 days followed by 0.4 mg/kg/day oral prednisolone × 27 days

- Month 2, 4, and 6: 2 mg/kg/day cyclophosphamide orally × 30 days
- Along with antiviral prophylaxis for *Pneumocystis jirovecii* (trimethoprim-cotrimoxazole and valganciclovir)

c. Rituximab, monoclonal antibody to CD20 antigen 375 mg/m^2 intravenously weekly × 4 doses. Maintenance dose should be given every 6 months.

d. Calcineurin inhibitor:
- Tacrolimus 0.025–0.40 mg/kg twice daily in divided doses × 6 months
- Cyclosporine
- Chlorambucil
- Mycophenolate mofetil

CASE 54

A 65-year-old diabetic for >8 years, chronic heavy smoker for 25 years, and hypertensive for only 1 year but poorly controlled male has come to medicine clinic for checkup. He had history of percutaneous transluminal coronary angioplasty (PTCA) 5 years ago to treat coronary artery disease. He has no history of symptoms related to retinopathy and neuropathy, hematuria, and frothy urine.

Physical examination demonstrated pulse rate 96 beats/min. All the peripheral pulse had good volume, but left dorsalis pedis, popliteal, and posterior tibial arteries are feeble. His both upper limbs blood pressure is 220/105 mm Hg, right lower limb 220/115 mm Hg but left lower limb 150/85 mm Hg. On auscultation, there are bruits in the both carotids, left femoral and left renal arteries. Systemic examination revealed cardiomegaly, but has grade II retinopathy.

1. **What is the most likely diagnosis?**
2. **What are the points in favor of this diagnosis?**
3. **In which other conditions, secondary hypertension will be suspected?**
4. **Where is the site of auscultation of renal bruit?**
5. **Is renal bruit heard in all the cases of renal artery abnormality?**
6. **What are the differences of blood pressure between upper and lower limbs?**
7. **What are the points indicating hemodynamic significance of the etiology?**
8. **What are the indications of revascularization in this case?**
9. **Mention the different techniques in case of renal artery stenosis?**
10. **What are the indications of salvageability of kidney on revascularization?**
11. **Mention the indications of nephrectomy in this case.**

Answers

1. This patient has been suffering from secondary hypertension due to renal artery stenosis along with type 2 diabetes mellitus and hypertensive retinopathy.
2. Following are the points in favor of secondary hypertension:
   a. Age is >55 years.
   b. Presence of uncontrolled hypertension
   c. History of smoking for >65 years
   d. Past history of coronary artery disease for which PTCA had been done.
   e. On examination, there are the evidences of atherosclerotic vascular disease.
   f. Presence of bruit in the left renal artery along with other arteries
   g. Absence of pedal edema and no urinary complaints
   h. Absence of diabetic involvement of the retina
3. In the following conditions, secondary hypertension should be suspected:
   a. Age is either <25 or >55 years.
   b. Presence of systolic blood pressure is >200 mm Hg.
   c. Resistant hypertension
   d. Weakness of muscles due to hypokalemia
   e. Presence of flush pulmonary edema
   f. Presence of:
      - Papilledema
      - Coronary artery disease
      - Cerebrovascular disease
      - Abnormal renal function

    g. Paroxysmal hypertension with facial flushing

    h. Unexplained declining renal function

4. Renal arterial bruit can be heard 1 cm above and lateral to the umbilicus.

5. Renal artery bruit cannot be auscultated in following conditions:

    a. If the stenosis is >80%.

    b. If the stenosis is <30%.

6. Blood pressure differences:

    a. Between both the upper limbs if >10 mm Hg—it is significant.

    b. If lower limb blood pressure is lower than 20/10 mm Hg, as compared to upper limbs—it is significant.

    c. Any blood pressure in the lower limb is lower than that in the upper limbs is significant.

7. Following are the factors determining the hemodynamic significance of renal artery stenosis:

    a. Hypokalemia

    b. Renal artery bruit

    c. Captopril renogram is positive.

    d. Fall in glomerular filtration rate with ACEI or ARBs

    e. Doppler study critical stenosis indicating >80% stenosis

    f. If the pressure gradient across the stenosis is >40%.

8. Following are the indications of revascularization in renal artery stenosis:

    a. Resistant hypertension

    b. Flush pulmonary edema

    c. Solitary functioning kidney with reticular activating system

    d. Refractory congestive heart failure in case of bilateral renal artery stenosis

    e. Rapid declining in the renal function in case of high-grade stenosis

9. Following are the techniques in this case:

    a. Endarterectomy

    b. Nephrectomy

    c. Autotransplantation through anastomosis the same kidney to another site of the aorta where there is less atherosclerosis.

    d. Bypass procedures:

      • In this case, splenorenal shunt

      • On right side, hepatorenal shunt

      • Iliorenal bypass

      • Mesentericorenal bypass

10. Following are the indications of the salvageability selected for revascularization:

    a. Size of the kidney is >9 cm.

    b. No feature of chronicity in histopathology

    c. Functional kidney as detected by intravenous urography or diethylenetriaminepentaacetic acid (DTPA) renogram

    d. Filling of distal renal artery through the collateral circulation by angiography

11. Following are the indications of nephrectomy in this case:

    a. If the size of the kidney is <8 cm.

    b. If glomerular filtration rate is <10%.

    c. Absence of collaterals in angiography

    d. Presence of occlusion after attempted revascularization

    e. Evidence of glomerulosclerosis and tubulo-interstitial fibrosis in the biopsy

CASE 55

A 55-year-old nondiabetic nonsmoker female having history of essential hypertension on amlodipine, 5 mg of metolazone, and 25 mg of chlorthalidone in divided doses to reduce the pedal admitted with alteration of sensorium for 48 hours prior to admission. He had no history of fever, vomiting, and loose motion in last 1 month.

On examination, the patient was nonresponding to verbal command, Glasgow Coma Scale 13, pulse rate 112 beats/min, regular, respiratory rate 24 breaths/min, blood pressure 100/60 mm Hg, and cold clammy extremities. Other systemic examinations including neurological were normal.

Laboratory examination demonstrated hematological examination was normal, liver function tests, serum sodium 116 mEq/L, potassium 3 mEq/L, chloride 95 mEq/L, bicarbonate 2 mEq/L, blood sugar 95 mg/dL, urea 55 mg/dL, creatinine 1.3 mg/dL. Arterial blood gas analysis demonstrated pH 7.48, PO_2 92 mm Hg, and PCO_2 33 mm Hg. MRI brain and chest X-ray was normal.

1. **What is the most likely diagnosis?**
2. **What are the points in favor of your diagnosis?**
3. **What is the cause of low sodium in the blood?**
4. **What is the mechanism of action of thiazide diuretic?**
5. **What is the mechanism of metolazone?**
6. **What are the correction factors in hyponatremia in diabetic patient?**
7. **Mention the normal serum osmolality and how can you calculate it in this patient.**
8. **What is fractional excretion of sodium or FeNa?**
9. **Mention the disadvantages of fractional excretion of sodium.**
10. **During treatment of this condition, how can you calculate rate of rise in sodium?**
11. **What do you mean by artifactual hyponatremia?**

Answers

1. The most likely diagnosis is metabolic encephalopathy due to hyponatremia induced by chlorthalidone and thiazide diuretics.

2. Following are the points in favor of this diagnosis:
   a. History of hypertension on high dose of two diuretics.
   b. Presence of ankle edema
   c. Absence of focal neurological deficit
   d. Absence of stigmata of chronic liver disease
   e. Mildly elevated urea with normal creatinine in serum
   f. Glasgow Coma Scale of 13
   g. Metabolic alkalosis
   h. Normal PO_2 and PCO_2
   i. Low sodium
   j. Low potassium

3. Hyponatremia is due to administration of two diuretics.

4. Thiazide blocks the thiazide-sensitive sodium-chloride symporter in the distal convoluted tubule leading to inhibition of the sodium and chloride thereby increasing the excretion of these electrolytes in the urine. Hence, this drug is saliuretic.

5. Metolazone acts on the distal convoluted tubule to decrease the absorption of sodium and chloride thereby increasing the excretion of these electrolytes through the urine.

6. Following are the correction factors to assess the fall in the serum sodium level in case of hyperglycemia:
   a. For each 100 mg/dL rise in the blood glucose over the serum blood glucose of 100 mg/dL, serum sodium decreases by 1.6 mEq/L
   b. In case of serum glucose of >400 mg/dL, for each rise over 100 mg/dL, serum sodium decreases by 2.4 mEq/L.

For example:
- If the serum glucose is 300 mg/dL and serum sodium is 132 mEq/L, so, should be added (2 × 1.6) or 3.2 mEq/L with 132 mEq/L to get real sodium level which will be 135 mEq/L.
- If the blood glucose is 700 mg/dL and serum sodium is 128 mEq/L, so, should be added (3 × 2.4) or 7.2 mg/dL with 128 mEq/L which will be 135.2 mEq/L, it is the real serum sodium level.

7. Normal serum osmolality is 284–294 mOsm/kg. Calculation of serum osmolality:
   Plasma osmolality:

   $$2 \times \text{serum sodium in mmol/L} + (\text{glucose in mg/dL/18}) + (\text{serum urea in mg/dL/6})$$

   So in this patient, the calculated osmolality:

   $$[(2 \times 116) + (95/18)] + (55/6)$$
   $$= (232 + 5.3) + 9.1 = 246.4$$

8. Fractional excretion of sodium is the percentage of filtered sodium that is excreted through the urine which helps to assess the efficiency of the tubule to reabsorb sodium.
   Following is the calculation of fractional excretion of sodium:

   $$(\text{Urine sodium/plasma sodium}) \times (\text{plasma creatinine/urinary creatinine}) \times 100$$

   If the fractional excretion of sodium is <1% in patient with oliguria, it indicates that tubules are intact to reabsorb sodium well.
   If the fractional excretion of sodium is >2%, it indicates that tubules are damaged.

9. The fractional excretion of sodium is not reliable in case of acute renal failure in those patients:
   a. Who are receiving the diuretics
   b. Whose volume status is normal.

10. The following formula is used to calculate the rate of rise in sodium:

$$\text{Rate of rise in sodium} = \frac{[(\text{Infusate sodium} - \text{patient's serum sodium}) \times \text{total body weight}]}{(\text{total body weight} + 1)}$$

If potassium-containing fluid is given, infusate (sodium + potassium) has to be used.

11. Following are the causes of pseudohyponatremia:
    a. Hyperlipidemia
    b. Hyperglobulinemia

    High lipid and protein content decrease the fluid content of the liquid. If flame photometry is used, it will measure the sodium in liquid phase. So, obviously the serum sodium level will be low. But, ion selective electrode is used. It will assess the sodium in total liquid. Hence, it will give proper estimation of serum level of sodium.

CASE 56

A 70-year-old type 2 diabetic on insulin for 12 years, stress incontinence for last 2 years, and two episodes of urinary tract infections with two separate organisms in late 1 year came to medical emergency with high rise of temperature with chill and rigor and vomiting for last 3 days prior to admission.

On examination, patient is conscious, temperature 103°F, pulse rate 120 beats/min, blood pressure 120/70 mm Hg, and left renal angle was tender. Other systemic examination was normal. Per vagina uterus was atrophic and no bleeding per vagina.

Routine urine examination demonstrated white blood cells casts and minimal proteinuria. Routine blood examination demonstrated white blood cell count 16,000/cc, polymorphonuclear leukocytosis, blood urea 90 mg/dL, creatinine 1.6 mg/dL, and blood sugar 220 mg/dL.

Ultrasound of the kidney demonstrated enlarged left kidney with increased echogenicity and normal pelvicalyceal system and thickened wall of the urinary bladder with residual volume of 100 mL.

1. **What is the most likely diagnosis?**
2. **How can you justify this diagnosis?**
3. **What are the diseases having overlap of symptoms with this disease?**
4. **What are the criteria of diagnosis of urinary tract infection by urine culture?**
5. **According to new guideline, what are the current definitions of different types of urinary tract infections?**
6. **What are the conditions responsible for complicated urinary tract infection?**
7. **What are the risk factors for recurrence of urinary tract infection in this age?**
8. **How does the nonsecretor status predispose to recurrence of urinary tract infection?**
9. **What are the adhesion factors of the bacteria implicated in the pathogenesis of this infection in women?**
10. **What are the normal mechanisms of defense in the urinary tract?**
11. **In case of recurrent urinary tract infection, how can you treat acute cystitis?**

Answers

1. The most likely diagnosis is acute left-sided pyelonephritis in a patient with type 2 diabetes mellitus in a patient of recurrent urinary tract infection.

2. Following points are in favor of your diagnosis:
    a. Long-standing uncontrolled diabetes mellitus
    b. Past history of recurrent urinary tract infection
    c. History fever with chill and rigor
    d. Tender left renal angle
    e. Ultrasonographic features of enlarged kidney

3. Following other diseases have major symptoms that overlap with urinary tract infection:
    a. Urinary calculi
    b. Menopausal syndrome of genitourinary tract
    c. Vulvar dermatitis
    d. Vulvodynia
    e. Interstitial cystitis
    f. Noninfectious vulvovaginitis
    g. Hypertonic pelvic floor muscle dysfunction.

4. Following are the criteria for diagnosis of urinary tract infection based on urine culture:

Method of collection	Quantitative criteria
Voided specimen	
In women, symptomatic cystitis	$\geq 10^3$
In women, acute pyelonephritis	$\geq 10^4$
In male, symptomatic urinary tract infection	$\geq 10^3$
In children, urinary tract infection	$\geq 10^5$
Collection in the external condom	$\geq 10^5$
Collection through the catheter	
In and out catheter	$\geq 10^2$
Suprapubic collection of urine	Any bacterial count is significant

5. According to the American Urology Association 2019:
   a. Acute bacterial cystitis: A culture-positive infection of the urinary tract with a bacterial pathogen associated with acute-onset symptoms like dysuria in conjunction with variable degrees of increased urinary urgency as well as frequency, hematuria, and new onset or worsening of incontinence.
   b. Uncomplicated urinary tract infection: It is characterized by an infection of urinary tract in a healthy patient with an anatomically as well as functionally normal urinary tract and no known factors which would make the patient susceptible to develop urinary tract infection.
   c. Complicated urinary tract infection: It is characterized by any episode of urinary tract infection that cannot be classified as "uncomplicated". An infection in a patient in which one or more complicating factors may put her at higher risk for development of urinary tract infection and potentially decrease the efficacy of therapy.
   d. Recurrent urinary tract infection: It means two separate culture-proven episodes of acute bacterial cystitis and associated symptoms within 6 months or three episodes within 1 year.
   e. Asymptomatic bacteriuria: It is characterized by the presence of bacteria in the urine that causes no illness or symptoms.

6. Following are the conditions responsible for complicated urinary tract infection:
   a. All male persons
   b. Pregnant women
   c. Renal diseases
   d. Anatomical abnormalities in the urinary tract such as diverticulum or vesicoureteral reflux
   e. Neurogenic bladder
   f. Stones
   g. Indwelling catheter
   h. Stents
   i. Fungal disease

7. Following are the risk factors for urinary tract infection in this patients:
   a. Lack of estrogen
   b. Incontinence
   c. Nonsecretor status
   d. Postvoidal residual urine
   e. Vitamin D deficiency
   f. Prior urinary tract infection
   g. Prior catheterization
   h. Urogenital surgery
   i. Cystocele
   j. Prolapse of pelvic organ

8. Nonsecretor status predisposes to recurrence of urinary tract infection by the following methods:
   a. Secretors will secrete ABO blood group antigen in the saliva, tear, urine, breast milk, and semen of the patient.
   b. Nonsecretor of the histo-blood group demonstrates increased affinity for binding of *E. coli* with uroepithelial cells.
   c. Unique nonsecretors are associated with glycolipid in the uroepithelial and vaginal cells that help in binding with specific *E. coli* adhesions. It is increased with age and hormonal status.
   d. Women having B and AB blood group has high risk of urinary tract infection.

9. Following are the adhesion factors of the bacteria implicated in the pathogenesis of this infection in women:
   a. Type 1 fimbria: It will bind to uroplankin resent on the surface of the bladder epithelium.
   b. P fimbria: It is a main factor in the bacteria leading to pyelonephritis and associated with severity of infection.
   c. Dr adhesin: These factors are responsible for adhesion of the different bacteria with the susceptible mucosal surface.
   d. F1C fimbria: It will adhere to the epithelium in the distal and collecting tubule.
   e. S fimbria: It helps in adhesion of the bacteria.

10. Following are the normal mechanisms of defense in the urinary tract:
    a. Anatomical features of urinary tract:
       - Continuous urinary flow
       - Absence of stasis during flow
       - Urinary bladder mucosa is covered with protective cells.
       - In the distal urethra, presence of normal microbial flora
    b. Physical properties of urine:
       - pH is acidic as most of the organisms are inhibited in this medium.
       - Osmolality: It will not favor bacterial overgrowth.
       - Low oxygen tension
       - There is high concentration of urea. It is bacteriostatic.
    c. Urinary proteins:
       - Tamm–Horsfall protein: It will bind to type 1 fimbriated *E. coli*.
       - IgA and IgG

    - Lactoferrin: It will chelate iron by its bactericidal activity.
    - Lipocalin: It will limit availability of iron through attacking the expressed siderophores in the bacteria.
    - Defensins:
       - α-defensins: It is secreted from the neutrophils.
       - β-defensins: It is secreted from the local renal epithelium.
    - Cathelicidins: It has direct bactericidal action.

11. Treatment of acute cystitis in patient with recurrent urinary tract infection:
    a. Administration of short case of antibiotics for 7 days
    b. 100 mg nitrofurantoin twice daily for 5 days
    c. Trimethoprim-cotrimoxazole DS 1 tablet twice daily for 3 days
    d. Fosfomycin 3 g in a single dose
    e. In case resistance to all the antibiotics described above, parenteral antibiotics for 7 days

CASE 57

A 70-year-old type 2 diabetic on insulin for 12 years, stress incontinence for last 2 years, and two episodes of urinary tract infections with two separate organisms in late 1 year came to medical emergency with high rise of temperature with chill and rigor and vomiting for last 3 days prior to admission.

On examination, patient is conscious, temperature 103°F, pulse rate 120 beats/min, blood pressure 120/70 mm Hg, and left renal angle was tender. Other systemic examination was normal. Per vagina uterus was atrophic and no bleeding per vagina.

Routine urine examination demonstrated white blood cells casts and minimal proteinuria. Routine blood examination demonstrated white blood cell count 16,000/cc, polymorphonuclear leukocytosis, blood urea 90 mg/dL, creatinine 1.6 mg/dL, and blood sugar 220 mg/dL.

Ultrasound of the kidney demonstrated enlarged left kidney with increased echogenicity and normal pelvicalyceal system and thickened wall of the urinary bladder with residual volume of 100 mL.

1. **What is the most likely diagnosis?**
2. **What are the nonantibiotic measures that should be taken in this case?**
3. **What are mechanisms of estrogen deficiency in this postmenopausal woman?**
4. **What are the options of vaginal therapy in this patient?**
5. **What are the contraindications to the estrogen therapy in this patient?**
6. **What is the effect of D-mannose in this patient?**
7. **What is the role of methenamine hippurate in this case?**
8. **What are the upcoming immunomodulators for this disease?**

Answers

1. The most likely diagnosis is acute left-sided pyelonephritis in a patient with type 2 diabetes mellitus and in a patient of recurrent urinary tract infection.

2. Following are the nonantibiotic measures that should be taken in this case:
   - Cranberry
   - Immunostimulants
   - Vitamin D
   - D-mannose
   - Vaginal vaccines
   - Use of probiotics
   - Instillation of hyaluronic acid and chondroitin sulfate

3. Following are the mechanisms of estrogen deficiency in this postmenopausal woman:
   a. Estrogen deficiency leads to:
      - Atrophy of epithelium of vulva, vagina, and lower urinary tract
      - Declining function of the detrusor muscles
      - Fibrosis of the bladder walls
      - Increase in the post-voidal residue
      - Loss of strength of musculature of the pelvic floor
      - Reduction in sensory threshold of the bladder
      - Increased sensitivity to neurotransmitters
   b. pH of the vagina increases above 5 due to decreased level of glycogen in the epithelial cells resulting in increased colonization of *E. coli* in the vagina
   c. Change of flora from *Lactobacillus* species to *Anaerococcus*, *Peptoniphilus*, and *Prevotella* as well as gram-negative fecal flora.
   d. Reduction of the volume of vaginal muscles leading to:
      - Slackness of the ligament that is responsible for holding the pelvic floor as well as the bladder.
      - Prolapse of the internal genitalia

4. Options of the vaginal therapy with estrogen are as follows:

Formulation	Composition	Dosage
Vaginal tablets	Estradiol	10 µg daily × 2 weeks followed by 10 µg 2–3 times weekly
Vaginal rings	17β-estradiol	2 mg ring will release 7.5 µg daily × 3 months
Vaginal cream	17β-estradiol	2 g daily × 2 weeks followed by 1 g 2–3 times weekly

Continued

Continued

Formulation	Composition	Dosage
	Conjugated estrogen from equine	0.5 grab daily × 2 weeks followed by 0.5 g twice weekly

5. Following are the contraindications for estrogen therapy:
   a. Absolute contraindications:
      - Breast carcinoma
      - Endometrial carcinoma
      - Liver disease
      - Thromboembolic disorders
   b. Relative contraindications:
      - Hypertension
      - Diabetes mellitus
      - Presence of gallstones

6. Effect of D-mannose in this patient: D-mannose after rapid absorption will be excreted in the urinary tract. Its structure is similar to the binding sites in the uroepithelial receptors. D-mannose in the urine will saturate H adhesins in the type 1 pili of uropathogenic *E. coli* thereby binding to mannosylated host proteins will be prevented.

7. In the acidic environment of urine, methenamine is hydrolyzed into ammonia and formaldehyde. Formaldehyde being bacteriostatic inhibits the bacterial cell division as well as synthesis of methionine in the bacteria.

8. Following are the upcoming immunomodulators:
   a. Oral immunostimulant:
      - It is the extract of 18 different types of the uropathogenic *E. coli* which is killed by heat.
      - Oral capsule OM-89 and OM-89S: First one is recommended by the European Association of Urology (EAU) guideline.
      - Increase in the neutrophil and phagocytosis of the macrophages will lead to stimulation of innate immunity.
   b. Vaginal vaccine:
      - Solco-Urovac
      - It is vaginal cream or suppository or pessary.
      - It contains 10 uropathogenic bacterial strains killed by heat
      - It will induce humoral immunity in the urogenital tract.
   c. Uromune:
      - It is sublingual preparation.
      - It contains selective strains of *E. coli*, pneumoniae, *Proteus vulgaris*, and *Enterococcus faecalis*.
      - It will generate TH1, TH17, and interleukin-10 to secrete T cells.

CASE 58

A 56-year-old nonhypertensive and nondiabetic, nonalcoholic, and nonsmoker man had history of polycythemia rubra vera 22 years ago for which he was treated with therapeutic phlebotomy along with hydroxyurea administration. About 12 years ago, he developed proteinuria and serum creatinine was 8.5 mg/dL. Kidney biopsy demonstrated focal glomerulosclerosis and diagnosed as chronic kidney disease with end-stage renal failure and under maintenance hemodialysis.

For kidney transplantation, he was selected for ABO incompatible kidney transplant from his wife. For this, he took rituximab 200 mg on the 14th pretransplant day followed by 10 sessions of plasmapheresis to reduce the anti-A antibody titer from 1:296 to 1:12. Post-transplant period, he received tacrolimus, steroid along with basiliximab, and was symptom free. On examination, he has pallor, pulse rate 84 beats/min and blood pressure 140/80 mm Hg. Other systemic examinations were normal. On auscultation, there was no bruit.

1. **What is the most likely diagnosis?**
2. **If the pretreatment was not performed, what will happen in this type of transplant?**
3. **Is there any role of splenectomy in this ABO-incompatible transplant?**
4. **What is the current protocol for desensitization in case of ABO-incompatible transplant?**
5. **What are the methods of extracorporeal removal of antibodies?**
6. **What are the types of assays for measuring anti-A and anti-B antibodies?**
7. **What are the various causes of thrombotic microangiopathy in case of biopsy of transplanted kidney?**

Answers

1. This is a case of polycythemia rubra vera being suffered from biopsy proved focal glomerulosclerosis leading to chronic kidney disease underwent ABO-incompatible renal transplant, but there was post-transplant rejection of kidney transplant due to anti-A antibodies.

2. ABO blood group antigens are present on the red blood cells as well as vascular endothelium involving glomerular and peritubular capillaries and veins. As a result, large amount of antibodies when developed in the patients with kidney transplant will lead to antigen-antibody reaction in the grafted renal blood vessels resulting in acute rejection of the grafted kidney. There are marked thrombi within the glomeruli, mesangiolysis and peritubular capillaritis, neutrophilic and lymphocytic infiltration, and in severe cases, there are interstitial hemorrhages.

3. Previous splenectomy was used prior to transplant but it led to severe infection after transplantation. Hence, this splenectomy has been replaced by administration of CD20 monoclonal antibody rituximab which depletes B cells.

4. Current protocol for desensitization in case of ABO-incompatible transplant:
   a. CD20 antibody 375 mg/m² or rituximab 100 mg 2 weeks prior to renal transplantation
   b. Next, reduction of the antibody titer by following methods:
      - Plasmapheresis
      - Double-filtration plasmapheresis
      - ABO column like glycosorb

   Pre-treatment antibody titer should be checked to 1 in 8 but in some cases 1 in 32.
   c. Post-transplant induction by:
      - Antithymic globulin
      - Interleukin-2 receptor antibody like basiliximab
      - Subsequent immunosuppression as per protocol

5. Following are the methods of extracorporeal removal of antibodies:
   - Plasmapheresis
   - Double-filtration plasmapheresis
   - ABO column like glycosorb

   Pre-treatment antibody titer should be checked to 1 in 8 but in some cases 1 in 32

6. Following are the types of assays for measuring anti-A and anti-B antibodies:
   a. Tube test, where hemagglutination is measured by addition of serum-containing antibodies from the recipient with the antigen-containing red blood cell blood group.
   b. ABO column assay: The results are expressed as IgG and IgM titers in 1 in 2, 1 in 4, or 1 in 64, etc.

7. Various causes of thrombotic microangiopathy in case of biopsy of transplanted kidney are as follows:
   a. Recurrence of the disease due to mutation of the complement factors

b.   Antiphospholipid syndrome

c.   Post-transplant thrombotic microangiopathy de novo:

- Related to class of donor and procurement and preservation of the organ:
    - Ischemia reperfusion of injury
    - Activation of complement due to donation after brain death or after cardiac death

- Associated with the post-transplant events:
    - Drugs
    - Fungal infection
    - Viral infection—*Cytomegalovirus* and parvovirus
- Causes unrelated to transplant:
    - Malignancy
    - Pregnancy
    - Drugs like vascular endothelial growth factor

CASE 59

A 46-year-old woman having past history of dry conjunctiva for 1 year came to emergency department with fatigue, generalized muscle weakness leading to difficulty in walking for last 2 weeks. She experienced similar episodes in last 6 months. She had no history of vomiting, diarrhea, intake of drugs, and hematuria.

Physical examination demonstrated heart rate 76 beats/min, blood pressure 120/70 mm Hg, and respiratory rate 22 breaths/min. She has hypotonia and absent plantar reflexes bilaterally. Other physical examinations are normal.

Laboratory investigation demonstrated renal function test normal. Urine analysis demonstrated urine pH 7.8, red blood cell 2–3/HPF, absent cast, and presence of calcium oxalate crystals.

Serum electrolytes demonstrated chloride 128 mmol/L, potassium 2 mmol/L, and bicarbonate 15 mmol/L. ANA is negative, but anti-SSa (Ro) and anti-SSb (La) are positive.

Arterial blood gas analysis demonstrated pH 7, bicarbonate 7 mmol/L, and chloride 127 mmol/L. Urinary anion gap is 13.6 mmol/L. Ultrasound of the abdomen demonstrated bilateral hyperechoic foci in the kidney indicating presence of stones.

1. **What is the most likely diagnosis?**
2. **What are the points in favor the diagnosis?**
3. **What is the mechanism of this disease after transplantation of kidney?**
4. **What are the laboratory investigations in this disease?**
5. **What are the calcium, phosphorus, and citrate in the urine?**
6. **Which stone is very common in this disease and why?**
7. **In case of idiopathic variety of this disease, what are the additional tests required?**
8. **How can you differentiate this disease from diarrhea in case of hyperchloremic acidosis?**
9. **How can you differentiate between the incomplete and complete variety of this disease?**
10. **What is the furosemide test in this disease?**
11. **What do you know by bicarbonate load test?**
12. **What is fractional bicarbonate excretion?**
13. **What are the consequences of this disease?**
14. **What should be the dietary advice to be given in this disease?**
15. **What are the prognoses in this disease?**

Answers

1. The most likely diagnosis is distal renal tubular acidosis in patient suffering from Sjögren's syndrome leading to normal anion gap metabolic acidosis resulting in hypokalemia.

2. Following are the points in favor of this diagnosis:
   a.   Normal renal function
   b.   Hyperchloremic metabolic acidosis in arterial blood gases
   c.   Severe acidemia

d. Urine pH > 5.5
e. Absence of history of diarrhea
f. Presence of nephrocalcinosis in ultrasound
g. Presence of Sjögren's syndrome

3. In case of renal transplant:
   a. Defective excretion of ammonium
   b. Generalized distal tubular dysfunction resulting from chronic rejection

4. Following are the laboratory investigations in distal renal tubular acidosis:
   a. Urine pH < 5.5
   b. Excretion of ammonium decreased
   c. Hypokalemia
   d. Hyperglobulinemia
   e. Citrate concentration of urine is low.
   f. Absence of Fanconi syndrome
   g. Positive anion gap
   h. Spontaneous metabolic acidosis
   i. Hypercalciuria
   j. Nephrocalcinosis and nephrolithiasis

5. In distal tubular acidosis, there are hypercalciuria and hyperphosphaturia due to:
   a. Increased release of calcium and phosphate from the bone to buffer the excess hydrogen ion
   b. Direct effect of this disease on the reabsorption of these ions in the tubules

   If the urinary level of calcium is >4 mg/kg/day, it is known as hypercalciuria.

   In distal renal tubular acidosis, there is hypocitraturia resulting from:
   a. Increased utilization of citrate in the proximal tubule due to intracellular acidosis leading to increased gradient for the reabsorption from the tubule
   b. Increased high intraluminal pH which will convert citrate to readily reabsorbable citrate. If the level of citrate in urine is <2 mg/kg/day, it is known as hypocitraturia.

6. In case of distal renal tubular acidosis, hypercalciuria and hypocitraturia along with metabolic acidosis and alkaline urine lead to increased chance of stone formation. These stones are either calcium oxalate or calcium phosphate. So, combination of hypercalciuria, hyperphosphaturia and hypocitraturia will lead to nephrocalcinosis and nephrolithiasis.

7. In case of idiopathic variety of distal renal tubular acidosis, following additional tests are required:
   a. Hearing evaluation should be done this disease may be associated with sensorineural deafness though it develops in late.
   b. Systemic lupus erythematosus
   c. Sjögren's syndrome
   d. Chronic hepatitis

8. In case of hyperchloremic acidosis, the etiology whether it is diarrhea or distal renal tubular acidosis can be differentiated by the following methods:
   a. Fractional excretion of sodium:
      - ≤1% in diarrhea
      - >2% in distal renal tubular acidosis
   b. Urinary anion gap (sodium + potassium – chloride):
      - Positive anion gap in distal and proximal renal tubular acidosis
      - Negative anion gap in case of diarrhea

9. In case of incomplete renal tubular acidosis:
   a. There is renal tubular acidosis without spontaneous metabolic acidosis.
   b. There is impaired response to acidify urine maximally in response to exogenous administration of exogenous acid.

   In case of complete renal tubular acidosis:
   a. There is spontaneous non-anion gap metabolic acidosis.
   b. There is low excretion of ammonium.
   c. There is less than maximal urinary pH.

10. Effect of furosemide administration: It will increase the delivery of sodium ion in the distal tubule and generate luminal electronegativity which leads to increased secretion of hydrogen and potassium ion in the collecting duct. So, the secretory capacity of distal hydrogen and potassium ion capacities can be estimated. So, this test can determine the mechanism and site of defect in distal renal tubular acidosis.

Defect		Urine pH		Urinary potassium excretion	
	During acidosis	After administration of furosemide	Baseline	After administration of furosemide
Normal	<5.5	More decreased	Normal	Increased
Hypokalemic distal renal tubular acidosis	>5.5	There is no change	Increased	More increased

Continued

Continued

Defect	Urine pH		Urinary potassium excretion	
	During acidosis	After administration of furosemide	Baseline	After administration of furosemide
H+ ATPase defect—medullary collecting duct alone	>5.5	<5.65	Normal	Increased
H+ ATPase defect—cortical collecting duct alone	>5.5	>5.5	Normal	Increased
Voltage defect—cortical collecting duct	>5.5	>5.5	Decreased	Unchanged

11. Bicarbonate load test: This test can characterize the type of renal tubular acidosis.
12. Fractional excretion of HCO_3 is an important index of proximal renal tubular handling of bicarbonate ion. It can be calculated as:

$$FE_{HCO3} = (U_{HCO3} \times P_{Cr})/(P_{HCO3} \times U_{Cr}) \times 100$$

    a. Normally proximal tubule absorbs almost all the bicarbonates from the tubule leading to excretion of <5% in the urine
    b. In case of proximal tubular acidosis, fractional excretion of bicarbonate is >15%.
    c. In case of distal renal tubular acidosis, fractional excretion of sodium is <5%. But, it may vary according to urinary pH as per Henderson–Hasselbalch equation.
    d. In hyperkalemic distal renal tubular acidosis, fractional excretion of bicarbonate is 5–10%.
13. Following are the consequences of this type I renal tubular acidosis:
    a. Progression to chronic kidney disease
    b. Bone disease resulting from acidosis and hypercalciuria
    c. In children stunted growth
    d. Nephrocalcinosis
    e. Nephrolithiasis

    f. Severe hypokalemia
    g. Recurrent or refractory pyelonephritis
    h. Nephrogenic diabetes insipidus
14. Following dietary advices should be given to this patient:
    a. Increased intake of citrus fruit
    b. Increased intake of fluid
    c. Restriction of intake of:
       • Sodium
       • Oxalate
       • Fructose
       • Animal protein
    d. Normal intake of calcium
    e. Avoidance of aluminum utensils during cooking if the patient is on Shohl's solution.
15. Following are the prognoses in this disease:
    a. Prognosis is good if the patient is on lifelong therapy with alkali as it will normalize the serum bicarbonate level in distal renal tubular acidosis. Dose is 1–3 mEq/kg/day in divided doses. It will:
       • Improve renal phosphate clearance
       • Subside hypercalciuria
       • Improve potassium homeostasis
       • In case of children, there is restoration of growth

CASE 60

A 40-year-old male having history of hypertension on three antihypertensive drugs came to medical clinic with painless hematuria, fever with chill and rigor, and nonradiating abdominal pain having no aggravating or relieving factors.

His 24 hours urine demonstrated 1 g/day protein and microscopy demonstrated 12–15 red blood cells/HPF. Blood count demonstrated 22,000/cc white blood cells with neutrophilic leukocytosis. Blood urea was 120 mg/dL and creatinine 8 mg/dL.

Ultrasonogram of abdomen demonstrated both the kidneys are enlarged in size with multiple cysts bilaterally in the kidney.

1. **What is the most likely diagnosis?**
2. **What type of genetic disorder this patient has been suffering from and why?**
3. **What are the renal manifestations in this patient?**
4. **How can you differentiate this disease from urinary tract infection?**
5. **How can you detect the cyst infection in this patient radiologically?**
6. **What are the causes of hematuria in this patient?**

7. **How can you manage the cyst infection in this patient?**
8. **What is the management of intracystic hemorrhage?**
9. **What are the extrarenal manifestations in this disease?**
10. **What are the causes of loin pain in this disease?**
11. **If this patient will undergo peritoneal dialysis, what will be the possible complications?**
12. **What are the indications of nephrectomy in this patient?**
13. **What are the indications of genetic testing in this patient?**

Answers

1. This patient has been suffering from ADPKD with drug-resistant hypertension leading to chronic kidney disease.

2. Patient with PKD2 is less severe as compared to PKD1 phenotype. If there is family history of end-stage kidney disease (ESRD) before 55 years of age, the patient may suffer from PKD1 mutation. On the other hand, if there is history of ESRD after 70 years of age, the patient obviously suffers from mutation of *PKD2* gene. As the age of the patient is 40 years, this patient should have mutation of *PKD1* gene.

3. Following are the renal manifestations of ADPKD:
   a. Hypertension:
      - Increased sympathetic tone
      - Increased activity of renin-angiotensin activation system
      - Primary vascular dysfunction
   b. Cyst infection
   c. Cyst hemorrhage
   d. Nephrolithiasis cyst wall calcification:
      - Increased urinary stasis
      - Reduced urinary pH
      - Hypocitraturia
      - Decreased excretion of ammonia
   e. Kidney pain:
      - Associated with uric acid nephrolithiasis
      - Hypocitraturic calcium oxalate nephroli-thiasis
      - Distal acidification defect
   f. Renal cell carcinoma
   g. Chronic kidney disease

4. Following can differentiate cyst infection from urinary tract infection:
   a. Tenderness in the loin is diffuse in pyelonephritis whereas tenderness is discrete in cyst infection.
   b. In pyelonephritis, white blood cell cast and urine culture is positive. In case of cyst infection, urine culture is negative and absence of white blood cell cast.

5. MRI can detect the infection in the cyst with 100% specificity:
   a. Intracystic signal by diffusion-weighted MRI
   b. Cyst wall thickening

6. Causes of hematuria are as follows:
   a. Spontaneous bleeding
   b. Cyst infection
   c. Stones
   d. Subcapsular hematoma
   e. Retroperitoneal hematoma
   f. Malignancy
   g. Current use of anticoagulant and antiplatelet drugs

7. Management of cyst infection:
   a. Medical management:
      - Drugs are:
         - Fluoroquinolones
         - Trimethoprim-cotrimoxazole
         - Chloramphenicol
      - Oral drugs should be continued for 2–3 weeks.
      - If there is no response to oral drugs after administration of oral drugs for 5 days then parenteral antibiotics should be given.
   b. Surgical management:
      - If the fever will persist after 2 weeks of antibiotic therapy:
         - Surgical aspiration percutaneously in case of single cyst
         - In case of multiple cyst, laparoscopic or fenestration of the cyst through lumbotomy or flank incision
         - In case of patients with end-stage renal failure on dialysis, nephrectomy should be considered.

8. Management of cyst hemorrhage:
   a. Episodes of hemorrhage are usually self-limited and will be resolved within 7 days.
   b. This should be maintained by:
      - Bed rest
      - Analgesic

- Adequate hydration
- Supportive care

c. If bleeding continues for >7 days, malignancy should be ruled out.

d. Patient should be hospitalized if:
- Bleeding is >7 days.
- Subcapsular hematoma
- Retroperitoneal hematoma

This patient should undergo:
- Embolization of segmental artery
- Nephrectomy

9. Extrarenal manifestations in this disease are as follows:

a. Central nervous system manifestation:
- Intracranial aneurysm
- Arachnoid cyst
- Spinal meningeal cyst

b. Cardiovascular system:
- Pericardial effusion
- Dissecting aneurysm of:
  ○ Ascending aorta
  ○ Coronary arteries
- Mitral valve prolapse
- Mitral regurgitation
- Aortic regurgitation
- Tricuspid regurgitation

c. Respiratory system: Bronchiectasis

d. Abdomen:
- Multiple renal cyst
- Dissecting aneurysm of splenic arteries
- Pancreatic cysts
- Diverticular disease of the colon
- Abdominal hernias

e. Genitourinary system:
- Male fertility
- Cysts in the seminal vesicle

10. Following are the causes of loin pain in this disease:

a. Renal cyst due to:
- Distention of the stretching and traction of the renal capsule
- Traction of the renal pedicle
- Muscular pain due to large cyst

b. Hemorrhage in the cyst—there is acute pain in the loin.

c. Infection in the renal cyst—presents with acute pain in the loin, high-grade fever with chill, and local tenderness

d. Pyelonephritis: Patient presents with bilateral diffuse loin pain.

e. Nephrolithiasis: Patient presents with acute or recurrent pain in the loin radiating to groin and hematuria.

f. Malignancy

11. Following are the possible complications in this patient and the patient will undergo peritoneal dialysis:

a. Abdominal hernia

b. Inguinal hernia

c. Pericatheter leak

d. Intestinal perforation

e. Renal injury

f. Gram-negative peritonitis

g. Abdominal pain

h. Effective surface area in the peritoneum will decrease leading to inadequate clearance.

12. Following are the indications of unilateral or bilateral nephrectomy in this patient:

a. Presence of intractable renal pain

b. Recurrent infection

c. Symptomatic nephrolithiasis

d. Marked limitation of the daily activities

e. Severe malnutrition

f. Suspected cancer

g. Extension of the native kidney into the potential pelvic surgical site

h. Uncontrollable renal hemorrhage

i. Failure to embolize intra-arterially

j. Development of ventral hernia due to massively enlarged kidney

13. Following are the indications of genetic testing in this patient:

a. Uncertain results of imaging with need for a definite diagnosis

b. Atypical presentations:
- Early and severe disease presentation
- Renal failure without significantly enlarged kidneys
- Markedly discordant disease within the family
- Marked asymmetry in the disease severity in-between the kidneys
- No family history with sporadic onset
- Syndromic features
- Reproductive counseling before renal transplantation

CASE 61

A 28-year-old man having history of steroid-resistant focal segmental glomerulosclerosis for last 7 years developed end-stage renal failure with creatinine level of 10 mg/dL and according to the advice of the nephrologist live-related renal transplant from his mother was performed without any induction therapy. On the third day, his serum creatinine decreased to 2.5 mg/dL. But on the fourth postoperative day, patient developed decreased urination with increase in weight and creatinine raised to 4 mg/dL. There was no fever or burning sensation during micturition. His urgent Doppler study demonstrated no abnormality.

1. **What is the most likely diagnosis?**
2. **What are the causes of this disease?**
3. **In this acute deterioration of the transplanted kidney function, what should be the line of management?**
4. **What are the types in this acute type?**
5. **What may be the most serious complication in this patient?**

Answers

1. The most likely diagnosis is acute graft dysfunction.
2. The causes of acute graft dysfunction are as follows:
   a. Early within 3 months:
      - Prerenal causes:
        - Volume depletion
        - Hypotension
        - Vascular thrombolysis
        - Drugs: NSAIDs and calcineurin inhibitors
      - Intrinsic renal causes:
        - Acute tubular necrosis due to preoperative and perioperative hypotension
        - Cellular, humoral, or both types of immunity-mediated hyperacute or accelerated rejection of the graft
        - Pyelonephritis in the graft
        - Thrombotic microangiopathy due to calcineurin inhibitors, infection like *Cytomegalovirus*.
        - Focal segmental glomerulosclerosis
      - Postrenal obstruction:
        - Obstruction in the ureter due to stricture, kinking, and blood clot
        - Enlarged prostate due prostate hypertrophy and prostate cancer
        - Obstruction in the Foley catheter
        - Neurogenic bladder
        - Perinephric collection of fluid
3. In this acute deterioration of the transplanted kidney function, following should be the line of management:

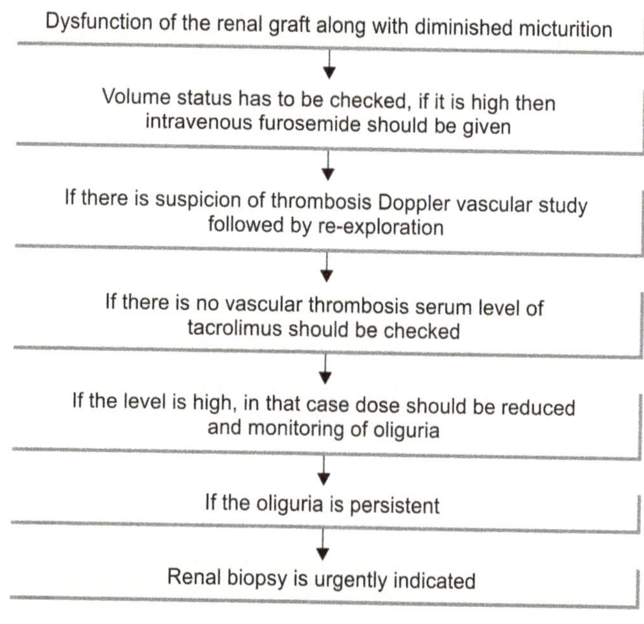

4. Acute rejection occurs in early and late post-transplant period. It can be mediated by:
   a. Acute cellular rejection through T cell mediated
   b. Acute antibody-mediated rejection through the preformed antibodies

   Acute rejection can be subdivided into three types based on the severity as well as time of rejection:
   a. Hyperacute rejection: It is characterized by rejection on the table due to preformed antibodies to HLA or ABO blood groups, but it is nowadays rare due to pretransplant crossmatching.
   b. Accelerated acute rejection: It is characterized by rejection due to antibody occurring in the sensitized recipients within 24 hours.

c. Acute cellular rejection: It occurs within few months of transplantation induced by T cell-mediated rejection. Nowadays, its incidence has been reduced due to administration of the T cell-depleting induction drugs.

5. Following are the transplant-specific factors that are involved in the pathogenesis of the thrombosis in the graft in addition to thrombophilia that contributes to the thrombosis in the vessels:

a. If the recipients are in the pediatric age group:
   - Dehydration
   - Mismatch in the size of the donor-recipient vessels

b. Technical errors:
   - Injury to the vascular clamps
   - Kinking of the vessels
   - Injury to the perfusion cannulation

c. Vascular rejection

d. Abnormality in the vessels in the donor kidney like thrombosis

e. Cadaveric pediatric "en-bloc" transplantation

f. If the patient is on intravenous methylprednisolone in high dose with OKT3 as this may activate tissue factor or factor VII pathway.

g. Hypercoagulable state like antiphospholipid syndrome

h. If the donor is elderly because hypotension in the donor along with reperfusion injury may lead release of procoagulant factors from the cytokines.

CASE 62

An 18-year-old child having history of end-stage renal failure was on continuous peritoneal dialysis with dextrose-based solution, three exchanges daily for 3 years. But, patient noticed swelling of lower limbs, reduction of ultrafiltration from 1,300 to 300 mL/day for last 3 months.

On examination, there was edema, blood pressure 160/105 mm Hg, pulse rate 116 beats/min, bilateral pedal edema, and basal crackles in the both lung bases. Then the patient started taking hemodialysis.

1. **What is the most likely diagnosis?**
2. **How can you define this case?**
3. **What are the causes of dialysis-related fluid overload?**
4. **Which important features have to look for during physical examination in this patient?**
5. **What are the investigations should be done in this patient?**
6. **What is the mechanism of ultrafiltration through the peritoneal membrane?**
7. **What are the different types of this disease?**

Answers

1. The patient has been suffering from ultrafiltration failure leading to fluid overload as this patient has been suffering from chronic kidney disease with end-stage renal failure.

2. Ultrafiltration failure can be defined as failure to achieve net ultrafiltration of at least 400 mL during 4 hours dwell with 4.25% dextrose.

3. Causes of dialysis-related fluid overload are as follows:

a. Noncompliance with salt as well as restriction of water

b. Noncompliance with prescription of fluid of peritoneal dialysis

c. Inappropriate prescription of peritoneal dialysis
   - Concentration of the fluid of peritoneal fluid is inappropriate.
   - If the dwelling time is too long with fluid containing dextrose
   - If the prescription of ambulatory peritoneal dialysis is not matched with the status of membrane transporter.

d. Loss of residual function of the kidney

e. Mechanical complications:
   - Leak in the peritoneum
   - Pericatheter leak
   - Communication between the pleural and peritoneal cavity
   - Leak in the abdominal wall

f. Malfunction of the membrane

g. If the hyperglycemia is uncontrolled

4. Important features have to look for during physical examination in this patient:

a. Examination of the patient to see any evidence of fluid overload:
   - Other signs of involvement which is not related to chronic kidney disease and peritoneal dialysis.

- Severity of fluid overload
- Evidence of mechanical complications should be searched.
  b. Evidences of physical examination include:
    - Pitting edema—its extent and its distribution
    - Evidence of structural heart disease
    - Evidence of pulmonary hypertension
    - Examination of catheter and its sites of introduction
    - Examination of peritoneal fluid like turbidity
5. Following investigations should be done in this patient:
   a. 2D echocardiography:
      - Left ventricular dysfunction
      - Pulmonary hypertension
      - Right ventricular dysfunction
   b. Serum albumin estimation in case of hypoalbuminemia
   c. Serum glucose in case of hyperglycemia
   d. Ultrasound of the catheter tunnel in case of pericatheter leak
   e. CT scan with iodinated contrast added in the peritoneal dialysate in case of peritoneal leak
   f. Cell count and culture of the peritoneal fluid in case of peritonitis
6. In the peritoneal membrane, there are two types of pores like small and ultrasmall pores. 60% ultrafiltration occurs through small pores and 40% through the ultrasmall pores.
   a. Small pores through which water and dissolved solids transport along the osmotic and hydrostatic gradient for the first 90 minutes or more during the dwelling time.
   b. Free water only transport through the ultrasmall port mediated through the aquaporin 1
7. There are four types of ultrafiltration failure:
   a. Type 1 ultrafiltration failure: It results from inflamed peritoneal membrane leading to increased vascularity resulting in rapid absorption of glucose and faster diminution of the osmotic gradient; as a result, fluid movement will be reduced within the peritoneal cavity. So if the duration of the peritoneal dialysis is longer, there is more chance of developing this type of ultrafiltration failure.
   b. Type 2 ultrafiltration failure: It is characterized by low osmotic conductance of glucose. The normal value of osmotic conductance of the peritoneal membrane is 50–100 μL/min/mm Hg. In this failure in spite of glucose remaining within the peritoneal cavity, glucose fails to exert osmotic conductance.
   c. Type 3 ultrafiltration failure: Here, there is decrease in the surface area of the peritoneal membrane due to structural abnormality of this membrane like acquired intrinsic insufficiency of ultrafiltration.
   d. Type 4 ultrafiltration failure: It is characterized by high rate of loss of total peritoneal fluid along with increased reabsorption of fluid through the lymphatics and the peritoneal tissues.

CASE 63

A 40-year-old male having history of ADPKD and bilateral renal calculi for last 7 years associated with hydronephrosis due to stone and stricture in the urethra (for which endoscopic dilatation done) leading to end-stage renal failure was undergone live renal transplantation from his wife as a donor and induced with basiliximab followed by immunosuppression with triple drugs. Patient developed post-transplant diabetes mellitus for which he was being treated with insulin. Though immediately after transplant, creatinine level was gone down to 1.2 mg/dL, but from 8th postoperative day onward, he developed recurrent urinary tract infection with different bacteria each time and treated with different antibiotics according to the culture and sensitivity. Retrograde cystourethrogram demonstrated grade III reflux into the graft. These repeated dysfunctions of the graft led to graft dysfunction. His serum creatinine was raised to maximum 2.2 mg/dL for last 1 year.

1. **What is the most likely diagnosis?**
2. **What are the risk factors present in this case?**
3. **What are the types on urinary tract infections occur in this patient?**
4. **What is the definition of renal transplant?**
5. **What is asymptomatic bacteriuria in renal transplant?**

6. **Define uncomplicated urinary tract infection in renal allograft?**
7. **How can you evaluate the case of recurrent urinary tract infection?**
8. **What is BK virus infection in this renal allograft?**
9. **What are the risk factors present in this case which will induct BK virus?**
10. **How can you diagnose BK virus infection?**

Answers

1. This patient has been suffering from postrenal transplant graft dysfunction (on immunosuppression with triple drug therapy) due to recurrent infection of the urinary tract as he suffered from ADPKD with multiple renal calculi and urethral stricture.

2. Following are the risk factors in this patient:
    a. Urethral stricture
    b. New-onset diabetes mellitus
    c. Prior urological procedure
    d. Immunosuppression
    e. Altered anatomy of the genitourinary tract
    f. Infection in the cyst
    g. Presence of renal stones in the native kidney

3. Following are the types of infection occur in this patient:
    a. Different types of bacteria
    b. Mycobacterial infection
    c. Fungal infection
    d. Asymptomatic bacteriuria

4. Symptomatic urinary tract infection in renal transplant: It can be defined as presence of bacteria of $>10^5$ colony forming unit/mL in the urinary sample in patients with dysuria, flank pain in the allograft and dysuria, and fever with chill and rigor.

5. Asymptomatic bacteriuria in renal allograft:
    a. In male: Presence of one bacterial species in single clean-catch voided urine specimen having colony count of $\geq 10^5$ colony forming unit/mL in absence of symptoms.
    b. In female: Presence of same bacterial strains at $\geq 10^5$/mL in two consecutive voided urine specimen in absence of clinical features of urinary tract infection.

6. Uncomplicated urinary tract infection in renal allograft can be defined as outgrowth of bacteria of $>10^5$ colony forming unit/mL in a properly collected clean-catch urine sample from a patient with symptoms of dysuria, urinary frequency, and urinary urgency.

7. Following are the line of evaluation in this case:
    a. In the graft and native kidney for calculi:
        -   CT scan
        -   Ultrasound
        -   X-ray of kidney, ureter, and urinary bladder
    b. To detect complex cysts in the kidneys: CECT in the kidney, ureter, and bladder
    c. To detect in infection in the cyst in the polycystic kidney PET-CT scan
    d. To detect reflux of urine micturating cystourethrogram
    e. To detect dysfunction of the urinary bladder:
        -   Uroflowmetry
        -   Cystoscopy
        -   Urodynamic studies
    f. To detect transplant ureteric obstruction, renal dynamic scan

8. BK virus is a double-stranded polyoma virus which replicates in the nuclei of the host. This infection is characterized by tubulointerstitial disease leading to ureteral stricture resulting in obstructive disease occurring after 2–4 months of renal transplant looking like mimicking rejection.

9. Following are the risk factors present in this patient:
    a. Use of steroid pulses to prevent rejection
    b. New-onset diabetes mellitus
    c. Antithymocyte globulin

10. By following methods BK virus infection can be diagnosed:
    a. Polymerase chain infection in the blood and urine—viral load of $>1,000$ copies is strongly associated with this infection-related nephropathy.
    b. Presence of "decoy cells" in the urine samples—cells having enlarged nuclei and single basophilic inclusion
    c. Gold standard method is biopsy of the renal graft demonstrating:
        -   Tubulointerstitial inflammation
        -   Intranuclear viral inclusions

CASE 64

A 52-year-old male having history of chronic kidney disease with end-stage renal failure as a consequence of ADPKD and family history of type 2 diabetes mellitus was undergone renal transplant from living donor, his wife and then induction with antithymic globulin followed by triple drug for immunosuppression was continued. He developed post-transplant hepatitis C and was treated effectively. But after 6 months of post-transplant, he developed increased micturition.

Laboratory investigation during 6 months post-transplant demonstrated fasting blood sugar of 96 mg/dL, creatinine 1.6 mg/dL, and postprandial sugar was 220 mg/dL, and HbA1c 7.4%.

1. **What is the most likely diagnosis?**
2. **What are the current criteria of diagnosing this disease?**
3. **What are the risk factors for developing this disease?**

Answers

1. This patient has been suffering from post-transplant diabetes mellitus.
2. The current criteria for the diagnosis of post-transplant diabetes mellitus are as follows:
   a. Symptoms of diabetes and random plasma glucose > 200 mg/dL
      Or,
   b. Fasting plasma glucose ≥ 126 mg/dL
      Or,
   c. 2 hours postprandial glucose > 200 mg/dL during an oral glucose tolerance test
3. Following are the risk factors in this patients:
   a. Modifiable risk factors:
      - Obesity
      - Steroids
      - Calcineurin inhibitors
      - Infections:
        - Hepatitis C
        - *Cytomegalovirus* infection
   b. Nonmodifiable factors:
      - Age: Usually >50 years
      - Ethnicity
      - Race
      - Sex: Male sex is vulnerable.
      - Family history
      - Impaired glucose tolerance
      - Adult polycystic kidney disease

CASE 65

A 40-year-old female referred to nephrology clinic with persistent bilateral pedal edema and frothy urine for 3 months. On investigation, urine protein +++, no red blood cells in urine, and only white blood cells are 0–1/HPF. Serum creatinine was 0.8 mg/dL. Kidney biopsy done that demonstrated:

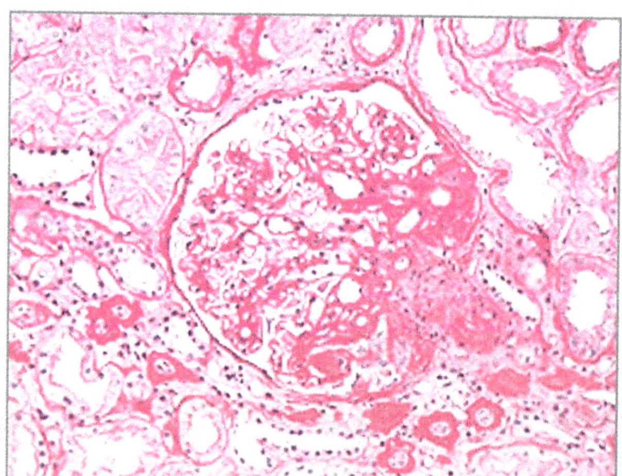
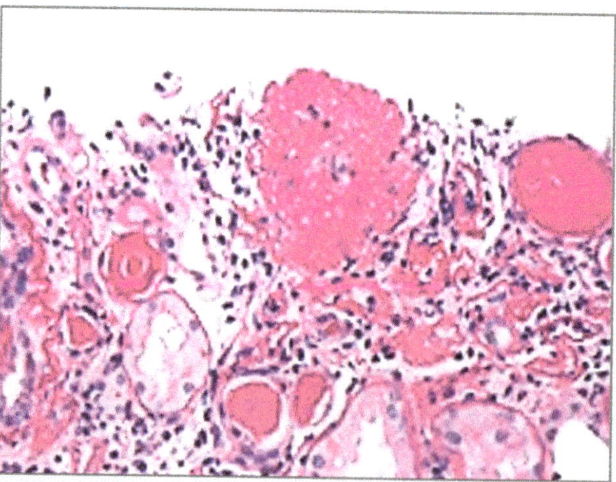

1. **What is the above histology demonstrated?**
2. **What is your diagnosis?**
3. **What are the types of this disease?**

Answers

1. Above pictures demonstrates:
   a. Left hand picture demonstrates:
      - Some part of the glomeruli is affected.
      - Mesangial expansion with hypercellularity
      - Glomerular sclerosis
      - There is also effacement of podocytes.
   b. Right hand picture demonstrates:
      - Hyperplasia and hypertrophy of the visceral epithelial cells of the glomerulus
      - Collapse of the glomerular tuft
2. This is a case of focal segmental glomerulosclerosis.
3. There are four types of focal segmental glomerulosclerosis:
   a. Tip variant: In this variant, disease involves tubular pole in the glomerulus occurring in white. There is effacement of podocytes. Creatinine level will not be increased, good response to treatment.
   b. Cellular variant: It is characterized by:
      - Hypercellular glomerulus
      - Endocapillary hyperplasia
      - Glomerular epithelial cell hyperplasia
      - Diffuse effacement of foot process
      - Full-blown nephrotic syndrome
   c. Collapsing variant:
      - Hypertrophy and hyperplasia of the glomerular epithelial cells
      - Collapse of the glomerular tuft
      - It occurs in:
        - Parvovirus B19 infection
        - *Cytomegalovirus* infection
        - HIV infection
        - Drugs such as interferon and pamidronate
   d. Perihilar variant:
      - It involves the vascular pole of the glomerulus
      - It is the adaptive changes as a result of increased pressure in the glomerulus
      - Mild foot process effacement
      - Subnephrotic range of proteinuria
      - Normal serum level of albumin

CHAPTER 12

Respiratory Medicine

CASE 1

A 34-year-old female having history of hypothyroidism and insomnia, mother of two male children, came to medical outdoor with history of productive cough, common cold, and sore throat for last 8 days following the recovery of her child from running nose, fever, and sore throat.

On examination, her temperature was 98.8°F, respiratory rate 16 breaths/min, pulse rate 84 beats/min, and blood pressure 120/80 mm Hg.

Laboratory serology was negative, antinuclear antibody (ANA) negative, total count 8,800/cc, renal, liver function tests negative, electrolytes normal, and glucose 88 mg/dL. Rapid test for influenza is negative.

1. **What is the most likely diagnosis?**
2. **How can you differentiate this disease from mild upper respiratory tract infection?**
3. **What are the specific criteria by the American College of Chest Physicians when chest X-ray is advised?**
4. **Where is the spirometry required?**
5. **What are the organisms involved in the pathogenesis in this disease?**
6. **What are the complications in this disease?**
7. **Why in this case guaifenesin is used?**
8. **How can you define the chronic type of this disease?**

Answers

1. The most likely diagnosis is acute bronchitis.
2. In mild upper respiratory tract infection, the infection involves upper respiratory tract and will be resolved within few days, whereas in acute bronchitis, the symptoms will persist for more than a week along with the involvement of lower respiratory tract.
3. Following are the specific criteria by the American College of Chest Physicians when chest X-ray is advised:
   a. Heart rate > 100 beats/min
   b. Respiratory rate > 24 breaths/min
   c. Oral body temperature surpassing 38ºC
   d. Chest X-ray findings of egophony or fremitus
4. Spirometry is not required usually but in case of suspected lung cases it may be required:
   a. Chronic obstructive pulmonary disease (COPD)
   b. Interstitial lung disease (ILD)
   c. Asthma
5. Following organisms are responsible:
   a. In 85% cases of respiratory viruses:
      - Rhinoviruses
      - Respiratory syncytial viruses
      - Influenza A and B
      - Parainfluenza viruses
      - Coronaviruses
   b. 10% cases of bacteria are involved:
      - *Bordetella pertussis*
      - *Chlamydophila pneumoniae*
      - *Mycoplasma pneumoniae*
6. Following are the complications in this disease:
   a. Acute respiratory distress syndrome
   b. Secondary pneumonia
   c. Prolonged symptoms

d. Spontaneous pneumothorax
e. Spontaneous pneumomediastinum
7. Guaifenesin is used in this case because:
   a. It reduces frequency of coughing significantly
   b. It reduces the thickness of the sputum

8. Chronic bronchitis can be defined as presence of cough and production of sputum lasting for 3 months or longer for 2 consecutive years or more.

CASE 2

A 32-year-old male, working as shipbuilder, has been admitted in the respiratory unit with productive cough, pricking type of pain in the right lower part of the chest and respiratory distress, and low-grade fever for 5 days.

On examination, there was clubbing, decreased movement of right side of the chest, shifting of trachea to the left side, stony dull percussion from right fourth space downward, breath sound, vocal resonance was decreased on the right side of the chest.

1. **What is the most likely diagnosis?**
2. **What are the general features that should be searched to detect the etiology of this disease?**
3. **What are the causes of the dullness at the right lower part of the chest?**
4. **How can you differentiate the causes of dullness in the right lower part of the chest?**
5. **What are the differentiating points in exudate and transudate?**
6. **What is the minimum amount of fluid required to detect the effusion?**
7. **Mention the conditions of pleural fluid pH and glucose level that are low but high lactate dehydrogenase (LDH) levels.**
8. **Mention the importance of measuring the pleural fluid pH and glucose.**
9. **How can the pleural fluid cytology diagnose the etiology of this disease?**
10. **What is the significance of pleural fluid amylase levels?**
11. **What are the causes where pleural exudates are negative for cytology but there is lymphocytosis?**
12. **What are the earliest radiological features of pleural fluid detection?**
13. **In case of doubt of pleural effusion, how can you confirm it?**
14. **What is the use of ultrasonography in this case?**
15. **What are the complications in this disease?**
16. **How can you differentiate thickened pleura from this disease?**
17. **What are the causes of recurrence in this disease?**

Answers

1. The most likely diagnosis is right-sided moderate pleural effusion.
2. The general features for detecting the etiology of the disease are as follows:
   a. Clubbing: Bronchogenic carcinoma
   b. Nicotine staining: Smoker having bronchogenic carcinoma
   c. Lymph nodes: Infection, collagen disease, and carcinoma
   d. Raised jugular venous pressure—cardiac failure
   e. Deformities in the proximal interphalangeal (PIP) and metacarpophalangeal (MCP) joint—rheumatoid arthritis
   f. Butterfly rash: Systemic lupus erythematosus (SLE)
3. Following are the causes of dullness in the right lower part of the chest:
   a. Pleural effusion
   b. Pleural thickening
   c. Consolidation
   d. Collapse of the lung
   e. Raised diaphragm
4. Following are the differentiating points:
   a. In pleural effusion:
      • Decreased movement on the affected side
      • Shifting of trachea to the opposite side
      • Stony dullness
      • Egophony at the upper border of pleural effusion
   b. Pleural thickening:
      • No deviation of trachea

- Woody dull percussion
- Breath sound is heard

c. Consolidation:
- Diminished movement on the affected side
- No deviation of the trachea
- Woody dull percussion note
- Bronchial breath sound
- In late phase, presence of crackles

d. Collapse of the lung:
- Diminished movement on the affected side
- Deviation of the trachea to the same side
- Woody dull percussion note
- Diminished breath sound, there may be bronchial breath sound.

5. The differentiating points in transudate and exudate are as follows:
   a. Ratio of pleural fluid to serum protein is >0.5.
   b. Ratio of pleural fluid to serum protein LDH is >0.6.
   c. Pleural fluid LDH is more than two-thirds of upper limit of normal of serum LDH.

6. At least 500 mL of fluid is required in the pleural cavity to detect pleural effusion.

7. In the following conditions, pleural fluid pH and glucose level are low but high LDH levels:
   a. Empyema
   b. Malignancy
   c. Rheumatoid arthritis
   d. Tuberculosis
   e. Esophageal rupture
   f. SLE

8. The importance of measuring the pleural fluid pH and glucose:
   a. If the pH is <7.3 and glucose level below 60 mg/dL, the life expectancy of the patient will be low, i.e., 2.1 months.
   b. If the pH is low, there will be extensive pleural involvement as diagnosed by thoracoscopy.
   c. If the pH is low, the failure of pleurodesis rate will be very high.

9. Following diagnosis can be made from the pleural fluid cytology:
   a. Normally pleural fluid contains 1,500 cell/cc with mononuclear cell predominance
   b. Cell count > 50,000/cc—parapneumonic effusion
   c. If the cell count is <1,000/cc, transudative pleural effusion.

d. If the eosinophil count is >10% of total cells in pleural fluid:
- Benign disease
- Asbestos-related effusion
- Pneumothorax
- Post-hemithorax

e. Pleural fluid lymphocytosis:
- One-third of transudate
- Malignancy
- Tuberculosis
- Lymphoma
- Collagen vascular disease
- Sarcoidosis

10. Significance of pleural fluid amylase levels:
    a. If the pleural fluid amylase is greater than serum amylase:
    - Pancreatitis
    - Bacterial pneumonia
    - Carcinoma
    - Esophageal rupture
    - In case of malignant pleural effusion, cytology if fails to differentiate the adenocarcinoma from mesothelioma, in that case pleural fluid amylase will be higher in adenocarcinoma.

11. Following are the causes where pleural exudates are negative for cytology but there is lymphocytosis:
    a. Tuberculosis
    b. Collagen vascular disease
    c. Tumors
    d. Lymphoma

12. Earliest radiological features of pleural fluid detection are as follows:
    a. In anteroposterior view, there is blunting of the costophrenic angle.
    b. Loss of clear definition of the diaphragm on lateral view

13. In case of suspicion of pleural fluid in the cavity, the chest X-ray should be taken in the lateral decubitus position to show the layering of the fluid along the dependent chest wall.

14. In following cases, ultrasonography is necessary in case of pleural effusion:
    a. Loculated pleural effusion
    b. To guide thoracocentesis
    c. In case of closed pleural biopsy
    d. Insertion of chest drain
    e. To differentiate pleural effusion from pleural thickening

15. Complications of pleural effusion:
    a. Thickened pleura
    b. Empyema thoracis
    c. In long-standing cases, there may be nonexpansion of the lung
    d. Acute pulmonary edema
    e. Hydropneumothorax
    f. Cachexia
16. Differences between the thickened pleura and pleural effusion:

Thickened pleura	Pleural effusion
There may be retraction of the chest on the involved side	There is bulging of the chest on the affected side
Movement may be diminished	Movement of the affected side is markedly diminished

Continued

Continued

Thickened pleura	Pleural effusion
There is no shifting of the trachea	Trachea will be shifted toward opposite side
Woody dull percussion note	Stony dull percussion note
Diminished breath sound on the affected side	Breath sound will be absent on the affected side

17. Causes of recurrences of pleural effusion:
    a. Slow recurrences:
       - Tubercular effusion on the antitubercular drugs
       - Meigs syndrome
       - Collagen vascular disease
       - Congestive cardiac failure

CASE 3

A 35-year-old female presented with sudden onset of pricking type chest pain increased during inspiration as well as coughing.

On examination, there is scratchy sound heard in both phase of respiration and increased in intensity during pressure of the stethoscope on the affected area.

1. **What is the most likely diagnosis?**
2. **What do you expect in this case as compared to pneumonia?**
3. **What should be the changes in ECG in this case?**

Answers

1. The most likely diagnosis is pleural rub. It may be due to pulmonary embolism.
2. In case of pulmonary embolism, the perfusion is decreased but ventilation will be normal, whereas in case of pneumonia, both ventilation as well as perfusion will be decreased.
3. In case of pulmonary embolism:
    a. Sinus tachycardia
    b. Tall R wave in V1
    c. S wave in LI, LII, and LIII
    d. S wave in LI and Q wave and inverted T wave in LIII

CASE 4

A 40-year-old female gardener having history of asthma controlled by steroid inhaler and long-acting β_2-agonist and having a nasal polyp on nasal steroid developed respiratory distress which was very difficult to control. She had no pets.

Laboratory investigation demonstrated total leukocyte count 8,000/cc, absolute eosinophil count 3,200/cc, IgE *Aspergillus* RAST positive, and Aspergillus precipitins IgG 3 lines. Chest X-ray demonstrated:

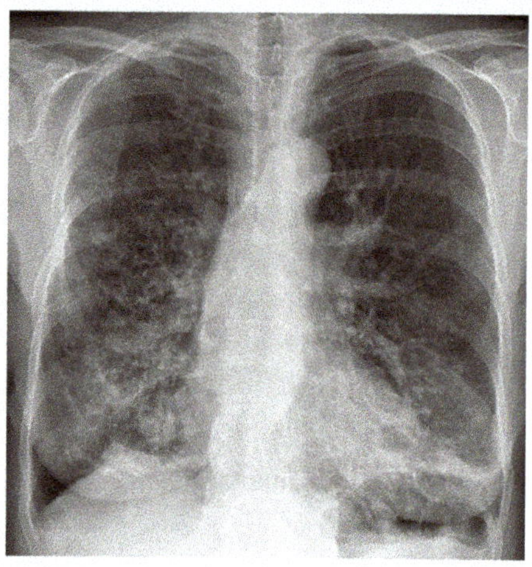 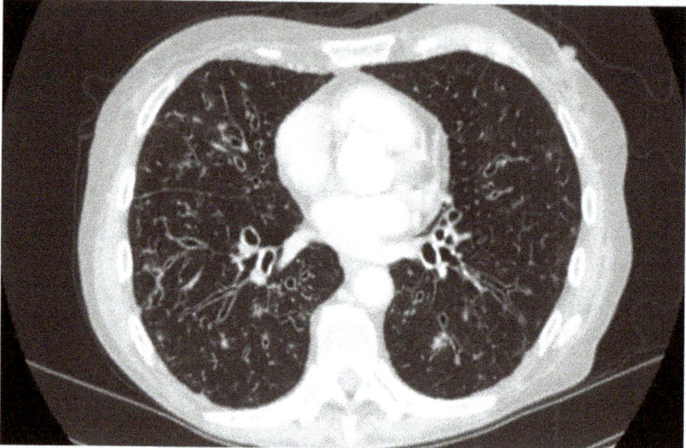

1. **What is demonstrated in the chest X-ray?**
2. **What is demonstrated in the CT scan of chest?**
3. **What are the causes of the sudden deterioration of the patient's condition?**
4. **What is the most likely diagnosis?**
5. **What are the causative organisms?**
6. **Who are vulnerable to this infection?**
7. **What are the differences in auscultation in the vulnerable patients?**
8. **What are the features suggestive of aspergillus infection?**
9. **What are the radiological shadows present in this disease?**
10. **What is the revised radiological classification of allergic bronchopulmonary aspergillosis (ABPA) based on high-resolution computed tomography (HRCT) of chest?**
11. **What are the Rosenberg–Patterson criteria in this disease?**
12. **Which monoclonal antibody is used in this case?**

Answers

1. Chest X-ray demonstrates:
   a. Hyper-extended lung field
   b. Widespread bronchiectatic changes
2. CT scan of the chest demonstrates:
   a. Dilated airways which are much larger as compared to blood vessels
   b. Presence of tree in bud nodularity
3. Following are the causes of sudden deterioration of the symptoms after very good control:
   a. Development of gastroesophageal reflux
   b. Weight gain
   c. New triggers of asthma:
      - House dust and mite
      - Pollen
      - Car-fur
      - Occupational exposure
   d. New psychological pressure
   e. New social pressure
   f. Associated other diagnosis, like:
      - Allergic bronchopulmonary aspergillosis
      - Churg–Strauss syndrome
4. The most likely diagnosis is ABPA.
5. The most likely causative organism is *Aspergillus fumigatus.* The others are:
   a. *Aspergillus niger*
   b. *Aspergillus flavus*
   c. *Aspergillus clavatus*
6. Patients with preexisting asthma and cystic fibrosis are vulnerable to develop ABPA.
7. In case of bronchial asthma, there is presence of rhonchi on auscultation. In case of patient with cystic fibrosis, there is crepitation due to bronchiectasis.

8. Following are the features suggestive of *Aspergillus* infection:
   a. Increased serum immunoglobulin E (IgE) of >1,000 IU/mL
   b. Specific IgE to *A. fumigatus*
   c. Increased serum IgG to *A. fumigatus*
   d. Peripheral blood eosinophilia
9. Following radiological shadows are present in this disease:
   a. Finger in glove opacity—indicates mucus plug in the dilated bronchi
   b. Tramline shadows—characterized by parallel line shadow extending from the hilar region along the bronchial distribution indicating edematous inflamed bronchi
   c. Toothpaste shadows—indicate impacted mucus in the bronchi
   d. Ring shadows—indicate dilated bronchi with inflamed bronchial wall
10. The revised radiological classification of ABPA based on HRCT of chest:
    a. ABPA-S, i.e., serological ABPA—where diagnostic criteria are fulfilled in absence of radiological features in HRCT thorax.
    b. ABPA-B, i.e., ABPA with bronchiectasis—where diagnostic criteria of ABPA are fulfilled in presence of bronchiectasis.
    c. ABPA-HAM, i.e., ABPA with high-attenuation mucus—where ABPA along with presence of high-attenuation mucus in HRCT thorax
    d. ABPA-CPF, i.e., ABPA with chronic pleuro-pulmonary fibrosis—ABPA along with at least two radiological features of fibrosis such as fibrocavitary lesion, pulmonary fibrosis, and pleural thickening in absence of mucoid impaction.
11. The Rosenberg–Patterson criteria in this ABPA are as follows:
    a. Eight major criteria:
       i. Asthma
       ii. Presence of transient pulmonary infiltrate
       iii. Immediate cutaneous activity of *A. fumigatus*
       iv. Elevated serum total IgE
       v. Precipitin antibodies against *A. fumigatus*
       vi. Peripheral blood eosinophilia
       vii. Elevated serum IgE and IgG to *A. fumigatus*
       viii. Central or proximal bronchiectasis with normal tapering distal bronchi
    b. Three minor criteria:
       i. Expectoration of golden brownish sputum plug
       ii. Positive sputum culture for *Aspergillus* species
       iii. Late or Arthus type skin sensitivity
12. Omalizumab: It is anti-IgE recombinant humanized monoclonal antibody which binds Fc-epsilon R1 receptor on the IgE present on the mast cells or basophils. It is used for treating uncontrolled bronchial asthma on the step-4 GINA guideline of treatment.

CASE 5

A 75-year-old housewife having past history of myocardial infarction on amiodarone, aspirin, and furosemide came to emergency department with progressively increasing breathlessness which was ultimately severe but no cough. She had no pets.

On examination, there was clubbing, central cyanosis, no edema, and normal jugular venous pressure. Auscultation demonstrated bibasilar crepitations and systolic murmur in the aortic area.

Laboratory investigation demonstrated hemoglobin 14.5 g/dL, total count 6,290/cc, erythrocyte sedimentation rate (ESR) 50 mm/1st hour, rheumatoid factor positive but ANA, antismooth muscle cell antibody, and antimitochondrial antibody were negative. α1-antitrypsin was normal. USG demonstrated hepatosplenomegaly.

Pulmonary function test demonstrated:

- FEV_1: 2.1 (131 predicted)
- FVC: 2.8 (144 predicted)
- FEV_1/FVC –
- TLC: 4.8 L
- RV: 1.9 L
- Gas transfer—reduced

Chest X-ray demonstrated:

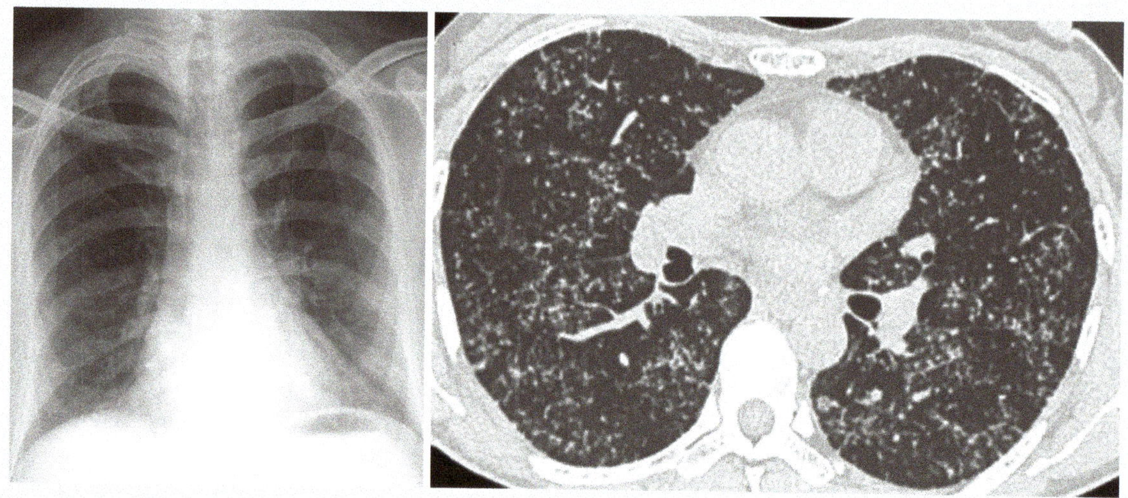

1. **What is the interpretation of pulmonary function test?**
2. **What are the features demonstrated in the chest X-ray?**
3. **Interpret CT scan of thorax.**
4. **What are the differential diagnoses?**
5. **What is the most likely diagnosis?**
6. **Why there is finger clubbing here?**
7. **Why gas transfer is low here?**
8. **What bedside test and what specific investigation should be done?**
9. **What are the complications of this disease?**
10. **What are the types of this disease?**
11. **What are the clinical features in this disease?**

Answers

1. Lung function test demonstrates:
    a. Supranormal dynamic lung volume
    b. No evidence of restrictive or obstructive lung disease
    c. Static lung volume is normal.
2. Chest X-ray demonstrates:
    a. Bilateral diffuse reticulonodular opacities
    b. Heart size and contour of mediastinum are normal
3. CT scan of thorax demonstrates:
    a. Diffuse moderate emphysematous changes
    b. Subpleural reticular changes
    c. Honeycomb changes at both the bases
4. The differential diagnoses are:
    a. Emphysema
    b. Interstitial lung diseases
    c. Hepatopulmonary syndrome in case of cirrhosis
    d. Thromboembolic disease in the lung

5. The most likely diagnosis is hepatopulmonary syndrome in a case of chronic liver disease.
6. Clubbing here is due to:
    a. Interstitial lung disease
    b. Chronic liver disease
7. In absence of restrictive or obstructive lung disease, isolated reduction of gas transfer is due to:
    a. Emphysema
    b. Early interstitial lung disease
8. Bedside test to investigate the postural changes in oxygen saturation, because in upright posture there is decrease in oxygen saturation which is known as orthodeoxia in case pulmonary arteriovenous malformation as compared to thromboembolic disease.

    Specific investigation should be chest CT pulmonary angiogram which demonstrates:
    a. Evidence of pulmonary emboli
    b. Evidence of increased nodularity at the periphery of the both lung bases—it is consistent with

pulmonary arteriovenous malformation secondary to hepatopulmonary syndrome.

9. Complications of hepatopulmonary syndrome as it is a fatal disease decreasing the life span:
   a. There is progressive vasodilatation with worsening of hypoxemia.
   b. Refractory hepatopulmonary syndrome as there are fails to improve oxygenation even after liver transplantation.
   c. Severe posttransplant hypoxemia
   d. Posttransplant portopulmonary hypertension

10. There are two types of hepatopulmonary syndrome based on locations of dilated pulmonary vessels:
    a. Type I hepatopulmonary syndrome: It is characterized by:
       - Dilated pulmonary vessels at the precapillary levels near the gas exchange units in the lungs
       - Supplemental oxygen improves PO_2
    b. Type II hepatopulmonary syndrome: It is characterized by:
       - Evidence of dilated vessels leading to development of arteriovenous shunt away from the gas exchange units in the lung
       - Supplemental oxygen fails to improve PO_2

11. Following are the important features in this disease:
    a. Central cyanosis
    b. Digital clubbing
    c. Diffuse telangiectasia
    d. Platypnea: There is worsening of dyspnea while supine from standing position.
    e. Orthodeoxia

CASE 6

A 43-year-old female having history of progressive dysphagia, dysphonia, and progressive increasing shortness of breathlessness. Pulmonary function tests demonstrated:

- FEV_1: 9 L—70% predicted
- FVC: 2.6 L—74% predicted
- FEV_1/FVC ratio –
- SPO_2: 92% at 4 L of oxygen
- TLC: 3.8 L—83% predicted
- Residual volume: 1.5 L—91% predicted

Following are the clinical features:

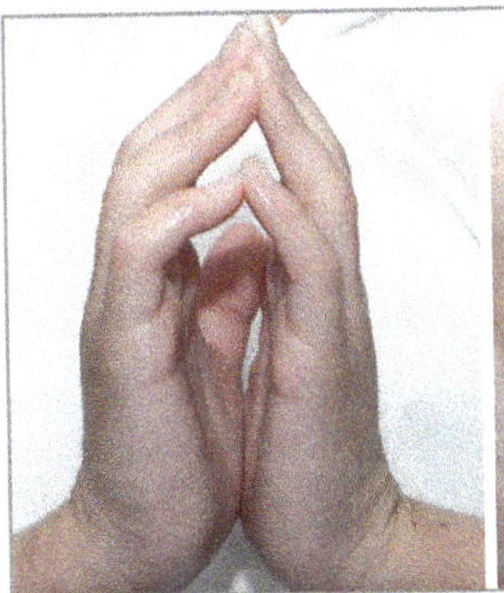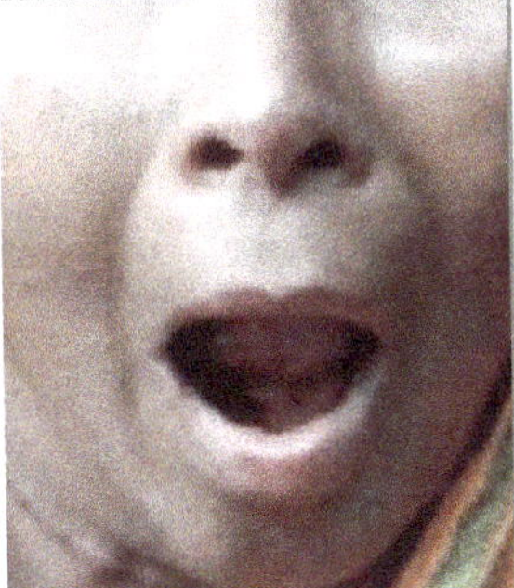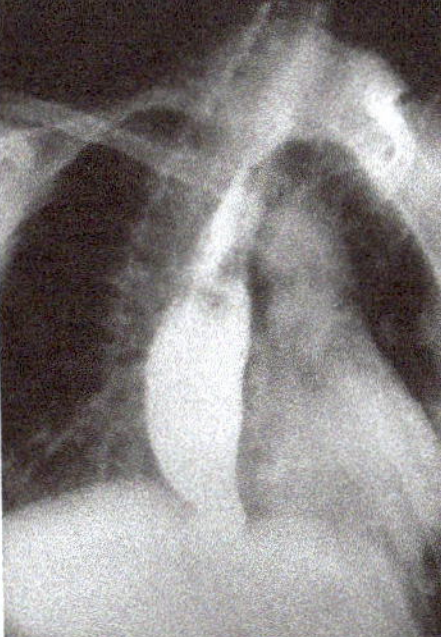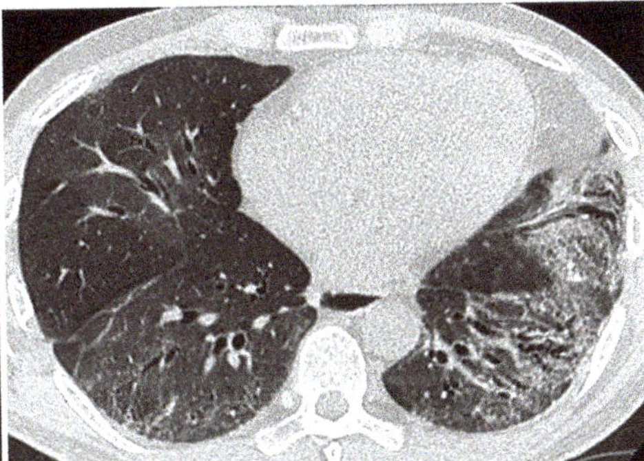

1. **Interpret pulmonary function test.**
2. **What do the clinical pictures demonstrate above?**
3. **What is your diagnosis?**
4. **How this patient can be monitored?**
5. **What is the treatment option?**

Answers

1. Pulmonary function test demonstrates:
   a. Reduction of FEV_1, FVC, and total lung capacity
   b. Residual volume but
   c. Increased FEV_1/FVC ratio

   Above points indicate restrictive lung disease.

2. The above clinical picture demonstrates:
   a. Skin tightening, induration as well as thickening around the fingers
   b. Fish-mouth appearance
   c. Dilatation of esophagus without any organic obstruction indicating esophageal dysmotility
   d. CT scan of thorax demonstrates:
      - Reticular and reticulonodular shadow throughout the lungs bilaterally
      - Ground-glass appearance bilaterally in the base of the lungs

3. This patient has been suffering from interstitial lung disease in a case of systemic sclerosis.

4. This patient can be monitored in the following ways—as this disease involves multiple organs such as lungs, heart, kidneys, hence, multidisciplinary follow-up is required such as pulmonary function test, echocardiography, renal function test, and pulmonary arterial pressure. Following factors promoting the initiation of treatment are:
   a. Deterioration in chest X-ray or pulmonary function test over 6–12 months
   b. Duration of the systemic disease is <5 years.
   c. Patient is anti-Scl-70 positive.
   d. Severe respiratory disease, like:
      - In CT, there is extensive disease.
      - Moderate-to-severe reduction in TL_{CO}
      - Restrictive ventilator defect

5. a. Immunosuppressive therapy:
      - Mycophenolate mofetil: It is the 1st line of action as it will improve the progression of the disease.
      - Cyclophosphamide: It will reduce the progression of decline in FVC and improving the respiratory distress.
      - Rituximab: Monoclonal antibody to CD20 + B cells. It is used as refractory cases to immunosuppressive therapies.
      - Tocilizumab: It is interleukin-6 receptor antagonist. It will stabilize the lung function.
   b. Antifibrotic therapy:
      - Nintedanib: It is tyrosine kinase inhibitor, slows the decline of FVC and useful in progressive lung fibrosis.
      - Pirfenidone: It is used in case of progressive pulmonary fibrosis.

CASE 7

A 40-year-old female having history of rhinitis and nasal polyp has been admitted with progressively increasing breathlessness which was exacerbated with exercise but improved with bronchodilator, cough with scanty, and thread-like sputum and fever.

On examination, the accessory muscles of respiration were active, tachycardia, tachypnea, and pulsus paradoxus. On auscultation, there was diffuse rhonchi throughout the chest bilaterally.

1. **What is your diagnosis?**
2. **What are the triggering factors in this disease?**
3. **Defined this disease.**
4. **Describe the anatomy of the bronchi.**
5. **What are the different types of asthma?**
6. **What do you mean by acute severe asthma?**
7. **What are life-threatening indicators in case of acute asthma?**
8. **What are the indicators of severe life-threatening attack in this patient?**

Answers

1. This patient has been suffering from acute bronchial asthma.
2. Following are the triggering factors in bronchial asthma:
   a. Viral infection
   b. Emotion
   c. Exercise
   d. Drugs like β-blockers
   e. External antigens
   f. Gastroesophageal reflux disease
   g. Chronic sinusitis

h. Tobacco smoking

i. Obesity

j. Chemical fumes

3. This disease is characterized by musical sound heard by the passage of air through the narrowed bronchi.

4. There are three types of bronchi:

   i. Cartilaginous bronchi

   ii. Membranous bronchi

   iii. Gas exchange bronchi including respiratory bronchioles and alveolar duct

Smallest nongas exchange bronchioles, i.e., terminal bronchioles have diameter of 0.5 mm.

Structure of the airways include:

- Mucosa consisting of epithelial cells responsible for specialized mucus production
- Basement membrane
- Smooth muscle cells extending to entrances of the airways
- Supports of connective tissue consisting of fibrocartilaginous tissue

Cellular elements include:

- Mast cells responsible for control of histamine and other mediators
- Basophils, eosinophils, neutrophils, and macrophages responsible for release of mediators extensively in early and distal phase of bronchial asthma.

5. Following are the types of asthma:

a. Allergic asthma

b. Extrinsic asthma

c. Intrinsic asthma

d. Brittle asthma

e. Seasonal asthma

f. Occupational asthma

g. Difficult asthma

h. Severe asthma

i. Atopic asthma

6. Features of acute severe asthma are as follows:

a. Inability of the patient to complete the sentence in one breath

b. Rate of respiration is >25 breaths/min.

c. Pulse is >112 beats/min, regular.

d. Peak expiratory flow rate is <50% predicted.

7. Following are the life-threatening indicators in case of acute asthma:

a. Exhaustion

b. Confusion

c. Coma

d. Peak expiratory flow rate is <33% of predicted.

e. Bradycardia or hypotension

8. Following are the indicators of very severe life-threatening attack:

a. Normal or increased carbon dioxide tension

b. Low pH

c. PO_2 is <60 mm Hg.

CASE 8

A 55-year-old smoker for >30 years came to emergency department with cough with yellowish expectoration for last 15 days and progressively increasing respiratory distress for 5 days.

On examination, patient was in flexed posture with pursued lip breathing, central cyanosis, raised jugular venous pressure, and edema feet. Respiratory system examination demonstrated barrel-shaped chest, intercostal suction, and excavation of the supraclavicular, infraclavicular, and suprasternal fossae. Palpation demonstrated diminished movement of the chest bilaterally and percussion was hyperresonance bilaterally. On auscultation, there is diminished breath sound with prolonged expiration, diminished vocal resonance, and absent-added sound.

1. **What is your diagnosis?**
2. **How can you define this disease?**
3. **What is chronic bronchitis with or without exacerbation?**
4. **What are the accessory muscles of respiration?**
5. **What factors will happen when respiratory movement is decreased?**
6. **What are the Global Initiative for Chronic Obstructive Lung Disease (GOLD) criteria of COPD?**
7. **What are the features of advanced COPD?**
8. **What are the bedside signs of emphysema?**
9. **What are the complications in this disease?**
10. **What is congenital lobar emphysema?**
11. **What is bullous emphysema?**

Answers

1. This patient has been suffering from COPD in a smoker having central cyanosis.

2. Chronic obstructive pulmonary disease can be defined as chronic progressive disorder having airflow obstruction, i.e., $FEV_1 < 80\%$ predicted and FEV_1/FVC ratio $< 70\%$ which will not be changed over several months.

3. Chronic bronchitis can be defined as cough with or without production of sputum on most of the days in a week for at least 3 months in 1 year for 2 consecutive years. Chronic bronchitis with exacerbation can be defined as acute exacerbation such as appearance of fever and production of persistent or recurrent mucopurulent sputum in absence of lung abscess or bronchiectasis.

4. Following are the accessory muscles of respiration:
   a. Alae nasi
   b. Sternocleidomastoid muscles
   c. Trapezius
   d. Serratus anterior
   e. Scaleni
   f. Latissimus dorsi
   g. Pectoralis
   h. Accessory muscles of respiration
   i. Abdominal muscles

5. Following factors will happen when respiratory movement is decreased:
   a. Reduced expansion of the chest
   b. Palpable length of the trachea will be reduced along with tracheal tug.
   c. Intercostal recession
   d. Hyperactive accessory muscles of respiration
   e. Widening of the subcostal angle
   f. Excavation of infraclavicular, supraclavicular fossae, and suprasternal notch.

6. GOLD criteria of chronic obstructive lung disease are as follows:

Gold stage	Severity	Symptoms	Spirometry
0	At risk	Chronic cough and production of sputum	Normal
I	Mild	With or without chronic cough and production of sputum	$FEV_1/FVC < 70\%$ $FEV_1 = 80\%$ predicted
II	Moderate	With or without chronic cough and production of sputum	$FEV_1/FVC < 70\%$ $FEV_1 = 50–79\%$ predicted
III	Severe	With or without chronic cough and production of sputum	$FEV_1/FVC < 70\%$ $FEV_1 = 30–49\%$ predicted
IV	Very severe	With or without chronic cough and production of sputum	$FEV_1/FVC < 70\%$ $FEV_1 = <30\%$ predicted

7. These are the signs of advanced airflow obstruction:
   a. Evidence of dyspnea or orthopnea with pursed lips
   b. Excavation of the suprasternal notch, supraclavicular, and infraclavicular fossa.
   c. Central cyanosis
   d. Barrel-shaped chest
   e. Pulsus paradoxus
   f. Reduction of the palpable tracheal length above the suprasternal notch
   g. Bounding pulses
   h. Flapping tremor
   i. Rhonchi on forced expiration

8. Following are the bedside signs of emphysema bilaterally:
   a. Pursed lip during breathing
   b. Chest shape is barrel-shaped.
   c. Apex beat is not palpable.
   d. Chest movement is diminished.
   e. Diminished expansion of chest
   f. Vocal fremitus and resonance diminished
   g. Percussion note is hyperresonant
   h. Diminished vesicular breath sound
   i. Muffled heart sound
   j. Cardiac as well as liver dullness will be obliterated.
   k. Palpable even in absence of hepatomegaly

9. Complications of COPD are as follows:
   a. Pneumothorax due to rupture of bulla
   b. Cor pulmonale
   c. Recurrent pulmonary infection
   d. Congestive cardiac failure
   e. Type 2 respiratory failure
   f. Hypoxia resulting in secondary polycythemia

10. Rarely infant develops this disease due to check valve mechanism in the bronchus leading to unilateral threatening overdistention of the alveoli.

11. Bulla can be defined as distention of the air spaces of >1 cm in diameter which may be congenital. But if this bulla appears in case of generalized emphysema or progressive fibrosis, it is known as bullous emphysema.

CASE 9

A 25-year-old man came to medical outdoor with spiky rise of temperature, pain in the left lower chest, cough with rusty sputum for 5 days, and respiratory distress for 2 days.

On examination, patient was toxic looking, pulse rate 112 beats/min, respiratory rate 28 breaths/min, and herpes labialis. Chest infection demonstrated trachea central, accessory muscles were active, and movement restricted on one side. Vocal fremitus increased and woody dull on percussion. On auscultation, bronchial breath sound, crackles, and friction rub over the left lower part of the chest.

1. **What is your diagnosis?**
2. **Why there is chest pain?**
3. **What are the stages in this disease?**
4. **In which persons, there is presence of consolidation in chest X-ray but asymptomatic?**
5. **What are the causes of consolidation of lung?**
6. **What are the features of viral etiology?**
7. **What are the extrapulmonary manifestations in this case?**
8. **Name the causes of recurrent pneumonia.**
9. **What is nonresolution and what are the causes?**
10. **What are the types of bacterial infection in this disease?**
11. **What are the atypical and typical form of this disease?**
12. **Name five features indicating the etiology in this disease.**
13. **What are the complications in this disease?**

Answers

1. The most likely diagnosis is acute lobar pneumonia.
2. Chest pain in this case is due to involvement of the pleura overlying the lesion resulting to development of friction in-between the pleura resulting in pleural friction rub.
3. There are four stages in this disease:
   a. Stage of congestion:
      - Diminished vesicular breath sound
      - Appearance of inspiratory crackles due to alveolitis
   b. Stage of red hepatization: All the signs of consolidation
   c. Stage of gray hepatization: All the signs of consolidation
   d. Stage of resolution:
      - Bronchial breathing is replaced by either bronchovesicular or vesicular breathing.
      - Presence of inspiratory and expiratory crackles

4. In following patients, features of consolidation are present but asymptomatic:
   a. Elderly
   b. Alcoholic
   c. Immunocompromised
   d. Neutropenia
5. Following are the causes of consolidation:
   a. Pneumonia
   b. Apical tuberculosis
   c. Bronchogenic carcinoma
   d. Massive pulmonary infarction
   e. Collagen vascular disease
6. Features of viral pneumonia are as follows:
   a. Constitutional symptoms
   b. There may be no respiratory symptoms.
   c. Cough with mucoid expectoration
   d. Hemoptysis
   e. Physical signs are lacking.
   f. Reticulonodular pattern in the chest X-ray

g. Evidence of spontaneous resolution

h. Normal white blood cell count

7. Extrapulmonary manifestations in this case are as follows:

a. Articular:
   - Arthritis
   - Arthralgia

b. Cardiac:
   - Myocarditis
   - Pericarditis

c. Blood: Autoimmune hemolytic anemia

d. Skin:
   - Erythema nodosum
   - Stevens–Johnson syndrome

e. Hepatitis

f. Glomerulonephritis

8. Causes of recurrent pneumonia are as follows:

a. Chronic bronchitis

b. Pharyngeal pouch

c. Bronchial tumor

d. Hypoglobulinemia

e. Gastroesophageal reflux disease

f. Achalasia cardia

9. Nonresolution can be defined as persistence of radiological findings in spite of 8 weeks of proper antibiotic therapy. The causes of nonresolution of the radiological features are as follows:

a. Inappropriate antibiotic therapy

b. Appearance of complication

c. Decreased immunity:
   - Diabetes mellitus
   - Alcoholism
   - Steroid therapy
   - Neutropenia
   - Acquired immunodeficiency syndrome (AIDS)
   - Hypogammaglobulinemia

d. Partial bronchial obstruction:
   - Bronchial tumor
   - Foreign body in the bronchus

e. Fungal infection

f. Pulmonary infarction

g. SLE

h. Gastroesophageal reflux disease

i. Achalasia cardia

10. Types of bacterial pneumonia are as follows:

a. Community-acquired pneumonia or CAP: It can be defined as infection of the lung tissue acquiring from the community or within 48 hours of hospital admission.

b. Hospital-acquired pneumonia or HAP: It can be defined as infection of the lung tissue in non-intubated patient after 48 hours of hospitalization.

c. Ventilator-associated pneumonia or VAP: It can be defined as the infection of the lung tissue develops in a patient 48 hours or more after intubation for mechanical ventilation.

d. Healthcare-associated pneumonia or HCAP: It can be defined as infection of the lung tissue acquiring from the healthcare personnel in nursing home, dialysis center, and outpatient department of patients having history of hospitalization.

11. Typical form of this disease can be cultured in the typical media. The causes of typical form of this disease are as follows:

a. *Streptococcus pneumoniae*

b. *Haemophilus influenzae*

c. *Staphylococcus aureus*

d. Group A streptococci

e. *Moraxella catarrhalis*

f. Anaerobes

g. Aerobic gram-negative bacteria

Atypical forms caused by:

a. *Legionella*

b. *Mycoplasma pneumoniae*

c. *Chlamydia pneumoniae*

d. *Chlamydia psittaci*

12. Following five features indicate the etiology of this disease:

a. Bradycardia: *Legionella*

b. Impaired gag reflex: Aspiration pneumonia

c. Bullous myringitis: *Mycoplasma*

d. Dental illness: Anaerobes

e. Cutaneous nodules: Nocardiosis

13. Complications in this disease are as follows:

a. Cavitation

b. Empyema

c. Lung fibrosis

d. Necrotizing pneumonia

e. Pulmonary abscess

f. Meningitis

g. Death

CASE 10

A 65-year-old female came to medicine outdoor with chest pain along with cough for 25 days and she was advised a course of antibiotic and chest X-ray. She also complained of change in the voice during this course. His chest X-ray demonstrated:

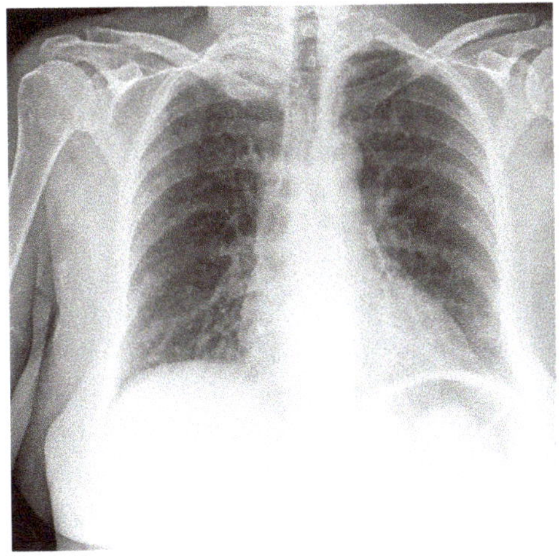

1. **What is the most likely diagnosis?**
2. **What will be the feature of the malignant consolidation?**
3. **Name the extrapulmonary manifestations in this disease.**
4. **What are the types of manifestations of this disease?**
5. **What are the indications of radiotherapy in this disease?**
6. **How can you evaluate this disease?**
7. **What are the complications in this disease?**

Answers

1. The patient has been suffering from bronchogenic carcinoma.
2. Following are the features of malignant consolidation:
   a. Elderly patient
   b. Smoker for long duration
   c. Progressively increasing dyspnea
   d. Hemoptysis
   e. Pleuritic chest pain
   f. Weight loss
   g. Malignant cachexia
   h. There may be shifting of trachea if there is associated collapse.
   i. Cervical lymphadenopathy
   j. Signs of consolidation
   k. Local spread to:
      - Pleura leading to pleural effusion
      - Hilar lymph nodes leading to dysphagia in case of compression to esophagus
      - Dysphonia in case of compression of recurrent laryngeal nerve
      - Paralysis of right dome of diaphragm due to involvement of right phrenic nerve
      - Superior vena cava syndrome
      - Monoplegia due to involvement of the brachial plexus
      - Horner syndrome due to compression on the cervical sympathetic nerve.
3. Extrapulmonary manifestations are as follows:
   a. Endocrine manifestations:
      - Adrenocorticotropic hormone (ACTH): Cushing's syndrome
      - Antidiuretic hormone (ADH): Hyponatremia
      - Parathyroid hormone (PTH): Hypercalcemia
      - Serotonin: Carcinoid syndrome
      - Erythropoietin: Polycythemia
      - Insulin-like peptide: Hypoglycemia
      - Sex hormone: Gynecomastia
   b. Dermatological manifestations:
      - Acanthosis nigricans
      - Pruritus
   c. Neurological manifestations:
      - Encephalopathy

- Polyneuropathy
- Myelopathy
- Myopathy
- Amyotrophy
d. Skeletal manifestation—digital clubbing
e. Muscular manifestations:
- Polymyositis
- Dermatomyositis
- Lambert–Eaton syndrome
f. Hematological manifestations:
- Hemolytic anemia
- Thrombocytopenia
g. Vascular manifestation: Migratory thrombo-phlebitis

4. Following are the types of pulmonary manifestations:
a. Partial bronchial obstruction leading to collapse of the lung
b. Solid mass leading to consolidation
c. Secondary degeneration and necrosis in the tumor leading to cavitation in the tumor
d. Compression of the mediastinal structures leading to:
- Superior vena cava syndrome
- Dysphonia
- Dysphagia
- Paralysis of diaphragm
- Intercostal neuralgia
- Pericardial effusion
- Chylous pleural effusion
- Monoplegia

5. Indications of radiotherapy in this disease are as follows:
a. Dysphagia
b. Hemoptysis
c. Bronchial obstruction
d. Pancoast tumor
e. Mediastinal compression
f. Before and after surgery

6. Evaluation of the lung cancer: Lung cancer can be evaluated by the following mechanisms:
a. Radiological imaging:
- Contrast-enhanced CT scan to evaluate:
  - Tumor-related atelectasis
  - Postobstructive pneumonitis
  - Intrathoracic metastasis
  - Extrathoracic metastasis
  - Coexisting lung disease
- Positron emission tomography-computed tomography (PET-CT) to detect the potential sites of metastasis.
b. Invasive staging:
- Bronchoscopic endobronchial ultrasound—transbronchial aspiration by needle
- Endoscopic transbronchial aspiration by needle
- Mediastinoscopy
- Thoracoscopy or video-assisted thoracoscopy

7. Complications in this disease are as follows:
a. Chemotherapy-induced nausea and vomiting
b. Fatigue
c. Weight loss
d. Anorexia
e. Neutropenia
f. Anemia
g. Nephrotoxicity
h. Neurotoxicity

CASE 11

A 29-year-old man admitted in the emergency department with high fever with chill and rigor, chest pain for 3 days, and progressively increasing breathlessness for 1 day. Chest X-ray demonstrated:

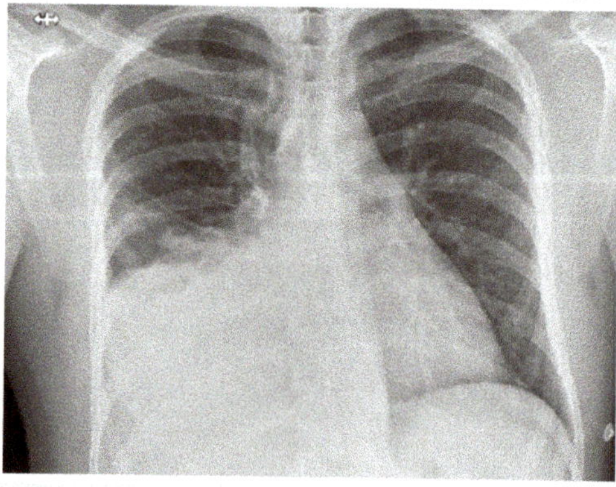

1. **What is your diagnosis?**
2. **What are the histories to be taken to diagnose this case?**
3. **How can you differentiate this disease from thickened pleura?**
4. **What are the differentiating points to differentiate this disease from pleural effusion?**

Answers

1. This patient has been suffering from empyema thoracis.
2. Histories are as follows:
   a. History of cough with purulent sputum:
      - Lung abscess
      - Bronchiectasis
   b. History of chest injury: Hemithorax
   c. History of aspiration in bedridden patient— aspiration pneumonia
3. Differences between the empyema thoracis and thickened pleura:

Thickened pleura	Empyema thoracis
There may be retraction of the chest on the involved side	There is bulging of the chest on the affected side
Movement may be diminished	Movement of the affected side is markedly diminished

Continued

Continued

There is no shifting of the trachea	Trachea will be shifted toward opposite side
Woody dull percussion note	Stony dull percussion note
Diminished breath sound on the affected side	Breath sound will be absent on the affected side
Presence of toxemia	Absence of toxemia
Absence of intercostal tenderness	Presence of intercostal tenderness

4. Following are the differentiating points of empyema thoracis as compared to pleural effusion:
   a. Toxemia
   b. Intercostal tenderness
   c. Clubbing of the fingers

CASE 12

A 50-year-old man having long-standing history of cough with recurrent copious expectoration for >5 years came to chest outdoor with high fever and cough with profuse fetid expectoration for 4 days.

On examination, he had retraction in the lower part of the chest. On auscultation, there was coarse crackles in the left lower bases. HRCT of chest demonstrated:

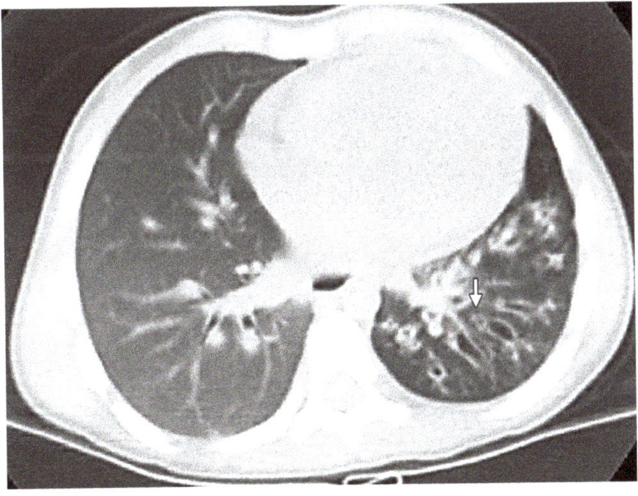

1. **What are the differential diagnoses?**
2. **After HRCT of chest, what is the diagnosis?**
3. **In case of bronchopulmonary aspergillosis, which part of the lung will be involved by this disease?**
4. **What is dry and wet form of the disease?**
5. **What are the abnormalities associated with this disease?**
6. **What are the complications in this disease?**
7. **What are the types in this disease?**
8. **What are the clinical features to detect the etiology in this disease?**
9. **What are the cardinal signs of bronchiectasis in CT scan?**
10. **What are the patterns of findings in this disease in CT scan of lung?**

Answers

1. The differential diagnoses are:
    a. Tubercular cavity with full of exudate
    b. Empyema thoracis with bronchopleural fistula
    c. Cystic fibrosis
2. HRCT of chest demonstrated several lower lobe cylindrical bronchiectasis, thereby the diagnosis is infective bronchiectasis.
3. In case of bronchopulmonary aspergillosis, proximal bronchi will be dilated leading to proximal bronchiectasis.
4. In case of wet bronchiectasis, there is chronic cough with massive purulent sputum mainly in the morning on lateral or lying down position along with dilated airways in the HRCT of thorax.

    In case of dry bronchiectasis, the patient may be asymptomatic or evidence of recurrent nonproductive cough along with hemoptysis and the upper lobe bronchi will be involved.
5. Following anomalies are associated with this disease:
    a. Congenital absence of bronchial cartilage
    b. Azoospermia
    c. Tracheobronchomegaly
    d. Congenital kyphoscoliosis
    e. Chronic sinopulmonary infection
    f. Situs inversus
6. Complications in this disease are as follows:
    a. Recurrent pneumonitis
    b. Cor pulmonale
    c. Secondary amyloidosis
    d. Bacteremia leading to septicemia
    e. Meningitis leading to brain abscess
    f. Pulmonary apoplexy due to massive hemoptysis
    g. Aspergilloma in the bronchiectatic cavity
7. Following are the types in this disease:
    a. Cylindrical bronchiectasis: Here, the bronchi are uniformly dilated.
    b. Varicose bronchiectasis: Here, the bronchi are irregular and beaded in appearance.
    c. Saccular bronchiectasis: Here, the bronchi are ballooned or cystic in appearance.
8. Clinical features to detect the etiology of this disease are as follows:
    a. Localized wheezing: Bronchial obstruction
    b. Widespread wheezing: Bronchopulmonary aspergillosis
    c. Connective tissue disease: Arthritis and rashes
    d. Cystic fibrosis: Recurrent sinus disease and infertility
9. The cardinal signs of bronchiectasis in CT scan are as follows:
    a. Bronchoarterial ratio of >1
    b. Lack of bronchial tapering
    c. Airway is visible within 1 cm of the pleural surface or abutting the mediastinal pleural surface.
10. Following are the features in CT scan of chest in bronchiectasis:
    a. Tram-track sign in case of cylindrical bronchiectasis
    b. Signet ring: This is characterized by dilated bronchi adjacent to branches of pulmonary artery giving ring appearance, i.e., internal diameter of bronchi is greater than that of adjacent pulmonary artery.
    c. Cystic or saccular where there are thin-walled cystic spaces.
    d. Varicose looks like nonuniform dilatation of bronchi
    e. Mosaic lung attenuation characterized by heterogeneous density of lung in the damaged segment in the lung due to tapping of air in geographical distribution
    f. Dilated bronchial arteries

CASE 13

A 40-year-old man came to chest outdoor with complaint of recurrent cough with copious production of sputum for several years. Also, he complained of recurrent abdominal pain along with greasy diarrhea for last several years. On examination, there was foul-smelling breath, clubbing of the fingers, and anemia. He had no issue.

1. **What is your most likely diagnosis?**
2. **What are the points in favor of your diagnosis?**
3. **What are the tests to be done to confirm the diagnosis?**
4. **What is cause of the "no issue" in this patient?**
5. **What is the cause of this type of stool in this patient?**
6. **In this patient, what are the organisms responsible for purulent sputum?**
7. **What is the significance of sweat testing in this disease?**
8. **Is there any risk of cancer in this patient?**
9. **What are the causes of death in this patient?**
10. **What are the investigations to be done in this disease?**

Answers

1. The most likely diagnosis is cystic fibrosis.
2. Following points are in favor of this diagnosis:
   a. Male patient
   b. Purulent massive amount of sputum
   c. Presence of steatorrhea
   d. Anemia
3. Following are the tests to be done in this case:
   a. Urine for sugar
   b. Fecal content of fat
   c. Sweat sodium
4. "No issue" is due to azoospermia which is the result of absent vas deferens.
5. Steatorrhea in this patient is due to blockage of the pancreatic duct by the abnormal mucus. There is also obstruction of the biliary tract.
6. Following organisms are responsible for purulent sputum:
   a. *Haemophilus influenzae*
   b. *Staphylococcus aureus*
   c. *Pseudomonas aeruginosa*
   d. *Burkholderia cepacia*
7. If the serum sweat concentration is >60 mmol/L, it indicates cystic fibrosis.
8. There is risk of malignancy of gastrointestinal tract. Hence, persistent symptoms of gastrointestinal tract should be treated very carefully.

9. The causes of death in this disease are the following:
   a. Pneumonia
   b. Pneumothorax
   c. Bronchiectasis
   All may lead to acute respiratory failure and death.
10. Following investigations should be done in this patient:
    a. Chest X-ray to demonstrate:
       - Apical bronchiectasis
       - Pneumonia
       - Prominence of the bronchovascular markings
       - Focal atelectasis
       - Round peripheral opacities
    b. CT scan for confirmation of the Chest X-ray findings
    c. Arterial blood gases analysis
    d. Pulmonary function test to detect the pattern of lung function
    e. Sputum for culture sensitivity
    f. Pilocarpine iontophoresis sweat test
    g. Nasal membrane potential difference
    h. Pancreatic exocrine function test
    i. Semen analysis to detect azoospermia or oligospermia
    j. Genotyping for genetic mutation

CASE 14

A 39-year-old coal miner worker came to emergency department with progressive exertional respiratory distress, dry cough for 2 months, and fever and weight loss for 2 weeks.

On examination, there was tachycardia, tachypnea, central cyanosis, and grade 3 clubbing. Chest examination demonstrated movement of the chest has been restricted bilaterally, active accessory muscles, on palpation, reduced vocal fremitus, reduced expansion of the chest, and on percussion lung bases were dull. On auscultation, there was diminished breath sound and end-expiratory crackles at both bases.

1. **What are the causes of basal crackles in patient with clubbing?**
2. **What is the most likely diagnosis?**
3. **What is Hamman–Rich syndrome?**
4. **What do you mean by respiratory bronchiolitis?**
5. **What are the types in this coal miner disease?**

Answers

1. The causes of crackles at the base of the lung with clubbing:
   a. Bronchogenic carcinoma
   b. Bronchiectasis
   c. Asbestosis
   d. Interstitial pulmonary fibrosis
   e. Fibrosing alveolitis
2. The most likely diagnosis is coal worker's pneumoconiosis.
3. Hamman–Rich syndrome is acute onset disease characterized by progressively increasing dyspnea, fever, dry cough, weight loss, and evidences of bilateral pulmonary fibrosis.
4. Respiratory bronchiolitis is an interstitial lung disease characterized by infiltration of the mononuclear cells as well as fibrosis due to accumulation of pigment laden macrophages in the respiratory bronchioles.
5. There are two types of coal worker pneumoconiosis:
   a. Simple coal worker pneumoconiosis is reversible nonprogressive disease radiologically characterized by presence of nodules without cavitation.
   b. Progressive massive fibrosis is irreversible and progressive disease characterized by radiologically single of multiple nodular masses with cavitation involving mainly upper lobes.

CASE 15

A 25-year-old male presented in the emergency department with fever with chill and rigor, cough with copious purulent foul-smelling expectoration increased more during lying down position for 5 days not responding to first-generation cephalosporin, and chest pain for 4 days and respiratory distress for 2 days. He had no history of tuberculosis.

On examination, the patient looked toxic, tachycardia, pallor, tachypnea, grade 3 clubbing, and no hepatomegaly. There was intercostal tenderness in the right lower chest.

Chest X-ray demonstrated:

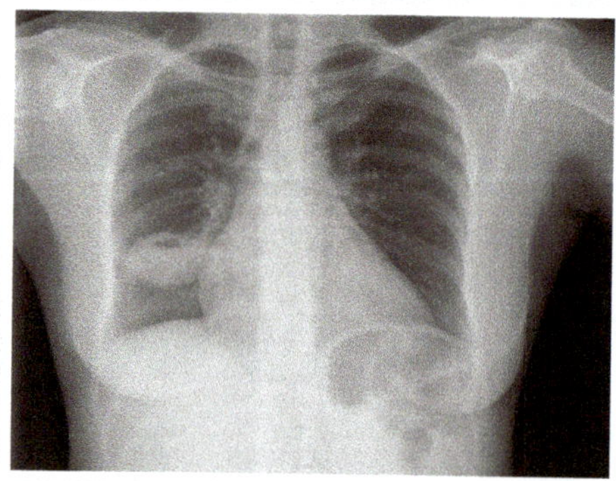

1. **What has been demonstrating in the chest X-ray?**
2. **What is the diagnosis?**
3. **What are the points in favor of your diagnosis?**
4. **What are the factors predisposing to lung abscess development?**
5. **What are the bronchogenic causes of lung abscess?**
6. **What are the causes of lung abscess?**
7. **What are the sites of the lung abscess?**
8. **If there is edema in this patient, what it will indicate?**
9. **Why it is not a case of loculated empyema?**

Answers

1. The straight X-ray demonstrated evidence of round lesion having well-circumscribed border and air-fluid level. It is a case of lung abscess.
2. This patient has been suffering from lung abscess.
3. Points in favor of the diagnosis are as follows:
   a. History of chest pain and spiky rise of temperature with chill and rigor
   b. Purulent fetid expectoration and amount is copious.
   c. Foul breath
   d. X-ray feature of lung abscess
4. Following are the predisposing factors:
   a. Immunocompromised host
   b. Posttransplantation
   c. Patients receiving immunosuppressive therapies
   d. Patients are at high risk of aspiration:
      - Seizures
      - Bulbar dysfunction
      - Alcohol intoxication
      - Cognitive impairment
5. Bronchogenic causes of lung abscess are bronchial obstruction due to:
   a. Tumor
   b. Foreign body
   c. Enlarged lymph nodes
   d. Congenital malformation
6. The causes of lung abscess are as follows:
   a. Primary abscess due to necrotizing pneumonia:
      - Pyogenic organism:
        o *Staphylococcus aureus*
        o *Klebsiella pneumoniae*
        o Streptococci
      - Tuberculous bacilli

- Fungi:
  o *Aspergillus fumigatus*
  o *Histoplasma capsulatum*
- Amebic liver abscess
   b. Secondary lung abscess:
      - Metastatic lung abscess
      - Bronchogenic carcinoma
      - Thromboembolism leading to cavitation in the lung
7. Sites of lung abscess are as follows:
   a. If the patient is lying down in position:
      - Right lung involving:
        o Posterior segment of upper lobe
        o Superior segment of lower lobe
      - If the patient is upright in position: Basal segment of both the lower lobes.
8. If there will be edema in the affected patient having lung abscess, the causes are:
   a. Hypoproteinemia as a result of loss of protein through the profuse expectoration
   b. Malnutrition
   c. Malabsorption
   d. Renal amyloidosis leading to nephrotic syndrome
9. Differences between loculated empyema and lung abscess:

Loculated empyema	Lung abscess
Shape is lenticular	Shape is round
Wall is uniformly enhanced thick wall	Wall is irregularly enhanced thick wall
Adjacent lung will be compressed	Surrounding lung is not compressed
Visceral and parietal layers of the pleura are separated	Visceral and parietal layers of the pleura are not separated
The angle with the chest wall is obtuse	The angle with the chest wall is acute

CASE 16

A 45-year-old male having past history of tuberculosis 15 years ago getting full course of antitubercular medications came to chest outdoor with the complaint of recurrent hemoptysis, chest pain and weight loss for last 6 months, and cough and purulent expectoration for last 1 week.

On examination, temperature was raised, pulse rate 112 beats/min, tachypnea, and grade 3 clubbing.

Chest examination demonstrated flattening of right upper chest and drooping of the right shoulder, and diminished movement in the same area. Trachea was shifted to the right. On auscultation, there was cavernous type bronchial breath sound and inspiratory and expiratory crackles in the right upper chest.

1. **What is your diagnosis?**
2. **What are the points in favor of your diagnosis?**
3. **What are the differential diagnoses?**
4. **What are the different types of this specific lesion seen in the lung?**
5. **How can you differentiate fluid-filled lesion from empty lesion?**
6. **What is pseudo form of this lesion?**

Answers

1. This patient has been suffering from posttubercular cavitary lesion in the right upper chest.
2. The following points are favor of this diagnosis:
   a. Reduced movement in the right upper part of the chest
   b. Drooping of the right shoulder
   c. Flattening of the right upper chest
   d. Shifting of the trachea to right
   e. Percussion note is dull.
   f. Cavernous type bronchial breath sound
   g. Inspiratory and expiratory crackles
3. Following are the differential diagnoses:
   a. Bronchiectasis
   b. Resolving consolidation
   c. Lung abscess
   d. Malignancy of the lung
4. There are two types of cavitary lesions in the lung:
   a. Thin-walled cavity, if:
      - It is shaggy and irregular—lung abscess and bronchogenic carcinoma
      - It is smooth and regular:
        - Tubercular cavity
        - Hydatid cyst
        - Fungal infection
5. Differentiating points between empty and fluid-filled cavity:
   a. Vocal fremitus and resonance—absent in fluid-filled cavity whereas increased in empty cavity
   b. Breath sound diminished in fluid-filled cavity but cavernous in empty cavity
   c. Whispering pectoriloquy is present in empty cavity but absent in fluid cavity.
   d. Posttussive crepitation present in case fluid-filled cavity but absent in empty cavity.
6. Pseudocavity is an area getting from the summation of shadow of the vessels, ribs, and calcifications.

CASE 17

A 65-year-old smoker male admitted with bovine cough with mucoid expectoration and night sweat with low-grade fever for 6 months, chest pain for 2 months, and progressive hoarseness of voice, and puffiness of the face for last 1 month.

On examination, face was puffy, suffused conjunctiva, engorged nonpulsatile neck vein, and palpable and matted cervical lymph nodes. Percussion of the chest demonstrated widening of the mediastinum. Chest examination demonstrated as described below:

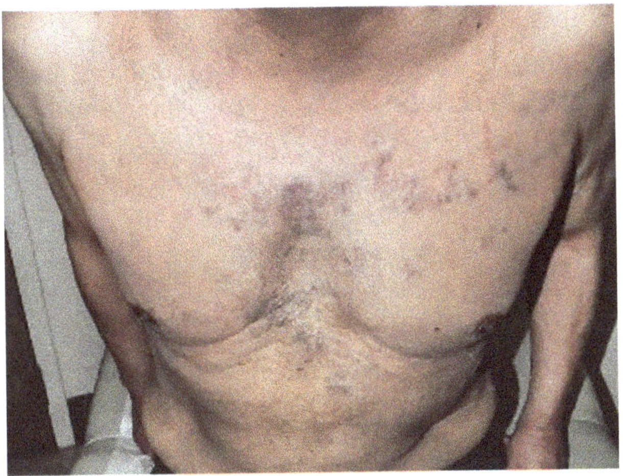

1. **What is the most likely diagnosis?**
2. **What are the points in favor of your diagnosis?**
3. **Mention the boundary of the superior mediastinum.**
4. **What are the structures present in the superior mediastinum?**
5. **Mention the causes of the compression of the superior mediastinum.**
6. **In case of compression of the superior mediastinum, what are the structures involved?**
7. **What do you mean by pneumomediastinum?**

Answers

1. The most likely diagnosis is compression of superior mediastinum by tubercular lymphadenitis.
2. Following points are in favor of the diagnosis:
    a. Suffused face
    b. Hoarseness of the voice
    c. Bovine cough
    d. Engorged nonpulsatile neck veins
    e. Engorged veins in the upper chest
    f. Widening of the mediastinum on percussion
3. Boundaries of the superior mediastinum are as follows:
    a. Above by thoracic inlet
    b. Below by the upper part of the heart and great vessels
    c. Anteriorly by sternum
    d. Posteriorly by spines
4. Structures present in the superior mediastinum:
    a. Lymph nodes
    b. Thymus
    c. Aortic arch
    d. Trachea
    e. Superior vena cava
    f. Esophagus
    g. Connective tissue
5. Following are the causes of compression of the superior mediastinum:
    a. Bronchogenic carcinoma
    b. Tubercular lymphadenitis
    c. Lymphoma
    d. Leukemia
    e. Aortic aneurysm
    f. Esophageal cancer
    g. Mediastinal fibrosis
    h. Pneumomediastinum
6. Following structures are involved in this syndrome:
    a. Esophagus: Dysphagia to both solid and liquid
    b. Trachea: Respiratory distress, stridor, and cough
    c. Nerves:
        - Recurrent laryngeal nerves: Hoarseness of voice and bovine cough

- Phrenic nerve: Diaphragmatic paralysis leading to respiratory paralysis and hiccup (hiccough)
- Cervical sympathetic nerve: Horner syndrome

d. Vessels:
  - Superior vena cava: Suffused face, visual disturbances, headache, and engorged nonpulsatile neck veins
  - Azygos vein: Right-sided pleural effusion
  - Lymphatics: Nonpitting edema in the upper thorax, there may be chylothorax.

7. Pneumomediastinum means collection of air within the mediastinum due to:
   a. Rupture of the alveoli leading to dissection of air into the mediastinum
   b. Perforation of trachea and esophagus
   c. Dissection of air into the mediastinum from neck or abdomen

CASE 18

A 32-year-old female having dust allergy came to chest outdoor with dry cough, low-grade fever, and recurrent breathlessness associated chest pain for 6 months. Blood pressure was normal but respiratory rate 28 breaths/min, and pulse rate 100 beats/min. Chest diffuse rhonchi and coarse crepitations throughout the chest bilaterally. Blood demonstrated eosinophilia:

1. **What is your diagnosis?**
2. **What are the points in favor of your diagnosis?**
3. **What is eosinophilia?**
4. **How can you classify this disease?**
5. **What is hypereosinophilic syndrome?**
6. **What are the clinical characteristics of Loeffler's syndrome?**
7. **What are the criteria of tropical pulmonary eosinophilia?**
8. **What are the histopathological changes in tropical pulmonary eosinophilia?**

Answers

1. It is a case of pulmonary eosinophilic syndrome.
2. Points in favor of this diagnosis are as follows:
   a. Presence of low-grade fever and recurrent breathlessness
   b. Presence of wheeze
   c. Presence of crepitations and rhonchi on auscultation
   d. Presence of blood eosinophilia
3. Normal absolute blood eosinophil count is 440/cc or 4% of total blood count of white blood cells. If the count is above 400/cc or >4% of total blood count, it is known as eosinophilia.
4. This disease can be classified into two types:
   a. Extrinsic types:
      - Helminth infestation:
        - Ascaris
        - Toxocara
        - Filaria
      - Fungi: *Aspergillus fumigatus*
      - Drugs:
        - Nitrofurantoin
        - PAS
        - Chlorpropamide
        - Imipramine
   b. Intrinsic types:
      - Eosinophilic pneumonia
      - Hypereosinophilic syndrome
      - Polyarteritis nodosa
      - Churg–Strauss syndrome
5. Hypereosinophilic syndrome is characterized by:
   a. Peripheral blood eosinophil count is >1,500/cc for at least 6 months.
   b. Absence of extrinsic causes of eosinophilia
   c. Absence of history of allergy
   d. Tissue infiltration by mature eosinophils
   e. Presence of bone marrow eosinophilia
6. Loeffler's syndrome is a benign acute idiopathic eosinophilic pneumonia caused by *Strongyloides stercoralis, Ancylostoma duodenale, Ascaris,* or *Toxocara* which is characterized by migratory pulmonary infiltrate along with cough, respiratory distress, and fever.

7. Criteria of pulmonary eosinophilia are as follows:
    a. Suggestive clinical picture such as fever, cough, and episodic wheezing with or without hematemesis
    b. History of prolonged stay in the endemic area
    c. Lack of microfilaria in the day and night samples of blood
    d. Eosinophil count in the peripheral blood is 3,000/cc.
    e. High titer of antifilarial antibodies
    f. In the chest X-ray, it demonstrates reticulo-nodular shadows
    g. Clinical response to diethylcarbamazine citrate

8. Histopathological changes are as follows:
    a. Histiocytic infiltration of the lung parenchyma
    b. Eosinophilic infiltration of the interstitium leading to formation of eosinophilic abscesses, eosinophilic granuloma as well as eosinophilic bronchopneumonia.
    c. Mixed cells reaction involving histiocytes, epithelioid cells, and lymphocytes at the 6 months to 2 years of onset
    d. If untreated, pulmonary fibrosis will develop.

CASE 19

A 56-year-old man having 118 kg in weight came to medicine outdoor with nighttime storing, daytime somnolence, morning headache, visual disturbances, and retrosternal burning pain.

On examination, his blood pressure was 160/100 mm Hg, pulse rate 100 beats/min, and central cyanosis. Chest examination demonstrated reduced movement of the chest and diminished breath sound. Apex beat was not palpable.

1. **What is your diagnosis?**
2. **Why there was central cyanosis?**
3. **What type of obstruction will occur in this disease and why?**
4. **Why there is hypoventilation?**
5. **What is the importance of neck circumference in this disease?**

Answers

1. The patient has been suffering from Pickwickian syndrome.
2. Central cyanosis occurred due to sleep-induced hypoventilation.
3. The patient has been suffering from obstructive sleep apnea caused by narrowing of the upper airway due to apposition of the tongue and palate against the posterior pharyngeal wall.
4. Alveolar hypoventilation results from:
    a. Blunted respiratory drive
    b. Increased mechanical load imposed on the chest wall muscles
5. Neck circumference acts as predictor of results of positive sleep test in obese patient:
    a. If the patient is hypertensive, 4 cm has to be added.
    b. In case of habitual snorer or if the patient gasps at night, 3 cm has to be added.
    Results:
    - If the circumference is <43 cm, low clinical probability.
    - If the circumference is between 43 and 48 cm, it indicates intermediate probability.
    - If the circumference is >48 cm, high probability.

CASE 20

A 54-year-old nonsmoker man presented with respiratory distress and nonproductive cough on long-standing steroid drugs. On examination, there was peripheral cyanosis, steroid purpura, and grade 4 clubbing but no stigmata of rheumatological diseases.

Chest examination revealed centrally placed trachea, reduced expansion bilaterally, at bases percussion note dull, reduced vocal fremitus, and find end-expiratory crackles.

1. **What is the most likely diagnosis?**
2. **What are the stigmata of the systemic disorders in this disease?**
3. **In case of lymphadenopathy, what will be the cause?**
4. **What are the respiratory causes of clubbing?**
5. **What are the special investigations to be done to detect the etiologies?**
6. **What should be the HRCT findings in this disease?**
7. **What are the causes of apical fibrosis?**
8. **What are the causes of basal fibrosis?**
9. **How can you classify this disease according to the American Thoracic Society?**
10. **What are the complication in this disease?**

Answers

1. The most probable diagnosis is idiopathic pulmonary fibrosis and the patient is on steroid therapy.
2. Stigmata of systemic disorders in this disease are as follows:
   a. Evidence of symmetrical deforming arthropathy and rheumatoid nodules—indicates rheumatoid arthritis
   b. Evidence of CREST phenomenon—indicates systemic sclerosis
   c. Presence of butterfly rash, arthropathy, livedo reticularis, and petechial rash—indicates SLE
   d. Evidence of Gottron's papules, heliotrope rash in the periorbital areas, and proximal myopathy—indicates dermatomyositis.
   e. Evidences of Café-au-lait spots and neurofibroma—indicate neurofibromatosis
   f. Absence of lumbar lordosis, stooped posture, and fixed kyphosis—indicates ankylosing spondylosis
   g. History of radiation therapy in the chest wall and erythema—indicates radiation therapy
   h. Presence of erythema nodosum, lupus pernio, lymphadenopathy, and maculopapular skin rash—indicates sarcoidosis
   i. Presence of slate-gray pigmentation and irregular pulse rate—indicates drugs like amiodarone
3. If there is lymphadenopathy, it indicates sarcoidosis.
4. Following are the respiratory causes of clubbing:
   a. Bronchiectasis
   b. Bronchogenic carcinoma
   c. Lung abscess
   d. Empyema
   e. Interstitial lung disease
   f. Cystic fibrosis
   g. Tuberculosis
   h. Mesothelioma

5. Following are the special investigations to be done to detect the etiology:
   a. Complete blood count:
      - Anemia: Vasculitis
      - Polycythemia: In case of hypoxia
      - Leukocytosis: Hypersensitivity pneumonitis
   b. Creatine phosphokinase (CPK)—increased in polymyositis and dermatomyositis
   c. Precipitating antibodies in case of hypersensitivity pneumonitis
   d. Serum angiotensin-converting enzyme—increased in sarcoidosis
   e. Autoimmune profile:
      - ANA
      - Extractable nuclear antigen
      - Antineutrophil cytoplasmic antibody
      - Antiglomerular basement membrane antibodies
   f. Rheumatoid factor
6. HRCT findings in this disease:
   a. Coarse reticular, linear opacities, and cystic air spaces—indicate fibrotic histopathological process
   b. Ground-glass opacities—indicate cellular inflammatory processes
7. Causes of apical fibrosis in the lung are as follows:
   a. Radiation
   b. Extrinsic allergic alveolitis
   c. Tuberculosis
   d. Silicosis
   e. Coal-worker pneumoconiosis
   f. Psoriasis
   g. Berylliosis
   h. Allergic bronchopulmonary aspergillosis
   i. Sarcoidosis
8. Causes of basal fibrosis in the lung are as follows:
   a. Asbestosis
   b. Idiopathic pulmonary fibrosis

c. Connective tissue disease
d. Rheumatic diseases except ankylosing spondylosis and psoriasis
e. Drugs

9. Classification of this disease according to the American Thoracic Society criteria:
   a. Acute interstitial pneumonia
   b. Usual interstitial pneumonia
   c. Nonspecific interstitial pneumonia
   d. Desquamative interstitial pneumonia
   e. Lymphoid interstitial pneumonia
   f. Cryptogenic organizing pneumonia
   g. Respiratory bronchiolitis—interstitial lung disease

10. Complications of this disease are:
    a. Recurrent chest infection
    b. Respiratory failure
    c. Pulmonary hypertension
    d. Bronchogenic carcinoma
    e. Cor pulmonale

CASE 21

A 55-year-old smoker came to emergency department with breathlessness at rest and wheeze heard from distance in unaided ear.

On examination, there was pursed-lip breathing, trachea central, and reduced cricoid notch distance. His accessory muscles are active and hyperresonant notes on percussion bilaterally. On auscultation, there was diminished breath sound with prolonged expiration and forced expiration time was >6 seconds.

1. **What is the most likely diagnosis?**
2. **How can you define chronic obstructive lung disease, chronic bronchitis, and emphysema?**
3. **What is the pathophysiology in this disease?**
4. **What are the common causes of this disease?**
5. **What are the types of emphysema?**
6. **What should be the chest X-ray features in this disease?**
7. **What are the findings in the blood indicating some pathology/etiology?**
8. **Mention the requirements for the long-term oxygen therapy in this patient.**
9. **What is the importance of α1-antitrypsin in this disease?**

Answers

1. The most likely diagnosis is COPD.
2. Definitions are:
   a. Chronic obstructive pulmonary disease: It is characterized by progressive as well as irreversible airflow obstruction as a result of chronic bronchitis and emphysema.
   b. Chronic bronchitis: It is characterized by coughing of productive sputum on most of the days for at least 3 months in the 2 consecutive years.
   c. Emphysema: This is characterized by permanently enlarged air spaces distal to terminal bronchioles along with the destruction of the walls of the alveoli in absence of fibrosis. It is pathological diagnosis.
3. Pathophysiology in this disease:
   a. In the large central airways, peripheral bronchioles and lung parenchyma activate neutrophils and macrophages liberate elastases that cannot be effectively neutralized by the antiproteases leading to destruction of the lung parenchyma.
   b. Smoking also releases elastases and neutrophil chemotactic factors
   c. Smoking also leads to increased oxidative stress due to formation of free radicals leading to cellular apoptosis and cellular death
   d. In chronic bronchitis:
      - There is hyperplasia of the bronchial wall smooth muscles.
      - Bronchial wall thickening due to edema
      - Ciliary abnormalities
      - Focal squamous metaplasia

      In the respiratory bronchiole, there is:
      - Additional plugging by mucus
      - Goblet cell metaplasia
      - Hyperplasia of the smooth muscle cells
      - Fibrosis

4. Common causes of this disease are the following:
   a. Smoking
   b. Coal dust
   c. $\alpha 1$-antitrypsin deficiency
   d. Centriacinar pattern
   e. Panacinar pattern
   f. Mixed centriacinar and panacinar pattern
5. Types of emphysema are the following:

Types	Involvement of airways	Pattern of damage
Centriacinar type	• Respiratory bronchioles • Central portion of acinus • Distal alveolar duct and alveoli are well-preserved	Upper lobes and apex are more involved as compared to lower lobes
Panacinar type	Whole acinus, entire alveolar duct distal to terminal bronchiole	Lower lobes are more as compared to upper lobes and apex

6. Chest X-ray demonstrates:
   a. Hyperinflated lung field
   b. Flattened diaphragm
   c. Tubular heart shadow
   d. Presence of bullae
   e. Hilar vasculature is prominent with peripheral pruning
   f. In lateral view there is increased retrosternal airspace.
7. Findings in the blood indicating the etiology:
   a. Increased white blood cell count indicating acute exacerbation of the disease
   b. Increased hemoglobin indicating secondary polycythemia
   c. Serum potassium as it will be decreased in case of long-standing bronchodilator.
   d. Liver function test indicating deficiency of $\alpha 1$-antitrypsin
   e. Inflammatory markers in case of acute exacerbations
   f. Serum $\alpha 1$-antitrypsin deficiency
8. Requirement of long-term oxygen therapy in this patient following the criteria:
   a. Patient who stops smoking, i.e., carboxy-hemoglobin is <3%.
      And
   b. $PaO_2 < 7.3$
      Or,
      PaO_2 = 7.3–8.0, when stable and one of the following is present:
      • Secondary polycythemia
      • Pulmonary hypertension
      • Peripheral edema (presence of cor pulmonale)
      • Nocturnal hypoxemia (SaO_2 is <90% for >30% of the time)
9. The importance of $\alpha 1$-antitrypsin deficiency: Normal serum level of $\alpha 1$-antitrypsin is >11 mmol/L which is protective. If this level is <9 mmol/L, the patient may develop emphysema. According to electrophoretic mobility, this enzyme is characterized as M (medium), S (slow), and Z (very slow). Phenotype ZZ and SS are associated with severe deficiency. This enzyme is synthetized in liver and after liberation from liver it will be distributed in the alveolar and interstitial fluid. So, genetic defect of this molecule prevents its release from the hepatocytes leading to lowering of its concentration in the serum as well as alveoli resulting in destruction of the lung tissue by the neutrophil elastase. Here, damage is panacinar and involves lower lobes. On the other hand, accumulation of the genetically defective $\alpha 1$-antitrypsin within the hepatocytes leads to destruction of these cells and chronic liver disease results. Cigarette smoking aggravates the progression of emphysema.

CASE 22

A 40-year-old nonsmoker female came to medicine outdoor with cachexia but no breathlessness, and no joint pain. On examination, no palpable lymph node, no clubbing, trachea central, reduced expansion of the right side of chest, and percussion note stony dull and reduced vocal fremitus. On auscultation, breath sound and vocal resonance are diminished, but bronchial breathing at the upper level of plural effusion.

1. **What is your diagnosis?**
2. **If the central venous pressure is increased then what should be the etiology of this disease?**
3. **If there is peripheral edema, what is the etiology of this disease?**
4. **What are the physical examinations required to detect the etiology of this disease?**
5. **What are the drugs producing this disease?**

6. How can you specifically diagnose the suspected pleural effusion?
7. Mention the normal composition of pleural fluid.
8. What are the mechanisms responsible for formation of pleural effusion?
9. Mention the causes if there is hemorrhage in the pleural cavity.
10. If LDH, the pleural fluid is >1,000 IU/L, what are the causes?
11. If the glucose content of the pleural fluid is low, what are the causes?
12. If the amylase content of the pleural fluid is high, what are the conditions responsible?
13. In case of malignant etiology if the pH of pleural fluid is low, what are the conditions?
14. What are the complications of drainage of pleural fluid?

Answers

1. The most likely diagnosis is right-sided pleural effusion.
2. If the central venous pressure is increased, the etiology is pulmonary hypertension which may be due to pulmonary disease or congestive cardiac failure.
3. If there is peripheral edema, the etiologies are either due to congestive cardiac failure or hypoalbuminemia.
4. Following physical examinations are required to detect the etiologies of pleural effusion:
   a. If clubbing with or without pulmonary hypertrophic osteoarthropathy, nicotine staining in the fingers in the hand, lymphadenopathy—bronchogenic carcinoma and mesothelioma.
   b. Presence of lymphadenopathy and hepatosplenomegaly—it indicates lymphoma
   c. Presence of bilateral symmetrical arthropathy involving the MCP or PIP, rheumatoid nodules, and deformities of the hands indicates rheumatoid arthritis
   d. Presence of butterfly rash, purpura, livedo reticularis, petechial skin rash, and arthropathy indicates SLE
   e. Presence of jaundice, hepatomegaly, ascites, pedal edema, and peripheral signs of hepatic failure indicates chronic liver disease
   f. Presence of breast lump, lymphadenopathy, or past history of breast lump resection—indicates carcinoma breast
   g. Generalized edema, cachexia, and poor nutritional status indicate hypoalbuminemia
   h. Increased central venous pressure, third and fourth heart sound, and peripheral edema indicate congestive cardiac failure
5. Following are the drugs producing the pleural effusion:
   a. Procarbazine
   b. Practolol
   c. Methotrexate
   d. Bromocriptine
   e. Nitrofurantoin
   f. Methysergide
6. Specific investigations to diagnose a case of pleural effusion are as follows:
   a. If suspicion of tuberculosis or malignancy, pleural biopsy
   b. If suspicion of pulmonary embolism, CT angiography of pulmonary artery
   c. If there is lymphoproliferative disorder or bronchogenic carcinoma, CT scan of chest.
   d. Bronchogenic carcinoma—bronchoscopy
   e. If cardiac failure, echocardiography
   f. Mammogram in case of suspicion of breast cancer
   g. In case of suspected gastrointestinal malignancy, renal cancer, or lymphoproliferative disorder
7. Normal composition of pleural fluid is:
   a. Color: Clear
   b. pH: 7.6–7.64
   c. Protein: 1–2 g/L
   d. White blood cell count < 1,000/cc
   e. Lactate dehydrogenase < 50% of plasma concentration
   f. Glucose level is same as that of plasma.
8. Following are the mechanisms of pleural effusion:
   a. Altered permeability in the pleural membrane:
      - Inflammation
      - Neoplasia
      - Pulmonary embolism
   b. Increased capillary permeability:
      - Inflammation
      - Trauma
      - Infection
      - Neoplasia
      - Pancreatitis

- Drug hypersensitivity
- Uremia

c. Oncotic pressure is decreased:
- Cirrhosis
- Hypoalbuminemia
- Nephrotic syndrome

d. Increased capillary hydrostatic pressure:
- Congestive cardiac failure
- Superior vena cava obstruction

e. Decreased lymphatic drainage:
- Trauma
- Cancer

f. Increased fluid in the peritoneal cavity and migration across the diaphragm:
- Cirrhosis
- Peritoneal dialysis

9. Causes of hemorrhagic pleural effusion are as follows:
   a. Malignancy
   b. Pulmonary embolism
   c. Tuberculosis
   d. Trauma to the chest

10. The causes of high LDH > 1,000 IU/L in pleural effusion are as follows:
    a. Empyema
    b. Malignant effusion
    c. Collagen vascular disease
    d. Pleural paragonimiasis

11. Causes of low glucose concentration in the pleural fluid are as follows:
    a. Empyema
    b. Malignancy
    c. Systemic lupus erythematosus
    d. Tuberculosis
    e. Esophageal rupture
    f. Rheumatoid arthritis

12. Causes of high amylase content in the pleural fluid are as follows:
    a. Pancreatitis
    b. Malignancy
    c. Esophageal rupture
    d. Bacterial pneumonia

13. In case of malignant pleural effusion in the pH of pleural fluid is low, i.e., <7.3, the causes are the following:
    a. Pleural involvement is extensive.
    b. High yield in the pleural fluid cytology
    c. Life expectancy is shorter.
    d. Success rate of pleurodesis is decreased.

14. Complications of pleural fluid drainage are as follows:
    a. Hydropneumothorax
    b. Pneumothorax
    c. Hemothorax
    d. Hypovolemia
    e. Unilateral pulmonary edema

CASE 23

A 40-year-old man came to medicine outdoor with productive cough and exertional breathlessness.

On examination, there was grade II clubbing, no nicotine staining, normal central venous pressure, and no lymphadenopathy.

Chest examination demonstrated normal inspection, palpation and percussion, and vocal fremitus normal. Auscultation in the right base demonstrated inspiratory crackles which is altered with coughing along with expiratory wheeze.

1. **What is the most likely diagnosis?**
2. **In case of lymphadenopathy, what may be the cause?**
3. **If the percussion note is dull, what are the causes of bronchiectasis?**
4. **What are the causes of scattered wheeze in this case?**
5. **What are the differential diagnoses in this case?**
6. **What is the pathophysiology of this disease?**
7. **How anatomical distribution of the bronchiectasis can help to diagnose the etiology?**
8. **What are the organisms involved in this case?**
9. **What is yellow nail syndrome?**
10. **What is Kartagener's syndrome?**
11. **What is Mounier–Kuhn syndrome?**

Answers

1. The most likely diagnosis is left basal bronchiectasis.
2. If there is lymphadenopathy, the diagnoses are the following:
   a. Bronchogenic carcinoma
   b. Sarcoidosis
   c. Tuberculosis
3. If the percussion note is dull, the causes of bronchiectasis are as follows:
   a. Fibrosis
   b. Collapse
   c. Consolidation
4. The causes of scattered wheeze in this case are obstruction airway and obstruction may be due to:
   a. Compressibility of the bronchial wall leading to destruction of the muscular as well as elastic component of the bronchial walls
   b. Malignant masses, lymph nodes, and granuloma leading to obstruction of the airways
   c. Coexistent obstructive airway disease
5. Following are the differential diagnoses in this patient:
   a. Bronchiectasis
   b. Bronchogenic carcinoma
   c. Lung abscess
   d. Pulmonary fibrosis
6. Due to destruction of the bronchial smooth muscles and elastin, components of the bronchial wall leading to transmural inflammation, edema, scarring, and ulceration of the bronchial wall resulting in dilatation and destruction of the bronchi.
7. Following anatomical distribution of the disease can help to diagnose the etiology:
   a. Infection can involve:
      - Lower lobe
      - Right middle lobe
      - Lingula
   b. Obstruction can involve right middle lobe.
   c. Chronic fungal infection and tuberculosis can involve upper lobe.
   d. In case of ABPA:
      - Proximal bronchiectasis central bronchi in upper lobes
      - Other bronchiectasis involving distal bronchial segments
8. Following organisms may be involved in this case:
   a. *Haemophilus influenzae*
   b. *Staphylococcus aureus*
   c. *Pseudomonas aeruginosa*
   d. *Streptococcus pneumoniae*
   e. *Klebsiella pneumoniae*
   f. *Aspergillus fumigatus*
9. Yellow nail syndrome is characterized by:
   a. Slowly growing excessive longitudinally as well as transverse curved nail
   b. Pleural effusion
   c. Bronchiectasis
   d. Sinusitis
   e. Lymphedema
10. Kartagener's syndrome is characterized by:
    a. Autosomal disorder
    b. Immobile cilia syndrome
    c. Dextrocardia
    d. Situs inversus in of 50% cases
11. Mounier–Kuhn syndrome:
    a. Multiple tracheal diverticula
    b. Marked dilatation of trachea
    c. Bronchiectasis
    d. Recurrent respiratory tract infection

CASE 24

A 76-year-old smoker came to medicine outdoor with respiratory distress and productive cough, progressively increasing respiratory distress.

On examination, there was nicotine staining in the fingers, left supraclavicular lymphadenopathy, grade 3 clubbing, trachea central, and normal cricoid-notch distance.

Chest examination demonstrated reduced chest expansion on inspection and palpation, stony dull on percussion absent breath sound and absent vocal resonance, and bronchial breathing. Just above the area of dullness—all the features are on the right mid and lower zone.

1. **What is the most likely diagnosis?**
2. **What are the types of this disease?**
3. **What are the risk factors in this disease?**

4. **What are the characters of the fluid in this disease?**
5. **What are the blood tests that can be a clue to the etiology in this disease?**
6. **What are the modalities of palliative care to be given to the patient?**

Answers

1. The patient has been suffering from right-sided pleural effusion probably from bronchogenic carcinoma.
2. Following are the types of the disease:
   a. Small cell carcinoma:
      - It is also known as oat cell carcinoma.
      - It arises from amine precursor uptake and decarboxylation
      - It secretes many polypeptide hormones
   b. Nonsmall cell carcinoma—it is subdivided into following types:
      - Adenocarcinoma: It is most common type and occurs in both smoker and nonsmoker. It arises from peripheral areas of the lung.
      - Bronchoalveolar carcinoma: It occurs from multiple sites and spreads along the preexisting alveolar cells.
      - Squamous cell carcinoma: It is also known as "epidermoid carcinoma." It may cavitate.
      - Large cell carcinoma: It is least common type, also known as "undifferentiated carcinoma."
3. The risk factors are:
   a. Smoking
   b. Radiation
   c. Asbestos
   d. Iron oxide
   e. Interstitial lung disease
   f. Coal tar
   g. Radon
   h. Arsenic
   i. Chromium

4. Following are the characters of the pleural fluid:
   a. Hemorrhagic
   b. Low pH
   c. Low glucose
   d. Exudate
   e. Cytology
   f. Increased amylase
5. Following are the blood tests required:
   a. Full blood count:
      - Anemia of chronic disease
      - Thrombocytopenia
   b. Clotting profile:
      - Blood gas analysis: Syndrome of inappropriate antidiuretic hormone secretion (SIADH) in hypokalemic alkalosis
      - Calcium: Hypercalcemia in case of bony metastasis or increased parathormone production.
   c. Liver function test:
      - Deranged in hepatic metastases
      - Increased alkaline phosphatase in bony metastases
6. Following are the modalities of palliative care:
   a. Antidepressants
   b. Steroids
   c. Pain killer
   d. Anxiolytics
   e. Radiotherapy in case of bone pain, hemoptysis, or intractable cough
   f. In case of inoperable intraluminal tumor, endobronchial laser therapy
   g. Stent: Tracheobronchial

CASE 25

A 45-year-old nonsmoker having history of thoracotomy came to medical outdoor for routine checkup.

On examination, there was no peripheral edema, lymphadenopathy, and venous prominence, but grade III clubbing. Chest examination demonstrated tracheal deviation to the left and thoracotomy scar on the left chest. Left lower ribs were pulled in. Apex beat was pulled to the left. Diminished movement in the lower left part of chest, percussion note dull, diminished breath sound in the same area.

1. **What is the most likely diagnosis?**
2. **In this patient what may be the causes of this operation?**
3. **Why is inspection of the chest very much required in this patient?**
4. **What are the possible indications of this operation?**
5. **What should be the typical findings in the chest after the operation?**

Answers

1. This patient has been suffering from left-sided lower lobectomy.
2. In this patient, the causes of operation are as follows:
   a. Bronchiectasis
   b. Interstitial lung disease
   c. Bronchogenic carcinoma
3. Chest expansion is required because the chest expansion is reduced locally corresponding the area of lobectomy.
4. Following are the possible indications of this operation:
   a. Bronchiectasis
   b. Nonsmall cell lung cancer
   c. Solitary pulmonary nodule
   d. Tuberculosis
   e. Cystic fibrosis
   f. Lung abscess
5. Following are the findings in this case:
   a. Lower ribs are pulled in.
   b. Trachea will be shifted to the left side.
   c. Left lower part of the chest will be less expanded.
   d. Breath sound in the left lower part of the chest is reduced.

CASE 26

A 45-year-old nonsmoker having history of thoracotomy came to medical outdoor for routine checkup.

On examination, there was gross tracheal deviation to the left and scar on the left side of the chest. There was gross flattening of the left chest, apex beat to the left, grossly reduced movement of the left side of chest, percussion note dull, and breath sound absent on the same area. But bronchial breathing in the left upper zone.

1. **What is the most likely diagnosis?**
2. **What are the possible indications of this operation?**
3. **How can you differentiate this operation from the lobectomy on the same side clinically?**

Answers

1. The most likely diagnosis is left-sided pneumonectomy.
2. The possible indications of pneumonectomy are as follows:
   a. Bronchiectasis
   b. Pulmonary tuberculosis
   c. Bronchogenic carcinoma
3. Differentiation between left-sided pneumonectomy and left upper and lower lobectomy:

Features	Left pneumo-nectomy	Left lower lobectomy	Left upper lobectomy
Movement of chest wall	Left chest wall flattening	Left lower ribs are pulled in	Left upper ribs pulled in

Continued

Features	Left pneumo-nectomy	Left lower lobectomy	Left upper lobectomy
Deviation of trachea	Grossly deviated to the affected side	Central position or mildly deviated to affected side	Deviated to right
Expansion	Absent on the affected side	Reduced	Reduced
Breath sound	Absent	Reduced in the affected part	Reduced in the affected part

Continued

CASE 27

A 35-year-old nonsmoker male came to medicine outdoor with cough and production of yellowish sputum but no respiratory distress.

On examination, there was no clubbing, tachycardia, and no venous prominence.

Chest examination demonstrated tracheal shifting to the left, flattening left upper chest with reduced movement, and percussion note dull with bronchial bleeding with increased vocal resonance in the same area.

1. **What is your diagnosis?**
2. **What are the possible differential diagnoses?**
3. **How can you exclude the above diagnoses?**
4. **Name five other causes of this type of lesion?**
5. **Who are at risks of tuberculosis?**
6. **What are the types of manifestations of tuberculosis in the chest X-ray in this disease?**

Answers

1. The most likely diagnosis is left apical fibrosis probably due to old pulmonary tuberculosis.
2. The differential diagnoses are the following:
   a. Consolidation of left upper lung
   b. Collapse of left upper lobe of the lung
   c. Bronchogenic carcinoma involving the left upper lobe
3. Exclusion of the diagnoses:
   a. In case of consolidation: No shifting of trachea
   b. In case of collapse of left upper lobe: Bronchial breathing is not associated with collapse, if present, it is due to deviated trachea.
   c. In case of bronchogenic carcinoma:
      - There is associated clubbing.
      - History of smoking
      - Presence of lymphadenopathy
      - Features of Horner syndrome may be present.
4. Five important causes of left apical fibrosis are as follows:
   a. Asbestosis
   b. Allergic bronchopulmonary aspergillosis
   c. Silicosis
   d. Coal worker's pneumoconiosis
   e. Langerhans cell histiocytosis
5. Following are at high risks of tuberculosis:
   a. Elderly
   b. Asian immigrants
   c. Alcoholic
   d. Debilitated persons
   e. Immunocompromised subject
   f. Medical professionals
   g. Closed contact with the active patients
6. Following are the types of manifestations of tuberculosis in the chest X-ray:
   a. Fluffy confluent soft shadow
   b. Infiltration in the apical area of the lung
   c. Dense nodular opacities
   d. Fibrocaseous lesion
   e. Presence of tuberculoma
   f. Multiple miliary mottling shadows
   g. Presence of calcification in the lesion
   h. Presence of pleural effusion
   i. Upper zone bronchiectasis
   j. Enlarged hilar lymph nodes

CASE 28

A 45-year-old nonsmoker, no hypertensive male has come to emergency department as routine checkup after being intervened in the right chest.

On examination, there was no clubbing and no lymphadenopathy.

Respiratory examination demonstrated gross deviation of the trachea to the right and thoracotomy scar on the right posterior part. There is absence of the ribs superiorly. There is evidence of reduced chest expansion on the right upper part with dull percussion note but reduced vocal fremitus and coarse crepitations.

1. **What is the most likely diagnosis?**
2. **How can you differentiate it from pneumonectomy?**
3. **If there will be bronchial breath sound in the right apical part, what may be the cause?**
4. **What are the complications of the main disease?**
5. **What are the features in the chest X-ray in this disease if untreated?**
6. **Prior to the effective chemotherapy what are the methods of treatment in this disease?**

Answers

1. The most likely diagnosis is right thoracoplasty to treat tuberculosis prior to the day of antitubercular therapy.
2. The differentiating features between the pneumonectomy and thoracoplasty:

Clinical features	Left pneumonectomy	Left thoracoplasty
Deformity	It is less marked	It is more marked along with the evidence of resection of ribs in the superior part
Expansion of chest	Whole right chest expansion is reduced	Only the affected part is reduced
Percussion	Dull throughout the right chest	Dull, only the affected part of the chest
Breath sounds	Absent throughout the right chest	Absent in the upper part but normal in the lower part of the chest

3. If the bronchial breath sound can be heard in the right apical, it is due to gross shifting of the trachea.
4. Complications of this untreated disease, i.e., pulmonary tuberculosis:
   a. Acute complications:
      - Pleural effusion
      - Empyema
      - Collapse of the lung
      - Miliary tuberculosis
      - Pneumothorax
      - Acute respiratory distress syndrome
      - Respiratory failure
      - Laryngitis
      - Tubercular meningitis
   b. Chronic complications:
      - Pulmonary fibrosis
      - Aspergilloma
      - Reactivation of the tuberculosis

5. The findings in the chest X-ray in case of untreated tuberculosis are the following:
   a. Cavitation in the affected area
   b. Mediastinal lymphadenopathy
   c. Reactivation of the tuberculosis:
      - Posterior segment of the right upper lobe
      - Apicoposterior segment of the left upper lobe
      - Apical segment of the lower lobes
   d. Tuberculoma representing the old infection
   e. Miliary tuberculosis

6. Following are the methods of treatment prior to effective antitubercular chemotherapy:
   a. Thoracoplasty involving removal of 3–5 ribs in the upper part to make collapse of the affected part of the lung
   b. Plombage therapy involving insertion of plombe into the extrapleural space to make collapse of the affected lung. The plombage includes:
      - Solid paraffin wax
      - Lucite spheres
      - Plastic ping-pong balls
      - Sponges of the plastic material
      - Oil in the pleural cavity
   c. Artificial pneumothorax involving insertion of the air into the pleural cavity on the affected side in order to make collapse in the affected part of the lung
   d. Phrenicotomy involving crush of the phrenic nerve to produce the unilateral diaphragmatic paralysis and to make the affected lung relax
   e. Postural test where the patient should lie on the affected lung to reduce the movement of the affected lung.
   f. Shot bag method where a bag containing 1 pound of shot to be placed over the clavicle of the affected side in order to reduce the movement of that lung and the amount of weight should be increased gradually up to 5 pounds.

CASE 29

A 29-year-old nonsmoker male came to chest outdoor with progressively increasing respiratory distress and productive cough with yellow-colored sputum.

On examination, there was no lymphadenopathy, clubbing, venous engorgement, normal cricoid-notch distance, and no tracheal shifting.

Chest examination demonstrated diminished expansion and movement in the right lower chest, dull percussion, bronchial breathing, and increased vocal resonance in the same area.

1. **What is your most likely diagnosis?**
2. **In case of associated lymphadenopathy, what other diagnosis can be thought?**
3. **If there is tracheal shifting, what is the associated cause may be thought about?**
4. **If the cricoid-notch distance is reduced, what is the associated diagnosis?**
5. **What infection can be diagnosed from urine testing?**
6. **What is the importance of D-dimer in this case?**
7. **What are the causes of cavitary lesion?**
8. **What are the predisposing factors in case of Legionnaire's disease?**
9. **What are the sources of Legionnaire's infection?**

Answers

1. The most likely diagnosis is right basal consolidation due to most probably bacterial infection.
2. If the patient has associated lymphadenopathy, the patient may suffer from chronic bacterial infection or malignancy.
3. If there is associated tracheal shifting, the patient has associated absorption collapse.
4. If the cricoid-notch distance is reduced, the patient has associated COPD.
5. Following infections can be diagnosed from the urine testing:
   a. Pneumococcal antigen
   b. *Legionella* antigen
6. The importance of D-dimer is:
   a. D-dimer is elevated in infection as well as malignancy
   b. If the D-dimer is negative, associated pulmonary embolism should be excluded.
   c. If the D-dimer level is low, it cannot exclude pulmonary embolism.
7. Following are the causes of cavitary lesion:
   a. *Staphylococcus aureus*
   b. *Pseudomonas aeruginosa*
   c. *Klebsiella pneumoniae*
   d. Tuberculosis
   e. Aspergilloma
   f. Anaerobic infection
   g. *Histoplasma capsulatum*
   h. Noninfectious causes:
      - Cancer
      - Caplan's syndrome
      - Wegener granulomatosis
      - Pulmonary rheumatoid nodule
8. Predisposing factors for Legionnaire's disease are as follows:
   a. Debilitated individual
   b. Elderly
   c. Immunocompromised individual
   d. Alcoholism
   e. Smoking
   f. Chronic obstructive pulmonary disease
9. Sources of *Legionella* infection:
   a. Contaminated water pooling system
   b. Showers
   c. Non-serviced air-conditioning system.

CASE 30

A 51-year-old nonsmoker came to emergency department with sudden onset of respiratory distress. On examination, the central venous pressure was elevated, no clubbing and lymphadenopathy, normal cricoid-notch distance, and trachea in normal position. There was also tender swollen right calf.

Chest examination demonstrated reduced expansion and movement in the right lower part of the chest, dull percussion note, bronchial breathing with crepitations, and increased vocal resonance and pleural rub in the same area.

1. **What is your diagnosis?**
2. **In this case to detect the underlying cause, what are the other points which should be considered?**
3. **What are the extrapulmonary manifestations that may occur in this case?**
4. **What do you mean by CURB-65 criteria?**
5. **What should be the ECG features in this case?**
6. **What are the risk factors in this etiology?**

Answers

1. The patient has been suffering from right-sided basal consolidation with pulmonary hypertension along with right-sided deep venous thrombosis suggesting pulmonary embolism as an etiological factor.

2. To detect the underlying cause, following points should be investigated:
   a. Pneumonia:
      - Pyrexia
      - Hemoptysis
      - Purulent sputum
   b. Malignancy:
      - Cachexia
      - Digital clubbing
      - Nicotine staining
      - Lymphadenopathy
      - Productive calf
   c. Infarction:
      - Features of pulmonary hypertension
      - Deep venous thrombosis
      - Bruise—indicating the patient receiving anticoagulation

3. Extrapulmonary manifestations in this case are as follows:
   a. Cardiac:
      - Pericarditis
      - Myocarditis
   b. Neurological manifestations:
      - Meningitis
      - Aseptic meningitis
      - Bullous meningitis
      - Transverse myelitis
      - Guillain–Barre syndrome
      - Peripheral neuropathy
   c. Hematological manifestations:
      - Cold autoimmune hemolytic anemia
      - Thrombocytopenia
      - Disseminated intravascular coagulation (DIC)
   d. Rheumatological manifestations:
      - Myalgia
      - Arthralgia
      - Myositis
   e. Gastrointestinal features:
      - Vomiting
      - Diarrhea
      - Pancreatitis
      - Hepatitis
   f. Dermatological manifestations:
      - Erythema nodosum
      - Erythema multiforme
      - Stevens–Johnson syndrome
   g. Renal manifestations:
      - Interstitial nephritis
      - Glomerulonephritis
   h. Endocrine manifestation: SIADH

4. CURB-65 means:
   a. Confusion
   b. Urea > 7 mmol/L
   c. Respiratory rate of ≥30 breaths/min
   d. Blood pressure systolic < 90 mm Hg
   e. Age ≥ 65 years

   CURB-65 score is used to detect the prognosis, i.e.,
   a. Oral versus intravenous antibiotic administration
   b. Inpatient versus outpatient management

5. ECG features in the etiology are as follows:
   a. Sinus tachycardia
   b. Tall R wave in V1
   c. Right ventricular strain
   d. Right bundle branch block

6. Following are the risk factors in this pulmonary embolism:
   a. Malignancy
   b. Recent surgery
   c. Immobile patient
   d. Oral contraceptive pill
   e. Previous history of pulmonary embolism
   f. Pregnancy
   g. Protein C and protein S deficiency
   h. Antithrombin III deficiency

CASE 31

A 32-year-old nonsmoker came to emergency department with chest pain following severe bout of cough.

On examination, patient is tachypneic, no clubbing, lymphadenopathy, and normal venous pressure.

Chest examination demonstrated tracheal shifting to left, inflated right upper chest with tympanic on percussion and diminished breath sound, and diminished vocal resonance on auscultation.

1. **What is the most likely diagnosis?**
2. **If there is clubbing, what are the etiologies behind it?**
3. **If this disease is associated with raised venous pressure, what is the etiology?**
4. **Mention the pathophysiology of spontaneous pneumothorax.**
5. **What are the clinical signs of tension pneumothorax?**
6. **How can you manage the tension pneumothorax?**
7. **Mention the predictor of reexpansion pulmonary edema.**
8. **What is the rate of resolution of the spontaneous pneumothorax?**

Answers

1. The most likely diagnosis is spontaneous pneumothorax.
2. If the patient has clubbing, the causes of this disease are as follows:
   a. Bronchiectasis
   b. Cystic fibrosis
   c. Malignancy
   d. Interstitial lung disease
3. If the venous pressure is increased, the diagnosis is tension pneumothorax.
4. Pathophysiology of this disease: In tall and young individuals, rupture of the subpleural bleb underlying the visceral pleura in absence of any respiratory disease leading to formation of spontaneous pneumothorax.
5. Clinical signs of tension pneumothorax are the following:
   a. Deviation of trachea to the opposite side
   b. Raised venous pressure
   c. Mediastinal shifting to opposite side
6. Tension pneumothorax can be managed by:
   a. High-flow oxygen administration
   b. Insertion of the large bore needle into the second intercostal space in the midaxillary line in the affected side of the chest
   c. Insertion of intercostal drain promptly
7. If the lung will be collapsed for long time in case of spontaneous pneumothorax, there is greater chance of developing reexpansion pulmonary edema during taking out the air.
8. Rate of absorption of air is very slow, which is about 1.22–1.8% of the volume of hemithorax daily.

CASE 32

A 71-year-old smoker cachectic male came to medicine emergency department with respiratory distress.

On examination, there was finger clubbing, normal venous pressure, no pedal edema, supraclavicular lymphadenopathy, and tracheal deviation to the right.

Chest examination demonstrated chest expansion and movement was diminished in the left lower part of the chest along with dull percussion, decreased breath sound, and vocal resonance in the same area.

1. **What is your diagnosis?**
2. **What are the clinical signs in favor of the etiology in this patient?**
3. **What are the features to look for to detect the cause of the diagnosis?**
4. **What are the types in this disease?**
5. **What are the causes of central collapse of this disease?**
6. **How can you differentiate the different causes of the disease?**
7. **What are the features seen in the chest X-ray in this disease?**
8. **What are the complications in this disease?**

Answers

1. The diagnosis is left basal collapse due to malignancy in the lung.
2. The points in favor of the diagnosis are as follows:
   a. Smoking
   b. Finger clubbing
   c. Supraclavicular lymphadenopathy
   d. Cachexia
3. Following features should be sought to detect the etiology of the diagnosis:
   a. Cancer:
      - Finger clubbing
      - Cachexia
      - Smoking
      - Lymphadenopathy
   b. Tuberculosis:
      - Lymphadenopathy
      - Apical sign
   c. Hilar lymphadenopathy:
      - Erythema nodosum
      - Lupus pernio
      - Lymphadenopathy
      - Maculopapular rash
   d. Mucus plug in case of:
      - Bronchial asthma
      - Chronic obstructive lung disease
      - Bronchiectasis
4. There are two types of atelectasis:
   a. Obstructive atelectasis:
      - Malignancy
      - Tuberculosis
      - Extrinsic compression by hilar lymphadeno-pathy
      - Mucus plug in case of:
        - Asthma
        - Chronic obstructive lung disease
        - Bronchiectasis
      - Foreign body
      - Wrongly placed endotracheal tube
   b. Nonobstructive atelectasis:
      - Passive atelectasis:
        - Pleural effusion
        - Pneumothorax
        - Large bulla
   - Compression atelectasis:
     - Cancer
     - Loculated pleural effusion
   - Cicatrization:
     - Interstitial lung disease
     - Necrotizing pneumonia
   - Rounded atelectasis: Asbestos leading to pleural plaque
   - Adhesive atelectasis:
     - Adult respiratory distress syndrome
     - Pulmonary embolism
     - Radiation pneumonitis
     - Inhalation of smoke
     - Postoperative
5. Causes of central collapse are as follows:
   a. Inhaled foreign body
   b. Bronchial adenoma
   c. Enlarged tracheobronchial lymph node
   d. Mucus plugs
   e. Stricture or stenosis
   f. Pericardial effusion
   g. Aortic aneurysm
6. Differentiation between central and partial causes of collapse:

Clinical features	Central causes of collapse	Peripheral causes of collapse
Tracheal shifting	To the same side	Same side
Elevated dome of diaphragm	Same side	Same side
Breath sound	Absent on the involved side	Tubular breath sound
Vocal resonance	Absent or decreased	Increased with whispering pectoriloquy
CT scan of chest	Golden "S" sign characterized by collapse with loss of open bronchus	Collapse with open bronchus
Feature on the other side of chest	Compensatory hypertrophy characterized by hyperresonant note and diminished breath sound with prolonged expiration	Compensatory hypertrophy is absent

7. Features of collapsed lung in chest X-ray are as follows:
   a. Homogeneous opacity indicating collapsed lung
   b. Cardiac shadow and trachea will be shifted to the same side.
   c. Dome of the diaphragm will be elevated in the same side.
   d. In case of long time collapse, there is crowding of the ribs and reduction of the intercostal spaces.
   e. If the collapse is due to malignancy leading to development of pleural effusion, then this evidence can be seen.
   f. Radiological features of other causes of collapse such as mediastinal lymphadenopathy or foreign body can be seen.
8. Complications of collapse:
   a. Secondary infection
   b. Spontaneous pneumothorax

CHAPTER 13

Rheumatology

A 70-year-old woman having history of type 2 diabetes mellitus and congestive failure came to medical clinic with following dermatologic features:

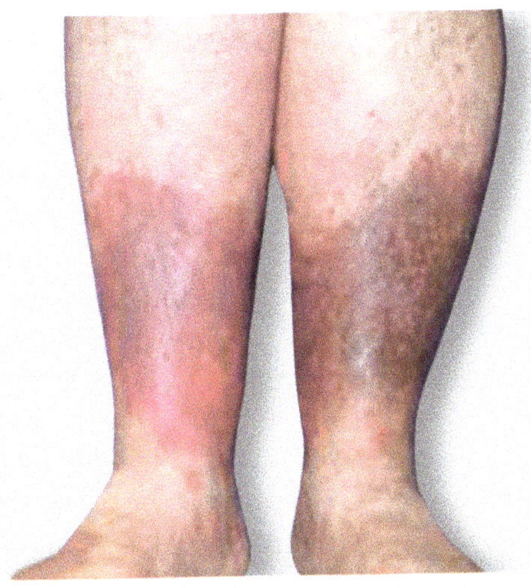

Her hematological features were within normal limit, viral serology was negative, antinuclear antibody (ANA), and extended ANA panel was negative.

1. **Describe the above dermatological picture.**
2. **What is the most likely diagnosis?**
3. **What are the points in favor of your diagnosis?**
4. **What are the other terms that can be used for this?**
5. **Define this disease.**
6. **What is the pathophysiology behind it?**
7. **What are the risk factors behind it?**
8. **What are the histopathological changes in this disease?**
9. **What are the complications in this disease?**

Answers

1. The above picture demonstrates localized single plaque reddish-brown in color involving the pretibial and medial aspect of the legs bilaterally.
2. The most likely diagnosis is acute lipodermatosclerosis.
3. Following are the points in favor of this diagnosis:
   a. Erythrocyte sedimentation rate (ESR) is mildly raised
   b. Hematological test is normal.
   c. Serology is negative.

4. Other terms used in this are as follows:
    a. Sclerosing panniculitis
    b. Hypodermitis scleroderma formis
5. Lipodermatosclerosis can be defined as development of subcutaneous fibrosis as well as induration of the skin in the lower extremities.
6. Pathophysiology behind it:

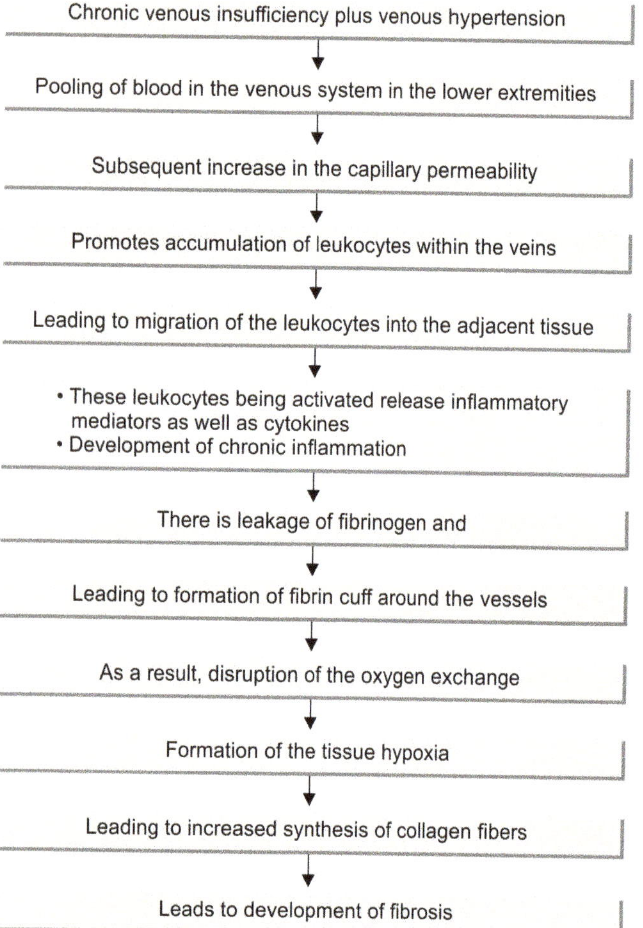

There is also decreased angiogenesis due to increased local response to vascular endothelial growth factor-1 as well as angiopoietin-2.

Increased activity of metalloproteinase and downregulation of angiogenesis will predispose ulceration in the lower extremities.

7. Following are the risk factors:
    a. Aging
    b. Obesity
    c. Prior history of deep venous thrombosis
    d. Family history of venous insufficiency
    e. Tobacco use
8. Histopathological changes are as follows:
    a. In acute stages:
        • Infiltration of the lymphocytes in the septa surrounding the fat lobules
        • Cystic fat necrosis
        • Capillary hemorrhage
        • Deposition of hemosiderin
    b. In chronic stage:
        • Lobular panniculitis
        • Mixed cellular infiltrate
        • Breakdown of the adipocytes
        • Lipomembranous changes leading to pseudocyst formation within the subcutaneous tissue
9. Following are the complications in this disease?
    a. Due to persistent inflammatory states and fibrosis, there is impaired wound healing.
    b. Increased propensity to ulceration
    c. Pain in the lower extremities: It may be acute and severe in acute case and continuous chronic pain in chronic case.

CASE 2

A 27-year-old man came to medical clinic with low back pain and pain around the left ankle. On enquiry, he complained of morning stiffness. On examination, there is tenderness in the left tendo Achilles. On laboratory examination, there is raised ESR and neutrophilic leukocytosis. His X-ray of the pelvis demonstrated:

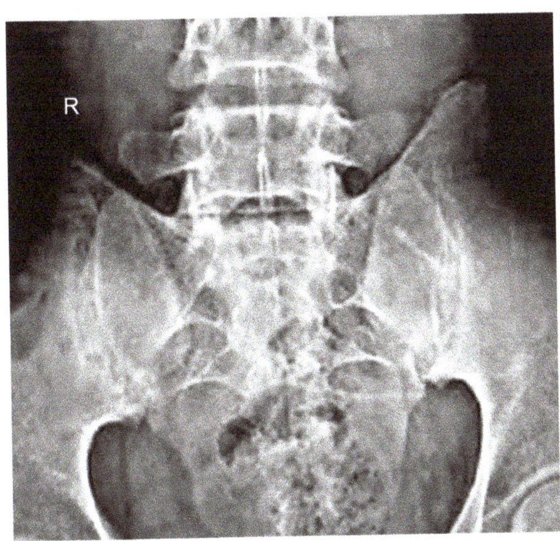
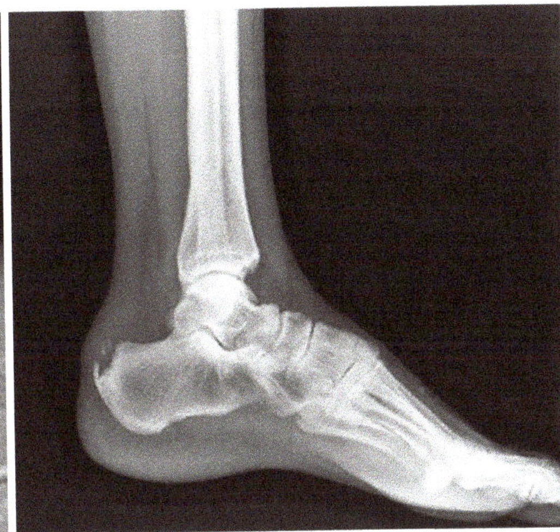

1. **Describe the above X-rays.**
2. **What is the most likely diagnosis?**
3. **What are the points in favor of this diagnosis?**
4. **How can you differentiate this disease from mechanical back pain?**
5. **How can you classify this disease according to the Assessment of Spondyloarthritis International Society (ASAS) classification criteria?**
6. **How can you grade sacroiliac joint involvement?**

Answers

1. Above X-ray demonstrates:
   a. Pelvic X-ray demonstrates inflammatory changes bilaterally
   b. X-ray of the ankle demonstrates thickening of the soft-tissue shadow of the tendo Achilles along with calcified foci
2. The most likely diagnosis is spondyloarthropathy with left Achilles tendinitis.
3. Following are the points in favor of this diagnosis:
   a. Involvement of sacroiliac joints in the form of sacroiliitis
   b. Increased inflammatory markers
4. Following are the differentiating points:

Parameter	Inflammatory back pain	Mechanical back pain
Onset	<45 years of age	Any age
Presence of morning stiffness	>60 minutes	<30 minutes
Nocturnal pain	Frequently occurs	Not present
Effect of exercise	Improves	Exacerbates

5. Following are the classifications of spondyloarthropathies according to ASAS criteria:

Axial spondyloarthritis		Peripheral spondyloarthritis	
Inflammatory back pain ≥3 months, age of onset <45 years and either column here		Arthritis, enthesitis, or dactylitis and either column here	
HLA-B27 and ≥2 other spondylo-arthritis features as below:	Sacroiliitis on imaging: Active inflammation on MRI	≥ Spondyloarthritis features as below:	≥2 other spondyloarthritis features as below:
Inflammatory back pain	Or	Psoriasis	Arthritis
Arthritis	Radiographic sacroiliitis (grade II if bilateral, grade III if bilateral)	Inflammatory bowel disease	Enthesitis
Enthesitis	And	Preceding infection	Dactylitis

Continued

Continued

Axial spondyloarthritis		Peripheral spondyloarthritis	
Uveitis	≥1 other spondyloarthritis feature	HLA-B27	Inflammatory back pain
Dactylitis		Sacroiliitis on imaging	Family history of spondyloarthritis
Psoriasis			
Inflammatory bowel disease			
Good response to nonsteroidal anti-inflammatory drugs (NSAIDs)			
Family history of HLA-B27			
Elevated C-reactive protein			

6. According to New York criteria gradation of sacroiliac joint:
   a. Grade 0: Normal features
   b. Grade 1: Suspicious changes
   c. Grade 2: Presence of minimal abnormality along with small areas of erosions or sclerosis without alteration of joint width
   d. Grade 3: Unequivocal abnormality—moderate or advanced sacroiliitis consisting of:
      - Erosions
      - Sclerosis
      - Widening
      - Narrowing
        And/or
      - Partial joint fusion (ankylosis)
   e. Grade 4: Severe abnormality in the form of total ankylosis

CASE 3

A 30-year-old female came to medical clinic with pain and deformity of the hands. On examination:

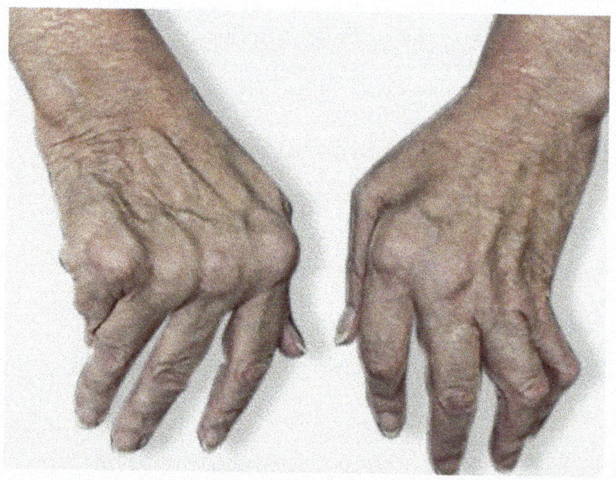
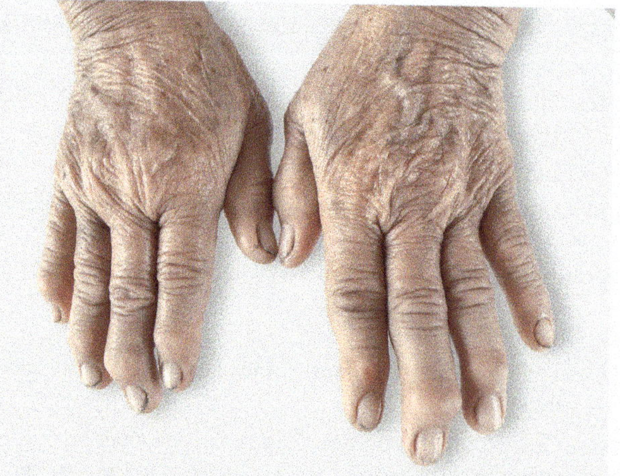

1. **Mention the deformities shown in the above pictures.**
2. **What is your diagnosis?**
3. **What are the antibodies specific in this case?**
4. **Why other antibody is not specific for this diagnosis?**
5. **What are the genetic associations in this disease?**

6. **What is the relation of smoking with this disease?**
7. **Why and which infections are associated with this disease?**
8. **How periodontitis may be responsible for this disease?**
9. **What are the protective factors for rheumatoid arthritis?**
10. **What are the provocative factors for rheumatoid arthritis?**

Answers

1. Following are deformities seen in the above pictures:
   a. Right hand picture demonstrates swan neck deformity in the both hands characterized by:
      - Flexion at the distal interphalangeal joints
      - Extension of the proximal interphalangeal joints
      - Ulnar deviation of the both hands at the metacarpophalangeal joints
   b. Left hand picture demonstrates swan neck deformity characterized by:
      - Flexion at the proximal interphalangeal joints
      - Extension of the distal interphalangeal joints
      - Extension of the metacarpophalangeal joints
      - Ulnar drifting of the both hands

2. This patient has been suffering from rheumatoid arthritis with fixed deformity.

3. Anticyclic citrullinated self-peptides are highly specific for the diagnosis of rheumatoid arthritis with sensitivity and specificity of 65 and 95%, respectively.

4. Other antibody like rheumatoid factor in high titer is 50% specific for the diagnosis of rheumatoid arthritis because low titer of antibody may be present in the following conditions:
   a. Bacterial endocarditis
   b. Hepatitis C
   c. Cryoglobulinemia
   d. Primary biliary cirrhosis

5. Following genetic associations are seen in this rheumatoid arthritis:
   a. There is three- to fourfold increased risk of association of rheumatoid arthritis with HLA-DR4 as compared to control.
   b. There is association of third hypervariable region of DRβ1 allele which is also known as "susceptibility epitope."
   c. Protein tyrosine phosphate 22
   d. Peptidylarginine deiminase 4

6. Smokers are susceptible to rheumatoid arthritis:
   a. Smoking is the stimulus for citrullination of the protein leading to generation of antibodies.
   b. Susceptibility epitope (HLA-SE) is increasingly susceptible to bind with citrullinated protein. Smoker has two copies of epitopes; hence, the chance of rheumatoid arthritis is 40-fold.
   c. After cessation of smoking, there is long latency nearly 40 years when the risk will come to nonsmoker level.

7. Following infections are associated with rheumatoid arthritis:
   a. Epstein–Barr virus
   b. Parvovirus B19
   c. Enteric bacteria
   d. *Mycoplasma*
   e. Chikungunya virus

   By the following mechanisms, the viruses are associated with rheumatoid arthritis:
   a. Direct invasion of the synovium
   b. Molecular mimicry
   c. Activation of toll-like receptors

8. Bacteria responsible for periodontitis, *Porphyromonas gingivalis*, produce citrullination of its own peptidylarginine deiminase (PADI) enzyme leading to development of rheumatoid arthritis.

9. Following dietary factors are protective against rheumatoid arthritis:
   a. Omega-3 fatty acids
   b. Consumption of fish oils
   c. Antioxidants in the fruits and vegetables:
      - Vitamin C
      - Vitamin E
      - Carotenoids
      - Lycopene

10. Following dietary factors provocative for rheumatoid arthritis:
    a. Deficiency of vitamin D
    b. Excessive consumption of coffee
    c. High salt intake

CASE 4

A 32-year-old woman came to eye clinic with pain in the eye with ciliary congestion. The eye surgeon found the following features. She was sent to medicine for further evaluation.

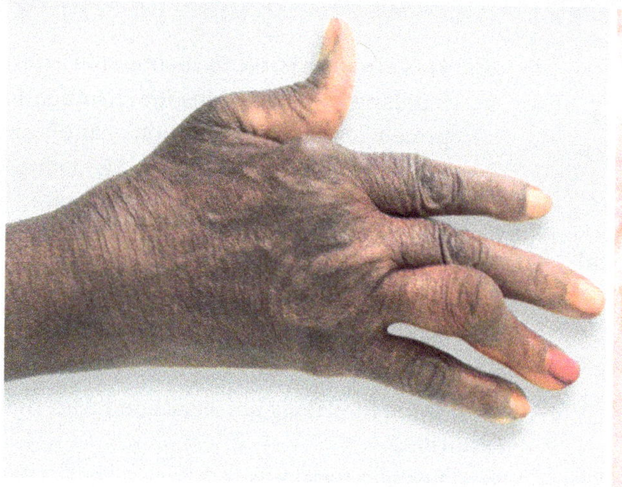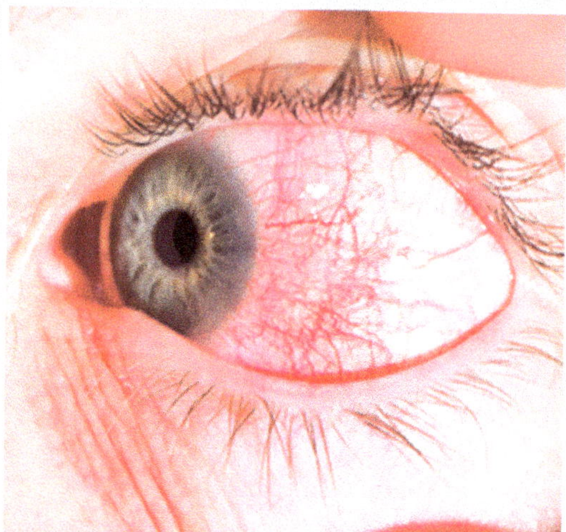

1. **What has been demonstrated in the above pictures?**
2. **What is the most likely diagnosis?**
3. **What are the other extraarticular manifestations in this disease?**
4. **Mention the classification criteria in this disease.**

Answers

1. Following are the deformities in the hand:
    a. Boutonniere deformity characterized by:
        - Flexion at the proximal interphalangeal joint
        - Hyperextension at the distal interphalangeal joint
        - Hyperextension at the metacarpophalangeal joint
    b. Z deformity of thumb—it is characterized by:
        - Flexion at the metacarpophalangeal joint
        - Hyperextension at the proximal and distal interphalangeal joints
    c. Ulnar drifting of all the fingers at the metacarpophalangeal joints.

        There is evidence of sclera congestion with dark red discoloration and tenderness.
2. This patient has been suffering from rheumatoid arthritis.
3. Following are the extra-articular manifestations:
    a. Eye:
        - Iridocyclitis
        - Episcleritis
        - Uveitis
        - Scleritis
        - Retinal vasculitis
    b. Psychiatric manifestations:
        - Anxiety
        - Depression
    c. Pulmonary Bronchiolitis obliterans:
        - Pleuritis
        - Interstitial lung disease
    d. Neurological manifestations:
        - Compressive neuropathy
        - Peripheral neuropathy
        - Carpal tunnel syndrome
    e. Cardiac: Pericarditis
    f. Hematologic manifestations:
        - Anemia
        - Lymphadenopathy

- Splenomegaly
- Hepatomegaly

g. Bone:
- Atlantoaxial dislocation
- Enthesitis

h. Rheumatic nodules
i. Vasculitis:
- Small vessel vasculitis
- Gangrene
- Purpura

j. Atherosclerosis
k. Amyloidosis

4. Following are the ACR/EULAR classifications criteria in this disease:

Joint involvement:
- 1 large joint: 0 points
- 2–10 large joints: 1 point
- 1–3 small joints (with or without large joint involvement): 2 points
- 4–10 small joints (with or without large joint involvement): 3 points
- 10 joints (at least 1 small joint): 5 points
  Large joints include shoulders, elbows, hips, knees, and ankles. Small joints include metacarpophalangeal (MCP), proximal interphalangeal (PIP), and metatarsophalangeal (MTP) joints.
- Serology (at least 1 test result is needed)
- Negative rheumatoid factor (RF) and anti-cyclic citrullinated peptide (anti-CCP): 0 points
- Low-positive RF or anti-CCP (above the upper limit of normal but ≤3 times): 2 points
- High-positive RF or anti-CCP (>3 times the upper limit of normal): 3 points
- Acute-phase reactants (at least 1 test result is needed)
- Normal C-reactive protein (CRP) and erythrocyte sedimentation rate (ESR): 0 points
- Abnormal CRP or ESR: 1 point

Duration of symptoms:
- <6 weeks: 0 points
- ≥6 weeks: 1 point

A score of ≥6 confirms RA, but lower scores may still warrant further evaluation

CASE 5

A 32-year-old female has come to dermatology clinic with following features:

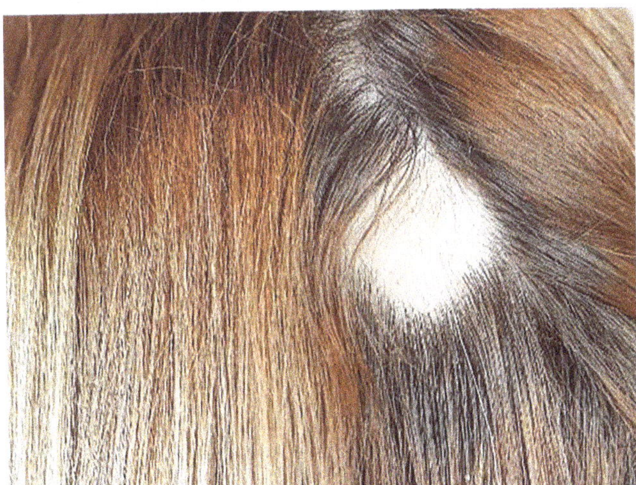

Her blood test demonstrated ESR 110 mm/1st hour, her ANA demonstrated 1 in 160 positive, and her double-stranded DNA was performed as it demonstrated:

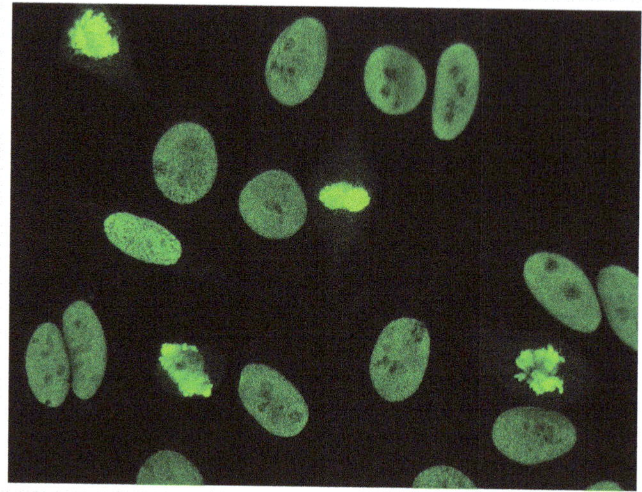

1.   **What do the above pictures demonstrate?**
2.   **How can you differentiate this immunofluorescence pattern from the pattern in systemic sclerosis?**
3.   **What is your diagnosis?**
4.   **What are the criteria for this diagnosis?**
5.   **What are the different types of rashes found in this disease?**
6.   **What are the genetic contributions in this disease?**
7.   **What are the environmental factors associated with this disease?**

Answers

1. The above pictures demonstrate:
    a. Scalp demonstrates bald patch of hair loss with evidence of scarring and broken hair in the central part
    b. Immunofluorescence microscopy demonstrates rim pattern of distribution of antibodies directed against the specific antigen
2. In systemic sclerosis, the antigen-antibody complexes distribution is in the form of centromere pattern.
3. The patient has been suffering from systemic lupus erythematosus.
4. According to classification criteria in 2012 American College of Rheumatology (ACR) for this disease:
    a. Clinical criteria:
        - Acute cutaneous lupus
        - Chronic cutaneous lupus
        - Oral or nasal ulcers
        - Nonscarring alopecia
        - Arthritis
        - Serositis
        - Renal
        - Neurologic
        - Hemolytic anemia
        - Leukopenia
        - Platelet count of <100,000/cc
    b. Immunological criteria:
        - ANA
        - Anti-dsDNA
        - Anti-Smith antibody
        - Antiphospholipid antibody (APLA)
        - Low level of complement such as C3, C4, and CH50
        - Direct Coombs test
5. Following are the different types of rashes found in this disease:
    a. Malar rash: It is characterized by erythematous flat or raised types of lesions seen over the malar prominence but sparing the nasolabial fold.
    b. Discoid rash: It is characterized by erythematous raised patches along with adherent keratotic scaling and follicular plugging with or without atrophic scarring in case of elderly.
    c. Photosensitive rash: It is characterized by erythematous skin rashes in response to sunlight which can be detected from either history or from clinical examination.
    d. Lupus nonspecific skin lesions include:
        - Bullous lesions are seen as blistering lesions in the skin.

- Periungual erythema: It is characterized by dilatation of capillaries demonstrated by dermoscopy seen at the base of the nails.
- Chilblain lupus: It is characterized by violaceous macules or plaques or both seen on the acral surfaces which will be worsened after exposure to humid and cold weather.
- Livedo reticularis: It is characterized by violaceous or erythematous reticular or net like lesion in the skin.

6. Following are the types of genetic contribution in this disease:
   a. High concordance rate of this disease in the monozygotic twins
   b. According to genome-wide association studies, following genomes are associated with this disease:
      - HLA-DR2 and HLA-DR3
      - Mutation of three prime repair endonuclease 1 (TREX1)

- Deficiencies of C1q, C4A, C4B, and C2
- Genes involving in the increased responsiveness to interferon-α.
  - STAT4
  - PTPN22
  - IRF5

7. Following environmental factors are associated with this disease:
   a. Viruses—*Cytomegalovirus* and Epstein–Barr virus
   b. High level of lipopolysaccharide: It is the component of cell wall in the gram-negative bacteria.
   c. In women, low ratio of Firmicutes to Bacteroidetes in the gut
   d. Exposure to ultraviolet ray triggers the cutaneous manifestations in this disease
   e. Drugs

CASE 6

A 40-year-old woman demonstrated the following skin lesion and echocardiographic feature. She has systolic murmur in the left lower sternal border with increased during inspiration.

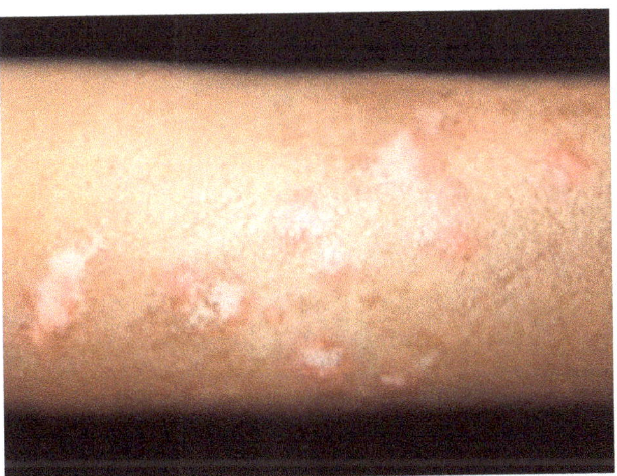

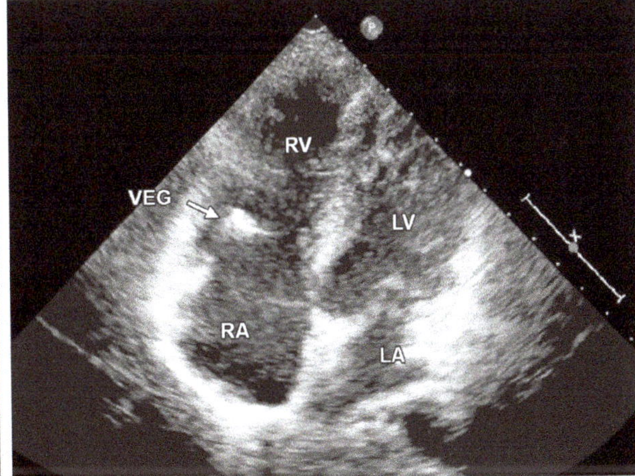

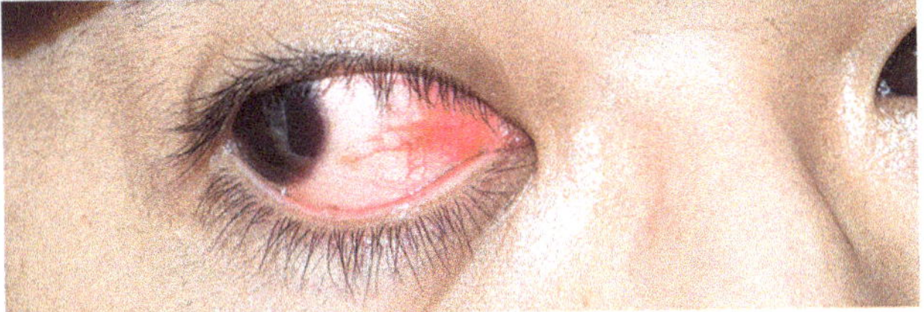

1. **What are the features seen in the above pictures?**
2. **What are the causes of this eye lesion?**
3. **What is the diagnosis?**
4. **What are the cardiological features in this disease?**
5. **What are the neurological features in this disease?**
6. **What are the eye lesions seen in this disease?**

Answers

1. Following features are seen in this disease:
   a. There are erythematous papules and plaques having adherent scales with central hypopigmented areas, peripheral hyperpigmented areas, and atrophic scarring.
   b. 2D echocardiography demonstrated subtricuspid vegetation
   c. There is evidence of edema of the cornea, infiltration of the cornea with inflammatory cells, and ciliary congestion involving the right eye.

2. Causes of keratitis:
   a. Infectious keratitis:
      - Bacteria: *Staphylococcus, Streptococcus, Pseudomonas, Nocardia,* and atypical mycobacteria
      - Protozoa: *Acanthamoeba*
      - Fungal: *Aspergillus, Candida, Fusarium,* Microsporidia, and *Alternaria*
      - Viral: Herpes simplex, herpes zoster, adenovirus
      - Helminths: Onchocercal keratitis
   b. Noninfectious keratitis:
      - Local causes:
        ○ Giant papillae
        ○ Foreign body in the sulcus subtarsalis
        ○ Trichiasis
      - Xerophthalmia
      - Neurotrophic ulcer in the cornea:
        ○ Herpes zoster ophthalmicus
        ○ Damage of trigeminal nerve due to tumor or trauma
      - Peripheral ulcerative keratitis:
        ○ Granulomatous polyangiitis
        ○ Rheumatoid arthritis
        ○ Polyarteritis nodosa
        ○ Systemic lupus erythematosus (SLE)

3. This patient most probably has been suffering from systemic lupus erythematosus.

4. Following are the cardiological features in this disease:
   a. Pericardium:
      - Acute pericarditis
      - Pericardial effusion
      - Cardiac tamponade
   b. Myocardium:
      - Global hypokinesia
      - Coronary artery disease due to atherosclerosis
      - Systolic murmur:
        ○ Functional murmur due to fever, tachycardia, and anemia
        ○ Mitral valve prolapse
      - Heart failure
      - Infectious endocarditis
   c. Endocardium:
      - Libman–Sacks endocarditis involving mitral and tricuspid valves
      - Valvular regurgitation

5. Following are the neurological features in this disease:
   a. Central features:
      - Headache
      - Disorders of mood
      - Seizure disorders
      - Aseptic meningitis
      - Cerebrovascular disease
      - Anxiety disorders
      - Psychosis
      - Myelopathy
      - Movement disorders
      - Demyelinating diseases
   b. Peripheral diseases:
      - Mononeuropathy
      - Polyneuropathy
      - Acute inflammatory demyelinating polyradiculoneuropathy
      - Cranial nerve involvement
      - Myasthenia gravis
      - Plexopathy
      - Autonomic disorders

6. Following are the eye lesions in this disease:
   a. Dry eye—keratoconjunctivitis sicca
   b. Anterior uveitis
   c. Keratitis
   d. Scleritis
   e. Episcleritis
   f. Retinal vasculopathy—cotton-wool exudates and hemorrhages
   g. Involvement of the optic nerve
   h. Iatrogenic glaucoma and cataract—due to administration of glucocorticoid
   i. Plaquenil retinopathy also known as "bull's eye maculopathy"

CASE 7

A 48-year-old female having history of stage 5 chronic renal failure came to surgical clinic to show breast pain and advised MRI with contrast-based gadolinium for evaluation. But after few days, she developed localized tightness in the front chest, blackening of the skin, and Peau d'orange color. Biopsy has been taken from the localized blackened area.

1. **What is the most likely diagnosis?**
2. **How can you define this disease?**
3. **What is the gadolinium-based contrast agent?**
4. **What should be the histological features?**
5. **What are the features in the peripheral blood of the patient?**
6. **What are the complications in this disease?**

Answers

1. This patient has been suffering from gadolinium-induced nephrogenic systemic fibrosis.
2. Nephrogenic systemic fibrosis is characterized by progressive multiorgan fibrosing condition due to exposure to gadolinium-based contrast in MRI and demonstrated as thickening of the skin as well as subcutaneous tissue along with systemic manifestations due deposition of gadolinium in the skin.
3. Gadolinium-based contrast agent consists of two types of chelating molecules:
    a. Linear molecules: These are less stable, link to the molecules weakly; hence, they are high-risk agent.
    b. Cyclic molecules: These are more stable, link to the molecules strongly, hence, they are low-risk agent.
4. Histology of the skin demonstrates:
    a. Increased cellularity consisting of:
        - Spindle-shaped fibroblast: It is expressed as procollagen type 1 and CD34.
        - Fibrohistiocytic cells
        - Fibroblast-like cells
        - Polygonal epithelioid fibroblast
    b. Increased amount of collagen arranged haphazardly
    c. Deposition of mucin
5. Following features may be present in the peripheral blood in this patient:
    a. Peripheral eosinophilia
    b. Antinuclear antibodies
    c. Hypercoagulability
    d. Anticardiolipin antibody
6. Following are the complications in this disease:
    a. Fibrosis of the following organs:
        - Lung—leads to pulmonary hypertension
        - Heart—leads to cardiomyopathy
        - Skeletal muscles—weakness of the skeletal muscles
        - Renal tubules leading to worsening of the already existent chronic kidney disease
    b. Thrombosis of the blood vessels leading to development of systemic hypertension resulting in decreased tolerance to hemodialysis
    c. Flexion contracture within weeks
    d. Frequent falls leading to fracture of the long bones

CASE 8

A 40-year-old female came to dermatology clinic with the following feature:

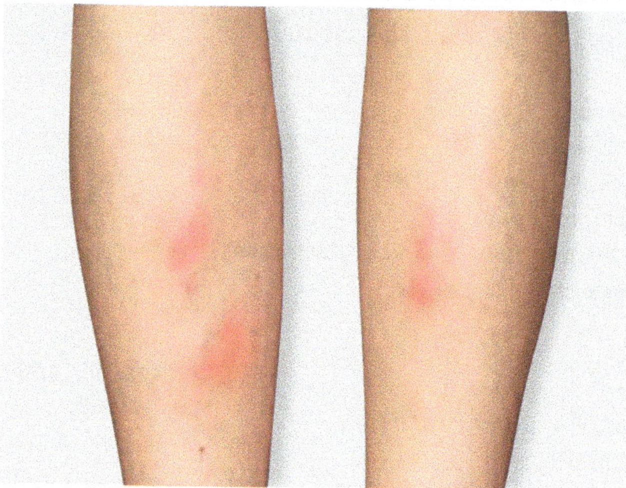

1. **What is the lesion?**
2. **What is the diagnosis?**
3. **What are the noninfectious causes of this lesion?**
4. **What are the stages in this lesion?**
5. **How can you evaluate this lesion?**

Answers

1. The lesion is characterized by painful firm, solid erythematous nodules localized on the extensor surface of the legs.
2. This is erythema nodosum.
3. Following are the noninfectious causes of erythema nodosum:
   a. Malignancy:
      - Leukemia
      - Lymphoma
      - Occult cancers
   b. Drugs:
      - Antibiotics: Penicillin and sulfonamide
      - Oral contraceptives
      - Iodides
      - Bromides
   c. Inflammatory bowel disease
   d. Miscellaneous causes:
      - Oral contraceptives
      - Sarcoidosis
      - Whipple's disease
      - Behçet's syndrome

4. There are three stages in this disease:
   a. Prodromal phase:
      - Nonspecific—from 3–6 days
      - Fever, joint pain, and abdominal pain
      - Nasopharyngeal infection
   b. Stable phase:
      - Settles within 1–2 days
      - Persistence or increase in the prodromal phase
      - Appearance of the nodules in the specific sites
      - Edema in the ankle
      - Hilar adenopathy
      - Pain in the lesion is increased by orthostatism.
   c. Regressive phase:
      - Spontaneous evolution by symptomatic treatment and rest
      - Evolution of the nodes in 10 days toward blue and yellowish contusiform followed by complete disappearance
5. Following are the evaluations in this lesion for diagnosis:
   a. For infectious cause—complete blood count, C-reactive protein (CRP), and vital signs

b. For tuberculosis and suspicion of Lofgren syndrome—chest X-ray, Mantoux test, and interferon-γ test

c. In case of suspected streptococcal infection, throat swab culture, rapid test, serology, antistreptolysin O (ASO) titer, and streptodornase test

d. Suspicion of viral infection—4 weeks interval, two samples for increasing titer in viral serology

e. In case of diarrhea or digestive problem, examination of stool

f. In case of doubt, cutaneous biopsy

CASE 9

A 48-year-old male came to medicine outpatient department with bilateral lower limb swelling and rash involving the lower extremities which were demonstrated below:

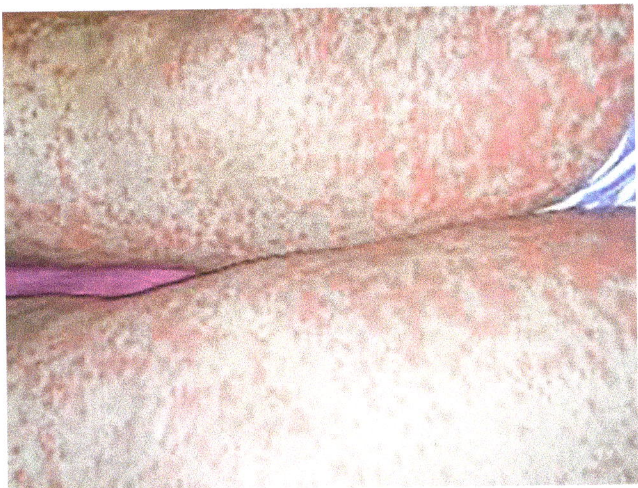

1. **Describe the feature in the above picture.**
2. **What is your diagnosis?**
3. **What type of immune complex disease is this?**
4. **Name the other causes of this immune complex disease.**
5. **What is the pathophysiology in this disease?**
6. **What are the histopathological and immunofluorescence microscopic findings in this disease?**

Answers

1. The above picture demonstrates erythematous macule and palpable papule size 1 mm to 1 cm in diameter being present in the lower extremities bilaterally in the dependent areas present in different stages.
2. The diagnosis is leukocytoclastic vasculitis.
3. This disease is small vessel vasculitis.
4. Following are the causes of small vessel vasculitis:
   a. Leukocytoclastic vasculitis or hypersensitivity vasculitis
   b. Cryoglobulinemic vasculitis
   c. Hypocomplementemic urticarial vasculitis
   d. Erythema elevatum diutinum
   e. Henoch–Schönlein purpura
   f. Sjögren's syndrome
   g. Rheumatoid arthritis
   h. SLE
   i. Paraneoplastic vasculitis
   j. Drug-induced vasculitis
   k. Infection-associated vasculitis

5. Description of the pathophysiology of this disease:

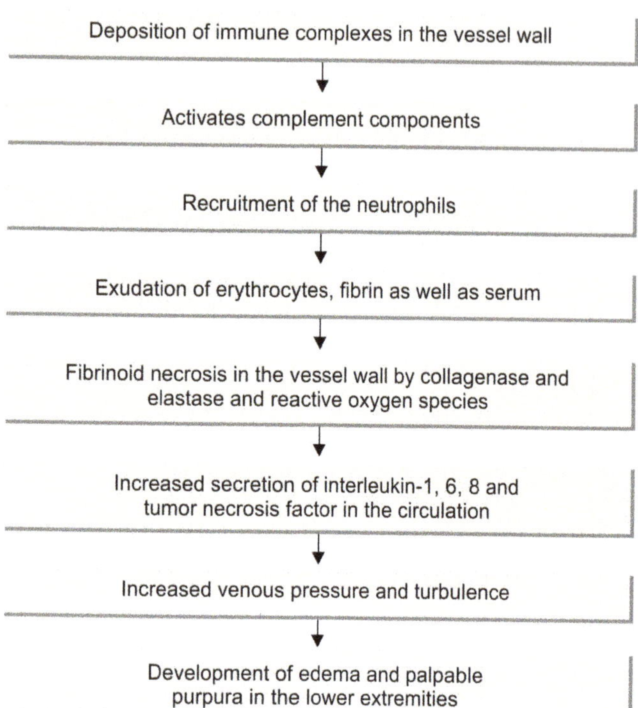

6. Following are the histopathological findings from the punch biopsy of the skin:
   a. Light microscopy demonstrates:
      - Destruction of the vessel wall
      - Infiltration of inflammatory cells around the vessel wall
      - Degeneration of the neutrophils known as leukocytoclasis with dust of nuclei known as karyorrhexis.
      - Presence of fibrinoid necrosis
      - Exudation f red blood cells in the dermis
      - In case of drug induced cases infiltration of eosinophils
      - If the lesion is more than 2 days, there is infiltration of lymphocytes.
   b. In the immunofluorescence microscopy demonstrates:
      - Deposition of IgA is specific of hypersensitivity vasculitis.

CASE 10

A 70-year-old man having long time history of tophaceous gout was undergone renal transplant 12 years back. He developed severe drug reaction after administration of allopurinol.

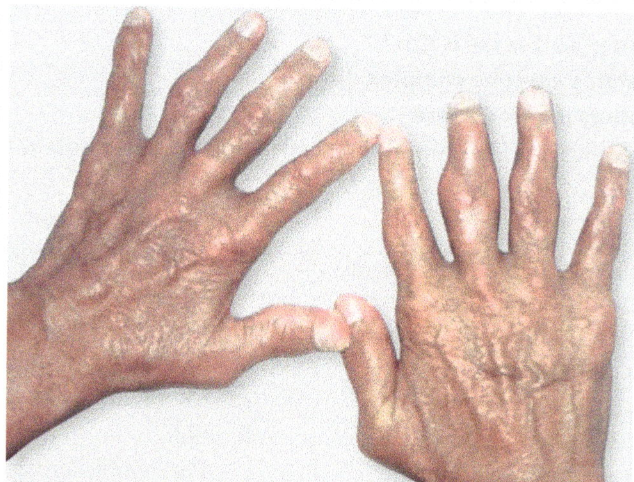

1. **Describe the above picture.**
2. **What is your diagnosis?**
3. **What are the physical findings in this case?**
4. **What are the complications in this case?**
5. **What are the erosions typical of this disease in radiology?**
6. **What are the ultrasonographic features specific for gout?**
7. **What is the use of uricase in this disease?**

Answers

1. The picture demonstrates multiple tophi present in the proximal interphalangeal joints of first, second, and third fingers of right and left hands.
2. The patient has been suffering from chronic tophaceous gout.
3. Physical findings in this case are the following:
   a. Most common involvement is single joint and may be multiple joints.
   b. Fever
   c. Evidence of posterior interosseous syndrome
   d. Presence of tophi in the soft tissue of helix, finger, toes, prepatellar bursa, and olecranon
   e. Involvement of the eye:
      - Conjunctival nodules containing crystals
      - Band keratopathy
      - Blurred vision
      - Scleritis
      - Anterior uveitis
4. Complications of tophaceous gout are as follows:
   a. Secondary infection
   b. Severe degenerative arthritis
   c. Renal stones
   d. Urate nephropathy
   e. Increased susceptibility to infection
   f. Involvement of spinal cord
   g. Fracture of the joints with tophi
5. Following are the erosions specific for gout:
   a. Joint space maintenance
   b. Periarticular osteopenia is absent.
   c. Erosion will be outside the joint capsule.
   d. Sclerotic border—cookie-cutter or punched-out border
   e. Erosions will be distributed asymmetrically but distal joints are most commonly involved.
6. Following features can be visible in the established cases of gout:
   a. "Double-contour sign": It is characterized by hyperechoic irregular line of monosodium urate crystals on the surface of the irregular cartilage which is overlying an adjacent hyperechoic bony contour.
   b. "Wet clumps of sugar" which is characterized by hypoechoic as well as hyperechoic materials having an anechoic rim.
   c. Presence of erosions adjacent to tophaceous gout
7. Uricase is recombinant porcine pegylated uricase or urase oxidase. It catalyzes the conversion of urate to soluble allantoin and uricase is absent in human being.

   Mg Pegloticase is given can be given as intravenous infusion every 2 weeks. Prior to administration serum uric acid should be checked to confirm.
   a. It sustains urate lowering efficacy, i.e., <6 mg/dL
   b. Absence of antibody to pegloticase
      This drug should be discontinued when the serum level is >6 mg/dL.

   It is contraindicated in case of glucose-6-phosphate dehydrogenase (G6PD) deficiency as there is risk of hemolysis.

CASE 11

A 28-year-old male came to emergency department with continuous high fever, pain in all the joints, backache, pain in the left side of chest and occasional vomiting, and weight loss for 2 months. He had no history of hemoptysis or hematemesis cough.

On examination, there was pallor, palpable discrete horizontal group of cervical glands, and hepatosplenomegaly. On auscultation, there was fine crepitation along with pleural rub in the left lower chest. Musculoskeletal examination demonstrated enlarged tender knee and shoulder and wrist joints bilaterally.

Laboratory examination demonstrated hemoglobin 8 g/dL, white blood cell count 35,000/cc, ESR 112 mm/1st hour, CRP 60 g/L, renal function test and electrolytes are within normal limit, serum glutamate-pyruvate transaminase (SGPT) 100 IU/L, and serum glutamate-pyruvate transaminase (SGOT) 120 IU/L. ASO titer 440 IU/L, serum ferritin level 1070 ng/dL, and citrullinated peptide (anti-CCP) antibody is negative.

Ultrasound demonstrates hepatosplenomegaly, mild ascites, and mesenteric lymphadenopathy.

1. **What extra and important history should be taken to clench the diagnosis?**
2. **What is the diagnosis if the above history is positive?**
3. **What should be the pattern of fever in this disease?**
4. **What are the criteria for this disease?**

5. **What are the two main differential diagnoses?**
6. **How can you exclude these diseases?**
7. **What is the definition of this disease?**
8. **What is the comment on the serum ferritin level?**
9. **In the biopsy of lymph node, what histological feature may be found?**
10. **What are the complications in this disease?**
11. **What is the prognosis in this disease?**
12. **What are the poor prognostic markers in this disease?**
13. **What are the factors associated with the good prognosis in this disease?**
14. **What is the rationale of treatment in this patient?**

Answers

1. History regarding rash that will appear during the onset of fever and disappear after defervescence of fever should be taken, this is known as "Salmon rash."

2. If the rash will be present, this patient would suffer from adult-onset Still's disease.

3. In adult-onset Still's disease, the pattern of fever should be:
   a. Quotidian fever, i.e., daily rise and daily fall Or,
   b. Double quotidian fever, i.e., twice a day with intervening afebrile period in-between the episode.

4. The Yamaguchi criteria for this disease are the following: Definite diagnosis requires at least two major and three minor criteria.
   a. Major criteria:
      - Fever ≥ 39°C for ≥1 week
      - Arthralgia or arthritis for ≥2 weeks
      - Characteristic of Salmon rash
      - Leukocytosis, i.e., total white blood cell count is >10,000/cc with predominant neutrophils.
   b. Minor criteria:
      - Pharyngitis
      - Lymphadenitis
      - Hepatomegaly/splenomegaly
      - Abnormal liver function test
      - Negative for ANA or rheumatoid factor

      Exclusion criteria:
      - Current infection
      - Malignancy mainly lymphoma
      - Active rheumatoid diseases

5. Following are the two main differential diagnoses:
   a. Lymphoma
   b. Systemic lupus erythematosus

6. Above two differential diagnoses can be excluded by following methods:
   a. SLE can be excluded by:
      - Negative ANA
      - High rise in CRP
   b. Lymphoma can be excluded by:
      - High rise in temperature
      - Presence of seronegative arthritis
      - Leukocytosis

7. Adult-onset Still's disease is characterized by:
   a. Inflammatory polyarthritis
   b. Quotidian pattern of fever
   c. Salmon-pink maculopapular rash
   d. Serum ferritin level > 1,000 ng/mL

8. Serum ferritin level must be >1,000 ng/dL, i.e., five times of the normal value. More common is the level between 3,000 ng/dL and 30,000 ng/dL. But the specificity of this value is poor because this level may be found in the following diseases:
   a. Neoplastic diseases
   b. Infections
   c. Gaucher's disease

9. Histological features in the lymph node biopsy are as follows:
   a. Typical or atypical paracortical hyperplasia
   b. Vascular proliferation
   c. Aggregation of histiocytes
   d. Exuberant immunoblastic reaction
   e. Follicular hyperplasia

10. Following are the complications in this disease:
    a. Macrophage activation syndrome
    b. Acute hepatic failure
    c. Cardiac tamponade
    d. Amyloidosis
    e. Myocarditis
    f. Disseminated intravascular coagulation

g. Interstitial lung disease

h. Pulmonary hypertension

11. Following are the types of prognoses in this disease:

    a. In 1/3rd of cases there may be the complete resolution in this disease.

    b. In 1/3rd of cases there is cyclic relapse and remit in this disease.

    c. In 1/3rd of cases disease becomes chronic and will evolve into rheumatoid arthritis.

12. Following factors are associated with poor prognosis:

    a. Disease becoming refractory to glucocorticoids

    b. Polyarthritis

    c. Persistently raised serum ferritin level

13. Following factors are associated with good prognosis:

    a. Prompt resolution of the clinical and laboratory features of the disease

    b. Absence of relapse after reduction of the dose of the steroid beyond 2–3 months period

14. Therapeutic decision should be taken based on the disease activity:

    a. Mild disease characterized by fever, arthralgia, and mild arthritis—they will respond to NSAIDs and low-dose glucocorticoids for better control of this disease.

    b. Moderate disease activity characterized by high-grade fever and involvement of the internal organs leading to life-threatening condition—in this patient, prednisolone should be started with 0.5–1 mg/kg/day prednisolone orally based on the severity of the disease.

    c. In case of life-threatening condition such as cardiac tamponade and severe hepatic involvement, 1 g methylprednisolone should be started intravenously for 3 days followed by oral prednisolone.

CASE 12

A 70-year-old female having no history of hypertension or diabetes mellitus came to emergency department with low-grade fever, anorexia, night sweat and weight loss for 6 months, and frequent unilateral temporal headache and pain in the knee joints, and difficulty in vision for 3 months.

On examination, there is mild pallor, vitals are normal, both knee joints are swollen, and left-sided temporal artery is tender on palpation.

Laboratory investigations demonstrated hemoglobin 9 g/dL, white blood cell count 11,000/cc with mild neutrophilic leukocytosis, eosinophils 8%, and ESR 140 mm/1st hour. Serology for ANA, rheumatoid factor (RF) and anti-CCP antibody are negative.

Routine urine demonstrated moderate proteinuria and few red and white blood cells.

Ultrasonography of abdomen and chest X-ay are normal. Blood and urine culture showed no growth.

1. **What is the most possible diagnosis?**
2. **What are the points in favor of this diagnosis?**
3. **What are the classification criteria in this disease?**
4. **What is the pathophysiology in this disease?**
5. **What are the characteristics of headache in this disease?**
6. **Why there is tenderness in the jaw?**
7. **What are the visual symptoms?**
8. **How large vessels are involved?**
9. **What is the invasive test that may be a clue to the diagnosis?**

Answers

1. The most possible diagnosis is giant cell arteritis or temporal arteritis.

2. Following features are in favor of this diagnosis:

    a. Unilateral headache

    b. Unexplained fever

    c. Sex predilection

    d. High ESR

3. Classification criteria in giant cell arteritis according to ACR are as follows: Three out of five criteria are required for making definite diagnosis of this disease:

    a. New headache

    b. At the onset of symptom age should be ≥50 years.

    c. ESR ≥ 50 mm/1st hour

d. Abnormalities in the temporal arteries such as tenderness or decreased pulsation

e. Abnormalities in the temporal artery biopsy such as vasculitis, predominance in the infiltration of mononuclear cells, formation of granulomatous inflammation, and presence of multinuclear giant cells

4. Pathophysiology in this disease:

```
Initial insult to the vascular endothelium by infection,
trauma, drug, and autoantigen
                    ↓
Dendritic cells present in the adventitia are activated
                    ↓
Activated dendritic cells release:
Chemokines that attract CD4+ helper cells as well as
macrophages in the arterial wall interleukin-6 and 18 that activate
T cells which in turn release interferon-γ
                    ↓
Interferon-γ:
Promotes inflammation
Activation of macrophages
Formation of granuloma

Secrete nitric oxide in the intimal layer will unite to form
syncytia leading to formation of "Giant cells"
                    ↓
Activated macrophages release oxygen free radicals and matrix
metalloproteinase and increase the systemic inflammation
through the release of interleukin-1 and 6
                    ↓
This leads to damage of endothelium and disruption of
internal elastic lamina
```

5. Characteristics of headache are as follows:

a. It occurs in elderly

b. It is insidious in onset and progressive in nature.

c. Resolve spontaneously, rarely

d. Headache is severe, resistant to over-the-counter analgesic.

e. During brushing the hair, there is tenderness in the scalp.

f. Focal tenderness of the temporal artery

6. There is pain in the jaw during chewing or talking. This is known as jaw claudication. It occurs due to decrease in supply of blood to the jaw muscles.

7. Following are the visual symptoms:

a. Amaurosis fugax: It is monocular visual loss and temporary due to ischemia in the ophthalmic artery. This will lead to transient ischemia in the optic nerve, retina, and choroid. Symptoms will be visual blurring and diplopia, to start with it is unilateral, but later on, if untreated both eyes are involved.

b. Anterior ischemic optic neuropathy following episode of amaurosis fugax due to complete cessation of blood flow through posterior ciliary artery leading to acute optic nerve head ischemia.

c. Posterior ischemic optic neuropathy occurs due to cessation of blood flow through retrobulbar portion of the optic nerve. Blindness is the presenting feature.

d. Diplopia resulting from:
   - Injury to the oculomotor system
   - Injury to the extraocular muscles
   - Paresis of ocular motor nerves
   - Brainstem disease

e. Bitemporal hemianopia—it results from compromise of the artery supplying the optic chiasma

f. Homonymous hemianopia—it results from the compromised vessels supplying the retrochiasmal portion of visual sensory pathways

g. Visual hallucination resulting from:
   - Glucocorticoid-associated psychosis
   - Charles Bonnet syndrome: It occurs in psychologically normal patients resulting from loss of vision in case of any lesion in the peripheral or central visual pathway.

8. Large vessels are involved in younger patients:

a. Aortic arch syndrome: It occurs due to involvement of subclavian or axillary artery:
   - Claudication of arms
   - Absent pulses
   - Asymmetric pulses in both the hands

b. Aortitis:
   - Active lesion mainly involves ascending aorta and may lead to aortic valve dilatation.
   - Aneurysm, mainly thoracic part of aorta
   - Dissection, mainly in case of chronic aortitis

9. Temporal artery biopsy is the gold standard in the diagnosis of this disease. It will demonstrate:

a. Infiltration of lymphocytes and macrophage

b. Disruption of internal elastic lamina

c. Luminal narrowing

d. Proliferation of the intima

e. Fibrinoid necrosis

CASE 13

A 35-year-old patient came to medicine outpatient department with neck pain and pain in the hands for 4 years (demonstrated below). He had history of morning stiffness which was recovered by activity. He had history of skin lesion which demonstrated below:

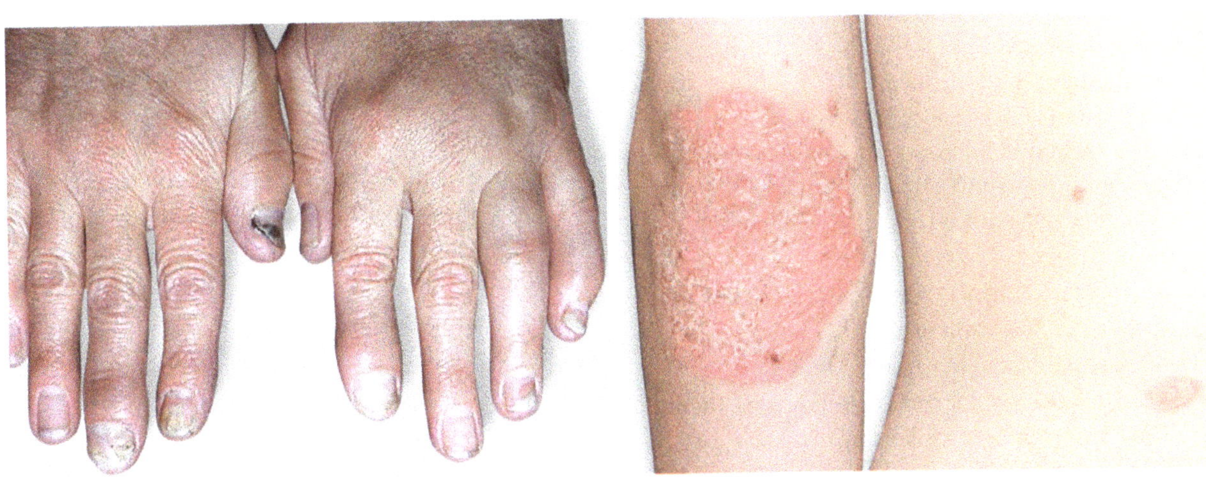

1. **What do the above pictures demonstrate?**
2. **What is your most likely diagnosis?**
3. **What is the genetic association with this disease?**
4. **What are the extra-articular manifestations in this disease?**
5. **What are the periarticular features seen in this disease?**
6. **What are the specific radiological features in this disease specific to psoriatic arthritis?**
7. **Mention the criteria for psoriatic arthritis.**
8. **What are the radiological features seen in this disease?**
9. **According to ACR criteria, classify the active psoriatic arthritis.**
10. **Classify the biologics used in this disease.**

Answers

1. The above pictures demonstrate:
   a. There is swelling of the distal interphalangeal joints of all the fingers of both hands. There is also evidence of pitting in the nails in both the hands.
   b. Skin lesion demonstrated plaque-like well-circumscribed lesion with silvery scales with some bleeding points seen on the extensor aspect of the elbow of left upper limb. There is also small evolving lesion seen on the lower aspect of the back.
2. The most likely diagnosis is psoriatic arthritis.
3. Following genetic association seen in this disease:
   a. *HLA-B*08:01*—associated with peripheral arthritis, asymmetric polyarthritis, damage of the joints, and ankylosis.
   b. *HLA-B*27:05*—axial involvement, symmetric sacroiliitis, dactylitis, and enthesitis
   c. *HLA-B*38:01*—polyarthritis
   d. *HLA-B*39:01*—polyarthritis
   e. *HLA-B*44:02*—it is protective, milder disease.
   f. *HLA-B*57:01*
   g. *HLA-C*06:02*
   h. Non-HLA gene: *IL-23R*—this gene produces proteins which is responsible for immune-mediated inflammation.
4. Following extra-articular manifestations seen in this disease:
   a. Psoriatic skin lesions
   b. Pitting on the nails and onycholysis—there severity of the nail manifestation directly correlates with the severity of the skin and joint diseases
   c. Posterior uveitis

5. Following are the periarticular features seen in this disease:
   a. Enthesitis
   b. Dactylitis
   c. Tenosynovitis
6. Following radiological features specific for this disease:
   a. Bone destruction
   b. Pathologic new bone formation
7. CASPAR criteria for classification of psoriatic arthritis: Presence of an inflammatory articular disease (joint, spine, or entheseal) plus ≥ 3 points from the following:
   a. Evidence of psoriasis (one of the following):
      - Current psoriasis (2 points)
      - Personal history of psoriasis (1 point)
      - Family history of psoriasis (1 point)
      - Psoriatic nail dystrophy (1 point)
      - Negative test for rheumatoid factor (1 point)
   b. Dactylitis (one of the following):
      - Current dactylitis (1 point)
      - History of dactylitis by a rheumatologist (1 point)
      - Radiological evidence of juxta-articular new bone formation (1 point)
8. Following radiological features seen in this disease:
   a. Erosive changes
   b. Growth of new bone in the distal joints
   c. Pencil-cup erosion
   d. Lysis of the terminal phalanges
   e. Periostitis
   f. Growth of new bone at the sites of enthesitis
9. According to ACR guideline, classification of the active psoriatic arthritis includes one or more of the following:
   a. Swollen joints
   b. Tender joints
   c. Dactylitis
   d. Enthesitis
   e. Axial disease
   f. Active axial/nail involvement
   g. Extra-articular inflammatory manifestations such as uveitis or inflammatory bowel disease.
10. Classification of biologics in the treatment of psoriatic arthritis:
    a. Anti-tumor necrosis factor (anti-TNF) agents:
       - Adalimumab
       - Certolizumab
       - Etanercept
       - Golimumab
       - Infliximab
    b. Anti-interleukin-17 agents:
       - Ixekizumab
       - Secukinumab
    c. Anti-interleukin-12/interleukin-23 agents: Ustekinumab
    d. Phosphodiesterase 4 (PDE4) inhibitor: Apremilast
    e. T-cell modulator: Abatacept
    f. Janus kinase inhibitor: Tofacitinib

CASE 14

A 56-year-old nonhypertensive, nondiabetic woman came to medical outpatient department with fever, generalized backache, myalgia, anorexia for 6 months, and difficulty during deglutition, skin color changes during exposure to clod and exertional respiratory distress for last 1 month.

On examination, there is moderate anemia, blood pressure 110/65 mm Hg, pulse rate 100 beats/min, and arthralgia.

Laboratory investigation demonstrates hemoglobin 10 g/dL, white blood cell count 14,500/cc, ESR 120 mm/1st hour, serum electrolytes are normal, bilirubin 0.6 mg/dL, SGPT 110 IU/L, alkaline phosphatase 300 IU/L, and serology demonstrated rheumatoid factor positive.

1. **What is the most probable diagnosis?**
2. **What is most common differential diagnosis in this disease?**
3. **What are the antibodies present in this disease?**
4. **What are the infective agents that act as triggering factor for this disease?**
5. **What are the poor prognostic factors in this disease?**
6. **Mention the complications in this disease.**
7. **What are the muscle enzymes elevated in this disease?**
8. **What are the electromyographic findings in this disease?**
9. **From which muscles biopsy can be done and what are the features in this biopsy?**
10. **What are the diagnostic criteria in this disease?**

Answers

1. The most probable diagnosis is polymyositis.
2. The most common differential diagnosis in this disease is polymyalgia rheumatica. This can be excluded if following are present:
   a. High muscle enzyme
   b. Rheumatoid factor positivity
   c. Positive ANA
   d. Positive anti-Jo-1
3. Following antibodies are present in this disease:
   a. Myocyte-specific antibodies:
      - Nuclear Mi-2 protein
      - Aminoacyl transfer ribonucleic acid synthetase (anti-Jo-1)
      - Components of the signal recognition particle
   b. Myositis-associated antibodies:
      - Nuclear Ku antigen
      - PM/Scl nucleolar antigen
      - Small nuclear ribonucleoprotein
      - Cytoplasmic ribonucleoprotein
4. Following infective agents act as triggering factor for this disease:
   a. Human immunodeficiency virus (HIV)
   b. Coxsackievirus B1
   c. Hepatitis B virus
   d. Echovirus
   e. Adenovirus
   f. Influenza virus
5. Following are the poor prognostic markers in this disease:
   a. Female sex
   b. Advanced age
   c. Race—African American
   d. Interstitial lung disease
   e. Presence of anti-Jo antibodies
   f. Dysphonia
   g. Dysphagia
   h. Associated malignancy
   i. Delayed treatment
   j. Inadequate treatment
   k. Cardiac involvement
6. Following are the complications in this disease:
   a. Pulmonary causes:
      - Aspiration pneumonia
      - Interstitial lung disease
      - Pneumonia
      - Carcinoma of the lung
   b. Cardiac involvement:
      - Pericarditis
      - Congestive heart failure
      - Heart block
      - Arrhythmias
      - Myocardial infarction
   c. Gastrointestinal causes:
      - Malabsorption
      - Dysphagia
   d. Infection
   e. Carcinoma of breast
   f. Steroid-induced myopathy
7. Following muscle enzymes are elevated in this disease:
   a. Lactate dehydrogenase
   b. SGOT
   c. SGPT
   d. Aldolase
   e. Creatine phosphokinase (CPK)
8. Following are the electromyographic features found in this disease:
   a. Evidences of:
      - Membrane instability
      - Increased insertional activity
      - Fibrillation potential
      - At rest, positive sharp waves
   b. Evidences of:
      - Myopathic changes of motor unit action potential
      - Decrease in amplitude and duration
      - Increased polyphasic potential
      - Bizarre, high-frequency repetitive discharges
   c. Chronic changes include features of denervation-reinnervation
9. From deltoid and quadriceps femoris muscles biopsy can be taken. Histological changes include:
   a. Early changes include:
      - Focal endomysial infiltration with mononuclear cells containing CD8+ T lymphocytes and widespread expression of minimum histocompatibility complex class I antigen
      - Obliteration of the capillaries
      - Damage of the endothelial cells
      - Increased amount of connective tissue
   b. Late changes include:
      - Degeneration of the muscle fibers
      - Evidence of fibrosis
      - Regeneration of muscle fibers

10. Diagnostic criteria in this disease are as follows:
    a. Typical clinical history
    b. Laboratory evidence of increased muscle enzymes
    c. Feature in the electromyography
    d. Evidence of muscle biopsy

CASE 15

A 31-year-old nondiabetic woman came to medicine outpatient department with quotidian pattern of fever, burning sensation during micturition, dysuria and lower abdominal pain for 15 days, and sudden appearance of painful swelling of the left knee joint along with spiky fever along with rashes in the body for 3 days.

On examination, her pulse rate was 120 beats/min, regular, blood pressure 120/70 mm Hg, temperature 104°F, and lower abdomen is tender.

Laboratory investigation demonstrated white blood cell count 19,000/cc with polymorphonuclear leukocytosis. Routine urine demonstrated turbid urine with plenty of pus cells/HPF, protein +, and crystal absent. Culture and sensitivity demonstrated no growth.

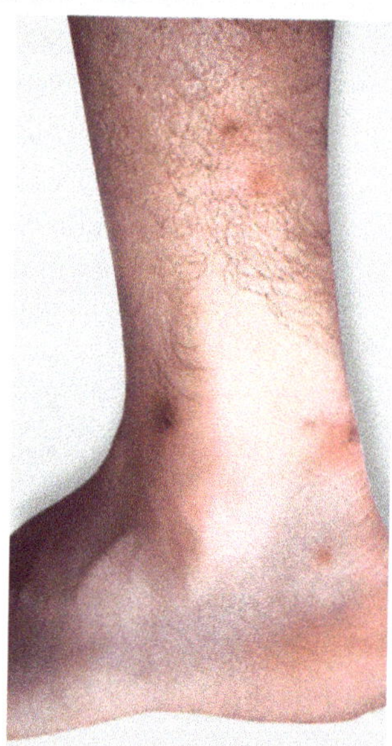

1. **Describe the rash in the above picture.**
2. **What is the most likely diagnosis?**
3. **What are the clinical forms in this disease?**
4. **What are the factors that help in development of this disease?**
5. **What are diagnostic features of the clinical forms of this disease?**
6. **How can you evaluate specifically for this disease?**
7. **What are the differential diagnoses?**
8. **Mention the complications in this disease.**
9. **What should be the preferred treatment in this case?**

Answers

1. Above picture demonstrates the evidence of maculopapular, pustular, and hemorrhagic rashes in the lateral side of the left leg.

2. The most probable diagnosis is gonococcal arthritis.

3. There are two clinical forms of this disease:
   a. Arthritis-dermatitis syndrome
   b. Localized septic arthritis

4. Following factors are responsible for this disease:
   a. Host factors:
      • Deficiency of the complement
      • Pregnancy

- Menstruation
- History of pelvic surgery
- Intrauterine devices

b. Organism virulence factors:
  - Specific outer membrane protein of gonococcus known as "porin 1A" which:
    - ○ Promotes resistance
    - ○ Diminishes host inflammatory response
    - ○ Promotes invasion to the host cells
    - ○ Provides specific substrate for growth

5. Following are the specific features in the clinical forms of this disease:
   a. Arthritis-dermatitis syndrome: The specific triad in this form is:
      - Tenosynovitis: It can be demonstrated by tenderness on the flexor tendon during passive extension affecting fingers, wrist, and toes.
      - Polyarthralgia
      - Dermatitis
        Associated constitutional symptoms such as fever, malaise, and body ache
   b. Localized septic arthritis: It is characterized by monoarthritis or asymmetric oligoarthritis or polyarthritis affecting knee, ankle, elbow, and wrist.

6. By following methods, we can evaluate this disease:
   a. Laboratory studies:
      - Two sets of blood culture prior to administration of the antibiotics
      - Inflammatory markers:
        - ○ White blood cell count
        - ○ ESR
        - ○ CRP
      - Serum prolactin > 0.5 ng/mL—it is more specific and less sensitive.
      - Culture from cervix, urethra, and rectum
      - Nucleic acid amplification testing of urine specimen in both men and women and vaginal swab in women.
      - Serum lactate dehydrogenase
   b. Imaging:
      - Plain radiograph for evaluation of:
        - ○ Joint destruction
        - ○ Bony involvement
        - ○ Effusion
        - ○ Erosions
        - ○ Chondrocalcinosis
        - ○ Extent of the disease
      - Magnetic resonance imaging to detect osteomyelitis and adjacent abscess
      - Echocardiography for evaluation of septic emboli
   c. Arthrocentesis should be done in case of monoarticular joint pain along with effusion:
      - Presence of crystals cannot exclude the infection
      - White blood cell count of >50,000/cc with predominant polymorphonuclear leukocytosis
      - Gram stain of the synovial fluid to detect gram-negative bacteria
      - Polymerase chain reaction of the synovial fluid for detection of gonococcal DNA

7. Following are the differential diagnoses:
   a. Septic arthritis: It can be differentiated by microbiological identification in the synovial fluid and its culture.
   b. Poststreptococcal arthritis: Here, the rash is neither vesicular nor pustular.
   c. Crystal arthropathy: It can be differentiated by analysis of synovial fluid.
   d. Other inflammatory arthritis such as rheumatoid arthritis and psoriatic arthritis by clinical and radiological features.

8. Following are the possible complications in this disease:
   a. Meningitis
   b. Joint damage
   c. Periarthritis
   d. Endocarditis
   e. Osteomyelitis

9. Following should be the preferred treatment:
   a. Ceftriaxone 1 g intravenously daily along with 100 mg doxycycline orally twice daily to cover superinfection with *Chlamydia trachomatis* for 7 days
   b. After 2–3 days of clinical improvement ceftriaxone should be given 250 mg intramuscularly daily for 7–14 days.

CASE 16

A 50-year-old nondiabetic, nonhypertensive female came to medical outpatient department with 5 months history of recurrent high fever, pain in the ear along with progressively increasing loss of hearing which was recovered within 7 days each time with analgesics. In the last 3 months, she also complained of recurrent pain and blockage of nasal passage along with hoarseness of voice and pain in the eye which was recovered with analgesics also.

On physical examination, there was anemia, pulse rate 110 beats/min, and blood pressure 120/70 mm Hg.

Laboratory investigation demonstrated hemoglobin 8.5 g/dL and white blood cell count 14,000/cc with polymorphonuclear leukocytosis. Serum creatinine was 1.2 mg/dL and urea was 35 mg/dL. Electrocardiography demonstrated sinus tachycardia.

1. **What is the most likely diagnosis?**
2. **What are the points in favor of your diagnosis?**
3. **Define this disease.**
4. **What is the main pathophysiology behind it?**
5. **What are the genetic associations in this disease?**
6. **What are the associated conditions that may be found in this disease?**
7. **What are criteria behind this diagnosis?**
8. **What should be the possible treatment in this case?**

Answers

1. The most likely diagnosis is relapsing polychondritis.
2. Following points are in favor of this diagnosis: Involvement of the cartilage of ear, nasal passage, and tracheal cartilage.
3. Relapsing polychondritis can be defined as the autoimmune condition where there is recurrent inflammation of auricular, tracheal, and nasal cartilage leading to pain and swelling of these cartilages resulting in diminished hearing, hoarseness of voice, and nasal blockage, respectively.
4. Pathophysiology in this disease:
   a. Affected cartilaginous tissues are infiltrated with CD4+ T cells, plasma cell, macrophages, and neutrophils leading to release of degrading enzymes.
   b. Proinflammatory cytokines are released during flares like monocytes chemoattractant protein-1, macrophage inflammatory protein-1β as well as interleukin-8 leading to recruitment of macrophages and monocytes.
   c. Autoantibodies against collagen type II, IX, and XI and matrilin, an extracellular matrix, found in tracheal cartilage and cartilage oligomeric protein
   d. Serum collagen type II autoantibodies will correlate with the severity of the disease.
   e. Serum antimatrilin antibody is increased in this patient during nasal flares.

5. Following genetic associations found in this disease:
   a. *HLA-DR4*
   b. *HLA-DRB1*16:02*
   c. *HLA-B*67:01*
   d. *HLA-DQB1*05:02*
6. Following associated conditions may be found in this disease:
   a. Myelodysplastic syndrome
   b. Behçet's disease
   c. Systemic vasculitis
   d. Rheumatoid arthritis
   e. Systemic lupus erythematosus
   f. Psoriatic arthritis
   g. Inflammatory bowel disease
7. Following are the Michet's diagnostic criteria behind this diagnosis. This diagnosis requires two major or one major and two minor criteria for this diagnosis.
   a. Major criteria:
      - Auricular chondritis
      - Nasal chondritis
      - Laryngotracheal chondritis
   b. Minor criteria:
      - Ocular inflammation:
         ○ Conjunctivitis
         ○ Keratitis
         ○ Episcleritis
         ○ Uveitis
      - Loss of hearing

- Vestibular dysfunction
- Seronegative inflammatory arthritis

8. Possible treatment in this case:
   a. In case of involvement of nasal, laryngeal, and auricular cartilage, colchicine or dapsone and if required low-dose glucocorticoids.
   b. In case severe symptoms such as sensorineural hearing loss and laryngotracheal involvement, intravenous methylprednisolone 1 g daily for 3 days followed by oral prednisolone 1 mg/kg daily along with immunosuppressive therapy such as methotrexate, cyclophosphamide, azathioprine, or cyclosporine.
   c. Biologics in case of polychondritis is infliximab. But, adalimumab, abatacept, and etanercept can be given

CASE 17

A 30-year-old nondiabetic, nonhypertensive female admitted in emergency department with severe and persistent postpartum bleeding for 1 month. She complained of weakness, headache, malaise, and continuous high-grade fever for last 15 days. She had also history of pain in the left lower limb.

On examination, there is pallor, pulse rate 120 beats/min, blood pressure 110/70 mm Hg, temperature 103°F, lower limb calf muscles are tender, reddened, and swollen.

Laboratory investigations demonstrated hemoglobin 5 g/dL, white blood cell count 16,000/cc with neutrophil 70%, microcytic hypochromic type red blood cells, and platelet count 110,000/cc.

Routine analysis of urine demonstrated protein ++, plenty of pus cells but no RBC, and culture was negative. ECG demonstrated low voltage tracing.

Chest X-ray demonstrated the following features:

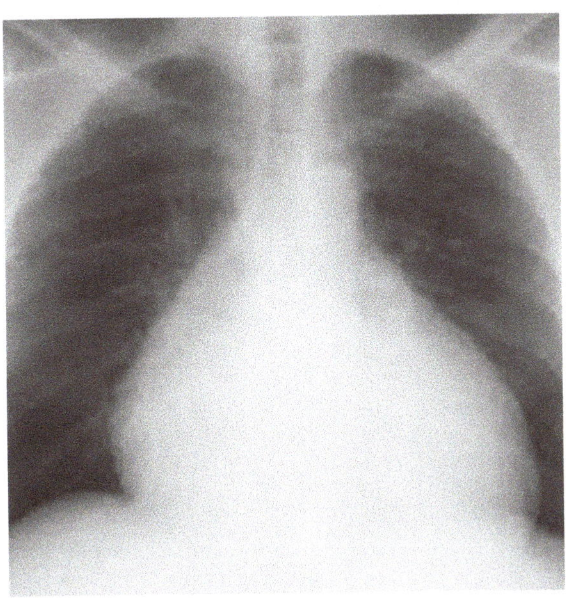

1. **What has been demonstrated in the chest X-ray?**
2. **What is your diagnosis?**
3. **What are the clues to the diagnosis?**
4. **Is there any associated feature suggesting another diagnosis?**
5. **What are the antibodies that can be found in the blood of the patient suffering from the associated disease?**
6. **What are the genetic associations in this associated condition?**
7. **What are the infections induct APLA?**
8. **What are the drugs induct APLA production?**
9. **Mention the criteria of APLA syndrome.**

Answers

1. Above X-ray demonstrated:
   a. Cardiomegaly
   b. Oligemic lung field
2. The diagnosis is systemic lupus erythematosus.
3. Following are the clues to the diagnosis:
   a. High ESR
   b. Elevated leukocyte count
   c. Low platelet count
   d. Pericardial effusion with oligemic lung field
   e. Low voltage wave tracing
4. The associated diagnosis is APLA syndrome suggesting from the following features:
   a. Persistent postpartum bleeding
   b. Deep venous thrombosis in the left lower limb
5. Following antibodies are found in this patient suffering from APLA syndrome done by enzyme-linked immunosorbent assay (ELISA):
   a. Anticardiolipin antibodies IgG and IgM
   b. Anti-β2-glycoprotein-1 antibodies
   c. Lupus anticoagulant
6. Following genetic associations are found in APLA syndrome:
   a. *HLA-DR4*
   b. *HLA-DR7*
   c. *DRw53*
   d. *DQw7*
   e. *C4*
7. Following infections induct APLA:
   a. *Borrelia burgdorferi*
   b. Treponema
   c. Leptospira
   d. HIV
8. Following drugs induct APLA production:
   a. Procainamide
   b. Chlorpromazine
   c. Quinidine
   d. Phenytoin
9. Criteria for the diagnosis of this APLA syndrome:
   a. Clinical criteria: One of the following clinical features should be confirmed to diagnose APLA:

- Vascular thrombosis: ≥1 events of arterial or venous thrombosis confirmed by appropriate imaging or histopathology. For histopathology, thrombosis must be present without any inflammation in the vessel wall.
  - Past thrombotic episode can be included as a criterion as long as it was appropriately confirmed by specific diagnostic methods and there is no other cause of thrombosis.
  - Superficial venous thrombosis should not be included in this criterion.
- Pregnancy morbidity:
  - ≥1 unexplained fetal death of morphologically normal fetus that is confirmed by ultrasound and clinical examination ≥10 weeks of gestation
  - ≥1 premature birth of morphologically normal neonate before 34th weeks of gestation. This prematurity is secondary to preeclampsia, eclampsia, or insufficiency of the placenta.
  - ≥3 consecutive spontaneous abortions prior to 10th weeks of gestation after ruling out any anatomical or hormonal abnormalities in the mother and placental chromosomal causes.

   b. Laboratory criteria: ≥1 laboratory findings should be confirmed to diagnose APLA syndrome:

- Lupus anticoagulant can be detected in ≥2 occasions in ≥12 weeks apart.
- IgG or IgM antiphospholipid antibodies can be detected in the serum or plasma in moderate or high titers (>40 GPL or >99th percentile) as measured by standard ELISA on ≥2 occasions at ≥12 weeks apart.
- IgG or IgM anti-β2-glycoprotein antibodies can be detected in serum or plasma in moderate-to-high titers (>99th percentile) as measured by ELISA test on ≥2 occasions at ≥12 weeks apart.

CASE 18

A 25-year-old female was admitted with weakness, high continued fever, headache for nearly 1 month and small bruise throughout the body, and backache for 1 week.

On examination, there is pallor, pulse rate 110 beats/min, blood pressure 100/70 mm Hg, and spleen is palpable four fingers below the left costal margin.

Laboratory investigations demonstrated hemoglobin 9.5 g/dL, microcytic and hypochromic RBC, white blood cell count 12,000/cc, and ESR 65 mm/1st hour.

Urine routine analysis demonstrated protein ++ and few pus cells.

1. **What are the differential diagnoses?**
2. **What is your most likely diagnosis?**
3. **What are the investigations that should be done to clench the diagnosis?**

Answers

1. The differential diagnoses are:
   a. Idiopathic thrombocytopenic purpura
   b. Systemic lupus erythematosus
2. The most likely diagnosis is systemic lupus erythematosus as splenomegaly is absent in idiopathic thrombocytopenic purpura and ESR will not be so high.
3. Following investigations should be done to clench the diagnosis:
   a. ANA
   b. dsDNA

CASE 19

A 32-year-old female came to medical outpatient department with pain and swelling of the both knee joints, low-grade continuous fever as well as weakness for >4 months.

On examination, there was pallor, discrete nontender cervical lymphadenopathy, and just palpable spleen.

Laboratory investigation demonstrated hemoglobin 11 g/dL, platelet count 120,000/cc, and ESR 70 mm/1st hour. Serology demonstrated rheumatoid factor positive, venereal disease research laboratory (VDRL) positive, and ASO titer 600 IU/L.

1. **What is the possible diagnosis?**
2. **What are the genetic associations in this disease?**
3. **What are the complement deficiencies seen in this disease?**
4. **What is the importance of positivity in VDRL?**
5. **What is the importance of ASO titer positivity?**
6. **What are the histological features found in the lymph node?**
7. **If the patient will become pregnant, what are the complications that may occur in this patient?**
8. **What are the differential diagnoses in this case and how can you exclude those diseases?**

Answers

1. The most likely diagnosis is systemic lupus erythematosus.
2. Following genetic associations are seen in this disease:
   a. *HLA-DRB1*
   b. *HLA-DR2*
   c. *HLA-DR3*
   d. *HLA-DRX*
   e. *TNFAIP3*
   f. *STAT4*
   g. *STAT1*
   h. *TLR-7*
   i. *IRAK1/MECP2*
3. Following complements are deficient in this disease:
   a. C1q: >0%
   b. C1r: >90%
   c. C1s: >90%

    d.   C4: 50%

    e.   C2: 20%

    f.   TREX1

4. In case of SLE, VDRL is false positive. In the following cases, VDRL is positive:

    a.   Old age

    b.   Narcotic abuse

    c.   Leprosy

5. ASO positivity indicates prior infection with *Streptococcus*.

6. Following histological features found in the lymph node in this disease:

    a.   Follicular hyperplasia

    b.   Giant cell infiltration

    c.   Plasma cell infiltration in the interfollicular zones

    d.   Necrosis in the paracortical T-cell zones

7. Following complications may occur in this patient if the patient will become pregnant:

    a.   Spontaneous abortion

    b.   Preeclampsia

    c.   Fetal loss

    d.   Maternal thrombosis

    e.   Anti-Ro and anti-La can cross the placenta leading to development of:
- Fetal heart block
- Neonatal lupus who may present with photosensitive rash.

    f.   Flaring of lupus, if the disease was uncontrolled in the last 6 months prior to pregnancy

    g.   Increased mortality during pregnancy if the patient has been suffering from severe manifestations of SLE.

8. Differential diagnoses:

    a.   Rheumatoid arthritis: In this disease, SLE-specific autoantibodies and hypocomplementemia are absent.

    b.   Drug-induced lupus: In this case, there is resolution of symptoms after withdrawal of the drug.

    c.   Adult-onset Still's disease: Here, SLE-specific autoantibodies, no malar rash, and no other organ involvement.

    d.   Behçet's disease: Here, there is absence of serological feature and no organomegaly.

    e.   Sarcoidosis: Here, there is bilateral hilar lymphadenopathy, which is rare in SLE.

CASE 20

A 25-year-old nonhypertensive and nondiabetic female admitted in the medicine emergency department with the history of transient unconsciousness along with left-sided hemiparesis. She had past history of recurrent nasal bleeding.

On examination, all the vitals were normal. Neurological system examination demonstrated features of upper motor neuron weakness on the right side. Other systemic examinations were within normal limit.

Laboratory investigation demonstrated hemoglobin 8 g/dL, microcytic and hypochromic, platelet count 80,000 cc, ESR 130 mm/1st hour, INR 1.5, activated partial thromboplastin time two times the control, and serum fibrinogen was normal.

1. **What is the most likely diagnosis?**
2. **What are the pathophysiologies behind this disease?**
3. **What are the vessels involved in this case?**
4. **What are the risk factors responsible for adverse outcome in pregnancy?**
5. **What are the adverse pregnancy-related complications in this disease?**
6. **What are the dermatological manifestations to be searched in this disease?**
7. **In the severe form of this disease what treatment should be given?**

Answers

1. The most likely diagnosis is APLA syndrome.

2. Pathophysiology behind this disease: APLA antibody affects the coagulation and thrombosis through the separate mechanisms:

    a.   APLA antibody binds to platelet leading to:
- Upregulation of the production of thromboxane A2
- Expression of glycoprotein IIb/IIIa

    b.   APLA binds to endothelial cells and monocytes leading to increased production of the tissue factors

    c.   APLA binds to endothelial cells leading to increased expression of adhesion molecules

       The above interactions favor thrombosis.

    d.   APLA activates complement leading to initiation of the inflammatory cascade resulting in thrombosis.

e. Disruption of protein C by APLA leading to initiation of thrombosis

f. Antibodies to naturally occurring anticoagulant β2-glycoprotein lead to prothrombotic state

g. In case of early pregnancy, APLA has inhibitory effect on the proliferation of trophoblast cells.

h. In late pregnancy, the complication arises from:
- Remodeling of spiral arteries
- Reduced proliferation as well as invasion of extravillous trophoblast
- Inflammation at the maternal-fetal interface

3. Artery and veins are involved in this case:

a. Following arteries are involved in this disease:
- Deep veins in the leg
- Pelvic vein
- Renal vein
- Mesenteric vein
- Hepatic vein
- Portal vein
- Axillary vein
- Ocular vein
- Sagittal vein
- Inferior vena cava

b. Following arteries are involved in this disease:
- Cerebral arteries
- Retinal artery
- Brachial artery
- Mesenteric artery
- Coronary artery
- Peripheral arteries

4. Following are the risk factors for the adverse outcome in the pregnancy:

a. Triple positivity:
- Lupus anticoagulant
- Anticardiolipin antibodies
- Anti-β2-glycoprotein-1 antibodies

b. History of previous loss of pregnancy

c. History of thrombosis

d. SLE

5. Following are the adverse pregnancy-related complications in this disease:

a. Pregnancy loss

b. Preeclampsia

c. Fetal distress

d. Premature birth

e. Intrauterine growth retardation

f. Placental insufficiency

g. Abruptio placentae

h. HELLP syndrome: It is characterized by hemolysis, elevated liver enzymes, and low platelet count.

6. Following dermatological manifestations to be searched for in this disease:

a. Livedo reticularis

b. Splinter hemorrhages

c. Skin infarct

d. Leg ulcers

e. Superficial thrombophlebitis

f. Blue toe syndrome

g. Raynaud's phenomenon

h. Necrotizing purpura

7. In the severe variety of this disease, following treatment should be given:

a. Treatment of the precipitating factor like infection and SLE flare

b. Intravenous heparin followed by oral anticoagulation

c. 1 g methylprednisolone intravenously for 3 days followed by oral prednisolone 1 mg/kg daily

d. Plasma exchange with or without 400 mg/kg intravenous immunoglobulin for 4–5 days.

e. If the treatment is ineffective, following drugs should be given in specific cases:
- Cyclophosphamide in patient with SLE flare
- Rituximab in patient having autoimmune hemolytic anemia or thrombocytopenia

CASE 21

A 50-year-old nondiabetic, nonhypertensive female came to medical outpatient department with pain and swelling in the multiple joints in the body, weakness, anorexia, weight loss, myalgia for 4 years, and progressively increasing difficulty in deglutition for 8 months.

On examination, there was pallor, emaciated, tender and swollen elbow and knee joints and muscles, few painful ulcers in the mouth, the eyelids, hair, and chest X-ray demonstrated:

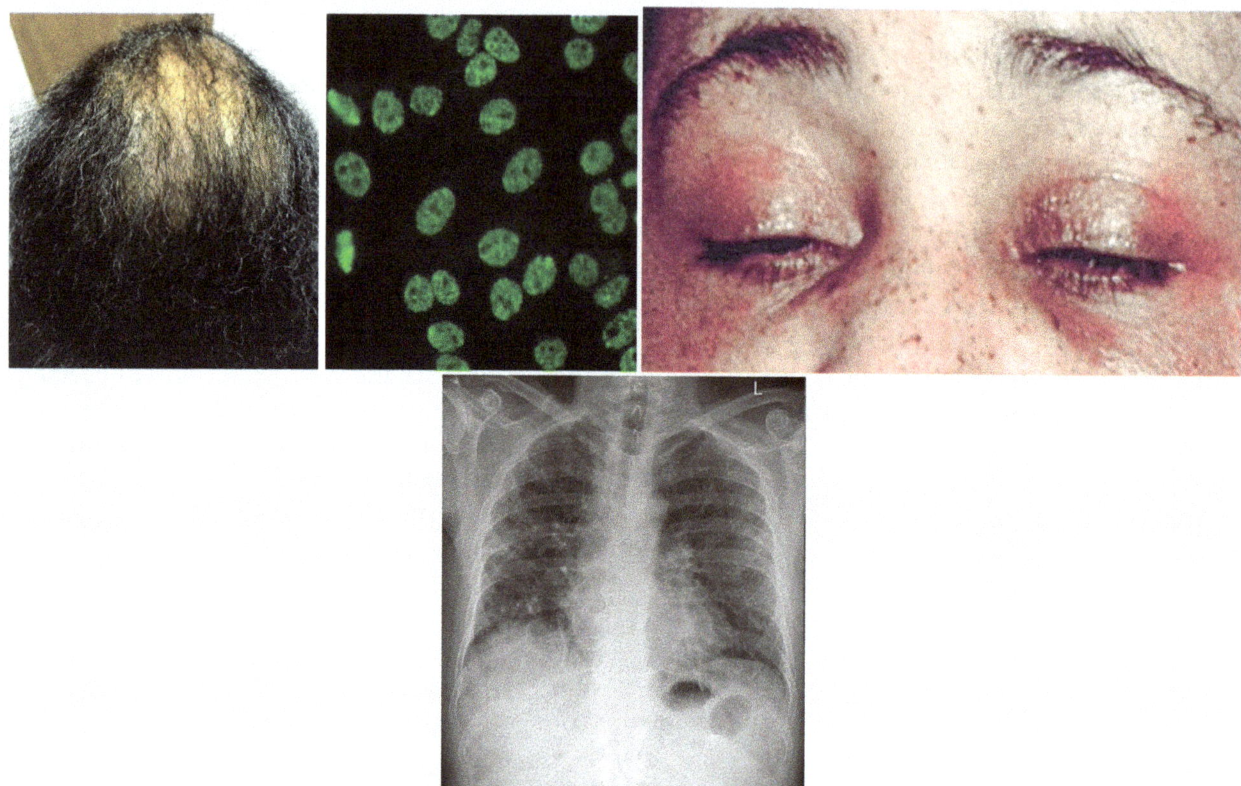

Laboratory investigations demonstrated ESR 120 mm/1st hour, white blood cell count 12,000/cc, anti-RNP antibody is positive, anti-Scl antibody is positive, and ANA showed above 2nd middle.

1. **What do the above pictures demonstrate?**
2. **What is the most probable diagnosis?**
3. **Define this disease.**
4. **What are the specific features related to the specific disease that are present in this case?**
5. **What are the complications in this disease?**
6. **What are the features in ECG?**
7. **What are the CT scan features in the lung in this disease?**
8. **What are the vascular features in this disease?**

Answers

1. Description of the above pictures:
   a. First picture demonstrated the cicatricial alopecia involving the center of the head.
   b. Second picture demonstrated immuno-fluorescent image showing ANA.
   c. Third picture demonstrated heliotropic erythema covering both the eyelids.
   d. Fourth picture demonstrated reticular and reticulonodular pattern in both the lungs field.
2. The most likely diagnosis is mixed connective tissue disease.
3. Mixed connective tissue disease can be defined as systemic connective tissue disease having overlapping feature of at least two connective tissue diseases of:
   a. Systemic lupus erythematosus
   b. Systemic scleroderma
   c. Rheumatoid arthritis
   d. Polymyositis
   e. Dermatomyositis
   Along with serological features of:
   a. Anti-RNP antibody
   b. Other specific antibody specific for the disease.
4. In this case, features of the following diseases are present:
   a. Heliotropic erythema over the eyelid—dermatomyositis
   b. Severe muscle pain—polymyositis
   c. Cicatricial alopecia, arthritis, raised ESR, and positive ANA—systemic lupus erythematosus
   d. Anti-Scl antibody positive—scleroderma

e. Anti-RNP antibody—sine qua non of mixed connective tissue disease

5. Following are the complications in this disease:
   a. Life-threatening complications:
      - Thrombotic thrombocytopenic purpura
      - Renal crisis
      - Malignant hypertension
      - Pulmonary hypertension leading to respiratory failure
   b. Cardiovascular complications:
      - Dilated cardiomyopathy
      - Cardiac tamponade
      - Coronary sclerosis
      - Ischemic cardiomyopathy
      - Arrhythmias
   c. Malignancies
   d. Infections
6. ECG features in this disease are as follows:
   a. Hemiblock
   b. Bundle branch block
   c. Atrioventricular block
   d. Low voltage complexes in cardiomyopathy and pericardial effusion
7. Following are the CT scan findings in the lung in this disease:
   a. Ground-glass opacities
   b. Linear opacities
   c. Subpleural nodules
   d. Septal thickening
   e. Traction bronchiectasis
   f. Peripheral and lower lobe predominance
   g. Less common features:
      - Honeycomb appearance
      - Airspace consolidation
      - Emphysema
      - Centrilobular nodules
8. Following are the vascular features in this disease:
   a. Raynaud's phenomenon
   b. Digital ulcers
   c. Vasculitis

Treatment of these vascular features:
   a. Gloves and warm clothing
   b. Cessation of smoking
   c. Use of calcium channel blockers
   d. Topical nitroglycerin
   e. Low-dose aspirin
   f. Phosphodiesterase-5 inhibitors
   g. Direct arterial vasodilators:
      - Bosentan
      - Prostaglandin infusion therapy

CASE 22

A 17-year-old girl has come to medical outpatient department with history of progressively increasing polyarthralgia, weight loss, anorexia, evening rise low-grade continuous fever with night sweat, and painful ulcers in the mouth for 2 years. He was given empirical full course of antitubercular therapy by the village doctor but without any effect.

On examination, there was pallor, cervical lymphadenopathy, and just palpable spleen.

Lymph node biopsy demonstrated reactive hyperplasia. Her echocardiography was performed which demonstrated:

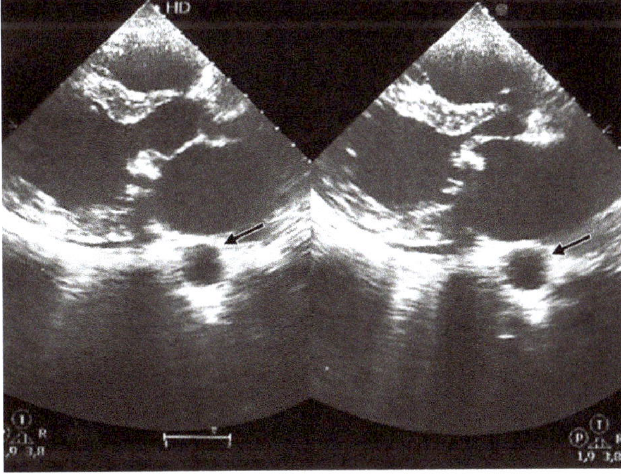

1. **What does the above picture demonstrate?**
2. **What are the causes of this finding?**
3. **What should be the histological features in this finding?**
4. **What are the valves that may be involved in this case?**
5. **What is your diagnosis?**
6. **What are the common causes of this picture in this patient?**

Answers

1. Doppler echocardiography demonstrated the evidence of vegetation on the mitral valve diagnostic of Libman-Sacks endocarditis or marantic endocarditis.
2. Following are the causes of this finding:
   a. Systemic lupus erythematosus
   b. Malignancies of pancreas, colon, ovary, lung, biliary channels, and prostate
   c. Antiphospholipid syndrome
   d. Rheumatoid arthritis
   e. Sepsis
   f. Disseminated intravascular coagulation
3. The most likely diagnosis is systemic lupus erythematosus.
4. Following are the histological features in this disease:
   a. Active verrucae—it consists of:
      - Clumps of fibrin with foci of necrosis
      - Plasma cells
      - Lymphocytes
   b. Combination of active and healed lesion—consists of combined necrotic as well as healed lesion
   c. Healed lesion—it consists of dense fibrous, vascularized, and scar tissue
5. Following valves are involved in this case:
   a. Mitral valve
   b. Aortic valve
   c. Tricuspid valve
6. As the patient's age is only 17 years, the common causes are either systemic lupus erythematosus or antiphospholipid syndrome:
   a. In case of antiphospholipid syndrome, there should be history of evidences of arterial or venous thrombosis, anticardiolipin antibody IgG and IgM, and lupus anticoagulant positivity.
   b. In case of SLE as there should be history of polyarthralgia, skin rash, splenomegaly, lymphadenopathy, positive ANA, and dsDNA.

CASE 23

A 15-year-old male came to medical outpatient department with complaint of polyarthritis involving wrists then elbows followed by knees bilaterally along with weakness, weight loss, and low-grade fever for 6 months. For the last 15 days, he felt neck stiffness along with recurrent sore throat.

On examination, there was bilateral nontender discrete cervical lymphadenopathy, tenderness of the involved joint, and palpable spleen.

Laboratory investigation demonstrated hemoglobin 8.5 g/dL, white blood cell count 12,000/cc, ESR 100 mm/1st hour, ASO titer 350 IU/L, and CRP 46 mg/dL.

1. **What is the most probable diagnosis?**
2. **What are the other probabilities?**
3. **Define this disease.**
4. **What are the human leukocyte antigen (HLA) varieties associated with rheumatoid factor positive and rheumatoid factor negative juvenile idiopathic arthritis (JIA)?**
5. **What are the categories of JIA?**
6. **What is the pathophysiology in this disease?**
7. **What are the radiographic signs of arthritis?**

Answers

1. The most likely diagnosis is JIA or Still's disease.
2. The other possibilities are:
   a. Acute leukemia
   b. Lymphoma
   c. Disseminated tuberculosis
   d. Infection
   e. Systemic lupus erythematosus
3. Juvenile idiopathic arthritis is a heterogeneous condition characterized by low-grade fever, polyarthritis, lymphadenopathy, neck stiffness, hepatosplenomegaly, and leukocytosis.
4. Following HLA varieties are associated with rheumatoid factor negative JIA:
   a. HLA-A2
   b. HLA-DRB1:11
   c. HLA-DRB1:08
   Following HLA varieties are associated with rheumatoid factor positive JIA:
   a. HLA-DRB1:01
   b. HLA-DRB1:04
5. According to the International League of Associations of Rheumatology, there are seven categories of JIA:
   a. Oligoarthritis
   b. Rheumatoid factor-positive polyarthritis
   c. Rheumatoid factor-negative polyarthritis
   d. Systemic arthritis
   e. Psoriatic arthritis
   f. Enthesitis-related arthritis (ERA)
   g. Undifferentiated arthritis
6. The pathophysiology in this disease:

Imbalance between the Th1 and Th17 of adaptive immunity

↓

Induces matrix metalloproteinase and proinflammatory cytokines

↓

Lead to joint damage resulting in monoarthritis, polyarthritis, and psoriatic arthritis

In case of ERA, crucial cytokine, interleukin-23 results:
   a. Inflammation through tumor necrosis factor and interleukin-17
   b. Formation of new bone through interleukin-22
7. Following are the indirect radiographic signs in arthritis:
   a. Swelling of the soft tissues
   b. Increased density of the soft tissues
   c. Dislocation of the fat folds in surrounding the joints

CASE 24

A 60-year-old hypertensive but nondiabetic female having past history of bronchial asthma on salbutamol inhaler came to emergency department with dry cough, severe respiratory distress, and continuous low-grade fever for 10 days.

On physical examination, blood pressure 165/90 mm Hg, pulse rate 112 beats/min, regular, and normal jugular venous pressure. On auscultation, occasional rhonchi in the both lung field was heard.

Laboratory investigation demonstrated hemoglobin 8 g/dL, white blood cell count 12,000/cc, ESR 120 mm/1st hour, eosinophil 17%, neutrophil 61%, creatinine 4.6 mg/dL, urea 45 mg/dL, sodium 130 mEq/L, potassium 5 mEq/L, chloride 70 mEq/L, and bicarbonate 7.34 mEq/L.

Urine analysis demonstrated ++ protein and few red blood cells. Chest X-ray and paranasal sinuses demonstrated:

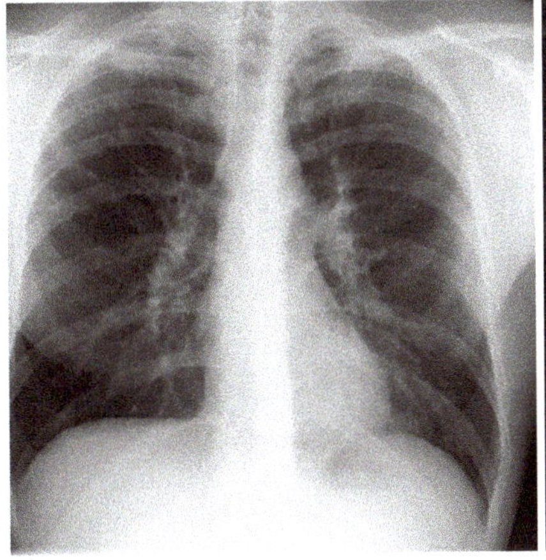 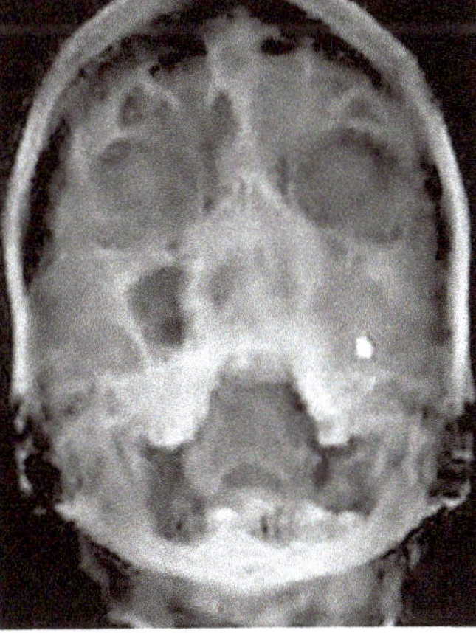

Ultrasonography demonstrated enlarged kidneys bilaterally.

1. **What do the above pictures demonstrate?**
2. **What is the most likely diagnosis?**
3. **What are the diagnostic criteria in this disease?**
4. **In this case, what are the points in favor of this diagnosis?**
5. **What are the phases of development in this disease?**
6. **What are the treatment strategies in this disease?**
7. **What are the risk factors associated with high mortality?**

Answers

1. The above pictures demonstrate:
   a. Bilateral infiltrates in the both lungs
   b. Opacity of the left maxillary sinus
2. The most likely diagnosis is eosinophilic granulomatosis with polyangiitis.
3. According to ACR, the diagnostic criteria: Presence of at least four of the following six criteria is required:
   a. Asthma
   b. Eosinophilia > 10%
   c. Mononeuropathy or polyneuropathy attributable to a systemic vasculitis
   d. Migratory or transient infiltrates on chest radiography
   e. Paranasal sinus abnormality (acute or chronic paranasal pain or radiographic opacification of paranasal sinuses)
   f. Extravascular eosinophils on biopsy
4. Following are the points in favor of this diagnosis in this case:
   a. Bronchial asthma
   b. Eosinophil count is >10%.
   c. Transient infiltrate in the chest radiography
   d. Opacification of the left maxillary sinus
5. Following are the phases of presentation in this disease:
   a. First phase is prodrome, starting in the childhood, and lasts for 30 years. Features are:
      - Nasal polyposis
      - Sinusitis
      - Allergic rhinitis
      Asthma develops after the age of 35 years.
   b. Second phase: This phase is characterized by peripheral blood and tissue eosinophilia. Features are:
      - Loeffler's pneumonia
      - Chronic eosinophilic pneumonia
      - Eosinophilic gastroenteritis

   c. Third phase: It is characterized by small vessel vasculitis which started 3 years after development of asthma.
6. Treatment strategies are as follows:
   a. Induction of remission:
      - Without poor prognosis:
        - 1 mg/kg prednisolone orally daily for 3 weeks followed by tapering at 5 mg every 10 days to 0.5 mg/kg followed by tapering at 2.5 mg at every 10 days to minimal effective dose or until complete withdrawal of the drugs
          Or,
        - 1 g methylprednisolone intravenously for 3 days followed by prednisolone as previously described
      - Relapse:
        - 2 mg/kg azathioprine orally daily × at least 6 months
          Or,
        - 600 mg cyclophosphamide in pulse every 2 weeks orally for 1 month followed by every 4 weeks
      - With poor prognosis:
        - 15 mg methylprednisolone intravenously × 3 days + oral prednisolone as previous dose regimens
          Plus
        - 600 mg cyclophosphamide in pulse every 2 weeks orally for 1 month followed by every 4 weeks
          Or,
        - Cyclophosphamide 2 mg/kg orally for 3 months or 600 mg cyclophosphamide in pulse every 2 weeks orally for 1 month followed by every 4 weeks, this is followed by 2 mg/kg azathioprine orally for 1 year or more.
   b. Maintenance of remission:
      - 10–25 mg methotrexate orally weekly

- 1.5–2.5 mg/kg/day cyclosporine A
- 2 mg/kg/day azathioprine

c. In refractory cases:
- Plasma exchange
- 0.4 mg/kg intravenous immunoglobulin daily × 3 days
- 3 million IU interferon-α thrice weekly subcutaneously.
- Tumor necrosis factor such as infliximab, etanercept, or adalimumab
- Rituximab 325 mg/m^2 × 4 weeks

7. Following risk factors are associated with high mortality:
   a. Proteinuria of >1 g daily
   b. Cardiomyopathy
   c. Involvement of gastrointestinal tract
   d. Renal insufficiency—serum level of creatinine is >1.58 mg/dL.
   e. Involvement of central nervous system

CASE 25

A 40-year-old female presented to medicine outpatient department with history of recurrent low-grade fever, sneezing, epistaxis, pain in the ear, and progressively increasing hoarseness of voice for 1 year. During this time, she also lost weight and weakness.

On examination, pulse rate was 100 beats/min, regular, blood pressure 110/60 mm Hg, respiratory rate 24 breaths/min, and purpuric spots in the both legs. Nasal examination demonstrated hypertrophied turbinate with presence of crust.

Laboratory investigation demonstrated hemoglobin level 10 g/dL, white blood cell count 20,000/cc, platelet count 400,000/cc, and ESR 75 mm/1st hour. Chest X-ray demonstrated bilateral apical opacities. Chest X-ray of paranasal sinuses demonstrated as below. Renal function test and serum electrolytes are within normal limit.

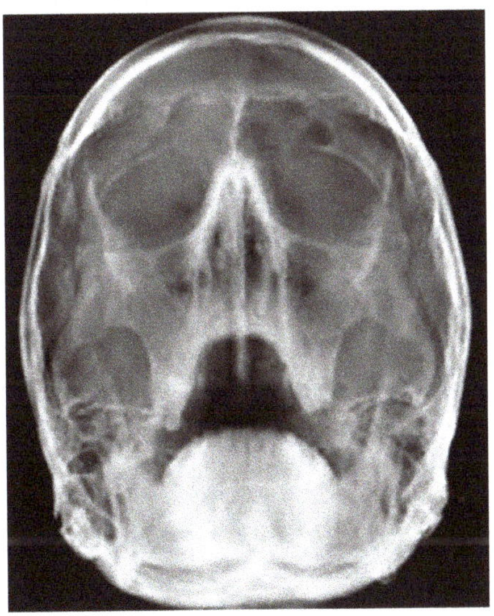

1. **What does the above picture demonstrate?**
2. **What is the most probable diagnosis?**
3. **Define this disease.**
4. **How can you classify this disease according to the severity?**
5. **Mention the diagnostic criteria of this disease.**
6. **In patient having hemoptysis but clear X-ray, what are the chest findings in the CT scan?**
7. **What are the genetic associations in this disease?**
8. **What are the infections responsible for exacerbations of this disease?**
9. **What should be the histopathological findings in the lung biopsy?**
10. **Which specific diagnostic feature supports the diagnosis?**
11. **What are the complications in this disease?**

Answers

1. The above picture demonstrates mucosal thickening in the both maxillary sinuses.

2. The most probable diagnosis is Wegener granulomatosis.

3. Wegner granulomatosis is a small medium-sized vessels necrotizing granulomatous vasculitis involving the blood vessels in nose, sinuses, lungs, throat, and kidneys resulting in upper and lower respiratory tract infection, destruction of the nasal cartilage, and glomerulonephritis leading to renal failure.

4. This disease can be classified according to the severity:
   a. Localized disease: Localized involvement of the upper and lower respiratory tract infection in absence of any systemic involvement or any constitutional symptoms.
   b. Early systemic disease: In absence of organ-threatening or life-threatening disease.
   c. Generalized disease: It is characterized by renal or other organ-threatening disease with serum creatinine level is <4.5 mg/dL.
   d. Severe disease: This disease is characterized by renal or other vital organ failure with serum creatinine level ≥5.6 g/dL.
   e. Refractory disease: It is a progressive disease that is unresponsive to glucocorticoid alone and cyclophosphamide (uncommon).

5. According to ACR, the diagnostic criteria: At least two of the four following criteria should be present:
   a. Nasal or oral inflammation (painful or painless ulcers, purulent, or bloody nasal discharge)
   b. Abnormal chest radiograph (nodules, fixed infiltrate, or cavities)
   c. Five red blood cells per high power field or red cell cast in the sediment of urine
   d. Pathologic evidence of granulomas, leukocytoclastic vasculitis, and necrosis

6. In patient having hemoptysis but clear X-ray, following are the CT scan of the chest findings:
   a. Small areas of cavitations
   b. Nodules
   c. Interstitial lung disease

7. Following are the genetic associations in this disease:
   a. Defective alleles for $\alpha 1$-antitrypsin
   b. Proteinase 3 gene
   c. Cytotoxic T lymphocyte associated protein 4
   d. Major histocompatibility complex class II, DP α-1 gene
   e. Certain types of FC γ receptor III b present on the surface of the neutrophils and macrocytes/monocytes.

8. Following infections exacerbate the disease process:
   a. Bacteria: Colonization with *Staphylococcus aureus*
   b. Viral infection:
      - *Cytomegalovirus*
      - Hepatitis C virus
      - Parvovirus B_{19}
      - Epstein–Barr virus

9. Following are the histopathological findings in the lung biopsy:
   a. Granulomas which are surrounded by the palisading histiocytes and giant cells.
   b. Liquefaction and coagulative necrosis containing numerous eosinophils and multinucleated giant cells.
   c. Angiitis of the arteries and venules by:
      - Neutrophils
      - Plasma cells
      - Eosinophils
      - Scanty lymphocytes
      - Plasma cells

10. The specific diagnostic test is serum anti-PR3 antibodies that support the diagnosis of this disease.

11. Following are the complications in this disease:
    a. Complications due to disease itself:
       - Permanent vision loss
       - Loss of hearing
       - Mononeuritis multiplex
       - Saddle-nose deformity
       - Septal perforation
       - End-stage renal disease
       - Acute hypoxic respiratory failure due to diffuse pulmonary hemorrhage
    b. Complications due to immunosuppressive therapies:
       - Infections
       - Infusion reaction
       - Death
       - Lymphoma
       - Myelodysplastic syndrome

CASE 26

A 40-year-old female came to medicine outpatient department with painful oral ulcers and pain and swelling in the large joints for 1 year, pain in the lower abdomen with bloody loose motion along with painful ulcers in the scrotum for 15 days.

On examination, there were multiple aphthoid painful ulcers on the tongue, gum and scrotum, and red eyes. Both the knee and elbow joints are swollen and tender. Following lesions were seen on the legs.

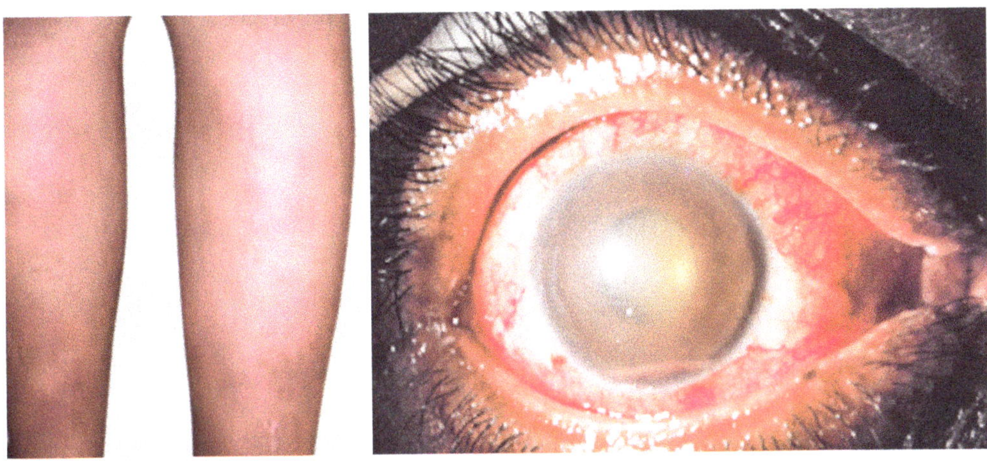

1. **What was demonstrated in the above pictures?**
2. **What is the most likely diagnosis?**
3. **Define this disease.**
4. **What are the genetic associations with this disease?**
5. **What are the protective genes in this disease?**
6. **What are the proposed International criteria for Behçet's disease 2013?**
7. **What is pathergy test?**
8. **What are the cutaneous manifestations in this disease?**
9. **What is the treatment of the above skin lesion?**

Answers

1. Above pictures demonstrate:
   a. Multiple erythematous nodules seen on the anterior surface of the lower legs bilaterally that is tender to touch.
   b. Right eye demonstrates circumlimbal congestion; pupil is slightly irregular due to posterior synechia.
2. The most likely diagnosis is Behçet's syndrome.
3. Behçet's syndrome is an autoimmune condition characterized by mucocutaneous features like recurrent oral and genital ulcers, chronic relapsing uveitis and systemic vasculitis involving all-sized arteries and veins and malignant aphthosis.
4. Following genetic associations are associated with this disease:
   a. *HLA-B51*
   b. *HLA-B15*
   c. *HLA-B27*
   d. *HLA-B57*
   e. *HLA-B26*

   Non-HLA association in this disease:
   a. Endoplasmic reticulum aminopeptidase 1
   b. Interleukin-23R
   c. Interleukin-12RB2
   d. Interleukin 10
5. Following are the protective genes in this disease:
   a. *HLA-B49*
   b. *HLA-A03*
6. The proposed International criteria for Behçet's disease 2013 are:

   Patient present with the following manifestations whose total points are ≥4 can be classified as Behçet's syndrome:

Criteria	Points
Oral aphthosis	2
Genital aphthosis	2
Ocular lesions	2
Skin manifestations	1
Involvement of central nervous system	1
Vascular lesions	1
Pathergy test (optional)	1

7. Pathergy test is specific but less sensitive:
   a. It is considered positive if an erythematous papule of >2 mm will be formed within 48 hours.
   b. Blunt needle produces more positive reaction
8. Following are the cutaneous lesions:
   a. Erythema nodosum
   b. Superficial thrombophlebitis
   c. Deep vein thrombosis
   d. Acneiform or pseudofolliculitis
   e. Pyoderma gangrenosum-like lesion
   f. Pustular vasculitis lesion
   g. Small vessel vasculitis
   h. Sweet syndrome-like lesion
9. Treatment of the erythema nodosum:
   a. Combination of 40–60 mg prednisolone daily orally plus 50 mg azathioprine daily orally
   b. If the dose of azathioprine is well tolerated, the dose can be increased to 50 mg every 4 weeks.
   c. Target dose is 2.5 mg/kg/day.
   d. Every 2 weeks complete blood count should be done till the maximum tolerated dose, then monitoring should be done every 6–12 weeks.
   e. Prednisolone should be continued at targeted dose for 1 month, then the dose should be tapered gradually to complete the total course within 3–4 months.

CASE 27

A 30-year-old female suffering from systemic lupus erythematosus at her third trimester of pregnancy developed sudden convulsion and was brought to emergency immediately and lower uterine cesarean section was performed. After birth, the neonate did not cry. On examination, pulse rate was 42 beats/min and regular. Immediate ECG was done that demonstrated features of complete heart block.

1. **What is the cause of this heart block here and why?**
2. **How can you treat this patient?**
3. **What investigation should be done in any patient who is suspected to be SLE patient?**

Answers

1. The cause of the congenital complete heart block is presence of anti-Ro antibody which will cross the placental barrier and produced this feature. It occurs in <3% of patients.
2. As this heart block is permanent, this block should be treated by permanent insertion of pacemaker.
3. So in any patient suffering from systemic lupus erythematosus and wants to be pregnant, anti-Ro antibody should be done. So that the pregnant woman becomes cautious about future of the baby.

CASE 28

A 50-year-old hypertensive, diabetic female on antihypertensive medications recently started atorvastatin for her severely deranged LDL level. After 15 days, she had pain in the muscles, difficulty in standing from sitting position, and combing her hair.

On examination, proximal muscles were tender, and proximal muscle power and tone normal.

Laboratory investigations demonstrated CPK 1056 IU/L, urea 90 mg/dL, and creatinine 3.6 mg/dL.

1. **What is the most likely diagnosis?**
2. **What are the clinical spectra in this disease?**
3. **What are the proposed mechanisms in this disease?**

4. **What are the risk factors responsible for this disease?**
5. **Why thyroid-stimulating hormone (TSH) should be checked in this disease?**
6. **Are all these types of etiological agents may lead to this disease?**
7. **Why were urea and creatinine raised in this case?**
8. **How can you manage this disease?**

Answers

1. The most likely diagnosis is statin-induced myopathy.
2. The clinical spectra in this disease are:
    a. Myalgia
    b. Myositis
    c. Rhabdomyolysis
    d. Asymptomatic increase in the serum CPK
3. Following are three proposed mechanisms that may produce this disease:
    a. Impaired cholesterol synthesis may lead to changes in the cholesterol in the membrane of the myosite leading to changes in the behavior of the membrane.
    b. Impaired synthesis of a compound in the pathway of cholesterol synthesis particularly deficiency of coenzyme Q_{10} leading to impaired activity of enzyme in the mitochondria.
    c. Depletion of the product in the HMG-coenzyme A reductase pathway, isoprenoids leading to increased apoptosis of myofibers.
4. Following are the risk factors in this disease:
    a. Age > 80 years
    b. Female sex
    c. Low body mass index
    d. Vigorous exercise
    e. Diabetes mellitus
    f. Diseases affecting the liver and kidney function
    g. Untreated hypothyroidism
    h. Excess alcohol
    i. Intercurrent infections
    j. Major surgery
    k. Major trauma
    l. Diet:
        - Excessive cranberry juice
        - Excessive grapes
    m. Genetic factors:
        - Polymorphism in the cytochrome P450 isoenzymes
        - Inherited defect in the muscle metabolism
    n. Drug interactions with those drugs that inhibit cytochrome P450 isoenzyme pathway:
        - Nicotinic acids
        - Fibrate
        - Cyclosporine
        - Amiodarone
        - Warfarin
        - Antifungal
5. TSH should be checked as hypothyroidism may lead to hypercholesterolemia and increased CPK in the blood.
6. Lyophilized statins such as atorvastatin, simvastatin, and lovastatin are more likely to produce this type of symptom as compared to hydrophilic drugs such as rosuvastatin, pravastatin, and fluvastatin because the former drugs will penetrate the muscle membrane leading to myotoxic effect.
7. Myositis leads to release of myoglobin which passes through the kidney leading to renal failure.
8. Statin should be stopped immediately.

CASE 29

A 45-year-old nonhypertensive female admitted in the chest department nonproductive cough and breathlessness. On examination, there were grade 3 clubbing, central cyanosis, and presence of Velcro crepitations in the lungs bilaterally.

1. **What is your diagnosis?**
2. **What are the histories you have to take in this case?**
3. **What are the causes of this disease?**
4. **What are the diagnostic tests in this case?**

Answers

1. The most likely diagnosis is interstitial lung disease.
2. Following history should be taken mainly in female:
   a. Skin rashes
   b. Polyarthritis
   c. Raynaud's phenomenon
   d. History of drug ingestion
   e. Occupation
3. The causes are:
   a. Collagen vascular disease:
      - Rheumatoid arthritis
      - SLE
      - Scleroderma
      - Dermatomyositis
   b. Occupational lung disease.
      - Asbestosis
      - Silicosis
      - Coal worker pneumoconiosis
   c. Drugs:
      - Busulfan
      - Bleomycin
      - Methotrexate
      - Nitrofurantoin
      - Amiodarone
   d. Extrinsic alveolitis
   e. Mitral valve disease
   f. Hemosiderosis
4. High-resolution CT scan can confirm the diagnosis.

CASE 30

A 21-year-old male suffering from pulmonary tuberculosis came to outpatient department with following features:

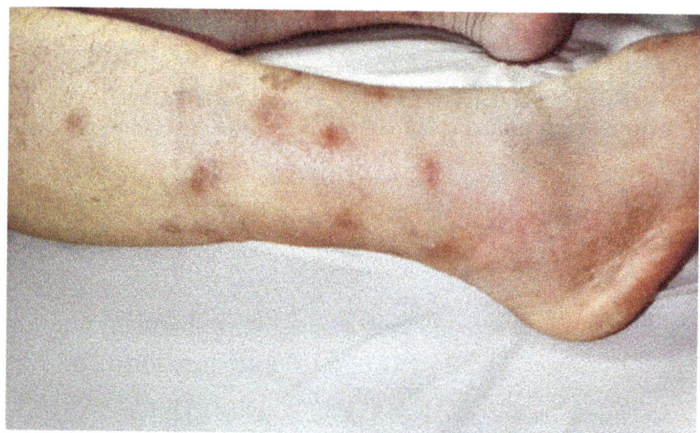

1. **What has been demonstrated in the above picture?**
2. **What is the most likely diagnosis?**
3. **What are the types of this lesion?**

Answers

1. Abode picture demonstrates:
   a. The presence of tender ulcerated nodules in the calf of the right lower limb
   b. The limb is edematous.
   c. Nodules are ulcerated having bluish border.
2. The most likely diagnosis in the background of tuberculosis is Bazin's disease.
3. There are two types of this lesion:
   a. Erythema induratum of Bazin type: It is associated with tuberculosis.
   b. Erythema induratum or Whitfield type: It is not associated with tuberculosis.

CASE 31

A 45-year-old female came to medical outpatient department with following features:

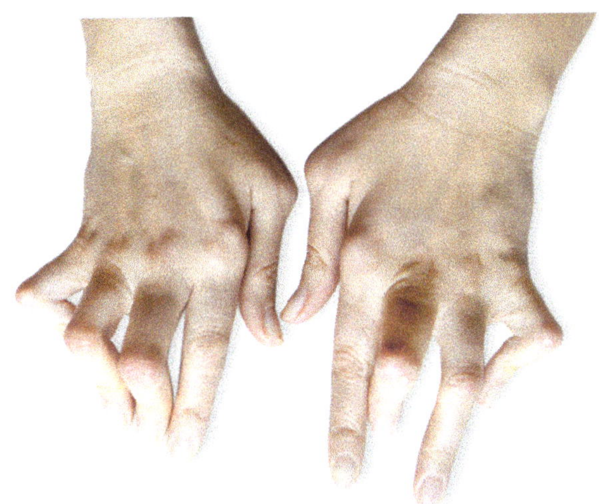

1. **What is the deformity shown here?**
2. **What is the most likely diagnosis?**
3. **What are the other types of deformities present in this case?**
4. **What are the extra-articular manifestations in this disease?**
5. **What are the causes of anemia in this disease?**
6. **What is palindromic variety of this disease?**

Answers

1. Following are the types of deformities shown in the above picture:
   a. Hyperflexion of the proximal interphalangeal joints and hyperextension of the distal interphalangeal joints in both the hands—Boutonniere deformity
   b. Hyperextension of the interphalangeal joint and flexion of metacarpophalangeal joint along with exaggerated adduction of first metacarpal—suggests Z deformity
2. The most likely diagnosis is rheumatoid arthritis producing symmetrical bilateral polyarthritis involving all the small joints.
3. Other deformities in this disease are:
   a. Swan neck deformity: This is characterized by hyperextension of the proximal interphalangeal joints and hyperflexion of the distal interphalangeal joints.
   b. Subluxation of metacarpophalangeal joints due to dorsal displacement of head of the metacarpal and volar and proximal displacement of head of the proximal phalanx leading to chronically swollen metacarpophalangeal joint.
   c. Ulnar deviation of the hand occurs due to erosion and laxity of the tendon of extensor carpi ulnaris overlying the styloid process of ulna
   d. Subluxation of wrist
   e. Piano key sign or floating ulnar styloid
   f. Vaughan–Jackson deformity occurs due to rupture of the extensor tendon of third, fourth, and fifth digits leading to inability to extend the fingers.
4. Following are the extra-articular manifestations in this disease:
   a. Ocular:
      - Scleritis
      - Episcleritis
      - Iridocyclitis
      - In case of associated Sjögren's syndrome keratoconjunctivitis sicca
   b. Pulmonary manifestations:
      - Fibrosing alveolitis
      - Rheumatoid nodules
      - Caplan syndrome
      - Small airway disease
      - Pleuritis and pleural effusion

c. Cardiovascular features:
- Pericarditis
- Pericardial effusion
- Mitral regurgitation
- Aortic regurgitation
- Myocarditis

d. Neurological manifestation:
- Mononeuritis multiplex
- Peripheral neuropathy
- Entrapment neuropathy
- Subluxation of the atlantoaxial joints

e. Soft-tissue manifestations:
- Rheumatic nodules
- Tenosynovitis
- Bursitis
- Muscle wasting

5. Causes of anemia in this disease are as follows:
   a. Anemia of chronic disease
   b. Deficiency of folate
   c. Hypersplenism in case of Felty syndrome
   d. Drugs leading to depression of the bone marrow

6. Palindromic variety of rheumatoid arthritis is characterized by recurrent episodes of arthritis involving the individual joint lasting for few hours to few days.

CASE 32

A 55-year-old patient came to outpatient department with this posture. The patient had history of back pain and stiffness for >10 years and gradual restriction of the movements in the back. On eye examination, following was demonstrated:

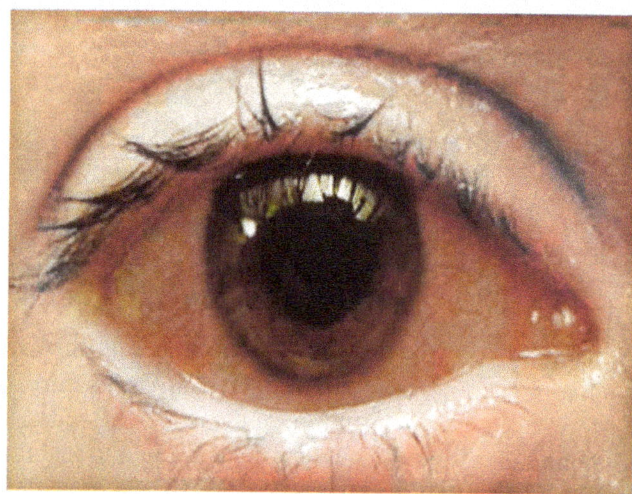
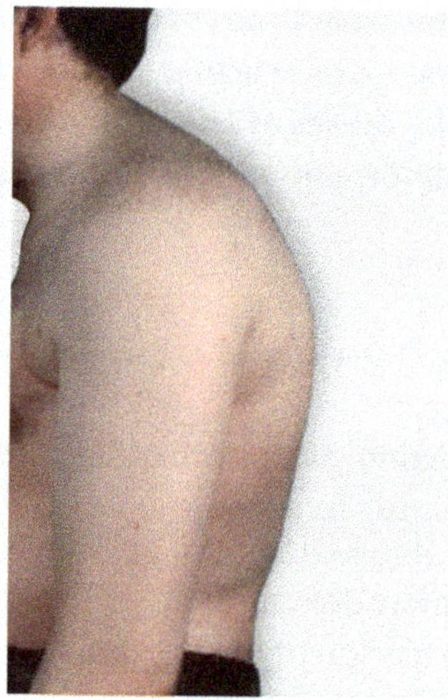

1. **What does the above posture demonstrate?**
2. **What is your diagnosis?**
3. **What should be the classical components in the history in this patient?**
4. **What are the extra-articular manifestations in this disease?**
5. **What are the maneuvers to be done in this case?**
6. **What are the complications of this disease?**
7. **Which HLA variety is associated with this disease?**
8. **What are the common features in this HLA variety?**
9. **What are the diagnostic criteria in this disease?**
10. **What are the agents that should be given in this disease?**

Answers

1. Above pictures demonstrate:
   a. Eye showing congestion in the ciliary region suggestive of iridocyclitis
   b. Typical "question mark" posture due to loss of lumbar lordosis and increased kyphosis
2. The patient has been suffering from ankylosing spondylitis.
3. Classical components of the symptoms are as follows:
   a. Pain occurs at night
   b. Symptoms will be improved with exercise.
   c. Symptoms will start before the age of 40 years.
   d. Insidious onset of the low back pain
   e. Rest cannot relieve the symptom
4. Extra-articular manifestations in this disease are the following:
   a. Eyes—iridocyclitis
   b. Cardiovascular:
      • Aortic regurgitation
      • Various conduction defect
   c. Pulmonary:
      • Fibrosing alveolitis
      • Restrictive lung disease
   d. Central nervous system: Quadriplegia
   e. Foot:
      • Achilles tendinitis
      • Plantar fasciitis
5. Following maneuvers are done for diagnosis:
   a. The patient is asked to look in either side—here the whole body of the patient will be turned to that side during trying.
   b. The patient is asked to stand on his heel and back against the wall; here the occiput of the head cannot touch the wall due to limitation of the spine.
   c. Schober test—it can measure the flexion of the lumbar spine.
6. Complications in this disease:
   a. With minor trauma spinal fracture
   b. Cauda equina syndrome
   c. Pulmonary fibrosis
   d. Aortic regurgitation
   e. Amyloidosis
7. HLA-B27 is associated with this disease.
8. Following are the common characteristics in the HLA-B27-positive arthritis:
   a. Asymmetric involvement of the distal joints
   b. Low back pain
   c. Familial aggregation
   d. Anterior uveitis
   e. Other extra-articular manifestations
   f. Seronegativity
   g. X-ray demonstrates features of sacroiliitis
9. Following are the diagnostic criteria in this disease:
   a. Clinical criteria:
      • Low back pain and stiffness for >3 months that is not relieved by rest but improves with exercise.
      • Sideways and frontal plane limitation of the spinal movement
      • Chest expansion limitation relative to normal values that is correlated for age and sex
10. Following drugs are used in this disease:
    a. NSAIDs
    b. Sulfasalazine
    c. Tumor necrosis factor—α-inhibitors:
       • Infliximab
       • Adalimumab
       • Etanercept
       • Golimumab
       • Certolizumab
    d. Corticosteroids
    e. Janus kinase inhibitors:
       • Tofacitinib
       • Upadacitinib
    f. Interleukin-17 inhibitors:
       • Secukinumab
       • Ixekizumab

CASE 33

A 67-year-old female came to orthopedic clinic with pain in the knee joints and difficulty in climbing upstairs and getting up from the sitting position, increased after a period of inactivity and pain will be decreased in the evening after increased activity. The picture of the hand has been depicted here:

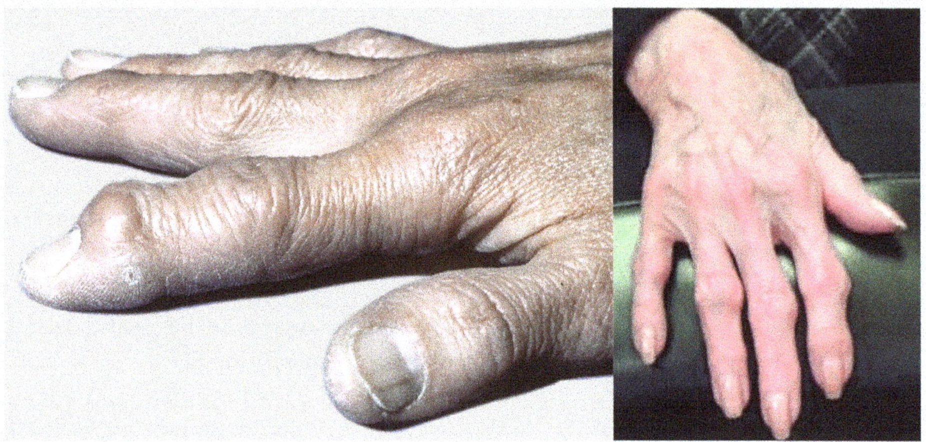

1. **Describe the above pictures.**
2. **What is the diagnosis?**
3. **Which are the joints commonly involved?**
4. **What are the causes of this disease?**
5. **Mention the risk factors in this disease.**
6. **What are the specific radiological hallmarks in this disease?**
7. **What do you know about the nodular variety of this disease?**
8. **What is the role of aggrecan in this disease?**

Answers

1. The above pictures demonstrate:
   a. First picture demonstrates bony swellings over the proximal interphalangeal joints—Heberden's nodes
   b. Second picture demonstrates bony swelling over the distal interphalangeal joint
2. This patient has been suffering from osteoarthritis.
3. Following joints are commonly involved:
   a. Knee
   b. Hip
   c. Feet
   d. Hand
   e. Ankle
   f. Lumbar spine
   g. Cervical spine
4. Causes of the disease:
   a. Primary
   b. Secondary:
      - Congenital:
         ○ Hypermobility
         ○ Congenital dysplasia
      - Structural disease: Perthes disease
      - Trauma and mechanical factors
      - Inflammatory arthropathies:
         ○ Rheumatoid arthritis
         ○ Septic arthritis
      - Neuropathic joints:
         ○ Diabetes
         ○ Syringomyelia
         ○ Tabes dorsalis
      - Endocrinal:
         ○ Hyperparathyroidism
         ○ Hypothyroidism
         ○ Acromegaly
      - Metabolic changes:
         ○ Hemochromatosis
         ○ Chondrocalcinosis
5. Following are the risk factors in this disease:
   a. All the secondary causes
   b. Obesity

c. Old age
d. Osteoporosis
e. Trauma
f. Occupation
g. Injury during sports

6. Radiological hallmarks in this disease are the following:
   a. Reduction of joint space
   b. Sclerosis of the subchondral bone
   c. Formation of subchondral cyst
   d. Osteochondral bodies
   e. Osteophytosis

7. Nodular variety of osteoarthritis is primary osteoarthritis having following characteristics:
   a. Middle-aged women are affected.
   b. Autosomal dominance
   c. Polyarticular involvement of the interphalangeal joints
   d. Presence of Heberden's nodes and Bouchard's nodes
   e. Arthritis may be acute.
   f. Square deformity of the hand.
   g. Later on, other big joints are involved.

8. Loss of aggrecan in the joint fluid is the primary event leading to destruction of the cartilage in osteoarthritis. Three enzymes are responsible for the degradation of this enzyme:
   a. ADAMTS1
   b. ADAMTS4
   c. ADAMTS5

These enzymes will play an effective role in the treatment of this disease.

CASE 34

A 28-year-old male presented to medicine department with severe pain and swelling over the right great toe.

On examination, the following features were found:

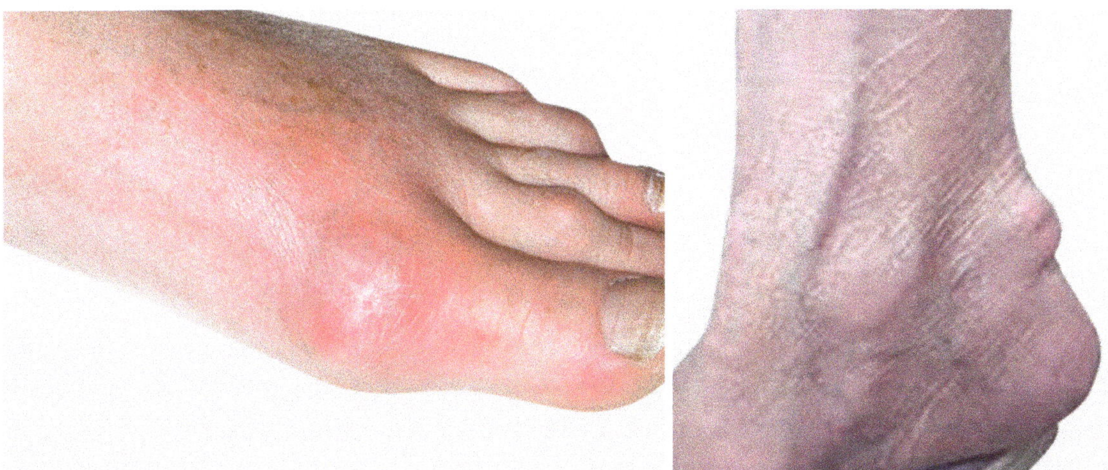

1. **What are features demonstrated in the above pictures?**
2. **What is the most likely diagnosis?**
3. **What are the clinical spectra of presentation in this disease?**
4. **Name the precipitants in gout.**
5. **What are the complications of this disease?**
6. **What are the characteristic erosions in radiography in this disease?**
7. **What are the ultrasonographic findings in this disease?**
8. **How can you demonstrate the underexcretor of uric acid in this disease?**
9. **What do you know about the pseudovariety of this disease?**

Answers

1. In the above pictures demonstrate:
   a. There is swelled reddened area over the ball of great toe and proximal interphalangeal joint of second toe.
   b. In the second picture, there is evidence of tophi over the lateral malleolus of right ankle joint.
2. The most likely diagnosis is acute tophaceous gout.
3. The clinical spectra of the disease are as follows:
   a. Asymptomatic hyperuricemia
   b. Acute gouty arthritis
   c. Chronic erosive and deforming arthritis
   d. Chronic tophaceous gout
   e. Gouty nephropathy with hypertension and renal stone
4. The precipitating factors of gout are as follows:
   a. Intake of alcohol
   b. Dehydration
   c. Surgery
   d. Food rich in purine:
      - Liver
      - Kidney
      - Sweet bread
   e. Drugs like thiazides
5. Complications of gout are as follows:
   a. Severe degenerative arthritis
   b. Urate nephropathy
   c. Increased susceptibility to infection
   d. Renal stones
   e. Nerve and spinal cord impingement
   f. Fracture in joints with tophaceous gout
6. Following are the characteristic erosions seen in gout radiologically:
   a. Maintenance of joint space
   b. Absence of periarticular osteopenia
   c. Location outside the capsule of the joint
   d. Sclerotic borders (cookie-cutter, punched-out)
   e. Asymmetric distribution among the joints having strong predilection for the distal joints
7. Following are the ultrasonographic findings in gout:
   a. "Double-contour" sign: It is characterized by hyperechoic irregular line of monosodium urate crystals on the surface of articular cartilage overlying adjacent hyperechoic bony contour.
   b. Erosions of the bones adjacent to tophi
   c. Wet clumps of sugars: It is characterized by tophaceous materials, described as hyperechoic and hypoechoic heterogeneous materials having an anechoic rim.
8. Patients having 24 hours uric acid urinary excretion <800 mg/day—can be confirmed as underexcretor and less producer. If it is >800 mg/day, they can be described as high uric acid producers.
9. Pseudogout is characterized by deposition of calcium pyrophosphate dehydrate crystals in the articular cartilage and periarticular tissue, the causes being:
   a. Hyperparathyroidism
   b. Hypothyroidism
   c. Hemochromatosis
   d. Wilson's disease

CASE 35

A 45-year-old diabetic woman came to diabetic clinic with progressively increasing painless swelling of the right ankle joint which is depicted below:

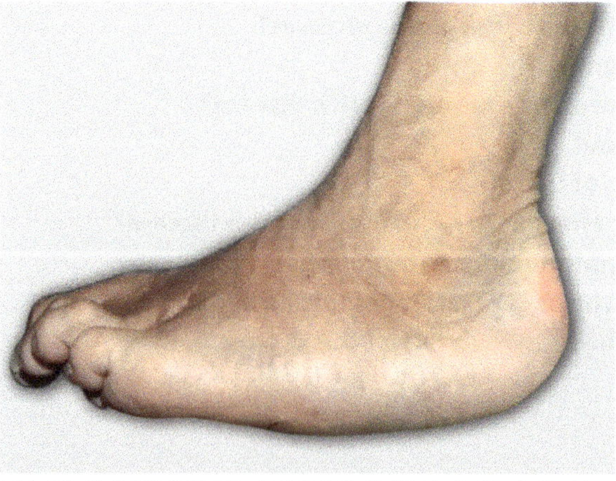

1. **Describe the joint.**
2. **What are the palpatory features in this joint?**
3. **What are the causes of this type of joint?**
4. **How can you conclude that this joint is hypermobile?**
5. **What are the stages of Charcot joint?**
6. **What are the complications in this joint disease?**

Answers

1. Joint is swollen, red but painless with restriction of movement at the ankle joint.
2. During palpation, there is no tenderness, hypermobile joint, and there may be palpatory crepitus on the swelling.
3. Causes of Charcot joint:
   a. Diabetes mellitus
   b. Tabes dorsalis
   c. Leprosy
   d. Syringomyelia
4. Hyperextensibility of the ankle joint >90° is indicative of hyperextensibility.
5. Following are the stages of Charcot joint:
   a. Stage 0 or pre-Charcot or prodromal stage:
      - Clinically, it is red, hot, and swollen foot, but no deformity
      - There is no change in radiograph.
   b. Stage 1 development/destruction:
      - Clinically, there is erythema, edema of the foot, raised temperature but no pain.
      - Radiologically:
        ○ Bony debris in the joints,
        ○ Fragmentation of subchondral bone
        ○ Subluxation of joints
        ○ Fracture and/or dislocation
   c. Stage 2 coalescence:
      - Clinically, there are decreased signs of inflammation.
      - Radiographically:
        ○ Worsening of stage 1 features
        ○ Absorption of bony debris
        ○ New bone formation
        ○ Coalescence of large fragments with sclerosis of ends of the bones
   d. Stage 3 consolidation:
      - Clinically, there is resolution of inflammation. There is change in the bony architecture due to underlying final bony remodeling as a result new pressure points arise leading to ulcer formation.
      - Radiologically, there is remodeling of the affected joints and bones.
6. Complications in this joint disease are as follows:
   a. Deformities of the foot:
      - Flat foot
      - Rocker bottom foot
      - Hammertoes
      - Ankle equinus
   b. Bony prominences lead to:
      - Ulceration
      - Infection
      - Loss of limbs
   c. Recurrence of Charcot joint

CASE 36

A 32-year-old diabetic female came to emergency department with spiky fever and severe painful swelling of the right elbow joint following operation of the bursa in that joint.

1. **What is your diagnosis?**
2. **What are the other causes of swollen and tender elbow joint?**
3. **What are the causes of single joint involvement?**
4. **What are the predisposing factors in this disease?**
5. **What are the organisms in adult may be responsible for this disease?**
6. **What may be the complications in this case?**

Answers

1. The patient has been suffering from acute septic monoarthritis.
2. Following are the causes of tender elbow joint:
   a. Trauma to elbow
   b. Acute osteoarthritis
   c. Acute rheumatoid arthritis
   d. Acute gouty arthritis
   e. Acute septic arthritis
   f. Acute hemarthrosis
3. Following are the causes of monoarticular arthritis:
   a. Reactive arthritis
   b. Bacterial arthritis
   c. Acute gout
   d. Acute pseudogout
   e. Traumatic arthritis
   f. Sarcoidosis
   g. Acute hemarthrosis
   h. Acute rheumatoid arthritis
4. Following are the predisposing factors of septic arthritis:
   a. Immunocompromised individual
   b. History of trauma
   c. History of surgery
   d. Neuropathic joint
   e. History of rheumatoid arthritis
5. Following bacteria are responsible for septic monoarthritis:
   a. *Staphylococcus aureus*
   b. *Streptococcus pneumoniae*
   c. *Salmonella* in case of sickle cell anemia
   d. *Pseudomonas* in case of trauma
   e. *Neisseria gonorrhoeae*
6. Complications in this case are as follows:
   a. Osteomyelitis
   b. Sepsis
   c. Chronic pain
   d. Osteonecrosis
   e. Discrepancies in the leg length

CHAPTER 14

Toxicology

A 25-year-old female after a severe quarrel and fight with her husband closed the door of her room. Her husband went out of West Bengal for business. After 3 days, he returned and broke the closed door and found his wife drowsy and scattered amount of vomitus.

On examination, the patient was drowsy, blood pressure 90/60 mm Hg, pulse rate 120 beats/min, abdomen is tender, SpO_2 95%, and other systemic examinations were normal except Glasgow Coma Scale 12/15.

Laboratory investigation demonstrated hemoglobin 10 g/dL, white blood count 12,000/cc, bilirubin 9.5 mg/dL, serum glutamate-pyruvic transaminase (SGPT) 1200 IU/L, serum glutamate-oxaloacetic transaminase (SGOT) 800 IU/L, international normalized ratio (INR) 2.1, urea 120 mg/dL, creatinine 1.9 mg/dL, sodium 127 mEq/L, potassium 3.1 mEq/L, and glucose is 65 mg/dL.

Toxicology in urine demonstrated acetaminophen level was positive.

1. **What is your diagnosis?**
2. **In what stage of this disease, the patient was found?**
3. **What are the stages of this disease?**
4. **What is the mechanism of action of the etiological agent?**
5. **What is the lethal dose of this etiological agent?**
6. **What are the factors on which the prognosis of the patient depends?**
7. **What is the definite treatment in this case as the liver enzymes are raised?**

Answers

1. The most clinical diagnosis is acute acetaminophen poisoning leading to acute hepatocellular and renal failure.
2. This patient was in the third stage of the disease as this patient was in drowsy stage, renal dysfunction, and hypoglycemia.
3. There are four stages in this poisoning:
   a. Stage 1: This stage is within 0–24 hours. Symptoms are nausea, vomiting, and anorexia.
   b. Stage 2: Duration is between 24 and 36 hours. Laboratory investigation demonstrates raised SGOT and SGPT and coagulation tests are abnormal.
   c. Stage 3: Duration is between 72 and 96 hours. Features are spectrum of fulminant hepatotoxicity such as encephalopathy, coagulopathy, renal dysfunction, and hypoglycemia leading to shock.
   d. Stage 4: Duration is more than 96 hours. In this stage, patient will either recover or die with normalization with resolution of hepatic architecture within 3 months.
4. Mechanism of action of this drug:
   a. Liver and kidney injury will occur through the generation of N-acetyl-p-benzoquinone, a toxic metabolite, by cytochrome P450 mixed function oxidase in the setting of increased hepatic glutathione.
   b. In case of alcoholism, there is decreased store of glutathione or induction of CYP2e1, an enzyme may lead to acetaminophen toxicity.

5. The lethal dose is >153 mg/L regardless of time of gestation.

6. Prognosis depends upon the following criteria:
   a. Serum creatinine is >3.4 mg/dL.
   b. Development of grade 3–4 encephalopathy.
   c. Arterial pH is <7.3 in spite of adequate hydration with fluid.
   d. INR is >6.5 or prothrombin time is 1.8 times the control.

7. Specific treatment in this acute hepatocellular failure:
   a. In case of no bleeding, coagulopathy may not be corrected but if there is bleeding, vitamin K or the blood products should be given.
   b. Monitoring of serum ammonia as it will prognosticate this disease.
   c. For maintaining normocapnia, ventilation should be started.
   d. In case of hypoglycemia, administration of glucose
   e. In case of hyponatremia, administration of sodium
   f. In case of normocapnia, ventilation should be started.
   g. In case of acute hepatocellular failure due to acetaminophen poisoning, lever transplantation should be done following the "modified King's College Criteria":
      - pH is <7.3
        Or,
      - Serum lactate is >3.0 mmol/L after resuscitation with fluid after 12 hours of admission.
      - Arterial lactate concentration is >3.5 mmol/L after early resuscitation (4 hours).

CASE 2

A 72-year-old lady immediately after verbal conflict with her son-in-law consumed two tablets of aluminum phosphide. She started vomiting; hence, she was taken to emergency department.

On examination, the patient was found irritable, spontaneous breathing, blood pressure 90/60 mm Hg, SpO_2 92% in room air, pulse rate 110 beats/min, regular, pupil constricted, and no evidence of external injuries. Systemic examination demonstrated diffusely tender abdomen and other systems were normal.

Laboratory examination demonstrated, PaO_2 82, $PaCO_2$ 22, pH 7.3, and HCO_3 11 mmol/L. Renal, liver function, coagulation tests, complete blood count, urine analysis, ECG, and chest X-ray were normal. Urine toxiscreen was positive for phosphide.

1. **What is your diagnosis?**
2. **Interpret the arterial blood gases?**
3. **What are the mechanisms of toxicity?**
4. **What is the lethal dose of phosphine gas in human beings?**
5. **What are the types of clinical features?**
6. **How can you treat this patient?**

Answers

1. The patient has been suffering from acute aluminum phosphide poisoning.

2. The arterial blood gas demonstrated metabolic acidosis with respiratory alkalosis.

3. The mechanisms of toxicity are:

After oral ingestion of aluminum phosphide will release phosphine gas in the stomach in presence of hydrochloric acid

↓

This phosphine gas will be absorbed from the mucosa in the gastrointestinal tract

↓

After absorption phosphine will be oxidized into oxyacid.

↓

Phosphine affects mitochondria and inhibits cytochrome C oxidase

↓

Forms highly reactive hydroxyl radicals

↓

This oxidized phosphine affects heart, liver, lung, and kidney

↓

Development of different cardiac arrhythmias, pulmonary edema, and intractable shock

↓

Some amount of phosphine will be excreted in the urine and lung in unchanged form

After inhalation or postingestion exhalation, it will damage the alveolar-capillary membrane leading to acute lung injury.

4. Permissible exposure limit of phosphine in the working atmosphere is <0.3 ppm.
    - More than 50 ppm is dangerous to life.
    - 400–600 ppm is lethal within half an hour.

5. Following are the types of clinical features:
    a. Mild type of poisoning: Clinical features are—
        - Abdominal pain
        - Nausea
        - Continuous vomiting
        - Headache
        - Tachycardia
    b. Moderate-to-severe poisoning: Clinical features are—
        - Jaundice
        - Nervous system:
            o Dizziness
            o Headache
            o Paresthesia
            o Numbness
            o Tremor
            o Weakness in the muscles
            o Diplopia
        - Cardiovascular system:
            o Tightness in the chest
            o Arrhythmias
        - Hepatic: Jaundice

6. Management in this patient:
    a. Gastric decompression and lavage with 1:10,000 potassium permanganate as it will oxidize phosphate to nontoxic phosphate.
    b. Gastric lavage with coconut oil:
        - It will make a protective layer on the gastric mucosa so that phosphine gas gets absorbed from the mucosa.
        - It will help in diluting hydrochloric acid.
        - It also inhibits breakdown of the phosphide from the tablets
    c. Administration of the sodium bicarbonate inhibits phosphine release by:
        - Neutralizing the hydrochloric acid
        - Decreasing the catalytic reaction of the phosphide with the hydrochloric acid
    d. Activated charcoal should be given if the patient will come within 1 hour of the ingestion to prevent the absorption of the phosphide.
    e. Tissue perfusion and oxygenation should be adequately maintained.
    f. 100 mEq sodium bicarbonate should be given intravenously followed by 75 mEq in 500 mL of half-strength normal saline at a rate of 100 mL/hour.
    g. For maintaining blood pressure norepinephrine, β-receptor agonist such as dopamine or dobutamine should be given.

CASE 3

A 25-year-old female after getting report of her unsuccessful results in the medicine took 20 tablets of alprazolam in her hostel room. After 3 hours, she was found drowsy in her bed by her friend and was taken to the emergency department at once.

On examination, her Glasgow Coma Scale was E3M6V4, blood pressure 100/60 mm Hg, pulse rate 64 beats/min, regular, respiratory rate 16 breaths/min, random blood glucose 110 mg/dL, SpO_2 98% in room air, and pupil constricted.

1. **What is the urgent and definite test that should be done?**
2. **What is your likely diagnosis?**
3. **What is the mechanism of action of this drug?**
4. **What are the neurological features found in this patient?**
5. **How can you manage this patient?**
6. **What is the specific antidote to this drug?**
7. **What are the toxicities of this antidote?**

Answers

1. Urine for toxiscreen to get the drug benzodiazepine.
2. This student has been suffering from benzodiazepine overdose.
3. The mechanism of actions: Benzodiazepine enhances γ-aminobutyric acid (GABA)-mediated neurotransmission through the frequency of opening of chloride channel.
4. Following are the neurological features in this disease:
   a. Dizziness
   b. Confusion
   c. Drowsiness
   d. Blurred vision
   e. Unresponsiveness
   f. Anxiety
   g. Ataxia
   h. Nystagmus
   i. Hallucination
   j. Slurred speech
   k. Amnesia
   l. Paradoxical agitation
   m. Respiratory depression
   n. Hypotension
5. Management:
   a. Supportive care and monitoring of the patient
   b. Maintenance of airway, breathing, and circulation
   c. Foley catheter to relieve urinary retention
6. Specific antidote to this drug is flumazenil, a competitive benzodiazepine antagonist. It can be given at 0.1 mg over 1 minute to maximum 1 mg until:
   a. Therapeutic effect is achieved.
   b. Toxicity will be developed.
7. Toxicities of this antidote are:
   - Withdrawal
   - Seizure

CASE 4

A 70-year-old male after discussion regarding a family dispute with his wife went for sleep. His wife had osteoarthritis for which she was on salicylate off and on for last 1 year. In the next morning, he complained of blurring of the vision and tinnitus.

On examination, patient was hyperventilating, confused, respiratory rate was 32 breaths/min, blood pressure 120/85 mm Hg, and pulse rate 110 beats/min. Other systemic examinations were normal.

Arterial blood gas analysis demonstrated pH 7.03, PCO_2 16 mm Hg, PO_2 92 mm Hg, potassium 2 mEq/L, and serum salicylate level was 50 mg/dL. ECG, MRI of the brain, and chest X-ray were normal.

1. **What is the most likely diagnosis?**
2. **What is the mechanism of action of this drug?**
3. **What is the acid–base abnormality in this case?**
4. **What is the lethal dose of this drug?**
5. **What are the features in this acute poisoning?**
6. **What are the investigations that should be done in the urine?**
7. **What should be the treatment?**
8. **What are the indications of hemodialysis in this patient?**

Answers

1. The most likely diagnosis is salicylate poisoning.
2. The mechanism of this drug:
   a. It will uncouple oxidative phosphorylation leading to interference with the cellular respiration.
   b. As salicylates cross the cell membranes easily, it will become more toxic when the blood pH become acidic.
   c. This stimulates respiratory center in the medulla leading to respiratory alkalosis
   d. When salicylate enters the cells affecting mitochondria leading to metabolic acidosis
   e. Loss of water, sodium, and potassium through the kidney and water loss through the lung during hyperventilation leading to dehydration
   f. Excretion of salicylate will be increased in acidic urine.
3. Arterial blood gases demonstrated severe metabolic acidosis with respiratory alkalosis.

4. Following are the lethal dose of salicylate:
   a. >125 mg/kg of body weight—mild toxicity
   b. >250 mg/kg of body weight—moderate toxicity
   c. >500 mg/kg of body weight—severe toxicity
5. Features of acute poisoning are the following:
   a. Initially, nausea, vomiting, and hyperactivity leading to hyperventilation and tinnitus
   b. In the later stage, fever, confusion, hyperactivity, and convulsion
   c. Lastly, rhabdomyolysis leading to acute renal failure
6. Following investigations should be done in the urine:
   a. Myoglobin
   b. Toxiscreen
7. Management of the patient:
   a. Gastric decompression with activated charcoal
   b. If the bowel sound is present, activated charcoal should be repeated every 4 hours until the charcoal will appear in the urine.
   c. Alkaline diuresis with the potassium chloride to prevent renal failure until the urinary PH is ≥8.

   d. Hypokalemia should be prevented by potassium infusion.
   e. Glucose should be infused to prevent hypoglycemia.
   f. Seizure should be prevented with benzodiazepine.
   g. 150 mEq of sodium bicarbonate along with 40 mEq potassium chloride in 1 L of 5% dextrose to maintain the resuscitation of the patient.
   h. External cooling and cold sponging should be done to treat fever.
   i. Intake and output chart should be maintained to monitor the balance of the fluid.
8. Following are the indications of hemodialysis in this patient:
   a. Severe neurologic impairment
   b. Renal dysfunction
   c. Respiratory insufficiency
   d. Acidemia in spite of all the supportive measures
   e. If the serum salicylate level is >100 mg/dL in this case.

CASE 5

A 40-year-old male after his daily usual works went to a bar with his colleague to take "a beer" and at the end of the party while he was outside the bar, felt unconscious on the sidewalk.

On examination, patient is drowsy, responded to painful stimulus, blood pressure 100/60 mm Hg, pulse rate 64 beats/min, pupil constricted, respiratory rate 10 breaths/min, SpO$_2$ 90%, blood sugar 100 mg/dL, Glasgow Coma Scale E2V3M5, and no evidence of external injuries.

Urine toxiscreen demonstrated positive for opioids.

1. **What is the most possible diagnosis?**
2. **What are the causes of opioid overdose?**
3. **What is the risk of overdose increases?**
4. **What are the receptors that mediate the effect of opioid?**
5. **How can you manage opioid overdose?**

Answers

1. The most probable diagnosis is opioid overdose.
2. Following are the causes of opioid overdose:
   a. Complications of substance abuse
   b. Unintentional overdose
   c. Intentional overdose
   d. Therapeutic drug error
3. Risk of overdose increases in the following:
   a. Those taking escalating doses
   b. Male gender
   c. Return to use after cessation
   d. Age between 20 and 40 years
   e. White non-Hispanic race
   f. Combining the opioid with other sedative medications
   g. Patient suffering from following diseases:
      - Human immunodeficiency virus (HIV)
      - Depression
      - Lung disease
      - Liver diseases

4. Following receptors mediate the effects of opioid:
   a. Mu receptors: It will mediate—
      - Analgesia
      - Euphoria
      - Sedation
      - Respiratory depression
      - Gastrointestinal dysmotility
      - Physical dependence
      - Medullary diminished response to hypercarbia
      - Decreased hypoxia-related respiratory response
   b. Kappa receptors: It mediates-
      - Analgesia
      - Dysphoria
      - Miosis
      - Diuresis
   c. Delta receptors: It mediates—
      - Analgesia
      - Inhibition of the release of dopamine
      - Suppression of cough
   d. Sigma receptors: When it will be stimulated, it mediates:
      - Dysphoria
      - Hallucination
      - Psychosis

5. Following are the management in this case:
   a. Control of airway and breathing
   b. If the respiratory rate is <12 breaths/min, naloxone is indicated.
   c. Naloxone, nalmefene, and naltrexone antagonize all the opioid receptors. Dose of naloxone is 0.4–2 mg in adult. Initial bolus dose is 0.05–0.1 mg intravenously or intramuscularly and should be repeated every minute until the restoration of ventilation.
   d. If the patient is tolerant to naloxone, high dose should be given, but the adverse effect is withdrawal effect that can be managed by antiemetics.

CASE 6

A 4-year-old child came to emergency department with three episodes of convulsions, with vomiting. The vomitus contains white particles and has smell of camphor. On further enquiry, his mother told that the child was in front of the camphor ball while she was keeping the clothes in the almirah.

On examination, the patient was drowsy, no focal neurological deficit, afebrile, and all the vital signs are normal. All the biochemical as well as hematological parameters were within normal limit.

1. **What is the most probable diagnosis?**
2. **What are the camphor-containing substances?**
3. **What is the mechanism of action of this camphor?**
4. **What is the lethal dose for developing convulsion?**
5. **What are the clinical features occur in this patient?**
6. **How can you manage this patient?**

Answers

1. The most likely diagnosis is camphor poisoning.
2. Following are the camphor-containing substances:
   a. Vicks VapoRub
   b. Camphor phenol oral rinse
   c. Rubs containing emu oil
   d. Vicks inhaler
   e. Mothballs
3. The mechanism of actions of camphor:
   a. Site of action is intraneuronal.
   b. It strongly activates and desensitizes the transient receptor potential vanilloid channel subtype 1 in vanilloid-independent process.
4. The lethal dose to develop neurological manifestations is ingestion of >30 mg/kg camphor-containing product.
5. Following are the clinical features in the camphor poisoning:
   a. Neurological manifestations:
      - Acute seizures preceded by:
         - Muscle fasciculation
         - Delirium
         - Confusion
         - Hallucination
         - Restlessness
   b. Respiratory complications after seizures may occur.

c. Gastrointestinal:
  - Nausea
  - Vomiting
  - Epigastric pain
d. Cardiovascular:
  - Cardiomyopathy
  - Prolonged QT

6. The patient can be managed by the following processes:
  a. Skin should be thoroughly washed in case of skin contamination.
  b. Benzodiazepines should be given to treat seizures.

CASE 7

A 52-year-old nonhypertensive and nondiabetic old man was brought to emergency department with low level of consciousness. On further query from his party, the doctor came to know that the patient brought marijuana from the market silently.

On examination, blood pressure was 130/90 mm Hg, pulse rate 50 beats/min, SpO_2 97% in room air, Glasgow Coma Scale on auscultation and there was diminished breath sound.

Patient has been admitted in intensive care unit and intubated.

1. **What is the most likely diagnosis?**
2. **What are the types of preparations of this toxic product?**
3. **What is the primary psychoactive compound?**
4. **What is the mechanism of action?**
5. **What are the clinical features?**
6. **What are the different types of doses in this poison?**
7. **How can you manage in this patient?**

Answers

1. The most likely diagnosis is cannabinoid poisoning.
2. Following are the types of cannabinoid preparation:
   a. Marijuana: It is a part or extract of the plant to induce therapeutic or psychometric effect.
   b. *Ganja*: It is crushed leaves and inflorescences of the female plants and can be smoked in the pipes or cigarettes.
   c. *Bhang*: It is made of concoction from buds as well as leaves of cannabis which will be ground into paste.
   d. Hashish or *charas* is made of dried resin that has been collected from flower tops.
   e. Sinsemilla: It is seedless plant.
   f. Marijuana "blunts": It is cheap cigars which will be sliced open and packed with cannabis followed by reseal.
   g. Cannabis tea: It is made of adding of saturated fat with the hot water along with small amount of cannabis.
3. The main primary psychoactive compound in cannabis is tetrahydrocannabinol.

4. Mechanism of action: They have—
   a. Sympathomimetic action
   b. Antiemetic properties
   c. Augmentation of release of dopamine
5. Clinical features in this patient may occur:
   a. Central nervous system:
     - Incoordination
     - Ataxia
     - Sedation
     - Depression of central nervous system
     - Coma
   b. Psychiatric features:
     - Euphoria
     - Anxiety
     - Agitation
     - Time disorientation
     - Hallucination
     - Delusion
     - Acute psychosis
   c. Cardiovascular:
     - Tachycardia
     - Orthostatic hypotension
   d. Respiratory: Rarely pneumothorax

6. Following are the types of lethal doses of cannabinoid:
   a. Low dose (50 µg/kg):
      - Mild sedation
      - Mild disorientation
      - Euphoria
      - Disinhibition
   b. High dose (250 µg/kg):
      - Tachycardia
      - Postural hypotension
      - Anxiety
      - Perceptual disturbances
      - Depression of central nervous system
7. Management in this patient:
   a. In case of low Glasgow Coma Scale, intubation and ventilation should be done.
   b. If the patient is agitated, diazepam should be given at a dose of 2.5–5 mg every 5 minutes intravenously until sedated.
   c. Hypotension and tachycardia should be treated by intravenous fluid.
   d. Cannabinoid hyperemesis syndrome should be treated by:
      - Hot showers
      - Intravenous fluids
      - Antiemetics
   e. Naloxone—µ-opioid receptor inverse agonist at the same time κ-receptor and δ-receptor antagonist.

CASE 8

One mechanical worker was brought to emergency department with severe cough and respiratory distress with inhalation burn injury in the face following inhalation of gas from burning motor bike while he was sleeping in the garage with half opened door.

On physical examination, blood pressure 130/85 mm Hg, pulse rate 120 beats/min, respiratory rate 32 breaths/min, SpO_2 86% in room air, and Glasgow Coma Scale 15/16. There was burn over the face, nose, singing of the nasal hair, and chest and abdomen. On auscultation of the chest, there were bilateral basal crepitations and occasional rhonchi.

1. **What is the most likely diagnosis?**
2. **What are the sources of this gas?**
3. **What are the various components of smoke?**
4. **What are the mechanisms of actions of this agent?**
5. **What are the clinical features in this poisoning?**
6. **What are the possible complications in this poisoning?**
7. **How can you treat this patient?**
8. **In which conditions of this patient, hyperbaric oxygen should be considered?**
9. **What are the complications of administration of hyperbaric oxygen?**

Answers

1. This patient has been suffering from carbon monoxide poisoning.
2. Following are the sources of this gas:
   a. Automotive exhaust
   b. Motorboat exhaust
   c. Propane-fueled heaters
   d. Wood or coal burning stoves or heaters
   e. Furnaces
   f. Generators
3. Various components of smoke are as follows:
   a. Carbon monoxide
   b. Phosgene
   c. Hydrogen sulfide
   d. Ammonia
   e. Sulfur dioxide
   f. Hydrogen cyanide
   g. Formaldehyde
   h. Acrylonitrile

4. Mechanisms of action of carbon monoxide are as follows:
   a. Carbon monoxide having 230–270 times greater affinity to bind with hemoglobin as compared to oxygen will bind very strongly and shift the hemoglobin dissociation curve toward left thereby unloading of oxygen from the hemoglobin into the tissues.
   b. Carbon monoxide interferes with the cellular respiration through the inactivation of mitochondrial cytochrome oxidase.
   c. Reduced oxygen-carrying capacity due to formation of carboxyhemoglobin leading to development of cardiac arrhythmias
   d. Severe hypotension is seen in this poisoning due to:
      - Activation of guanylyl cyclase that is responsible for relaxation of smooth muscles.
      - Displacement of nitric oxide from the platelets leading to vasodilatation
   e. There is alteration in the myelin basic protein leading to alteration of the immune response resulting in precipitation of neurological dysfunction.
5. Following are the clinical features in this poisoning:
   a. Mild cases:
      - Headache
      - Nausea
      - Vomiting
      - Dizziness
      - Blurred vision
   b. Moderate cases:
      - Syncope
      - Confusion
      - Dyspnea
      - Chest pain
      - Tachycardia
      - Tachypnea
      - Rhabdomyolysis
   c. Severe cases:
      - Dysrhythmias
      - Palpitations
      - Myocardial ischemia
      - Hypotension
      - Cardiac arrest
      - Respiratory arrest
      - Pulmonary edema
      - Convulsion
      - Coma
6. Following are the possible complications in this poisoning:
   a. Amnesia
   b. Psychosis
   c. Irritability
   d. Dementia
   e. Parkinson's disease
   f. Depression
   g. Loss of memory
   h. Deficit of speech
   i. Cortical blindness
7. Treatment of the patient:
   a. Immediately the patient should be removed from that area.
   b. FiO_2 should be maintained to 1.0.
   c. Cardiac monitoring
   d. Patient should be given high-flow oxygen through the nonbreathing mask.
   e. Hyperbaric oxygen should be given at three times of the atmospheric level can decrease the half-life of carboxyhemoglobin from 6 hours to only 24 minutes.
8. Hyperbaric oxygen should be considered in patients with the following conditions:
   a. Pregnant patients
   b. Decreased consciousness levels
   c. Significant neurologic deficit
   d. Chest trauma
   e. Noncooperative patients
   f. Signs of ischemia
   g. Metabolic acidosis
9. Following are the complications in application of hyperbaric oxygen:
   a. Decompression sickness
   b. Rupture of tympanic membrane
   c. Oxygen toxicity
   d. Treatment of coexistent cyanide toxicity
   e. Checking of ischemic complications as well as neurologic sequelae

CASE 9

A 40-year-old male after retiring from the office took leaf of Oduvanthalai mixed with whisky at night and went to bed. Next day at 3 AM, he started vomiting and abdominal pain and respiratory distress for which he was brought to emergency department.

On examination, blood pressure 80/50 mm Hg, pulse rate 88 beats/min, respiratory rate 36 breaths/min, and patient is drowsy, but afebrile. Systemic examination revealed diffuse abdominal tenderness.

Arterial blood gases demonstrated pH 7.18, PaO_2 60 mm Hg, $PaCO_2$ 90 mm Hg, lactate 1.8 mmol/L, urinary pH 7.1, urine is red colored and demonstrated myoglobin, serum sodium 129 mmol/L, and potassium 2.8 mmol/L. liver function test was normal.

1. **What is your diagnosis?**
2. **What are the metabolic abnormalities occurred in this patient?**
3. **What is the toxic principle in the leaf?**
4. **What is the lethal dose of this toxic principle?**
5. **What is the fatal period in this poisoning?**
6. **What are the clinical features in this poisoning?**
7. **What is the specific antidote in this poisoning?**

Answers

1. This is a case of Oduvanthalai poisoning.
2. Following are the metabolic abnormalities in this poisoning:
   a. Lactic acidosis with respiratory acidosis
   b. Distal renal tubular acidosis
   c. Type 2 respiratory failure
   d. Rhabdomyolysis leading to myoglobinuria resulting in renal failure
3. Toxic principle of the leaf is arylnaphthalene lignan lactones—it is diphyllin and its derivative.
4. The lethal dose of this toxic principle is 10.5 g/kg of body weight/200–400 leaves.
5. The lethal period is 1–3 days.
6. Following are the clinical features:
   a. Headache
   b. Vomiting
   c. Abdominal pain
   d. Palpitation
   e. Tachycardia
   f. Tachypnea
   g. Neuromuscular weakness
   h. Respiratory distress
   i. Hypotension
   j. Renal failure
   k. Acute respiratory distress syndrome
   l. Shock
   m. Cardiac dysrhythmias
7. The specific antidotes for this poisoning are:
   a. N-acetylcysteine: For decontamination, dose is 150 mg/kg for 1 hour, 50 mg/kg over 4 hours, then 100 mg/kg for 16 hours.
   b. L-cysteine
   c. Melatonin
   d. Thiol-containing compound

CASE 10

A 42-year-old man was brought to emergency department with irritable behavior and in agitation following several episodes of vomiting 3 hours ingestion of three cyanide tablets. On further enquiry, patient's copartner told about his tensed behavior due to his sudden financial crisis.

On examination, blood pressure was 100/60 mm Hg, pulse rate 124 beats/min, regular, respiratory rate 36 breaths/min, SpO_2 96%, systemic examination normal, arterial blood gases demonstrated mild metabolic acidosis, and other hematological and biochemical examinations were within normal limit.

1. **What is the lethal dose of cyanide?**
2. **What is the dose of cyanide associated with seizures or death?**

3. **What are the mechanisms of toxicities?**
4. **What should be the level of lactate indicative of cyanide poisoning?**
5. **Where is the cyanide found?**
6. **What are the antidotes of cyanide?**
7. **What are the routes of cyanide absorption?**

Answers

1. The lethal dose of cyanide is 150–200 mg.
2. Cyanide concentration of ≥ 2.5 µg/mL is associated with seizures, coma, or death.
3. The mechanisms of toxicities are as follows:
   - Cyanide is attached with the ferric ions found in terminal oxidative respiratory enzyme. Cytochrome oxidase is found in the mitochondria.
   - As a result, due to uncoupling of mitochondrial oxidative phosphorylation, cellular respiration will be inhibited resulting in histotoxic anoxia.
   - So, there is anaerobic cellular metabolism leading to development of lactic acidosis.
4. Serum lactate level is 8 mmol/L and is 94% sensitive and 74% specific of cyanide poisoning.
5. Cyanide is found in:
   a. In the industries during the extracting process to recover gold and silver
   b. Electroplating
   c. Case hardening of steel
   d. Dyeing
   e. Printing
   f. Photography
   g. Synthesis of inorganic and organic chemicals
   h. Production of chelating agents
6. The antidotes of cyanide are:
   a. Hydroxycobalamin—5 g intravenously over 15 minutes
   b. Sodium thiosulfate—12.5 g in 50 mL of distilled water and to be given intravenously over 30 minutes
   c. Sodium nitrite—10 mg/kg intravenously over 3–5 minutes
7. There are two routes of cyanide absorption:
   a. Gastrointestinal tract
   b. Skin

CASE 11

A 42-year-old male was brought to emergency department with agitation and uncontrolled behavior while he was traveling from Kovalam to Hyderabad.

On examination, his blood pressure was 100/70 mm Hg, pulse rate 124 beats/min, regular, respiratory rate 32 breaths/min, SpO_2 98% in room air, and capillary blood glucose 170 mg/dL.

ECG demonstrated supraventricular tachycardia. CT abdomen and chest and brain were normal.

All hematological and biochemical examinations were normal except toxiscreen was positive for cocaine.

1. **What are the dose-related side effects in cocaine poisoning?**
2. **What is the effect in infants in case of cocaine overdose?**
3. **What is the pathophysiology in this cocaine poisoning?**
4. **What are the effects of cocaine in the body?**
5. **What are the features of cocaine toxicity?**
6. **What are the stages of cocaine toxicity?**
7. **What are the complications of cocaine poisoning?**

Answers

1. The dose-related side effects in cocaine poisoning are as follows:
   a. 1–3 mg/kg is safe dose of local anesthetics.
   b. 20–30 mg is the recreational dose.
   c. >1 g is the lethal dose.
2. Cocaine is secreted in the breast milk. So, it can lead to cocaine intoxication and withdrawal syndrome.

3. Pathophysiological effect in case of cocaine poisoning: Cocaine binds and blocks the monoamine reuptake transporter at the nerve endings leading to accumulation of increased amount of monoamines resulting in prolonged sympathetic effects.
4. Cardiovascular effects:
   a. Stimulation of α- and β-1 receptor stimulations leading to increased:
      - Heart rate
      - Myocardial contractility
      - Blood pressure
   b. Vasoconstriction of the epicardial coronary arteries leads to decreased myocardial oxygen supply resulting in myocardial ischemia.
   c. Due to α-adrenergic and adenosine diphosphate (ADP)-mediated increased aggregation of platelets leading to activation of platelets and formation of thrombus.
   d. As local anesthetic, it will block the sodium channels leading to interference of impulse propagation resulting in risk of conduction disturbances and tachyarrhythmias.
5. Following are the clinical features:
   a. Neurological side effect:
      - Euphoria
      - Anxiety
      - Dysphoria
      - Agitation
      - Aggression
      - Paranoid psychosis
      - Visual hallucination
      - Tactile hallucination
      - Hyperthermia
      - Myoclonic movement
      - Seizures
   b. Cardiovascular effects:
      - Tachycardia
      - Pretension
      - Arrhythmia
      - QT prolongation
      - Conduction disturbances
      - Acute coronary syndrome
      - Acute pulmonary edema
   c. Gastrointestinal:
      - Nausea
      - Vomiting
      - Diarrhea
      - Abdominal pain
   d. Eye:
      - Blurring of vision
      - Corneal lesion
      - Vision loss
   e. Pruritus
6. Stages of cocaine toxicity are as follows:
   a. Stage 1:
      - Central nervous system:
        - Headache
        - Nausea
        - Mydriasis
        - Vertigo
        - Twitching
        - Pseudohallucination
      - Skin—hyperthermia
      - Lung—tachypnea
      - Vascular—increased blood pressure, ectopic beat
   b. Stage 2:
      - Central nervous system:
        - Seizures
        - Encephalopathy
        - Incontinence
        - Increased deep tendon reflexes
      - Skin—hyperthermia
      - Lung:
        - Tachypnea
        - Gasping
        - Apnea
        - Irregular breathing
      - Cardiac:
        - Arrhythmias
        - Hypertension
        - Peripheral cyanosis
   c. Stage 3:
      - Central nervous system:
        - Areflexia
        - Coma
        - Loss of vital function
        - Fixed and dilated pupils
      - Lung:
        - Apnea
        - Respiratory failure
        - Agonal breathing
        - Cyanosis
      - Cardiac:
        - Ventricular fibrillation
        - Hypotension
        - Cardiac arrest

7. Complications of cocaine poisoning are as follows:
   a. Thrombophlebitis
   b. HIV infection
   c. Cellulitis
   d. Hepatitis
   e. Pulmonary emboli
   f. Endocarditis
   g. Aneurysms

CASE 12

A 30-year-old farmer took some amount of yellow cow dung powder following a quarrel in his house and was brought in unconscious state following several episodes of vomiting to the emergency department.

On examination, patient is deeply unconscious and not responding to painful stimuli. The pupil is constricted, reacting to light equally. His vitals were normal and other systemic examinations were normal. All hematological and blood biochemistry were normal except liver function test such as SGOT 127 IU/L and SGPT 145 IU/L.

1. **What are the types of cow dung powder and types of toxic product in them?**
2. **What is the cause of raised liver enzymes?**
3. **What are the eye complications in this case?**

Answers

1. Two types of cow dung powder:
   a. Yellow cow dung powder—contains auramine O diarylmethane dye
   b. Green cow dung powder—contains malachite green triphenylmethane dye
2. Auramine causes centrilobular necrosis of the liver resulting in the raised liver enzymes
3. Following are the eye complications:
   a. Conjunctival edema
   b. Hyperemia of conjunctival mucosa
   c. Purulent discharge
   d. Total opacification of cornea

CASE 13

A 28-year-old motor garage worker developed severe bouts of vomiting following consumption of 150 mL break oil followed by drowsiness and was brought to emergency department.

On examination, blood pressure was 180/100 mm Hg, pulse rate 120 beats/min, regular, respiratory rate 32 breaths/min, SpO_2 98% in room air, and other systemic examination was normal.

Serum creatinine level increased to 1.3 mg/dL, glomerular filtration rate decreased to 60 mL/meter/min, arterial blood gases demonstrated anion gap metabolic acidosis, and increased level of lactate with PCO_2 level of 18 mm Hg.

1. **What are the mechanisms of toxicity?**
2. **When does nephrotoxicity start and why?**
3. **Which investigation can detect this toxic product?**
4. **Mention the criteria for starting the antidote.**
5. **What are the indications of hemodialysis in this patient?**
6. **What are the criteria for administering the ethanol?**

Answers

1. Following are the mechanisms of toxicity:
   a. Ethylene glycol is oxidized in the liver by alcohol dehydrogenase to glycolaldehyde which is responsible for nephrotoxicity.
   b. Glycolaldehyde is metabolized by aldehyde dehydrogenase to glycolic acid leading to generation of metabolic acidosis resulting in Kussmaul breathing along with profound obtundation.

c. Glycolic acid is then metabolized to glyoxylic acid by glycolic acid oxidase or by lactate dehydrogenase due to its resemblance with lactate. This oxalic acid combines with calcium to form calcium oxalate resulting in hypocalcemia producing:
- Tetany
- Nerve palsies
- Seizures
- Arrhythmias

2. 12 hours after intoxication, nephrotoxicity develops leading to increased creatinine and precipitation of the crystal in the proximal tubules resulting in nephropathy.

3. Gas chromatography is the most common method that can detect the serum ethylene glycol.

4. Criteria of starting the antidote in this poisoning are as follows:
   a. Serum ethylene glycol > 20 mg/dL
      Or,
   b. Documented recent history of ingestion of toxic amounts of ethylene glycol and an osmolar gap of >10 mOsmol/L
      Or,
   c. Suspected ethylene glycol ingestion and at least two of the following:
      - Arterial pH < 7.3
      - Serum bicarbonate < 20 mmol/L
      - Osmolar gap > 10 mOsmol/L
      - Oxalate crystalluria

5. Hemodialysis is indicated in the following patients with ethylene glycol poisoning:
   a. Severe acidosis
   b. Ethylene glycol level in the serum >50 mg/dL
      Or,
   c. Evidence of end-organ damage, i.e., renal failure

6. Ethanol should be given in the following patents as per current criteria:
   a. If the serum ethylene glycol is >20 mg/dL
   b. Known case of recent ethylene glycol poisoning with osmolar gap of >10 mmol
      Or,
   c. Strong clinical suspicion with three of the following:
      - Arterial pH < 7.3
      - Serum bicarbonate <20 mmol/L
      - Urinary oxalate crystals

CASE 14

A 25-year-old female was brought to the emergency department with history of ingestion of 150 mL of toilet cleaning agent Harpic at her residence following quarrel and fight with her husband, which was immediately followed by vomiting.

In the emergency department, all the vitals were normal, other systemic examination was normal, and hematological and biochemical tests were normal. Patient was shifted to intensive care unit.

1. **What are the types of this poison?**
2. **What are the sites of action?**
3. **What are the clinical features of this poisoning?**
4. **What are the complications of this poisoning?**
5. **What is the treatment of this poisoning?**

Answers

1. Pyrethroids are of two types:
   a. Type 1: This has no cyano group, less severe. Example is permethrin.
   b. Type 2: It always contains cyano group, more severe. Examples are cypermethrin and fenvalerate.

2. Following are the sites of actions:
   a. At as low as 10^{-10} M, pyrethroids alter sodium and chloride channels
   b. At concentration of 10^{-7} M, it acts as membrane stabilizer and produces apoptosis
   c. It acts on GABA receptor
   d. It also acts on nicotinic and acetylcholine receptors
   e. It acts on peripheral benzodiazepine receptor

3. Clinical features of this poisoning are as follows:
   a. In case of type 1 poisoning:
      - Fine tremor
      - Reflex
      - Hyperexcitability

b. In case of type 2 poisoning:
- Severe salivation
- Hyperexcitability
- Choreoathetosis

c. Other features are:
- Dizziness
- Headache
- Fatigue
- Vomiting
- Diarrhea
- Stinging
- Burning
- Irritability to sound
- Itching
- Tingling and numbness

d. Immediate features:
- Erosions in the gastrointestinal tract leading to bleeding as reflected by hematemesis
- Swelling of the tongue
- Laryngospasm
- Drooling
- Hypersalivation
- Irritation to the eyes

e. In severe cases:
- Pulmonary edema
- Seizures
- Coma

f. Delayed features:
- Esophageal stricture
- Esophageal cancer
- Gastric stenosis

4. Following are the complications in this poisoning:
   a. Esophageal perforation leading to mediastinitis
   b. Bowel perforation leading to peritonitis
   c. Respiratory tract injury leading to laryngeal soreness and aspiration pneumonia

5. Treatment of this poisoning is as follows:
   a. As pyrethroids are volatile, there is chance of paresthesia affecting the face and eyes; hence, vitamin E is effective in preventing the paresthetic reaction.
   b. Eye contamination can be treated immediately by flushing with large amount of saline water.
   c. Endoscopy should be done within 24–48 hours of ingestion.
   d. Administration of intravenous fluid
   e. Airways should be secured.
   f. Surgery should be done in case of any chronic complication.

CASE 15

A 30-year-old man professional worker as potter in the department of pottery came to emergency department with severe abdominal pain, vomiting, and diarrhea. His mouth examination demonstrated as below the picture:

On examination, blood pressure was 110/70 mm Hg, pulse rate 110 beats/min, regular, and respiratory rate 28 breaths/min. Complete blood count demonstrated as below. Rest of the blood biochemistry and serology were negative.

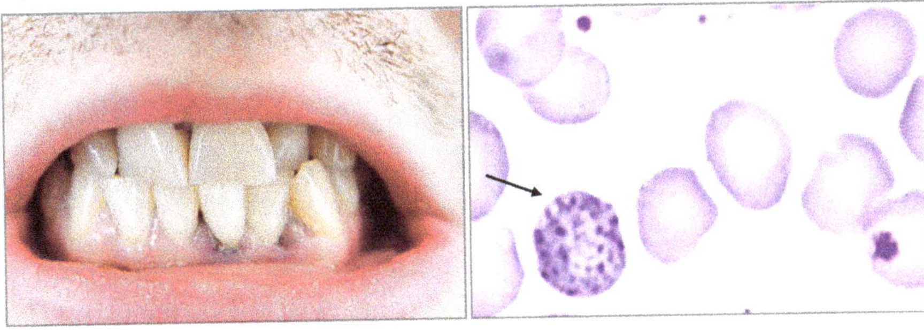

1. **What do the above pictures demonstrate?**
2. **What is your diagnosis?**
3. **What are the sources in which this poison is found?**
4. **What is the pharmacodynamics of lead?**
5. **What are the neurological, musculoskeletal, and gastrointestinal manifestations in this poisoning?**
6. **What are the chelating agents required in this poisoning?**
7. **What is the blood level of his poison indicative of this poisoning?**
8. **What are the hematological abnormalities occurring in this poisoning?**

Answers

1. The above pictures demonstrate:
   a. Blue line in the gum
   b. Peripheral blood picture demonstrates basophilic stippling
2. The most likely diagnosis is lead poisoning.
3. The sources of lead are as follows:
   a. Dietary supplements
   b. Ayurvedic medication
   c. Traditional remedies
   d. Cosmetics
   e. Metallic charms
4. Lead is primarily absorbed from the respiratory mucosa and mucosa of the gastrointestinal tract. After absorption, lead binds to red blood cells and will be distributed into two major components:
   a. Soft tissue that includes liver, bone marrow, kidney, and brain
   b. Bone

   10–15% of the absorbed lead will be excreted in the urine and bile.
5. Following are the systemic manifestations in this poisoning:
   a. Neurological:
      - Seizures
      - Cerebral edema
      - Encephalopathy
      - Psychiatric disturbances
      - Learning disabilities
      - Peripheral motor neuropathy
   b. Gastrointestinal:
      - Nausea
      - Vomiting
      - Diarrhea
      - Abdominal pain—colicky type
      - Lead line on the gingival line
      - Pancreatitis
      - Hepatitis
   c. Musculoskeletal:
      - Lead line due to increased deposition of calcium at the epiphyses.
      - Decreased growth and strength of the bone
6. Following are the chelating agents:
   a. Dimercaprol:
      - In mild case: 3 mg/kg injection deep intramuscularly 6 hourly for 3–5 days.
      - In severe case: 4 mg/kg intramuscularly 6 hourly for 5 days
   b. Edetate calcium disodium: Continuous intravenous infusion of 50 mg/kg/day.
   c. Succimer: 10 mg/m^2 orally 8 hourly for 5 days followed by 12 hourly for 14 days.
   d. Penicillamine can be used when the blood level is 25–40 µg/dL.
7. Blood level of lead if >10 µg/dL, it suggests lead poisoning.
8. Hematological abnormalities are the following:
   - As lead inhibits the enzymes responsible for synthesis of hemoglobin; hence, erythropoietic protoporphyria and zinc protoporphyrin will be increased in case of acute lead poisoning.
   - Hypochromic microcytic anemia
   - Basophilic stippling
   - Ferritin level: It can distinguish lead poisoning from iron-deficiency anemia.

CASE 16

A 75-year-old male having history of bipolar disorder and hypertension came to medicine department with slowness of speech and difficulty in the concentration during talking. On enquiry, patient was found to take 300 mg lithium thrice daily.

On examination, his blood pressure was 130/80 mm Hg, pulse rate 60 beats/min, respiratory rate 18 breaths/min, and SpO$_2$ 98% in room air. Systemic examination was normal. ECG revealed signs of bradycardia, ST depression in the precordial leads, and prolonged QT.

Laboratory investigation demonstrated serum creatinine 2.9 mg/dL, urea 70 mg/dL, lithium level 3.4 mEq/L, and sodium 150 mEq/L.

1. **What is the most likely diagnosis?**
2. **What are the causes of increased level of lithium?**
3. **What are the neurological and renal abnormalities that may occur in this case?**
4. **What are the ECG abnormalities in this case?**

Answers

1. The most likely diagnosis is lithium overdose.
2. The causes of increased lithium level in the blood are as follows:
   a. Excessive intake leading to acute or acute on chronic overdose poisoning
   b. Impaired excretion: Depletion of sodium or volume will lead to increased resorption of lithium in the kidneys in the following conditions:
      - Vomiting
      - Diarrhea
      - Febrile illness
      - Excessive exercise
      - Renal insufficiency
      - Restriction of water
      - Excessive sweating
      - Congestive heart failure
      - Low-sodium diet

3. Neurological features:
   a. Coarse
   b. Hyperreflexia
   c. Nystagmus
   d. Ataxia
   e. Mild confusion to coma

   Renal complications:
   a. Impaired ability to concentrate the urine
   b. Nephrogenic diabetes insipidus
   c. Sodium-losing nephritis
   d. Nephrotic syndrome

4. Following are the ECG features of lithium overdose:
   a. Flattening of T wave
   b. Sinus node dysfunction
   c. QT prolongation
   d. Intraventricular conduction defect
   e. U wave

CASE 17

A 40-year-old woman came to emergency department with severe abdominal pain, fever, and diarrhea after taking inhalation of the mercury fume when it was taken from the thermometer and allowed to vaporize on the heating stove.

On examination, blood pressure was 145/90 mm Hg, pulse rate 110 beats/min, temperature 101°F, and SpO$_2$ 98% in room air.

Laboratory examination was normal. Chest X-ray and CT scan of abdomen were normal.

1. **What are the types of mercury?**
2. **What are the sites of absorption of mercury?**
3. **What are the potentially serious presentations?**
4. **What are the clinical features of acute mercury poisoning?**
5. **What should be the level associated with neuropsychiatric disturbances?**
6. **How can you decontaminate the mercury in case of poisoning?**
7. **What are the antidotes mercury?**

Answers

1. There are two types of mercury:
   a. Elemental mercury: It is found in—
      - Thermometer
      - Barometer
      - Paints
      - Pigments
   b. Organic mercury: It is alkoxyalkyl mercury, alkyl mercury, and methyl mercury.
2. Mercury is absorbed from two sites:
   a. Elemental mercury is minimally absorbed from the gastrointestinal tract. But, mostly absorbed from the respiratory tract.
   b. Organic mercury is absorbed from both gastrointestinal and respiratory tract.
3. Following are the potentially serious presentations:
   a. Inhaled mercury or vapor during heating mercury or through the aerosol from vacuuming a broken thermometer results pulmonary edema and neurological manifestations.
   b. Ingestion of the mercury in the form of mercury salts leads to gastrointestinal hemorrhage, acute kidney injury, and shock
4. Clinical features of acute mercury poisoning:
   a. Acute exposure to elemental mercury: It occurs through the inhalation.

- Headache
- Nausea
- Vomiting
- Fever with chills
- Salivation
- Visual disturbances
- Respiratory distress
- Dry cough

b. Acute exposure to inorganic mercury salts through the ingestion:
- Severe gastrointestinal hemorrhage
- Local oropharyngeal pain
- Metallic taste
- Nausea
- Vomiting
- Diarrhea

c. Acute exposure to organic mercury:
- Respiratory distress
- Dermatitis
- Tremor
- Renal tubular dysfunction
- Over weeks to months delayed neurotoxicity

5. 24 hours urinary mercury level associated with neuropsychiatric disturbances is >100 µg/L.
6. Process of decontamination of mercury in case of mercury poisoning:
a. Environmental:
- Cleaning up of the mercury spills
- Contaminated carpets or surfaces should be discarded.

b. Elemental mercury:
- Clothing should be removed.
- Mercury should be removed from the skin.
- Oral polyethylene glycol should be administered.
- Subcutaneous deposits should be removed surgically.

c. Organic mercury: Activated charcoal should be administered.

7. Antidotes of mercury are the following:
a. Dimercaprol
b. Penicillamine
c. Succimer

CASE 18

A 35-year-old male came to emergency department with vomiting following intake of crushed four seeds in dub water.

On examination, all the vitals were normal.

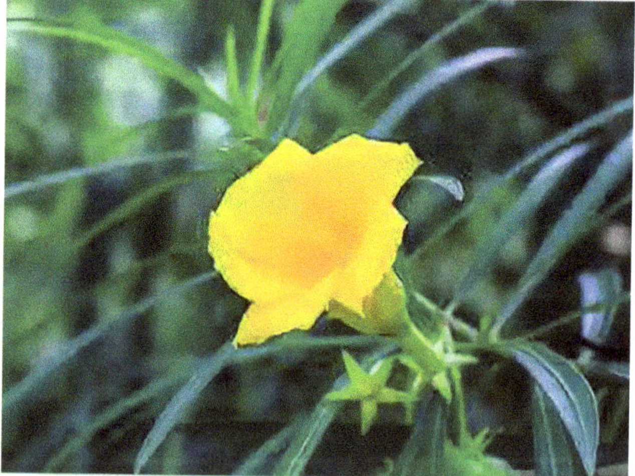

1. **What is the flower?**
2. **What are the cardiac glycosides present in this yellow oleander?**
3. **What is the fatal dose of this poisoning?**
4. **What are the clinical features in this poisoning?**
5. **How can you treat the atrioventricular (AV) block in this patient?**

Answers

1. This is the flower of yellow oleander.
2. The cardiac glycosides include:
   a. Oleandrin
   b. Nerioside
   c. Digitoxigenin
   d. Thevetin
   e. Vetoxin
3. The fatal dose of yellow oleander is 8–10 seeds and 15–20 g of root.
4. The clinical features are:
   a. Bradycardia
   b. AV block
   c. Hypertension
   d. Lethargy
   e. Dizziness
   f. Gastrointestinal distress
   g. Convulsion
   h. Electrolyte disturbance
   i. Coma
   j. Blistering or dermatitis in case of sap of yellow oleander
5. AV block can be treated by 0.6 mg atropine as intravenous infusion and it should be repeated until the clinical effects are achieved.

CASE 19

A 40-year-old female came to emergency department with irritability, confusion, vomiting, and restlessness following intake of 100 mL of that poison as shown in the picture below:

On examination, blood pressure was 150/80 mm Hg, pulse rate 64 beats/min, regular, respiratory rate 32 breaths/min, pinpoint pupil, and excessive secretions through the mouth.

1. **What does the picture demonstrate here?**
2. **What is the most likely diagnosis?**
3. **What is the mechanism of action in this poison?**
4. **What are the various modes of intoxication of the organophosphorus compound?**
5. **What are the clinical features in this poisoning?**
6. **What is the intermediate syndrome?**
7. **How do you treat this patient?**

Answers

1. The picture demonstrated here is an organophosphorus pesticide dichlorvos.
2. The most likely diagnosis is organophosphorus poisoning.
3. The mechanism of action of this poison is that it will inhibit irreversibly cholinesterase and pseudocholinesterase, i.e., butyrylcholinesterase enzymes which hydrolyze the neurotransmitter acetylcholine into choline and acetic acid leading to accumulation of acetylcholine at the neural synaptic junction. As a result, there is overstimulation of the central nervous system and myoneural junctions.
4. Following are the various modes of intoxication of the organophosphorus compound:
   a. Accidental ingestion through the gastrointestinal tract

b. Dermal absorption through the breach in the skin

c. Absorption through the conjunctiva as well as buccal mucosa

d. Inhalation through the respiratory tract

5. Following are the features of intoxication:

a. Muscarinic effect:
- Salivation
- Lacrimation
- Urination
- Defecation
- Nausea/vomiting
- Bronchorrhea
- Bronchospasm
- Bradycardia
- Miosis

b. Nicotinic effects:
- Fasciculation in the muscles
- Cramping
- Diaphragmatic paralysis
- Weakness of muscles

c. Autonomic effects:
- Hypertension
- Tachycardia
- Pallor
- Anxiety
- Emotional liability
- Restlessness
- Ataxia
- Tremor
- Seizures
- Coma

6. This intermediate syndrome is characterized by paralysis of the bulbar, respiratory, and proximal muscles paralysis following acute cholinergic phase within 24–96 hours of exposure which will be resolved within 1–3 weeks requiring mechanical ventilation. There may be complications such as infections and cardiac arrhythmias.

7. Treatment of this poisoning:

a. In case of mild exposure, 2–5 mg atropine intramuscularly should be administered to block muscarinic receptors followed by waiting for 10–15 minutes to take its effect. After this time, if the patient will not develop symptoms further, no further atropine injection is recommended.

b. In case of severe symptoms, 2 mg atropine should be administered intravenously at every 3–5 minutes till the patient will be fully atropinized.

c. Glycopyrrolate to prevent muscarinic effect: 0.2 mg glycopyrrolate should be administered intravenously per 1 mg of neostigmine or 5 mg of pyridostigmine in the same syringe to reduce salivary, pharyngeal, or tracheobronchial secretion.

d. Pralidoxime: 1–2 g should be infused intravenously over 15–30 minutes to block nicotinic receptors and has to be repeated within 1 hour if required and should be repeated after 12 hours. Pralidoxime binds with the organophosphate thereby reactivating the phosphorylated acetylcholinesterase. As it will not depress the respiratory center, it can be given with the atropine.

CASE 20

A 42-year-old patient working in the electroplating industry was brought to the emergency department following ingestion of potassium dichromate dissolved in water within 1 hour after warm talk with his parents.

On examination, all the vitals were normal and systemic examinations were normal.

1. **What is potassium dichromate?**
2. **What are the types of biotransformation in this chromium?**
3. **Which bioform is used in the industry?**
4. **What is the pathophysiology of this poison?**
5. **What are the chelating agents for this poison?**

Answers

1. Potassium is an oxidizing agent in case of laboratory and industrial applications.

2. There are two types of biotransformation in chromium:
   a. Hexavalent chromium
   b. Trivalent chromium

3. Uses of chromium:
   a. Chromite—trivalent chromium is present.
   b. Hexavalent chromium is used in the following industry:
      - Electroplating
      - Aircraft building
      - Building of ship
      - Dye casting
      - Match industry
      - Metal cleaning
      - Tanning
4. Pathophysiology of potassium chromate:
   a. Hexavalent chromium:
      - Injury to gastrointestinal tract
      - Hepatic failure
      - Renal failure
      - Cellular toxicity leading to mitochondrial injury and lysosomal injury
   b. Trivalent chromium has reduced the level of toxicity.
5. Chelating agents are:
   a. D-penicillamine
   b. N-acetylcysteine
   c. Dimercaprol
   d. Dimercaptopropanesulfonic acid (DMPS)

CASE 21

A 38-year-old female was brought to emergency department with severe vomiting for several times after taking rodenticide in the form of white phosphorus mixed with water 5 hours before. On further enquiry, we came to know that her husband badly behaved with her.

On examination, her pulse rate was 110 beats/min, blood pressure 100/70 mm Hg, SpO_2 98% in room air, pupil is normal in size and reacting to light, abdomen was normal. Other systemic examinations were normal.

1. **What is the mechanism of actions of this poisoning?**
2. **What is the lethal dose of this poison?**
3. **What are the other rodenticides present?**
4. **What are the types of clinical presentation in this patient?**
5. **How can you evaluate the different types of rodenticides by investigation?**
6. **What are the complications may occur in this patient?**

Answers

1. White phosphorus is absorbed through the following routes:
   a. Ingestion
   b. Inhalation
   c. Dermal absorption
   It will:
   a. Affect function of ribosomes
   b. Affect protein synthesis
   c. Impair glucose homeostasis
   d. Impair triglyceride and lipoprotein metabolism
   All the above will lead to fatty degeneration of liver, kidney, and brain.
2. Lethal dose of this rat killer is 1 mg/kg.
3. The other rodenticides are as follows:
   a. Thallium
   b. Sodium monofluoroacetate
   c. Fluoroacetamide
   d. Strychnine
   e. Zinc phosphide
   f. Aluminum phosphide
   g. Elemental phosphorus
   h. Arsenic
   i. Barium carbonate
   j. Tetramethylenedisulfotetramine
   k. Aldicarb
   l. α-chloralose
   m. Pyriminil
4. Following are the clinical presentations in this patient:
   a. Initially, the patient is symptomatic.
   b. First stage, i.e., within 24 hours:
      - Gastrointestinal symptoms such as abdominal pain, nausea, vomiting, and smoky stool.
      - Cardiovascular collapse leading to cardiac failure

- • Diarrhea leading to loss of electrolytes
- • ECG features:
  - ○ Dysrhythmias
  - ○ Wide QRS complexes
  - ○ ST segment depression
- • Early death due to above causes

c. Second stage, i.e., 1–3 days: Features of toxic hepatitis, i.e., elevation of liver enzymes

d. Third stage in >3 days:
- • Acute liver failure
- • Acute renal failure
- • Encephalopathy
- • Arrhythmia
- • Coagulopathy
- • Hypotension
- • Bone marrow toxicity

e. In the late stage: Changes in the central nervous system such as confusion, psychosis, hallucination, coma, and death.

5. Following are the methods of evaluation:

a. Blood glucose:
- • Hypoglycemia: Pyriminil
- • Hyperglycemia: Zinc phosphide or aluminum phosphide

b. Complete blood count:
- • Anemia: Zinc phosphide

c. Basic metabolic panel:
- • Hypocalcemia: White phosphorus and fluoroacetamide

- • Elevated blood urea nitrogen (BUN): Arsenic, thallium, white phosphorus, zinc phosphide, and aluminum phosphide

d. Serum phosphorus: Hyperphosphatemia—white phosphorus

e. Liver function test: Elevated liver enzymes—thallium, white phosphorus, arsenic, zinc phosphide, and aluminum phosphide

f. Creatinine phosphokinase: increases in strychnine poisoning.

g. Prothrombin time and INR: Increased in case of anticoagulant

h. Troponin: Increased in case of zinc phosphide and aluminum phosphide

i. Lipases: Increased

j. Arterial blood gases: Metabolic acidosis—fluoroacetamide

k. ECG changes:

l. QTc prolongation—white phosphorus, arsenic, and fluoroacetamide

m. Chest X-ray and abdominal X-ray: Radiopaque shadow—arsenic, thallium, and barium carbonate

6. Complications are as follows:

a. Hepatic failure

b. Renal failure

c. Type 1 diabetes

d. Permanent neurological damage

CASE 22

A 2-year-old baby suddenly arouse from deep sleep and started crying. It was found that there was sudden swelling and reddening of the left forearm. While searching around, the following insect was found.

On examination, blood pressure was 90/60 mm Hg, pulse rate 132 beats/min, respiratory rate 36 breaths/minute. Other systemic examinations were normal.

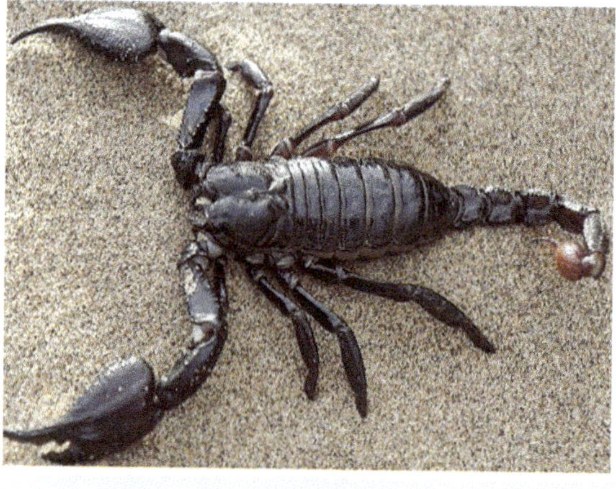

1. **What is your diagnosis?**
2. **What are the species of scorpion?**
3. **Mention the gradation of envenomation?**
4. **What are the complications?**
5. **What is the antivenom found against scorpion sting?**

Answers

1. The diagnosis is scorpion sting poisoning.
2. Following are the species of scorpion:
    a. Neuromuscular poison: *Centruroides* and *Parabuthus*
    b. Cardiovascular poison: *Buthus*, *Mesobuthus*, and *Androctonus*
3. Gradation of envenomation:
    a. Grade 1:
        - At the local site, there is pain and paresthesia.
        - Tap test: It can be done by tapping on the area of the sting while distracting the patient's attention produces pain.
    b. Grade 2: Presence of pain in the local site as well as proximal region.
    c. Grade 3:
        - Addition of the cranial nerves:
            o   Increased oral secretion
            o   Blurred vision
            o   Rapid movement of the tongue
            o   Nystagmus
        - Skeletal muscular dysfunction:
            o   Tetanus-like arch on the back
            o   Flailing of the extremities
    d. Grade 4: Here, both the cranial nerves and skeletal muscular dysfunctions may occur:
        - Hyperemia
        - Pulmonary edema
        - Multiorgan failure
4. Following are the complications:
    a. Cardiac involvement in the form of:
        - Tachycardia progressing to bradycardia
        - Premature beats
        - Arrhythmias
        - Gallop rhythm
        - Congestive cardiac failure
        - Pulmonary edema
5. The specific antivenom against scorpion sting is purified antivenom F(ab')2: As the venom spreads from the local site into the circulation is 10–20 minutes and its duration of action will be maximum 30 minutes. So, this antivenom should be given as early as possible. Dose is three vials in 20–50 mL normal saline and should be given over 30 minutes.

CASE 23

A 40-year-old female suddenly developed progressively increasing vomiting and fever but not associated visual blurring or headache of dizziness. She was brought to the hospital emergency department. On enquiry from the patient, she told that while she was working in the storeroom, she saw few creatures were roaming in the floor as demonstrated below.

On examination, her blood pressure was 90/60 mm Hg, pulse rate 72 beats/min, respiratory rate 28 breaths/min, and SpO_2 98% in room air. There was a bite mark on the right foot. Other systemic examinations were normal. Laboratory investigation demonstrated platelet count 85,000/cc.

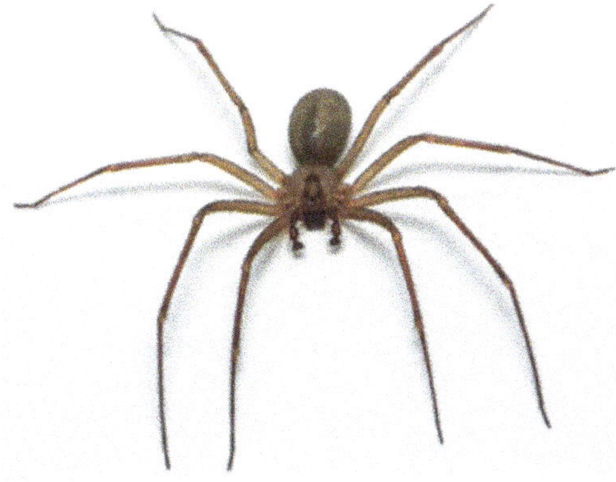

1. **What does the above picture demonstrate?**
2. **What is the diagnosis?**
3. **What are the clinical features in this spider bite?**
4. **What is the effect of bite?**
5. **What should be the treatment?**

Answers

1. The above picture demonstrates brown recluse spider.
2. The patient has been suffering from brown spider bite poisoning.
3. Following are the clinical features in this spider bite:
   a. Nausea
   b. Vomiting
   c. Fever
   d. Disseminated intravascular coagulation
   e. Thrombocytopenia
4. Effects of the bite:
   a. On the first day, the site of bite is mildly red.
   b. On the third day, there is presence of necrosis of the surrounding of the skin and subcutaneous fat.
   c. On the ninth day, there is severe destructive necrosis.
   d. Within few weeks, the lesion will be resolved.
5. Treatment should be:
   a. Analgesics
   b. Antibiotic to treat secondary infection
   c. Prophylaxis against tetanus
   d. Supportive measures

CASE 24

A 25-year-old male was brought to emergency department 2 hours after ingestion of 2 g of strychnine with respiratory distress and severe agitation.

On examination, his blood pressure was 95/65 mm Hg, pulse rate 112 beats/min, regular, but peripheral pulses were feeble. In the emergency department, he developed sudden generalized tonic-clonic convulsion.

1. **What is strychnine?**
2. **What is the mechanism of action of strychnine?**
3. **What is the lethal dose?**
4. **What investigation should be done to evaluate strychnine poisoning?**

Answers

1. Strychnine is a toxin alkaloid found in the seeds of *Strychnos* nux-vomica tree, which is native to India.
2. Strychnine competitively inhibits the glycine receptors mainly in the spinal cord which is primarily inhibitory neurotransmitter. This inhibition of the glycine receptors will lead to stimulation of postsynaptic neurons in uncontrolled fashion leading to diffuse involuntary contraction of the muscles. As it has no effect on the higher motor neuron centers, this severe muscle contraction looks like seizures without any postictal period.
3. The median lethal dose of strychnine is 1.5 mg/kg.
4. Thin layer chromatography should be performed on the gastric aspirate to evaluate strychnine poisoning.

CASE 25

A 28-year-old male 2 hours after taking tea from the tea shop became delirious, agitated in his house, and was brought to emergency department. After going to that tea shop, some seeds were found in one pot. The tea maker was arrested on that spot, and on enquiry, he confessed regarding giving the seeds as below:

On examination, his blood pressure was 140/90 mm Hg, pulse rate 120 beats/min, respiratory rate 32 breaths/min, the patient becomes irritated, hallucinated, mouth was dry, pupils were dilated, not reacting to light or accommodation, bladder palpated above the symphysis pubis, SpO_2 90% in room air, temperature 100°F, and skin was warm and dry.

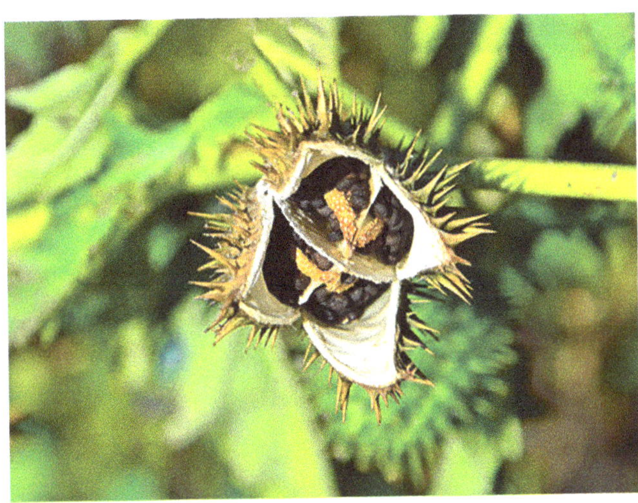

1. **What is shown in the above picture?**
2. **What is the diagnosis?**
3. **What is the mechanism of action of this poison?**
4. **What is the lethal dose of this poison?**
5. **What is the composition of the seeds?**
6. **What are the medicinal uses of these components of the active compounds?**
7. **How accidental poisoning can occur?**
8. **What is the antidote for this poisoning?**

Answers

1. The above picture is the *Datura* seeds.
2. The patient has been suffering from *Datura* poisoning.
3. The mechanism of action: The active compounds act to the central muscarinic as well as peripheral muscarinic receptors as competitive antagonist.
4. The lethal dose of this seed: 50–100 seeds
5. The active compounds of the seeds are:
   a. Scopolamine
   b. Atropine
   c. Hyoscyamine
   d. Other tropanes
6. Medicinal uses of *Datura* alkaloids are the following:
   a. Atropine:
      - Treatment of vagal syncope and bradycardia
      - To reduce salivary and bronchial secretions
      - Antidotes for carbamates, organophosphates, and certain mushrooms
      - To treat iriocyclitis
   b. Hyoscine:
      - Antispasmodic
      - Preanesthetic medication
      - Treatment of motion sickness
      - Aids to endoscopic examination

7. Accidental poisoning can occur in the following processes:
   a. Patient can take it thinking as it is capsicum seed.
   b. Therapeutic misadventures
   c. Foraging children in the countryside chewing seeds out of the curiosity
   d. Overenthusiastic use as antidote organo-phosphate poisoning

8. The antidote for *Datura* poisoning is physostigmine: Dose is 0.1–0.3 mg intravenously every 3 minutes to maximum 2 mg to reduce the incidence of the cardiovascular side effect.

CASE 26

A 30-year-old male was found unconscious in his room and was taken to the emergency department of a hospital. On enquiry, it was found that after a dispute with his father regarding the marriage of his girlfriend. During the search in the room a bottle was found.

On examination, his blood pressure was 120/80 mm Hg, heart rate 120 beats/min, and SpO_2 was 99%. Serum creatinine was 2.1 mg/dL and urea 78 mg/dL.

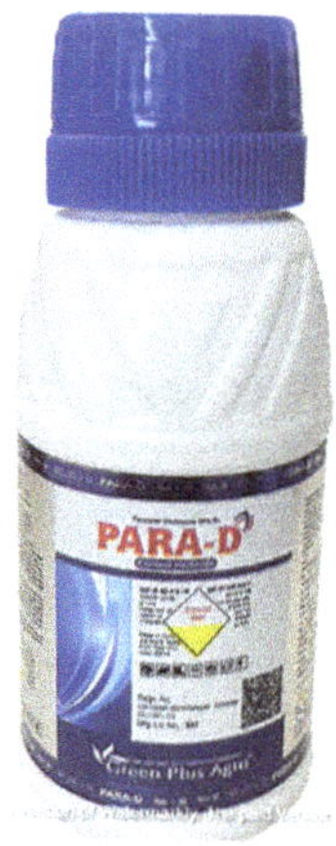

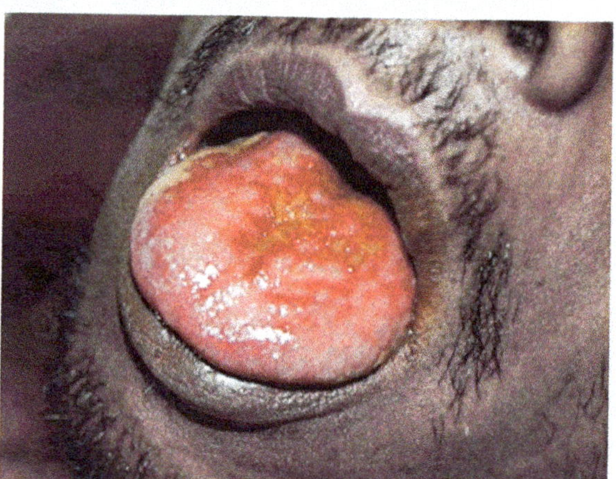

1. **What do the above pictures demonstrate?**
2. **What is the mechanism of action of paraquat?**
3. **Which is the primary target organ in this toxicity and what is the pathophysiology occurs in this organ?**
4. **What are the other organs involved in this poisoning?**
5. **What is the clinical course in this poisoning?**
6. **What are the gastrointestinal manifestations in this poisoning?**

Answers

1. Above pictures demonstrate:
   a. Paraquat bottle
   b. Paraquat tongue: It can be classically described as ulceration and blooding involving dorsum of the tongue.

2. Paraquat is able to undergo redox-cycling and generation of reactive oxygen species leading to development of:
   a. Lipid peroxidation
   b. Mitochondrial toxicity
   c. Oxidation of nicotinamide adenine dinucleotide phosphate hydrogen (NADPH)
   d. Activation of nuclear factor κβ
   e. Apoptosis

3. The primary target organ is lung.
   a. Destructive phase where patients with type I and II pneumocytes demonstrate swelling, vacuolation, disruption of mitochondria and endoplasmic reticulum leading to sloughing of alveoli resulting in pulmonary edema.
   b. Proliferative phase where the alveoli is filled up with mononuclear profibroblast which will be transformed into mature fibroblast within weeks.
   c. Phase of lung fibrosis

4. Other organs involved are as follows:
   a. Kidney: Here, there is large vacuolation of the proximal convoluted tubules leading to necrosis of the tubules.
   b. Liver: Here, there is hepatocellular injury associated with degranulation of rough and smooth endoplasmic reticulum and mitochondrial damage occurring within hours to days.
5. Following are the clinical courses in this poisoning:
   a. If there is ingestion of 50–100 mL of paraquat, patient develops following fulminant organ failure leading to death within few days:
      - Pulmonary edema
      - Cardiac failure
      - Renal failure
      - Hepatic failure
      - Convulsion due to involvement of central nervous system
   b. If the ingestion is <50 mL, two organs are involved and toxicities will be developed within 2–6 days.
      - Kidney
      - Lung: It is involved in two phases:
         i. Acute alveolitis over 1–3 days
         ii. Secondary fibrosis
6. Gastrointestinal manifestations in this poisoning are as follows:
   a. Paraquat tongue
   b. Mucosal lesions in the:
      o Esophagus
      o Stomach
      o Pharynx
   c. Esophageal perforation leading to mediastinitis

CASE 27

A 24-year-old man was brought with ptosis and local swelling and blistering at the site of bite after a bite of a snake 3 hours ago.

On examination, the blood pressure was 110/70 mm Hg, pulse rate 112 beats/min, respiratory rate 28 breaths/min, and neurological examination demonstrated evidence of external ophthalmoplegia. At the local site, there were features of blistering and swelling.

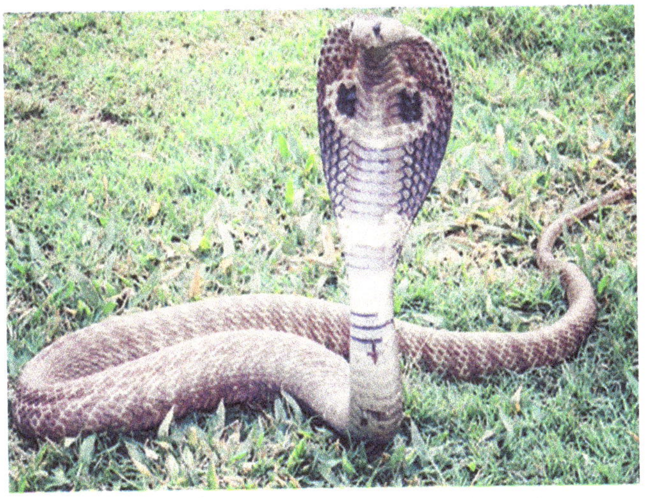

1. **What is the snake?**
2. **What other snake is responsible for local swelling?**
3. **What are the features present in this case?**
4. **In which family this snake belongs to?**
5. **What are the toxins along with mechanism of actions in this venom?**
6. **What is the lethal dose of the venom in this snake?**

Answers

1. This snake is cobra.
2. The other snakes responsible for local swelling is Russell's viper.
3. The features in this case are as follows:
   a. At the local site, there is swelling, then blistering followed by necrosis.
   b. Nausea and vomiting to start with
   c. Early neurological features are:
      - Elevation of the eyebrows due to contraction of the frontalis muscles
      - Ptosis
      - External ophthalmoplegia
      - Blurred vision
      - Loss of visual accommodation due to mydriasis
      - Perioral paresthesia
   d. Late neurological features are:
      - Dysphagia
      - Dysphasia
      - Paralysis of jaw and palatal muscles
      - Paralysis of tongue
      - Respiratory muscle paralysis within minutes to hours
      - Muscles weakness in the limb
   e. Autonomic dysfunction:
      - Salivation
      - Nausea
      - Vomiting
      - Abdominal pain
   f. Alteration of the mental status such as drowsiness and euphoria
   g. Chest pain or chest tightness
   h. Eye pain and blurring of vision
4. This snake belongs to the family Elapidae.
5. Following are the toxins along with the mechanism of actions:
   a. α-neurotoxins also known as three-fingered toxins. Kit will block the postsynaptic nicotinic acetylcholine receptors thereby block depolarization leading to paralysis.
   b. Cardiotoxin: It produces—
      - Irreversible depolarization of the muscle cells leading to lysis of cells
      - Dysfunction of the platelet aggregation
      - Inhibition of the protein kinase C
      - Inhibition of Na-K-ATPase leading to different types of arrhythmias
   c. Complement activating proteins activate alternate pathway complement without formation of antigen-antibody complex
   d. Enzymes:
      - Phospholipase A2: It will damage hematocytes, mitochondria, skeletal muscles, and vascular endothelium.
      - Hyaluronidase: It will degrade extracellular matrix leading to dispersion of the tissues.
      - L-amino acid oxidase: It is responsible for characteristic yellow coloration.
      - Acetylcholinesterase will terminate the cholinergic neurotransmission leading to impairment of muscle contraction.
6. Lethal dose of venom of Indian cobra, i.e., Naja naja, is 0.29 mg/kg.

CASE 28

A 24-year-old man was brought with ptosis after a bite of a snake 3 hours ago.

On examination, the blood pressure was 110/70 mm Hg, pulse rate 112 beats/min, respiratory rate 28 breaths/min, and neurological examination demonstrated evidence of external ophthalmoplegia. At the local site, there is no tissue reaction or blistering.

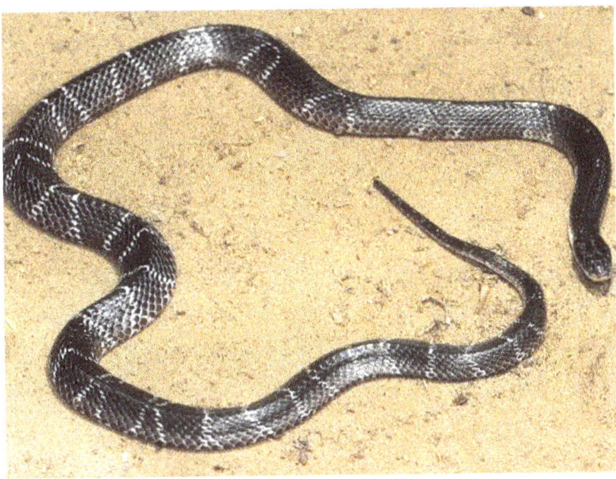

1. **What snake does the above picture demonstrate?**
2. **In which family does this snake belong?**
3. **What should be the classical signs in this case?**
4. **What is the venom required in this case?**

Answers

1. The above picture demonstrates common krait.
2. This snake belongs to family Elapidae.
3. The classical signs are the following:
   a. Mild case: Local signs without systemic signs or symptoms
   b. Moderate case:
      - Extension of swelling with systemic features:
        - Nausea
        - Vomiting
        - Paresthesia
        - Diarrhea
        - Fatigue
        - Lightheadedness
        - Sweating
        - Chills
      - ± Laboratory investigations
   c. Severe case:
      - Swelling extension to all the limb muscles
      - Systemic features:
        - Respiratory failure
        - Shock
        - Bleeding
        - Loss of consciousness
        - Fasciculation
        - Seizures
        - Pulmonary edema
      - Several laboratory blood tests
4. Following are the doses of venom:
   a. In mild case, 3–5 vials
   b. In moderate case, 6–10 vials
   c. In severe case, 11–20 vials

CHAPTER 15

Medical Ethics

CASE 1

A 45-year-old obese man came to outdoor with complaint of confined himself within the house, not interested to talk with his friend, difficulty in going to sleep. His friends married, but he was sole and not interested in marrying because he felt worthlessness.

1. **What is your next course of action?**
2. **What are the criteria of this disease?**
3. **What actions you should take in this patient?**

Answer

1. Patient should be screened for major depression.
2. Diagnostic criteria of major depression are as follows:
   a. S: Disturbances in sleep
   b. I: Decreased interest in the activities
   c. G: Sensation of guilt
   d. E: Energy will be decreased.
   e. C: Difficulty to concentrate
   f. A: Decreased appetite
   g. P: Psychomotor retardation
   h. S: Thought of suicide

   Depressed mood along with four of the above criteria for at least 2 weeks suggests that this patient has been suffering from major depression.
3. Following actions should be taken in this patient:
   a. Identification of the source of stressors such as finances and relationship
   b. Try to avoid making relationship with this patient outside the professional settings
   c. Treatment of obesity as this will be associated with many serious medical conditions.
   d. Correction of depression as this makes him to commit suicide.

CASE 2

A 5-year-old baby was taken to emergency department with fracture of the right forearm as a result of fall from distance by his babysitter. On examination, the pulses were normally palpable. The concerned doctor as well as babysitter tried to contact his parents by repeated phone but failed to contact.

1. **What is the next course of action?**
2. **Is babysitter the legal guardian?**
3. **As there is no deformity and all the peripheral pulses were palpable, what should be the next course of action?**

Answers

1. The doctor concerned and the babysitter always should try to contact repeatedly because the fracture of the right forearm is not life-threatening, because legal consent is required from the parents or legal guardian.

2. Babysitter is not the legal guardian.

3. Since all the peripheral pulses were palpable, X-ray of the fractured area as well as the legal consent should be taken prior to corrective treatment.

CASE 3

A 28-year-old pregnant woman having past history of syphilis was offered to perform human immunodeficiency virus (HIV) serology in the third trimester as a part of antenatal care, but she refused to do it despite several attempts through the discussion of its importance in the early detection and its future risk to unborn child.

1. **Is it mandatory to perform this test in this pregnant woman?**
2. **What is the role of physician in this case?**
3. **Is there any role of father to convince her wife?**
4. **If the test is done against her will and the test is positive, what will happen to the patient?**
5. **In what condition this test can be done against her will by a physician?**

Answers

1. It is not mandatory to perform this test in the pregnant woman because the unborn child should not have same right as that in adult individual.

2. The physician should educate this patient, encourage test but cannot force her to perform this test as the baby is unborn.

3. The father has no role to convince her wife if she refuses this test.

4. If this is done against her will and she will be accidentally positive, she can use a case against the physician as this is done against her will or without her knowledge.

5. The test can be done against her will or without her knowledge when the doctor tries to prevent harm to another person.

CASE 4

A 56-year-old hypertensive, diabetic male having history of coronary artery disease came to emergency department with respiratory distress due to sepsis-induced severe acute renal injury. On investigation, the potassium was 7.5 mmol/L, total count 23,000/cc with leukocyte preponderance. The patient in this condition filled up the form "do not resuscitate (DNR)" and "do not intubate" and patient told the authority to keep this form in front of the bedsheet.

1. **In this condition, this patient should be admitted in which category of bed?**
2. **Is there any role of the patient's surrogate or power of attorney in this condition?**
3. **Is palliative care the same as that in DNR?**

Answers

1. If the patient is severe and if you think that this high level of potassium can stop the heart, you have to admit this patient in intensive care unit (ICU) as this may require cardiopulmonary resuscitation like intravenous antiarrhythmic drugs, defibrillation, etc. So, withholding this treatment will be inappropriate and it is independent of DNR.

2. In this condition, you should not surrogate or make a power of attorney because there is no reason to suspect that this patient is not able to make his decision by himself.

3. Palliative care may or may not be associated with intubation or resuscitation. Hence, the patient can be admitted in the ICU for palliative care.

CASE 5

A 75-year-old female has been admitted with suspected lung cancer. Her biopsy report was pending. Her relatives are very anxious of lack of cure. They told that the result of the biopsy should not be disclosed to the patient as they think that she may be upset with this type of report which is at all required.

1. **What is your first and foremost duty?**
2. **What is therapeutic privilege?**
3. **When will you disclose the information to the patient?**
4. **What is the best way in this case?**
5. **In which condition of the patient, he or she can give his or her decisions?**
6. **When can ethical committee involve in this case?**

Answers

1. The first and foremost duty of a doctor in this case is to inform fully regarding her disease.
2. By therapeutic privilege, the doctor has every right not to disclose the information from the patient if he or she believes that this information may do enormous psychological harm to the patient.
3. The doctor can disclose this information to the patient first not to her party if he or she thinks that:
   a. This patient cannot commit suicide.
   b. The patient is mentally stable.
4. The best way is to first discuss with the patient and her party prior to testing and if a positive response can be found from both sides, then this should be done and the results should be conveyed to both sides.
5. Fully awakened patient can give his or her decision without consulting his or her surrogate, power of attorney.
6. Ethical committee can be involved in the following circumstances:
   a. If the patient is not able to hive his or her decisions.
   b. If the family members are not satisfied with the decisions.
   c. Patient is not also sure about the patient's best interest.

CASE 6

A 40-year-old male has history of generalized epilepsy for which he is on the antiepileptic drugs for 6 months without any further convulsion. He went to the doctor's clinic. He is a newly appointed Lorry-driver. As he should not drive further, but according to the patient as there is no further convulsion and he is on treatment, and he is completely cured.

1. **Why there is restriction in this profession?**
2. **What will be the initial course of action?**
3. **What should the patient be advised?**
4. **What are the consequences of violating confidentiality?**
5. **What should be the physician's report?**
6. **When will the physician report to department of motor vehicle (DMV) regarding the medical condition of the patient?**

Answers

1. The aim of the restriction in this profession is to protect the public safety.
2. The best initial course of action is:
   a. Open discussion with the patient
   b. Discuss and make understand his situation
   c. The rationale should be explained.
   d. He should be aware of all the potential risks.
   e. Conversation with full disclosure of what may happen in the patient cannot handle this situation in proper way.
3. The patient should be advised to discuss fully regarding his medical history with the employer.

4. Violation of the confidentiality:
   a. Carry the serious consequences
   b. Limit the effectiveness of the physicians
5. In some countries, the physician's report is voluntary, whereas in few countries such as Nevada and New Jersey, there are mandatory reporting laws. So, the physician will be liable if the patient is involved in any accident.

6. Physician should report to DMV regarding the medical condition of the patient which may hinder the safe driving according to the American Medical Association when:
   a. Substantial impairment of driving will be a strong threat to both patient and public safety.
   b. Advice of the physician has been disregarded.
   c. Reporting of the impaired driver will not be mandated by law.

CASE 7

A 28-year-old male has been admitted in ICU with head injury following motor vehicle accident, in spite of intensive treatment the patient declared brain dead. The responsible doctor being long-standing resident due to its close family relationship with the patient's party wants to take consent regarding the donation of the organs.

1. **Can a family person give consent to donate organ of the dead patient?**
2. **Who will obtain consent for the transplantation of the organ?**
3. **What is the next course of action of the person who is authorized to obtain consent?**

Answers

1. The patient's party cannot give consent for organ donation because it will create the conflicting situations in the family.
2. The hospital authority where the patient has been died should inform local organ procurement organization of each patient who already died or near to death.
3. After getting information from the authority, the coordinator of the procurement organization will take the consent from the next kin.

CASE 8

After being pregnant for the first time, 30-years-old female in the third week got a news from the laboratory that her human chorionic gonadotropin (hCG) level has been gradually decreasing. She knew this is indicative of miscarriage. So, she was very depressed and cried "God has been given punishment".

1. **What should be the most appropriate response in this situation?**
2. **Is there any indication of sending the patient to chaplain?**
3. **Is there any chance of giving hope of continuation of that pregnancy?**
4. **What question can the physician ask to this woman?**

Answers

1. Firstly, allow the patient for some period of silence so that during the period she will process the hurtful news. After that the physician should educate regarding the results and at the same time educate regarding the options present in future.
2. If the patient understands the situation very well and sends your condolences, even after that if the patient cannot refrain herself from anxiety, then she should be referred to chaplain.
3. The doctor should not give false hope that she can have successful pregnancy as the patient may severely suffer from the false hope.
4. Physician should ask why she thought that the God is giving punishment in this method. Rather he or she reassures that this miscarriage is not the fault on the part of the patient.

CASE 9

A 32-year-old woman suffering from pulmonary tuberculosis gave birth to a baby. She asked about whether she can feed her baby with mother's milk because she knows the mother's milk is the best ever milk for any baby.

1. **What is the response of the treating doctor to the mother?**
2. **What are the diseases or drugs that will prevent the breastfeeding to the baby?**

Answers

1. Firstly, the doctor should tell the woman not to breastfeed her child because it is not advisable. But, if she argues in this matter, she has to explain her that if she tries to breastfeed her baby. There is a great chance of her child contracting tuberculosis.

2. Following diseases and drugs that will prevent breastfeeding to the baby:
   a. HIV-positive patients
   b. Untreated active tuberculosis
   c. Patients on chemotherapy
   d. Patients on radiotherapy
   e. Use of illicit drugs

CASE 10

A 40-year-old woman came to emergency department with right lower quadrant pain and vomiting. She was taken to operating theater for urgent operation. But after opening the area, it was found that appendix was normal, but a mass attached with the right ovary.

1. **What should be the immediate line of action for the surgeon?**
2. **Who will take the decision regarding the line of treatment in this case?**
3. **What should be the next line of action to be taken by the doctor?**
4. **If the patient is unconscious for some duration, in that case who will give the judgment?**
5. **If during operation of ovarian tumor, appendix seen inflamed, what should the immediate decision?**

Answers

1. The surgeon has to stop the operation immediately.
2. The patient herself will give consent including the refusal to treatment as she is well competent.
3. The doctor will take the fully informed consent from the patient after informing the following:
   a. Description of the procedure
   b. Nature of the procedure
   c. Rationale of the treatment
   d. Benefits of the treatment
   e. Risks of the disease as well as risk of operation
4. If the patient is unconscious for the time being, during that time her husband should give his decision under the doctrine "substituted judgment," but if she wakes up, she can change his decision.
5. If the patient is on elective surgery for ovarian tumor and during operation the appendix seen inflamed, the surgeon can do appendectomy without any consent of the patient or her party because inflamed appendix can be turned into appendicular abscess or appendicular perforation. This is a case of true emergency; hence, surgeon can be permitted to operate without the repeat consent again.

CASE 11

A 16-year-old girl was taken to emergency department by her parents with complaint that she was sexually active with her 17-year-old boyfriend and insisted for genital examination and urine for pregnancy test. The girl was the student of higher living with her parents. So, she cannot say anything.

1. **What is your opinion regarding the pelvic examination in this patient?**
2. **Since the patient is an adolescent, what should be your opinion?**
3. **What are the factors for which parental consent is not required for minors?**

Answers

1. You have to give respect the wishes of the minor and without her consent anything cannot be done.
2. If the patient is child and he or she refuses care, parent will override their decision; so, there will not be any problem. But if he or she is adolescent and they refuse care regarding any issue such as sexually transmitted disease (STD), pregnancy, or contraception, this cannot be performed and this is supported by State Law.
3. Following are the factors for which parental consent is not required in minors:
   a. Sex: Sexually transmitted disease, pregnancy, or contraception
   b. Substance drug abuse
   c. Rock and Roll: Cases of emergency and trauma

CASE 12

A 46-year-old female was referred to orthopedic surgeon with a diagnosis of carpal tunnel syndrome for treatment, in exchange that surgeon gave 15% of his income from that patient to that colleague as a referral.

1. **What do you mean by referral?**
2. **Is it a proper step for referral?**
3. **What is the medical code of ethics in this regard?**

Answers

1. Referral means fee splitting which is nothing but sharing of the professional fees that is taken from the patient will be shared between the doctor colleagues.
2. This referral is not the proper step because it will corrupt the decision-making process in the diagnosis because it will break the basic trust of the patient that will lead to ultimately break the doctor-patient relationship.
3. The code of medical ethics states that "payment by or to a physician solely for the referral of a patient is fee splitting and is unethical".

CASE 13

An illegally undocumented emigrant patient has been suffering from tuberculosis. The patient was afraid that he may be deported to his own country by the Government of Health.

1. **What is your role in this case?**
2. **Is there any role of Government of Health in this case?**
3. **Is it mandatory to report the treatment of tuberculosis to the health department?**
4. **What will be done in case of noncompliant patient?**

Answers

1. The doctor should provide medical care to the patient ethically.
2. Department of Health or physician will not report regarding the immigration status to the Government.
3. It is not mandatory to report the Government before, during, or after the treatment of tuberculosis regarding his immigration status.
4. Noncompliant patient may be incarcerated against his will for taking antitubercular drugs, but for this health reason he will not face deportation.

CASE 14

A 60-year-old man has been admitted with ST elevation myocardial infarction of 2 hours duration. So, urgent intervention is needed. But, the interventional cardiologist explained the benefits of this intervention at the same time the risks of this intervention like coronary rupture or hematoma. So, the patient refused to go for intervention and only allowed the medical treatment. But, ultimately that patient developed cardiac arrest. His sons did a lawsuit against that doctor.

1. **Is the doctor liable for the death in this case?**
2. **What is the legitimate consent?**

Answers

1. The doctor here is of course liable because he did not explain the risk of not allowing to perform the coronary intervention. So, the victim will not be aware of the risk of death without this intervention.

2. To make the consent legitimate following points should be included:
   a. The nature of intervention
   b. Most significant risks of this procedure
   c. Benefits of this intervention
   d. Risks of not performing this procedure
   e. The possible alternatives to this intervention

CASE 15

A 55-year-old man admitted with right-sided weakness which was healed within 24 hours and diagnosed as transient ischemic attack and CT scan of brain was normal. So, the doctor discussed with neurologist regarding the patient and he only advised closed follow-up as outpatient after discharge. But within 1 day, this patient developed a complete stroke. So, the patient filed a lawsuit against this physician as he did not inform the alternative to outpatient management of transient ischemic attack.

1. **Is it right to file a lawsuit against the doctor in this case?**
2. **In this case, what is the judgment of the court?**

Answers

1. This doctor is of course liable because he did not inform the patient or the party, the alternative to outpatient management such as MRI brain and Doppler ultrasound of carotid artery and vertebral arteries that can prevent the stroke.

2. The Supreme Court has given the judgment "any physician who treats a patient to inform the patient about the availability of all alternatives, viable medical modes of treatment, including diagnosis as well as benefits and risks of such treatment".

CASE 16

A 39-year-old male on routine checkup suddenly saw that he has very high cholesterol level and after taking history he was diagnosed as familial hypercholesterolemia. He was divorced and has two children. Since this disease is autosomal dominant. His children are at high risk. But since both the children are in the custody of his wife, he refused to inform this risk.

1. **Is there any role of confidentiality on the part of the male person?**
2. **Is there any role of health department to notify this disease?**
3. **What has been emphasized in the code of medical ethics?**

Answers

1. Rights of confidentiality of the patient ends when it comes into the conflict with the safety of the other people. In this case, the children have every right to know whether they will be affected by the genetic diseases. According to the agreement of the divorce, each and every parent must inform the other parent regarding the genetic diseases that can affect their children.

2. Health department never notifies the genetic disease rather this department notifies the transmissible diseases such as HIV, tuberculosis, STDs, and water and food borne diseases to population at risk.

3. According to the code of medical ethics, physicians must inform all the patients requiring genetic testing of the circumstances and under this they notify biological relatives who are at high risk of diseases.

CASE 17

A 65-year-old man has been admitted with gunshot wound in collapsed condition. His blood pressure was 80/50 mm Hg and pulse rate 120 beats/min with a low volume. Doctor decided to give blood transfusion, but at that moment, the wife of the patient arrived and told that blood transfusion is against their religion's belief, Jehovah's Witness "do not accept blood transfusion" has been written on his shirt also. But as there was severe blood loss and the patient may die without it.

1. **What do you mean by Jehovah's Witness "do not accept blood transfusion"?**
2. **What is the duty of the attending doctor at this stage?**

Answers

1. Jehovah's Witness "do not accept blood transfusion" means "abstinence from blood," any form of blood should not be accepted.
2. This type of patients should carry the cards carrying the belief of the religion which indicates the directive of refusal of blood. But there are a large number of possibilities that will dissuade the doctor from obeying the command of the wife and stopping the blood transfusion to save the precious life and allowing him to die. So, the blood transfusion should be given to the patient.

CASE 18

A 23-year-old female came to a doctor with the report of positive test for pregnancy in the urine. She told that, in the intoxicated state, unprotected intercourse with her husband happened and as she was studying then, and she does not want to carry the pregnancy further. But, her husband opposed this abortion.

1. **What should be the legal obligation?**
2. **What is the rule of the Supreme Court?**

Answers

1. According to the court of law, the rights of the woman to abort should never be vetoed by her ex-boyfriend, partner, or even her legal husband, and it is not necessary to notify the legal husband regarding the abortion that her wife already accepted.
2. The rule of the Supreme Court is, "It cannot be claimed that the father's interest in the fetus's welfare is equal to the mother's protected liberty".

CASE 19

A 50-year-old man came to emergency department with cardiac arrest, as you are an attending doctor, you gave him cardiopulmonary resuscitation, and pulse rate was regained. His wife at once gave you a cheque of ₹ 5 lacs. But after 2 months, suddenly you have received a legal notice which made you shocked to see that the patient developed pneumothorax as a result of overenthusiastic chest compression.

1. **Is it right to send you the legal notice?**
2. **Is it right to take the compensation by any doctor on duty?**
3. **Who is a Good Samaritan?**

Answers

1. Yes, it is correct to send a legal notice to the doctor because he already accepted compensation.
2. If the on-duty doctor accepts compensation or sends the bills, it will complicate the issue because you are on-duty doctor, so it might revoke your Good Samaritan immunity.
3. While going from Jerusalem to Jericho a person was attacked by robber and left the man by the side of the road. When a priest saw the wounded man while passing, he passed by the other side of the road. But a Samaritan while passing the wounded man, came upon him, gave the primary care, and took him to an inn for proper care. Next day before leaving inn he gave two silver coins to the inn-keeper and told that if he will spend much more than this, he will repay on his way back.

CASE 20

In absence of your colleagues, you are advised to treat a patient presenting with low back pain treated by painkiller medications but without any result. You tried to refer this patient to neurologist, but your friend told you not to do it. So, you gave the patient naproxen, the patient told you that you are better qualified than your colleague.

1. **What is your opinion?**

Answer

1. The main aim of mine is to make him understand that the regular doctor is similarly qualified and encourage him to bring up his concerns with him. If he is still unsatisfied, he can visit to a different doctor. But, always he should encourage open communication with the resident doctor regarding his problem.

CASE 21

A 13-year-old patient has been admitted with right lower limb pain, subsequent X-ray of right tibia demonstrated suspected swelling and biopsy demonstrated features of osteosarcoma. Everything regarding the biopsy results has been told to his parents. Then, the doctor went to the patient to see whether the pain has been subsided or not. But immediately the patient asked the doctor "regarding result of the biopsy, whether surgery is required or not or he can be discharged or not".

1. **What should be your next response?**
2. **What should be the rule if the child is minor?**
3. **What should the doctor ideally do?**
4. **In what condition, the doctor may follow suit?**

Answers

1. The doctor will ask the patient whether his parents have been told anything or not.
2. If the patient is minor or below the age of 18 years, in that case the parents will take the decisions after knowing the result of biopsy and the process of management.
3. Ideally, the doctor will go to the patient along with his parents to inform him regarding his condition, and what will be the next step of management?
4. If for any reason, the parents tell the doctor not to inform the child, the doctor must follow the suit.

CASE 22

A 55-year-old man was admitted in unconscious state with severe bleeding due to self-inflicted gunshot wound. By seeing this the resident doctor immediately called surgeon for immediate management because his blood pressure was nearly 80/50 mm Hg. But in the bed ticket record, the doctor discovered that already the "DNR" and DNI".

1. **What is the importance of DNR or DNI in this case?**
2. **In postmortem analysis, what are the conditions found to be associated with suicidal attempt?**
3. **What type of mental illness may suffer these patients who attempt suicide?**
4. **What should be the opinion of the American Society of Bioethics regarding DNR in case of suicide?**
5. **In case of natural death, where DNR or DNI should be carried out?**
6. **In which case, suicidal attempt will be a good option?**
7. **In this case, what the resident doctor will do?**

Answers

1. In case of attempted suicide, the decision to override the request of "do not resuscitate" is a conflict between the patient's autonomy, beneficence, and nonmaleficence. Usually, a large number of suicidal attempts are:
   a. Irrational acts
   b. The victim does not possess the decision-making capacity as this type of patients may suffer from severe mental illness which will impair the capacity to judge.
2. In postmortem analysis, following conditions found to be associated with suicidal attempt:
   a. Major depression
   b. Psychosis
   c. Substance abuse
3. The patients attempting suicide usually suffer from treatable mental illness and that illness can be treated effectively so that they will never want to commit suicide in future.
4. According to the American Society of Bioethics DNR/DNI will be nullified in case of suicidal attempt and utmost effort should be made to revive this patient.
5. In case of natural death, DNR/DNI should be carried out when:
   a. Resuscitation attempt will not be successful.
   b. This resuscitation may cause harm to this patient in future if the patient will survive.
6. Suicidal attempts will be a good option where there is unbearable physical pain or suffering.
7. The resident doctor will exert his full effort to save the life of the patient with resuscitation equipment. Even after full attempt, the doctor will notice and diagnose that the patient is brain dead, in that case DNR order will allow the resuscitation equipment to disconnect from the patient and to allow the patient to go for natural death.

CASE 23

A 70-year-old male has been admitted with progressive jaundice and ultimately diagnosed as metastatic pancreatic cancer. Patient after came across the report, he just cried to doctor "I came to know the bad news".

1. **What is the response of the doctor?**
2. **What is real in this case?**

Answers

1. Patient has every right to know the result of the test. But if there is evidence that the patient may commit suicidal attempt after hearing the news, in that case the result of the report can be withheld.
2. In this case, the answer of the patient showed that the patient is not doing self-harm. So, here the patient should not make a mislead by false reassuring the good results in this case.

CASE 24

A 45-year-old female insisted his doctor-friend to prescribe weight-losing drug phentermine, also told him that she took this drug before. As she was new in this area, hence she already fixed appointment with the new physician.

1. **What is the response of the doctor-friend in this case?**
2. **In which cases, this type of prescription is permissible?**

Answers

1. In any area, coworkers will approach to the physician to prescribe any antibiotic or controlled substance. Most of the medical boards discourage this type of prescription, if it is necessary, it requires proper documentation.

2. In the following conditions, this type of prescription is permissible:
   a. In case of emergencies
   b. In the settings where no qualified physicians are available.

CASE 25

A 45-year-old man came to emergency department with history of hematemesis. Immediately after arrival, the sister produced intravenous access and then administered intravenous fluid. After the introduction of nasogastric tube, bright red blood was suctioned. Gastroenterologist while on the way to hospital agreed to see and perform the upper gastrointestinal endoscopy in the attending physician would take the consent within the transit of him.

1. **What is the best response?**
2. **What is informed consent?**
3. **Can the attending doctor be eligible to take the consent regarding the endoscopy procedure?**

Answers

1. The gastroenterologist should obtain consent once he entered the hospital.
2. According to the AMA, the informed consent is the communication between the patient and the physician regarding the specific medical intervention such as specifics of the procedure, risk, benefit, and complications of the procedures.
3. The attending doctor is not eligible to take the consent of the upper gastrointestinal endoscopy and discuss the risk, benefits, and complications of this procedure.

CASE 26

A 70-year-old diabetic and hypertensive female on antidiabetic and antihypertensive medications having no prior history of suicidal tendency found unconscious in her home and taken to emergency department.

1. **What are the risk factors for successful suicidal completion?**

Answer

1. Following are the risk factors:
   a. Prior attempts of suicide
   b. Drug abuse
   c. Alcohol abuse
   d. Access to firearms
   e. Unmarried
   f. Lacking social support
   g. Depression
   h. Use of three or more prescribed medications
   i. Age—young or elderly
   j. Female attempts more but male dies of it

CASE 27

A 67-year-old male came to ophthalmologist with complaint of progressively increasing loss of vision for last 8 months. After checking, he was diagnosed for closed-angle glaucoma. So, he was advised not to do drive the car or any type of vehicle. But he continued. Within few months he failed to read the traffic signs.

1. **What is the advice of the doctor to the patient?**
2. **What is the duty of the doctor to prevent damage of the community?**
3. **Why should it be reported to DMV?**

Answers

1. Due to loss of vision, he may be in danger to himself as well as to the community, so he is advised to select an alternative transportation.
2. As the doctor has no right to remove the driving license from the patient, his ethical duty is to report DMV so that this authority can take the decision that his license should be removed.
3. According to the law, it must be reported to DMV because restriction of the driving privileges can prevent injury as well as death of the patient and the third parties and it cannot be ignored.

CASE 28

A 72-year-old female came to orthopedic outpatient department with feature of osteomyelitis of foot and advised amputation of foot under cover of intravenous antibiotic. But the patient refused because the patient thought that he may die after the operation. But during the period, he developed respiratory tract infection leading to sepsis and he was intubated. Her family advised to perform amputation of foot to prevent the spread of infection and to save her life.

1. **What should be the exact course of action?**
2. **You have to follow the direction of the patient—why?**
3. **What is autonomy?**
4. **What are the requirements of autonomy?**

Answers

1. The exact course of action is to treat the patient with intravenous antibiotics rather not to ampute the feet.
2. The doctor has to follow the decision of the patient as this is autonomy, and it is more important rather than the substituted judgment.
3. Autonomy can be defined as respect to the rights of the patient to make his or her own decision in respect of the medical care.
4. Even if the autonomy of the patient is unwise, but you have to respect the decision of the patient. This autonomy is possible when there is ability of the patient to make his or her decisions. Following are the components of autonomy:
   a. Understanding the diagnosis as well as prognosis of a disease
   b. Understanding of the recommendation as well as alternative management of the disease
   c. Each and every risk and benefit of the alternative management can be acknowledged.
   d. Use of local reasoning for making the decisions
   e. The decision must be stable not fluctuate.

CASE 29

A 27-year-old female patient came to you with history of trying to get pregnancy for last 1 year but without any result. You referred her to a gynecologist in her infertility clinic. Next day, her husband came to you and confessed that he had vasectomy 1 year back that was not told to her wife till now.

1. **Is it necessary to tell the wife regarding this?**
2. **What is confidentiality?**
3. **What is your next action of the doctor?**

Answers

1. You have no obligation to tell everything about her husband to his wife, this should be confidential.
2. Confidentiality can be defined as preservation of the authorized restriction on access as well as disclosure including the protection of personal privacy as well as proprietary information.
3. It is not mandatory one spouse must know everything of the medical care received by the other. So, it is the duty of the doctor to perform the test and at the same time encourage the husband to inform his wife regarding the vasectomy.

CASE 30

A mother took her 2-months-old baby to a pediatric doctor for routine vaccination schedule and told mercury and thimerosal used in the vaccine may be liable to develop autism in her baby in future, whether these vaccines are safe or not?

1. **What is the opinion of the doctor?**
2. **What is the actual thought regarding this vaccine?**
3. **Is it a fact that thimerosal is responsible for autism?**

Answers

1. According to the doctor, though there is link between these vaccines and autism, all the organizations recommend these vaccinations in the vaccination schedule.
2. Although the mother's viewpoint is recognized, all the major societies still recommend these vaccines in the immunization schedule. The alternative vaccination schedule has been proposed, but in this schedule the duration between the different vaccinations is increased over a longer period of time; hence, level of protection will be decreased and hence this schedule till today is not endorsed officially.
3. Thimerosal, a preservative, has been reduced and, in some vaccines, it has been removed from 2001. In spite of that there is no recent decrease in the incidence of autism in this child. Hence, it has been concluded that exposure to thimerosal in childhood is not the primary cause of autism.

EU GSPR Authorised Reprsentative
Logos Europe, 9 rue Nicolas Poussin
1700, La Rochelle, France
Phone: +33 (0) 6 67 93 73 78
E-mail: contact@logoseurope.eu

www.ingramcontent.com/pod-product-compliance
Ingram Content Group UK Ltd.
Pitfield, Milton Keynes, MK11 3LW, UK
UKHW060046170726
7214IPUK00037B/382